CRITICAL CARE MANUAL:

Applied Physiology and Principles of Therapy

CRITICAL CARE MANUAL:

Applied Physiology and Principles of Therapy

Second Edition

Robert Francis Wilson, M.D.
Professor of Surgery
Wayne State University School of Medicine
Detroit, Michigan
Chief of Surgery
Director, Trauma Services
Director, Surgical Intensive Care Units
Detroit Receiving Hospital
Detroit, Michigan

F. A. DAVIS COMPANY • Philadelphia

Published in 1979 by Upjohn under the title Upjohn's Critical Care Manual.

Printed in the United States of America

Last digit indicates print number: 10 9 8 7 6 5 4 3 2

acquisitions editor: Robert G. Martone
production editor: Gail Shapiro
cover design by: Steven Ross Morrone

As new scientific information becomes available through basic and clinical research, recommended treatments and drug therapies undergo changes. The author(s) and publisher have done everything possible to make this book accurate, up to date, and in accord with accepted standards at the time of publication. The authors, editors, and publisher are not responsible for errors or omissions or for consequences from application of the book, and make no warranty, expressed or implied, in regard to the contents of the book. Any practice described in this book should be applied by the reader in accordance with professional standards of care used in regard to the unique circumstances that may apply in each situation. The reader is advised always to check product information (package inserts) for changes and new information regarding dose and contraindications before administering any drug. Caution is especially urged when using new or infrequently ordered drugs.

Library of Congress Cataloging-in-Publication Data

Wilson, Robert F. (Robert Francis), 1934–
    Critical care manual : applied physiology and principles of
therapy / Robert Francis Wilson. — 2nd ed.
      p.   cm.
    Includes bibliographical references and index.
    ISBN 0-8036-9355-9 (softbound : alk. paper) : $60.00 (est.)
    1. Critical care medicine—Handbooks, manuals, etc.   I. Title.
    [DNLM: 1. Critical Care. 2. Emergencies.   WB 105 W752c]
RC86.8.W56 1992
616'.028—dc20
DNLM/DLC
for Library of Congress   92-9898
                                                                CIP

Introduction

Perhaps the most important factor in improving the care of seriously ill or injured patients over the past 25 years has been the development of special care units. These units have shown that careful, constant monitoring of critically ill patients by highly skilled personnel provides earlier and more accurate diagnosis and treatment of a multitude of problems, particularly cardiovascular and respiratory failure. Emphasis has progressively shifted from better management of established disorders to earlier diagnosis and treatment, and finally to recognition of trends in the patient's condition and laboratory values which suggest that problems are developing or are likely to occur. Thus, therapy may be started early, frequently as a prophylactic measure, when it is more likely to be effective.

Appreciation of the value of intensive monitoring has stimulated the development of increasingly sophisticated equipment and techniques, which require that nurses and health care professionals working in critical care units develop more and more expertise and knowledge in the pathophysiology of organ failure.

As trauma continues to be a leading cause of death and disability, and as more and more individuals live long enough to develop cardiac, pulmonary, and other organ failure, hospitals have been compelled to enlarge their critical care facilities to meet these needs. Concomitantly, more and more physicians, nurses, and paramedical personnel are needed to provide the necessary services in their critical care units.

Consequently, the knowledge required by those caring for critically ill and injured patients has expanded rapidly. This has created an increasing need for continuing education of the entire staff in all critical care areas. Recognition of this need has prompted the publication of this manual as a practical source of information based on teaching and clinical experience. In easily accessible form, the manual covers relevant topics, from the basic pathophysiology of the more frequently seen problems in acutely ill patients to an orderly, practical approach to diagnosis and treatment. For maximum usefulness, each chapter begins with a comprehensive outline and ends with a summary of the most important points.

While this manual is not intended to supplant standard textbooks or journals, it is our hope that it will be found useful in training of critical care personnel, for review, and as a readily available reference.

ROBERT FRANCIS WILSON

Acknowledgments

I wish to acknowledge Jacqueline A. Wilson, M.S., R.N., reviewing editor, for her contributions and Bernadette Daley for her invaluable editorial assistance.

Contents

List of Abbreviations

A-aDO$_2$	alveolar-arterial oxygen difference
ACG	apex cardiogram
ADH	antidiuretic hormone
AMI	acute myocardial infarction
AOC	arterial oxygen content
AP	anteroposterior
ARDS	adult respiratory distress syndrome
ARF	acute respiratory failure
ATP	adenosine triphosphate
AVRIO	artioventricular
A-V	arteriovenous
BUN	blood urea nitrogen
CAO	chronic airway obstruction
CBC	complete blood count
CCU	coronary care unit
CHF	congestive heart failure
CI	cardiac index
CNS	central nervous system
CO	cardiac output
COPD	chronic obstructive pulmonary disease
CPAP	continuous positive airway pressure
CPK	creatine phosphokinase
C$_S$	static compliance
CSF	cerebrospinal fluid
C$_T$	total compliance
CVP	central venous pressure
DIC	disseminated intravascular coagulation
G/W	glucose and water
EKG	electrocardiogram
EPP	equal pressure point
ERV	expiratory reserve volume
F	rate of airflow
Fl	fluid
f	frequency per minute
FEV$_{1.0}$	first-second forced expiratory volume
FiO$_2$	fraction of inspired oxygen
FRC	functional residual capacity
FVC	forced vital capacity
IABP	intra-aortic balloon pumping
IC	inspiratory capacity
ICU	intensive care unit
IMV	intermittent mandatory ventilation
IPPB	intermittent positive pressure breathing
IRV	inspiratory reserve volume
KCG	kinetocardiogram

LAH	left anterior hemiblock
LBBB	left-bundle branch block
LDH	lactic dehydrogenase
LMWD	low molecular-weight dextran
LPH	left posterior hemiblock
LVEDP	left ventricular end-diastolic pressure
M^2	square meters of body surface area
MDF	myocardial depressant factor
MMFR	maximum midexpiratory flow rate
MOC	maximum oxygen content
NPO	nothing by mouth
P	pressure
$P(A-a)O_2$	alveolar-arterial oxygen difference
P_ACO_2	alveolar carbon dioxide tension
P_aCO_2	arterial carbon dioxide tension
P_AO_2	alveolar oxygen tension
P_aO_2	arterial oxygen tension
PAT	paroxysmal atrial tachycardia
PaR	pulmonary arteriolar resistance
P_{AW}	pressure to overcome airway resistance
P_B	barometric pressure
P_C	capillary hydrostatic pressure
PCO_2	carbon dioxide partial pressure
P_{CW}	pressure to overcome chest wall resistance
$P\bar{e}CO_2$	average carbon dioxide tension in expired gases
PEEP	positive end-expiratory pressure
PiO_2	inspired oxygen pressure
PH_2O	water vapor pressure
P_L	pressure required to overcome lung resistance
PMN	polymorphonuclear leukocytes
PN_2	partial pressure nitrogen
PND	paroxysmal nocturnal dyspnea
PO_2	partial pressure oxygen
P_t	tissue or pericapillary hydrostatic pressure
π_p	plasma oncotic pressure
π_t	tissue or interstitial oncotic pressure
PVC	premature ventricular contraction
$P_{\bar{v}}CO_2$	carbon dioxide tension in mixed venous blood
$P_{\bar{v}}O_2$	oxygen tension in mixed venous blood
PAWP	pulmonary artery wedge pressure
Q	flow
Q_s/Q_t	physiologic shunting in the lung
R	resistance
R_{AW}	airway resistance
RBBB	right-bundle branch block
R_{CW}	chest wall resistance
RISA	radioiodinated serum albumin
R_L	lung resistance
R_Q	respiratory quotient
R_S	static resistance
R_V	residual volume
SA	sinoatrial
SaO_2	arterial oxygen saturation
SGOT	serum glutamic oxaloacetic transaminase
SRS	slow-reacting substance
TLC	total lung capacity

TTI	tension-time index
V	volume
V_A	alveolar ventilation
$\dot{V}_A$	alveolar ventilation per minute
V_d	dead space
V max	maximum velocity of contraction
VOC	venous oxygen content
$\dot{V}/\dot{Q}$	alveolar ventilation perfusion ratio
V_t	tidal volume
WPW	Wolff-Parkinson-White (syndrome)

PART ONE

THE CARDIOVASCULAR SYSTEM

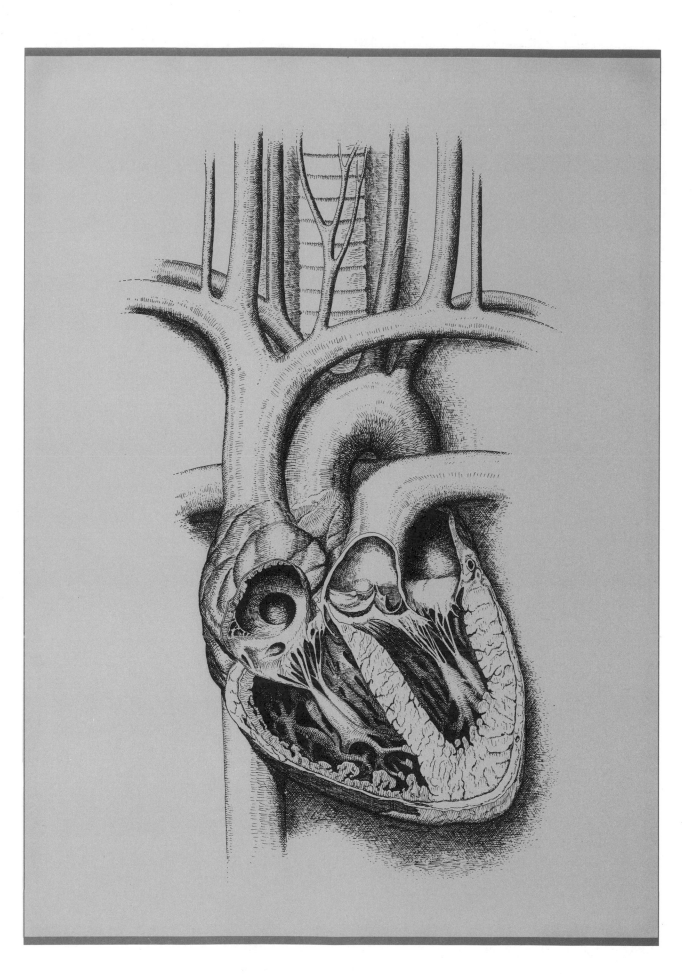

PART ONE

THE CARDIOVASCULAR SYSTEM

CHAPTER 1

Cardiovascular Physiology

I. FUNCTIONAL ANATOMY OF THE HEART

The heart is composed primarily of interlacing fibers of specialized muscle that have many of the characteristics of skeletal muscle. Externally, the muscle (myocardium) is covered by a serous membrane referred to as the epicardium. Internally, the myocardium is lined by the endocardium, which is a layer of endothelium reinforced by fibrous connective tissue.

The heart is normally about the size of an individual's clenched fist. In an average-sized adult, it is about 12.5 cm (5 in) long and about 8.5 cm (3½ in) wide at its greatest diameter. It weighs about 300 g in the average adult male and 250 g in the average adult female, or about 2 g for each pound of ideal body weight.

A. ATRIA

Both atria are thin-walled structures located behind, slightly above, and to the right of their corresponding ventricles. They act as reservoirs and booster pumps for filling the ventricles. While the ventricles are contracting, the atria act as reservoirs. During the early phase of ventricular diastole, blood flows passively from the atria into the ventricles, but during the later phase of ventricular filling, the atria contract, pumping in an additional quantity of blood, which accounts for 20% to 30% of the filling of the ventricles. Loss of atrial systole in an otherwise normal heart has only minimal effect, but if there is any impediment to left ventricular filling, such as with mitral valve stenosis, left atrial systole becomes very important and may account for more than 50% of left ventricular filling.

AXIOM
Atrial fibrillation can dramatically reduce cardiac output and may cause pulmonary edema in patients with significant mitral stenosis.

1. Right Atrium

The superior and inferior venae cavae enter the dorsum of the right atrium, and the coronary sinus enters somewhat anteriorly and superiorly to the entrance of the inferior vena cava. The auricle, a small ear-shaped appendage of the atrium, is attached to the right atrium anteriorly just below the entrance of the superior vena cava. Also opening into the right atrium are numerous small thebesian veins, which drain some of the venous blood from the myocardium directly into the right heart rather than through the coronary sinus.

2. Left Atrium

The pulmonary veins, usually four in number, empty into the left atrium posteriorly. In contrast to the right atrium, which has multiple, prominent muscular bands on its inner surface, the interior of the left atrium is smooth except within its auricle. The left atrium is above and behind the left ventricle. Since it is the most posterior chamber of the heart, it might be more appropriately called the posterior atrium. When it becomes dilated, as it does with chronic mitral valve disease, it tends to displace the esophagus posteriorly, and as it continues to enlarge, it bulges to the right and upward. If the left atrium becomes greatly dilated, it may form the right border of the heart on x-ray and compress the left lower lobe bronchus, causing left lower lobe atelectasis.

B. VENTRICLES

The force to circulate blood through the lungs and the rest of the body is supplied by the right and left ventricles, respectively. The wall of the left ventricle is much thicker (8 to 12 mm) than that of the right ventricle (3 to 4 mm) and it must push against a systemic vascular resistance (mean pressure, 90 mm Hg), which is normally at least six times that present in the pulmonary circuit (mean pressure, 8 to 15 mm Hg) (Table 1.1).

Although the normal upper limit of systolic pressure in the right ventricle and pulmonary artery is often said to be 25 mm Hg, in young adults it is normally 12 to 15 mm Hg. The normal right ventricle cannot achieve a pressure greater than 40 mm Hg without going into acute failure. In like manner, the normal left ventricle cannot achieve an aortic pressure greater than 180 to 200 mm Hg without developing some failure.

AXIOM

If aortic systolic pressure exceeds 150 to 160 mm Hg, the left ventricular end diastolic pressure (LVEDP), even in a normal heart, often doubles, and the left ventricle may dilate and go into failure.

The left ventricle is posterior and lateral to the right ventricle, and has the shape of a narrow cone. The left ventricle tends to squeeze blood out as it contracts, whereas the crescent-shaped right ventricle has a pumping action similar to a bellows. Under ordinary circumstances, each ventricle will eject about 70 to 80 ml of blood with each contraction. This is about 60% to 70% of the normal left ventricular end-diastolic volume (100 to 150 ml) and 50% to 60% of the normal right ventricular end-diastolic volume (125 to 175 ml).

C. CARDIAC VALVES

The aortic and pulmonary valves are often referred to as the semilunar valves because of the half-moon shape of their valve leaflets. Each valve has three thin, delicate leaflets that are somewhat thickened along their free edges. At their bases they are attached to a thick, fibrous ring called the annulus.

The atrioventricular valve on the right (the tricuspid valve) has three leaflets and three papillary muscles. The mitral valve on the left has two leaflets (a larger anteromedial leaflet and smaller posterior leaflet) and two papillary muscles. The leaflets of both valves are attached to two or more papillary muscles of the ventricle by thin, fibrous bands called chorda tendineae. The leaflets extend into the ventricles in a funnel shape during ventricular diastole and are spread out into the shape of a parachute during systole. This helps prevent prolapse of the leaflets into the atria while the ventricle is contracting.

Table 1.1

PRESSURE AND OXYGEN SATURATION IN VARIOUS CHAMBERS IN THE HEART	Pressure (mm Hg)	O₂ Saturation, %
Superior vena cava	0–5	70–75
Inferior vena cava	0–5	75–80
Coronary sinus	—	30–40
Right atrium	0–5	70–75
Right ventricle	12–25/0–5	70–75
Pulmonary artery	12–25/5–10 (8–15)*	70–75
Pulmonary capillaries	6–12	98–100
Left atrium	5–10	95–98
Left ventricle	120/0–5	95–98
Aorta	120/80 (90)	95–97

*Parentheses refer to mean pressure.

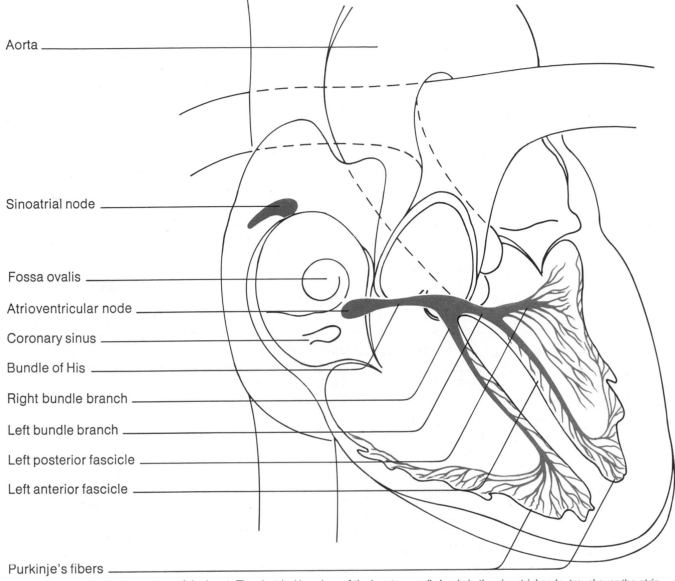

Aorta

Sinoatrial node

Fossa ovalis

Atrioventricular node

Coronary sinus

Bundle of His

Right bundle branch

Left bundle branch

Left posterior fascicle

Left anterior fascicle

Purkinje's fibers

Figure 1.1 Conducting system of the heart. The electrical impulses of the heart normally begin in the sinoatrial node, travel over the atria to the AV node, and then down the bundle of His and its branches to the terminal Purkinje fibers.

D. CONDUCTING SYSTEM

The conducting system (Fig. 1.1) of the heart is made up of atypical cardiac muscle myofibrils that have abundant sarcoplasm, which is very rich in glycogen. This specialized tissue has the capability of rhythmic electrical impulse formation and can conduct impulses much more rapidly than typical cardiac muscle. Proper function of this conducting system makes it possible for the atria and ventricles to contract in proper sequence, and for the muscle fibers in each chamber to contract in an efficient, coordinated manner.

1. The Sinoatrial Node

The electrical impulses in the heart normally begin at the sinoatrial (SA) node, which is the main regulator of the heart rate. This narrow band (1 to 2 cm long) of special conducting tissue is found at the junction of the superior vena cava and right atrium, anterior to the right auricle. The sinus node artery comes off the proximal 2 cm of the right coronary artery in 60% of patients and the proximal 1 cm of the left coronary artery in 40% of patients.
Under normal basal conditions, the SA node discharges an electrical im-

7

pulse to the rest of the heart 70 to 80 times per minute. The impulse from the SA node spreads over the atria to stimulate atrial contraction and along special upper, middle, and lower internodal tracts to the atrioventricular (AV) node. During sleep, in some athletes, and with increased vagal stimulation, the rate may be less than 50 per minute with little change in cardiac output by the normal heart. However, if stroke volume is limited by disease or the pulse rate gets below 40 per minute, cardiac output may fall sharply.

AXIOM

In infants, the elderly, and patients with diseased hearts, stroke volume may be relatively fixed. Therefore, cardiac output will be directly proportional to heart rate and a bradycardia may be extremely deleterious.

2. The Atrioventricular Node

The atrioventricular (AV) node is located in the floor of the right atrium, at the interatrial septum in front of the coronary sinus, near the membranous portion of the interventricular septum. The AV node has an intrinsic discharge rate of only 40 to 60 beats per minute. Thus, if the SA node is not functioning, the heart rate at rest will tend to be slower. The impulses picked up or generated by the AV node are transmitted along the AV bundle of His to the Purkinje fibers and then to the myocardium. In 90% of patients, the area of the AV node is supplied by the posterior descending branch of the right coronary artery; in the other 10% it is supplied by the posterior descending branch of the left circumflex coronary artery. The area of the AV node is richly supplied by vagal fibers, and ischemia in this area may cause bradycardia with nausea and vomiting.

AXIOM

If an older patient with nausea and vomiting has bradycardia, one should look for posterior myocardial ischemia.

3. Bundle of His

The bundle of His is a continuation of the AV node. It is 10 to 20 mm long and 2 to 4 mm wide. It runs in the inferior border of the membranous portion of the interventricular septum down to the muscular portion of the interventricular septum, where it divides into right and left bundles. The left bundle divides after a short distance into a long, thin anterior branch and a shorter, thicker posterior branch. The right bundle usually continues on to the right ventricle as a single main branch. These three fascicles then subdivide to ramify over their respective ventricles just under the endocardium in terminal branches called Purkinje's fibers.

4. Purkinje's Fibers

Purkinje's fibers not only act as the terminal portion of the conduction system, but also can function as a backup intrinsic pacemaker for the heart. However, their discharge rate is only 20 to 40 beats per minute. Thus, they seldom initiate a heartbeat except when there is a complete AV block and complete absence of AV nodal impulses.

AXIOM

Unusual ventricular complexes in a patient with a very slow heart rate may represent escape beats (not premature ventricular contractions).

5. Accessory Fibers

Accessory fibers can serve as conduction pathways to bypass the normal AV conduction system. These fibers form the anatomic and physiologic basis for the arrhythmias associated with the pre-excitation syndromes. Mahaim fibers, which connect the sinus node and the AV junction, may be particularly important.

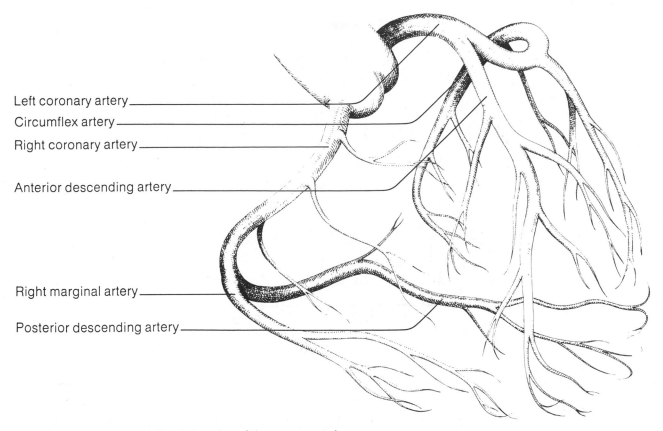

Left coronary artery

Circumflex artery

Right coronary artery

Anterior descending artery

Right marginal artery

Posterior descending artery

Figure 1.2 The distribution of main branches of the coronary arteries.

E. CORONARY ARTERIES

1. Anatomy

The heart's blood supply is often described in terms of three vessels: the right, the left anterior descending, and the left circumflex coronary arteries (Fig. 1.2). The right coronary artery (RCA) arises from the right aortic sinus of Valsalva and runs between the right atrium and ventricle, back to the posterior interventricular groove, where it becomes the posterior descending artery. One or more acute marginal branches supply the lateral portion of the right ventricle.

The left coronary artery (LCA) arises from the left aortic sinus of Valsalva and divides within 1.0 to 2.5 cm into the left anterior descending (LAD) coronary artery and the left circumflex (LCF) coronary artery. The LAD runs in the anterior interventricular groove, supplying the anterior portion of the interventricular septum and the anterior surfaces of the right and left ventricles. The LCF runs posteriorly between the left atrium and ventricle, giving off obtuse marginal (OM) branches before it descends on the posterior surface of the left ventricle. The posterior circumflex artery supplies the lateral and posterior portions of the left ventricle.

2. Normal Coronary Blood Flow

Coronary blood flow in an adult male at rest averages about 250 to 300 ml/min which is about 1.0 ml/g of heart muscle, or 4% to 5% of the total cardiac output. During systole, blood flow through the capillaries in the left ventricular myocardium, especially in the deep subendocardial layers, falls to very low levels because the contracting cardiac muscle compresses these vessels (Fig. 1.3). During diastole, the cardiac muscle relaxes and no longer obstructs the capillaries; therefore, myocardial blood flow is rapid in this phase of the cardiac cycle. The thickness of the myocardium and force of contraction of the right ventricle are far less than that of the left ventricle; thus, changes in the amount of blood flow

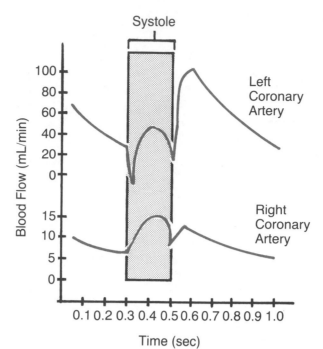

Figure 1.3 Blood flow during the cardiac cycle.

in the right coronary artery during systole and diastole are relatively mild compared with those in the left coronary artery.

3. Control of Coronary Blood Flow

a. Autoregulation

Blood flow through the coronary arteries is determined almost entirely by local autoregulation in response to the metabolic needs of the myocardium. This mechanism works well even if the nerves to the heart are severed. Extraction of oxygen by the myocardium normally is greater than in any other tissue. Coronary sinus blood has the lowest Po_2 (18 to 20 mm Hg) and lowest saturation (30% to 35%) of any venous blood in the body. Thus, even in the normal resting state, 65% to 70% of the oxygen present in arterial blood is removed as blood passes through the heart. Therefore, there is no so-called oxygen reserve in coronary blood.

AXIOM
If increased oxygen is required by the heart, it cannot extract any more from the blood; additional oxygen can be supplied only by increasing coronary blood flow.

The heart is one of the few organs that can utilize lactate for fuel, and therefore coronary venous lactate normally is lower than arterial lactate.

AXIOM
Increased coronary sinus lactate is usually a good indicator of myocardial ischemia.

b. Neurogenic Influences

Direct sympathetic stimulation of the coronary arteries tends to cause slight vasoconstriction. However, sympathetic stimulation also greatly increases both force and rate of contraction of the heart muscle, thereby increasing myocardial oxygen needs, which tends to cause vasodilation. Thus, the direct vasoconstriction effect of sympathetic stimulation is generally overridden by its effects on cardiac muscle, which indirectly can cause tremendous coronary artery vasodilation.

Parasympathetic stimulation has no direct effect on the coronary arteries, but it may decrease myocardial oxygen consumption (MVo_2) by up to 50%, primarily by reducing heart rate and to a certain extent by reducing contractility.

c. Effects of Various Drugs

Norepinephrine, epinephrine, and sympathetic nervous system stimulation all indirectly cause coronary vasodilation by increasing myocardial oxygen demand. They can also increase coronary blood flow in patients in shock by causing peripheral vasoconstriction, thereby increasing the central aortic and coronary perfusion pressures. Nitrates and papaverine, on the other hand, can cause direct coronary vasodilation. However, since they also cause peripheral vasodilation, they reduce the diastolic pressure used to perfuse the coronary arteries. This could reduce coronary blood flow, but at the same time, the pressure against which the heart must pump is reduced, thereby decreasing the metabolic demands of the heart.

d. Atherosclerosis

Atherosclerotic involvement of the coronary arteries is usually greatest in the more proximal portions. Smaller vessels (less than 1.0 mm in diameter) are involved relatively infrequently, particularly if they are within the myocardium. Thus, surgical bypass grafts to the smaller portions of the coronary arteries often have a fairly normal distal runoff.

Development of collateral vessels after coronary occlusion can be an important prognostic factor. There are, however, relatively few communications among the larger coronary arteries except around the apex of the heart. Nevertheless, anastomoses among the smaller arteries (approximately 200 to 250 μm in diameter) may occasionally develop into significant collaterals if a large proximal vessel becomes gradually occluded. There has been some concern that beta-adrenergic blocking agents, by reducing myocardial oxygen demand, might reduce the development of collateral blood vessels in the myocardium.

F. CARDIAC NERVES

The sympathetic system innervates the heart through nerves arising from the cervical and upper thoracic ganglia of the sympathetic trunks and by the parasympathetic nervous system through the vagus nerves. Stimulation of the sympathetic nervous system releases the hormones norepinephrine (at the sympathetic nerve endings) and epinephrine (from the adrenal medulla). Epinephrine has about 50% alpha and 50% beta effects, whereas norepinephrine has about 90% alpha and 10% beta effects. The beta-adrenergic effect increases the rate of SA nodal discharge, increases the excitability of all portions of the heart, and increases the force of contraction of all cardiac musculature, both atrial and ventricular. The alpha-adrenergic effect causes vasoconstriction of most blood vessels, particularly the arterioles.

The beta-adrenergic effect is apparently produced by increasing the production of adenyl cyclase in the effector tissue. Adenyl cyclase, in turn, stimulates increased production of 3',5'-cyclic adenosine monophosphate (cAMP), which then acts as a second messenger in the myocardium. The alpha-adrenergic effect acts through adenosine triphosphatase (ATPase) and is very prominent in most vessels, especially in the skin, but has little or no effect on cerebral vessels.

Stimulation of the vagus nerves causes the hormone acetylcholine to be released at its nerve endings. This causes a decreased rate of discharge of the SA node and decreased excitability of the AV junctional fibers, thereby slowing conduction in the ventricles.

G. PERICARDIUM

The pericardium is a fibroserous sac surrounding the heart and roots of the great vessels. It is continuous with the epicardium. The space between the serous membranes of the epicardium and pericardium is called the pericardial cavity. Normally, the pericardial cavity contains only a few milliliters of fluid. If the volume of fluid rapidly accumulates to more than 100 to 200 ml, the excess fluid can cause pericardial tamponade with impaired filling of the heart.

II. CARDIAC CONTRACTILITY

A. BASIC PHYSIOLOGY OF MUSCLE CONTRACTION

1. Microscopic Functional Anatomy

All striated muscle, including skeletal and cardiac muscle, is made up of numerous muscle fibers about 10 to 100 μm in diameter, which, in turn, are made up of several hundred to several thousand myofibrils (Fig. 1.4). The myocardial cell is demarcated from adjacent cells by sarcolemma and intercalated disks. Each cell contains an energy generation system (the mitochondria), an intracellular transportation and storage system for calcium and other ions (the transverse tubular system and sarcoplasmic reticulum), and an electromechanical apparatus (the myofibrils) that converts chemical energy into mechanical work. A relatively small proportion of the myocardial cell is allocated to the cytoplasm. However, glycolytic enzymes in the cytosol provide an important alternate energy source that helps maintain membrane integrity during anaerobic conditions. Each myofibril contains about 1500 myosin and about 3000 actin filaments, which run parallel to each other. These large, polymerized protein molecules, which are responsible for muscle contraction, are suspended within the sarcoplasm.

2. Changes with Stimulation and Contraction

Depolarization is initiated by a short duration increase in the permeability of the cell membrane to Na^+ and Ca^{2+}. Two specific transmembrane channels for inward movement of these ions have been described. The fast channel permits initial rapid entry of Na^+ into the cell. The slow channel allows a slower entry of Ca^{2+} slightly later.

The rapid flow of Na^+ down its concentration gradient into the cell produces rapid depolarization and is termed phase 0 of the action potential. It

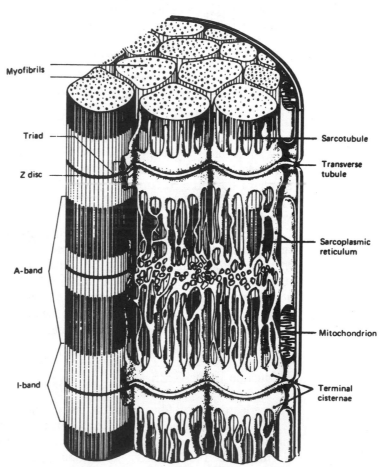

Figure 1.4 Skeletal muscle. (From Bloom, W and Fawcett, DW: A Textbook of Histology, ed 8. WB Saunders, Philadelphia, 1969, with permission.)

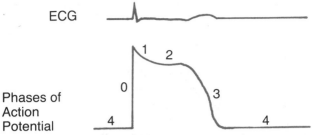

Figure 1.5 Phases of the action potential in myocardial cells showing relationship to the ECG.

coincides with the QRS complex of the surface electrocardiogram (Fig. 1.5). Closure of the fast Na^+ channels and an influx of chloride ions results in phase 1 of the action potential. This phase is very brief and is associated with rapid, but only partial, return of the membrane potential. During phase 2, calcium entry by the slow channel keeps the cell isoelectric but still depolarized as K^+ leaves the cell at approximately the same rate. This corresponds in time to the ST segment of the surface electrocardiogram. During phase 3, continuing and increasing K^+ efflux from the cell returns the membrane potential of the cell to the resting level of -90 mV. Although repolarization is complete at this point, the normal ionic gradients, especially for Na^+ and K^+ across the cell membrane are not yet re-established. During phase 4, specialized membrane-bound enzyme systems, especially the sodium-potassium ATPase pump, remove Na^+ from the cell and return K^+ back into the cell. This process is energy dependent and requires an abundant supply of adenosine triphosphate (ATP).

The action potential developed at one site on the surface of a muscle fiber spreads inward rapidly through specialized structures referred to as T-tubules. The T-tubules connect with the terminal cisternae of the sarcoplasmic reticulum. Flow of the electric current through the terminal cisternae promotes release of sodium and calcium into the surrounding sarcoplasm and then into the myofibrils to initiate contraction.

The main substances involved in muscle contraction are the two contractile proteins, actin and myosin, and two regulatory proteins, troponin and tropomyosin. Each myosin molecule has two heads that extend laterally to connect with thinner filaments of actin during systole. These actomyosin bridges push the actin fibers toward the center of the sarcomeres so that the muscle fibers shorten and tense (Fig. 1.6). The fibrous protein called tropomyosin prevents actomyosin from bridging except with proper stimulation. Troponin is a globular protein that binds to tropomyosin and has a strong avidity for calcium ions. Ionized calcium initiates contraction by binding to troponin, thereby producing conformational changes in tropomyosin, which then allows actomyosin bridges to form (Fig. 1.7). Calcium not only relieves tropomyosin inhibition, but also activates ATPase so that ATP hydrolysis and actomyosin bridging can occur simultaneously. Calcium also mediates glycogenolysis, which provides a burst of energy in the form of ATP. After contraction is completed, calcium is almost immediately resorbed into the longitudinal tubules. This resorption of calcium is also an active process requiring ATP.

ATP seems to function as a relaxing agent as well as an energy source for contraction. When bound ATP is hydrolyzed to adenosine diphosphate (ADP) and inorganic phosphate, energy is released, and muscle contraction occurs. After ATP binds to the myosin heads, actomyosin bridging is inhibited and the muscle relaxes. Since unbridled ATPase activity would lead to a state of continual contraction, this enzyme's regulation by ionized calcium assumes great importance. These events can, at least, partially explain the effects of certain clinical states. A reduction in plasma-ionized calcium levels to less than two-

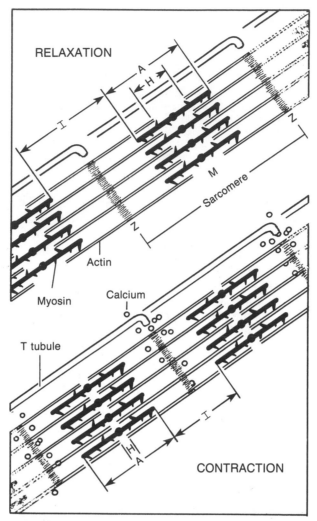

Figure 1.6 Arrangement of thin (actin) and thick (myosin) filaments in muscle relaxation and contraction. These two sets of filaments ''slide'' past each other as ''bridges'' are formed between the myosin heads and actin-binding sites. As the filaments overlap, fiber shortening, or contraction, occurs. (From Dolan, JT: Critical Care Nursing. FA Davis, Philadelphia, 1991, p 733, with permission.)

thirds normal tends to inhibit myocardial relaxation and decrease myocardial contractility. Acidosis produces the same effect, presumably by competing with calcium for binding sites on troponin. Catecholamines increase contractility by increasing calcium transport through a cAMP-mediated mechanism. They may do this in part by enhancing relaxation through increased activity of the sarcoplasmic reticulum. This would explain why catecholamines that increase cAMP (beta-adrenergic agonists) also tend to relax vascular smooth muscle to cause vasodilation.

3. Differences between Cardiac and Skeletal Muscle

The microscopic anatomy of cardiac muscle fibers and the basic mechanism of contraction are very nearly the same as that in skeletal muscle. However, cardiac muscle fibers are formed from a series of distinct cells connected at junctures called intercalated disks. These intercalated disks slow conduction of action potentials to rates as low as 0.5 m/sec, which is about one tenth that found in skeletal muscle. This allows better coordination of myocardial contraction, producing a more prolonged squeezing effect rather than just a rapid twitch.

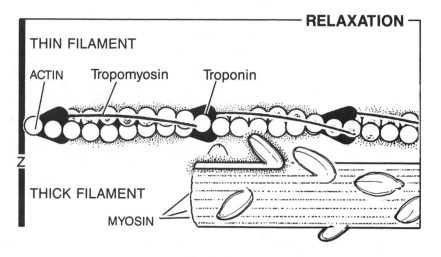

RELAXATION

THIN FILAMENT

ACTIN   Tropomyosin   Troponin

Z

THICK FILAMENT

MYOSIN

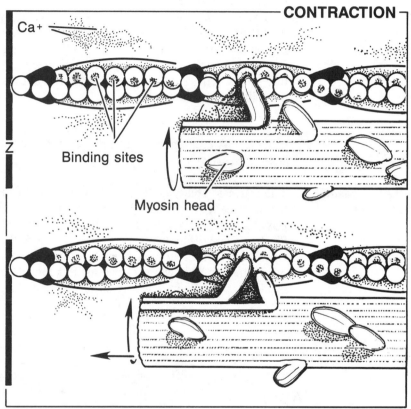

CONTRACTION

Ca+

Z

Binding sites

Myosin head

Figure 1.7 Initiation of muscle contraction by calcium. During relaxation, interaction between thin filaments (actin) and thick filaments (myosin) is blocked by the troponin-tropomyosin complex. Contraction occurs when, in response to an electrical impulse, calcium is made available to bind with troponin, which, in turn, induces a conformational change in tropomyosin, thereby exposing actin-binding sites. "Cross bridges" or links are formed between the protuberant myosin heads and the exposed actin-binding sites, which, when repeated many times over, "slide" the thin filaments toward the center of the sarcomere, thereby causing the muscle to shorten, or "contract." (From Dolan, JT: Critical Care Nursing. FA Davis, Philadelphia, 1991, p 732, with permission.)

Also, cardiac muscle fibers are arranged in large latticework formations called functional syncytiums, so that impulses transmitted over the membrane of any single fiber can spread relatively easily to all the other fibers of that chamber.

The action potential in skeletal muscle lasts less than 0.01 second, whereas the action potential in cardiac muscle has a duration of about 0.15 second in the atria and 0.30 second in the ventricles. During this entire period, the chemical process for eliciting contraction continues. Thus, cardiac muscle remains contracted 150 to 300 times longer than most skeletal muscle.

Perhaps the greatest difference between cardiac and skeletal muscle is that cardiac muscle is intrinsically self-excitable. Its membrane is considerably more permeable to sodium than that of skeletal muscle. This allows the heart muscle membrane potential to discharge periodically, providing a rhythmic, slow heartbeat if it is not stimulated by the conduction system.

B. FACTORS AFFECTING CARDIAC FUNCTION

The main factors that affect cardiac function and cardiac output include preload (filling of the heart during diastole), afterload (resistance against which the heart must pump), contractility of the heart, coordinated pattern of contraction, and heart rate.

1. Preload

Preload refers to the load or tension on a muscle as it begins to contract. In the heart, this term refers primarily to the stretch or length of myocardial fibers, which in turn is determined by the quantity of blood in the ventricle at the end of diastole (Fig. 1.8). Thus, when the contractility of the left heart is evaluated with cardiac function curves, the stroke-work index is usually plotted against the pulmonary artery wedge pressure (PAWP), which is thought to reflect left atrial pressure and left ventricular preload. However, it is now clear that PAWP will not reflect left ventricular end-diastolic volume accurately if left ventricular compliance is abnormal.

PITFALL
Assuming that the left ventricular diastolic volume is increased because the PAWP is high.

a. Effects of Increased Filling of the Heart

The intrinsic ability of the heart to adapt itself to increasing loads of inflowing blood is called Starling's law of the heart. E. H. Starling, the great English physiologist, focused his 1918 Linacre lecture on this phenomenon. Basically, Starling's law of the heart states that the more the heart is filled during diastole (within certain physiologic limits), the greater the quantity of blood it will pump out. Stated another way, an increase in ventricular fiber length during diastole is associated with an increase in cardiac work during systole. This form of intrinsic

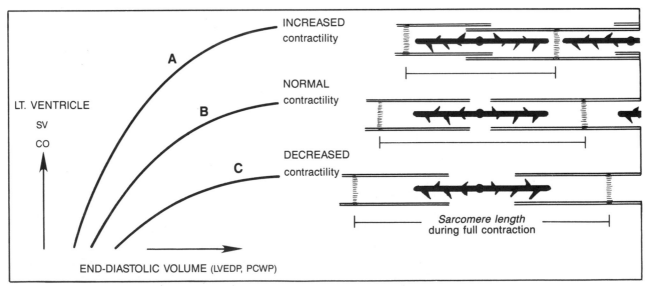

Figure 1.8 The end-diastolic volume determines the end-diastolic length of myocardial fibers and is proportional to the stroke volume and cardiac output. (From Dolan, JT: Critical Care Nursing. FA Davis, Philadelphia, 1991, p 739, with permission.)

autoregulation of the heart (in which the size of the ventricular chamber determines the amount of ventricular activity on contractility) has been referred to as heterometric autoregulation. In contrast, hemometric autoregulation refers to changes in ventricular activity due to alterations in heart rate (Bowditch effect) or aortic pressure (Anrep effect) without any change in diastolic ventricular fiber length. Thus, increased filling of the heart, increased pulse rate, or increased aortic pressure all tend to increase myocardial contractility.

Although often described separately, these effects are all somewhat interrelated. For example, increased filling of the heart increases the resting heart rate (Bainbridge reflex) at the same time that it increases pumping effectiveness. The Bainbridge reflex appears to be initiated primarily by receptors in the walls of the right atrium or venae cavae that transmit impulses to the vasomotor center by way of vagal afferent fibers.

Although a sudden 30% increase in blood volume may more than double cardiac output, this effect usually lasts only a few minutes. Cardiac output then gradually returns to normal because (1) increased cardiac output increases hydrostatic pressure in the capillaries so that fluid moves out of the capillaries into the tissues, thereby decreasing blood volume; and (2) increased pressure in the veins causes them to distend, thereby increasing venous capacity and reducing venous return.

Increased blood volume also increases atrial distention, which in turn causes increased secretion of atrial natriuretic peptide (ANP), primarily by the left atrium. ANP is a potent natriuretic diuretic and vasodilating substance. The resultant loss of salt and water in the urine and dilatation of vessels act to reduce cardiac filling. Patients with increased cardiac filling pressure and congestive heart failure usually have significantly elevated plasma levels of immunoreactive ANP.

AXIOM
Use of post end-expiratory pressure during ventilatory assistance will reduce the net distending pressure of the atria, thereby reducing ANP secretion when it may be needed to reduce an increased blood volume and excess cardiac filling.

b. Measurement of Filling Pressures in the Heart

Filling of the heart is determined primarily by the transmural cardiac filling pressure, which represents the difference between the pressure inside and outside the heart. If the extravascular pressure in the chest increases, as with a tension pneumothorax or positive pressure ventilation with positive end-expiratory pressure (PEEP), the transmural (distending) pressure is reduced by the amount of the increased extravascular pressure. In contrast, with negative extravascular pressure in the chest (as during deep spontaneous inspiration), transmural pressure increases and, therefore, tends to dilate the heart and major blood vessels, and venous return into the right heart increases. Currently, central venous pressure (CVP) is used to obtain information concerning the filling of the right heart and the PAWP reflects filling pressures in the left heart.

(1) Central Venous Pressure

Central venous pressure (CVP) is the pressure present in the central systemic veins of the chest, including innominate veins, superior vena cava, and right atrium. Unless there is stenosis of the tricuspid valve (which is very rare), the CVP is approximately equal to the diastolic, or filling pressure, in the right ventricle. However, blood volume is not the only factor that affects the CVP. The CVP also tends to rise if there is right heart failure, peripheral venoconstriction, increased blood volume, or increased pulmonary vascular resistance.

PITFALL
Assuming that right heart filling is adequate if the CVP is high.

(a) Normal values

The normal CVP is most physiology books is written as 0 to 5 mm Hg (Table 1.1). Actually, the CVP in normal, healthy young adults outside the hospital probably averages about 0 to 2 mm Hg, and during inspiration the CVP may fall to −3 to −5 cm H_2O. In hospitalized patients, particularly those in an intensive care unit (ICU), the "normal" or average CVP is usually somewhat higher, in the range of 3 to 6 mm Hg or 4 to 8 cm H_2O.

AXIOM
If the CVP is less than 4 to 8 cm H_2O in an ICU patient, one should be concerned that the patient may be hypovolemic.

(b) Factors affecting CVP

The main factors affecting the CVP include blood volume, function of the right heart, and the amount of pulmonary and systemic vasoconstriction.

(i) Blood volume

Any increase in blood volume tends to increase venous return to the right heart and thereby raise the CVP. However, in the severely hypovolemic patient, rather large amounts of fluid can usually be administered rapidly with relatively little increase in the CVP. On the other hand, rapid administration of fluid to a patient who is already overloaded with fluid usually causes a precipitous rise in the CVP.

AXIOM
The rate of rise of the CVP as fluid is rapidly given during a fluid challenge is a better gauge of right ventricular filling than the CVP level itself.

(ii) Right ventricular function

Any factor that interferes with the ability of the right ventricle to pump out the blood brought to it tends to raise the CVP. The distended neck veins classically associated with right heart failure are usually just a reflection of the high CVP present in such circumstances.

AXIOM
Distended neck veins should make one suspicious of volume overload, cardiac failure, tension pneumothorax, and pericardial tamponade.

In most instances in which right heart failure occurs, it is secondary to left heart failure. When left ventricular end-diastolic pressure and then left atrial pressure rise, pulmonary artery pressure tends to increase correspondingly. This may place a considerably greater-than-normal pressure load on the right ventricle. However, as long as the pulmonary arterial systolic pressure does not exceed 40 mm Hg, the normal right ventricle can usually continue to empty satisfactorily with only a slight rise in right-atrial pressure. However, if pulmonary arterial pressure suddenly exceeds 40 mm Hg, the normal right ventricle begins to fail and there is a progressive increase in right ventricular diastolic and right-atrial pressure. If the rise in pulmonary artery resistance is gradual, the right ventricle may have time to hypertrophy and rarely may even become able to achieve pressures exceeding systemic levels.

AXIOM
If the pulmonary artery pressure exceeds 40 mm Hg, the patient probably has a hypertrophied right ventricle from prior exposure to an increased pulmonary vascular resistance.

(iii) Pulmonary vascular resistance

Anything that interferes with blood flow through the lungs will tend to raise the CVP. Some of the more common causes in ICU patients include sepsis, use of high levels of PEEP, chronic obstructive lung disease, and pulmonary emboli. These are probably the most frequent reasons that the CVP may be deceptively high in hypovolemic patients.

| (iv) Systemic vasoconstriction | Systemic vasoconstriction tends to involve both arteries and veins. Constriction of the larger veins increases the CVP because it reduces vascular capacity and increases venous return. If vascular capacity is reduced and blood volume remains constant, the physiologic effect is almost the same as keeping vascular capacity constant and increasing blood volume. In other words, reducing vascular capacity tends to cause a relative hypervolemia with increased venous return.

Arterial vasoconstriction increases the resistance against which the left heart must pump. This tends to reduce cardiac output and raise intracardiac pressures. As the end-diastolic pressure in the left ventricles rises, left atrial pressure, pulmonary artery pressure, and then right heart pressures will tend to rise.

(c) Using the CVP clinically

PITFALL
Relying on water manometer CVP readings in a patient requiring high-ventilatory pressures.

Whenever possible the CVP should be measured electronically, rather than with a manometer. A water manometer does not react rapidly to pressure changes; therefore, it tends to provide a reading somewhere between the peak and mean CVP developed during the ventilatory cycle.

In many ICUs, great care is taken to measure the CVP with the patient flat in bed and spontaneously breathing (because positive-pressure ventilation may increase the CVP). Certainly, such maneuvers increase the accuracy of the CVP reading, but these steps are usually unnecessary.

AXIOM
The response of the CVP to a fluid challenge is far more informative than individual CVP readings.

Correlation between the CVP level and the blood volume in critically ill or injured patients is often extremely poor, and the response of the CVP to a rapid fluid load (20 ml/min) is generally far more reliable than the absolute value. The correlation between CVP levels and the amount of fluid needed to correct hypovolemia is also often quite poor.

AXIOM
Patients with severe sepsis or respiratory failure, because of increased pulmonary vascular resistance, tend to have high CVP readings, even when hypovolemic.

(d) Venous pressure waves

The mean CVP and pulmonary artery wedge (occlusion) pressures are the standard clinical measurements of cardiac filling. Additional information can often be obtained by examining the pressure waves that are developed in the atria and great veins during the cardiac cycle (Figs. 1.9 and 1.10). The venous pressure waves occurring at various phases in the cardiac cycle are referred to as the A, C, and V waves. The A wave is caused by atrial contraction, and the z descent immediately follows. The z point which follows the onset of ventricular contraction is the point at which atrial and ventricular pressures are transiently equal and also indicates the beginning of the C wave. The C wave occurs at the beginning of ventricular contraction as pressure is rising in the ventricle. It is caused partly by elevation and bulging of the AV valves into the atria and partly by pressure waves transmitted from large adjacent arteries. As the rapid ejection of systole comes to an end, the AV valve falls away from the atria, producing a fall in the venous pressure called the x descent. The V wave which follows reflects increased pressure in the atria as they fill during the phase of isometric relaxation of the ventricle. The y descent represents rapid emptying of the atria immediately after the AV valves open. With tricuspid stenosis, the right-atrial y descent will be more gradual than normal. If the AV valve is incompetent, the |

Aortic pressure

Left atrial pressure
Left ventricular pressure

EKG

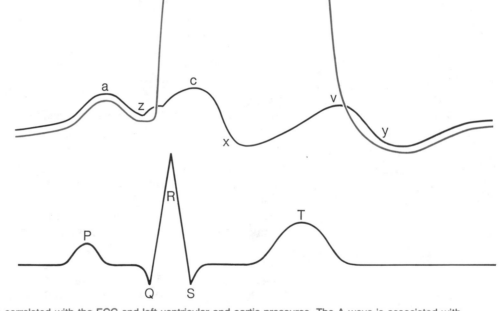

Figure 1.9 Venous pressure waves correlated with the ECG and left ventricular and aortic pressures. The A wave is associated with atrial systole, the C wave with early ventricular systole and bulging up of the AV valves, and the V wave is due to filling of the atria during ventricular systole.

combined C-V wave due to regurgitant flow into the atrium may be extremely high.

(e) Peripheral veins

If a CVP line is not available, the venous pressure can be estimated rather simply by observing the distention of the neck veins. For example, in the sitting position the neck veins are seldom visibly distended in the normal person. However, when the right atrial pressure exceeds 10 mm Hg (13.6 cm H_2O), the internal jugular veins in the lower neck of a sitting patient usually become quite obvious. When the right atrial pressure exceeds 15 mm Hg (20 cm H_2O), the veins in the neck usually become even more distended and venous pulse waves may become prominent.

AXIOM

Prominent pressure waves in distended neck veins often reflect some tricuspid valve incompetence due to overfilling or failure of the right ventricle.

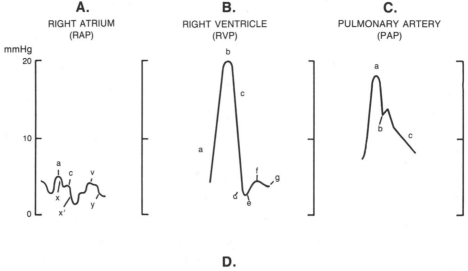

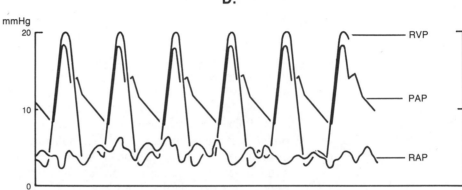

Figure 1.10 (*A*) Normal right atrial pressure (RAP) waveform showing an A wave, a C wave, and a V wave, followed by the x, x', and y descents. (*B*) Normal right ventricular pressure (RVP) waveform showing (a) isovolumetric contraction, (b) rapid ejection, (c) reduced ejection, (d) isovolumetric relaxation, (e) early diastole, (f) atrial systole (atrial kick), and (g) end distole. (*C*) Normal pulmonary artery pressure (PAP) waveform showing (a) systole (b) dicrotic notch and (c) end diastole. (*D*) Shows all three pressures (RAP, RVP, and PAP) superimposed on one another. All three pressures reflect low-pressure systems of right heart and pulmonary circulation (From Dolan, JT: Critical Care Nursing. FA Davis, Philadelphia, 1991, p 836, with permission.)

(f) Peripheral venous pressure

Since there is some resistance to venous return from the peripheral veins into the central (intrathoracic) veins, peripheral venous pressure (PVP) may be more than 5 to 10 cm H_2O higher than CVP. Therefore, if the PVP is high, the CVP may be high or low. However, if the PVP is low, the CVP must also be low. With these potential errors in mind, the response of peripheral venous pressure to a fluid load can occasionally be of some help. The height to which the hands of the patient must be raised above the heart (tricuspid valve) can also provide a rough indication of the CVP.

(2) Pulmonary Artery Wedge (Occlusion) Pressure

The pulmonary artery occlusion pressure (usually referred to as the pulmonary artery wedge pressure, or PAWP) usually provides fairly accurate information on the filling pressures of the left ventricle. The Swan-Ganz catheter is a soft catheter with a balloon near its top. After the catheter has been advanced into the right atrium, the balloon is inflated with about 0.8 cc of air. The flow of blood in the heart then carries the balloon and attached catheter into the right ventricle and out into a pulmonary artery. The balloon is then deflated and passed a bit further out into a smaller branch of the pulmonary artery. When the balloon is inflated enough to occlude the pulmonary artery, the tip will be exposed to a "wedge pressure" which reflects left atrial filling pressures relatively well.

Prior to the development of pulmonary artery balloon catheters, the only available measurements of left atrial pressure were obtained by (1) catheters inserted directly during cardiac surgery, (2) catheters passed into the right atrium and through the interatrial septum into the left atrium, or (3) pulmonary artery catheters passed out so far into the pulmonary arterial system that the tip of the catheter was "wedged" in a small pulmonary artery and arterialized blood could be aspirated from it. The Swan-Ganz catheter has provided the opportunity to measure PAWP in most patients easily and rapidly. As a result, it has become increasingly clear that there are many situations in which the filling pressures of the right and left heart are quite disparate. Furthermore, the filling pressures of the left heart as reflected by PAWP obviously has a much greater effect on the systemic circulation than does the CVP.

Recently, Stork, Muller, and Piske reported on the use of transmitral pulsed-Doppler echocardiography (tpDE) to determine PAWP. The correlation was extremely good ($r = 0.98$). However, tpDE was of limited value for assessing systolic ventricular function.

(a) Normal values

The mean pressure in the left atrium and the major pulmonary veins normally averages 5 to 10 mm Hg, and the PAWP, which is usually only 1 to 2 mm Hg higher, averages 6 to 12 mm Hg (Table 1.1). The pressure in the left atrium is usually greater than the pressure in the right atrium for three reasons: (1) the left ventricle has far greater force than the right ventricle, resulting in much more ventricular thrust against the left atrium than the right; (2) part of the pulse pressure in the pulmonary arteries is transmitted through the capillaries into the pulmonary veins; and (3) the compliance of the pulmonary veins, left atrium, and left ventricle is considerably less than the compliance of the right ventricle, right atrium, and large systemic veins.

(b) Factors affecting PAWP

PAWP is altered by the same factors that affect the CVP. However, increased blood volume often raises the CVP earlier than the PAWP. On the other hand, isolated ventricular failure is more apt to occur on the left than on the right.

(c) Errors in measuring PAWP

PAWP is either unobtainable or read somewhat incorrectly in 10% to 40% of cases. If the tip of the catheter is not at least 2 to 3 cm below the mitral valve, it can provide a falsely high reading, especially if PEEP is being used. In addition, if the pulmonary artery lumen is only partially occluded when the balloon is inflated, the pressure recorded will be somewhere between the mean PAP and the true PAWP.

AXIOM

The pulmonary artery diastolic pressure (PADP) is normally at least 1 to 2 mm Hg higher than the left atrial pressure or PAWP. If the PAWP really did exceed PADP, blood would tend to flow backward in the lung during diastole.

Whenever the PAWP is higher than the PADP, the accuracy of the PAWP reading should be questioned, and the catheter placement and balloon inflation should be checked. If the PADP exceeded PAWP appropriately initially, but later it appeared that PAWP exceeded PADP, one must suspect that the catheter tip has changed position, severe mitral insufficiency has developed, or the alveolar inflation pressures now exceed PVP in the portion of the lung containing the tip of the catheter.

If high ventilatory pressures are being used, the PAWP recorded on digital readouts is an average and often will not reflect the true end-expiratory pressure of each beat.

If the PADP is more than 5 mm Hg greater than the PAWP, excess pulmonary vasoconstriction with a higher-than-normal pulmonary vascular resistance is likely to be present. In ICU patients, this often is associated with a mortality rate exceeding 60% to 70%.

AXIOM

An increasing PADP-PAWP gradient implies increasing pulmonary hypertension and a much worse prognosis.

(d) Using PAWP clinically

With normal left ventricular function, the mean left atrial pressure and PAWP are usually less than 10 mm Hg. However, in critically ill patients, fluid can generally be given safely as long as the PAWP remains below 15 to 18 mm Hg. In patients with adult respiratory distress syndrome (ARDS), there is a definite advantage to keeping the PAWP less than 12 to 16 mm Hg. If the PAWP exceeds 22 mm Hg, particularly if it rises rapidly with a fluid load, some degree of left heart failure is present; if the PAWP exceeds 25 to 35 mm Hg, acute pulmonary edema is apt to occur. However, if pulmonary capillary permeability is increased, as in ARDS, pulmonary edema can occur with a PAWP less than 10 to 15 mm Hg.

AXIOM

Increasing clinical evidence of pulmonary edema in a patient with a normal or low PAWP should make one assume that sepsis or some other cause of increased pulmonary capillary permeability is present.

In patients with normal lungs, changes in the CVP reflect changes in the filling pressure in the left ventricle relatively well. However, several situations exist in which the CVP does not adequately reflect the left ventricular end-diastolic pressures. In patients with severe sepsis or respiratory failure, the CVP may be quite high because of increased resistance to flow in the pulmonary vessels even if the PAWP is quite low. In contrast, patients with an isolated left ventricular failure due to acute myocardial infarction may have a high PAWP and relatively low CVP, at least transiently.

(e) Complications

Although pulmonary artery catheters can provide extremely important information about the cardiovascular system, they can also cause complications. Arrhythmias frequently occur during insertion; however, these are seldom more than a few premature ventricular beats. Nevertheless, the catheter has caused ventricular fibrillation in a few patients, especially in the presence of an acute myocardial infarction or severe hypoxia or acidosis. If a left heart block is present, one must be extremely cautious and have a temporary pacemaker available because insertion of a PAWP catheter under these circumstances has about a 2% to 3% chance of producing a complete heart block. Pulmonary infarction and even exsanguinating hemorrhage due to excessive balloon pressure or prolonged inflation of the balloon has also been reported.

2. Afterload

An increase in systemic vascular resistance, or the pressure against which the heart must pump (as may be caused by a vasopressor) tends to increase ventricular contractility, but stroke volume and cardiac output tend to fall.

A fall in cardiac output is often seen with increasing age in adults and averages about 0.1 to 0.2 liters $\cdot$ min^{-1} $\cdot$ m^{-2} (Table 1.2). In a teenage boy, the cardiac index will tend to be about 3.5 to 3.8 liters $\cdot$ min^{-1} $\cdot$ m^{-2}. In a "normal" 50-year-old man, the cardiac index is apt to be about 3.1 to 3.4 liters $\cdot$ min^{-1} $\cdot$ m^{-2}. A fall in cardiac output is also often seen when vasopressors are used to correct hypotension. In such circumstances, these agents raise blood

Table 1.2

CHANGES IN BLOOD
PRESSURE, CARDIAC OUTPUT,
AND PERIPHERAL VASCULAR
RESISTANCE WITH AGE

Age (Years)	Blood Pressure (mm Hg)			Blood Flow		Peripheral Vascular Resistance†	
	Systolic/ Diastolic	Mean	Cardiac Index* $(L \cdot min^{-1} \cdot m^{-2})$	Cardiac Output (L/min)	$mm\,Hg \cdot L^{-1} \cdot min^{-1}$	$dyne \cdot sec \cdot cm^{-1}$	
10	90/60	70	3.7	4.4	14.7	1180	
20	110/70	83	3.5	6.0	13.0	1040	
30	115/75	88	3.4	5.8	14.3	1140	
40	120/80	93	3.3	5.6	15.7	1260	
50	125/82	96	3.2	5.4	16.9	1350	
60	130/85	100	3.0	5.1	18.6	1480	
70	135/88	104	2.9	4.9	20.2	1600	
80	140/90	107	2.8	4.8	21.3	1700	

*Assuming a body surface area of 1.2 m² at age 10 and 1.7 m² thereafter.
†Assuming a CVP of 5 mm Hg.

pressure but they can also increase the systemic vascular resistance (SVR) so much that the cardiac output falls and peripheral tissue perfusion is reduced.

PITFALL
Failing to recognize that drugs that increase blood pressure also tend to reduce cardiac output and tissue perfusion.

An important extrinsic mechanism relating myocardial activity to blood pressure is the so-called carotidoventricular, pressoreceptor, or baroreceptor reflex. Hypotension in the carotid sinus causes a reflex stimulation of the sympathetic nervous system, which, in turn, tends to increase the rate and force of myocardial contraction and also the degree of peripheral vasoconstriction. In contrast, an increased blood pressure tends to decrease the stimuli from the carotid sinus to the vasomotor center. This reduces sympathetic stimulation of the heart, thereby decreasing ventricular contractility and peripheral vasoconstriction. Vagal tone may also increase when blood pressure rises, thereby slowing the heart rate.

3. Cardiac Contractility

A heart that is hypertrophied or strongly stimulated by sympathetic impulses is capable of pumping greater quantities of blood than normal against a standard amount of resistance and may be considered to have increased myocardial contractility. Hypertrophy of the heart usually occurs in response to a chronic increased load, such as in long-distance runners or patients with hypertension or aortic stenosis.

4. Coordinated Contraction

Even if all the individual muscle units in the heart are functioning properly, failure of these units to beat in a coordinated fashion can greatly impair cardiac function. Some of the more frequent causes of uncoordinated myocardial contraction include (a) ischemia or trauma to the conduction system of the heart, producing various types of bundle-branch blocks; (b) ischemia or trauma to portions of the myocardium causing slower and/or weaker contraction than normal adjacent muscle; (c) arrhythmias; and (d) excessive dilatation of the ventricle.

5. Heart Rate

If the pulse rate is less than 50 or greater than 150 per minute, cardiac output often falls and the tendency to arrhythmias increases. However, in well-trained athletes, it is not unusual for the resting pulse rate to be less than 50 and greater than 180 during maximal exertion. Heart rates in adults average about 70 to 80 per minute. In children, pulse rates tend to be slightly higher, but rates less than 60 per minute are considered to be bradycardia and rates greater than 100 per minute are considered to be tachycardia.

If venous return is reduced or stroke volume is limited, bradycardia may cause a severe reduction in cardiac output and an excessive rise in the left ventricular end-diastolic pressure. In many critically ill or injured patients, the highest cardiac output with the best cardiac function is often obtained at pulse rates of 100 to 120 per minute.

PITFALL
Progressive attempts to reduce heart rates to less than 100 per minute in patients with sepsis or an increased oxygen consumption.

When the heart rate is excessively fast, several physiologic alterations occur. The ratio of myocardial oxygen consumption/myocardial oxygen delivery (MVo_2/MDo_2) falls, and myocardial hypoxemia is more apt to occur. Due to reduced diastolic time, left ventricular coronary blood flow is decreased. In addition, the tachycardia results in relatively more time in systole and increased myocardial contractility, both of which cause an increased myocardial oxygen consumption.

It should also be noted that there may be an important teleological advantage to an increased contractility when the pulse rate rises. To empty the heart properly in a shorter period of time requires a more rapid rate of rise of intraventricular pressure. This decreases the duration of the ejection period, which, in turn, increases the duration of diastole during which virtually all of the left coronary blood flow occurs. Furthermore, if ventricular contraction and relaxation are both more rapid, diastolic ventricular filling will be increased.

AXIOM
Although an increased heart rate may increase cardiac output and contractility, in patients with coronary artery disease, this tends to increase myocardial oxygen demand more than coronary blood flow and can cause myocardial ischemia.

6. Other Factors

Other factors that may influence cardiac function include hypoxia, anemia, and the concentrations of various cations.

a. Hypoxia

Mild hypoxia may cause a moderate increase in sympathetic stimulation, which, in turn, may increase cardiac contractility. However, severe hypoxia will tend to impair myocardial function. These changes are due to several effects that hypoxia can have on the circulation. For example, hypoxia tends to cause peripheral vasodilation, which, by reducing afterload, increases cardiac output. Thus, with mild-to-moderate hypoxemia, cardiac output may increase up to double normal resting values. However, if hypoxia becomes very severe (Pao_2 less than 45 to 50 mm Hg), myocardial function may deteriorate, and severe hypotension may develop.

b. Anemia

Anemia decreases the viscosity of the blood, which, in turn, decreases the resistance to blood flow. Severe anemia may also cause some tissue hypoxia with resultant dilatation of peripheral vessels. This further reduces the resistance against which the heart must pump. As a result, cardiac output tends to increase in an almost linear fashion as hematocrit falls. Consequently, the total amount of oxygen transported to the tissue may remain relatively constant despite fairly marked anemia. Once the hematocrit falls below 15%, however, cardiac output has to rise disproportionately and may not be able to keep pace with the fall in arterial oxygen content.

At the other extreme, patients with polycythemia (Hct >50%) tend to have a reduced cardiac output because of reduced need for blood flow and because of the increased viscosity and resistance to flow. Once the hematocrit exceeds 55%, viscosity increases almost geometrically, causing cardiac output to fall rather markedly, often with production of peripheral cyanosis.

c. Effects of Various Cations

Hyperkalemia (particularly above 7.0 to 7.5 mEq/liter) may produce AV block and cardiac standstill. An excess of potassium ions in the extracellular fluid (ECF) decreases the resting membrane potential of the myocardium, thereby decreasing the intensity of the action potential. As a result, with hyperkalemia or hypocalcemia, contraction of the heart becomes progressively weaker and slower. In contrast, a decrease in plasma potassium or a rise in ionized calcium concentrations tends to increase myocardial contractility. Calcium ions oppose the action of potassium and increase the force and duration of myocardial contraction. Both hypokalemia and hypercalcemia also increase the sensitivity of the heart to digitalis.

Shock and sepsis increase the movement of ionized calcium into, and potassium out of, myocardial cells and may thereby reduce myocardial function. Administering calcium may temporarily improve myocardial function; however, 30 to 45 minutes later, if cell membrane function is still impaired and cytoplasmic free calcium levels have risen, myocardial function may deteriorate below the baseline values.

C. MEASUREMENTS OF CARDIAC CONTRACTILITY

Numerous techniques have been developed to evaluate the contractility or functional capability of the heart. Some of these include (1) construction of cardiac function curves, (2) calculation of ejection fractions, (3) estimates of the velocity of muscle contraction, and (4) various noninvasive techniques.

1. Ventricular Function Curves

One of the best ways to express the functional ability of the heart is with ventricular function curves (Fig. 1.11). As ventricular diastolic filling pressure or volume increases, stroke work (stroke volume times mean pressure) also increases until it reaches a limit above which the ventricle begins to fail. The shape of the curve formed by plotting these parameters can then be used to evaluate myocardial contractility.

Left ventricular stroke work index (LVSWI) is calculated by the formula:

$$LVSWI = mBP \times \frac{SV}{BSA} \times 1.36 \times 10^{-2}.$$

Thus, if the mean blood pressure (mBP) is 90 mm Hg, stroke volume (SV) is 68 ml, and body surface area (BSA) is 1.7 m²,

$$LVSWI = 90 \times \frac{68}{1.7} \times 1.36 \times 10^{-2} = 49 \; \frac{g \cdot m}{m^2}.$$

On the normal curve in Figure 1.11, this would fall at a PAWP of about 11 mm Hg. If the patient were given enough fluid to raise the PAWP to 15 mm Hg, one would expect the LVSWI to rise to about 59 $g \cdot m \cdot m^{-2}$ by raising mBP, SV, or both. A number of other hemodynamic variables are also used to evaluate cardiac function (Table 1.3).

2. Ejection Fraction

Determination of end-systolic volume (ESV), end-diastolic volume (EDV), and ejection fraction (EF) is now possible using special right ventricular catheters, angiography, or echocardiography. The EF for each ventricle can be readily calculated from the ESV and EDV by the following formula:

$$EF = \frac{EDV - ESV}{EDV} = \frac{SV}{EDV}.$$

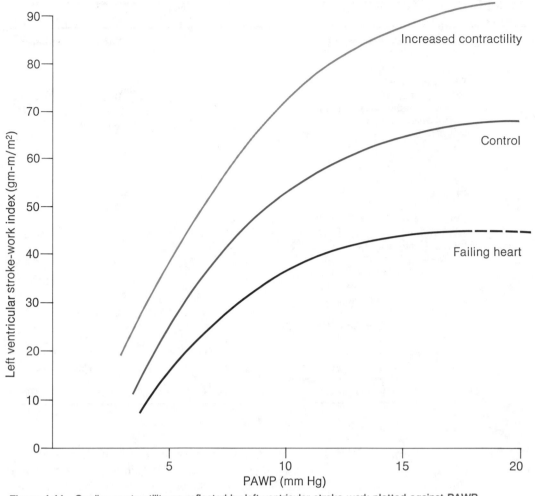

Figure 1.11 Cardiac contractility as reflected by left ventricular stroke work plotted against PAWP.

The normal EF for the left ventricle is 60% to 70%. The normal EF for the right ventricle is about 50% to 60%. In sepsis, although cardiac output may be high, EF is often lower than normal.

3. Noninvasive Methods

Several noninvasive techniques currently available for estimating cardiac function include echocardiography, apex cardiography, and measurements of systolic time intervals.

a. Echocardiography

Echocardiography can provide valuable data on the performance of the heart by evaluating (1) the motion of the left ventricle at its internal minor axis just above the plane of the mitral valve, (2) the thickness of the left ventricular wall, and (3) the synchrony and extent of muscle contraction from the mitral valve to the apex. These studies correlate rather well with the results from invasive techniques.

b. Systolic Time Intervals

Using simultaneous recordings of the echocardiogram, phonocardiogram, and carotid arterial pulse, the duration of the pre-ejection and ejection phases of the cardiac cycle can be estimated fairly accurately. Left ventricular dysfunction tends to lengthen the pre-ejection phase and shorten the ejection time.

Thus, the ratio of pre-ejection time to left ventricular ejection time (which is

Table 1.3

RELEVANT HEMODYNAMIC VARIABLES	Abbreviation/Name/Formula	Unit	Normal	Preferred
	Measured Parameters			
	HR — Heart rate	beats/min	60–100	<100
	BP — Blood pressure	mm Hg	120/80	>90<14
	CVP — Central venous pressure	mm Hg	1–6	>3<15
	PAP — Pulmonary artery pressure	mm Hg	12–25/5–10	
	PCWP — Pulmonary capillary wedge pressure	mm Hg	6–12	>6<18
	CO — Cardiac output	L/min	4–6	>5
	Derived Parameters			
	CI — Cardiac index = CO/body surface area	$L \cdot min^{-1} \cdot m^{-2}$	2.5–4.0	>35
	SVI — Stroke-volume index = (CI)(1000)/HR	$ml \cdot beat^{-1} \cdot m^{-2}$	33–47	>35
	LVSWI — Left-ventricular stroke-work index = (SVI) (mBP) (0.0136)	$g \cdot m \cdot m^{-2}$	44–68	>55
	RVSWI — Right-ventricular stroke-work index = (SVI) (PAP mean) (0.0136)	$g \cdot m \cdot m^2$	4–8	
	LCWI — Left-cardiac work index = (CI)(mBP) (0.0136)	$kg \cdot m \cdot m^{-2}$	3.0–4.7	
	RCWI — Right-cardiac work index = (CI)(PAP mean) (0.0136)	$kg \cdot m \cdot m^{-2}$	0.4–0.6	
	SVRI — Systemic vascular resistance index = 80 (mBP − CVP)/CI	$dyne \cdot sec \cdot cm^{-5} \cdot m^{-2}$	0.0–2750	>1700
	PVRI — Pulmonary vascular-resistance index = 80 (PAP mean − PAWP)/CI	$dyne \cdot sec \cdot cm^{-5} \cdot m^{-2}$	45–225	<200

normally about 0.35 ± 0.04 SD) tends to increase as the heart begins to fail. Changes in this ratio correlate well with other measurements of left ventricular function, but may not be able to distinguish changes in contractility from changes in preload or afterload. These measurements may also be much less reliable when conduction or valvular abnormalities are present.

c. Impedance Cardiography

Since the pioneering days of the early 1960s, the use of changes in thoracic electrical impedance to evaluate peripheral blood flow, thoracic fluid volume, cardiac output, and myocardial contractility has gradually increased. Numerous validation studies have, in general, confirmed the earlier work. More recently, impedance cardiography has been increasingly utilized in clinical medicine to evaluate SV and cardiac output.

Of particular interest are preliminary reports that a left ventricular ejection fraction (LVEF) index can be obtained from the thoracic electrical impedance cardiogram. Impedance cardiography would appear to be an ideal technique with which to repeatedly assess cardiac function, since it is noninvasive, simple to use, reproducible, and relatively inexpensive. Once LVEF and SV are obtained, left ventricular EDV and ESV can be determined and, with adjustments in preload, a Frank-Starling curve can be constructed. Such information would be particularly helpful in identifying types of cardiac dysfunction in patients and for serial assessments of therapeutic progress.

However, in a recent study by Miles, Gotshall, and Golden, it was found that there was no agreement between EFs measured by nuclear angiography and those determined by impedance studies. Thus, the possible role of impedance cardiography in evaluating myocardial function is questionable at this time.

D. ENERGY REQUIREMENTS OF THE HEART

Energy imparted to the blood ejected by the heart consists of kinetic energy of motion and potential energy in the form of pressure. Ordinarily, 96% to 98% of the work output of the left ventricle is in the form of pressure. Only 2% to 4%

1. Kinetic and Potential Energy

of the work output of the heart is used to create the kinetic energy associated with blood flow out of the heart. However, in certain conditions (such as aortic stenosis), as much as 50% of the total work output may be required to create the kinetic energy of blood flow.

2. Heat Production

During muscular contraction of the heart, most of the chemical energy used is converted into heat and only a small portion into work. The ratio of cardiac work output to the energy expenditure is called the efficiency of cardiac contraction. The efficiency of the heart under normal circumstances is only about 5% to 10%. However, during maximum work output it may rise to 15% to 20%.

3. Systolic Tension-Time Index (STTI)

Multiple studies have attempted to correlate myocardial oxygen consumption (MVo_2) with various measurements of cardiac function. From Sarnoff's studies on isolated hearts, it is now generally agreed that the MVo_2 correlates best with the calculated STTI. The STTI is equal to the average tension developed by the left ventricle during systole multiplied by the duration of systole per minute. Since the tension developed in the ventricular wall during systole is a function of systolic pressure and ventricular volume, the greater the systolic pressure and volume of the ventricle, the greater the MVo_2. As the pulse rate increases, the amount of time that the heart is in systole each minute also increases and causes the MVo_2 to rise. On the other hand, if a vasodilator is given, stroke volume increases, but the mean ventricular pressure is decreased. Thus, if the pulse rate remains constant, a vasodilator can cause cardiac output to increase without increasing MVo_2.

4. Pulse-Pressure Product

The pulse-pressure product (PPP) calculation can be used clinically to estimate changes in MVo_2. For example, if the systemic BP is 120/80 and the pulse rate is 70 per minute, the PPP is 120 × 70 or 8400. If the BP rises to 140/90 and the pulse rate rises to 120 per minute, the new PPP is 16,800 and the MVo_2 has probably doubled.

Calculations of the triple pulse-pressure product (TPPP) has been used by some investigators to estimate MVo_2 more accurately when the PAWP is available. If everything else is held constant, an increased PAWP is associated with an increased diameter of the ventricle at the end of diastole and, consequently, an increased MVo_2. The TPPP is calculated by the following formula:

$$TPPP = \text{pulse rate} \times \text{systolic BP} \times PAWP.$$

A normal TPPP might be 70 × 120 × 6 = 50,400. If the BP is 140/90, the pulse rate 120 per minute, and the PAWP 18 mm Hg, the TPPP is 302,400, or about six times normal. The TPPP probably overestimates changes in MVo_2. Using the square root of the PAWP rather than the PAWP itself is probably more accurate. Nevertheless, using these same numbers, the TPPP would increase from a normal of 20,576 to 71,276, or about 3.5 times normal.

AXIOM
Relatively minor increases in systolic BP, heart rate, and ventricular filling can cause great (geometric) increases in myocardial oxygen consumption.

5. Increased Contractility

Other factors that increase energy expenditure by the heart include fever or stimulation of the heart with epinephrine, norepinephrine, isoproterenol, dopamine, digitalis, and thyroxine. All these factors increase the metabolic activity of the cardiac muscle fibers themselves, which, in turn, increases the rate of oxygen usage.

E. PHASES OF THE CARDIAC CYCLE

The phases of the cardiac cycle are generally described in relation to changes in pressure and volume in the left ventricle during ventricular filling (diastole) and ventricular contraction (systole) (Fig. 1.12).

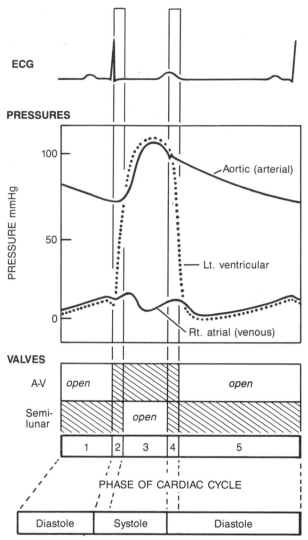

ECG

PRESSURES

PRESSURE mmHg

100

50

0

Aortic (arterial)

Lt. ventricular

Rt. atrial (venous)

VALVES

A-V   open   open

Semi-lunar   open

1 2 3 4 5

PHASE OF CARDIAC CYCLE

Diastole   Systole   Diastole

Figure 1.12 Phases of the cardiac cycle illustrating the relationship between electrical (ECG) and mechanical (aortic, left ventricular, and right atrial pressures, and valve opening and closure. (From Vander, A, Sherman, J, and Luciano, D: Human Physiology: The Mechanisms of Body Function, ed. 4. McGraw-Hill, New York, 1985, p 325, with permission.)

1. Ventricular Filling (Diastole)

If the heart rate is 75 per minute, diastole lasts about 0.53 second and systole about 0.27 second (Table 1.4). Thus, with a normal pulse rate, diastole takes up about two thirds of the cardiac cycle. By the time diastole is completed, the volume of blood inside the ventricle normally increases from about 40 to 50 ml to about 100 to 120 ml. During exercise, however, the volume of blood in the heart at the end of systole may fall to 30 ml or less and the diastolic volume may rise to 150 to 200 ml or more.

a. Protodiastole

The first phase of diastole, referred to as the protodiastole, is extremely short and lasts only 20 to 60 ms. During this period, occurring just after ventricular systole, ventricular pressure falls abruptly and the aortic valve closes.

b. Isometric Relaxation

The next phase, usually referred to as the period of isometric relaxation, lasts about 60 to 100 ms, and is characterized by continued muscle relaxation without any change in intraventricular volume. Ventricular pressure continues to fall rapidly until it is exceeded by the atrial pressure, and the mitral valve opens.

Table 1.4

PHASE OF THE CARDIAC CYCLE		Duration (msec)*
Diastole		530
Protodiastole	20–60	
Isometric relaxation	60–100	
Rapid filling	100–120	
Diastasis	160–220	
Atrial systole	120–180	
Systole		270
Isometric contraction	40–60	
Rapid ejection	80–100	
Reduced ejection	120–140	———
Total		800

*Assuming heart rate of 75 per minute = 800 msec/beat.

During isometric relaxation, pressure in the atrium rises, producing the rising limb of the venous V wave because of blood accumulating in the atria, and also because the base of the heart rises during relaxation, compressing the atria.

c. Rapid Filling

Immediately after the AV valve opens, blood flows rapidly into the ventricle. Pressure in the atria falls quickly, producing the so-called y descent in the venous-pressure tracing. During this period of rapid filling, which lasts about 100 to 120 ms, approximately 60% to 70% of ventricular filling occurs.

d. Diastasis

Filling of the ventricles during the next 160 to 220 ms becomes progressively slower. During this relatively prolonged period, often referred to as slow filling or diastasis, only 10% to 20% of ventricular filling occurs.

e. Atrial Systole

During the terminal phase of ventricular diastole, which generally lasts about 120 to 180 ms, the rate of ventricular filling is increased again because of atrial systole. This atrial "kick" is normally responsible for about 20% to 30% of ventricular filling. However, under normal demands in an otherwise normal heart, the atria can become completely nonfunctional as a result of atrial fibrillation or heart block, and the ventricles will still operate almost normally. In contrast, during exercise or in the presence of mitral stenosis, atrial systole can be extremely important and may account for 30% to 50% of the blood flow into the ventricle.

2. Ventricular Emptying (Systole)

a. Isometric Contraction

During the initial phase of systole, the left ventricular muscle is contracting but the pressure within the ventricle has not become high enough to open the aortic valve; consequently intraventricular volume is unchanged. This phase, often called the period of isometric contraction, generally lasts only about 40 to 60 ms.

b. Maximal Ejection

When the pressure inside the ventricle exceeds aortic pressure, the aortic valve opens and blood is ejected from the ventricle. Ventricular pressure continues to rise, and blood is rapidly ejected from the heart. By the time ventricular pressure reaches its peak, most of the blood that will leave has left the ventricle. This period of maximal ejection or rapid emptying generally lasts about 80 to 100 ms.

c. Reduced Ejection

After ventricular pressure reaches its peak, ejection of blood decreases rapidly, and the pressure in the aorta begins to fall as blood flow out of the distal end of the arterial system begins to exceed the inflow from the ventricle. This period of reduced ejection persists for about 120 to 140 ms and then, as the ventricular muscle begins to relax, pressure in the ventricles falls rapidly.

F. RELATIONSHIP OF HEART SOUNDS TO THE CARDIAC CYCLE

Left-ventricle contraction usually begins before and continues after that of the right ventricle. However, actual ejection of blood from the right ventricle (which has less pressure to overcome) starts before the left ventricle and persists after left ventricular ejection has ceased. Consequently, the usual sequence of valve movement at the onset of systole is mitral valve closure (MC), tricuspid valve closure (TC), pulmonary valve opening (PO), and aortic valve opening (AO). At the onset of diastole, the usual sequence of valve motion is aortic valve closure (AC), pulmonary valve closure (PC), tricuspid valve opening (TO), and mitral valve opening (MO). In other words, the tricuspid valve stays open longer than any other valve and the aortic valve is closed longer than any other valve (Fig. 1.13).

1. First Heart Sound

The first heart sound (S_1), which is normally low-pitched and of relatively long duration, is heard as the ventricles initially contract and the mitral and then the tricuspid valves close. Ejection sounds, which have a sharp clicking quality, may occasionally be heard during the initial phases of systole if there is hypertension in the pulmonary artery or aorta or if these vessels are significantly dilated. By auscultation alone, it may be difficult to differentiate a split first sound from ejection clicks. However, since ejection clicks may indicate more serious pathology, the sounds should be considered as ejection clicks until proven otherwise.

2. Second Heart Sound

The second heart sound (S_2), which is normally rapid and sharp, occurs at the beginning of isometric relaxation as the aortic and then pulmonary valves close. During expiration, aortic valve closure (A_2) normally occurs about 0.02 to 0.04 seconds before pulmonic valve closure (P_2), producing a split, second heart sound (Fig. 1.14). During inspiration, when the left heart is relatively less full and the right heart is more full than during expiration, A_2 tends to occur slightly earlier and P_2 slightly later so that the split is slightly wider (0.04 to 0.06 seconds). Conditions such as atrial septal defects (that result in increased pulmonary flow and later pulmonic valve closure) or mitral insufficiency (that results in early aortic valve closure) may increase the duration of the A_2-P_2 split. A right bundle-branch block (RBBB) will also tend to increase the split, whereas a left bundle-branch block (LBBB) decreases the split or may even cause a paradoxical split.

3. Third Heart Sound

With careful auscultation, a third heart sound (S_3) of low intensity and frequency occurring early in diastole can be heard in most children and in some young, healthy adults (Fig. 1.15). However, an S_3 in older patients often indicates left heart failure. The intensity of S_3 may also be increased with mitral insufficiency and pericardial effusion, which alter the distensibility of the ventricle. It is generally thought that the S_3 is produced during the period of rapid filling by abrupt limitations of ventricular distensibility producing tensing of the valve and its chordae.

4. Fourth Heart Sound

A fourth heart sound (S_4) can be heard with careful auscultation in many children and adults just prior to ventricular systole. This S_4 is also of low pitch and frequency and occurs during atrial systole. Its etiology, like that of S_3, is probably related to altered distensibility of the ventricle. The significance of S_4 has been debated extensively. In adults, it is often associated with ventricular abnormalities, particularly coronary artery disease or hypertension; in children, an S_4 is usually normal.

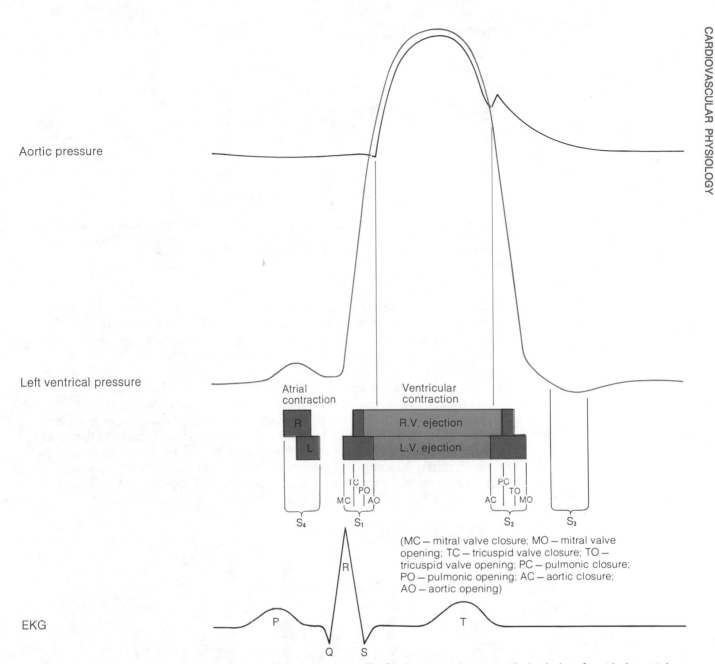

Aortic pressure

Left ventrical pressure

Atrial contraction

Ventricular contraction

R.V. ejection

L.V. ejection

TC
PO
MC AO

PC
TO
AC MO

S_4 S_1 S_2 S_3

(MC — mitral valve closure; MO — mitral valve opening; TC — tricuspid valve closure; TO — tricuspid valve opening; PC — pulmonic closure; PO — pulmonic opening; AC — aortic closure; AO — aortic opening)

EKG

R

P   T

Q S

Figure 1.13 Mechanical and electrical correlates of the heart sounds. The first heart sound occurs at the beginning of ventricular systole with closure of the mitral and tricuspid valves. The second heart sound occurs near the end of systole with the closure of the aortic and pulmonic valves. Note that the left ventricular contraction begins before and ends after right ventricular contraction.

5. Gallop Rhythm

The term gallop rhythm refers to a three-sound sequence or cadence consisting of S_1 and S_2 followed by a gallop sound representing an intensified S_3 or S_4. Three types of gallop rhythms have been described: (1) a protodiastolic gallop in which the gallop sound occurs very early in diastole, (2) a presystolic gallop in which the gallop sound occurs just before systole, and (3) a summation gallop in which the gallop sound consists of an intensification of both S_3 and S_4. Gallop rhythms generally indicate a failing left ventricle.

G. CARDIAC OUTPUT

Cardiac output is usually the most important factor to consider in relation to the circulation. Normal cardiac output for the young, healthy male adult averages about 5 to 6 liters/min or about 3.0 to 3.5 liters $\cdot$ min^{-1} $\cdot$ m^{-2}. Cardiac output of

PHYSIOLOGICAL SPLITTING

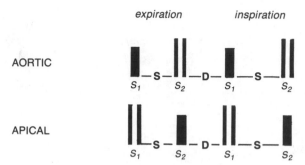

Figure 1.14 Auscultation of heart sounds: physiologic splitting as heard over the aortic and apical auscultatory areas during inspiration and expiration. S = systole, D = diastole. (From Dolan, JT: Critical Care Nursing. FA Davis, Philadelphia, 1991, p 765, with permission.)

females, who generally have less muscle and more fat, is about 10% less than that of males of the same body size or about 2.7 to 3.2 $liters \cdot min^{-1} \cdot m^{-2}$. Other factors that alter the so-called normal cardiac output include age and metabolism. The cardiac index (CI) averages about 3.5 $liters \cdot min^{-1} \cdot m^{-2}$ at 20 years of age. After that, the CI falls by about 0.1 to 0.2 $liters \cdot min^{-1} \cdot m^{-2}$ per decade so that at 80 years it averages about 2.8 $liters \cdot min^{-1} \cdot m^{-2}$ (Table 1.2).

Probably the greatest determinant of cardiac output is the overall body metabolism. That is, the greater the degree of activity of the muscles and other organs, the greater the cardiac output. Other factors that increase cardiac output above normal are those that either increase oxygen utilization, such as thyrotoxicosis, exercise, shivering, and so forth, or those that are associated with decreased removal of oxygen from the blood, such as sepsis, AV fistulas, and anemia. The

NORMAL VARIATIONS

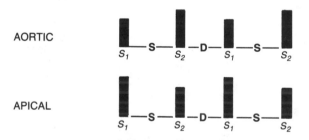

EXTRA HEART SOUNDS

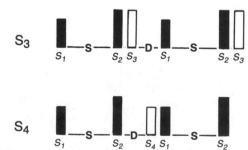

Figure 1.15 Auscultation of heart sounds: normal variations in heart sounds (S_1 and S_2) and extra heart sounds (S_3 and S_4) as heard over the aortic and apical auscultatory areas. S = systole, D = diastole. (From Dolan, JT: Critical Care Nursing. FA Davis, Philadelphia, 1991, p 764, with permission.)

second major determinant of cardiac output is the afterload. As a general rule, if SVR falls by 50%, the cardiac output will double and vice versa.

Although cardiac output can often fall by a third before there is a significant drop in systolic blood pressure, an abrupt fall to less than one-half normal may be life-threatening. In critically ill and injured patients, cardiac output should usually be maintained at levels that are about 50% greater than normal. If cardiac output less than two-thirds of normal is allowed to persist for more than a few hours, the critically ill or injured patient is apt to die.

III. PULMONARY CIRCULATION

A. ANATOMY

The lung has a double blood supply consisting of the pulmonary and bronchial arteries. The pulmonary arteries are a high-flow, low-pressure system that brings virtually the entire cardiac output from the right ventricle to the alveoli. The bronchial arteries are a low-flow, high-pressure system that supplies the supporting structures of the lung. In contrast, the pulmonary arterioles and venules have relatively little smooth muscle in their walls; therefore, changes in their diameter are largely due to pressure changes in the vessels. Pulmonary vessels are innervated by both vagal and sympathetic fibers, which are responsible for many of the vascular changes that occur in the lung.

Normally, the two-to-four bronchial arteries supply the supporting tissues of the lungs with about 50 to 100 ml of blood per minute. In cyanotic heart disease, the bronchial artery flow tends to be much greater than normal. Blood flowing in the bronchial arteries is oxygenated, in contrast to the mixed venous blood in the pulmonary arteries. However, some of the bronchial venous blood that is partially desaturated, empties into the pulmonary veins, lowering the average Po_2 in this otherwise fully oxygenated blood. This accounts for much of the 3% to 5% of the cardiac output that is normally physiologically "shunted" through the lungs without being fully oxygenated.

B. FACTORS AFFECTING PULMONARY VASCULAR RESISTANCE

The pulmonary arterial system is very compliant, and blood flow in the lungs may increase threefold to fourfold before the pulmonary artery pressure (normally 12 to 25/5 to 10 mm Hg) rises appreciably. Although the pulmonary arteries can tolerate increased flow quite well, if these vessels are subjected to a sustained increase in pressure, they begin to hypertrophy and pulmonary vascular resistance may rise rapidly.

1. Autonomic Nervous System

The autonomic nervous system has only a slight influence on the pulmonary vasculature. Vagal stimulation to the lungs causes a slight decrease in pulmonary vascular resistance. Sympathetic stimulation has the opposite effect.

2. Hypoxia

Hypoxia causes pulmonary arteries to constrict. If the hypoxia becomes severe, pulmonary vascular resistance may increase so much that cardiac output may fall. If a portion of a lung becomes atelectatic, pulmonary arterial constriction due to local hypoxia diverts blood flow from the poorly ventilated areas of the lung to other areas that are better aerated. It should be noted that this constrictive (autoregulatory) effect of a low Po_2 on the pulmonary arteries is opposite to the effect normally observed in systemic vessels. Failure of this autoregulatory mechanism during sepsis and after trauma and shock may cause much of the ventilation-perfusion (V/Q) mismatching that occurs in ARDS. Atelectasis by itself also has a pulmonary vasoconstricting effect, even without hypoxia, on a purely mechanical basis. Because of the elasticity of the lungs, collapse of alveoli in lobules causes tissue around the blood vessels in the atelectatic area also to collapse around the blood vessels, further reducing blood flow to atelectatic lung tissue. In ARDS, if the cardiac output is low, blood flow in the lung will preferentially go to the best-ventilated dependent alveoli. However, if the cardiac output is high, some of the blood will go to less well-ventilated alveoli. As a consequence, the arterial Po_2 will tend to drop and the calculated shunt (Qs/Qt) will increase. Thus, inotropes and/or vasodilators can increase the degree of hypoxemia.

3. Other Factors

a. Pulmonary Emboli

Large pulmonary emboli can produce a significant increase in pulmonary vascular resistance by mechanical blockade of arteries and arterioles. It has been thought that serotonin (5-hydroxytryptamine) released from platelets in the emboli may contribute to the problem by causing pulmonary vascular constriction. However, although serotonin can cause a severalfold increase in pulmonary resistance in animals, it has relatively little effect clinically.

b. Emphysema

Pulmonary emphysema is characterized by overexpansion of alveoli and destruction of many of the alveolar septal walls. Although total lung capacity may increase, loss of the alveolar septa and their capillaries decreases the size of the pulmonary capillary bed and reduces the total alveolar surface area of the lungs. This not only decreases gas exchange between the alveoli and the blood, but also increases the pulmonary dead space (areas that are ventilated, but not perfused).

As the emphysema gets worse and there is increasing destruction of the pulmonary capillaries and constriction of the arterioles by interstitial fibrosis, pulmonary arterial resistance progressively rises, increasing the strain on the right heart. In addition, the poor exchange of air in the excessively enlarged emphysematous alveoli results in alveolar hypoxia, which causes even more pulmonary vasoconstriction.

c. Diffuse Pulmonary Fibrosis

A number of pathologic conditions, such as the pneumoconioses, are associated with excessive fibrosis in the supportive tissues of the lungs. This fibrous tissue, like scar tissue anywhere, tends to gradually contract down around the vessels, increasing pulmonary vascular resistance. In the early stages, pulmonary arterial pressure is normal as long as the person is not exercising. However, with exercise, sepsis, or any other stress, the pulmonary arterial pressure may rise abruptly because these vessels cannot expand properly to accommodate the increased blood flow.

d. The Blood Volume of the Lungs

The amount of blood in the lungs at any one time is approximately 500 to 700 ml in an average adult male, or about 10% to 15% of the total blood volume. About 100 ml of this is in the pulmonary capillaries; the remainder is divided almost equally among the pulmonary arteries and veins.

C. DISTRIBUTION OF BLOOD FLOW IN THE LUNGS

The distribution of blood flow in the lungs is largely determined by gravity. While a patient is standing or sitting upright, the basilar portions of the lung get much more blood flow than the apices. The vessels in the basilar portions of the lower lobes may have a pressure 15 to 25 cm H_2O higher than at the apex.

The hydrostatic and resultant pleural pressures in the lung decrease the alveolar distending pressures in the inferior portions of the lung. This decreases the average size of the alveoli in the basilar segments and places them in a more favorable position on the pressure-volume curve for alveoli. Thus, for a given intrabronchial pressure change, there is more inflation of lower-lobe alveoli. However, the increased hydrostatic pressure in the dependent portion of the lung also increases the tendency to atelectasis. Patients with atelectasis or pneumonia should be turned frequently, at least once every 1 to 2 hours, and the side of the chest with abnormal lung tissue should be elevated as much of the time as possible. This reduces congestion in the diseased or damaged lung, decreasing its tendency to interstitial edema and atelectasis.

D. CAPILLARY BLOOD FLOW IN THE LUNGS

When cardiac output is normal, blood remains in the pulmonary capillaries for only about 1 second. During exercise, when cardiac output may increase threefold to fourfold, this transit time may decrease to less than 0.4 second. However, red blood cells must be in contact with ventilated alveoli for at least 0.4 second to be adequately oxygenated. If it were not for the fact that additional pulmonary capillaries open up to accommodate the increased blood flow when cardiac output rises, severe hypoxia might develop during stress or exercise.

E. FLUID SPACES IN THE LUNGS

The distribution of fluid between the capillary and interstitial fluid spaces depends on the local balance between osmotic and hydrostatic pressures. The colloid osmotic pressure (COP) of the blood is normally 22 to 28 mm Hg, which is far greater than the 6 to 8 mm Hg average hydrostatic pressure in the pulmonary capillaries. However, if heart failure develops so that the pulmonary capillary pressure rises above 25 mm Hg, the pulmonary lymphatics may not be able to remove the interstitial fluid as fast as it forms. This fluid accumulates initially in peribronchial interstitial spaces and later around alveoli in the more peripheral portions of the lung.

In the basilar portions of the lung, where the capillary pressure may be as much as 10 to 15 mm Hg greater than in the apex, damaged pulmonary capillary endothelium may allow fluid to leak into the interstitial tissue very rapidly at low hydrostatic pressures. This increased pulmonary capillary permeability, with resultant interstitial edema, appears to be the most important etiologic factor in the development of ARDS.

IV. SYSTEMIC CIRCULATION

A. BLOOD FLOW

1. Vessel Size

Blood flow through a vessel occurs because of a pressure gradient between its two ends. It must be emphasized that it is the difference in pressure between the ends of the vessel, not the absolute pressure, that determines the rate of flow. As blood flows through the vessel, a certain resistance or impedance to flow will be encountered. The relationship between flow (Q), the change in pressure (P), and the resistance (R) can be expressed mathematically as:

$$Q = \frac{P}{R}.$$

As the aorta and large proximal arteries progressively divide and become smaller in diameter, the total cross-sectional area of the vessels becomes progressively larger. The largest total cross-sectional area is in the capillaries. It then decreases again as veins become larger (Table 1.5).

The velocity of blood in systemic vessels varies inversely with their cross-sectional area. For example, the velocity of blood flow in the aorta is about 30 to

Table 1.5

CHARACTERISTICS OF VARIOUS TYPES OF BLOOD VESSELS IN HUMANS

	Lumen Diameter	Wall Thickness	Approximate Total Cross-Sectional Area (cm²)	Percentage of Blood Volume Contained*
Aorta	2.5 cm	2 mm	4.5	2
Artery	0.4 cm	1 mm	20	8
Arteriole	30 um	20 um	400	1
Capillary	5 um	1 um	4500	5
Venule	20 um	2 um	4000	4
Vein	0.5 cm	0.5 mm	40	45
Vena cava	3 cm	1.5 mm	18	5

*In systemic vessels. There is an additional 8% to 12% in the heart and 14% to 18% in the pulmonary circulation.
Source: Data from Gregg, DE: In Best, CH and Taylor, NB (eds): The Physiological Basis of Medical Practice, ed 8. Williams & Wilkins, Baltimore, 1966.

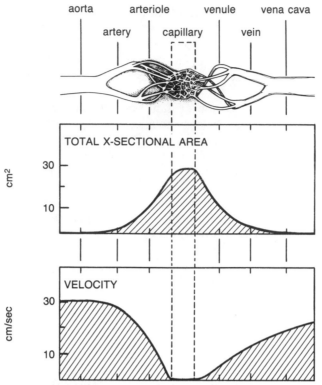

aorta   arteriole   venule   vena cava
artery   capillary   vein

TOTAL X-SECTIONAL AREA

cm²

30

10

VELOCITY

cm/sec

30

10

Figure 1.16 Relationship between total cross-sectional area and velocity of blood flow in the various vessels comprising the systemic circulation. (From Dolan, JT: Critical Care Nursing, FA Davis, Philadelphia, 1991, with permission.)

35 cm/sec, whereas the velocity of blood flow in the capillaries is about 0.5 mm/sec. Since the average capillary is 0.5 to 1.0 mm long, blood remains in the capillaries for only 1 to 2 seconds (Fig. 1.16).

The cross-sectional area in veins is about four or more times that in the associated or adjacent arteries; thus, flow in the veins is correspondingly reduced.

The equation determining blood flow in various vessels is known as Poiseuille's law:

$$Q = \frac{Pr^4}{8nl}.$$

It relates blood flow (Q) to the change in pressure (P), the radius (r), the length (l) of the vessel, and the viscosity (n) of the fluid. Since the rate of blood flow in a vessel is proportional to the fourth power of its radius, the size of a blood vessel plays the greatest role in determining the rate of flow.

Distribution of blood flow through tissues depends primarily on the size of the arteriolar lumen, which, in turn, is dependent on its muscle tone. In the smallest arterioles, small changes in muscle can have a great effect on local blood flow. The precapillary and postcapillary sphincters also have a high degree of intrinsic tone which can act independent of nerve impulses or humoral stimulation. Autoregulation to meet the metabolic needs of a tissue is the main determinant of the amount of precapillary and postcapillary vasoconstriction and local blood flow.

Several studies have been made of the blood flow to various organs in man under basal conditions (Table 1.6). The skeletal muscle of the body comprises about 35% to 40% of the total body mass. However, in the inactive state, blood flow to skeletal muscle is only 15% to 20% of the total cardiac output.

Table 1.6

APPROXIMATE BLOOD FLOWS TO VARIOUS ORGANS UNDER BASAL CONDITIONS	*Percent*	*ml/min*
Liver	25–30	1200–1500
Kidneys	20–25	1000–1250
Muscle	15–20	750–1000
Brain	12–15	600–900
Skin	8–10	400–500
Heart	4–5	200–250
Other	5–6	250–300
Total	100	4500–5500

2. Blood Viscosity

Blood viscosity can play a major role in blood flow, but its effect is often overlooked. Within most circumstances, there is a direct correlation between the hematocrit and the viscosity of the blood. However, when hematocrit rises about 55%, viscosity rises more rapidly. The resultant decrease in blood flow may increase the tendency to form intravascular thrombi, which will further impair blood flow in the involved vessels.

3. Red Blood Cell Deformability

Red blood cells have a diameter that allows them just barely to squeeze through most nutrient capillaries. Red cells that are deficient in ATP or are present in many patients with severe arteriosclerosis are stiffer than normal, thereby reducing capillary blood flow.

4. Metabolic Autoregulation of Blood Flow

The term autoregulation refers to the regulation of blood flow through a tissue in response to its need for nutrients and oxygen, independent of any influence by the nervous system. The precise mechanisms for autoregulation are not known, but it appears that the concentration of oxygen and carbon dioxide in tissues is very important. Experimental studies have shown that isolated small arteries respond to increased local oxygen and decreased carbon dioxide by constricting, and to decreased local oxygen or increased carbon dioxide by dilating. The smaller the artery, the greater the intensity of this effect. Although an increase in CO_2 tends to cause local vasodilation, if arterial blood becomes hypercarbic, it stimulates the vasomotor center to cause vasoconstriction in most tissues, but not the brain.

PITFALL
Failure to recognize that new hypertension in a critically ill patient might be due to CO_2 retention.

Oxygen is the most nearly "flow-limited" substance normally transported in the blood. For example, blood flow can fall by 90% in some tissues and still provide adequate quantities of amino acids, glucose, and fatty acids. However, if the blood flow is decreased by more than 70%, oxygen utilization may be decreased enough to jeopardize the viability of the tissue.

Another metabolic factor that may influence local blood flow is the availability of nutrients relative to their metabolism in the tissue. The greater the rate of metabolism and the less the availability of nutrients, the greater the rate of formation of vasodilator substances, such as lactic acid or bradykinin. These substances may diffuse or circulate back to the precapillary sphincters, meta-arterioles, and arterioles, causing vasodilation.

5. Neurogenic Control

Although metabolic autoregulation is an important determinant of blood flow at the tissue level, the nervous system is essential when large circulatory alterations are necessary. This occurs almost entirely through the autonomic nervous system, particularly the sympathetics. Strong sympathetic stimulation increases cardiac output and causes vasoconstriction in the kidneys and nonvital tissues such as the skin, thereby increasing blood flow to the heart, brain, and muscles as part of a "fight-or-flight" response. The parasympathetic nervous system has relatively little effect on blood flow except indirectly by its tendency to slow the heart rate.

The vasomotor tone of the arterioles tends to constrict the vessels. This is opposed by the hydrostatic pressure inside the arterioles, which tends to dilate the vessels. If hydrostatic pressure falls progressively lower and lower, it finally reaches a point at which the pressure inside the vessel is no longer capable of keeping the vessel open and maintaining flow. This pressure is called the critical closing pressure.

The law of Laplace helps to explain the closure of vessels at certain critical pressures. A variation of this law states that the distending force (F) tending to stretch the muscle fibers in the vascular wall is proportional to the diameter (D) of the vessel times the pressure (P), that is, F = DP.

B. BLOOD PRESSURE

Systolic pressure represents the highest pressure and diastolic pressure the lowest pressure in an artery with each contraction of the heart. Systolic pressure is affected by multiple factors that may be divided into those that regulate diastolic pressure and those that regulate pulse pressure.

Diastolic pressure is primarily determined by the amount of vasoconstriction present in the small arteries and arterioles. Pulse pressure (which is the difference between systolic and diastolic pressure) is determined mainly by SV and the elasticity of the aorta and its larger branches. With age, increased resistance in the aorta and its major branches tends to make the pulse pressure rise.

An acute drop in pulse pressure, as may occur with decreased SV because of hypovolemia, tends to be compensated for by an increase in diastolic pressure. Thus, systolic pressure often does not fall below 80 to 90 mm Hg in otherwise normal individuals until there is a 25% blood volume deficit. The mBP represents the average pressure through a cardiac cycle and, depending on the shape of the pressure curve, it will usually be equal to the pulse pressure multiplied by 0.3 plus the diastolic blood pressure. Thus, a patient with a blood pressure of 120/80 has a pulse pressure of 40 mm Hg, and a mBP of (40)(0.3) + 80, or 92 mm Hg.

1. Factors Affecting Arterial Pressure

As noted previously, the blood pressure (P) in the arterial system is determined primarily by the quantity of blood flow (Q) and the resistance in the arterioles (R):

$$P = QR.$$

Thus, any factor that increases cardiac output or total peripheral vascular resistance will increase blood pressure. In general, blood pressure is maintained at a relatively constant level so that a decrease or increase in cardiac output is associated with an opposite change in total peripheral resistance (R).

The three main mechanisms affecting systemic vascular resistance include the autonomic nervous system, the kidneys, and the endocrine system.

a. Nervous System

(1) Anatomy

(a) Central centers and receptors

The vasomotor center, the portion of the nervous system that has greatest control of the circulation, is located bilaterally in the reticular substance of the lower third of the pons and upper two thirds of the medulla. This center detects signals from vascular receptors in all parts of the body and then transmits impulses through the spinal cord and peripheral vasoconstrictor fibers to virtually all the blood vessels.

The hypothalamus can exert powerful excitatory or inhibitory effects on the vasomotor center. The posterolateral portions of the hypothalamus cause mainly excitation, whereas the anterior part can cause either excitation or inhibition, depending on the precise part of the anterior hypothalamus stimulated.

Several pressoreceptors or baroreceptors have been identified in the walls of large thoracic and neck arteries, particularly in the arch of the aorta and at the origin of the internal carotid arteries. These receptors are stimulated when the arterial walls are stretched by an increased blood pressure. Impulses from these baroreceptors inhibit the vasomotor center, resulting in a drop in blood pressure back toward normal.

Pressure on the neck over the baroceptors in the carotid sinuses decreases sympathetic nervous system activity and may increase vagal activity. As a result, the pulse rate tends to decrease and the arterial pressure may fall more than 20 mm Hg, even in a normal individual. In some individuals with a hypersensitive carotid sinus, a tight collar can occasionally cause arterial pressure to fall low enough to product fainting. If calcified arteriosclerotic plaques are present, simultaneous pressure on both the right and left carotid sinuses can cause such a strong negative pressoreceptor response that the resultant hypotension can cause a cardiac arrest.

PITFALL
Performing carotid artery massage without simultaneously evaluating heart rate and blood pressure.

Several chemoreceptors have been identified in the bifurcation of the common carotid arteries and along the aortic arch. These small chemoreceptors, 1 to 2 mm in size, are called the carotid and aortic bodies, respectively. They are most sensitive to decreases in the arterial Po_2. The carotid chemoreceptors send impulses along Hering's nerves, and the aortic bodies send impulses along the vagus nerves, eventually reaching the vasomotor and respiratory centers. By stimulating the vasomotor center, they elicit a vasoconstrictor response increasing blood flow to central vital organs.

The chemoreceptors are also stimulated to a certain extent by increases in the Pco_2 in the arterial blood. However, the effect of carbon dioxide on the vasomotor center itself is about 10 times as strong as the effect it produces by stimulating the chemoreceptors. Therefore, loss of the chemoreceptor response to CO_2 generally has little or no effect on the central vasoconstriction response to hypercarbia.

The peripheral nerves to blood vessels are predominately for vasoconstriction, but some vasodilator fibers are also present in certain tissues, particularly skeletal muscle. These vasodilator fibers release acetylcholine, which relaxes vascular smooth muscle. Sympathetic vasoconstrictor impulses are also transmitted to the adrenal medulla, which secretes both norepinephrine and epinephrine into the blood.

(b) Sympathetic nervous system

(i) Anatomy

The preganglionic neurons of the sympathetic nervous system have their cell bodies in the anterolateral gray matter of the thoracic and lumbar spinal cord from T1 through L3. The preganglionic axons travel in the anterior nerve root to the sympathetic ganglia, where they synapse with the postganglionic neurons. There are 22 pairs of sympathetic ganglia lying in the paravertebral chain situated on either side of the vertebral column. These chains are interconnected and also contain rami, which communicate with the spinal nerves (Fig. 1.17).

(ii) Physiology

The predominant neurochemical effector for the sympathetic nervous system is norepinephrine, which is released from the sympathetic nerve terminals. Epi-

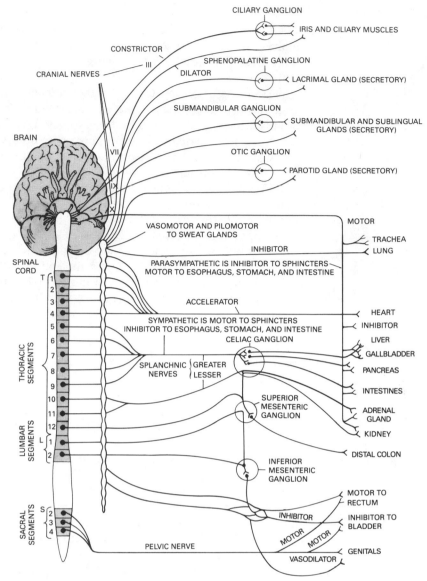

Figure 1.17 The sympathetic nervous system. [Modified from Thomas, CL (ed): Taber's Cyclopedic Medical Dictionary, ed. 16. FA Davis, Philadelphia, p 170, with permission.]

nephrine is the major vasoactive substance released from the adrenal medulla. The effects of sympathetic nervous stimulation are designed to facilitate fight or flight. Ventilation is increased by both a central effect on the ventilatory centers and by bronchodilation. The perfusion of vital organs is increased by an increased cardiac output and by constriction of vessels to nonvital organs. Function of both the gastrointestinal and genitourinary systems is decreased as a result of a relaxation of their peristaltic smooth muscle and contraction of their sphincters. Gastrointestinal secretory activity is also inhibited.

Metabolism is generally directed by sympathetic stimulation to provide more fuel for bodily function in the form of glucose and fatty acids through the action of epinephrine, cortisol, and glucagon. Epinephrine stimulates lipolysis (releasing fatty acids and glycerol) and glycogenolysis in the liver and muscle (releasing glucose), and inhibits insulin secretion and activity. Cortisol increases gluconeogenesis (new glucose formation) from protein. Glucagon stimulates hepatic glycogenolysis (releasing even more glucose). All of these metabolic responses increase blood glucose levels for fight or flight.

(c) Adrenergic receptors

Ahlquist and others characterized sympathetic stimulation as being predominately mediated through alpha or beta receptors. Beta-receptor activity is divisible into at least two forms, and more recently two separate alpha-receptor mechanisms have also been delineated. The beta$_1$-receptor mechanism is primarily involved in cardiac effects, inhibition of insulin secretion, and increased release of fatty acids, while the beta$_2$ receptors are primarily responsible for smooth-muscle relaxation, and increased gluconeogenesis and glycogenolysis in muscle and liver resulting in hyperglycemia (Table 1.7).

Both norepinephrine and epinephrine, possess alpha- and beta-receptor stimulating activity. Although norepinephrine has minimal beta$_2$-receptor activity, epinephrine can strongly stimulate both beta$_1$- and beta$_2$-receptors.

The density of the receptors varies from tissue to tissue and under different circumstances. For example, continued beta-adrenergic stimulation causes a decrease in receptor density, while prolonged administration of beta-receptor antagonists results in an increase in the number of receptors. Denervation, whether chemical or surgical, also results in an increase in the number of receptors.

(i) Beta-receptor physiology

The initial binding of a beta-agonist to its receptor converts the receptor to the active state. This allows the receptor to couple to the nucleotide regulator (N) protein. This complex then promotes the dissociation of guanine diphosphate (GDP) from its tightly bound position on the N protein. This vacated binding site then becomes occupied by a molecule of guanine triphosphate (GTP), which is stimulatory. The interaction of GTP with the N protein has two effects. First, it catalyzes the inactive form of adenylate cyclase to the active form, with the resultant breakdown of ATP to cAMP. Second, it converts the receptor into its inactive state again. The cAMP stimulates a series of protein kinases, eventually resulting in membrane phosphorylation and a stimulatory effect on that organ. Antagonists have affinity for both the inactive uncoupled and the active coupled form of the receptors. The receptor is thereby maintained in a relatively inactive state, and considerably more agonist than usual is required to unbalance the equilibrium.

The state of the receptor complexes may be changed by various environmental and pathophysiologic situations. For example, the desensitization process, which has been referred to as *tolerance* or *tachyphylaxis,* is now known to

Table 1.7

EFFECTS OF RECEPTOR STIMULATION*

Receptor	Location	Effect
Alpha$_1$	Postsynaptic effector cells; primarily arterioles	Vasoconstriction
	Cardiac	
Alpha$_2$	Presynaptic membranes	Inhibition of NE release†
Alpha$_{2a}$	Platelets	Aggregation
Beta$_1$	Myocardium	Increased contractivity
	Sinatrial node	Accelerated atrial rate
	Atrioventricular node	Enhanced conduction
Beta$_2$	Arterioles	Vasodilation
	Bronchioles	Bronchodilation
Beta (other)	Adipose cells	Lipolysis
Dopamine$_1$	Renal and mesenteric arteries	Vasodilation
		Natriuresis
		Inhibition of aldosterone
Dopamine$_2$	Presynaptic membrane (?)	Inhibition of NE release

*Additional types of receptors with pharmacologic properties distinct from alpha, beta, and dopaminergic subtypes have also been proposed.
†NE = norepinephrine.

be due to decreased density and responsiveness of receptors, and this is referred to as *down-regulation* by pharmacodynamicists. The opposite effect with increased density and responsiveness of receptors is referred to as *up-regulation.*

(ii) Alpha-receptor physiology

Alpha-receptor-mediated activity is responsible for most of the sympathetically induced smooth-muscle contraction throughout the body. Alpha-receptor stimulation also causes decreased pancreatic insulin secretion.

The need to differentiate the alpha-receptor into alpha$_1$ and alpha$_2$ initially revolved around a negative feedback mechanism found in the sympathetic nervous system. The secretion of norepinephrine from sympathetic nerve terminals is accompanied by a feedback inhibition of subsequent norepinephrine secretion (Fig. 1.18). As various alpha-receptor antagonists were developed, some of these drugs were found to act by decreasing norepinephrine release from the presynaptic nerve terminal. Hence, the alpha$_2$ receptor appeared to be predominately presynaptic and acted by decreasing norepinephrine release from the nerve terminal, whereas the major effects of alpha-adrenergic agonist were postsynaptic.

In contrast to the beta receptors whose central nervous system (CNS) distribution and importance is still not understood, the alpha$_2$ receptors appear to be important in central nervous sympathetic mediation. Specifically, alpha$_2$ agonists reduce sympathetic outflow from the CNS and hence act as sympathetic nervous system inhibitors, whereas alpha$_2$-antagonist drugs tend to have the opposite effect, that is, they tend to stimulate CNS sympathetic nervous outflow. Furthermore, it now appears that there are also postsynaptic alpha$_2$ receptors in the periphery.

In general, vascular tissue innervated by the sympathetic nervous system responds predominately to alpha$_1$ agonists, whereas vascular tissue not inner-

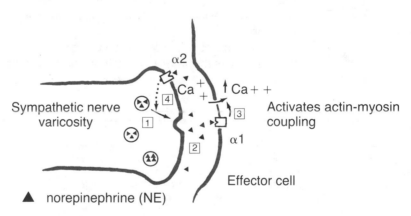

▲ norepinephrine (NE)

1. Depolarization of the sympathetic nerve produces NE vesicle fusion and release
2. The NE crosses the synaptic cleft to act at the α 1 receptor
3. Stimulation of the α 1 receptor increases Ca + + flux into the effector cell which then causes actin-myosin coupling
4. Released NE also acts at the α 2 receptor to inhibit further NE release

Figure 1.18 Peripheral circulatory control via α-adrenergic receptors. The sequence of events includes sympathetic nerve stimulation, norepinephrine effect at the postsynaptic effector cell, calcium influx, and feedback inhibition of further norepinephrine release (steps 1–4 described above). [From Zaritsky, A and Chernow, B: Catecholamines, sympathomimetics. In Chernow, B and Lake, CR (eds): The Pharmacologic Approach to the Critically Ill Patient. Williams & Wilkins, Baltimore, 1983, p 484, with permission.]

vated by the sympathetic nervous system responds primarily to alpha$_2$ agonists (which are blood borne). Interestingly, norepinephrine appears to have predominantly beta$_1$- and alpha$_1$-agonist activity, whereas epinephrine appears to have beta$_1$-, beta$_2$-, alpha$_1$-, and alpha$_2$-agonist activity. These effects, however, appear to be dose related, in that high doses of an alpha agonist primarily stimulate alpha$_1$ receptors, while low doses tend to stimulate alpha$_2$ receptors. Norepinephrine at low doses has predominantly a beta$_1$ effect but at high doses has a very strong alpha$_1$ effect, resulting in very severe vasoconstriction. The responses of the more commonly used catecholaminelike drugs at their usual doses is shown in Table 1.8.

At the cellular level, a second messenger cascade system, called the phosphatidylinositol/protein kinase C cascade, has been described. Binding of alpha-adrenergic agents activates phospholipase, which causes hydrolysis of lipids known as polyphosphoinositides to yield diacylglycerol and inositol triphosphate (IP$_3$). The diacylglycerol increases the affinity of protein kinase C for intracellular calcium. The IP$_3$ mobilizes calcium from intracellular stores. The resultant increase in calcium activates protein kinases, which catalyze the phosphorylation of myosin which initiates actomyosin coupling and, intimately, causes smooth-muscle contraction resulting in vasoconstriction. All these processes are calcium dependent and are affected by the actions of calcium channel blockers and by systemic hypocalcemia (Fig. 1.19).

(iii) Dopamine receptors

Dopamine is an important CNS neurotransmitter. However, even though peripheral dopamine receptors exist, especially in renal and intestinal vascular beds and the parathyroid, there is no unifying role for these peripheral dopamine receptors at present. Clinically, dopamine at low doses (1 to 3 $\mu g \cdot kg^{-1} \cdot min^{-1}$) primarily stimulates dopaminergic receptors in splanchnic vessels, causing them to dilate. At intermediate doses (5 to 10 $\mu g \cdot kg^{-1} \cdot min^{-1}$), dopamine has primarily positive inotropic effects, and at higher doses, dopamine causes increasing vasoconstriction. Dobutamine at 5 to 10 $\mu g \cdot kg^{-1} \cdot min^{-1}$) is a mild pulmonary and systemic vasodilator and has a positive inotropic effect. It also usually causes less tachycardia than dopamine.

(2) Nervous System Responses

(a) Effect of exercise and stress

When the cerebral cortex becomes active during stress of any type, nerve impulses are transmitted not only to skeletal muscles, but also directly along the corticospinal tracts to the preganglionic neurons of the sympathetic nervous system. These impulses excite sympathetic fibers throughout the body, thereby causing tachycardia and vasoconstriction with a rise in arterial pressure.

Table 1.8

SELECTIVITY OF CATECHOLAMINES FOR ADRENERGIC RECEPTORS*	Alpha$_1$	Alpha$_2$	Beta$_1$	Beta$_2$	DA$_1$	DA$_2$
Phenylephrine	++	0†	0	0	0	0
Norepinephrine	+++	++	+++	+	0	0
Epinephrine	+++	+++	+++	++	0	0
Isoproterenol	0	0	+++	+++	0	0
Dopamine	0 to +++	0 to +	0 to +++	0 to ++	+++	++
Dobutamine	0 to +	0	+++	++	0	0
Fenoldopam	0	0	+	++	++	++
Dopexamine	0	0	+	++	++	++

*+ to +++ = relative amounts of stimulation; these are not necessarily to scale between drugs. Some agents, particularly dopamine, have dose-dependent effects with alpha activity increasing at higher doses.
†0 = no stimulation.
DA = dopaminergic.

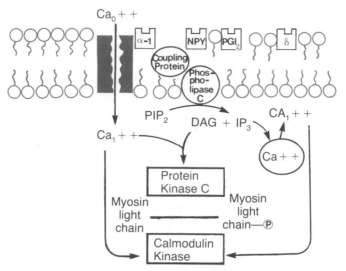

Figure 1.19 The phosphatidylinositol/protein kinase C cascade. The external cell membrane accommodates receptors fro a_1, and also neuropeptide Y (NPY), prostaglandin I_2 (PGI_2), and the delta opioid peptide receptor (δ). Extracellular calcium (Ca_o ++) moves into the cell via the calcium channel. Effects that are mediated through coupling proteins include hydrolysis of phosphatidylinositol 4,5-biphosphate (PIP_2), generation of diacylglycerol (DAG), and inositol 1,4,5-triphosphate (IP_3). The increase in intracellular calcium (Ca_i ++) allows vasoconstriction to occur. [From Chernow, B and Roth, BL: Pharmacologic support of cardiovasculature in septic shock. In Sibbald, WJ and Spring, CL (eds): New Horizons: Perspectives on Sepsis and Septic Shock. Society of Critical Care Medicine, Fullerton, CA, 1986, pp 173–202, with permission.]

Sympathetic stimulation stress increases BP and muscle blood flow by increasing cardiac output and causing vasoconstriction in nonvital tissues and vasodilation in muscle. Exercise and increased metabolism also cause vasodilation in muscle blood vessels. The combination of sympathetic stimulation and increased local metabolism can cause a tremendous increase in muscle blood flow. If an alpha-adrenergic blocker has been given, dilatation of blood vessels in muscles during strenuous activity can cause a severe drop in arterial pressure. The increased heat and lactic acid in active muscle also shift the oxygen dissociation curve to the right, thereby increasing oxygen availability to the tissues.

(b) Pressoreceptor reflexes

An increase in arterial pressure stimulates pressoreceptors, especially in the carotid sinus. These, in turn, transmit impulses that inhibit the vasomotor center. As a consequence, sympathetic tone throughout the body is decreased, dilating peripheral vessels and decreasing the activity of the heart, thereby causing the BP to fall back toward normal.

In addition, if hypertension occurs because the sympathetic nervous system is strongly and continuously stimulated for a period of several days, the responsiveness of these receptors is gradually reduced, and the blood pressure begins to return to normal. Likewise, sudden blockade or destruction of the sympathetic nervous system causes immediate vasodilatation, decreased heart rate, and a decrease in mean arterial pressure to about 50 mm Hg. Several days later, however, these will often return to normal. This follows Cannon's law of denervation, which states that if a structure can be stimulated by both nerve-borne and blood-borne stimuli, and if the nerve supply to the structure is destroyed, the structure becomes more sensitive to blood-borne stimuli.

(c) Central nervous system ischemic responses

If intracranial pressure (ICP) rises so high that blood flow to the vasomotor center in the brain is reduced, the vasomotor center becomes exceedingly active, transmitting powerful sympathetic vasoconstrictor impulses to vessels throughout the body and cardiac accelerator impulses to the heart until the arterial pressure rises to a level that provides adequate blood flow to the brain. This sympathetic response, sometimes referred to as the Cushing reflex, is one of the most powerful vascular reflexes and may be several times as great as responses related to the carotid sinus. It helps protect the brain's blood supply, but ordinarily it is not activated until the cerebral perfusion pressure (mBP-ICP) falls below 50 to 60 mm Hg.

b. Renal Regulation and Blood Pressure

Within a few minutes after the onset of renal hypoperfusion or decreased delivery of sodium to the distal tubule lumen, renin is released from the juxtaglomerular apparatus. Renin catalyzes the conversion of a plasma glycoprotein called angiotensinogen into a substance called angiotensin I. Within another minute or so, angiotensin I is converted into angiotensin II by an enzyme in the blood called angiotensin-converting enzyme. Angiotensin II persists for 5 to 20 minutes but is gradually inactivated by a number of different blood enzymes collectively called angiotensinase. Angiotensin II can raise arterial pressure by causing vasoconstriction of the systemic arterioles throughout the body and by increasing the production of aldosterone in the adrenal cortex. Aldosterone causes the kidneys to retain salt and water and excrete potassium.

Some of the mechanisms whereby sodium retention might cause an increase in arterial pressure include (1) sensitization of the arterioles by sodium so that they respond more powerfully to sympathetic impulses; (2) a direct effect of sodium on arterioles, causing increased constriction; or (3) penetration of the walls of the arterioles by sodium, increasing the water content of the arteriolar walls, thereby decreasing arteriolar compliance and/or constricting the lumen. However, a much more likely cause of the hypertension following salt retention is the associated increase in blood volume. An increase in extracellular fluid volume or blood volume can cause a rise in arterial pressure, even if sodium concentration decreases.

c. Vascular Lumen and Resistance

Although the total cross-sectional area of the arteries is much greater peripherally than proximally, resistance to blood flow increases rapidly in the very small arterioles, causing the systolic blood pressure to drop from 120 mm Hg in the aorta to approximately 85 mm Hg at the beginning of the arterioles. Within the arterioles, which account for one half to two thirds of all systemic vascular resistance, systolic pressure will decrease by another 55 mm Hg, or more. Thus, the hydrostatic pressure of blood as it enters the capillaries may be only 20 to 30 mm Hg at the arteriolar end and about 10 mm Hg at the venous end (Table 1.5). Various units have been used to quantitate vascular resistance. In the metric system, the units for pressure (P) are dynes/cm^2 and for flow (Q) are cm^3/sec. Since resistance (R) = P/Q,

$$R = \frac{dynes/cm^2}{cm^3/sec} = \frac{dynes}{cm^2} \times \frac{sec}{cm^3}$$

$$= \frac{dyne \cdot sec}{cm^5} = dyne \cdot sec \cdot cm^{-5}.$$

If pressure is expressed in millimeters of mercury and flow in liters per minute, the result is multiplied by 80 to convert mm Hg·liter^{-1}·min^{-1} into dyne·sec·cm^{-5}.

Age has a profound influence on vascular resistance, primarily because of arteriosclerotic changes. For example, the total peripheral systemic vascular resistance may increase from about 1000 at age 20 years to almost 2000 dyne·sec·cm^{-5} at 80 years of age. Although SV falls with age, the increasing resistance in the aorta and its major branches tends to cause pulse pressure to rise (Table 1.2).

d. Endocrine Regulation

(1) Catecholamines

Epinephrine and some norepinephrine are secreted by the adrenal medulla, whereas only norepinephrine is released from the nerve ending of sympathetic nerve fibers when the sympathetic nervous system is stimulated. These hormones generally act as an accessory part of the nervous regulation of circulation, particularly in tissues that are relatively resistant to ischemia and hypoxia, such as the skin.

(2) Renin-Angiotensin-Aldosterone

Aldosterone plays a major role in regulation of the cardiovascular system by its effects on extracellular fluid. The primary action of aldosterone is to increase the resorption of sodium and water from the renal tubules. This, in turn, tends to reduce the volume of urine and increase the volume of extracellular fluid. The resultant increase in blood volume tends to elevate arterial pressure and may also increase cardiac output, particularly if the patient was previously hypovolemic.

(3) The Kinins

Several vasoactive polypeptides (kinins) that can cause vasodilation have been isolated from blood and tissue fluids. The kinins are normally present as inactive kininogens, which are kinins attached to an alpha$_2$ globulin. An enzyme of particular importance is kallikrein, which is present in the blood and tissue fluids in an inactive form known as prekallikrein. When kallikrein becomes activated, it acts immediately on the alpha$_2$ globulins to release the kinins.

One of the kinins is bradykinin, which increases capillary permeability and is a very powerful vasodilator. For example, injection of 1 μg of bradykinin into the brachial artery of a man can increase the blood flow in that arm sixfold. The main other kinin is myocardial depressant factor (MDF). MDF comes primarily from an ischemic pancreas. In addition to its cardiac depressant effects, it also causes splanchnic vasoconstriction. Once formed, the kinins persist for only a few minutes because they are rapidly broken down by the enzyme carboxypeptidase. The activity of kallikrein can also be rapidly curtailed by a kallikrein inhibitor present in body fluids.

(4) Serotonin

Serotonin (5-hydroxytryptamine) is present in large concentrations in platelets and in chromaffin tissue in the intestine. Animal experiments have shown that serotonin is an amphibaric substance, because it can have either a vasodilator or a vasoconstrictor effect, depending on the underlying muscle tonus of the vessel when serotonin is administered. If the vessel bed is vasoconstricted, serotonin can act as a vasodilator. However, it is usually considered to be a vasoconstrictor. In the past, it had been thought that serotonin caused significant pulmonary vasoconstriction in patients with large pulmonary emboli. It is now generally agreed that most of the vascular obstruction, at least in humans, is caused mechanically by the emboli themselves.

(5) Histamine

Histamine can be released from almost every tissue of the body as a result of trauma, ischemia, or sepsis. Some histamine is "performed" histamine, which is released from eosinophils and mast cells in which it is stored. The majority of histamine, however, is probably "induced" histamine, which is produced or induced in the damaged cells themselves at the time of the insult, as demonstrated by a local increase in histidine decarboxylase, the enzyme that converts inactive histidine to histamine.

Histamine is a powerful arteriolar vasodilator and venous constrictor. The role of histamine in normal regulation of the circulation is unknown. In some pathologic conditions the intense arteriolar dilatation and venous constriction caused by histamine increases the capillary pressure so much that a tremendous quantity of edematous fluid leaks out of the circulation into the damaged or irritated tissues. Recently, some work has shown that the histamine/norepinephrine ratio in blood vessels can rise and may help to relieve the severe vasoconstriction that would occur in shock with norepinephrine alone.

e. Chemical Regulation

Acidosis tends to cause a local direct vasodilation, but this may also stimulate the vasomotor center indirectly to increase vascular tone. A mild alkalosis tends to cause arteriolar constriction, but severe alkalosis tends to cause dilatation. Hypercarbia tends to promote a local vasodilatation. However, carbon dioxide, acting on the vasomotor center, has an extremely powerful vasoconstrictive effect which overrides the local vasodilator effect in all tissues except the brain.

2. Methods of Measuring Blood Pressure

The most frequently used technique for measuring BP is the auscultatory cuff technique with a sphygmomanometer. Pressure in the cuff is raised to a level expected to occlude the major artery under the cuff, and then the pressure is gradually reduced. When the cuff pressure falls to a certain level, blood will begin to flow through the area of the vessel constricted by the cuff. As blood flows through the area of narrowing, vibrations are produced. If the vibrations are strong enough, noises referred to as Korotkoff's sounds will be heard when one listens with a stethoscope over the major vessel just below the cuff. The pressure at which these sounds are first heard is considered the systolic pressure. The pressure in the cuff is then decreased until there is little or no compression of the vessel so that the blood flow becomes more laminar and the vibrations produced in the area are greatly decreased. The pressure at which the vibrations and sound decrease markedly or disappear is considered the diastolic BP.

Unfortunately, errors in measuring the BP with the auscultatory technique are frequent. This is particularly true if the SV is very low. The vibrations and sounds may then be so reduced that Korotkoff's sounds cannot be heard except with a Doppler instrument. With the so-called unobtainable cuff pressure, the systolic pressure is usually less than 50 mm Hg; but in perhaps 5% of patients with an unobtainable cuff pressure, the intra-arterial pressure is actually normal or high, but blood flow in that area is not great enough to produce audible vibrations.

PITFALL
Assuming that the central aortic BP is always very low if the BP is unobtainable with the standard cuff technique.

Insertion of an intra-arterial line to obtain an accurate BP may be extremely important in patients with an unobtainable BP, particularly if there is any thought of administering a vasopressor to correct the apparent severe hypotension. However, one must also remember that the intra-arterial systolic pressure in the radial or dorsalis pedis artery may be 20 to 30 mm Hg or more higher than the central aortic pressure because of the build-up of pressure waves proximal to the small arterioles (Fig. 1.20).

3. Blood Pressure Changes with Age

The arterial BP in term newborn infants averages 65 ± 8 systolic and 32 ± 4 diastolic. The BP then gradually rises to about 100/65 by 10 years of age. Newborn infants of pre-eclamptic mothers have somewhat higher mean BPs at birth. The increase in arterial pressure in older age (Table 1.2) is usually associated with increased resistance in the arterioles (raising diastolic blood pressure) and an increased stiffness of the aorta and its major branches (raising pulse pressure).

4. Arterial Pressure Curves

a. Central versus Peripheral Pressures

Ejection of blood from the heart into large arteries causes their lumens to dilate and the pressure in the arterial system to rise. At the end of systole, the elastic stretch of the arterial walls maintains a high pressure in the arteries. The aortic valve closes when aortic pressure exceeds ventricular pressure. In aortic pressure tracings, the abrupt fall in BP as ventricular systole ceases is called the incisura or dicrotic notch. This is followed by a brief rise in BP again as soon as the aortic valve closes.

Because of its many elastic fibers, the aorta can function as a reservoir and

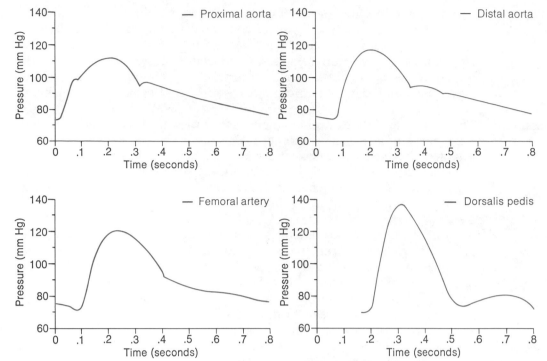

Figure 1.20 Note that although mean pressure tends to remain constant throughout the arterial tree, the pulse pressure tends to widen. The further one is from the heart.

compression chamber for blood as it is rapidly ejected from the heart. Blood stored in the distended elastic aorta and large arteries can then continue to flow during diastole through the peripheral vessels to the capillaries and then to the veins. The contour of the pressure waves found in various portions of the arterial tree are quite different (Fig. 1.20). As the pressure wave moves from the aorta to the peripheral vessels, the ascending portion of the pressure wave becomes steeper, the systolic pressure rises, and the anacrotic notch tends to occur later and lower on the pressure contour curve.

Although systolic pressures tend to be higher (20 to 30 mm Hg) in the more peripheral arteries, diastolic pressures tend to be about 10 mm Hg lower and the mean BP is relatively constant. This increasing rise in systolic pressure peripherally in vessels further from the heart is due to a buildup of pressure waves just proximal to the small arterioles. As blood is ejected into the aorta, a rapidly moving pressure pulse wave is also created. The velocity of transmission of this pressure pulse wave is about 3 to 5 m/sec, which is about 10 to 15 times faster than the actual blood flow. As the pressure wave moves peripherally, its velocity increases until it approaches 15 to 35 m/sec in the smaller arteries. This pressure pulse wave increases the apparent pulse pressure peripherally.

AXIOM

When evaluating changes in blood pressure, it is important to compare blood pressures taken at similar sites with similar techniques.

Systolic pressure in the radial artery is often 10 to 20 mm Hg higher than in the aorta. The systolic BP at the ankle is even higher so that the "ankle-arm" index or ratio of systolic BP at the ankles and the arm is usually 1.10 to 1.25. This is largely due to an increase to the rise in pulse pressure caused by pressure-wave augmentation. The increased pulse pressure in peripheral arteries appears to result from a combination of three factors. At least part of the pressure augmentation is due to a conversion of the kinetic energy of the blood into potential or pressure energy when it reaches the distal, less-compliant portions of the large arteries. The second factor is related to a backward deflection of pressure waves from the peripheral arteries. Since the first portion of the pressure wave is reflected back before the end of the same wave reaches the peripheral arteries, the first portion summates with the latter portion, causing higher pressures than would otherwise be expected. A third factor is related to transmission of the high-pressure portion of the pulse waves more rapidly than the low-pressure portions. This causes crowding together of the pressure waves and "peaking" of the pressure pulse peripherally. More marked amplifications of systolic and pulse pressure are found in children with peripheral vasoconstriction, particularly in pedal arteries.

(1) Problems with Intra-arterial Pressure Monitoring

Deceptively high or low pressure readings can be caused by various problems with intra-arterial catheters and the recording systems. Bedside monitoring systems are generally second-order, underdamped systems with numerous artifacts. To reproduce the pressure signal faithfully, the system should be optimally damped and the natural resonant frequency of the plumbing system should be at least 10 times the fundamental frequency of the signal being measured. This can be accomplished by:

1. Minimizing the distance between the transducer and the catheter.
2. Minimizing the number of stopcocks used.
3. Using very stiff, high-pressure tubing in the system.
4. Carefully removing all air bubbles from the system at the time of setup and periodically during the monitoring period.
5. Continuously flushing the catheter to discourage formation of blood clots.

A low natural frequency of the plumbing system can result in either accentuation or damping of the pressure signal. The dynamic response of the system should be checked at the bedside with the "snap-test," which provides a sudden increase and decrease in pressure, activating a fast-flush for approximately 1 second and then sharply releasing it. With an optimally damped system, the produced square wave should show a sharp rise in pressure followed by a rapid decrease in pressure with a quick return to baseline (Fig. 1.21).

In an overdamped system, there is no reverberation of the pressure after a fast flush. The systolic BP reading may be falsely low. In an underdamped system, there are multiple reverberations of the pressure after a flush; in such a system, the systolic BP readings tend to be falsely high.

In addition to the plumbing and monitoring equipment, certain physiologic factors can affect the accuracy of hemodynamic data and require special consideration. One major factor affecting the recorded hemodynamic pressure is the intrapleural pressure surrounding the heart and great vessels. Measurement of all hemodynamic pressures at end-expiration, when there is no air flow and the intrapleural pressure is unchanging, minimizes the effect of changes in intrapleural pressure on recorded hemodynamic pressures. However, determination of the point of end-expiration may, at times, be difficult. Use of a paper printout with a marker indicating end-expiration is the most valid way to obtain these data. The digital display value is inaccurate because most monitors simply average a certain number of beats, regardless of respiratory phase, and thus should not be relied on. However, newer monitoring systems have addressed this issue and now include an algorithm to identify the end-expiratory pressure.

AXIOM
Blood pressures obtained with an intra-arterial catheter tend to be higher than pressures taken indirectly with a cuff.

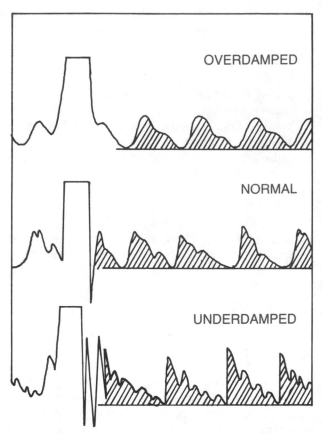

Figure 1.21 Square waves produced in response to a rapid change in pressure initiated by activating the fast flush device. (From Tilkian, A and Daily, EF: Cardiovascular Procedures. CV Mosby, St. Louis, 1986, p 90, with permission.)

b. Factors Affecting Pulse Pressure

Pulse pressure is largely determined by the SV, the compliance or distensibility of the arterial tree, and the character of ejection from the heart during systole. Any factor that increases SV, such as a decrease in pulse rate or an increase in cardiac output, also increases the pulse pressure. A decrease in compliance or distensibility of the arterial tree also tends to increase pulse pressure. In old age, much of the elastic tissue in the arterial walls is replaced by fibrous tissue. This greatly decreases the compliance of the arterial system and tends to increase pulse pressure, even though SV is often significantly reduced.

The rate of ejection of blood from the heart also affects pulse pressure. If the duration of ejection is prolonged, a larger portion of the SV runs off into the more distal portions of the systemic circulation while the remainder is still being ejected into the aorta; thus, the pulse pressure is not as high.

c. Abnormal Pressure Pulse

(1) Water-Hammer Pulse

In patients with aortic regurgitation or a large patent ductus arteriosus, SV may be very large and diastolic pressure very low. The extremely high pulse pressure that results may produce a powerful bounding (water-hammer) pulse which collapses almost completely between beats.

(2) Weak Pulse

The strength of a pulse on palpation is largely determined by the pulse pressure, not the systolic BP. A weak pulse at the radial artery usually indicates that SV is lower than normal (because of a rapid pulse rate or decreased cardiac output). The pulse in an extremity will also be weak if the arteries and arterioles in the extremity are so severely constricted or diseased that there is relatively little flow through the vessel being palpated.

(3) Pulsus Paradoxus

During inspiration, pressure in the thoracic cavity becomes more negative, and venous return to the right heart is increased. However, at the same time, the pressure in the lungs relative to the left atrium tends to fall, reducing the quantity of blood returning to the left side of the heart. As a result, left ventricular SV falls and systemic BP normally decreases by up to 10 mm Hg during inspiration. During expiration, the opposite effect occurs. Venous return to the right heart is decreased, but venous return to the left heart is increased (Fig. 1.22). In patients with constrictive pericarditis, pericardial tamponade, or right-ventricular infarction, diastolic filling of the left heart is further decreased. Consequently, during inspiration, patients with pericardial tamponade may have their systolic blood pressure fall by 15 mm Hg or more. Thus, pulsus paradoxus is not "paradoxical" but, rather, an exaggeration of a normal physiologic phenomenon. Obstructive pulmonary disease is the most common cause of a paradoxic pulse.

(4) Pulse Deficit

With arrhythmias such as atrial fibrillation, two beats of the heart may come so close together that there is very little diastolic filling pressure for the second beat. Under such circumstances, the second heart beat may be felt or heard over the precordium, but the SV may be too small to cause a palpable peripheral pulse. This difference between the pulse rate obtained by examining the heart directly and that obtained by palpating the pulsations in a peripheral vessel is referred to as a pulse deficit.

(5) Pulsus Alternans

In certain conditions, the heart beats strongly with one beat and then weakly with the next. This causes an alternation in the strength of the peripheral pulses, a condition called pulsus alternans. This is a relatively infrequent problem but may be strong evidence of left ventricular failure.

5. Patterns of Vascular Responses

In many situations, particularly severe stress, the entire vasomotor center acts as a unit, stimulating the heart, adrenal medulla, and vasoconstrictor system simultaneously. This "mass action" response increases cardiac output as well as

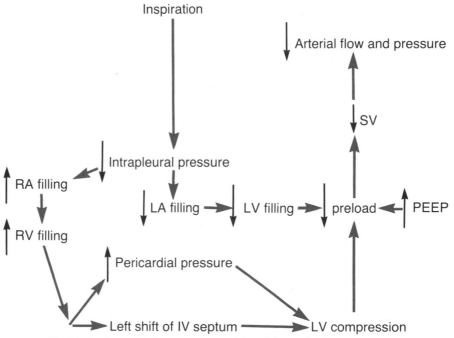

Figure 1.22 Mechanisms of pulsus paradoxus. RA = right atrial, RV = right ventricular, LV = left ventricular, IV = interventricular, SV = stroke volume, PEEP = end-expiratory pressure.

a. "Mass Action" Effect

peripheral vascular resistance, thereby greatly elevating the arterial pressure. Impulses are also transmitted simultaneously through the CNS to cause a state of generalized excitement and attentiveness, which seems to prepare the individual for fight or flight.

b. Emotional Fainting

Some people faint easily after an intense emotional experience, such as a sudden, severe fright. In such individuals, vessels throughout the body can become so vasodilated by the anterior hypothalamic vasodilator center that vascular capacity in the muscles increases severalfold. This causes arterial blood pressure and then cerebral blood flow to drop abruptly with resultant loss of consciousness.

c. Temperature Control

A discrete area in the preoptic region of the anterior hypothalamus is probably the major center for control for body temperature. Heating this center stimulates it to transmit impulses into the posterior hypothalamus, thereby inhibiting vasoconstrictor sympathetic fibers and causing dilatation of subcutaneous blood vessels. This increases subcutaneous blood flow and warms the skin, allowing it to give off body heat. Cooling the temperature control center induces vasoconstriction of the skin vessels, so that heat from the interior of the body is retained.

Increased body heat also tends to cause sympathetic excitation of the sweat glands. This in turn releases an enzyme called kallikrein which causes dilatation of the skin vessels. Kallikrein also splits globulins off vasoactive peptides in the interstitial fluid to release bradykinin and other powerful vasodilators.

d. Effect of Carbon Dioxide on the Vasomotor Center

The intensity of vasoconstrictor activity by the vasomotor center increases almost directly in proportion to the concentration of carbon dioxide in the blood. This systemic vasoconstrictor response to CO_2 is extremely powerful. However, if an alpha-adrenergic blocker such as dibenzyline is given, the CO_2 will cause a severe generalized vasodilation.

AXIOM

Administration of an alpha-adrenergic blocking agent can cause severe sudden hypotension if the arterial PCO_2 is high or rises.

e. Cushing Reflex

The so-called Cushing reflex is a type of CNS ischemic response that may result from increased cerebrospinal fluid pressure reducing the blood supply in the brain. This can cause a great increase in sympathetic nervous system activity with an abrupt rise in BP, usually with a simultaneous decrease in pulse rate. The respiratory rate may also fall, at least initially.

PITFALL

Failing to recognize that a rise in BP in a patient with head trauma may be a sign of increased ICP.

f. Vasodepression Due to Severe CNS Ischemia

If severe cerebral ischemia is allowed to persist, neuronal cells in the medullary, respiratory, and vasomotor centers begin to suffer metabolically and may become totally inactive. Apnea then occurs, followed by a fall in systolic arterial pressure to about 40 to 50 mm Hg (the level to which the blood pressure falls when all tonic vasoconstrictor activity is lost).

AXIOM

One should not blame hypotension in an injured patient on increased ICP unless the patient is apneic.

If the patient is trying to breathe, the hypotension has another etiology.

g. Reflexes from the Left Ventricle

Certain conditions associated with damage to the left ventricle or occlusion of coronary arteries are followed by a mild-to-moderate reflex decrease in arterial pressure. Injection of drugs referred to as veratrine alkaloids into the coronary system, for example, causes stimulation of certain nerve fibers in the ventricles, followed by a decrease in arterial pressure. This reflex, called the Bezold-Jarisch reflex, may also be caused by injection of glass or plastic spheres into the coronary arteries. It has been postulated that, by a similar mechanism, thromboses in the coronary arteries during a heart attack might cause a fall in arterial pressure. Thus, death might occasionally occur from the reflex fall in blood pressure rather than directly from the reduction in coronary blood flow.

h. Axon Reflex

The axon reflex is a special neuron reflex that utilizes only a single neuron and is the simplest reflex that can control circulation. When a small area of skin is damaged, pain receptors are stimulated and impulses are transmitted through pain nerve fibers into the spinal cord. Before reaching the spinal cord, some impulses also travel downward into other branches of the same nerve fiber. These returning retrograde impulses can cause a local vasodilation and hyperemia in the skin for 5 to 10 mm on either side of the damaged skin.

In the past, it was believed that sensory nerve endings secreted histamine or acetylcholine, which, in turn, caused the vasodilation. However, agents that block the actions of these two substances do not block the axon reflex. It has also been suggested that an adenosine phosphate compound or one of the kinins might be released by the pain nerve endings to cause the vasodilatation.

i. Vasomotor Waves

It has been noted that BP tends to rise 10 to 20 mm Hg and then fall again in a rhythmic fashion every 15 to 40 seconds. These oscillations in blood pressure have been called vasomotor waves, Mayer waves, or Traube-Hering waves. The cause of these vasomotor waves is not clear but may be related to oscillations in the sensitivity of the pressoreceptors and chemoreceptors.

C. THE VENOUS SYSTEM

The venous system functions primarily as a conduit to return blood from the capillaries to the heart, but it can also act as a reservoir for over 50% of the total blood volume.

1. Venous Return

Veins have only a small amount of muscle, and changes in their diameter are largely passive responses to the volume of blood present. Agents or situations that cause constriction of veins do, however, increase the rate at which blood will return to the heart.

An increase in vascular tone throughout the systemic circulation without a similar increase in pulmonary circulation often causes large volumes of blood to shift out of the peripheral vessels into the lungs and heart. This response is especially important during hemorrhage because it allows the circulation to continue to operate relatively normally, even when 15% to 25% of the total blood volume has been lost.

If the venous system were a passive set of tubes without valves, venous return, while standing, would be a serious problem. When a person is standing, pressure in the right atrium remains 0 to 5 mm Hg, but because of the effect of gravity, pressure in the veins of the feet rises to about 90 mm Hg. This hydrostatic pressure also affects peripheral pressures in the arteries: when standing, a person who has an arterial pressure of 100 mm Hg at the level of his heart has an arterial pressure in his feet of about 190 mm Hg.

Venous valves (which allow flow only toward the heart) and muscle contraction in the extremities are extremely important for maintaining venous return. Every time people move their legs, the contracting muscles compress the leg veins and blood is forced away from the areas of compression. Because the venous valves allow blood flow only toward the heart, blood is "pumped" centrally rather effectively by this mechanism.

AXIOM

Failure to contract leg muscles frequently and strongly enough while standing at "attention" for prolonged periods may reduce venous return enough to cause fainting.

2. Venous Reservoirs

About 50% to 60% of the blood in the circulatory system is normally present in veins that act as a reservoir for the circulation. Vasodilators may increase vascular capacity by 2 to 3 liters or more while vasoconstrictors may reduce vascular capacity by 1.0 to 1.5 liters. With even mild reductions in blood volume, sympathetic nervous stimulation tends to cause some constriction of the veins and arteries. Most of the contraction of capacitance veins occurs secondary to hypovolemia; however, it is probably a largely passive rather than an active muscle-constricting phenomenon.

D. CAPILLARIES

Only about 5% of the total capillary bed, especially in skeletal muscle, is open at any one time. However, diffusion of substances through the capillary membrane occurs so rapidly that, even though blood remains in the capillaries for only 1 or 2 seconds, the tissues normally receive all the oxygen and nutrients they require.

Vane, Anggard, and Botting have recently reviewed the regulatory functions of vascular endothelium. One of its main functions is maintaining the liquidity of blood. The vascular endothelium, which envelops the circulating blood in a continuous monolayer, is mainly responsible for this function.

Over the past 20 years other important functions of endothelium have been discovered. For instance the outer surface of the endothelial cell contains an angiotensin-converting enzyme. This same enzyme (also called kininase II) inactivates bradykinin, a potent vasodilator. Specific carrier mechanisms operate in the cell membrane to transport serotonin and adenosine into the endothelial cells, where they are metabolized by monoaminase oxidase and adenosine deaminase.

To maintain the patency of the blood vessels and the fluidity of blood, the endothelial cells synthesize large molecules, such as fibronectin and heparin sulfate, interleukin-1, tissue plasminogen activator, and various growth-promoting factors, and smaller molecules such as prostacyclin, endothelium-derived relaxing factor (EDRF), platelet-activating factor, and endothelin-1.

Stimulation of muscarinic receptors on endothelial cells from all species triggers the release of EDRF because it relaxes the underlying vascular smooth muscle. Later, it was observed that EDRF relaxed vascular smooth muscle by elevating cyclic guanosine monophosphate levels. EDRF was then shown to stimulate purified soluble guanylate cyclase, and the possible identity of EDRF as nitric oxide was pointed out simultaneously by Khan and Furchgott and Ignarro and associates.

In addition to the relaxing factors (prostacyclin and EDRF-nitric oxide), at least three vasoconstrictor substances are released by the vascular endothelium. These have been named endothelin-1 (formerly procine or human endothelin), endothelin-2, and endothelin-3 (formerly rat endothelin). The most striking property of endothelin-1 is its long-lasting hypertensive action. Endothelin-1 is the most active pressor substance yet discovered, with a potency 10 times that of angiotensin II. The kidney is about 10 times more sensitive than other vascular regions to the vasoconstrictor effects of endothelin-1. However, when endothelin-1 is infused intravenously into rats, its pressor activity is strongly limited by the release of prostacyclin and EDRF-nitric oxide.

The widespread distribution of specific high-affinity binding sites for endothelins in the blood vessels, brain, lungs, kidneys, adrenal glands, spleen, and intestines suggests that endothelins are involved in more than just regulation of cardiovascular tone. For example, endothelins may be involved in the maintenance of bronchoconstrictor tone in the lung and neurotransmission in the brain and spinal cord. One of the most interesting properties of endothelin-1 is its mitogenic action, which has been demonstrated in cardiovascular smooth-muscle cells, fibroblasts, and mesangial cells.

F. INTERSTITIAL FLUID

Movement of fluid back and forth between the capillaries and the interstitial fluid space is determined largely by the balance between the hydrostatic or filtration pressures in the capillaries and the balance between the COP of the blood and interstitial fluid. The relationship between these factors is described by the Starling equation (Fig. 1.23). It is generally assumed in systemic capillaries that the hydrostatic (filtration) pressure tending to push fluid out of the capillary is about 25 to 30 mm Hg at the arteriolar end of the capillary and 5 to 10 mm Hg at the venous end of the capillary. The interstitial fluid pressure is −5 to −10 mm Hg. Since the interstitial fluid pressure is negative, it tends to "pull" fluid out of the capillary into the interstitial fluid space. The interstitial COP is about 4 to 5 mm Hg and tends also to pull fluid into the interstitial space. The plasma COP, which is generally thought to be about 22 to 28 mm Hg, tends to be the major factor pulling fluid back into the capillary at its venous end.

The reflection coefficient is an index of how impermeable the capillary is to protein. If the value is 1.0, it is completely impermeable to protein, and if the value is 0.0, it is completely permeable to protein. Its normal value in systemic capillaries is probably close to 1.0 (Fig. 1.24). If the capillary filtration (hydrostatic pressure) rises or if the integrity of the capillary endothelium is impaired, fluid tends to move out of the vascular system into the interstitial fluid space. On the other hand, if the capillary filtration pressure falls due to hypovolemia, fluid tends to move into the capillaries from the interstitial space to re-expand blood volume.

Civetta has explored the reasons that, although the Starling equation is a simple mathematical expression, interpretation of the equation in different areas of the body has caused much controversy. These include (1) use of different measurement techniques, which often produce different values for each of the factors; (2) variability from tissue to tissue; (3) species differences; (4) different physiological states; and (5) the presence of other factors, such as lymph flow, that determine the status of the interstitial fluid space.

Pressure relationships in the interstitial space depend to a great extent on total tissue pressure, which represents the sum of forces exerted by (1) collagen fibers, (2) the gel in the interstitial space, and (3) cells abutting each other. The interstitial pressure (ISP) is also affected by (1) the rate of water passing into interstitial fluid (ISF) space from capillaries and, (2) the rate of evacuation of ISF by lymph flow. Most studies using implanted spheres or wicks report ISP values in the lung to be in the range of −5 to −7 mm Hg.

1. Interstitial Pressure and Volume Relationships

When ISP is negative, very slight increases in interstitial volume cause rapid increases in ISP. However, once atmospheric pressure is reached, large increases in interstitial volume are necessary to create any further increases in ISP.

2. Solid and Gel-State Considerations

Approximately 99% of all the ISF exists in a gel form. Gels not only help maintain the shape of the body, but they can also swell and incorporate large quantities of additional fluids. Nevertheless, diffusion is permitted to occur in an unrestricted fashion with the small amount of nongel fluid that is present. Thus,

$$J_V = K_F[(P_C - P_T) - \delta(\Pi_C - \Pi_T)]$$

Figure 1.23 A mathematical expression of the Starling equation. J_v = net volume flow; K_f = filtration coefficient; P_c = pulmonary microvascular pressure; P_T = interstitial pressure; δ = Staverman reflection coefficient; π_c = capillary oncotic pressure, π_T = tissue oncotic pressure.

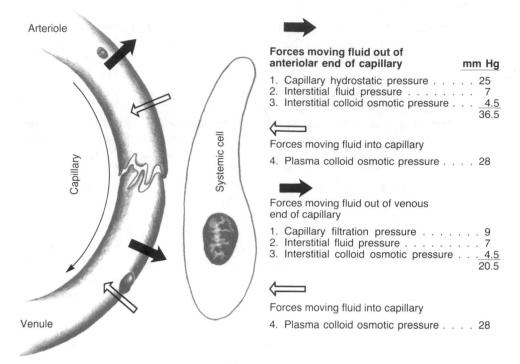

Arteriole

Capillary

Systemic cell

**Forces moving fluid out of
anteriolar end of capillary**   **mm Hg**

1. Capillary hydrostatic pressure 25
2. Interstitial fluid pressure 7
3. Interstitial colloid osmotic pressure . . . 4.5
                                          36.5

Forces moving fluid into capillary

4. Plasma colloid osmotic pressure 28

Forces moving fluid out of venous
end of capillary

1. Capillary filtration pressure 9
2. Interstitial fluid pressure 7
3. Interstitial colloid osmotic pressure . . . 4.5
                                          20.5

Forces moving fluid into capillary

4. Plasma colloid osmotic pressure 28

Venule

Figure 1.24 Movement of fluid into and out of capillaries.

shape is maintained while the distribution of fluid, electrolytes, and nutrients is not impeded.

Pressures exerted by the gel contribute to solid tissue pressure. These pressures result from the presence of fluid inside the gel, surface tension, and the Donnan effect of the charged particles. The gel possesses an abundance of negative charges that attract positive ions. These positive charges act to increase total osmotic pressure, which in turn attracts free fluid into the gel.

Although increases in ISF volume can be accommodated by changes in the gel volume and lymph flow, accumulations of large amounts of ISF eventfully increase free ISF. This will result in changes in the distribution of ISF volume according to the pull of gravity and can cause peripheral edema. Thus, once the safety factors of the gel and increased lymph flow are exhausted, free interstitial fluid accumulates, rather than causing further increases in intravascular pressures.

3. Interstitial Oncotic Pressure

In the lung, the interstitial oncotic pressure (IOP) is probably 70% to 80% of the serum value. This is quite different from the 15% to 20% of serum level felt to exist in peripheral tissues. If the normal plasma oncotic pressure is 20 to 25 mm Hg, then the oncotic gradient across the lung is only 4 to 6 mm Hg.

The Staverman reflection coefficient is a mathematical expression of the permeability of a membrane to any substance. For instance, if a membrane is totally impermeable to a particular substance, its reflection coefficient would be described as 1.0. However, if the membrane was completely permeable, its reflection coefficient would be 0. Numerous techniques, including histochemical and radioimmune assays and anatomical studies, have confirmed that the pulmonary capillaries are reasonably permeable to albumin, with a reflection coefficient in the range of 0.6 to 0.8. Thus, as pulmonary microvascular pressure increases and more ISF is formed, a simultaneous decrease in IOP will occur. This "interstitial protein washout" acts as an important safety mechanism because increases in the pressure gradient will be offset by an increase in the oncotic gradient. If plasma oncotic pressure remains the same, the IOP decreases and the total oncotic gradient increases.

4. Lymphatics

Not only does the ability to increase lymph flow provide a great margin of safety to accommodate increases in fluid flow from the capillary into the interstitial space, but it is also the main cause of a negative ISF pressure. If fluid accumulation increases to a point that ISP reaches 0 (atmospheric pressure), lymph flow can increase up to 20-fold. The fact that a 20-fold increase in lymph flow can occur with relatively small ISP changes (0 to 4 mm Hg) emphasizes the dynamic characteristics of lymphatic function. In addition, a 300% increase in pulmonary capillary pressure (4 to 12 mm Hg) can occur without any increase in ISF volume.

F. BLOOD FLOW THROUGH SPECIAL AREAS

1. Cerebral Blood Flow

The normal blood flow through the brain averages about 600 to 900 ml/min or 12% to 18% of the total cardiac output. The rate of blood flow through the brain is regulated primarily by the concentration of CO_2 in cerebral tissues. An increase in the $Paco_2$ tends to cause cerebral vasodilatation. Each 1.0-mm Hg rise in the $Paco_2$ increases cerebral blood flow by 2% to 4%. Hypoxia can also increase cerebral blood flow if the Po_2 falls below 50 to 60 mm Hg, but it is not nearly as effective as hypercarbia. Arterial BP under normal conditions has relatively little effect on cerebral blood flow, and minimal changes occur until the cerebral perfusion pressure (which is equal to the mBP minus the ICP) falls below 50 or 60 mm Hg. The sympathetic and parasympathetic systems have relatively little effect. Transection of these nerves causes little or no change in cerebral blood flow, except indirectly as a result of changes in extracranial blood flow.

2. Splanchnic Blood Flow

Approximately 1200 to 1800 ml of blood, or 25% to 30% of the cardiac output, enters the liver each minute. Of this total, about 1000 to 1200 ml is portal venous blood and 300 to 400 ml is hepatic artery blood; however, each of these vessels supplies about 50% of the oxygen used by the liver. Portal venous blood drains the stomach, intestine, spleen, and pancreas into the liver. About 70% to 80% of the portal venous blood comes from the intestines and 20% to 30% from the spleen and pancreas. After meals, the intestinal component tends to be greatly increased.

Hepatic arterial blood maintains the nutrition of connective tissues and bile ducts and then empties into the hepatic sinuses to mix with portal venous blood. It was thought for some time that interruption of hepatic artery flow for prolonged periods would almost invariably be fatal; however, there are now numerous cases of trauma in which bleeding from a severely torn liver was successfully controlled by ligation of a hepatic artery to one of the lobes, with maintenance of normal or near-normal liver function.

The hepatic sinuses are lined with an endothelium, which is much more permeable than most capillaries, so that even proteins can easily diffuse back into the sinuses.

The reticuloendothelial system of the liver is comprised largely of macrophages called Kupffer cells. These act as an extremely efficient remover of bacteria, bacterial products, and various vasoactive substances. Portal venous blood often contains a few bacteria from the gut; however, systemic blood is almost invariably sterile in the normal individual.

The primary factor that controls the rate of blood flow through the gastrointestinal tract is the rate of local metabolism. Parasympathetic stimulation has essentially no effect on gastrointestinal blood flow. However, it may increase smooth-muscle contraction, which may temporarily constrict intramural blood vessels and thereby decrease local blood flow. The circumferential arrangement of blood vessels around the intestine is extremely important. If the intestine becomes greatly distended, the blood vessels may be compressed and stretched sufficiently to occlude capillaries and then veins. If the gut becomes extremely distended, even arterial blood flow may cease.

Numerous extremely powerful vasoactive and proteolytic agents are constantly being formed by bacteria in the intestinal lumen. If the intestinal mucosa is not supplied with an adequate quantity of blood, proteolytic digestion of the mucosa and then bacterial invasion of the gut wall can occur rapidly. Thus, excessive distention of the intestines can result in gangrene and rupture within 24 to 48 hours or less.

Because of resistance at hepatic sinusoids, the pressure in the portal vein averages about 5 mm Hg higher than the pressure usually found in the inferior vena cava. If portal venous pressure rises abruptly, the splanchnic vessels can rapidly become severely congested. In cirrhosis, a large amount of fibrous tissue develops within the liver. Eventually, contraction of this fibrous tissue and expansion of new liver cells can compress the hepatic venules, thereby raising portal venous pressure to 25 to 30 mm Hg or higher. A similar elevation of portal venous pressure can occur if the proximal portal vein becomes thrombosed.

If the portal venous system is blocked suddenly, the patient often dies within a few hours because of ischemic damage to the bowel and fluid loss into splanchnic tissues. If portal blood flow is gradually occluded over a period of many months, large collateral channels to the systemic venous system may develop. The most important collaterals include anastomoses between (1) the splenic, gastric, and esophageal veins; (2) sigmoid and hemorrhoidal veins; and (3) intestinal veins through the peritoneal reflections to the posterior wall of the abdomen. However, even after major collateral channels have developed following portal venous blockade, pressure in the portal system remains elevated above normal. As a consequence, many cirrhotic patients develop ascites due to leakage of fluid through the hepatic capsule into the peritoneal cavity.

3. Muscle Blood Flow

During rest, blood flow through skeletal muscle averages 750 to 1000 ml/min, or about 15% to 20% of cardiac output. The arterioles of resting skeletal muscle exhibit an intense degree of vasomotor tone, independent of nervous stimuli, so that blood flow at rest is normally about one-twentieth the maximum that can occur with exercise.

The skeletal muscles are also provided with sympathetic vasoconstrictor and sympathetic vasodilator fibers. When maximally stimulated, sympathetic vasoconstrictor fibers can decrease blood flow through the muscles to about one-fourth normal. Sympathetic vasodilator fibers to the skeletal muscles secrete acetylcholine and, on maximal stimulation, can increase blood flow fivefold. These vasodilator fibers are activated by a special neurologic pathway that begins in the cerebral cortex close to the motor areas and passes downward through the hypothalamus and brain stem into the spinal cord, occasionally causing psychogenic fainting.

4. Blood Flow in the Skin

Circulation through the skin maintains its nutrition and conducts heat from the internal structures of the body to the surface so that it can be removed from the body. To accomplish this, the skin has two types of vessels. In addition to the usual nutrient arteries, capillaries, and veins, there are extensive subcutaneous venous plexuses with proximal AV anastomoses. These plexuses can hold large quantities of blood that can warm the surface of the skin and allow heat to be lost from the body. The AV anastomoses can also greatly reduce blood flow to the venous plexus, thereby reducing heat loss from the body. The AV anastomoses are found principally in the volar surfaces of the hands and feet, lips, nose, and ears, (i.e., the areas of the body most often exposed to maximal cooling).

At ordinary temperatures, the amount of blood flow in the skin to regulate body temperatures in an average adult is about 400 to 500 ml/min, which is 10 times as much as is needed to supply its nutrition. With severe sympathetic stimulation, as during hypovolemic shock, blood flow to the skin may decrease to as little as 10% of normal.

SUMMARY POINTS

1. Atrial fibrillation (with loss of atrial systole) can dramatically reduce cardiac output and may cause pulmonary edema in patients with significant mitral stenosis.

2. Normal systolic pulmonary artery pressure is only 12 to 15 mm Hg in young patients and 25 mm Hg or less in the elderly. A pulmonary artery pressure exceeding 25 to 40 mm Hg usually indicates pre-existing pulmonary disease and right-ventricular hypertrophy.

3. If aortic systolic pressure rises to 150 to 180 mm Hg in a patient who has been previously normotensive, the LVEDP often doubles, and if the increased LVEPD is persistent, it may cause the left ventricle to dilate and go into failure.

4. The normal ejection fraction is 60% to 70% for the left ventricle and 50% to 60% for the right ventricle.

5. In infants and patients with diseased hearts, SV may be relatively fixed. Therefore, cardiac output will be directly proportional to heart rate, and a bradycardia may be extremely deleterious.

6. If an older patient with nausea and vomiting has bradycardia, one should look for posterior myocardial ischemia.

7. Unusual ventricular complexes in a patient with a very slow heart rate may represent escape beats (not premature ventricular contractions).

8. Blood flow to the left ventricular myocardium, especially the subendocardial layers, is greatly reduced during systole. Consequently, tachycardia (which limits the amount of time in diastole) is deleterious if coronary artery flow is limited.

9. If increased oxygen is required by the heart, it cannot extract any more from the blood; the increased oxygen can be supplied only by increasing coronary blood flow.

10. An adequately perfused heart uses arterial lactate for fuel. Consequently, increased coronary sinus lactate is usually a good indicator of myocardial ischemia.

11. The main factors determining cardiac function and cardiac output are preload, afterload, contractility, cardiac rhythm, and heart rate.

12. It is an error to assume that left-ventricular diastolic volume is increased because the PAWP is high.

13. The CVP may be elevated by an increased blood volume, venous constriction, increased pulmonary vascular resistance, or right heart failure.

14. Use of PEEP during ventilatory assistance will reduce the net distending pressure of the atria, thereby reducing atrial natriuretic factor secretion when it may be needed to reduce an excess blood volume and pulmonary capillary pressure.

15. It is an error to assume that right heart filling is adequate if the CVP is high.

16. If the CVP is less than 4 to 8 cm H_2O in an ICU patient, one should be concerned that the patient may be hypovolemic.

17. The rate of rise of the CVP as fluid rapidly given (during a fluid challenge) is a better gauge of right ventricular filling than isolated CVP levels.

18. Distended neck veins should make one suspicious of volume overload, cardiac failure, tension pneumothorax, and pericardial tamponade.

19. One should not rely on a high water-manometer CVP reading to determine the patient's fluid status if the patient is on a ventilator, especially if the patient requires high-ventilatory pressures.

20. Patients with severe sepsis or respiratory failure, because of increased pulmonary vascular resistance, tend to have high CVP readings, even when hypovolemic.

21. Prominent pressure waves in distended neck veins often reflect some tricuspid valve incompetence due to overfilling or failure of the right ventricle.

22. The PAWP, when the catheter is properly positioned in West's zone III (where $Pa > P_v > P_A$), reflects left atrial filling pressures relatively well.

23. Whenever the PAWP is higher than the PADP, the accuracy of the PAWP reading should be questioned, and the catheter placement should be checked.

24. Increasing clinical evidence of pulmonary edema in a patient with a normal or low PAWP should make one assume that sepsis or some other cause of increased pulmonary capillary permeability is present.

25. The normal CI (cardiac output ÷ body surface area) in a healthy young adult is about 3.5 L/min per m² and falls about 0.1 to 0.2 L/min per m² per decade thereafter.

26. Since BP tends to rise with age, the calculated SVR which is equal to [(mBP − CVP) ÷ cardiac output], rises fairly rapidly in older individuals.

27. It is important to recognize that drugs that increase BP by causing vasoconstriction also tend to reduce cardiac output and tissue perfusion.

28. One should not aggressively attempt to reduce heart rates to less than 100 per minute in patients who are septic or have an increased oxygen consumption.

29. Although an increased heart rate may increase cardiac output and contractility, in patients with coronary artery disease this tends to increase myocardial oxygen demand more than coronary blood flow and can cause myocardial ischemia.

30. Myocardial oxygen consumption (MVO_2) is largely determined by the STTI, which is equal to the mean systolic BP developed by the heart multiplied by the average radius of the heart at the beginning of systole and the amount of time that the heart is in systole each minute.

31. Relatively minor increases in systolic BP, heart rate, and ventricular filling can cause major (geometrical) increases in MVO_2.

32. The first heart sound (S_1) is due primarily to closure of the mitral and then the tricuspid valves. The second heart sound (S_2) is primarily due to closure of the aortic and then the pulmonary valves.

33. A third heart sound (S_3) heard early in diastole is normal in children, but often is a sign of heart failure in older adults. A fourth heart sound (S_4) heard late in diastole also may be normal in children and is often associated with coronary artery disease or hypertension in adults.

34. Pulmonary vascular resistance rises with hypoxia or pulmonary disease.

35. The muscular layer of pulmonary arterioles tends to thicken and reduce lumen size if the vessel is exposed to chronically increased PAP (as with a ventricular septal defect).

36. Blood flow in the lung is largely determined by gravity and is primarily directed to its most dependent portions.

37. The cross-sectional area of the systemic circulation increases as blood moves from the heart to the capillaries and decreases again as the individual veins progressively increase in diameter closer to the heart.

38. The main factor determining the rate of blood flow in a vessel is described by Poiseuille's law as being the radius, and flow is proportional to the fourth power of the radius.

39. The main factor determining blood flow in nutrient capillaries is autoregulation, which relates the flow according to the metabolic needs of that tissue.

40. One should recognize that new hypertension in a critically ill patient may be due to CO_2 retention, pain, or anxiety.

41. Applying external pressure to the baroreceptors in the carotid sinus is interpreted centrally as an increased BP. The vasometer center responds by reducing sympathetic tone, which results in slowing of the heart rate and vasodilation.

42. One should not perform carotid artery massage without simultaneously and continuously evaluating heart rate and blood pressure.

43. Postsynaptic alpha$_1$-adrenergic receptors respond to norepinephrine released from the nerve terminal by causing vasoconstriction. Alpha$_2$ receptors are presynaptic and tend to decrease norepinephrine release from the nerve terminal, thereby decreasing vasoconstriction.

44. The beta$_1$-adrenergic receptors are primarily involved in the rate and force of myocardial contraction. Beta$_2$-receptor stimulation tends to cause smooth-muscle relaxation (dilatation) in bronchi and blood vessels.

45. One should not assume that the central aortic BP is always very low if the BP is unobtainable peripherally by the standard cuff technique.

46. When evaluating changes in BP, it is important to compare BP taken at similar sites using similar techniques.

47. The mean BP in the aorta is normally about the same as in the wrist or ankle. However, the systolic BP tends to be higher and the diastolic BP lower the further the pressure is measured from the heart.

48. Blood pressures obtained with an intra-arterial catheter tend to be at least 10 to 20 mm Hg higher than pressures taken indirectly with a cuff on the upper arm.

49. Pulsus paradoxus is an exaggeration of a normal phenomenon in which systolic BP falls by more than 10 to 15 mm Hg during inspiration, because of a reduced venous return to the left heart.

50. Pulsus paradoxus is usually due to pericardial tamponade, bronchospasm or hypovolemia.

51. Carbon dioxide tends to be a local vasodilator, but it acts centrally on the vasomotor center to cause peripheral vasoconstriction through alpha-adrenergic stimulation in almost all tissues except the brain.

52. Administration of an alpha-adrenergic blocking agent can cause severe, sudden hypotension if the arterial PCO_2 is high or rises.

53. A rise in BP in a patient with head trauma may be a sign of increased ICP.

54. Vasodilators reduce BP not only by causing arterial dilation, but also by dilating veins and thereby reducing venous return.

55. The flow of water between capillaries and the ISF space is expressed mathematically by Starling's equation:

$$J_v = K_f [(P_c - P_l) - (\pi_c - \pi_l)],$$

which relates intravascular pressure (P_c), ISF pressure (P_l), the protein reflection coefficient (sigma = σ), plasma COP (π_c), and interstitial COP (π_l).

BIBLIOGRAPHY

1. Albert, NR, et al: Heart muscle mechanics. Annu Rev Physiol 41:521, 1979.
1a. Ahlquist, RP: The adrenergic receptor. J Pharm Sci 55:359, 1966.
2. Barany, M and Barany, K: Phosphorylation of the myofibrillar proteins. Annu Rev Physiol 42:275, 1980.
3. Barrett, D and Wilson, RF: Alveolar-arterial oxygen difference in shock and respiratory failure. Circulation 40:40, 1969.
4. Beeson, PB and McDermott, W: Textbook of Medicine. WB Saunders, Philadelphia, 1975, pp 1107–1122.
5. Bergofsky, EH: Humoral control of the pulmonary circulation. Annu Rev Physiol 42:221, 1980.
6. Borgstrom, P, et al: An evaluation of the metabolic interaction with myogenic vascular reactivity during blood flow autoregulation. Acta Physiol Scand 122:275, 1984.
7. Chernow, B and Lake, CR: The pharmacologic approach to the critically ill patient. Williams & Wilkins, Baltimore, 1983.
8. Chernow, B and Roth, BL: Pharmacologic manipulation of the peripheral vasculature in shock: Clinical and experimental approaches. Circ Shock 18:141, 1986.
8a. Civetta, JM: A new look at the Starling equation. Crit Care Med 7:84, 1979.
9. Cohn, JN: Blood pressure measurements in shock, mechanism of inaccuracy in auscultatory and palpatory methods. JAMA 199:118, 1967.
10. Culver, BH and Butler, J: Mechanical influence of the pulmonary microcirculation. Annu Rev Physiol 42:187, 1980.

11. Daily, EK: Hemodynamic monitoring. In Dolan, JT (ed): Critical Care Nursing: Clinical Management through the Nursing Process. FA Davis, Philadelphia, 1991, pp 828–854.

12. Daveport, AP, et al: Autoradiographical localization of binding sites for porcine endiothelin-1 in humans, pigs, and rats: Functional relevance in humans. J Cardiovasc Pharmacol 13 and S166, 1989.

13. Dawson, CA: Role of pulmonary vasomotion in physiology of the lung. Physiol Rev 64:544, 1984.

14. Donald, DE and Shephert, JT: Automatic regulation of the peripheral circulation. Annu Rev Physiol 42:429, 1980.

15. Dorbin, PB: Mechanical properties of arteries. Physiol Rev 58:397, 1978.

16. Durling, BR and Klitzman, B: Local control of microvascular function: Role in tissue oxygen supply. Annu Rev Physiol 42:373, 1980.

17. Eisenberg, E and Green, LE: The relation of muscle biochemistry to muscle physiology. Annu Rev Physiol 42:293, 1980.

18. Ellis, D: Na-Ca exchange in cardiac tissues. Adv Myocardiol 5:295, 1985.

19. Fabiato, A and Fabiato, F: Calcium and cardiac excitation-contraction coupling. Annu Rev Physiol 41:473, 1979.

20. Fishman, AP: Vasomotor regulation of the pulmonary circulation. Annu Rev Physiol 42:211, 1980.

21. Gastaldo, J, et al: Relationship between peripheral blood flow and tissue gases. Int Surg 59:521, 1974.

22. Gevers, W: Protein metabolism of the heart. J Mol Cell Cardiol 16:3, 1984.

23. Gil, J: Organization of microcirculation in the lung. Annu Rev Physiol 42:177, 1980.

24. Goldberg, LI: Dopamine and new dopamine analogs: Receptors and clinical applications. J Clin Anesth 1:66, 1988.

25. Gotshall, RW and Miles, DS: Noninvasive assessment of cardiac output by impedance cardiography in the newborn canine. Crit Care Med 17:63, 1989.

26. Gray H: Anatomy of the human body. Goss CM (ed). WB Saunders, Philadelphia, 1971, Chap 4.

27. Guyton, AC: An overall analysis of cardiovascular regulation. Anesth Analg 56:761, 1977.

28. Guyton, AC and Jones, CE (eds): Physiology Series One: Cardiovascular Physiology, Butterworth & Co and University Park Press, Baltimore, 1974.

29. Hayes, DF, et al: Effects of traumatic hypovolemic shock on renal function. J Surg Res 16:490, 1974.

30. Haddy, FJ: The role of humoral Na^+, K^+-ATPase inhibitor in regulating precapillary vessel tone. J Cardiovasc Pharmacol (Suppl 2)6:S439, 1984.

31. Hert, JA: Cardiovascular response to stress in man. Annu Rev Physiol 46:177, 1984.

32. Higgins, TL: Current concepts in inotropic support. Hosp Formul 25:967, 1990.

33. Hoffman, BB and Lefkowitz, RJ: Adrenergic receptors in the heart. Annu Rev Physiol 44:475, 1982.

34. Hugh, JMB: Pulmonary circulatory and fluid balance. Int Rev Physiol 14:135, 1977.

35. Ignarro, LJ, et al: Endothelium-derived relaxing factor (EDRF) released from artery and vein appears to be nitric oxide (NO) or a closely related radical species (abstract). Fed Proc 46:644, 1987.

36. Ikemoto, N: Structure and function of the calcium pump protein of sarcoplasmic reticulum. Annu Rev Physiol 44:297, 1982.

37. Inoue, A, et al: The human endothelin family: three structurally and pharmacologically distinct isopeptides predicted by three separate genes. Proc Natl Acad Sci USA 86:2863, 1989.

38. Johansson, B: Vascular smooth muscle reactivity. Annu Rev Physiol 43:359, 1981.

39. Josephson, ME and Singh, BN: Use of calcium antagonists in ventricular dysfunction. Am J Cardiol 55:81B, 1985.

40. Judy, WW, Hall, JH, and Demeter, RJ: The contribution of passive and active diastolic filling on hemodynamics (abstract). Fed Proc 44:1735, 1985.

41. Khan, MT and Furchgott, RF: Similarities of behavior of nitric oxide (NO) and endothelium-derived relaxing actor in perfusion cascade bioassay system (Abstract). Fed Proc 46:385, 1987.

42. Kon, V, et al: Glomerular actions of endothelin in vivo. J Clin Invest 83:1762, 1989.

43. Langer, GA: Sodium-calcium exchange in the heart. Annu Rev Physiol 44:435, 1982.

44. Levy, MN: The cardiovascular physiology of the critically ill patient. Surg Clin North Am 55:483, 1975.

45. McDonald, TF: The slow inward calcium current in the heart. Annu Rev Physiol 44:425, 1982.

46. Martonosi, AN: Mechanisms of CA^{2+} release from sarcoplasmic reticulum of skeletal muscle. Physiol Rev 64:1240, 1984.

47. Meijler, FL: Atrioventricular conduction versus heart size from mouse to whale. J Am Coll Cardiol 5:363, 1985.

48. Miles, DS, Gotshall, RW, and Golden, JC: Accuracy of electrical impedance cardiography for measuring cardiac output in children with congenital heart defects. Am J Cardiol 61:612, 1988.

49. Miller, FC, et al: Heart rate and blood pressure in infants of pre-eclamptic mothers during the first hour of life. Crit Care Med 11:532, 1983.

50. Morgan, DL and Proske, U: Vertebrate slow muscle: Its structure, pattern of innervation, and mechanical properties. Physiol Rev 64:103, 1984.
51. Ng, ML, Levy, MN, and Zieske, HA: Effects of changes of pH and carbon dioxide tension on left ventricular performance. Am J Physiol 213:115, 1967.
52. O'Rourke, MF: Vascular impedance in studies of arterial and cardiac function. Physiol Rev 62:670, 1982.
53. Park, MK, Rosenbaum, JL, and German, VF: Systolic pressure amplification in pedal arteries in children. Crit Care Med 11:286, 1983.
54. Poelaert, JIT, et al: Hemodynamic effects of dopexamine in patients following coronary artery bypass surgery. J Cardiothorac Anesth 3:441, 1989.
55. Power, RF, et al: Autoradiographic localization of endothelin-1 binding sites in the cardiovascular and respiratory systems. J Cardiovasc Pharmacol 13:S50, 1989.
56. Rakugi, H, et al: Endothelin stimulates the release or prostacyclin from rat mesenteric arteries. Biochem Biophys Res Commun 160:924, 1989.
57. Randall, WC (ed): Nervous Control of Cardiovascular Function. Oxford University Press, New York, 1984.
58. Rippe, JM, et al: Intensive Care Medicine. Little, Brown & Co, Boston, 1985.
59. Rubanyi, GM, and Vanhoutte, PM. Hypoxia releases a vasoconstrictor substance from the canine vascular endothelium. J Physiol 364:45, 1985.
60. Rueter, H: Ion channels in cardiac cell membranes. Annu Rev Physiol 46:473, 1984.
61. Rosen, AL, Gilbert, H, and Moss, GS: Methods of evaluating myocardial function. Surg Clin North Am 55:81, 1975.
62. Rothe, CF: Reflex control of veins and vascular capacitance. Physiol Rev 63:1281, 1983.
63. Rowell, LB: Reflex control of regional circulations in humans. J Auton Nerv Syst 11:101, 1984.
64. Schatz, IJ and Wilson, RF: Cardiovascular failure following trauma. In Walt, AJ and Wilson, RF (eds): The Management of Trauma: Practice and Pitfalls. Lea & Febiger, Philadelphia, 1975, p 554.
65. Staub, NC: Pulmonary edema due to increased microvascular permeability. Annu Rev Med 32:291, 1981.
66. Stiles, GL, et al: Beta-adrenergic receptors: Biochemical mechanisms of physiological regulation. Physiol Rev 64:661, 1984.
67. Stork, TV, Muller, RM, and Piske, GJ: Noninvasive determination of pulmonary artery wedge pressure: Comparative analysis of pulsed Doppler echocardiography and right heart catheterization. Crit Care Med 18:1158, 1990.
68. Sutton, RN, Wilson, RF, and Walt, AJ: Differences in acid-base levels and oxygen-saturation between central venous and arterial blood. Lancet 2:748, 1967.
69. Swan, HJC: The role of hemodynamic monitoring in the management of the critically ill. Crit Care Med 3:83, 1975.
70. Tregear, RT and Marston, SB: The crossbridge theory. Annu Rev Physiol 41:723, 1979.
71. Vane, JR, Anggard, EE, and Botting, RM: Regulatory functions of the vascular endothelium. N Engl J Med 323:27, 1990.
72. Vary, TC, et al: Control of energy metabolism of heart muscle. Annu Rev Physiol 43:419, 1981.
73. Veigl, VL and Judy, WV: Reproducibility of hemodynamic measurements by impedance cardiography. Cardiovasc Res 1983:17:728.
74. Weissler, AM: Noninvasive methods for assessing left ventricular performance in man. Am J Cardiol 34:111, 1974.
75. Wilson, RF (ed): Critical Care Medicine. Upjohn, Kalamazoo, 1976.
76. Wilson, RF, Sarver, E, and Birks, R: Central venous pressure and blood volume determinations in clinical shock. Surg Gynecol Obstet 132:631, 1971.
77. Wilson, RF, et al: Cardiopulmonary resuscitation. In Walt, AJ and Wilson, RF (eds): The Management of Trauma: Practice and Pitfalls. Lea & Febiger, Philadelphia, 1979, p 149.
78. Wilson, RF, et al: Physiologic shunting in the lung in critically ill or injured patients. J Surg Res 12:571, 1970.
79. Winegrad, S: Regulation of cardiac contractile proteins: Correlations between physiology and biochemistry. Circ Res 55:565, 1984.
80. Winegrad, S: Calcium release from cardiac sarcoplasmic reticulum. Annu Rev Physiol 44:451, 1982.
81. Yoran, C, Covell, JW, and Ross, J, Jr: Structure basis for ascending limb of left ventricular function. Circ Res 32:297, 1973.
82. Zachariah, PK, et al: Atrial natriuretic peptide in human essential hypertension. Mayo Clin Proc 62:782, 1987.
83. Zak, R and Rabinowitz, M: Molecular aspects of cardiac hypertrophy. Annu Rev Physiol 41:539, 1979.
84. Zeigler, MG: Postural hypotension. Annu Rev Med 31:239, 1980.
85. Zinner, SH, et al: Factors affecting blood pressures in newborn infants. Hypertension 2:1, 1980.

CHAPTER 2

Acute Myocardial Infarction

I. INTRODUCTION

Each year approximately 2.0 to 2.5 million individuals in the United States suffer acute myocardial infarctions (AMI), and about 30% to 40% of these patients will die of their infarction. About two thirds of these deaths occur before the patient reaches a hospital. Of those who reach the hospital alive, up to 15% to 25% die within the next 4 weeks as a result of an extension of the infarction or from complications.

II. ETIOLOGY

Narrowing of coronary arteries is almost invariably atherosclerotic in origin. Other, but very infrequent, causes of occlusion or narrowing include trauma, emboli from various sources, periarteritis associated with collagen disease, or narrowing of the coronary artery ostia due to aortic valvular disease. In 5% to 15% of cases, an acute myocardial infarction occurs without significant underlying coronary artery disease. In such circumstances, it is assumed that the blood flow relative to the needs of the myocardium was greatly decreased, either because of greatly increased demands caused by severe work or stress and/or decreased coronary blood flow caused by coronary artery spasm or an arrhythmia.

PITFALL

Failure to pay adequate attention to the prevention of Valsalva maneuvers in patients with severe coronary artery disease.

Severe bearing down as when attempting to defecate (especially when constipated) may be extremely hazardous. An exaggerated Valsalva maneuver such as this will increase afterload on the heart and also reduce venous return and coronary blood flow at a time when the myocardium's need for blood and oxygen may be greatly increased. Heavy meals and sleep may also be associated with decreased coronary blood flow. Postprandially, cardiac output may increase while blood flow tends to be diverted to splanchnic areas. During sleep, cardiac output tends to fall and consequently blood pressure (BP) may fall below the critical closing pressure of diseased coronary vessels. During rapid eye movement (REM) sleep, an increased sympathetic discharge can increase myocardial oxygen demand at a time when coronary blood flow is reduced.

III. PATHO-PHYSIOLOGY

A. CORONARY BLOOD FLOW

The left ventricle and its portion of the septum weighs approximately 1.0 to 1.2 g/lb of body weight and has a blood flow of about 150 to 200 ml/min. Total coronary blood flow at rest is about 250 ml/min or 0.8 to 1.2 $ml \cdot min^{-1} \cdot g^{-1}$ of myocardium.

AXIOM

If the heart needs more oxygen, it must come from increased coronary blood flow. There is no oxygen reserve in coronary artery blood.

During severe exercise or stress, the coronary arteries can dilate enough to increase coronary flow more than fivefold. Even at rest, the myocardium normally extracts nearly all the oxygen available in the blood. The venous Po_2 in the coronary sinus is about 18 to 20 mm Hg, with an oxyhemoglobin saturation of 30% to 35%.

AXIOM

Myocardial oxygen demand is determined primarily by the systolic tension time index.

The main determinant of coronary artery blood flow is the metabolic requirement of the heart. According to Sarnoff, this can be determined by the systolic tension-time index (STTI). The STTI is equal to the mean systolic pressure developed by the ventricle multiplied by its radius (tension = pressure $\times$ radius) multiplied by the fraction of each minute that the heart is in systole. Thus, the oxygen needs of the heart increase with increased systolic pressure, increased diameter (dilatation) of the left ventricle, and tachycardia, which increases the amount of time per minute that the heart is in systole. Newer work suggests that at a constant heart rate, the initial stretch of the myocardial fiber, rather than the arterial BP or cardiac output (CO), is the main determinant of myocardial oxygen consumption.

AXIOM

Blood flow to the myocardium depends largely on diastolic aortic pressure, left ventricular diastolic pressure, the resistance to blood flow in the coronary arterioles, and the amount of time in diastole.

In the left ventricular myocardium, intramyocardial tension during systole is often higher than aortic pressure. Consequently, there is little or no blood flow in the innermost (subendocardial) myocardium except during diastole. In contrast, blood flow to the right ventricular myocardium may continue throughout the cardiac cycle. Even here, however, coronary flow is greater during diastole.

AXIOM

A low aortic diastolic BP and high left ventricular diastolic pressure can greatly reduce blood flow through the left ventricle.

Normally, the transmyocardial pressure gradient is 70 to 80 mm Hg. However, if the aortic diastolic blood pressure (BP) is low and left ventricular (LV) diastolic pressure is high, the LV transmyocardial pressure gradient is greatly decreased. A patient with an arterial BP of 120/80 and LV diastolic BP of 5 mm Hg has a transmyocardial pressure gradient of 75 mm Hg. This is almost four times that of a patient whose aortic BP is 80/40 and LV diastolic pressure is 20 mm Hg.

AXIOM

Tachycardia increases myocardial oxygen requirements and decreases the time for coronary blood flow.

Since an increased heart rate decreases the amount of time in diastole, tachycardia can cause a significant reduction in coronary blood flow. Certain vasopressor drugs such as norepinephrine, metaraminol, and methoxamine tend to cause direct coronary vasoconstriction. However, by increasing the left ventricular work and myocardial metabolism, these indirectly dilate the coronary arteries. Unfortunately, this autoregulatory mechanism does not work well in atherosclerotic coronary vessels.

B. CORONARY ATHEROSCLEROSIS

Atherosclerosis is a disease affecting primarily the intima of blood vessels. The intima is narrow in normal arteries, and is composed of a continuous layer of endothelial cells that form the interface between the blood and vessel wall. The endothelial cells are attached to a layer of connective tissue called the basement membrane. The rest of the intima contains loose connective tissue and occasional smooth-muscle cells. Outside this layer is a band of elastic tissue, the internal elastic membrane, which separates the rather acellular subintimal tissue from the adjacent medial or muscle layer. The medial layer consists predominantly of concentrically arranged layers of smooth-muscle cells.

In atherosclerosis, the intimal layer undergoes marked thickening caused by deposition of fat and increases in the amount of connective-tissue matrix. It is not certain why this occurs. One hypothesis states that the thickening is a response to injury which interrupts the endothelial lining and exposes the underlying connective tissues to formed elements of the blood. It is further proposed that blood platelets adhere to and aggregate on the exposed connective tissue, form a temporary plug, and in doing so release their contents into the arterial wall. A small cationic protein that is released from aggregated platelets has been demonstrated to be mitogenic as well as chemotactic for arterial smooth-muscle cells. According to this postulate, in response to injury, smooth-muscle cells migrate into the intima, multiply, and synthesize connective tissue. This may be the initial phase of an atherosclerotic lesion. It has also been found that smooth-muscle cells from diseased human arteries can secrete substances with mitogenic activity. This capacity to produce an endogenous, potentially self-stimulatory (autocrine) growth factor may help to explain how replication of smooth-muscle cells can begin early in atherogenesis, even while the endothelial barrier remains intact.

The possible role of proteoglycans in coronary atherogenesis has also been studied. Proteoglycans are one component of connective tissue known to influence cell adhesion, migration, and proliferation during morphogenesis. Thus, they seem well suited to be involved in the pathogenesis of atherosclerosis. The major sources of arterial proteoglycans are arterial endothelium and smooth muscle. Cell cultures have demonstrated that endothelium and smooth-muscle cells can synthesize at least three different families of proteoglycans.

At a later stage in coronary atherosclerosis, lipid-filled macrophages begin to accumulate in focal areas in the subintimal layer, which is further thickened by a localized fibrous reaction to the lipid material (Fig. 2.1.). Eventually these macrophages disappear, but the lipid material remains behind and becomes amorphous. This atheroma can then crystalize, ulcerate, and/or calcify with further increase in the surrounding fibrous-tissue formation. Four possible complications may then develop: (1) narrowing of the lumen by the atheromatous process, (2) hemorrhage into the wall of the vessel, (3) luminal thrombosis, or (4) embolism of the atheromatous material or attached clot.

In the coronary arteries, the atheromatous process is located mainly in the proximal portions of the vessels. Intramyocardial arteries, less than 1.0 to 1.5 mm in diameter, appear to be involved much less frequently than the larger, more proximal epicardial portions of the vessels. Atherosclerotic changes also occur only rarely in the portion of a coronary artery that is completely surrounded by myocardium.

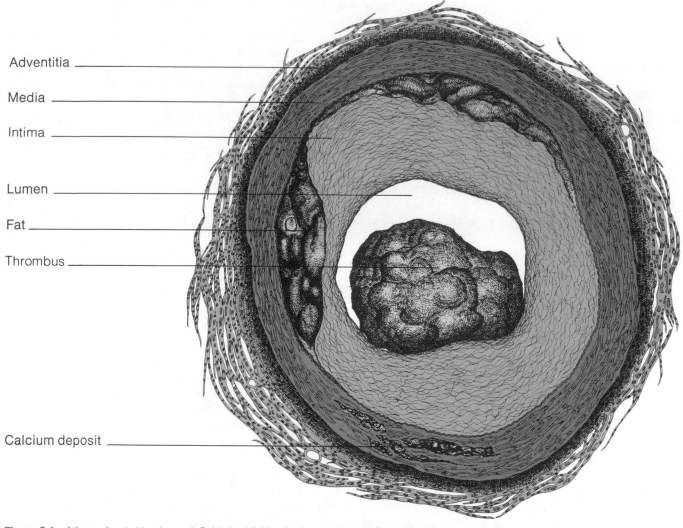

Adventitia

Media

Intima

Lumen

Fat

Thrombus

Calcium deposit

Figure 2.1 Atherosclerotic blood vessel. Subintimal lipid collections or thrombi formed in the vessels may narrow or occlude the lumen.

The great majority of acute myocardial infarctions appear to be associated with an acute thrombosis of a diseased coronary artery. Krusteal, using fibrin and fibrinogen-related antigens, suggested that in patients with unstable angina or an acute myocardial infarction there is an active, ongoing thrombotic process that might be prevented by antiplatelet or anticoagulant therapy.

C. PATHOLOGIC CHANGES IN THE MYOCARDIUM

An AMI may be defined as necrosis or death of myocardium due to ischemia. Left ventricular wall damage by an acute myocardial infarction tends either to be transmural (involving the entire thickness of the muscle in the damaged area) or localized to the subendocardial myocardium. Subendocardial infarcts are particularly apt to occur in patients with left ventricular hypertrophy. As the myocardium thickens in ventricular hypertrophy, the vessels to the endocardium become longer and thinner, increasing the vulnerability of the subendocardial myocardium to any ischemic process.

D. EVOLUTION OF THE INFARCTION

The pathologic stages occurring in an acute myocardial infarction generally follow an orderly and progressive pattern. Early in the ischemic process, the myocardial cells stop contracting and, as these cells lose adenosine triphosphate (ATP), they become stiff with edema. Although few histologic changes are noted during the first 12 hours, the involved area may grossly appear slightly darker or bluer than normal, and microscopically the involved fibers may appear somewhat eosinophilic. After 12 hours a "wave front of death" can be noted proceeding from the endocardium out toward the epicardium. This is followed by increasing proteolysis caused initially by lysosomal enzymes and superoxides from the dead and dying myocardial cells. The process is continued later by similar substances from scavenging macrophages.

At 18 hours, the involved myocardium may still appear relatively normal on gross examination. Microscopically, however, the cytoplasm of the dead or dying muscle fibers begins to clump, local capillaries dilate, and leukocytes (particularly neutrophils) begin migrating into the area.

At 24 hours, the infarcted area grossly appears yellow with a border of reddish-purple tissue representing the marginally ischemic myocardium. Microscopically, the leukocytic infiltrate is now quite prominent, particularly at the junction of the involved and noninvolved tissue.

At 48 hours, fibroblasts appear and the infarcted area tends to become grayer, thinner, and depressed. Microscopically, the leukocytic infiltrate has increased, the nuclei of the muscle fibers become indistinct, and the cross striations of the muscle fibers become coarser.

After 96 hours, beginning at the periphery of the infarct, the dead muscle progressively disintegrates and disappears. After the seventh day, capillaries and connective tissue begin to grow into the dead tissue, and the infarcted area becomes firmer.

At the beginning of the third week, the involved area is usually thinner, and scar formation becomes apparent as the involved tissue takes on a ground-glass, gray appearance. Microscopically, the disappearing muscle is replaced by fibroblasts and increasing bands of collagen.

By 2 to 3 months the avascular scar of fibrous tissue is complete. However, if the scar is transmural, it may progressively stretch and form a ventricular aneurysm.

IV. DIAGNOSIS

A. ACUTE MYOCARDIAL INFARCTION

AXIOM

The diagnosis of an acute myocardial infarction is fairly secure if two of the following criteria are present: (1) typical history of chest pain, (2) typical electrocardiographic (ECG) changes, or (3) typical enzyme (CPK-MB) changes.

1. Signs and Symptoms

Pain is the presenting symptom in most patients with an AMI who live long enough to reach a hospital. In addition, many of these patients have had previous episodes of angina pectoris (Table 2.1).

Table 2.1

CHARACTERISTICS OF TYPICAL ANGINA PECTORIS	1. Location
	  a. Substernal, but often extends anywhere from C3 to T6
	  b. Occasionally limited to jaw, shoulder, or arm
	  c. Unlikely to be discretely localized
	2. Quality
	  a. Pressure or constriction
	  b. Visceral rather than superficial
	3. Duration
	  a. 30 seconds to a few minutes
	  b. Gradual waxing and waning
	4. Inciting factors
	  a. Physical effort
	  b. Emotional excitement
	  c. Cold
	  d. Eating
	5. Patterns of relief
	  a. Within 2 to 10 minutes of rest
	  b. Within 2 to 5 minutes of nitroglycerin

AXIOM

Any new jaw, neck, or chest pain developing in an older patient, particularly after stress or effort of any type, should be considered to be due to angina or possible myocardial infarction until proven otherwise.

The site of pain is extremely variable. It may involve the chest, back, epigastrium, neck, shoulder, arms, or even the teeth. Often, the pain is described as crushing pressure or heaviness over the sternum (Table 2.2).

The pain of an acute infarction usually lasts 30 to 60 minutes, until it is relieved spontaneously or by analgesics. The diagnosis of infarction should be particularly considered when the patient describes anginalike pain that is much more severe than normal and persists in spite of two or more nitroglycerin tablets. Some patients will lie down or sit quietly while the pain persists, while others may be extremely anxious and restless. There may or may not be a history of previous chest pain. The pulse rate tends to be slightly or moderately increased.

AXIOM

Up to 70% of patients with myocardial ischemic episodes and 15% of patients with an acute myocardial infarction have no chest pain or related symptoms.

In some patients, the symptoms of their myocardial infarction may not be noted because it occurs during surgery or during a cerebrovascular accident. Many have only epigastric distress, "gas," nausea, or severe weakness without obvious cause, particularly if it is an inferior myocardial infarction. At the other extreme, the patient may present with a cardiac arrest or shock.

Although most patients with an AMI have a slight-to-moderate sinus tachycardia, sinus bradycardia is occasionally present, particularly immediately after posterior myocardial infarcts. Occasionally an atrial gallop and/or a paradoxically split-second heart sound is heard.

In a study of the routine clinical criteria for diagnosing myocardial infarction within 24 hours of hospitalization, Lee and associates found that most patients with a myocardial infarction seen in an emergency department had enzyme abnormalities. Most of the other patients with infarcts had a recurrence of their ischemic pain during that period. If the enzymes were normal and there was no recurrent pain, 98% of the patients did not eventually meet criteria for the diagnosis of an acute myocardial infarction.

Table 2.2

PRESENTATION OF ACUTE MYOCARDIAL INFARCTION	1. Typical: substernal heaviness or crushing discomfort, with or without radiation to the neck, arms, and/or back
	2. Atypical
	  a. Unusual location or character of pain
	  b. New onset of left-ventricular failure
	  c. Syncope
	  d. Strokelike signs or symptoms
	  e. Severe anxiety or nervousness
	  f. Sudden onset of mania or psychosis
	  g. Overwhelming weakness
	  h. Epigastric discomfort with belching and distention
	  i. Peripheral arterial embolism

2. Laboratory Studies

Within 12 to 36 hours of a myocardial infarction, the white blood count (WBC) usually rises to 12,000 to 15,000/mm³ with a shift to the left. Blood glucose levels may rise, particularly in diabetics. Serum glutamic oxaloacetic transaminase (SGOT) levels usually rise slightly or moderately in 6 to 8 hours, reach a peak in 24 to 48 hours, and return to normal in 4 to 8 days (Fig. 2.2). Lactic dehydrogenase (LDH), especially fraction 5, may rise within 12 hours and persist for up to 10 days. The creatinine phosphokinase (CPK), particularly the myocardial-brain (MB) fraction, will also rise within several hours, reach a peak at 18 to 24 hours and return to normal in 48 to 72 hours.

AXIOM

Because there are other causes of CPK-MB increases not associated with acute myocardial infarction (Table 2.3), CPK-MB elevations should not be the sole diagnostic indicator of acute myocardial infarction in patients with chest pain.

3. Electrocardiographic Changes

a. ST-Segment and T-Wave Changes

Occasionally, the ECG provides the only evidence that a myocardial infarction has occurred. The mildest abnormality following occlusion of a coronary artery often is simple T-wave inversion or depression of the J point, which is the point at which the QRS complex ends and the ST segment begins (Fig. 2.3). With increasing ischemia, this is followed by elevation of the ST segment as a manifestation of sublethal myocardial injury, with impaired repolarization of the involved tissue. When present with an infarction, these ST-segment and T-wave changes are felt to come from areas of ischemia and sublethal injury surrounding the infarct. In about 20% of patients with chest discomfort at rest, the presence of persistent ST-T changes and CPK-MB elevations allow one to diagnose a non-Q wave myocardial infarction (Table 2.4).

Although many physicians rely on ST-T-wave changes to make a diagnosis of infarction, they are not diagnostic by themselves. These changes are nonspecific and can also be caused by severe stress, medications, or abnormal electrolyte levels. In addition, T-wave abnormalities may be delayed for up to 3 to 10 days after the infarction.

b. Changes in the QRS Complex

When the actual muscle death (infarction) occurs, the most consistent abnormality is a change in the initial ventricular electrical forces, as represented by changes in the QRS complex. Loss of the electrical forces from the infarcted area causes an initial negative deflection (Q wave) over the area of infarction (Fig. 2.4).

ECG changes seen with an infarction vary with the location of the ECG leads relative to the infarction. The QRS reflects movement of the initial depo-

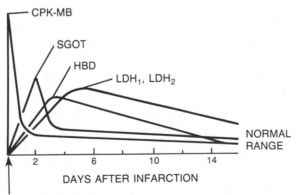

Figure 2.2 Evolution of enzyme changes after myocardial infarction. (From Dolan, JT: Critical Care Nursing. FA Davis, Philadelphia, 1991, p 901, with permission.)

Table 2.3

CAUSES OF CPK-MB INCREASES NOT ASSOCIATED WITH ACUTE MYOCARDIAL INFARCTION	Release of nonmyocardial CPK
	Trauma to muscle
	Crush injury
	Burns
	Electrical injuries
	Noncardiothoracic surgery
	Extreme exercise
	Grand mal seizures
	Various inflammatory and noninflammatory myopathies
	Chronic renal failure
	Hypothyroidism
	Chronic alcoholism
	Hyperthermia and hypothermia
	Cardiopulmonary resuscitation
	Defibrillation
	Intramuscular injections
	Cardiac injury other than acute myocardial infarction
	Cardiac contusions from trauma
	Cardiothoracic surgery
	Myocarditis
	Decreased clearance of serum CPK-MB
	Hypothyroidism and hyperthyroidism

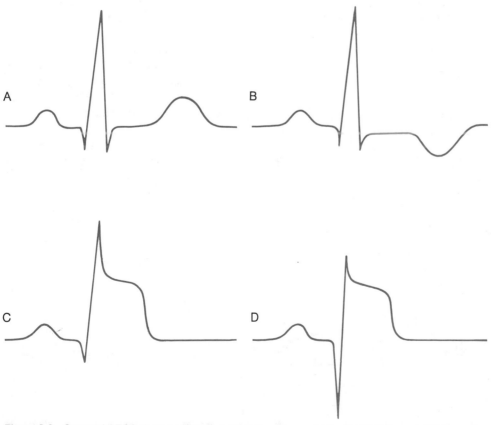

Figure 2.3 Sequential ECG changes following an acute coronary obstruction. (*A*) Normal. (*B*) Reversible ischemia; T-wave inversion and depression of the J point. (*C*) Injury pattern, elevation of the ST segment. (*D*) Infarction pattern, development of an abnormal Q wave.

Table 2.4

ACUTE ISCHEMIC HEART DISEASE SYNDROMES

History	ECG	Serum CPK-MB Enzymes	Diagnosis
Exertional chest discomfort	No changes or transient ST-T changes	Normal	Stable angina pectoris
Increasing chest discomfort with exertion or at rest	No changes or transient ST-T changes	Normal	Unstable angina pectoris
Chest discomfort at rest	Persistent ST-T changes	Elevated	Non-Q-wave myocardial infarction
Chest discomfort at rest	Q waves or loss of R waves	Elevated	Q-wave myocardial infarction

larization forces away from the infarct, the ST segments tend to be elevated toward the infarct, and the T waves tend to be directed away from the infarct. The lead directly over the infarction may show a QS pattern with an elevated ST segment. Over the injured area near the infarction, the QRS complex may be normal, but the T wave is often inverted.

PITFALL

Insisting on abnormal or typical ECG findings to make a diagnosis of an acute myocardial infarction.

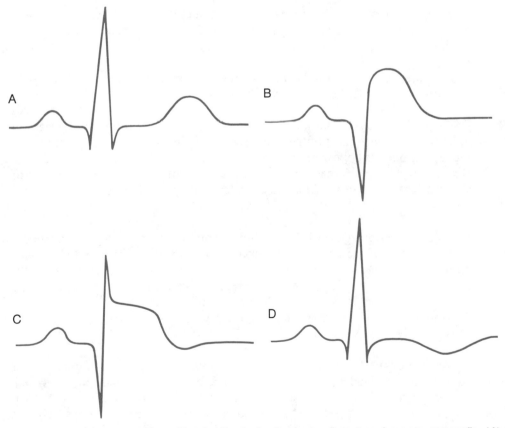

Figure 2.4 ECG abnormalities with infarction in the involved, adjacent, and remote myocardia. (*A*) Normal. (*B*) Directly over the infarction. (*C*) Adjacent to the infarction. (*D*) Over an injured area a slight distance from the infarction.

Development of Q waves or alterations in the R-wave amplitude and morphology can generally be regarded as diagnostic. However, if less than 1.0 cm³ of myocardium is infarcted, ECG changes will often be absent. Furthermore, certain portions of the left ventricle referred to as *silent* areas (such as endocardium, back of the left ventricle, papillary muscles, and posterior septum), right ventricle, and right atrium, may show little or no ECG changes in spite of significant damage. The ECG diagnosis of acute infarction in a patient who has had a previous myocardial infarction or a previous left bundle-branch block (LBBB) may be particularly difficult.

c. Time Sequences

The ST-segment elevation often appears almost immediately after an infarction and remains for a variable period of time ranging from as little as 12 hours to as long as 10 to 14 days (Figs. 2.5 and 2.6). If the ST segments remain elevated for a longer period, a ventricular aneurysm should be suspected. As the ST segments lower with time, the T-wave inversions deepen and become lowest when the ST segment finally returns to the baseline. T-wave inversion may not appear for 6 to 24 hours, but may persist for months or years. The QRS abnormalities, particularly a deep, wide Q and absence of an R wave in some leads, often persist indefinitely.

d. ECG Changes Associated with Location of Infarction (Table 2.5)

(1) Anteroseptal Myocardial Infarction

An anteroseptal myocardial infarction is characterized by a persistent QS pattern or absence of the usual progressive increase in the height of the R wave from V_1 through V_3 or V_4 (Fig. 2.7).

(2) Anterolateral Myocardial Infarction

An infarction that extends over the anterolateral portion of the left ventricle will cause the greatest ECG changes in leads I, aVL, and V_3 through V_6 (Fig. 2.5). Reciprocal changes may occasionally be seen in aVR.

(3) High Anterolateral Myocardial Infarction

A high anterolateral myocardial infarction will cause abnormalities in I and aVL and sometimes in II, but the V leads may show no or only minimal changes.

(4) Diaphragmatic (Inferior) Myocardial Infarction

Like the high anterolateral infarctions, the diaphragmatic (inferior) myocardial infarctions produce most of their changes in the limb leads. Usually only minimal abnormalities appear in the precordial leads except for some reciprocal ST changes in the early stages. The changes in the limb leads consist primarily of abnormal Q waves in II, III, and aVF, with more prominent R waves in I and aVL.

(5) Inferoposterior Myocardial Infarction

An inferoposterior myocardial infarction involving the diaphragmatic and posterior portions of the left ventricle produces Q waves in II, III, and aVR with more prominent R waves in I and aVL (as seen in inferior infarctions) (Fig. 2.8). It also produces tall R waves and upright T waves in V_1 through V_4 (i.e., reversing the usual R:S ratio). In V_5 and V_6 the R waves become smaller and there may be small Q waves and/or T-wave inversion.

(6) Posterior Myocardial Infarction

AXIOM

An isolated posterior myocardial infarction may produce few or no diagnostic ECG changes. A large posterior infarction may produce tall R waves and upright T waves in V_1 through V_3 or V_4 with a smaller R wave in V_6 with or without a small Q-wave and T-wave inversion in V_5 and V_6. The limb leads may show no change or relatively mild changes in II, III, and aVF (Fig. 2.9).

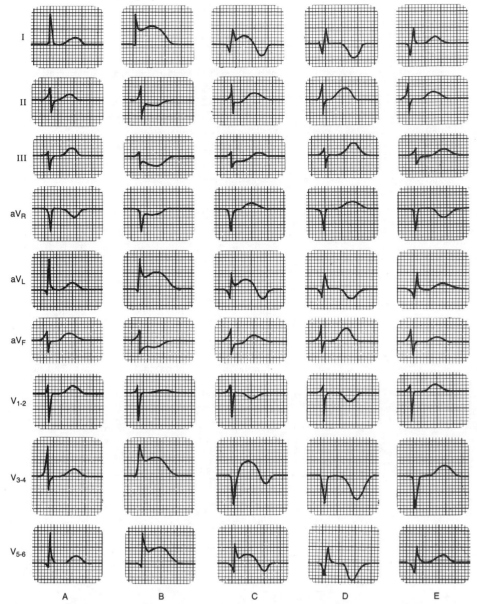

Figure 2.5 Diagrammatic illustration of serial electrocardiographic patterns in anterior-wall myocardial infarction. (*A*) Normal tracing. (*B*) Early pattern. There is ST-segment elevation in leads I, aVL, and V₃. V₆ and ST depression in leads II, III, and aVF (the ST depression might reflect inferior-wall ischemia or reciprocal depression). (*C*) Later pattern (hours to days). Q waves are present in leads I, aVL, and V₅ to V₆. QS complexes are present in leads V₃ and V₄ indicating that the major area of infarction underlies the area recorded by leads V₃ and V₄. ST-segment changes persist but to a lesser degree, and the T waves are beginning to invert in those leads in which ST-segment elevation is present. (*D*) Late (established) pattern (days to weeks). The Q waves and QS complexes persist. The ST segments are isoelectric. The T waves are deeply and symmetrically inverted in the leads that showed ST elevation and tall in the leads that showed ST depression. This pattern may persist for the remainder of the patient's life. (*E*) Very late pattern (months to years). The abnormal Q waves and QS complexes persist, but the T waves have returned to normal. Without the benefit of serial ECGs, it is not possible to determine when myocardial infarction occurred. Therefore, no conclusions should be drawn as to the age of the process on the basis of a single ECG (From Dolan, JT: Critical Care Nursing. FA Davis, Philadelphia, 1991, p 903, with permission.)

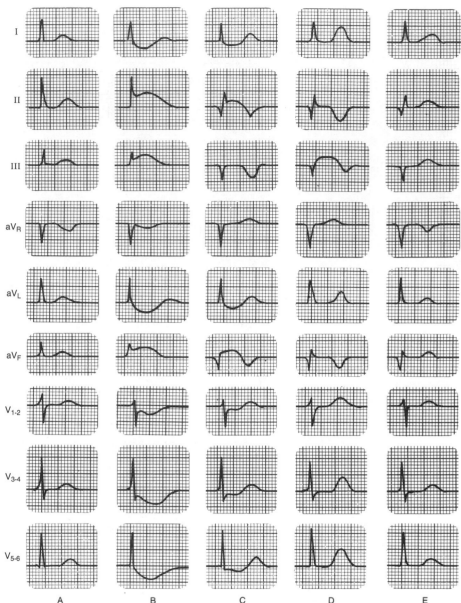

I

II

III

aV_R

aV_L

aV_F

V_{1-2}

V_{3-4}

V_{5-6}

A   B   C   D   E

Figure 2.6 Diagrammatic illustration of serial electrocardiographic patterns in inferior myocardial infarction. (*A*) Normal tracing. (*B*) Very early pattern (hours after infarction). There is ST-segment elevation in leads II, III, and aVF, and ST-segment depression in leads I, aVL, and aVR, as well as in the precordial leads. (*C*) Later pattern (hours to days). Abnormal Q waves have appeared in the inferior leads. There is less ST elevation in these leads and less ST depression in the anterior leads. The T waves are becoming inverted in leads II, III, and aVF. (*D*) Late (established) pattern (days to weeks). The ST segments are isoelectric. Deep, symmetrically inverted T waves are seen in leads II, III, and aVF. The T waves are abnormally tall and symmetric in leads I and aVL, and in the precordial leads. This pattern may persist for the remainder of the patient's life. (*E*) Very late (months to years) pattern. The abnormal Q waves persist, but the T waves have become normal. (From Dolan, JT: Critical Care Nursing. FA Davis, Philadelphia, 1991, p 904, with permission.)

(7) Inferolateral Myocardial Infarction

An inferolateral or inferoapical infarction will produce some of the changes characteristic of both inferior and anterolateral infarctions. The main changes will occur in II, III, and aVF, with Q and T abnormalities or only T-wave inversions in V_5 and V_6.

(8) Subendocardial Infarctions

Myocardial infarcts are often categorized as transmural or nontransmural (subendocardial) based on whether or not Q waves develop on the electrocardio-

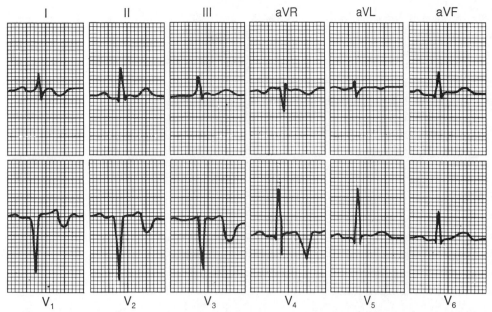

| I | II | III | aVR | aVL | aVF |
| V_1 | V_2 | V_3 | V_4 | V_5 | V_6 |

Figure 2.7 Stable anteroseptal myocardial infarction. QS complexes are seen in leads V_1 through V_3, with negative T waves in V_1 through V_4.

gram. A subendocardial infarction may have all of the clinical signs seen with the usual (transmural) infarctions.

On the ECG, ST-segment depression tends to be seen in leads I, II, V_5 and V_6. Morphologically the junction between the QRS and ST segment (J point) is often depressed and the depression is relatively uniform over the ST segment, in contrast to the sloping and sagging ST segment contours of left ventricular strain and digitalis effect.

The persistence over a period of days of the ECG picture of subendocardial injury developing in a setting similar to those for other infarctions is characteristic of the subendocardial injury. The lack of changes in the initial QRS forces is a remarkable feature of such infarcts; it may be explained by postulating a separate blood supply to the conduction tissue.

Although there has been much written about the differences between transmural (Q-wave) and subendocardial (non-Q-wave) infarctions, it is now known that Q waves may be seen with nontransmural infarctions and that transmural

Table 2.5

LOCATION OF INFARCT BY ECG LEADS	Infarct Area	ECG Leads	ECG Changes
	Anterior wall	V_1-V_6	QS pattern
			Poor R-wave progression
	Anteroseptal	V_1-V_3 or V_4	QS pattern
			Poor R-wave progression
	Anterolateral	I, aVL, V_1-V_6	Abnormal Q waves
	Inferior wall (diaphragmatic)	II, III, aVF	Abnormal Q waves
	Inferolateral	II, III, aVF, V_5, V_6	Abnormal Q waves
	Posterior wall	V_1, V_2	Tall, wide R wave
	Posteriolateral	V_1, V_2	Tall, wide R wave
		I, aVL, V_5, V_6	Abnormal Q waves
	Lateral wall	I, aVL, V_4, V_6	Abnormal Q waves

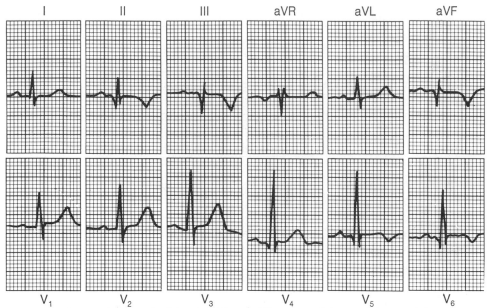

Figure 2.8 Stable inferoposterior infarction. Abnormal Q waves with inverted T waves in leads II, III, and aVF. Relatively large R waves and small S waves in leads V_1 through V_3 with upright T waves. Inverted T waves in V_5 and V_6.

infarctions do not always develop Q waves. Q-wave and non-Q-wave infarcts are the preferable terms, and the patient's clinical course and evolutionary changes in serial records are the main factors used to estimate depth of necrosis.

(9) Heart Rate Variability

Heart rate variability (HRV) has recently been noted by Zbilut and Lawson to be of some prognostic importance in acute myocardial infarction. In normal individuals there is much more variability in R-R intervals on continuous ECG tracings than in individuals with acute myocardial infarction or those who later experience significant dysrhythmia.

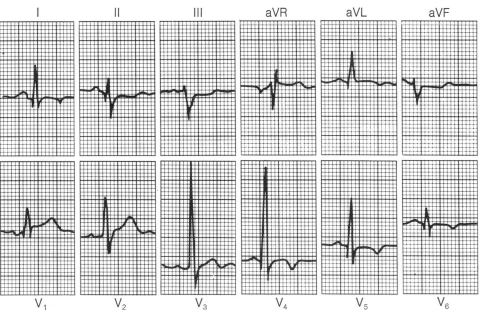

Figure 2.9 Posterior myocardial infarction. Relatively large R waves and small S waves in leads V_1 through V_3, with upright T waves. Inverted T waves in leads V_4 through V_6, I, and aVL.

B. DIFFERENTIAL DIAGNOSIS

Several clinical entities may produce symptoms very similar to those often seen with AMI. In some of these, the differential diagnosis may be extremely difficult.

1. Acute Anxiety

AXIOM

Patients with acute anxiety attacks can also have myocardial infarctions.

Acute anxiety may produce all of the classic symptoms of an AMI. In many instances, the only clue to this diagnosis is a history of multiple similar episodes with no objective findings. However, there may not be any objective laboratory or ECG changes in some patients with significant infarctions. Consequently, patients clinically suspected of having a myocardial infarction should be admitted to the hospital and observed for 48 to 72 hours.

2. Acute Pericarditis

Acute pericarditis is apt to be associated with a sharp or knifelike pain aggravated by deep breaths, coughing, or position changes. The early appearance of fever and a pericardial friction rub also suggest pericarditis rather than an acute infarction. ECG abnormalities include characteristic ST-segment elevation in two or three limb leads and all or most of the anterior precordial leads. Reciprocal depression usually is seen only in leads aVR and V_1. T-wave changes appear late, if at all. QRS changes do not occur except for occasional decreases in amplitude because of a pericardial effusion.

3. Dissecting Aortic Aneurysm

AXIOM

If a younger man has had severe chest pain but has normal coronary arteries, one should look for an aortic dissection.

The pain of aortic dissection often has its peak at onset, in contrast to the gradually increasing intensity of the pain often seen with myocardial infarction. The pain of aortic dissection often had a tearing quality and frequently radiates or, with time, moves down the back. Hypertension is usually, but not always, present, and a reduction in the systolic BP below 120 mm Hg will often dramatically relieve pain. Wide differences in the BP of the arms or loss of pulse in one arm are strongly suggestive of a dissection. An x-ray, if it reveals widening of the aortic shadow, may be almost diagnostic. If a diagnosis of dissection, particularly of the ascending aorta, is suspected, an aortogram should be performed as soon as the patient's condition has stabilized, in anticipation of early surgical correction. Dissections of the descending thoracic aorta can often be managed medically.

4. Pulmonary Embolism

A large pulmonary embolism can closely simulate myocardial infarction, and both conditions may be associated with significant reductions in coronary blood flow. Pulmonary emboli, however, are more apt to result in severe dyspnea and tachypnea and a more marked reduction in arterial Po_2. Likewise, elevated central venous pressure (CVP) and pulmonary artery (PA) pressures with a normal or low pulmonary artery wedge pressure (PAWP) may be seen with early pulmonary emboli, whereas the reverse may be seen in the early stages of myocardial infarction.

ECG changes characteristic of pulmonary emboli are rare but may include S waves in I and V_6 and Q waves in II, III, and aVF. A new right-bundle-branch block is much more frequent. The chest x-ray is often normal, except in patients with associated atelectasis, heart failure, or pulmonary infarction. Definitive diagnosis of moderate-sized or large emboli can be made either with pulmonary arteriograms, or on finding large or multiple areas of impaired perfusion on the lung scan in areas where the ventilation scan and chest x-ray are normal.

5. Biliary Colic

AXIOM

Older individuals with repeated "indigestion" actually often have myocardial ischemia.

Biliary colic often radiates from the right hypochondrium around to the right scapular area and is apt to be associated with nausea or vomiting. Tenderness in the right upper quadrant of the abdomen tends to favor the diagnosis of gallbladder disease, but similar signs can occur with acute right heart failure and hepatomegaly. Interestingly, gallbladder disease by itself may occasionally be associated with ECG changes that disappear following cholecystectomy. Demonstration of filling defects in the gallbladder or nonvisualization of the gall bladder on an oral cholecystogram, HIDA scan, or intravenous (IV) cholangiography are almost diagnostic of cholecystitis, but they do not rule out concomitant disease of the coronary arteries.

6. Pneumothorax

A spontaneous pneumothorax, usually due to rupture of one or more blebs may cause chest pain and dyspnea very similar to those seen with an acute myocardial infarction. However, with a pneumothorax, the onset of pain is usually more abrupt and pleuritic, and there is usually more tachypnea. A small-to-moderate sized pneumothorax may be missed on physical examination but can generally be seen readily on chest x-ray, particularly on films taken during deep expiration.

AXIOM

Upright chest x-rays should be obtained on all patients with chest or upper abdominal pain.

7. Perforated or Penetrating Peptic Ulcer

A perforated or deeply penetrating duodenal or gastric ulcer usually causes pain centering in the epigastric area with significant tenderness and rigidity of the abdomen. With a perforation, subdiaphragmatic air can usually (70%) be seen on a good upright or decubitus abdominal film. A previous history of ulcer disease can also help in diagnosis, but patients with coronary artery disease may also have a history of repeated bloating, belching, and abdominal discomfort.

8. Rupture of the Esophagus

Spontaneous rupture of the esophagus is seldom diagnosed when the patient is first seen. The most frequent initial diagnosis is that of an acute myocardial infarction. In most instances, rupture of the esophagus is preceded by vomiting or retching, which is often vigorous and repeated. The triad of vomiting or retching, chest pain, and free air in the neck or chest on physical examination or chest x-ray is virtually diagnostic of esophageal rupture. X-ray confirmation can often be obtained by a gastrographin swallow. However, 25% to 50% of gastrographin swallows may be falsely negative and should be followed with a barium study.

9. Necrotizing Pancreatitis

Necrotizing pancreatitis may cause substernal chest pain, hypotension, and ECG changes difficult to differentiate from those of acute myocardial infarction. A previous history of pancreatitis, radiation of pain straight through to the back, abdominal distention and tenderness (with or without rigidity), and elevated serum or urine amylase levels are helpful but not absolute differential points.

10. Pericardial Tamponade, Constrictive Pericarditis, and Cardiomyopathies

Cardiac tamponade, constrictive pericardial disease, and restrictive cardiomyopathy may all be difficult to differentiate from an acute myocardial infarction (especially a right ventricular infarction). Echocardiogram may be particularly helpful in ruling out tamponade or pericardial disease. Absence of typical ECG and CPK-MB changes may help rule out the cardiomyopathies.

Table 2.6

DETERMINING CARDIAC RISK OF SURGERY	Criteria	Points
	1. History	
	a. Age >70 years	5
	b. MI in previous 6 months	10
	2. Physical examination	
	a. S$_3$ gallop or jugular venous distension	11
	b. Important vascular aortic stenosis	3
	3. Electrocardiogram	
	a. Rhythm other than sinus or PACs on last preoperative ECG	7
	b. >5 PVCs/min documented at any time before operation	7
	4. General status (any of the following)	3
	PO$_2$ <60 or PCO$_2$ >50 mm Hg	
	K <3.0 or HCO$_3$ <20 mEq/L	
	BUN >50 or Cr >3.0 mg/dl	
	(Blood urea nitrogen)	
	Abnormal SGOT	
	Signs of chronic liver disease	
	Bedridden from noncardiac causes	
	5. Operation	3
	a. Intraperitoneal, intrathoracic, or aortic operation	
	b. Emergency operation	4
	Total possible	53

Source: Goldman, L, et al: Multifactorial index of cardiac risk in noncardial surgical procedures. N Engl J Med 297:845, 1977.

11. During Surgery

a. Risk Factors

The greatest risk of dying after many types of surgery, particularly those on portions of the cardiovascular system, are directly related to the risk of developing an AMI or severe heart failure. In 1977, Goldman and associates developed a grading system for assessing patients for their cardiovascular risk (Table 2.6).

The incidence of postoperative complications rises directly with the number of points in the cardiac risk index. Of the patients with 26 or more points, more than one half died postoperatively and another 22% had life-threatening complications (Table 2.7).

For many years physicians quoted the Mayo Clinic series reported by Tarhan and associates relating the incidence of perioperative myocardial infarction to the time since the previous infarction. As a consequence, elective surgery was generally put off, whenever possible, for at least 6 months after an acute myocardial infarction. A more recent series from Loyola, reported by Rao, Jacobs, and El-Etr, however, indicates that the risk is much less if careful

Table 2.7

	Class	Point Total	Life-Threatening Complications (%)	Cardiac Death (%)
CARDIAC RISK INDEX	I (N = 537)*	0–5	4 (0.7)	2 (0.2)
	II (N = 316)	6–12	16 (5)	5 (2)
	III (N = 130)	13–25	15 (11)	3 (2)
	IV (N = 18)	≥26	4 (22)	10 (56)

*N = number of patients studied.
Source: Goldman, L, et al: Multifactorial index of cardiac risk in noncardial surgical procedures. N Engl J Med 297:845, 1977.

Table 2.8

RISK OF PERIOPERATIVE RECURRENT MYOCARDIAL INFARCTION CORRELATED WITH TIME FROM PRIOR INFARCTION	Time Since Previous MI (mo)	Mayo Series (%)	Loyola Series (%)
	0–3	35	6
	3–6	18	2
	>6	5	2

monitoring is performed (Table 2.8). In the Rao series, the incidence of recurrent perioperative myocardial infarction fell to 5.8%, 2.3%, and 1.9% with surgery performed 0-3, 3-6, and >6 months after the first infarction (Table 2.8). The differences in the Loyola series were: (1) pulmonary artery catheters were used routinely, (2) patients were monitored in the intensive care unit (ICU) for at least 72 to 96 hours postoperatively, and (3) vasoactive drugs were used immediately to treat hemodynamic abnormalities.

AXIOM

As a general rule, any patient having major vascular surgery should have a preoperative coronary arteriogram if he has (1) a past history of a myocardial infarction; (2) angina, even if it is stable; or (3) ECG evidence of a previously unrecognized myocardial infarction.

b. Reducing Risk

In patients with an increased risk, careful monitoring of BP, cardiac output, filling pressures (especially PAWP), and blood gases is extremely important. Whenever possible, the patient's optimal filling pressure, using Starling cardiac function curves, should be determined preoperatively. These optimal filling pressures should be maintained intraoperatively and for at least 24 to 48 hours postoperatively.

12. Coronary Artery Surgery

Patients with increasing angina in spite of optimal medical management should, in the absence of other problems greatly increasing operative risk, have coronary artery bypass surgery. In some instances it may be appropriate first to attempt angioplasty of selected proximal stenoses. In otherwise good-risk patients, coronary artery surgery has a mortality of less than 1% or 2%. In addition, the relief of symptoms and survival rate in patients with unstable angina is much better with early surgery, rather than continued medical management.

V. MEDICAL TREATMENT OF ACUTE MYOCARDIAL INFARCTION

The initial management of patients with proven or strongly suspected AMI involves (a) initial stabilization, (b) careful monitoring for arrhythmias or development of heart failure, and (c) use of thrombolytic agents. The primary function of coronary care units (CCU) is the early detection and management of cardiac arrhythmias and other complications of an AMI. In addition, CCU treatment should include relief of pain, maintenance of adequate oxygenation, and rest.

A. PAIN RELIEF

Large doses of morphine [10 to 15 mg intramuscularly (IM)] or dilaudid (1 to 2 mg IM) are often required to relieve the pain of AMI. Meperidine is frequently inadequate and often causes nausea or vomiting.

PITFALL

Administration of narcotics to hypotensive or hypovolemic patients.

If there is a tendency to hypotension or respiratory depression, these medications should be given in multiple small IV doses after correction of any hypovolemia.

B. OXYGEN AND VENTILATION

AXIOM
Relief of anxiety may relieve pain better than a narcotic.

Any tendency to hypoventilation requires early consideration of ventilatory assistance, particularly if there is impaired cardiovascular function. Oxygen (preferably by mask if tolerated) may occasionally produce dramatic pain relief and may increase tissue Po_2 in marginally ischemic areas of myocardium.

C. THROMBOLYTIC THERAPY FOR CORONARY THROMBOSIS

1. Indications

The major indication for thrombolytic therapy in coronary artery disease lies in its potential for preventing a transmural infarction or reducing its size if given soon after an acute coronary artery occlusion. There is now abundant evidence that: (a) acute coronary thrombosis is present in most cases of acute transmural infarction, (b) clotted coronary arteries can be recanalized in about 65% to 75% of cases within 20 to 30 minutes by the local perfusion or IV infusion of streptokinase, urokinase, or tissue-type plasminogen activator (TPA), and (c) early restoration of coronary blood flow within the first few hours following the onset of chest pain has resulted in prevention of infarcts or reduction in their size. The reduction in infarct size has been demonstrated not only by thallium scanning, but also by improved function of previously ischemic areas of the myocardium. Results with high-dose, brief-duration, IV infusions are not quite as good, but this procedure should be considered if intracoronary thrombolysis is not rapidly available.

Plasminogen activators have a twofold action: (1) circulating plasminogen to plasmin with lysis of clots (fibrin) and (2) fibrinogenolysis, which reduces the risk of rethrombosis. The diffusion of the activator into the thrombus results in activation of the fibrin-bound plasminogen and the formation of plasmin bound to fibrin. Consequently, only the fibrin in the clot is available for the action of plasmin, and the selectivity of this process is further enhanced by the inability of plasma inhibitors to turn off the fibrinolysis rapidly.

Contrary to initial concerns, evidence now seems to indicate that there is no correlation between the extent of fibrinogenolysis and the incidence or severity of bleeding complications. In all thrombolytic therapy studies, the major cause of bleeding has resulted from the lysis of hemostatic plugs at sites of vascular injury.

There are several theoretical advantages to very low fibrinogen levels that fall into two categories: those relating to the process of rethrombosis and those influencing flow rates. Fibrinogen links the exposed glycoproteins on the surface of activated platelets with each other to allow platelets to aggregate. In the presence of extensive fibrinogenolysis, platelets do not aggregate well, blood is hypocoagulable, and clotting, when it occurs, is slow and frequently inadequate because of the presence of large amounts of fibrinogen breakdown products. This limits the likelihood of *rethrombosis*, an occurrence that has emerged as a major problem in thrombolytic therapy, particularly with an agent such as TPA.

In low flow states, blood viscosity can be a major factor in rethrombosis. Fibrinogen, the only eccentric molecule present in plasma in relatively high molar concentration, is the major determinant of plasma viscosity. When blood is moving slowly through vessels, red cell clumping becomes an even more important factor in determining whole blood viscosity than the hematocrit. Again, as with platelet aggregation, the fibrinogen molecule allows red cells to clump together.

Consequently, extensive fibrinogenolysis improves flow rates through the microcirculation, and in areas of slowly flowing blood, this likely to result in a reduction in afterload and cardiac strain.

Criteria for thrombolytic agents are somewhat variable, but the multicenter thrombosis in myocardial infarction (TIMI) study used the following: at least 30 minutes of ischemic pain, ST-segment elevation of at least 0.1 mV in at least two contiguous ECG leads, less than 7 hours from onset of symptoms, and 75 years of age or less. Thrombolytic therapy exclusion criteria included any recent surgery or trauma, pregnancy, bleeding, poorly controlled hypertension, prolonged cardiopulmonary resuscitation (CPR), or severe, advanced illness (Table 2.9).

2. Agents

a. Streptokinase

Streptokinase (SK) is an exogenous plasminogen activator that lyses thrombi by first complexing with plasminogen, and the resulting complex then converts other plasminogen to plasmin. Plasmin disrupts the thrombus by severing the fibrin strands into fragments known as fibrin degradation products. However, the plasmin produced by infusion of therapeutic doses of SK also destroys fibrinogen and coagulation factors V and VIII, causing a systemic lytic state.

The systemic lytic state lasts 24 to 36 hours after the SK infusion has been completed and exposes the patient to the risk of major bleeding complications. The IV dose of SK needed to effect thrombolysis is larger, usually 750,000 to 1,500,000 units, compared with the 150,000 to 400,000 units used during intracoronary treatment.

b. Urokinase

Urokinase (UK), which is either synthesized from human fetal kidney cell cultures or isolated from urine, exists in two forms with molecular weights of 54,000 and 3000 d. The larger molecule is believed to be the native form, while the latter is an active fragment. UK is a very active protease, and it directly cleaves plasminogen to plasmin. Although UK is a native human plasminogen activator, it is different from the activator(s) appearing in plasma following stimulation of the intrinsic or extrinsic mechanisms of fibrinolysis. This suggests that the UK found in urine is made by the kidney rather than just excreted from the plasma. The in-vivo half-life of UK in plasma is approximately 16 minutes. The most frequently used loading dosage to initiate a thrombolytic state is 2000 units per pound of body weight. Since the methods for standardizing UK and SK are different, their units are not the same. The in-vivo activity of 2 to 3 units of UK is comparable to 1 unit of SK.

UK has several theoretical advantages as a thrombolytic agent in clinical practice: (1) it is nonantigenic, and true allergy is not seen; (2) there are no anti-UK antibodies present to interfere with its action, but variability in the rates of inactivation and clearance of UK do occur; and (3) UK, as compared to SK,

Table 2.9

CONTRAINDICATIONS TO THROMBOLYTIC THERAPY

Absolute contraindications
  Active internal bleeding
  Cerebrovascular process, disease, or procedure within 2 months
Relative contraindications
  Conditions requiring fibrin strands and plugs for normal hemostasis or healing (fibrinolysis is usually contraindicated within 10 days or onset of these conditions)
  Major surgery, organ biopsy, or puncture of noncompressible blood vessel
  Postpartum period
  Cardiopulmonary resuscitation during presence of rib fractures
  Thoracentesis, paracentesis, or lumbar puncture
  Recent serious trauma
  Potentially serious bleeding
  Uncontrolled coagulation defects

has a greater affinity for fibrin-bound plasminogen than it does for plasma plasminogen. Theoretically, this increased attraction for fibrin-bound plasminogen should result in better clot lysis at lower levels of hyperplasmia. Nevertheless, it is generally felt that there is no significant difference between UK and SK in clinical efficacy or in the incidence of hemorrhagic complications.

PITFALL
Failure to adequately anticipate bleeding problems with thrombolytic agents.

Bleeding complications are most frequently due to the lysis of hemostatic plugs at the sites of recent invasive procedures, not to the hematologic changes. Nevertheless, one study from Germany noted 60% (30/50) patency after an IV bolus of 2 million units of UK and "no complications related to urokinase therapy."

3. Tissue-type Plasminogen Activator

Tissue-type plasminogen activator (TPA) is a naturally occurring serine protease present in endothelium, circulating blood, and human tissue. Originally TPA was obtained from tissue cultures from a human melanoma cell line. Advances in gene technology have made adequate amounts of recombinant TPA (RTPA) from a mammalian cell line available for use.

Unlike SK, which activates plasminogen systemically, RTPA is fibrin specific and activates only plasminogen that is incorporated into thrombus. This produces a local supply of plasmin at the clot site. In most patients, little circulating plasmin is produced by RTPA. Therefore, clotting factors are not depleted as much and the incidence and severity of the bleeding complications are reduced. Doses of 60 mg or less and an infusion for less than 2 hours have caused only mild fibrinogenolysis with only a 28% decline in fibrinogen levels.

Almost all studies of RTPA have shown that it is an extremely effective IV thrombolytic agent, with reperfusion rates of up to 75% to 80%. Initially there were difficulties with reocclusion during and after TPA administration, possibly due to the short half-life of the drug; however, higher doses and longer administration regimens plus therapeutic levels of IV heparin for 48 hours or longer have improved these results.

AXIOM
Because of the short half-life of TPA, it is essential to simultaneously anticoagulate the patient, using continuous IV heparin, for 48 hours or longer.

4. Newer Agents

Newer products include single chain urokinase plasminogen activator (SCU-PA or prourokinase) and acyl plasminogen-streptokinase activator complex (APSAC). These agents are designed to activate the plasminogen bound to fibrin with decreased hemostatic abnormalities and bleeding. All of these agents are highly clot selective, but they are very expensive, have short lives, and require simultaneous heparin therapy.

Anistreplase (Eminase) or anisoylated plasminogen-streptokinase activator complex (APSAC), was tailored to improve thrombolysis by prolonging the duration of action, stability in the circulation, fibrin-binding, and speed of thrombolysis in vivo. Compared with streptokinase, the duration of action of anistreplase has been quadrupled, the time of administration has been reduced from 60 minutes to 2.5 minutes, the stability in plasma has been significantly lengthened, fibrin binding has been improved, the speed of thrombolysis in vivo probably has been shortened, and yet the extent of fibrinogenolysis has remained unaffected.

Other newer mutants of RTPA and SCU-PA have also been developed. These "third-generation" thrombolytic agents possess increased fibrin affinities and have longer half-lives than the second generation drugs. Early work on molecules that are hybrids of RTPA and SCU-PA is also promising, and perhaps these entities will become the "fourth-generation" thrombolytic agents.

5. Techniques

a. Intracoronary Thrombosis

(1) Procedure

An intracoronary catheter is inserted through a catheter sheath in the femoral artery and the extent of the occlusion is determined by angiography. Although the incidence of coronary artery spasm due to the catheter is 5% or less, intracoronary or IV nitroglycerin is given prophylactically. SK or UK is then infused through the coronary catheter into the involved artery. Subselective infusion is rarely done. Streptokinase is given at a rate of 2000 to 4000 international units (IU) per minute, and UK is given at a rate of 6000 IU per minute. The infusion is usually given for at least 1 hour, and in some studies, intracoronary infusion has been continued for an additional 30 to 60 minutes following clot lysis. Clot lysis generally occurs within the first 30 minutes of infusion. Periodic injection of the involved artery with contrast dye is used to determine reperfusion. Patients with reperfusion are generally maintained on a systemic infusion of heparin at 800 to 1200 IU per hour for 2 to 7 days. The catheter sheath is usually left in place 24 hours to aid hemostasis at the puncture site.

(2) Results

Noninvasive signs of successful reperfusion of an occluded coronary artery include new or increased arrhythmias, rapid fall of elevated ST segments, and abrupt relief of chest pain. A sudden, early (within the first 13 hours) rise in CPK-MB levels (which are measured hourly) has also been used to indicate reperfusion.

Reperfusion occurs in about 65% to 75%. Early reocclusion occurs in about of 15% to 20%, and about 30% of the patients who are initially reperfused by thrombolytic agents require further interventions, such as angioplasty or early coronary artery bypass grafting. Significant bleeding (requiring transfusions) has occurred in an average of 5% of patients, usually at the site of catheter placement.

AXIOM

The time from onset of severe ischemia to achievement of reperfusion is the major determinant of the extent of myocardial salvage.

Significant salvage of myocardium, as indicated by recovery of contractile function or an improved regional myocardial perfusion (as demonstrated by uptake of thallium by functional cells), is usually seen in patients who were reperfused during the first 4 to 6 hours of myocardial infarction. In one study, if thrombolytic therapy was initiated within 2 hours of the onset of symptoms, wall motion improved in 82% (14/17). If treatment was started 2 to 5 hours after symptoms began, improved wall motion was seen in only 46% (24/52). Although 6 hours is generally thought to be the maximum duration of severe ischemia that will allow myocardial salvage with thrombolytic therapy, later reperfusion may also provide some benefit.

The Western Washington Randomized Trial, reported by Kennedy et al, studied the effect of thrombolysis on mortality. Of the 116 control patients, 13 (11%) died within the first 30 days. In contrast, only 5 (4%) of 134 SK-treated patients died (P<0.022). At six months, the mortality rate difference was even more significant (15% vs. 4%) (P<0.0025). At 1 year, the mortality rate was 2.5% (2/80) in completely reperfused patients and 17% (9/53) in patients who were not or only partially reperfused.

In another early study, the mortality rate at 28 days was 6% (16/269) in those with thrombolytic therapy and 12% (31/264) in controls. However, 1-year survival was 91% and 89%, respectively, and the incidence of nonfatal reinfarction was 14% (36/253) with SK and 7% (16/233) in controls.

In another study, acute recanalization occurred in 74% of 43 SK-treated patients and only 6% of 18 nitroglycerin-treated patients. However, comparable patency rates were found in both groups after 10 to 14 days.

D. INTRAVENOUS THROMBOLYSIS INFUSION FOR ACUTE MYOCARDIAL INFARCTION

Although intracoronary thrombolysis has been quite successful, the intracoronary procedure requires rapid access to specially trained personnel and complex equipment. Intravenous thrombolytics are much quicker and simpler to administer and may be as effective as later intracoronary perfusions. Also, brief administration of a high dose ensures high concentrations of SK in the coronary circulation and may reduce the risk of bleeding complications.

1. Indications

2. Procedure

An infusion pump is generally used, and hydrocortisone is given prior to SK to reduce the incidence and severity of reactions. When administered through a peripheral vein, SK is given in doses that have varied from 750,000 IU over 20 minutes to 1,500,000 IU over 60 minutes. Patients who achieve reperfusion should generally have coronary angiography to determine if bypass surgery or percutaneous transluminal coronary angioplasty is needed.

3. Results

Early reports suggested that high-dose brief-duration administration of SK could lyse intracoronary clots in acute myocardial infarction in at least 40% to 60% of patients. These initial studies also showed that early and sustained reperfusion was associated with significant improvement of ventricular function. In a study by Alderman et al, recanalization was achieved in 73% of patients given intracoronary SK therapy and in 62% of those treated intravenously. The time from the onset of symptoms to the start of the infusion was similar in the two groups. Thus, it appeared that IV SK infusion can establish coronary reflow in a substantial proportion of patients treated soon after the onset of myocardial infarction. This was thought to be very important because IV treatment may re-establish coronary flow sooner than intracoronary thrombolysis.

Ornato has recently emphasized that administration of thrombolytics by emergency physicians, without waiting for consultation from cardiologists, can greatly reduce the time delay to administration of these drugs. This theoretically could greatly improve the results of thrombolytic therapy.

AXIOM
The earlier thrombolytic therapy is started, the better the results.

Once an infarct has fully developed, functional improvement of the heart may be minimal even if the related artery is opened. Although an angiography of infarct-related coronary arteries 16 ± 5 days after infarct revealed IV SK opened 85% (22/26) versus 40% (8/20) in control patients, left ventricular ejection fraction at discharge was not improved in either group. At 13 ± 7 months follow-up, the mortality was 19% with SK and 21% in controls.

4. Tissue Plasminogen Activator

The initial reports on the use of IV TPA were glowing. IV infusion rates of 5 $\mu g \cdot kg^{-1} \cdot min^{-1}$ for 90 minutes re-established perfusion in occluded arteries in more than 80% of patients. In a large double-blind study, a total dose of 0.75 mg/kg of TPA given by IV infusion over 90 minutes opened the infarct-related vessel in 61% (38/82) versus 21% (13/62) controls. The circulating fibrinogen levels at the end of the catheterization were 52% ± 29% of control.

In a multicenter trial to assess reperfusion in AMI, Anderson and associates randomized patients to receive Eminase 30 units as an IV injection over 2 to 4 minutes or intracoronary SK 20,000 units as a bolus followed by 2000 units per minute for 60 minutes. Rates of reperfusion with 90 minutes were 55% (76/122) with Eminase and 64% (73/114) with SK ($P<0.16$). Bleeding was reported more frequently in the Eminase group with most episodes at the catheter insertion site; no episodes were intracranial.

Bonnier studied myocardial reperfusion following treatment with either Eminase 30 units by IV injection over 5 minutes, or SK 250,000 units by intracoronary infusion over 90 minutes. Reperfusion occurred in 64% (23/36) of Eminase-treated patients and 67% (25/37) of patients treated with SK. Repeat angiography at 24 hours showed that reocclusion occurred in 1 of 22 (5%) Eminase patients and 3 of 23 (13%) patients in the SK group. Adverse events reported were minor, with all three occurring in the Eminase group: hematoma at puncture site (2) and hypotension (1).

More recently, Bassand studied 180 patients randomly assigned to receive either Eminase 30 units or TPA 100 mg within 4 hours following the onset of acute myocardial infarction symptoms. Both treatment groups received aspirin 250 mg/d plus heparin 1000 units/h during hospitalization. Coronary angiography was performed between day 3 and day 7. Patency rates of the occluded arteries were 72% for Eminase and 76% for TPA.

In a multicenter randomized study, patients with clinical and electrocardiographic evidence of AMI were administered Eminase 30 units over 4 to 5 minutes or IV SK 1.5 million units over 60 minutes. The mean time to thrombolytic therapy after onset of symptoms was 2.7 and 2.8 hours for the Eminase and SK groups, respectively. Heparin was administered after the first angiogram, which was performed 90 minutes after initiation of therapy. Patency rates at that time were 71.8% (28/39) for the Eminase group and 55.8% (24/43) for the SK group. Severe bleeding (hematoma and hemorrhage) occurred in two patients on Eminase and four patients on SK.

5. Platelet and Thrombolytic Therapy

It has been known for some time that platelets play an important role in atherosclerosis and acute coronary ischemia. Trip and associates found that patients with increased spontaneous platelet aggregation (within 10 minutes) had a 5.4 times greater risk of death within 5 years than patients with a negative spontaneous platelet aggregation (no aggregation within 20 minutes).

Collier, in a recent review of the role of antiplatelet drugs with thrombolytic therapy, noted that the international study of infarct survival ISIS-2 data suggests that aspirin makes an important contribution to the beneficial effects on mortality produced by SK at the expense of only a moderate increase in the number of minor hemorrhages. In apparent contrast, a recent preliminary report from the Phase I Thrombosis in Myocardial Infarction group failed to find a significantly increased rate of reperfusion 18 to 48 hours after TPA therapy in a group given aspirin (87.8%) as compared with a group not given aspirin (81.9%). However, the high rate of reperfusion in the control group and relatively small number of patients made it difficult to establish a significant difference. In 1983, Uchida and associates and Blasko and coworkers reported that intracoronary prostacyclin-augmented thrombolysis in patients with myocardial infarction whose coronary arteries did not reperfuse with SK. In some patients, intracoronary prostacyclin led to reperfusion even without the thrombolytic agent. However, there were severe side effects with prostacyclin, including hypotension, arrhythmias, hematemesis, and hematuria. Sharma and associates gave intracoronary prostaglandin E_1 with intracoronary SK to patients with AMI. The patients given prostaglandin E_1 and SK had significant decreases in the time to reperfusion (61 vs. 24 minutes) and in the dose of SK required for reperfusion (600,000 IU vs. 210,000 IU); in addition, the percentage of vessels that were patent at 10 days was greater in the group given combined therapy (88% vs. 50%), and the ejection fractions of those successfully recanalized were significantly greater (61% vs. 48%). However, the dose of prostaglandin E_1 had to be carefully titrated against the blood pressure.

Topol and associates recently noted that combined use of IV TPA and a stable prostacyclin analogue (iloprost) in patients with AMI did not increase the rate of either reperfusion or reocclusion, but did decrease fibrinogenolysis. They speculated that the prostacyclin analogue speeds the metabolism of recombinant TPA and reduces its efficacy. These studies illustrate the difficulty of administering these agents systemically because of their lack of specificity for platelets.

6. Stabilization Following Either Intracoronary or Intravenous Coronary Thrombolysis

The incidence of reocclusion, as demonstrated by repeat angiogram 2 to 4 weeks after reperfusion by intracoronary SK, ranged from 9% to 29% in four studies, and the average incidence of reocclusion was 17 percent.

It is felt that all patients with early coronary reperfusion should be maintained on a continuous IV infusion of heparin (800 to 1200 units per hour) beginning when the accelerated Partial Thromboplastin Time (aPTT) has fallen to 50 seconds or less after the thrombolytic therapy. The specifics for optimal antithrombotic prevention of rethrombosis by anticoagulants or platelet-controlling drugs remain unclear.

E. COMPLICATIONS

1. Allergic Reactions

PITFALL
Failure to anticipate severe allergic reactions in patients receiving SK.

About 5% of patients have pre-existing high titers of SK antibody. In such patients, ordinary doses of SK can cause severe reactions and make therapy ineffective. Such patients should be treated with UK or TPA. Even without pre-existing high titers of streptokinase, antibody allergic reactions are frequent.

SK antibody titers rise rapidly after treatment with SK and are significant by day 7. They persist for 3 to 6 months, then decline. If SK is given again, such antibodies may interfere with its efficacy and may cause severe allergic side effects.

Fever occurs in up to 30% of SK treatments. Pretreatment with steroids can reduce this incidence to less than 5%. True allergic side effects such as angioneurotic edema, hypotension, and bronchospasm occur in 1% to 2% of cases. Milder allergic phenomena, including rash, urticaria, and flushing, occur in up to 10% of patients. These milder reactions can be almost completely abolished by premedication with 100 mg hydrocortisone, which is repeated at 6- to 12-hour intervals. Most investigators continue SK therapy despite the presence or persistence of minor reactions. In the unusual instance of an anaphylactoid reaction, therapy should be stopped. With UK, fever may occur in 1% to 2% of patients, but the mechanism is obscure. Allergy to UK or TPA is extremely unusual.

Mild-to-moderate rash, itching, and urticaria can be effectively managed with antihistamines and/or steroids and do not require that SK therapy be discontinued. Pyrexia is managed by a combination of nonaspirin antipyretics and steroids. However, anaphylactoid reactions require not only immediate cessation of the SK infusion, but also vigorous and immediate therapy with steroids and epinephrine.

2. Bleeding

a. Incidence

Bleeding is the most serious frequent complication associated with thrombolytic therapy. The incidence is variable and is largely dependent upon the investigator's definition of "bleeding." Some have defined bleeding as all bleeding episodes, including minor cutdown or venipuncture oozing; others count only transfusion-dependent episodes. Still others report only life-threatening episodes.

Bleeding requiring either transfusion or surgical repair of the site of arterial puncture occurred in 31 (5%) of 640 patients in nine early studies of intracoronary SK therapy. However, no patient died from bleeding or had major intracranial hemorrhage.

b. Prevention of Bleeding Problems

The best approach to the hemorrhage due to thrombolytic therapy is to prevent its occurrence. This is best achieved by proper patient selection and the avoidance of unnecessary invasive procedures.

Absolute contraindications to thrombolytic therapy include all active bleeding lesions. Disorders such as recent stroke, intracranial tumor, or uncontrolled severe hypertension, which have a potential for intracranial hemorrhage are also contraindications. Relative contraindications include major surgery less than 10 days previously, postpartum state, recent cardiopulmonary resuscitation, recent biopsy or needle puncture of poorly compressible areas, and concomitant hypocoagulable states.

Some studies of systemic IV thrombolytic therapy for AMI have excluded patients over 70 years of age, but such decisions should be based on physiological age, not chronological age.

Distal extremities should be used when either venous or arterial access is necessary since they provide easily compressible sites. The patient should be at bed rest to reduce the chances of dislodging the infusion catheter.

C. Treatment

Transfusion-dependent bleeding or bleeding into inaccessible sites (gastrointestinal, central nervous system, and retroperitoneum) requires immediate cessation of the thrombolytic agent. Although SK remains in the circulation for only a few hours, it often takes more than 18 to 24 hours for the body to remove the breakdown products of fibrinogen and fibrin and to synthesize the coagulation factors depleted by the therapy. Earlier return of hemostatic function can be obtained by administering fresh frozen plasma and cryoprecipitate. These are both excellent sources of fibrinogen and factors V and VIII. In catastrophic situations such as central nervous system hemorrhage, the effects of the thrombolytic agents can be immediately stopped with fibrinolytic inhibitors, such as epsilon-aminocaproic acid (Amicar). Anecdotal reports indicate that the use of such measures can restore hemostatic function to normal within 2 hours.

3. Arrhythmias

Lidocaine (Xylocaine), by bolus and then IV infusion of 2 mg/min, is generally initiated prior to thrombolysis in acute myocardial infarction and is continued for several hours following the therapy. Many patients have a transient period of ventricular irritability at the time of coronary recanalization; however, with lidocaine therapy, ventricular arrhythmias are not usually a serious problem and have not limited the therapy.

F. PERCUTANEOUS TRANSLUMINAL CORONARY ANGIOPLASTY OF THE CORONARY ARTERIES

Percutaneous transluminal coronary angioplasty (PTCA) can be used in many vascular beds and is considered by some physicians to be the method of choice in high-risk patients with obstructive vascular disease. This technique attempts to increase lumen size by application of a lateral internal force against the stenosed vessel wall by means of a distensible balloon. The resultant controlled vascular injury produces a wide array of histological changes that include compression and redistribution of atherosclerotic plaques as well as mural stretching and disruption of intima and media. Following the localized trauma, phagocytosis leads to removal of some of the exposed debris that had been previously walled off by a fibrous covering and endothelium.

Initially there were concerns that portions of the newly exposed plaque might embolize. However, intraoperative studies using millipore filters have shown that such emboli are not usually a problem, except with repeat dilatations. Healing and endothelialization of the dilated vascular segment have been demonstrated in many hemodynamic, angiographic, histological, and follow-up clinical studies.

The physiological benefits of PTCA have been documented by measurements of myocardial oxygen consumption and lactate extraction, improved ventricular performance, and increased work capacity. These changes have been repeatedly demonstrated by myocardial scintigraphy, serial exercise testing, and employment and recreation patterns after successful dilatation.

1. Patient Selection

PITFALL

Failure adequately to anticipate the possible need for an emergency coronary artery bypass in a patient proposed for PTCA.

While the criteria for patient selection for PTCA have been evolving over the past several years, some criteria remain unchanged. Foremost among these is the patient's overall suitability for surgery, if it becomes necessary to handle a complication. This is determined by the patient's clinical status, ventricular function, vascular anatomy, and willingness to have surgery if it is necessary.

Dilsizian, Rocco, and Freedman have recently pointed out the enhanced detection of ischemic but viable myocardium by the reinjection of thallium after stress-redistribution imaging. Using thallium exercise tomographic imaging and radionuclide angiography, they analyzed three sets of images (stress, redistribution 3 to 4 hours later, and reinjection). Of the 33% of patients who appeared to have irreversible ischemic myocardium on redistribution imaging, almost half demonstrated viable but jeopardized myocardium by an improved or normal thallium uptake after the second injection. These patients responded quite favorably to angioplasty, while those with persistent defects on thallium reinjection did not.

a. Clinical Considerations

In relation to symptoms, the ideal candidate has well-defined ischemic symptoms, preferably of short duration, despite good medical therapy. Long-standing angina is often associated with stenoses that are more difficult to dilate. While advanced age does not preclude dilatation, it should be recognized that elderly patients have somewhat higher morbidity and mortality rates if emergency coronary artery bypass surgery becomes necessary.

2. Types of Vessel Disease

a. Single-Vessel Disease

Isolated discrete proximal single-vessel disease is the best angiographic indication for PTCA. However, there are a number of other important anatomic considerations. The first of these concerns the demonstration of a fixed narrowing to a critical degree. If the stenosis does not cause a 70% reduction in vascular lumen, no increase in blood is apt to be demonstrated with PTCA. If the narrowing is due to spasm rather than fixed disease, the symptoms frequently persist after the dilatation and narrowing tends to recur. Second, most lesions in the distal one third of the coronary arteries are not accessible for dilatation. Third, despite their location, lesions at the origins (ostia) of the coronary arteries are typically resistant to dilatation and are associated with a high recurrence rate. In addition, stenoses of the left main coronary artery are unacceptable for dilatation unless the dilating catheter has a lumen, the vessel has been grafted distally, or the patient is on partial cardiopulmonary bypass so that some myocardial blood flow can be maintained during the balloon inflation. This is particularly important if the right coronary artery is also critically diseased. Furthermore, dissection of the left main coronary artery caused by the PTCA can be rapidly life threatening.

Extremely tight stenoses are associated with an increased risk of dissection from PTCA, particularly if they are long (>10 mm) or eccentric. Calcifications in the stenotic area also suggest a stenosis that is more resistant to dilatation and is more likely to be associated with significant intimal disruption; however, such calcifications do not preclude the procedure. The ideal lesion has a smooth-walled hourglass configuration without angiographic evidence of pre-existing intimal disruption or thrombus formation.

b. Double-Vessel Disease

Patients with significant two-vessel disease require a more cautious approach, particularly if there are high-risk lesions at both sites. Timing of the procedures is also of great importance, and the lesion whose location and severity is most ominous is dilated first. Any uncertainty as to the outcome of the first procedure should result in postponement of the dilatation of the second stenosis. This reduces the hazard of simultaneously jeopardizing two major vascular beds, unless the heart is being protected with partial cardiopulmonary bypass.

c. Occluded Vessels

Experience in recanalizing occluded vessels has grown rapidly, with success rates reported between 53% and 76% in selected cases. The involved vessel should be associated with viable but ischemic myocardium, which appears to be responsible for persistent symptoms. An additional consideration is the duration of the problem because occlusion for over 6 months is associated with significantly lower success rates. Other important angiographic parameters include visualization of the distal vessel to define the length of the occluded segment and, ideally, the presence of a "funnel-shaped" entrance so as to channel the guidewire along the original lumen. Extremely long (>15 mm) or eccentric occlusions are usually unacceptable for dilatation due to the high risk of dissection.

3. High-Risk Patients

The risk of PTCA to multiple vessels and left main lesions can be reduced by using simultaneous partial cardiopulmonary bypass assistance.

a. After Coronary Artery Bypass Grafting

Despite the efficacy of coronary artery bypass grafting, disease progression leads to recurrent or worsening symptoms in up to 5% of postoperative patients annually. In selected patents, PTCA represents an alternative to an often technically difficult second surgical procedure, particularly for (1) vessels not previously bypassed, (2) vessels jeopardized by graft closure, (3) lesions distal to implanted grafts, (4) lesions proximal to patent grafts but compromising flow to other branches, and (5) distal anastomoses (at the vein to coronary artery junction). Proximal anastomoses (saphenous vein to aorta junction) represent less favorable sites for PTCA due to technical difficulties with the catheter guide and higher recurrence rates. Higher recurrence rates are also seen with dilatation of stenoses developing in the portion of the vein between the two anastomoses. Although early studies demonstrated good initial success, long-term stenosis recurrence rates approach 50%.

4. Restenosis

One of the main problems with PTCA is the high incidence of restenosis. One technique to try to prevent this has been the use of self-expanding stents. However, Serruys and associates recently found that self-expanding coronary artery stents to prevent acute occlusion and late restenosis have not been very helpful. Of 117 stents inserted in 105 patients, 27 (23%) completely occluded (21 within 14 days), and significant restenosis occurred in 46% of the patent stents in a follow-up period of 5.7 ± 4.4 months. The mortality rate at 1 year was 7.6%.

Block in a recent editorial noted that, despite all of the clever mechanical devices at our disposal, the rate of restenosis after intracoronary interventions still remains between 25% and 45%.

5. Post-thrombolytic Therapy

Angiography after thrombolytic therapy frequently reveals patients who are in need of urgent definitive revascularization. Some groups, by combining PTCA with thrombolysis, have demonstrated a reduced risk of coronary reocclusion. The incidence of chest pain and ST-segment elevation during PTCA in a high proportion of patients who have had thrombolytic therapy suggests the presence of persistently viable, salvaged myocardium after successful thrombolysis. However, when possible, routine dilatation is usually postponed for at least 3 days after thrombolytic therapy.

Many studies have shown no significant advantage of early PTCA after thrombolytic therapy. For example, Topol and associates showed that the incidence of reocclusion after IV TPA and immediate angioplasty (11%) was essentially the same as for IV TPA and angioplasty delayed for 7 to 10 days (13%). However, in another study by Guerci, patients treated with IV TPA for acute myocardial infarction, who then had angioplasty on the third hospital day, had an increased ejection fraction with exercise (8.1 ± 1.4% vs. 1.2 ± 2.2%) and reduced incidence of postinfarction angina (19% vs. 5%). However, the ejection fraction at rest was not improved by the angioplasty.

6. Nonatherosclerotic Disease

Angioplasty has been successfully performed on a repeated basis in many vascular beds for segmental disease secondary to a variety of causes, including fibromuscular dysplasia and arteritis. With the presently available technology, PTCA should be considered as a therapeutic option in any individual with focal obstructive coronary disease regardless of its etiology.

7. Procedure

Selection of the sign of the dilating balloon is based on several considerations, the most important of which are the caliber of the vessel adjacent to the stenotic segment and the severity of the stenosis. The inflated diameter of the balloon should approximate the normal vessel diameter. However, if the vessel size falls between presently available catheters, slight undersizing is desirable. "Low-profile" dilatation catheters are particularly indicated for (a) severe stenoses, (b) a long history of angina, (c) poor guidewire catheter seating, (d) presence of calcium in the stenosis, (e) tortuous vessel proximal to the stenotic segment, (f) distal lesions, and (g) long stenosis (>10 mm).

Care is taken to note the deformity imposed by the lesion on the balloon to confirm correct positioning. Inflation pressure is increased in a stepwise fashion until an altered deformity of the balloon indicates a response. After complete deflation of the balloon has been ensured, the residual gradient is determined and a small injection of contrast is made to ensure good distal flow. Balloon inflations are repeated at appropriate intervals (to allow interim recovery) until no further stenosis is apparent·or until the pressure gradient across the stenotic area falls below 16 mm Hg.

8. Postangioplasty Care

PITFALL
Failure to monitor patients adequately for early reocclusion after PTCA.

Routine postangioplasty care is designed to monitor the patient closely for signs or symptoms of myocardial ischemia or arrhythmias. A 12-lead ECG is obtained, the patient is placed on telemetry for 18 to 24 hours, and blood is drawn for serial CPK-MB levels. If the procedure appears to be an angiographic success and the patient received the routine 10,000 units of heparin, the femoral sheaths are pulled approximately 2 hours after the procedure. If there is angiographic evidence of significant intimal disruption, anticoagulation in the form of a continuous heparin drip is maintained until the following morning. Routine medications for the immediate post-PTCA period include 80 or 325 mg of acetylsalicylic acid once or twice daily, sublingual and transdermal nitrates, and a calcium channel blocker.

9. Results

The initial results with PTCA have been extremely optimistic in selected cases when performed by experienced operators. Of Gruentzig's initial 50 cases, 32 (69%) were successfully dilated. Of these 32, five had an early restenosis corrected successfully by repeat PTCA in two cases and coronary artery surgery in three cases. Of 11 patients who had repeat angiograms at 5 years, eight (73%) had an excellent lasting effect and the renarrowing was mild in the other three.

If thrombolysis is combined with PTCA, good results are usually obtained. In one study, regional wall motion improved in 83% (19/23) of those who had both thrombolytic therapy and angioplasty, in 41% (7/17) of those with successful thrombolytic therapy but no angioplasty, and in 30% (6/20) of those who had no reperfusion after thrombolysis and no angioplasty. In a review of the PTCA registry of the National Heart, Lung, and Blood Institute, angiographic success rates were 88%, and the overall success rate (as indicated by a 20% reduction in all lesions attempted without death, myocardial infarction, or coronary bypass surgery) was 70%. The in-hospital mortality rate was 1.0%, and the nonfatal myocardial infarction rate was 4.3%.

PITFALL
Failure to adequately monitor patients for relatively asymptomatic late coronary occlusions after PTCA.

The restenosis rate as reflected by a loss of 50% of the original gain in luminal diameter occurs in about 30%. This restenosis appears to have five main factors: (a) the morphological features of the lesion (proximal versus distal, central versus eccentric, calcified versus noncalcified, etc.), (b) inadequate dilatation, (c) endothelial desquamation, (d) platelet and coagulation activation, and (e) smooth-muscle cell proliferation.

10. Complications

Overall complication rates in combined series have averaged about 21%, and the mortality rate is about 0.9%. The most frequent major complication of PTCA is an acute reduction in coronary blood flow. This problem is reported in approximately 5% of patients and is usually manifested as prolonged angina or coronary occlusion leading to infarction. The most common cause is coronary artery dissection due to the guidewire or the balloon inflation. Angiographic characteristics that are more likely to result in these complications include (a) high-grade obstructions (>90%), (b) eccentric stenoses, (c) excessively long stenoses (>15 mm), (d) a tortuous or bifurcating diseased segment, and (e) other "complicated" angiographic morphology. Any combination of these factors further increases the risk of dissection.

Mechanisms other than dissection of the stenotic segment may also cause myocardial ischemia. Coronary artery spasm has been reported in approximately 4% of cases. Other less common causes for diminished flow following PTCA include coronary embolization (plaque or air) and intimal trauma caused by the guide wire. Side-branch occlusion can occasionally cause ischemia, although the risk of such an event is small even when the branch is involved in the disease process. Ischemia arising in the first few hours after the effects of heparin have worn off is often due to thrombosis; however, spasm may play a role.

Appropriate management of the patient with an abrupt reduction in coronary flow following PTCA requires a careful but rapid assessment. Initial therapy includes oxygen administration, sublingual nifedipine, and, if needed, additional heparin. If the patient has already returned to the nursing unit, he or she should be taken back to the catherization laboratory immediately and a repeat angiogram obtained. In the event of coronary obstruction, intracoronary nitroglycerine can be given. If no response is obtained, repeat angioplasty should be attempted. If there is still persistent inadequate coronary perfusion with symptoms or other evidence of ischemia, prompt surgical revascularization should be considered.

The need for early aortocoronary bypass following unsuccessful PTCA is usually less than 5% to 10%. About two thirds have urgent surgery (within 24 hours of the PTCA) and a third have elective surgery. In one study, the rate of complications was 54% in those having urgent aortocoronary bypass and 19% in those having elective coronary surgery with mortality rates of 4.4% and 3.1%, respectively. Thus, although PTCA is a reasonable approach for many patients with ischemic heart disease, urgent aortocoronary bypass in post-PTCA patients carries an increased morbidity and mortality.

If urgent surgery is required, continuous infusion of IV nitroglycerin should be used empirically. If the hemodynamic status permits, IV propranolol may also help by reducing myocardial oxygen demand. If the patient develops cariogenic shock or a very low cardiac output, intra-aortic balloon pumping should be initiated early.

Other potential complications of percutaneous coronary angioplasty include (a) ventricular fibrillation (1%) which is most commonly encountered in right-coronary artery dilatation; (b) noncoronary vascular complications including hematoma formation, retroperitoneal blood loss, or development of a pseudoaneurysm; (c) central nervous system events; and (d) allergic reactions.

11. Recurrent Stenosis after Successful Dilatation

The specific cause of recurrent stenosis after PTCA is unknown but is probably due to fibrocellular proliferation. Restenosis usually manifests itself as recurrent angina, most often appearing 2 to 4 months after the procedure. Because of medical therapy and patient education, myocardial infarction is an uncommon presentation of recurrent disease. Routine follow-up in the asymptomatic patient should include exercise testing at approximately 3 months and a repeat angiogram at 6 months, or earlier if indicated.

Loss of greater than 50% of the initial gain in luminal diameter at 6 months is seen in 26% to 35% of the vessels dilated in most series. However, repeat PTCA can often be performed in the restenosed segment with good success and minimal complications. There is some concern, however, that emboli from repeated PTCAs can eventually impair myocardial function.

VI. PHARMACOLOGIC THERAPY

AXIOM
Beta-blockers should be begun as soon as possible after an acute myocardial infarction in patients who are not hypotensive, in heart failure, or bradycardic.

A. BETA-BLOCKERS

When given IV less than 12 hours from the onset of symptoms with an acute myocardial infarction, beta-blockers have been shown to reduce infarct size, complex ventricular arrhythmias, and early and late mortality rates. The effects of beta-blocker therapy on in-hospital mortality, reinfarction, and cardiac arrest have been examined in a total of 26 randomized trials involving more than 27,000 patients. Overall, patients treated with beta-blockers have had a 13% reduction in mortality, and the survival advantage is most evident during the first two postinfarct days. Patients treated with beta-blockers also had a 19% reduction in nonfatal reinfarctions and a 16% reduction in cardiac arrests.

The decreased mortality rate during the initial 48-hour postinfarction may be related to a reduction in the incidence of myocardial rupture. If this is true, beta-blockers may have an additional role in patients who receive thrombolytic therapy relatively late (> 12 hours) after symptom onset.

In the recently completed second Thrombolysis in Myocardial Infarction (TIMI-2) trial, a subgroup of 1,390 patients were randomly assigned to either immediate IV metoprolol followed by oral metoprolol or to oral metoprolol begun on postinfarct day 6. Although in-hospital and 42-day mortality rates were similar in both treatment groups, patients randomized to immediate beta-blockage had significantly fewer recurrent ischemic events and nonfatal reinfarctions. The patients treated within 2 hours of symptom onset derived the greatest overall benefits, experiencing significant reductions in recurrent infarctions and mortality rate at 42 days.

A trend toward less frequent intracranial hemorrhages has also been observed in patients receiving immediate beta-blocker therapy. In fact, no intracranial hemorrhagic events were observed among 631 patients treated with early IV metoprolol and 100 mg of TPA. Thus, the available data support the adjuvant use of beta-blockers in the treatment of patients with myocardial infarction receiving thrombolytic therapy.

1. Magnesium

AXIOM

Patients should probably be given some IV magnesium following an acute myocardial infarction, particularly if they are on diuretics, even if serum values are normal.

In patients with AMI, several studies have reported a transient decrease in serum Mg^{++} levels, apparently resulting from adrenergic stimulation and increased aldosterone secretion. Dyckner observed a 46% incidence of hypomagnesemia among 342 patients with AMI. In addition, patients with hypomagnesemia had an increased risk of ventricular arrhythmias. In three placebo-controlled double-blinded studies in patients with known or suspected AMI, Mg^{++} administration was associated with a 50% reduction in ventricular arrhythmias.

In one study, administration of magnesium within the initial 24 hours of a suspected AMI was associated with a significant reduction in 1 year mortality. Mechanisms underlying magnesium's benefits in AMI are probably related to its antiarrhythmic, antispasmodic, and antithrombotic properties. In addition, repeated IV isotonic $MgCl_2$ may decrease platelet-mediated vasoconstriction, vascular spasm, local thrombus formation, and distal arterial embolization.

Routine determination of Mg^{++} levels should be performed in patients with a high likelihood of hypomagnesemia, particularly those who are on diuretics for congestive heart failure or hypertension; however, serum levels of magnesium can be normal even in patients with significant total body deficits.

AXIOM

Even in the presence of normal serum Mg^{++} levels, patients can still have low intracellular levels.

In patients with torsades de pointes, ventricular tachycardia, or complicated myocardial infarction, Mg^{++} administration may be beneficial regardless of the serum Mg^{++} levels.

2. Nitrate Preparations

AXIOM

Patients with an evolving AMI should probably be given an IV drip of nitroglycerine; however, heparin dosage may have to be increased.

Intravenous nitroglycerine, in patients with an evolving AMI, can limit infarct size and decrease morbidity and mortality. These benefits are most likely due to an improved balance between myocardial oxygen supply and demand. Nitroglycerin also has platelet-inhibiting properties and, in standard doses, decreases adenosine diphosphate (ADP) and thrombin-mediated platelet aggregation, thereby improving the results with coronary thrombolysis.

In one study, IV nitroglycerin reduced anterior and inferior infarct size, especially in patients who were treated within 4 hours of onset of symptoms and were not hypotensive. It also reduced the frequency of infarct-related complications, including left ventricular thrombus formation, cardiogenic shock, and cardiac death. Although nitrate tolerance develops progressively during prolonged IV infusion, the tolerance is usually only partial and does not compromise the beneficial effects of therapy.

Current evidence suggests that nitroglycerin may stimulate guanylate cyclase, resulting in an increase in cyclic guanosine monophosphate. Patients receiving IV nitroglycerin function often require a larger heparin dose to achieve and maintain therapeutic levels of systemic anticoagulation.

3. Calcium-channel Blockers

AXIOM

One should consider giving diltiazem, beta-blockers, and aspirin to patients who have a non-Q-wave myocardial infarction and are not receiving thrombolytic therapy.

Although calcium antagonists should theoretically be beneficial in patients with an AMI, none of 22 clinical trials that have examined the effects of calcium antagonists (nifedipine, verapamil, or diltiazem) on clinical outcome in patients with either a threatened or confirmed myocardial infarction have shown an overall beneficial effect on infarct size, left ventricular function, progression to infarction, recurrent angina, rate of reinfarction, or mortality. The only benefit found was in the Diltiazem Reinfarction Study, which showed that at 14 days, patients sustaining a non-Q-wave infarction and receiving diltiazem had a significantly lower incidence of recurrent infarction, postinfarction angina, and angina with ST-T wave changes than patients given a placebo.

The ability of diltiazem to reduce systemic blood pressure, dilate coronary arteries, improve myocardial blood flow, reduce ventricular wall stress, and reduce the incidence of reinfarction with non-Q-wave infarctions suggests that it may possess antithrombotic properties as well.

Calcium antagonists, especially diltiazem, have been shown to decrease platelet nucleotide release, thromboxane A_2 generation, and aggregation in response to ADP, collagen, and epinephrine. Diltiazem has also been shown to inhibit platelet activating factor and increase vascular endothelial prostacyclin release. These effects appear to be enhanced in the presence of beta-blockers and low-dose aspirin. Probably because of these changes, patients receiving calcium antagonists at the time of their myocardial infarction had a fourfold increased risk of an intracranial hemorrhage after thrombolytic agents.

4. Angiotensin Converting Enzyme Inhibitor

AXIOM

Angiotensin converting enzyme (ACE) inhibitors may be of value in patients with an AMI, especially if they are hypertensive.

Locally generated vascular angiotensin is intimately involved in the regulation of coronary blood flow, and it also participates in the vascular response to injury by stimulating cellular proliferation, inflammation, and edema formation. ACE inhibitors antagonize the reninangiotensin system locally by preventing the synthesis of angiotensin II and by facilitating the generation of vasoactive mediators such as bradykinin, prostacyclin, and endothelium-derived relaxing factor. Patients receiving ACE inhibitors after a myocardial infarction are less likely to develop either infarct expansion or experience high-grade ventricular arrhythmias.

Experimentally, ACE inhibitors may improve ventricular contractile dysfunction and reduce malignant ventricular arrhythmias after reperfusion of ischemic myocardium. The mechanisms are probably multifactorial and include: (1) increased myocardial blood flow, (2) preservation of intracellular high-energy phosphates, and (3) attenuation of the renin-angiotensin system. ACE inhibitors may also act indirectly either as antioxidants or by altering the intracellular concentration of calcium.

B. RECOMMENDED ROUTINE CCU ORDERS FOLLOWING A SUSPECTED MYOCARDIAL INFARCTION

Strict bed rest should be required for the first 24 hours after a suspected myocardial infarction, and the patient is assisted in all matters of personal hygiene. The progression of activity thereafter will vary with the patient's response.

1. Bed Rest

2. Diet

Depending on the patient's condition, nothing by mouth (n.p.o.) or a full liquid diet may initially be ordered. Since an IV should be maintained and nausea may be present, oral intake is not necessary during the first 24 hours. Intake will progress to a diet that provides only a moderate sodium intake and about 1200 calories each day. Small, bite-sized, easily chewable food should be prepared. Fried foods, raw vegetables, and caffeinated, iced, and/or fatty beverages should be omitted.

3. Intake and Output

Intake and output and daily weights should be monitored. Constipation should be prevented.

4. Vital Signs

Vital signs should be monitored at least hourly for the first 4 to 6 hours and every 4 hours thereafter, as needed. A stable patient should not be awakened for these measurements.

5. Intravenous Line

A stable and adequate IV line with lumen equivalent to that of a 19-gauge needle should be inserted upon admission. Its patency should be maintained with a slow infusion of 5% glucose (dextrose)-in-water (D_5W).

6. ECG Monitoring

Continuous cardioscopic monitoring should be employed. In addition, a 12-lead diagnostic ECG should be taken upon admission and every morning thereafter. A 10-second ECG monitoring strip should be obtained (a) at the beginning of each nursing shift, (b) whenever monitor leads are applied or changed, and (c) whenever the rhythm or P, QRS, or T morphology changes. These strips should be marked and kept in the chart.

7. Antiembolic Precautions

A bed footboard and/or antiembolic hose should be used unless contraindicated.

8. Medications

A wide array of medications may be required by patients with angina or AMI. These will include analgesics, vasodilators, beta-blockers, and calcium channel blockers as needed to reduce myocardial oxygen demand.

Even if no arrhythmias are present, a syringe with 100 mg lidocaine should be kept at the patient's bedside during the first 48 hours. Other emergency drugs should also be readily available.

9. Rest

Mental, emotional, and physical rest are essential following an acute myocardial infarction. It is extremely important for physicians, nurses, and other personnel to provide the patient with such an environment. The cardiac care unit (CCU) personnel should ensure at least 2 hours of uninterrupted quiet in the morning and in the midafternoon to facilitate naps.

Straining while urinating or defecating should be discouraged or prevented. Valsalva maneuvers reduce venous return to the heart and increase afterload while at the same time greatly reducing cardiac output and coronary artery flow. A bedside commode is generally easier to use then a bedpan and should be provided unless the patient is hemodynamically unstable. Constipation must be prevented by providing adequate fiber, liquids, stool softeners, and/or laxatives.

10. Laboratory Studies

Routine laboratory studies upon admission should include complete blood count (CBC), urinalysis, serum electrolytes, multiphasic profile, SGOT, and serum LDH and CPK isoenzymes. CPK-MB activities should be obtained daily for 3 successive days in all cases of suspected AMI.

VII. COMPLI- CATIONS

Patients suffering an AMI can be divided into three main groups according to outcome: (a) those dying rapidly before they can obtain medical care, (b) those having an uncomplicated recovery, and (c) those having a course complicated by (1) arrhythmias, (2) pump failure, (3) major conduction defects, (4) persistent pain, (5) thromboembolism, (6) cardiac rupture, or (7) ventricular aneurysm.

A. ARRHYTHMIAS

About 85% of patients with AMI develop a cardiac arrhythmias, usually premature ventricular contractions (PVCs), at least transiently. Various factors, such as hypoxia, hypotension, and increased stress have been implicated in the etiology of these arrhythmias and should be corrected as soon as possible.

Ventricular tachycardia and ventricular fibrillation, the most dangerous of these arrhythmias, are often preceded by increasingly frequent PVCs. Similarly, multiple and/or multifocal premature atrial contractions often precede more dangerous atrial arrhythmias, such as atrial tachycardia, atrial flutter, or atrial fibrillation. Consequently, the philosophy of coronary care should be one of early recognition and prevention of serious arrhythmias. As an extension of this philosophy, it has been said that successful resuscitation of a patient with a cardiac arrest in a CCU should really be considered a "therapeutic failure." That is because, the patient, in order to be resuscitated, probably had ventricular fibrillation (rather than asystole) and probably had premonitory PVCs that were not recognized and treated adequately.

1. Ventricular Premature Beats

PITFALL

Failure to recognize that ventricular premature beats (VPBs) may be the first and only warning of impending ventricular fibrillation.

VPBs are the most frequent of the various arrhythmias seen after an acute myocardial infarction and are present in up to 88% of such patients. The presence of ischemia, hypoxia, and increased cathecholamines all increase myocardial excitability and the tendency to ventricular arrhythmias. If the excitability of the myocardium continues to increase, ventricular tachycardia will often develop, leading rapidly to ventricular fibrillation.

Indications for administering lidocaine to patients with an acute myocardial infarction and VPBs include:
- Frequent VPBs (more than 4 to 6 per minute)
- Multifocal VPB (VPBs having different configurations)
- Runs of VPBs (three or more VPBs in a row)
- VPBs encroaching on previous T waves
- Tachycardia

If any of these occur, a bolus of 100 mg of IV lidocaine should be given. VPBs that are persistent or recurring require a second or third bolus, along with an IV drip of 4 mg/min. If lidocaine does not adequately control the PVCs, procainamide IV in doses of 50 to 100 mg/min to a total of 500 mg (occasionally up to 1000 mg in severe cases) may be of benefit. If the PVCs increase rapidly, or if ventricular tachycardia develops, doses as high as 2 to 4 g may be given in 30 to 60 minutes. However, this very large dose may cause severe depression of myocardial function. Resistant cases may occasionally require quinidine and/or propranolol to obtain control.

Although treatment of potentially dangerous ventricular arrhythmias after myocardial infarction is important, the Cardiac Arrhythmia Suppression Trial (CAST) indicated that asymptomatic and minimally symptomatic arrhythmias in such patients may not require therapy, and certainly the use of encainide and flecainide, two classes of intracoronary antiarrhythmic agents, is associated with a substantial increase in the sudden death rate and total mortality.

2. Ventricular Tachycardia

The most frequent cause of sudden death following an acute myocardial infarction is ventricular fibrillation presumably originating at the junction of the infarct with the normal myocardium. Ventricular fibrillation apparently results from myocardial excitation from one or more ectopic ventricular foci, at a rate exceeding that to which the myocardium may rhythmically respond. Usually this increased excitation or irritability is first manifested by PVCs.

If ventricular tachycardia develops and causes hypotension or cardiac failure, immediate cardioversion plus IV lidocaine is the treatment of choice. Simultaneous vigorous efforts should be made to increase coronary blood flow and increased oxygenation of the blood. Acid-base balance and serum electrolytes should be kept at optimal levels.

If ventricular tachycardia is not associated with hemodynamic impairment, one can attempt conversion with drugs such as lidocaine, which should have been started when the PVCs developed. If lidocaine does not appear to be effective, procainamide may be given. Since these agents impair myocardial contractility if given in large doses, cardioversion should be attempted promptly if moderate doses do not rapidly correct the ventricular tachycardia.

3. Ventricular Asystole

In some instances of acute myocardial infarction, the infarction is so large (more than 70% of the left-ventricular myocardium) that cardiac output almost completely ceases. In most of these cases, asystole follows a period of ventricular fibrillation, but occasionally it occurs following a relatively normal rhythm. Successful resuscitation with so much dead myocardium is virtually impossible. With infarction of 40% to 70% of the left ventricular myocardium, cariogenic shock is often present and the added problem of ventricular tachycardia or fibrillation is frequently fatal.

4. Atrial Arrhythmias

About 15% to 20% of patients with AMI develop supraventricular tachyarrhythmias. Paroxysmal atrial contractions or atrial tachycardias can usually be controlled with quinidine (200 mg every 4 hours). Atrial fibrillation or flutter is associated with congestive heart failure in 75% to 80% of these patients and is best controlled with digitalis. Severe sinus bradycardia occasionally develops, particularly after posterior (inferior) myocardial infarctions. If the bradycardia does not respond to 1.0 mg of atropine $\times$ 2, an isoproterenol drip and/or temporary transvenous pacing may be required.

If the diagnosis of atrial flutter or fibrillation is not clear, one may have to confirm the diagnosis using carotid pressure and/or an intra-atrial electrogram. With atrial fibrillation, the ventricular rate can usually be controlled with IV digoxin. Propranolol and/or verapamil may be needed to help control the ventricular rate in a few cases. Occasionally cardioversion is necessary, particularly for patients who are hypotensive.

5. Causes of Persistent Arrhythmias

Persistent or recurrent arrhythmias after an acute myocardial infarction may be due to electrolyte imbalance, digitalis toxicity, or an irritable focus. Hypokalemia due to excessive use of diuretics and/or respiratory alkalosis is not infrequent. The ischemic myocardium appears to have an increased sensitivity to digitalis; thus, a maintenance dose of digitalis that was optimal before the ischemic episode may cause severe toxicity after an infarction. In some instances, improved oxygenation of the blood or increased coronary blood flow relative to demand may correct the tendency to arrhythmias.

AXIOM

With recurrent arrhythmias one must also look for mechanical problems such as hypovolemia, atelectasis, pericardial tamponade, and gastric dilation.

B. PUMP FAILURE

Left ventricular pump failure occurring after an acute myocardial infarction is associated with a greatly increased mortality rate which correlates with the amount of left ventricle that has become nonfunctional. As a general rule, dysfunction of 40% to 70% of the left ventricular myocardium causes shock or heart failure, and a loss of 70% or more is usually rapidly fatal.

Acute myocardial infarction shock continues to have a mortality rate of at least 60% to 80% in most hospitals. Of patients developing acute pulmonary edema, up to 60% to 70% die within 3 years. If the patient has x-ray evidence of acute cardiac enlargement, the mortality rate is at least 40% to 50%. The 3-year mortality rate even when there is no clinical or x-ray evidence of heart failure may be up to 20% to 25%.

1. Acute Myocardial Infarction Shock

a. Etiology

Death or dysfunction of 40% to 70% of the left ventricular myocardium will generally result in shock or death, because the heart is unable to supply adequate blood flow to maintain the function and viability of peripheral tissues and vital organs, including the heart itself. This complication occurs in about 15% of patients hospitalized with AMI. The patient with AMI shock usually has significant (70% to 80%) occlusion of the three main coronary arteries (right, left anterior descending, and left circumflex), and frequently he or she has had a previous myocardial infarction.

Acute myocardial infarction with shock occasionally may be due to an acute proximal aortic dissection occluding a coronary artery. This may be due to an intramural dissection or extravasation of blood into the perivascular tissues. An aortic dissection may also cause shock by exsanguination into the mediastinum or pleural cavity or by rupture into the pericardium, causing tamponade.

b. Clinical Manifestations

Acute myocardial infarction shock is characterized hemodynamically by left ventricular failure, low cardiac output, arterial hypotension, and peripheral vasoconstriction. The classic signs and symptoms include restlessness, cloudy sensorium, cold and clammy skin, tachycardia, weak and thready pulse, systolic blood pressure less than 90 mm Hg, and reduced urine output. Rarely, a patient develops hypotension without the other signs of clinical shock. Under such circumstances, the arterial blood pressure may be low, but cardiac output tends to be normal or only slightly decreased. Renal blood flow and urine volume may also remain relatively normal.

c. Treatment

(1) Fluid

Treatment of shock, regardless of its etiology, should follow certain logical steps (Table 2.10). When shock complicates AMI, maintaining a mean arterial pressure of at least 75 to 85 mm Hg to ensure adequate coronary blood flow is a necessity.

PITFALL

Delay in providing early ventilatory support in spite of marginal pulmonary function after an AMI because of concern about the discomfort of an endotracheal tube.

(2) Ventilation

Inadequate ventilation combined with poor tissue perfusion is highly lethal. Patients in shock, in spite of a normal or increased ventilation, often have reduced tidal volumes and a poor cough, resulting in an increased tendency to atelectasis, particularly at the lung bases. If there is any question about the adequacy of ventilation, early traumatic nasotracheal intubation and ventilatory assistance should be considered. Positive pressure ventilation may help prevent sudden, severe hypoxia or pulmonary edema and generally decreases the work of breathing.

(3) Oxygen

Even if the minute ventilation is adequate, oxygen may greatly improve oxygen delivery to the tissues and relieve pain due to myocardial ischemia. This is particularly important if the cardiac output is reduced. The oxygen is given by mask if the patient will readily tolerate it.

Interestingly, the tissue hypoxia seen with myocardial ischemia may be related to low triiodothyronine (T_3) levels. In fact, experimental data suggest that low T_3 levels may retard resumption of aerobic metabolism. Novitsky and

Table 2.10

AN OUTLINE OF TREATMENT OF SHOCK COMPLICATING ACUTE MYOCARDIAL INFARCTION	1. Oxygen, preferably by mask in high concentration, especially if the patient is cold, clammy, or cyanotic, or if the PaO$_2$ is less than 80 mm Hg.
	2. Nasotracheal intubation and positive-pressure ventilation if tidal volume or minute ventilation are inadequate, if the work of breathing is excessive, or if the patient is hypoxic in spite of 100% O$_2$ by mask.
	3. Fluids to correct hypovolemia, but without overloading. The PAWP should be increased to 15 to 18 mm Hg to ensure adequate left ventricular filling. The response to a fluid challenge is the best guide to fluid therapy.
	4. Inotropic agents:
	    Dogoxin—if there is evidence of heart failure or atrial fibrillation
	    Dopamine—to keep the mean arterial blood pressure at a minimum of 75 to 85 mm Hg
	    Dobutamine—to keep the cardiac index above 2.2 to 2.5 L·min^{-1}·m^{-2}
	    Isoproterenol—for bradycardia
	    GIK solution—glucose-insulin-potassium if poor response to above
	    Glucagon—last resort; may help increase contractility in patients on beta-blockers
	5. Correction of arrhythmias
	6. Correction of acid-base and electrolyte abnormalities (especially K and Ca).
	7. Vasopressors—increased dopamine or norepinephrine with phentolamine if mean BP is less than 75 mm Hg in spite of dopamine and other therapy.
	8. Vasodilators—should be administered very cautiously and only if severe vasoconstriction persists in a patient with an adequate blood pressure and intravascular volume. Intra-arterial BP and PAWP must be monitored closely.
	9. Diuretics—as needed to maintain a urine output of at least 30 ml/h (after adequate hydration).
	10. Corticosteroids—200 mg hydrocortisone IV bolus if still hypotensive to rule out subclinical adrenal insufficiency.
	11. Heparin—if evidence of deep venous thrombosis or pulmonary emboli.
	12. Mechanical cardiac assistance, such as intra-aortic balloon pumping, if shock due to power failure persists for more than 2 hours.

associates recently found that T$_3$ in doses of 0.2 μg/kg given in 6 doses 30 minutes apart significantly improved myocardial function after a 15-minute period of experimental cardiac ischemia. The biggest improvements were seen in cardiac index (CI) and maximum rate of pressure change (dP/dt max). It appears that T$_3$ can activate aerobic metabolism, enhance substrate metabolism, replenish high-energy phosphate stores, and correct myocardial lactic acidosis.

(4) Fluids

At least 20% of patients with AMI shock are hypovolemic due to prior diuretics or inadequate intake, and most of the others will benefit from a slightly higher left ventricular filling pressure.

(5) Pulmonary Artery Wedge Pressure

A pulmonary artery catheter should probably be inserted in all patients with AMI shock that persists for more than 5 to 10 minutes. The PAWP can provide important information on the quantity of fluid to give the patient. However, it is becoming increasingly clear that even the PAWP may not provide accurate information on optimal filling of the heart. It has been shown that end-diastolic volumes in the left ventricle with an acute infarct often correlate poorly with the PAWP because of changes in left ventricular compliance. For example, myocardial ischemia, right ventricular overload, or positive end-expiratory pressure (PEEP) will all tend to reduce left ventricular compliance, causing the PAWP to be higher than expected for a given left ventricular diastolic volume. Under such circumstances, the patient's response to a fluid challenge is often the best way to assess fluid status.

AXIOM
Most patients with AMI shock will benefit from cautious fluid loading.

An initial fluid challenge should be given very cautiously to correct hypovolemia that might be present with AMI shock. Although correction of hypovolemia is extremely important in these patients, it is also very easy to overload them with fluids. Fluid overloading is particularly apt to occur if the patient has a low CVP, which is mistakenly interpreted as evidence of hypovolemia. Occasionally an acute myocardial infarction produces an isolated left ventricular failure with a high PAWP (due to inadequate emptying of the left ventricle during systole and decreased left ventricular compliance). At the same time, the CVP may be low, at least temporarily, because the right ventricle is still functioning relatively well.

(6) Inotropic Agents

Digitalization is probably unnecessary in patients with an uncomplicated acute myocardial infarction. However, if cardiac failure or atrial fibrillation develops, digitalis may be beneficial. Digoxin is usually the best digitalis preparation to give under such circumstances. It should probably be given in multiple, small IV doses (0.25 to 0.50 mg) every 3 to 6 hours for a total dose of 1.0 to 1.5 mg, depending on the patient's electrolyte status and his or her clinical and ECG response.

PITFALL
Failure to adequately follow potassium and calcium levels in patients receiving digitalis preparations.

Hyperkalemia and hypocalcemia tend to decrease the sensitivity of the heart to digitalis. In contrast, hypokalemia, hypercalcemia, and shock tend to increase the sensitivity of the heart to digitalis.

Dopamine in doses of 5 to 15 μg$\cdot$kg$^{-1}\cdot$min^{-1} IV may help restore the mean arterial BP to levels of 75 to 85 mm Hg by its inotropic and vasoconstricting effects. Blood flow through cerebral and coronary vessels that have a 70% to 80% lumen stenosis depends largely on an adequate mean aortic pressure. Consequently, a very low blood pressure may cause the myocardial infarction to increase in size and further compromise the performance of residual viable myocardium. Although inotropic agents and vasopressors increase the oxygen demands of the heart, if more than 70% to 80% of the cross-sectional area of the coronary arteries is occluded, raising the mBP to 75 to 85 mm Hg tends to increase coronary blood flow more than it increases myocardial oxygen demands.

Dobutamine, like dopamine, at doses of 5 to 10 μg$\cdot$kg$^{-1}\cdot$min^{-1} tends to raise cardiac output; however, it also tends to cause some arterial vasodilation. Hence, it may be preferable to dopamine if the cardiac output is low and the BP is relative normal. Dobutamine is also more apt to be effective in patients with chronic heart failure because they tend to have myocardial catecholamine depletion, which interferes with dopamine's effectiveness.

Isoproternol is generally avoided in patients with acute myocardial infarction because it can increase myocardial oxygen demands much more than coronary blood flow. Nevertheless, in bradycardia patients, doses of 1 to 2 μg/min to raise the heart rate to 60 to 80 per minute may be of value. Atropine (in doses of 0.8 to 1.0 mg IV, which may be repeated once) or a transvenous pacemaker is often preferable to isoproterenol for managing bradycardias.

(7) Glucose-Insulin-Potassium Solutions

This *polarizing solution* may help stabilize cell membranes and thereby not only reduce the incidence of arrhythmias but also slightly increase cardiac output. The usual solution is 20% G/W with 40 units of insulin and 80 mEq of potassium per liter of solution. This is infused at 25 to 50 ml/h, depending upon the response.

(8) Recognition and Control of Arrhythmias

Early recognition and control of arrhythmias has provided the greatest improvement in the care of patients with acute myocardial infarction over the past two to three decades. However, since many of the drugs used to treat arrhythmias also depress myocardial contractility, they must be used with caution.

PITFALL

Failure to recognize that most antiarrhythmic agents also have negative inotropic and vasodilation effects that can cause hypotension, especially if the patient is hypovolemic.

(9) Correction of Acid-Base and Electrolyte Abnormalities

Acid-base and electrolyte abnormalities should be carefully corrected with proper regard to the patient's blood pressure and pH. Chronic abnormalities must not be corrected too abruptly. Highest priority must be given to correction of hypoxemia and volume deficits. The next priority is correction of the pH and potassium and calcium levels. Alkalosis (pH > 7.55), severe acidosis (pH < 7.15), severe hypocarbia ($Paco_2 < 25$ mm Hg) and hyperkalemia or hypocalcemia all may interfere with myocardial contractility.

(10) Vasopressors

It is important to maintain a mean arterial BP of 75 to 85 mm Hg in patients apt to have critical stenoses of coronary or cerebral vessels. If hypotension persists in spite of all of the above therapy including dopamine at doses exceeding 30 to 60 $\mu g \cdot kg^{-1} \cdot min^{-1}$, norepinephrine may be required. Although norepinephrine has a bad reputation for causing excessive vasoconstriction, a mixture of four ampules (total 16 mg) of norepinephrine with two ampules (total 10 mg) of phentolamine in 500 ml of 5% G/W given at 0.3 to 0.6 ml/min may raise BP with little or no decrease in cardiac output. Some physicians do not use phentolamine in the same solution with the norepinephrine, but if norepinephrine extravasates into perivascular tissues, the tissues are much less apt to slough if phentolamine is present.

(11) Vasodilators

Various vasodilators should be considered if the patient has severe, persistent vasoconstriction. Nitroprusside has a balanced vasodilating effect on both arteries and veins beginning at doses of 0.3 $\mu g \cdot kg^{-1} \cdot min^{-1}$ and gradually increasing the dose to 3.0 $\mu g \cdot kg^{-1} \cdot min^{-1}$ as needed. IV nitroglycerin in similar doses can directly dilate coronary arteries, and it causes a bit more vasodilation in systemic veins than in systemic arteries. Consequently, it has a greater effect on preload than on afterload. These agents should be avoided if the patient is hypovolemic.

AXIOM

An abrupt drop in BP when a vasodilator is started is generally a reliable indicator of hypovolemia.

(12) Diuretics

Diuretics, preferably in multiple small doses, should be given if the patient is overloaded with fluid or if the patient is oliguric in spite of all the therapy previously mentioned.

(13) Heparin

Heparin is often given to patients with an AMI. It probably has little effect on the coronary artery thrombosis, but it may be of value in preventing or treating deep venous thrombosis, pulmonary embolic, and left-atrial or left-ventricular thrombi.

AXIOM

Whenever one gives heparin, the platelet count should be followed to ensure that the patient does not develop heparin-induced thrombocytopenia syndrome.

**(14) Mechanical Cardiac
Assistance**

If cardiogenic shock persists in spite of adequate ventilation, oxygen, fluids, acid-base correction, inotropic agents, and control of arrhythmias, it can generally be assumed that the persisting shock is due to "power failure" resulting from inadequate functioning of the left ventricular myocardium. If shock due to power failure persists for more than 2 hours, the mortality rate approaches 100% and mechanical support of the circulation with intra-aortic balloon pumping (IABP) should be strongly considered.

IABP is designed to increase the endocardial viability ratio (EVR), which is the ratio of blood supply to the heart as indicated by the diastolic pressure time index (DPTI), and the oxygen demands of the heart as reflected by STTI.

$$\frac{DPTI}{EVR} = STTI.$$

The DPTI is equal to the left ventricular perfusion pressure (diastolic aortic pressure minus the left ventricular diastolic pressure) multiplied by the time (seconds) each minute that the heart is in diastole. IABP increases the blood supply to the heart by raising diastolic aortic pressure, reducing diastolic ventricular pressure (by allowing the heart to empty more), and slowing the pulse rate (increasing the time in diastole).

The STTI is equal to the systolic pressure developed by the left ventricle multiplied by the radius of the heart and by the amount of time each minute that the heart is in systole. IABP reduces oxygen demands of the heart by reducing systolic BP, reducing the radius of the heart (by emptying the heart more), and decreasing ejection time or the amount of time in systole.

PITFALL

Delay in instituting IABP in patients with persistent AMI shock.

If the IABP is begun before cardiovascular and other organ function has deteriorated irreversibly, a third or more of the patients may improve sufficiently to terminate IABP within 24 to 48 hours. A second third of the patients may improve temporarily but cannot be taken off IABP unless major mechanical problems (such as mitral insufficiency or ventricular septal defect) or major coronary occlusions are corrected. The remaining patients do not significantly improve with IABP and usually go on to die rapidly because of the large size of their ventricular infarction.

2. Heart Failure

The most frequent cause of heart failure after an acute myocardial infarction is dysfunction of a large portion of the myocardium by the ischemic process. However, one must also look for other possibly correctable causes (Table 2.11).

If the left ventricle cannot pump all the blood brought to it, blood will accumulate in the lungs, causing increasing pulmonary congestion. If pulmo-

Table 2.11

CAUSES OF HEART FAILURE DURING ACUTE MYOCARDIAL INFARCTION	Massive muscle necrosis
	Severe muscle ischemia with dysfunction ("stunning")
	Ventricular free-wall rupture
	Acute mitral regurgitation
	Papillary muscle dysfunction from ischemia
	Papillary muscle rupture from necrosis
	Formation of ventricular septal defect
	Pericardial effusion with cardiac tamponade
	Right ventricular infarction
	Unstable rhythms (e.g., sustained ventricular tachycardia, etc.)

nary venous and capillary pressures rise to 25 to 30 mm Hg or higher, pulmonary edema is apt to develop. With increased interstitial and intra-alveolar fluid, ventilation and oxygen exchange become progressively impaired and may cause death.

The heart failure following AMI initially may involve only the left side of the heart. Under such circumstances, the CVP may be temporarily normal despite the presence of pulmonary edema. Eventually, however, the right heart will also begin to fail, producing peripheral edema and hepatomegaly or ascites.

a. Diagnostic Evaluations

Because even mild degrees of congestive heart failure may exacerbate myocardial ischemia, prompt diagnosis and treatment are essential. Often the presence of heart failure can be assessed on clinical grounds and by examination of the chest roentgenogram. Clinical classifications, such as that developed by Killip and Kimbal, may be useful because of their relationship to prognosis (Table 2.12).

Similar clinical classifications can also be used to estimate the hemodynamic changes present (Table 2.13).

PITFALL
Assuming that one can accurately determine cardiac output and filling pressure by clinical means after an AMI.

Although these general guidelines may be helpful, they are not infallible. Approximately 25% of patients with cardiac indices less than 2.2 liters$\cdot$min$^{-1}\cdot$m^{-2} and 15% of patients with high pulmonary occlusion pressures ($>$18 mm Hg) are unrecognizable clinically. Thus, although hemodynamic monitoring is not always needed for diagnosis, it is required to ensure optimal titration of parenteral vasodilators and inotropic agents.

Pulmonary artery catherization facilitates aggressive, accurate management. Because one goal of catheterization is to guide rapid interventions, the catheter is usually required for only 24 to 48 hours or less. As a general rule, vasodilators combined with inotropes provide the best treatment of acute heart failure.

Amrinone is a recently introduced inotropic agent available for parenteral use. It exhibits potent phosphodiesterase inhibition resulting in positive inotropic and systemic and pulmonary vasodilating effects. It has been used primarily for patients with chronic congestive heart failure, but it may also be of some help if pulmonary hypertension is present.

If severe cardiac failure persists after acute myocardial infarction in spite of vigorous medical therapy (including digitalis, diuretics, salt and water restriction, etc.), one should look for mechanical cardiac defects that can be treated surgically. Correction or mitral regurgitation (due to papillary muscle dysfunction), ventricular septal defects, or ventricular aneurysms may dramatically relieve heart failure. Such surgery should be delayed as long as possible to allow

---

Table 2.12

RELATIONSHIP OF CLINICAL VARIABLES TO MORTALITY IN PATIENTS WITH ACUTE MYOCARDIAL INFARCTION	Killip Class	% of Patients	Mortality (%)
	I—no congestive heart failure	33	6
	II—mild-to-moderate congestive heart failure	38	17
	III—pulmonary edema	10	38
	IV—cardiogenic shock	19	81

Source: Killip, T III and Kimball, JT: Treatment of myocardial infarction in a coronary care unit: A two year experience with 250 patients. Am J Cardiol 20:457, 1967.

Table 2.13

RELATIONSHIP OF CLINICAL AND HEMODYNAMIC VARIABLES TO MORTALITY IN PATIENTS WITH ACUTE MYOCARDIAL INFARCTION (MEAN ± SD)	Clinical Class	Cardiac Index, L/min per m²	Wedge Pressure, mm Hg	Mortality
	1—no pulmonary congestion peripheral hypoperfusion	2.5 ± 0.5	12 ± 7	2.2%
	2—pulmonary congestion	2.3 ± 0.4	23 ± 5	10.1%
	3—peripheral hypoperfusion	1.9 ± 0.4	12 ± 5	22.4%
	4—pulmonary congestion and peripheral hypoperfusion	1.6 ± 0.4	27 ± 8	55.5%

Source: Forrester, JS, Diamond, GA, and Swan, HJ: Correlative classification of clinical and hemo-dynamic function after acute myocardial infarction. Am J Cardiol 65:241–271, 1990.

the scar tissue associated with these defects to mature, in order to facilitate suturing. However, if the heart failure continues to progress in spite of all medical therapy (including balloon pumping), emergency surgery may be required.

Surgery appears to have little role in correcting diffuse, severe left ventricular dysfunction due to an established infarct more than 6 to 8 hours old. However, there are a number of reports of improved ejection fractions after coronary artery bypasses, and use of thrombolytic agents or PTCA in such patients.

C. CONDUCTION DEFECTS

PITFALL
Delay in instituting temporary pacing in patients with major conduction defects after an AMI.

The role of artificial pacing in reducing the mortality rate associated with conduction defects following AMI has been widely discussed. It now seems clear that an AMI with loss of any two of the three main conduction fascicles (right bundle, left anterior bundle, or left posterior bundle) implies significant proximal coronary artery disease, usually in the left anterior descending coronary artery (Table 2.14).

The increased incidence of complete heart block and sudden death in patients with AV conduction defects may be greatly reduced by early or prophylactic pacing. Thus, even when infarction causes only a right bundle-branch block (RBBB), some cardiologists feel that it is an indication for prophylactic pacing. Initially, a temporary transvenous pacemaker is inserted (Table 2.15).

After 1 to 2 weeks, a decision concerning the need for permanent pacing should be made. If a bifascicular block (either an RBBB plus left anterior or

Table 2.14

BRADYCARDIA AND BLOCK: INFERIOR VERSUS ANTEROSEPTAL MYOCARDIAL INFARCTION	Characteristics	Inferior MI	Anterior MI
	Usual vessel occluded	Right coronary artery	Left anterior descending artery
	Mechanism of block	Increased vagal tone	Destruction of conduction system in the interventricular septum
	Block responsive to atropine	Yes	No
	Origin of escape rhythm	High-junctional conduction system	Peripheral Purkinje fibers
	Escape rate	40–50 beats/min	<30 beats/min
	Hemodynamic consequences of block	Mild	Severe
	Acute pacing required	Usually not	Yes, but outlook remains poor

Table 2.15

INDICATIONS FOR TEMPORARY PACING FOLLOWING ACUTE MYOCARDIAL INFARCTION	A. Prophylactic pacing

A. Prophylactic pacing
  1. Strongly indicated for
     a. New RBBB and LAHB*
     b. New RBBB and LPHB*
     c. Alternating BBB*
     d. Mobitz H 2° AVB*
     e. Complete heart block
  2. Possibly indicated for
     a. 1° AVB and old bilateral BBB
     b. 1° AVB and new BBB
B. Therapeutic
  2. Indicated pacing
     a. Medically refractory bradycardia with symptoms (CHF, chest pain, syncope)*
     b. Heart rate <50 beats/min
     c. AV dissociated rhythms with hemodynamic compromise

*RBBB = right bundle-branch block; LAHB = left anterior hemiblock; LPHB = left posterior hemiblock; BBB = bundle-branch block; AVB = atrioventricular block; CHF = congestive heart failure.

posterior hemiblock or a complete LBBB has developed during the course of an acute infarction, permanent prophylactic pacing is often warranted. Patients with complete block below the AV node (Mobitz type-II) should also receive permanent pacemakers.

D. PERSISTENT PAIN

Persistent or recurrent pain following an acute myocardial infarction must be treated aggressively. Judicious sedation not only can relieve pain directly, but may reduce myocardial oxygen demands. Antihypertensive agents can also reduce myocardial oxygen needs, but they must not be allowed to cause hypotension. Use of digitalis in these patients is controversial because it can increase myocardial oxygen demands and the incidence of arrhythmias. However, if overt heart failure is present, digitalis may reduce pain by decreasing heart size and thereby improving the balance between oxygen supply and demand. Intensive therapy with long- and short-acting nitrates, beta-adrenergic blockers, and calcium-channel blockers may also relieve pain. Experimental evidence suggests that if hypotension is avoided, these agents may reduce infarct size. Persistent angina in spite of aggressive medical therapy is a well-accepted indication for coronary arteriography and possible coronary artery bypass surgery or PTCA.

Chest pain after an AMI may occasionally be of pericardial or musculoskeletal origin. Pericarditis usually requires no special therapy unless the fever, pleuritic pain, or effusion is severe, in which case steroids may be of benefit. Musculoskeletal pain due at least partly to splinting or inactivity of chest or arm muscles should respond well to physiotherapy.

E. THROMBOEMBOLI

Anticoagulants are used in patients with AMI not only with thrombolytic therapy but also to reduce the incidence of venous thrombi (and subsequent pulmonary emboli) or systemic emboli (from thrombi forming on the endocardial surface of an infarction). Left-ventricular thrombi may form on the endothelial surface of myocardial infarctions, particularly if the infarction is transmural and involves the apical portion of the ventricle. These thrombi may detach and become systemic emboli. Even if the emboli are small, they may occlude an important coronary or cerebral vessel.

Patients who are particularly prone to venous thrombosis in the legs and development of subsequent pulmonary emboli include those who (1) are confined to bed, (2) have significant heart failure, (3) have a left ventricular aneurysm, or (4) have had previous thromboemboli. In such individuals, anticoagulation with coumarin seems to be appropriate. If acute deep venous thrombosis or acute pulmonary or systemic emboli are strongly suspected, IV heparin in full dosage should be started. Although intermittent heparin administration is used effectively in some centers, a loading dose of 5000 units followed by a constant infusion of 1000 ± 200 units/h to maintain clotting times at about two times normal is probably safer and more effective.

Although TPA may be more effective than SK or APSAC in acutely lysing thrombus, late vessel patency, improvement in ventricular function, survival benefits, and incidence of complications are comparable among all agents. Thrombolytic therapy improves the survival of patients with large or anterior infarctions. The improvement is less pronounced among patients with small or inferior infarctions. Thrombolytic therapy can reduce the risk of death from acute myocardial infarction in elderly patients, without excessively increasing the rate of bleeding complications. Patients with ST-segment depression and no ST-segment elevation on the initial ECG do not appear to benefit from thrombolytic drugs. Aspirin and β-blockers each enhance the benefit achieved with thrombolytic therapy; the optimal use of heparin is currently under investigation.

In a recent report, Turpie and associates studied 200 patients with anterior myocardial infarction who did not receive thrombolytic agents in the acute phase. These patients were randomized to receive subcutaneous administration of either 12,500 units of heparin every 12 hours or 5000 units every 12 hours (the amount conventionally given to prevent venous thrombosis). The larger dose of heparin reduced the incidence of left ventricular mural thrombi from 32% to 11%. In addition, the incidence of nonhemorrhagic strokes was reduced from 4% in the low-dose group to less than 1% in the high-dose group.

These new data support the use of short-term anticoagulant therapy in patients with acute transmural anterior myocardial infarction. Subcutaneous or IV heparin in a dosage sufficient to prolong the activated partial thromboplastin time to 1.5 to 2 times the control value is advocated, beginning immediately after the onset of infarction and continuing for approximately 10 days. In patients who by echocardiography have ventricular mural thrombi or large akinetic regions, it may be appropriate to follow the 10 days of heparin with 1 to 3 months of oral anticoagulation.

In an accompanying editorial, Fuster and Halperin noted that physicians treating AMI have a bit of a dilemma. Although aspirin may help prevent recurrent myocardial infarction, there is little reason to expect it to prevent cardiogenic emboli. On the other hand, although heparin may help protect against ventricular thrombi, it is generally thought to less protective than aspirin against recurrent myocardial infarction. Thus, a combination of these agents, probably in reduced dosage, might provide the best overall protection.

F. CARDIAC RUPTURE

Cardiac rupture is found at autopsy in 10% of acutely infarcted hearts. From the third to tenth day after infarction, the junction of the infarcted and normal tissue is particularly susceptible to rupture. It is thought that the rupture is caused by a shearing effect at the junction of the abnormal paradoxically moving myocardium and the normally contracting ventricular wall. Increased tension due to an increased diameter in the abnormal area of the heart also increases the likelihood of rupture. According to the Laplace relationship, the contracting ventricle subjects its wall to a tension (T) which is directly proportional to the pressure (P) and radius (r) of the cavity and inversely proportional to the thickness of the wall (h):

$$T = \frac{Pr}{2h}.$$

Thus, a thin bulging scar subjected to increased pressure is most apt to rupture. If a rupture does occur, the resulting massive hemopericardium is almost invariably rapidly fatal.

Although the clinical presentation of hypotension, distended neck veins and pulsus paradoxes with equalization of right atrial and PAWPs, is characteristic of pericardial tamponade, these findings may also be found in some patients with right ventricular infarction. Echocardiography or carbon dioxide angiography can help differentiate between these two entities. These two problems may also be differentiated by an inspiratory increase in right atrial pressure (Kussmaul's sign) which is common in right ventricular infarction, but is relatively uncommon in cardiac tamponade. Infarcted myocardium in the interventricular septum may also rupture, causing a ventricular septal defect. Rupture of an infarcted papillary muscle (usually the posteromedial muscle) of the mitral valve can result in massive mitral insufficiency.

Gradual bulging of a thin, weak fibrotic ventricular wall may result in the development of a clinically significant ventricular aneurysm. Such an aneurysm not only reduces the efficiency of myocardial contraction, but may also act as a site for intraventricular thrombosis or arrhythmia development.

G. PREVENTION OF RECURRENT MYOCARDIAL INFARCTION

Moss and Benhorin, in a recent review of the prognosis and management of patients after a first myocardial infarction, noted that age, ejection fraction, and infarct location (in decreasing order of importance) were identified by Ahnve and associates as independent predictors of cardiac mortality. Beta-blockers and aspirin have been shown to reduce the recurrence of coronary events. Routine prophylactic antiarrhythmic therapy is not recommended in this population.

Moss and Benhorin also identified the need for early (1-month postinfarction) and periodic exercise testing to identify the patients with jeopardized ischemic myocardium who are at high risk of another coronary event. These patients warrant further diagnostic evaluation with radionuclide techniques or coronary angiography in order to identify those who may benefit from medical treatment or revascularization procedures that would reduce the likelihood of a second coronary event. In patients with a normal response to exercise testing, the risk of cardiac mortality and morbidity is sufficiently low that no additional diagnostic testing is indicated.

Antiplatelet drugs may help to reduce the incidence of thrombosis in diseased coronary arteries. Aspirin may be of particular benefit in this regard. However, Smith, Arnesen, and Holme recently showed that long-term therapy with warfarin has an important beneficial effect and can be recommended in the treatment of patients who survive the acute phase after a myocardial infarction. It appears that a trial specifically designed to compare the results with aspirin and warfarin is needed to clarify this point.

The use of oral anticoagulation in the long-term treatment of survivors of AMI has been highly controversial for many years. In a recent study reported by Smith, Arnesen, and Holme, 1214 patients who had recovered from an AMI were randomized to treatment with warfarin (beginning an average of 27 days after the infarction) or a placebo with an average follow-up of 37 months. The use of warfarin resulted in a 24% reduction in mortality (15 vs. 20% death rate), a 34% reduction in the incidence of reinfarction (13.5 vs. 20.4%), and a 55% reduction in the number of total cerebrovascular accidents (3.3 vs. 7.2%). Thus, long-term therapy with warfarin has an important beneficial effect in patients who survive an acute myocardial infarction.

Two recent large, placebo-controlled trials have shown that verapamil routinely given 7 to 15 days after an AMI was beneficial in a subgroup of patients who had no signs or symptoms of congestive heart failure and had incomplete coronary occlusion or good collateral circulation. This is probably the best alternative for patients who cannot take beta-blockers because they have chronic obstructive pulmonary disease, asthma, peripheral vascular disease, diabetes mellitus, or sinus bradycardia.

SUMMARY POINTS

1. Acute myocardial infarction is usually due to thrombosis of a narrowed arteriosclerotic coronary artery.
2. A Valsalva maneuver increases myocardial oxygen demands but reduces venous return, cardiac output, and coronary blood flow.
3. One must make every effort to prevent constipation in patients with severe coronary artery disease.
4. Myocardial oxygen demand is primarily determined by the systolic tension-time index, which is equal to mean systolic pressure times the radius of the left ventricle and the amount of time in systole each minute.
5. Blood flow to the myocardium depends largely on diastolic aortic pressure, left ventricular diastolic pressure, the resistance to blood flow in the coronary arterioles, and the amount of time in diastole.
6. A low aortic diastolic BP and high left ventricular diastolic pressure can greatly reduce coronary blood flow to the left ventricle, especially the subendocardial myocardium.
7. Tachycardia increases myocardial oxygen requirements and decreases the time for coronary blood flow.
8. The diagnosis of an AMI is fairly secure if two of the following criteria are present: (a) typical history of chest pain, (b) typical ECG changes, or (c) typical enzyme (CPK-MB) changes.
9. Any new jaw, neck, or chest pain developing in an older patient (especially a man), particularly after stress or effort of any type, should be considered a possible myocardial infarction until proven otherwise.
10. Up to 70% of patients with myocardial ischemic episodes and 15% of patients with an acute myocardial infarction have no chest pain or related symptoms.
11. Gastrointestinal symptoms may be the main or presenting symptoms in many patients with an AMI, especially if the ischemia involves the inferior (diaphragmatic) myocardium.
12. Because there are other causes of CPK-MB increases not associated with AMI (Table 2.3), CPK-MB elevations should not be the sole diagnostic indicator of acute myocardial infarction in patients with chest pain.
13. Most patients presenting to an emergency department with chest pain will not have an AMI if the CPK-MB is not elevated and the pain is not recurrent.
14. A CPK-MB elevation by itself should not be the sole diagnostic indicator of AMI in patients with chest pain.
15. One should not insist on abnormal or typical ECG findings to make a diagnosis of an AMI.
16. An isolated posterior myocardial infarction may produce few or no diagnostic ECG changes.
17. The presence of chest pain at rest, CPK-MB increases, and persistent ST-T-wave changes without abnormal Q waves allow one to make a diagnosis of a non-Q-wave myocardial infarction.
18. The differential diagnosis of acute myocardial infarction includes acute anxiety attacks, acute pericarditis, dissecting aortic aneurysm, pulmonary embolism, biliary colic, pneumothorax, perforated or deeply penetrating peptic ulcer, rupture of the esophagus, pancreatitis, pericardial tamponade, constrictive pericarditis, and cardiomyopathies.

19. If a young man has had severe chest pain but has normal coronary arteries, one should look for an aortic dissection.
20. Older individuals with repeated "indigestion" actually often have myocardial ischemia.
21. Chest x-rays (including good posteroanterior and lateral views) should be obtained on all patients with chest pain as soon as the condition is stable.
22. The risk of a recurrent myocardial infarction is increased with the use of general anesthetic up to 3 to 6 months after an AMI.
23. As a general rule, any patient having major vascular surgery should have a preoperative coronary arteriogram, if he has (a) a past history of a myocardial infarction; (b) angina, even if it is stable; or (c) ECG evidence of a previously unrecognized myocardial infarction.
24. One should not administer narcotics to hypotensive or hypovolemic patients.
25. Use of a pulmonary artery catheter to optimize cardiac filling preoperatively and then maintaining the optimal PAWP intraoperatively and for 48 to 72 hours postoperatively can greatly reduce perioperative cardiac complications.
26. Thrombolytic therapy can reduce the morbidity and mortality of an AMI, and the sooner it is started, preferably within 2 to 4 hours, the better the results.
27. The main determinant of the amount of myocardium salvaged by thrombolytic therapy is the time between the onset of pain and the administration of the drug.
28. Streptokinase is quite antigenic and may cause severe allergic reactions.
29. Because of the short half-life of TPA, it is essential to simultaneously anticoagulate the patient, using continuous IV heparin, for 48 hours or longer.
30. Thrombolytic therapy can open up 60% to 80% of thrombosed coronary arteries. The reocclusion rate at 2 to 4 weeks is around 10% to 30%.
31. Thrombolytic agents can usually be given much earlier by the IV route, but the results are generally not quite as good as with intracoronary administration.
32. Contraindications to thrombolytic therapy include recent bleeding or surgery and any disease that increases the risk of strokes or bleeding at other sites.
33. Percutaneous transluminal coronary angioplasty (PTCA) probably should not be done on most individuals who cannot or will not have emergency coronary artery bypass graft (CABG) surgery if it is needed to handle a complication.
34. One must carefully monitor patients for early reocclusion after PTCA.
35. With thrombolytic therapy, bleeding complications occur in 1% to 5% and new strokes have occurred in about 0.5% to 2.0%.
36. When reperfusion occurs during thrombolytic therapy, severe ventricular arrhythmias may occur in spite of prophylactic lidocaine.
37. Early PTCA, within 2 to 3 days, after thrombolytic therapy shows no advantage over PTCA done 7 to 10 days later.
38. The most frequent cause of sudden death after an AMI is ventricular fibrillation.
39. Beta-blockers should begin as soon as possible after an acute myocardial infarction in patients who are not hypotensive, in heart failure, or bradycardia.
40. Patients should probably be given some IV magnesium following an acute myocardial infarction, particularly if they are on diuretics, even if serum values are normal.
41. Patients with an evolving acute myocardial infarction should probably be given an IV drip of nitroglycerine; however, heparin dosage may have to be increased.

42. One should consider giving diltiazem, beta-blockers, and aspirin to patients who have a non-Q-wave myocardial infarction and are not receiving thrombolytic therapy.
43. ACE inhibitors may be of value in patients with an acute myocardial infarction, especially if they are hypertensive.
44. Any tendency to inadequate ventilation in a patient with AMI shock should be treated with early endotracheal intubation and ventilatory support.
45. Up to 20% to 30% of patients with an AMI may have significant hypovolemia, and most patients with an AMI benefit from cautious fluid loading.
46. AMI shock therapy should be assisted with PAWP and intra-arterial monitoring.
47. Digoxin is probably contraindicated in patients with an uncomplicated AMI. However, if cardiac failure or atrial fibrillation develops, digoxin may be useful.
48. One should closely follow potassium and calcium levels in patients receiving digitalis preparations.
49. Dubutamine is usually the ideal agent to raise cardiac output in patients with AMI shock.
50. Isoproterenol is contraindicated in the treatment of AMI, unless the patient is severely bradycardic in spite of atropine and no pacemaker is readily available.
51. Antiarrhythmic agents also have negative inotropic and vasodilation effects that can cause hypotension, especially if the patient is hypovolemic.
52. An abrupt drop in BP when a vasodilator is started is generally a reliable indicator of hypovolemia.
53. Whenever one gives heparin, the platelet count should be followed to ensure that the patient does not develop heparin-induced thrombocytopenia syndrome.
54. If shock due to "power failure" persists for more than 2 hours in spite of good standard therapy, mechanical support with intra-aortic balloon pumping (IABP) should be strongly considered.
55. One cannot accurately estimate cardiac output and filling pressures by clinical means after an AMI.
56. The incidence of sudden deaths due to AV conduction defects may be greatly reduced by prophylactic cardiac pacing.
57. If a bifascicular Mobitz II or complete AV block persists for more than 2 weeks after an AMI, a permanent pacemaker should be inserted.
58. One should not delay instituting temporary pacing in patients with major conduction defects after an AMI.
59. The use of anticoagulants in patients with AMI may reduce the incidence of venous and intraventricular thrombi and systemic and pulmonary emboli.

BIBLIOGRAPHY

1. Abel, FL: Relative importance of cardiac output and arterial pressure in determining myocardial oxygen consumption and coronary blood flow. Circ Shock 24:85, 1988.
2. Ahnve, S, et al: First myocardial infarction: Age and ejection fraction identify a low-risk group. Am Heart J 116:925, 1988.
3. Alderman, EL, Jutzy, MR, and Berte, LE: Randomized comparison of intravenous versus intracoronary streptokinase for myocardial infarction. Am J Cardiol 1:14, 1984.
4. Alpert, JS: Myocardial infarction: General considerations. In Rippe, JM, Irwin, RS, and Dalen, JE (eds): Intensive Care Medicine. Little, Brown & Co, Boston/Toronto, 1985, p 297.
5. Anderson, JL, et al: A randomized trial of intracoronary streptokinase in the treatment of acute myocardial infarction. N Engl J Med 308:1412, 1983.
6. Anderson, JL, Rothbard, RL, Hackworthy, RA, et al: Multicenter reperfusion trial of intravenous anisoylated plasminogen streptokinase activator complex (APSAC) in acute myocardial infarction: Controlled comparison with intracoronary streptokinase. J Am Coll Cardiol 11: 1153, 1988.
7. Anderson, JL, Sorensen, SG, Moreno, FL, et al: Multicenter patency trial of intravenous

anistreplase compared with streptokinase in acute myocardial infarction. The TEAM-2 Study Investigators. Circulation 83:126, 1991.

8. Bassand, JP, Machecourt, J, Cassagnes, J, et al: Multicenter trial of intravenous anisoylated plasminogen streptokinase activator complex (APSAC) in acute myocardial infarction: Effects on infarct size and left ventricular function. J Am Coll Cardiol 13:988, 1989.

9. Becker, RC and Gore, JM: Adjunctive use of beta-adrenergic blockers, calcium antagonists, and other therapies in coronary thrombolysis. Am J Cardiol 67:25A, 1991.

10. Bergman, D: Assessment of intra-aortic balloon counterpulsation in cardiogenic shock. Crit Care Med 3:90, 1975.

11. Blasko, G, et al: Intracoronary administered prostacyclin and streptokinase for treatment of myocardial infarction. Adv Prostaglandin Thromboxane Leukotriene Res 11:385, 1983.

12. Block, PC: Coronary-artery stents and other endoluminal devices. N Engl J Med 324:52, 1991.

13. Bolooki, H, et al: Myocardial revascularization after acute infarction. Am J Cardiol 36:295, 1975.

14. Bonnier, JJ: Comparison of intravenous anisoylated plasminogen streptokinase activator complex with intracoronary streptokinase in acute myocardial infarction. Drugs 33:141, 1987

15. Cardiac Arrhythmia Suppression Trial (CAST) Investigators: Preliminary report: Effect of encainide and flecainide on mortality in a randomized trial of arrhythmia suppression after myocardial infarction. N Engl J Med 321:406, 1989.

16. Chatterjee, K and Swan, HJC: Vasodilator therapy in acute myocardial infarction. Mod Concepts Cardiovasc Dis 43:119, 1974.

17. Cintron, GB, et al: Bedside cognition incidence and clinical course of right ventricular infarction. Am J Cardiol 47:224, 1981.

18. Cohen, LS and Ross, AM: Long-term management of complicated myocardial infarction. Postgrad Med J (special issue) 57:17, 1975.

19. Collier, BS: Platelets and thrombolytic therapy. N Engl J Med 322:33, 1990.

20. Conti, CR: Large vessel coronary vasospasm: Diagnosis, natural history and treatment. Am J Cardiol 55:41B, 1985.

21. Daily, EK: Use of hemodynamics to differentiate pathophysiologic causes of cardiogenic shock. Crit Care Nurse Clin North Am 1:589, 1989.

22. Danish Study Group on the Verapamil in Myocardial Infarction: Effect of verapamil on mortality and major events after acute myocardial infarction. Am J Cardiol 66:779, 1990.

23. DeLuz, PL, et al: Oxygen delivery, anoxic metabolism and hemoglobin oxygen affinity (P_{50}) in patients with acute myocardial infarction and shock. Am J Cardiol 36:148, 1975.

24. Demling, RH and Wilson, RF: Specific Cardiovascular Disorders: Acute myocardial infarction. In Decision Making in Surgical Critical Care. BC Decker, Toronto/Philadelphia, 1988, p 93.

25. Dilsizian, V, Rocco, TP, and Freedman, NMT: Enhanced detection of ischemic but viable myocardium by the reinjection of thallium after stress: Redistribution imaging. N Engl J Med 323:141, 1990

26. Dyckner, T: Serum magnesium in acute myocardial infarction: Relation to arrhythmias. Acta Med Scand 207:59, 1980.

27. Eisenberg, PR and Jaffe, AS: Thrombolytic therapy. In Chernow, C (ed): The Pharmacologic Approach to the Critically Ill Patient. Williams & Wilkins, Baltimore, 1988, p 287.

28. Epstein, SE, et al: Dynamic coronary obstruction as a cause of angina pectoris: Implications regarding therapy. Am J Cardiol 55:61B, 1985.

29. Eukreja, RC, Kantos, HA, and Hess, MC: Captopril and enalapril do not scavenge the superoxide anion. Am J Cardiol 65:241–271, 1990.

30. Forrester, JS, Diamond, GA, and Swan, HJ: Correlative classification of clinical and hemodynamic function after acute myocardial infarction. Am J Cardiol 39:137, 1977.

31. Fox, AC: Infarction and rupture of the heart. New Engl J Med 309:551, 1983.

32. Fuster, V and Halperin, JL: Left ventricular thrombi and cerebral embolism. N Engl J Med 320:392, 1989.

33. Gertz, SD, et al: Effect of magnesium sulfate on thrombus formation following partial arterial constriction: Implications for coronary vasospasm. Magnesium 6:224–235, 1987.

34. Gibson, RS, et al: Prognostic significance and beneficial effect of diltiazem on the incidence of early recurrent ischemia after Q-wave myocardial infarction: Results from the Multicenter Diltiazen Reinfarction Study. Am J Cardiol 60:203–209, 1987.

35. Greenberg, H, et al: Effects of nitroglycerin on the major determinants of myocardial oxygen consumption: An angiograph on hemodynamic assessment. Am J Cardiol 36:426, 1975.

36. Greenberg, MA and Gitler, B: Left ventricular rupture in a patient with coexisting right ventricular infarction. New Engl J Med 309:539, 1983.

36a. Gruentzig, AR, et al: Long term follow-up after percutaneous transluminal coronary angioplasty. The early Zurich experience. N Engl J Med 316:1127, 1987.

37. Guerci, AD: Thrombolytic therapy for myocardial infarction. Md Med J 39:377, 1990.

38. Gunnar, RM and Loeb, HS: Use of drugs in cardiogenic shock due to acute myocardial infarction. Circulation 45:1111, 1972.

39. Honan, MB, et al: Cardiac rupture, mortality, and timing of thrombolytic therapy: A meta analysis. J Am Coll Cardiol 16:359, 1990.

40. Hutchins, GM: Pathological changes in aortocoronary bypass grafts. Annu Rev Med 31:289, 1980.
41. Jugdutt, BI and Warnica, JW: Tolerance with low dose intravenous nitroglycerin therapy in acute myocardial infarction. Am J Cardiol 64:581–587, 1989.
42. Katz, AM: Basic cellular mechanisms of action of the calcium channel blockers. Am J Cardiol 55:2B, 1985.
43. Kennedy, JW, et al: The Western Washington intravenous streptokinase in acute myocardial infarction randomized trail. Circulation 77:345, 1988.
44. Killip, T III and Kimbal, JT: Treatment of myocardial infarction in a coronary care unit: A two year experience with 250 patients. Am J Cardiol 20:457, 1967.
45. King, EG and Chin, WDN: Shock: An overview of pathophysiology and general treatment goals. Crit Care Clin 1:547, 1985.
46. Kones, RJ and Benninger, GW: Digitalis therapy after acute myocardial infarction. Heart Lung 4:99, 1975.
46a. Krusteal, JB, et al: Fibrin and fibrinogen-related antigens in patients with stable and unstable coronary artery disease. N Engl J Med 317:1361, 1987.
47. Kuhn, LA: The treatment of cardiogenic shock: The nature of cardiogenic shock. Am Heart J 74:578, 1967.
48. Lee, TH, et al: Ruling out acute myocardial infarction: A prospective multicenter validation of a 12-hour strategy for patients at low risk. N Engl J Med 324:1239, 1991.
49. Leon, MB, et al: Combination therapy with calcium-channel blockers and beta blockers for chronic stable angina pectoris. Am J Cardiol 55:69B, 1985.
50. Littman, D: Textbook of Electrocardiography, Harper & Row, New York, 1972.
51. Loeb, HS, et al: Effects of low-flow oxygen on the hemodynamics and left ventricular function in patients with uncomplicated acute myocardial infarction. Chest 60:352, 1971.
52. McAllister, RG, Jr, et al: Pharmacokinetics of calcium-entry blockers. Am J Cardiol 55:30B, 1985.
53. Mellion, BT, et al: Inhibition of human platelet aggregation by S-nitrothiols: Heme dependent activation of soluble guanylate cyclase and stimulation of cyclic GMP production. Mol Pharmacol 23:653–664, 1983.
54. Moss, AJ and Benhorin, J: Prognosis and management after a first myocardial infarction. N Engl J Med 322:743, 1990.
55. Mueller, HS: Treatment of acute myocardial infarction. In Shoemaker, WC, Thompson, WL, and Holbrook, PR (eds): Textbook of Critical Care. WB Saunders, Philadelphia, 1984, p 403.
56. Najafi, H, et al: Surgical management of complications of myocardial infarction. Med Clin North Am 57:205, 1973.
57. Norris, RM: Prognosis in myocardial infarction. Heart Lung 4:75, 1975.
58. Novitsky, D, et al: Triiodothyronine in the recovery of stunned myocardium in dogs. Ann Thorac Surg 51:10, 1991.
59. Ornato, JP: Role of the emergency department in decreasing the time to thrombolytic therapy in acute myocardial infarction. Clin Cardiol 13:48, 1990.
60. Ott, P and Fenster, P: Combining thrombolytic agents to treat acute myocardial infarction (editorial). Am Heart J 12:1583, 1991.
61. Paidipaty, BB, Husian, M, and Puri, VK: Right coronary artery occlusion after acute proximal dissection (hematoma). Crit Care Med 11:574, 1983.
62. Pfeffer, MA, Lamas, GA, and Vaughn, DE: Effect of captopril on progressive ventricular dilatation after anterior myocardial infarction. N Engl J Med 319:80–86, 1988.
63. Pratt, CM, Mahmarian, JJ, and Young, JB: Changing trends in the approach to acute myocardial infarction. In Civetta, JM, Taylor, RW, and Kirby, RR (eds): Critical Care. JB Lippincott, Philadelphia, 1988, p 909.
64. Rahimtoola, SH and Gunnar, RM: Digitalis in acute myocardial infarction: Help or hazard. Ann Intern Med 82:234, 1975.
65. Rahimtoola, SH, et al: Relationship of pulmonary artery to left ventricular diastolic pressures in acute myocardial infarction. Circulation 46:283, 1972.
66. Rao, TLK, Jacobs, KH, and El-Etr, AA: Reinfarction following anesthesia in patients with myocardial infarction. Anesthesiology 59:499, 1983.
67. Rasmussen, AS, et al: Intravenous magnesium in acute myocardial infarction. Lancet 1:234–236.
68. Report of the Holland Inter-university Niefedipine/Metoprolol Trial (HINT) Research Group: Early treatment of unstable angina in the coronary care unit: A randomized, double blind, placebo controlled comparison of recurrent ischemia in patients treated with nifedipine or metoprolol or both. Br Heart J 56:400–413, 1986.
69. Resnekov, L: Hemodynamic effects of acute myocardial infarction. Med Clin North Am 57:234, 1973.
70. Rigotti, NA, et al: Exercise and coronary heart disease. Annu Rev Med 34:391, 1983.
71. Ring, ME, Corrigan, JJ, and Fenster, PE: Antiplatelet effects of oral diltiazem, propranolol and their combination. Br J Clin Pharmacol 24:615–620, 1987.
72. Roberts, R and Marmor, AT: Right ventricular infarction. Annu Rev Med 34:377, 1983.

73. Roberts, R, et al: Specificity of elevated serum MB creatinine phosphokinase activity in the diagnosis of acute myocardial infarction: The stiff heart syndrome. Am J Cardiol 36:433, 1985.

74. Robertson, TL, et al: Aspirin, rt-PA, and reperfusion in AMI: A TIMI observational study (abstract). Circulation 78: Suppl II:128, 1988.

75. Ruskin, JN: The cardiac arrhythmia suppression trial (CAST) (editorial). N Engl J Med 321:386, 1989.

75a. Sarnoff, SJ, et al: Hemodynamic determinants of oxygen consumption of the heart with special reference to the tension time index. Am J Physiol 192:148, 1958.

76. Serruys, PW, et al: Angiographic follow-up after placement of a self-expanding coronary artery stent. N Engl J Med 324:13, 1991.

77. Shabetai, R, Fowler, NO, and Guntheroth, WG: The hemodynamics of cardiac tamponade and constrictive pericarditis. Am J Cardiol 47:224, 1981.

78. Sharma, B, et al: Addition of intracoronary prostaglandin E_1 to streptokinase improves thrombolysis and left ventricular function in acute myocardial infarction (abstract). J Am Coll Cardiol (Suppl A)11:104A, 1988.

79. Shepherd, JT and Vanhoutte, PM: Spasm of the coronary arteries: Causes and consequences (the scientist's viewpoint). Mayo Clin Proc 60:30, 1985.

80. Sherry, S: Unresolved clinical pharmacologic question in thrombolytic therapy for acute myocardial infarction. J Am Coll Cardiol 12; 2:519, 1988.

81. Sibbald, WJ and Driedger, AA: Right ventricular function in acute disease states: Pathophysiologic considerations. Crit Care Med 11:339, 1983.

82. Smith, P, Arnesen, H, and Holme, I: The effect of warfarin on mortality and reinfarction after myocardial infarction. N Engl J Med 323:147, 1990.

83. Spence, MI and Lemberg, L: Shock following acute myocardial infarction. Heart Lung 2:582, 1973.

84. Stone, HL, et al: Control of the coronary circulation during exercise. Annu Rev Physiol 45:214, 1983.

85. Swan, HJC: The role of hemodynamic monitoring in the management of the critically ill. Crit Care Med 3:83, 1975.

86. Talley, JD, Hurst, JW, King, SB III, et al: Clinical outcome 5 years after attempted percutaneous transluminal coronary angioplasty in 427 patients. Circulation 77:820, 1988.

87. Tarhan, S, Moffitt, EA, Taylor, WF, et al: Myocardial infarction after general anesthesia. JAMA 220:1451, 1972.

88. The TIMI Study Group: Comparison of invasive and conservative strategies after treatment with intravenous tissue plasminogen activator in acute myocardial infarction. N Engl J Med 320:618, 1989.

89. Topol, EJ, et al: Combined prostacyclin and tissue plasminogen activator therapy for acute myocardial infarction: Evidence for a new drug-drug interaction (abstract). Circulation (Suppl II)78:308, 1988.

90. Trip, MD, et al: Platelet hyperreactivity and prognosis in survivors of myocardial infarction. N Engl J Med 322:1549, 1990.

91. Turpie, AGG, et al: Comparison of high-dose with low-dose subcutaneous heparin to prevent left ventricular mural thrombosis in patients with acute transmural anterior myocardial infarction. N Engl J Med 320:352, 1989.

92. Uchida, Y, et al: Recanalization of obstructed coronary artery by intracoronary administration of prostacyclin in patients with acute myocardial infarction. Adv Prostaglandin Thromboxane Leukotriene Res 11:377, 1983.

93. Unger, T and Gohlike, P: Tissue renin angiotension systems in the heart and vasculature: possible involvement of the cardiovascular actions of converting enzyme inhibitors. Am J Cardiol 65:31–101, 1990.

94. Van Gilst, WH, et al: Differential influences of angiotensin converting enzyme inhibitors on the coronary circulation. Circulation (suppl I) 77:24–29, 1988.

95. Vohra, J: Beta-adrenergic blockade in arrhythmias of acute myocardial infarction. Heart Lung 2:662, 1973.

96. Webster, MAI, et al: Effect of enalapril on ventricular arrhythmias in congestive heart failure. Am J Cardiol 56:566–569, 1985.

97. Weisfeldt, L, Chandra N: Physiology of cardiopulmonary resuscitation. Annu Rev Med 32:435, 1981.

98. Wight, TN: Proteoglycans in pathological conditions: Atherosclerosis. Fed Proc 44:381, 1985.

99. Winniford, MD, et al: Calcium antagonists for acute ischemic heart disease. Am J Cardiol 55:116B, 1985.

100. Zelis, R and Flaim, SF: Calcium blocking drugs for angina pectoris. Annu Rev Med 33:465, 1982.

100a. Zbilut, JP and Lawson, L: Decreased heart rate variability in significant cardiac events. Crit Care Med 16:64, 1988.

CHAPTER 3

Arrhythmias

I. THE NORMAL ELECTRO-CARDIOGRAM

The electrocardiogram (ECG) is a graphic representation of the electrical activity of the heart. As the depolarization wave, also commonly called the cardiac impulse, passes through the heart, electrical currents spread out from the heart to the surface of the body. During the process of "depolarization," the normal negative potential inside the cell is lost and the membrane potential reverses and becomes slightly positive. If the net electrical force is toward a given electrode, the resultant deflection of the ECG by convention is positive (up). If it is away from the given electrode, the resultant deflection is negative (down).

The normal electrocardiogram is composed of a P wave, a QRS complex, and a T wave (Fig. 3.1). The QRS complex is a summation of three separate waves: the Q wave, the R wave, and the S wave.

A. P WAVE

The P wave, representing atrial depolarization, is normally up to 0.10 second wide and 3.0 mm tall. It is normally positive in all ECG leads except aVR. A positive P wave in aVR indicates that a junctional rhythm is present, the leads are misplaced, or the patient has dextrocardia. The PR interval from the beginning of the P wave to the beginning of the QRS complex represents conduction of the electrical impulse from the sinoatrial (SA) node to the atrioventricular (AV) node. It is normally 0.12 to 0.20 second wide. The PR segment is the isoelectric portion between the P wave and QRS complex. A prolonged PR interval indicates a first-degree heart block.

B. QRS COMPLEX

The QRS complex represents ventricular depolarization. The Q wave is normally a small initial downward deflection (before an R wave) after the PR segment. If the Q wave has a width of 0.04 second or greater and is at least one third the height of the QRS complex, it is considered to be abnormal. An abnormal Q wave is usually due to a myocardial infarction or a conduction abnormality.

AXIOM

The presence of abnormal Q waves should be considered evidence of myocardial infarction until proven otherwise.

The S wave is the first downward deflection after the R wave. Ventricular depolarization begins at the septum and proceeds from the left side of the septum to the right. Consequently, septal depolarization is reflected in a small initial upright deflection (R wave) in the right lateral precordial leads. Depolarization then proceeds simultaneously through both ventricles, from the endocardial to the epicardial surface.

Since the left ventricle has a larger mass than the right, the resultant electrical force of ventricular depolarization is the left. Thus, a normal-size heart that is in the correct position provides a small R wave and deep downward

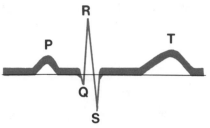

Figure 3.1 Typical ECG configuration.

deflection (S wave) in the early precordial leads (V_1 and V_2). In the lateral precordial leads (V_5 and V_6), the R waves become progressively taller and the S waves smaller.

The QRS complex is normally 0.06 to 0.10 second wide. A delay in ventricular conduction, such as right or left bundle-branch block results in a widened QRS complex. The QRS complex also tends to be wide if ventricular depolarization does not begin at the AV junction. The farther below the AV junction that the ventricular impulse originates, the wider the QRS complex and the slower the inherent heart rate. Impulses originating in the ventricle (so-called idioventricular beats) are characterized by a QRS complex of greater than 0.14 second in width with a bizarre shape and a rate of usually only 30 to 40 beats per minute. In addition, tachyarrhythmias can usually be diagnosed as being ventricular in origin if the QRS complex is widened to more than 0.12 second.

AXIOM

Repeated wide complexes may be an early warning of impending ventricular fibrillation.

The intrinsicoid deflection reflects the depolarization of muscle just beneath the recording electrode. It is measured by determining the time from the onset of the QRS to the peak of the R wave. In the right precordial leads (V_1V_2), the normal intrinsicoid deflection is 0.02 to 0.05 second.

C. INTERVAL

The QT interval, from the beginning of the Q wave to the end of the T wave, represents the refractory period of the heart. Its duration varies inversely with the heart rate and averages about 0.40 second. At 60 beats per minute the normal upper limit of the QT interval is 0.43 second and at 100 beats per minute, it is 0.35 second. It is generally thought that hypocalcemia is associated with a prolonged QT interval and that hypercalcemia is associated with a shortened QT interval. However, some investigators feel that such changes are related primarily to the heart rate. Other factors prolonging the QT interval are myocardial ischemia and quinidine. The QT interval can be shortened by digitalis, propranolol, and phenytoin.

PITFALL

Treating a prolonged QT interval with calcium in a relatively stable patient without first checking ionized calcium levels.

D. ST SEGMENT

The ST segment and T wave represent ventricular repolarization. Repolarization can be affected by a number of hemodynamic and metabolic factors as well as drugs and cardiac disease. For example, acute ischemia, increased intraventricular pressure, or increased thickness of the myocardial wall (such as with ventricular hypertrophy) may cause the ST segment and T wave to be inverted or negative. A scooped, pulled-down appearance of ST segment is characteristic of digitalis preparations. However, digitalis tends to shorten the QT interval and ischemia tends to prolong it.

PITFALL

Assuming that "nonspecific ST-T wave changes" are not important.

E. U WAVE

Although the U wave is often not seen on a normal ECG, it can be a normal component and may represent a ventricular afterpotential. It is most prominent in leads V_1 and V_2, and it is most likely to be seen in hypokalemia and coronary artery disease.

PITFALL

If the T wave is flat and the U wave is prominent, the ECG might be read as showing a prolonged Q-T interval (as with hypocalcemia) rather than hypokalemia, resulting in treatment opposite to that needed.

F. HIS BUNDLE ELECTRO-CARDIOGRAM

Conduction of impulses to the AV node, bundle of His, and Purkinje system can be studied with a special multiple-electrode catheter that is passed through a vein to the right side of the heart and manipulated into a position close to the tricuspid valve. The record of the electrical activity obtained with this catheter is called the His bundle electrogram (HBE). It normally shows an A deflection when the AV node is activated, an H spike during transmission through the His bundle, and a V deflection during ventricular depolarization (Fig. 3.2).

With the HBE and standard electrocardiographic leads, it is possible to accurately determine three intervals: (1) the PA interval, the time from the first appearance of atrial depolarization to the A wave in the HBE, which represents conduction time from the SA node to the AV node; (2) the AH interval, from the A wave to the start of the H spike, which represents the AV nodal conduction time; and (3) the HV interval, the time from the start of the H spike to the start of the QRS deflection in the ECG, which represents conduction in the bundle of His and the bundle branches out to the myocardium. The approximate normal values for these intervals in adults are PA 27 msec, AH 92 msec, and HV 43 msec.

G. PRINCIPLES OF VECTORIAL ANALYSIS OF ELECTRO-CARDIOGRAMS

Before it is possible to understand how cardiac abnormalities affect the contours of waves in the electrocardiogram, one must first become familiar with the concept of vectors and vectorial analysis as applied to electrical currents flowing in and around the heart. A vector is an arrow that points in the direction of current flow at a given instant in the cardiac cycle with the arrowpoint in the positive direction. Also, by convention, the length of the arrow drawn is proportional to the voltage generated by the current flow.

1. Use of Vectors to Represent Electrical Potentials

When a vector is directed horizontally toward the subject's left side, it is said that the vector extends in the direction of 0°. From this zero reference point, the scale of vectors rotates clockwise; when the vector is pointing straight down, it is said

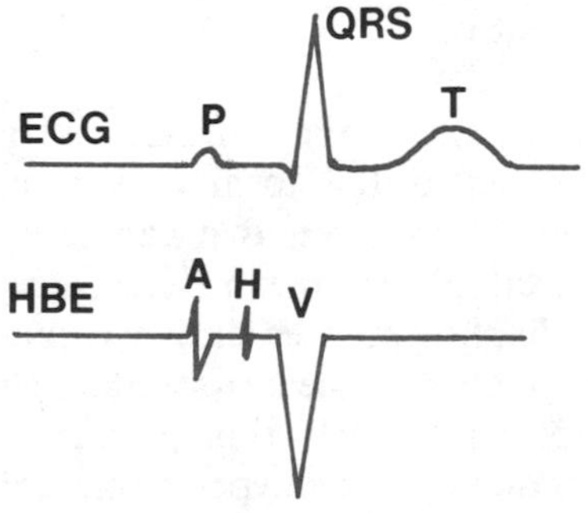

Figure 3.2 Diagram of simultaneous recordings of the surface electrocardiogram (ECG), the His bundle electrogram (HBE) which shows activity recorded from the atrium (A), the His spike (H), and the ventricle (V).

121

to have a direction of $+90°$; when the vector points horizontally to the right, it has a direction of $+180°$; and, when it extends straight upward, it is said to have a direction of $-90°$.

2. Denoting the Direction of a Vector in Terms of Degrees

In a normal heart the average direction of the vector of the heart during spread of the depolarization wave through the ventricles is called the mean QRS vector. This vector averages approximately $60°$. This means that during most of the depolarization wave, the apex of the heart remains positive with respect to the base of the heart.

Each of the three bipolar leads (I, II, III) and each of the three unipolar limb leads (aVR, aVL, aVF) actually represent the voltage gradient across a pair of electrodes connected to the body on opposite sides of the heart. The direction from the negative to the positive electrode is called the axis of the lead. Lead I is recorded from two electrodes placed on the two arms. Since the electrodes lie in the horizontal direction with the positive electrode to the left, the axis of lead I is $0°$. Lead II, obtained from electrodes on the right arm and left leg, is considered to have a vector of approximately $60°$.

By a similar analysis, lead III has an axis of approximately $120°$, lead aVR $210°$, aVF $90°$, and aVL $-30°$. The directions of the axis of all these different leads are shown in diagrams referred to as the hexagonal reference system (Fig. 3.3). When the cardiac vector is perpendicular to the axis of a lead, the voltage recorded in the electrocardiogram of that lead is very low. On the other hand, when the cardiac vector is in the same axis or direction as the lead, the entire voltage of the vector will be recorded on that lead.

3. Vectors Occurring during Depolarization of the Ventricles

When the cardiac impulse enters the ventricles through the bundle of His, the first part of the ventricles to become depolarized is the left endocardial surface of the septum. The depolarization then spreads rapidly to involve both endocardial surfaces of the septum. The wave of depolarization then continues along the endocardial surfaces of the two ventricles. Finally, it spreads through the ventricular muscle to the outside (epicardial surface) of the heart.

4. The Electrocardiogram during Repolarization

Once ventricular muscle has become depolarized, approximately 0.15 second elapses before sufficient repolarization is present to be observed in the electrocardiogram. Repolarization then proceeds throughout the ventricular muscle until it is complete about 0.35 to 0.40 second after the onset of the QRS complex. It is this process of repolarization that causes the T wave in the electrocardiogram.

The portion of ventricular muscle to repolarize first is the outer surface of the ventricles, especially near the apex of the heart. The endocardial areas normally repolarize last.

Because the outer and apical surfaces of the ventricles repolarize before the inner and basal surfaces, the positive end of the heart vector during repolarization is toward the apex of the heart. As a result, the T wave in the bipolar limb leads is normally positive.

5. Abnormal Ventricular Conditions That Cause Axis Deviation

Although the electrical axis of the ventricles averages approximately $60°$, it can swing to the right or left in the normal heart approximately $20°$. In addition, there are a number of conditions that can cause axis deviation beyond these normal limits. For example, the mean electrical axis of the heart tends to shift to the left when the diaphragm rises during expiration and when a person lies down. Likewise, angulation of the heart to the right can occur during inspiration when standing, especially in tall, thin persons whose hearts hang downward. When the muscle of one ventricle hypertrophies, the axis tends to deviate toward the hypertrophied ventricle.

When the left bundle branch is blocked, cardiac depolarization spreads

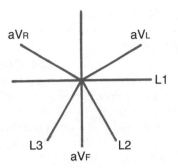

Note: After you have memorized the foregoing method of drawing the hexaxial system, the extensions to the negative electrodes should be put in as dotted lines; e.g.,

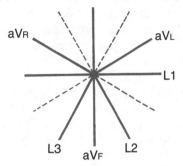

An entire lead on the hexaxial system stretches from the positive electrode through the electrical center to the negative electrode.

Then imagine a body superimposed on it with the arms slightly raised 30° and each leg 30° from the vertical.

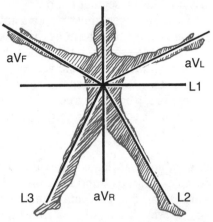

The hands and feet are the positive electrode sites.

Figure 3.3 The hexagonal reference system. (From Constant, J: Learning Electrocardiography, ed 3. Little, Brown & Co, Boston, 1987, p 40, with permission.)

through the right ventricle two to three times as rapidly as through the left ventricle. Thus, the right ventricle becomes electronegative while the left ventricle remains electropositive during most of the depolarization process. Consequently, a very strong positive vector projects from the right ventricle toward the left ventricle, producing intense left axis deviation. When the right bundle branch is blocked, the left ventricle depolarizes far more rapidly than the right ventricle so that intense right axis deviation occurs.

H. CONDITIONS THAT CAUSE ABNORMAL VOLTAGES OF THE QRS COMPLEX

The most common cause of high-voltage QRS complexes is increased muscular mass of the heart, usually from hypertrophy of the cardiac muscle in response to an excessive load, such as hypertension or aortic stenosis.

There are three major causes of decreased voltage in the electrocardiogram. These include (1) abnormalities of cardiac muscle that prevent generation of adequate quantities of current, (2) conditions around the heart reducing the ease with which current can be conducted to the surface of the body, and (3) rotation of the apex of the heart to point toward the anterior chest wall so that the electrical current of the heart flows mainly anteroposteriorly in the chest rather than in the frontal plane of the body.

I. CURRENT OF INJURY

Cardiac abnormalities, especially those that damage the heart muscle itself, can cause part of the heart to remain partially or totally depolarized all the time. When this occurs, current flows between the pathologically depolarized and the normal polarized areas, producing a so-called current of injury. The injured part of the heart is electronegative because it is depolarized and emits negative charges while the remainder of the heart is positive.

Some of the abnormalities that can cause a current of injury include (1) mechanical trauma, which makes the membranes remain so permeable that full repolarization cannot take place, (2) infectious processes that damage the muscle membranes, and (3) ischemia of local areas of muscle caused by coronary occlusion. Ischemia is by far the most common cause of a current of injury.

1. ST-Segment Changes

If one places the vector of the current of injury directly over the ventricles, the negative end of the vector points toward the permanently depolarized or "injured" area of the ventricles. When a current of injury occurs in one of the electrocardiographic leads, one finds that the ST segment and the TP segments of the electrocardiogram are not at the same potential levels in the record. Actually, it is the TP segment and not the ST segment that is shifted away from the zero axis. However, most persons are conditioned to consider the TP segment of the electrocardiogram as the reference potential level rather than the J point, which is the exact point at which the wave of depolarization completes its passage through the heart at the very end of the QRS complex. At that time, all parts of the ventricles are depolarized so that no current is flowing around the heart. Therefore, when a current of injury is evident in an electrocardiogram, it looks as if the ST segment is shifted from its normal level, and this is called an ST-segment shift (Fig. 3.4).

2. Q-Wave Changes

Usually an abnormal (large and wide) Q wave develops at the beginning of the QRS complex in leads I and aVL in established anterior infarctions because of transmural loss of muscle mass in the anterior wall of the left ventricle. In contrast, in established inferior transmural infarctions, an abnormal Q wave develops at the beginning of the QRS complex in leads II, III, and aVF because of loss of muscle in the inferior or diaphragmatic portion of the ventricle.

J. ABNORMALITIES IN THE T WAVE

The T wave is caused by repolarization of the epicardium at the apex of the heart before the endocardial surfaces of the bases of the ventricles. Consequently, it is normally positive in all of the standard bipolar limb leads. When conduction of the impulse through the ventricles is greatly delayed, the T wave is almost always of a polarity opposite to that of the QRS complex. Thus, if conduction does not occur through the Purkinje system, the rate of conduction is slowed, and the T wave is of opposite polarity to that of the QRS complex. This occurs whether the condition causing this delayed conduction is left bundle branch block, right bundle branch block, or premature ventricular contractions.

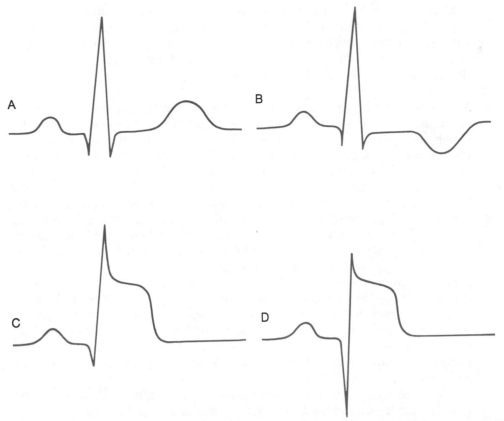

Figure 3.4 Sequential ECG changes following an acute coronary obstruction: (*A*) normal; (*B*) reversible ischemia, T wave inversion, and depression of the J point; (*C*) injury pattern, elevation of the ST segment; (*D*) infarction pattern, development of an abnormal Q wave.

II. ABNORMAL RHYTHMS

Abnormal cardiac rhythms can be caused by (1) abnormal rhythmicity of the SA pacemaker, (2) shift of the pacemaker from the SA node to the other parts of the heart, (3) blocks at different points in the transmission of the impulse through the heart, (4) abnormal pathways of impulse transmission through the heart, and (5) spontaneous generation of abnormal impulses in other parts of the heart.

A. ABNORMAL RHYTHMICITY OF THE SA PACEMAKER

The sick sinus syndrome is characterized as disorganized rhythms with multiple atrial ectopic beats along with periods of junctional rhythm or junctional premature beats with irregular P waves. However, it may be manifested by a wide variety of rhythm changes and may be intermittent so that 24-hour or longer Holter monitoring may be required for the diagnosis. It may also manifest itself as a sinus bradycardia and intermittent runs of atrial tachycardia or atrial fibrillation (so-called tachy-brady syndrome). This arrhythmia may be seen after cardioversion in patients with chronic atrial fibrillation and often indicates that atrial fibrillation is about to recur. Palpitations or fainting may occur, and if such symptoms are recurrent, an atrioventricular pacemaker may be required.

B. SHIFT OF PACEMAKER FROM SA NODE

Supraventricular tachycardia (SVT) is a regular rapid rhythm that arises from either a re-entry pathway or from an ectopic pacemaker above the AV node, in the AV node, or at its junction with the bundle of His. The SVT may be paroxysmal or nonparoxysmal. If P waves are seen before the QRS complex, the arrhythmia is considered to be an atrial tachycardia. If the P wave cannot be seen or occurs after the QRS, it is referred to as a junctional tachycardia.

C. HEART BLOCKS

A block between the atria and the ventricles can result from localized damage or depression of the AV node or the bundle of His. This may be caused by excessive vagal stimulation (which depresses conductivity in the junctional fibers), localized destruction of the AV bundle (as a result of a myocardial infarction), or depression of conduction caused by various drugs.

D. ABNORMAL PATHWAYS

Normally, when the cardiac impulse has traveled throughout the heart, the rest of the heart is temporarily refractory to repeat stimulation and the impulse simply disappears. The heart then remains quiescent until a new signal begins in the SA node. However, under certain conditions, the cardiac impulse travels around in a circuit in cardiac muscle or conduction fibers without stopping. This phenomenon is called re-entry or circus movement.

Three conditions that facilitate circus movement or the re-entry phenomenon include (1) increased length of the pathway around the circle, (2) decreased velocity of conduction, and (3) shortened refractory period of the heart muscle. These three conditions allow the impulse to stimulate responsive cardiac tissue again and begin another impulse. Thus, re-entry occurs when impulses encounter a slower or longer path of conduction with a one-way block so that when the impulses emerge, the cardiac tissue is ready to be stimulated again. This can occur with a variety of heart problems. For example, a long pathway frequently occurs in dilated hearts. A decreased rate of conduction frequently results from ischemia of muscle or high serum potassium levels. A shortened refractory period frequently occurs in response to drugs, such as epinephrine, or following repetitive electrical stimulation.

Two especially serious rhythms caused by circus movement or re-entrant impulses are flutter and fibrillation. Flutter means a rapid heart beat at rates of about 200 to 350 beats per minute but with reasonably coordinated contractions of the cardiac muscle. This type of rhythm occurs frequently in the atria but only rarely in the ventricles. Fibrillation is different from flutter in that it has an even higher rate and the contractions are uncoordinated. Because of these uncoordinated contractions, the involved portions of the heart fail to pump an adequate quantity of blood.

E. SPONTANEOUS GENERATION OF ABNORMAL IMPULSES

If a small area of the heart becomes much more excitable than normal, it can cause an abnormal impulse to be generated during the interval between normal impulses. This can occur in either the atria or the ventricles. This impulse starts a depolarization wave which spreads outward from the irritable area and causes a premature contraction of the heart. The point from which the abnormal impulse started is called an ectopic focus.

1. Premature Contractions — Ectopic Foci

Some of the more frequent causes of an ectopic focus include local muscle ischemia, overuse of stimulants such as caffeine or nicotine, lack of sleep, and anxiety. However, in many instances, especially when there is ischemia, the ectopic focus is caused by a re-entrant signal that comes around again after being delayed for a short period of time by slow transmission of the action potential in ischemic muscle. This signal then re-enters the ventricular muscle shortly after the heart muscle has repolarized from the previous beat.

2. Tachycardias

Sometimes an ectopic focus becomes so irritable that it establishes a rhythmic contraction of its own at a more rapid rate than that of the SA node. When this occurs, the ectopic focus becomes the pacemaker of the heart. In most such instances, the repetitive rhythm is caused by re-entrant signals that have been established as small circus movements out from the ectopic focus, into more normal muscle, and then back into the irritable area again. A common site for development of an ectopic pacemaker is the AV node itself, which can establish a re-entrant pathway within its own boundaries and cause a very rapid rate of contraction. The resulting rhythm has been referred to as paroxysmal supraventricular, AV nodal, junctional, or reciprocating tachycardia.

3. Afterdepolarizations

Under certain conditions, most notably intracellular calcium overload, oscillations in the transmembrane potential may occur. These "afterdepolarizations" may be recorded either during phase 3 (early afterdepolarizations) or during the early part of phase 4 (late afterdepolarizations). Should these afterdepolarizations reach threshold, a new action potential will be generated, and under appropriate conditions, it will be propagated to adjacent cells. Early and late afterdepolarizations may also be observed in response to hypothermia, electrolyte imbalance, catecholamine excess, or dilatation of a cardiac chamber.

III. SIGNIFICANCE OF ARRHYTHMIAS

The two most serious possible consequences of cardiac arrhythmias are sudden electrical death (due to ventricular fibrillation) or impaired cardiac function that leads to shock or heart failure. Various arrhythmias, such as PVCs, particularly in patients with myocardial ischemia, may suddenly become more frequent or multifocal. Such PVCs may quickly convert to a ventricular tachycardia and then ventricular fibrillation unless treated rapidly and aggressively. One of the main reasons that patients with an acute myocardial infarction (AMI) are placed in a coronary care unit (CCU) is so that premonitory ECG changes, such as increasing PVCs, can be diagnosed and treated promptly.

In otherwise normal individuals, cardiac output and organ blood flow can be maintained at relatively normal levels with pulse rates as low as 40 per minute or as high as 160 per minute. However, in patients with moderate to severe valvular disease (such as mitral stenosis) or significant (70% to 80%) coronary arterial occlusion, otherwise insignificant arrhythmias can decrease coronary blood flow below the critical levels necessary for myocardial function and/or viability.

Certain arrhythmias are more dangerous than others. For example, premature atrial or ventricular contractions may reduce carotid or coronary blood flow only by 8% to 12%, but atrial fibrillation, particularly if associated with a rapid ventricular response, may reduce cardiac output by as much as 20% to 40%. During ventricular tachycardia, coronary blood flow may fall as much as 60%.

Artucio and Pereira recently noted that 78% of 2820 consecutive ICU patients had arrhythmias. This ranged from 44% in trauma patients to 90% in patients with cardiovascular disease. The mortality rates with various arrhythmias was as follows: atrial tachyarrhythmias (40%), nodal rhythm (44%), ventricular bradyarrhythmias (77%), and ventricular rapid rhythms (51%). The relative risk of dying with these rhythms was increased 16% to 120% when compared to patients without arrhythmias.

IV. CLASSIFICATION OF ARRHYTHMIAS

Cardiac arrhythmias may be classified into two major categories: (1) disorders of pacemaker function and impulse formation, and (2) disorders of impulse conduction.

A. DISORDERS OF PACEMAKER FUNCTION

The SA node, which is located at the junction of the superior vena cava and right atrium, normally has the highest inherent rate of generating electrical cardiac impulses and will depolarize the slower pacemakers in the AV node or ventricle before they can develop their own beat. The exact mechanism by which these impulses are generated in the SA node is not known but is probably related to periodic spontaneous inward movements of sodium and calcium.

If the SA node does not generate impulses at a rapid enough rate, escape ectopic rhythms from lower pacemakers (junctional or idioventricular) with a slower intrinsic rate may appear. On the other hand, excessively rapid impulse formation from other areas of the heart may override the SA node and produce atrial, junctional, or ventricular tachycardias. Many of these tachyarrhythmias are produced because small areas of altered conductivity in the heart produce re-entry pathways or localized circus movements.

Proper treatment of an arrhythmia involves not only diagnosis of the abnormality and knowledge of the various forms of therapy, but also correction of possible etiologic factors. Excessive emotional or physical stress, coffee, tea, alcohol, or tobacco may increase the tendency for many arrhythmias. In addition, hypoxia, acidosis, alkalosis, potassium and calcium abnormalities, renal insufficiency, and disorders of the thyroid or adrenal glands may cause treatment to be ineffective or hazardous until they are corrected. Whenever an arrhythmia is present, a careful history for ingestion of drugs, such as digitalis, thyroid extract, and amphetamines, is particularly important.

1. Supraventricular Arrhythmias

a. Sinus Arrhythmias

Normal sinus rhythm is present when the impulses generated from the SA node occur at a regular rate of 60 to 100 per minute and are properly conducted (Fig. 3.5A). The heart rate in normal individuals is usually slightly irregular because of moment-to-moment variations in venous return, ventilation, and vagal tone. During inspiration, as the right heart distends because of an increased venous return, the heart rate tends to accelerate, and during expiration, it tends to slow.

When the difference in the time interval between the two fastest contiguous beats and two slowest contiguous beats is greater than 0.12 second, a sinus arrhythmia is said to exist. Sinus arrhythmias are common in young, healthy individuals but may have pathological significance in older individuals (Fig. 3.5B).

b. Sinus Bradycardia

A sinus rhythm of less than 60 per minute, referred to as sinus bradycardia, is usually caused by excessive vagal tone due to a variety of circumstances. It is most frequently seen in healthy, young athletes but may also be seen in myxedema and in some elderly patients with coronary atherosclerosis.

Sinus bradycardia is seldom less than 45 per minute and usually has little hemodynamic significance. However, if it occurs during the first few hours after an acute posterior myocardial infarction and if ventricular filling and/or stroke volume is reduced for any reason, the slow rate may reduce cardiac output to dangerously low levels (Fig. 3.6A).

Any circulatory reflex that stimulates the vagus nerve can cause the heart rate to decrease. Perhaps the most striking example of this occurs in patients with the carotid sinus syndrome. An arteriosclerotic plaque at the bifurcation of the common carotid artery causes excessive sensitivity of the pressure receptors (baroreceptors) located there. As a result, mild pressure on the neck may elicit a strong baroreceptor reflex, causing intense vagal stimulation of the heart and extreme bradycardia. Indeed, at times this reflex is so powerful that it can cause syncope or cardiac standstill (Fig. 3.6B).

PITFALL
Attempts to correct an asymptomatic bradycardia, especially in a patient who may have coronary artery disease.

c. Sinus Tachycardia

When the rate of normally conducted beats arising at the SA node exceeds 100 per minute, a sinus tachycardia is said to be present. Since the PR intervals tend to remain normal regardless of the heart rate, in a severe tachycardia the P waves can fall on the preceding T waves and obliterate the TP segment. Sinus tachycardia, in contrast to most of the other supraventricular tachyarrhythmias, seldom exceeds 160 per minute in adults at rest or 200 per minute in children (Fig. 3.7).

PITFALL
Attempting to slow a tachycardia without first determining its etiology.

Rate		Rhythm	Duration	
Ventricular	60–100	R-R regular	PR Interval .12–.20 sec	
Atrial	60–100	P-P regular	QRS Complex .06–.10 sec	

INTERVENTIONS: None

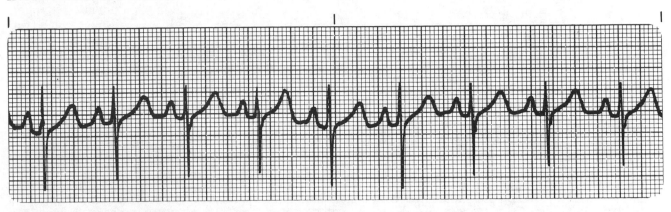

A   Lead II

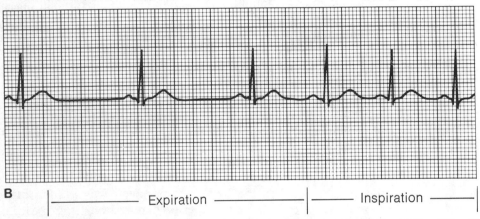

B |——————— Expiration ——————|—— Inspiration ——|

Figure 3.5 (*A*) Normal sinus rhythm. (From Dolan, JT: Critical Care Nursing. FA Davis, Philadelphia, 1991, p 807, with permission.) (*B*) Sinus arrhythmia. Note that the heart rate tends to rise during inspiraton and slow during expiration.

The most frequent cause of a sinus tachycardia is excessive sympathetic stimulation due to fear, pain, anxiety, exercise, or fever. As a general rule, each degree centigrade rise in temperature increases the pulse rate 18 per minute. Various drugs with atropine or catecholamine activity can also cause a sinus tachycardia.

When the rate is greater than 160 per minute, differentiation between tachycardias of sinus and atrial origin can be difficult. In sinus tachycardia, the heart rhythm tends to vary slightly with the ventilatory cycle. In contrast, abnormal atrial tachycardias tend to remain perfectly regular. Carotid sinus massage tends to produce only a gradual and temporary slowing of sinus tachycardias, but it will either have no effect on an atrial tachycardia or will cause it to cease abruptly. Treatment of sinus tachycardia primarily involves correcting underlying factors such as infection, pain, and hypoxia.

***d. Atrial Ectopic Beats
Rhythm Strip***

Any impulse arising in the atria outside the SA node is referred to as an ectopic atrial beat. With ectopic beats, the P wave occurs at a different time than the P wave that originates in the SA node, and it has a different shape. When it occurs as a premature beat, it is referred to as a premature atrial contraction (PAC). This is the most frequent form of atrial ectopic beat. The most common causes

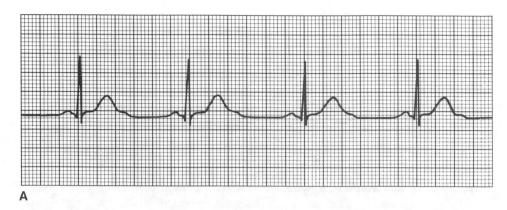

A

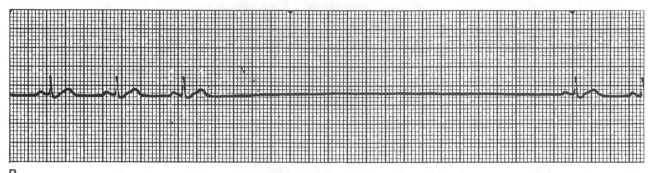

B

Figure 3.6 (*A*) Sinus bradycardia. (*B*) Sinus arrest (Part B from Brown, KR: Mastering Dysrhythmias. FA Davis, Philadelphia, 1988, p 41, with permission.)

of this arrhythmia include emotional stress, alcohol, coffee, digitalis, ischemia, or fluid overloads.

Atrial ectopic beats can usually be differentiated from those arising in the ventricles because the compensatory pause after an atrial ectopic beat is usually not complete unless the basic rate is rapid. This is in contrast to the full compensatory pause of ventricular premature beats (Fig. 3.8). In addition, the QRS complex seen with ectopic atrial beats is usually identical to those occurring with normal atrial conduction. Because aberrant ventricular conduction occurs, ectopic ventricular beats usually appear as wide, bizarre QRS complexes, completely different from normally conducted beats.

Atrial ectopic beats are seldom of hemodynamic significance, but they may prove troublesome to patients who are very concerned about their palpitations. The psychological symptoms in such patients can often be controlled by tranquilizers or sedatives. Nevertheless, if the premature atrial contractions are

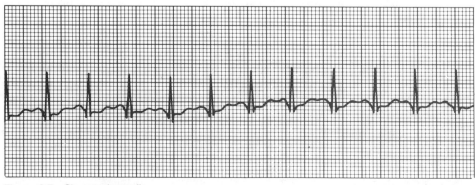

Figure 3.7 Sinus tachycardia.

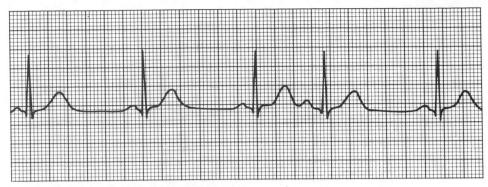

Figure 3.8 Atrial ectopic beats.

numerous or multifocal, problems such as atrial tachycardia, atrial flutter, or atrial fibrillation may develop. Quinidine can be given in an attempt to convert the rhythm to normal. If congestive heart failure is the underlying cause, treatment of the cardiac failure usually stops the arrhythmia.

e. Atrioventricular Junctional (Nodal) Premature Beats

Impulses arising prematurely in the area of the AV node are referred to as junctional or nodal premature beats. Although it has traditionally been taught that junctional impulses arise from within the AV junction, the pacemaker cells for most of the junctional rhythms actually probably lie in the bundle of His.

Junctional P waves may occur before (Fig. 3.9) or just after the QRS (Fig. 3.10) complex, or they may be absent. The P wave will be absent if atrial and ventricular activation is completed simultaneously or if there is a block of retrograde conduction in the atria.

The P wave in a junctional premature contraction is different from the P wave of normal sinus rhythm (Fig. 3.10). It is usually inverted in leads II, III, and aVF, and upright in leads I, aVR, and aVL. The PR interval with junctional beats is 0.12 second or less. Multifocal junctional premature contractions can also occur. In these, the P wave, PR interval, and possibly even the QRS complex will vary in configuration. There may or may not be a compensatory pause following a junctional premature contraction. The QRS complex is identical to that of a normally conducted beat unless aberrant ventricular conduction occurs or there is pre-existing bundle-branch block.

Junctional premature contractions may occur as isolated beats or in multiples of two, three, or more. They may occur in patients without heart disease, but tend to be associated with congestive heart failure, digitalis intoxication, coronary artery disease, or acute myocardial infarction, especially of the inferior wall.

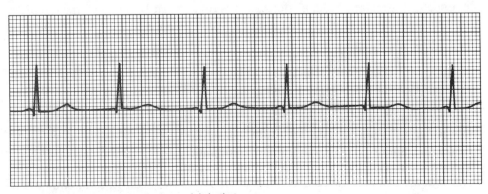

Figure 3.9 Upper atrioventricular nodal rhythm.

131

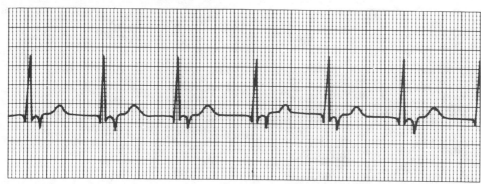

Figure 3.10 Lower nodal rhythm.

Treatment is directed to the underlying cause. If due to heart failure, the treatment is digitalis, diuretics, and fluid and salt restriction. If digitalis-induced, the drug must be stopped, and potassium and magnesium should generally be given. If the arrhythmia persists and causes symptoms, quinidine or procainamide may be helpful.

AXIOM

An arrhythmia developing while a patient is on a digitalis preparation should be considered as due to that drug until proven otherwise.

f. Nodal Rhythm

If the SA node persistently fails to form impulses or if the impulses are not transmitted to the AV node, the AV node may take over the pacemaker function of the heart at a slightly slower rate of about 50 to 70 beats per minute. Such a rhythm may occur following an acute posterior myocardial infarction or after various surgical procedures that cause excessive vagal tone. The ECG changes seen are similar to those found with the AV junctional (nodal) premature beats.

Treatment varies with the cause and symptoms. If the patient is asymptomatic, treatment is unnecessary. If the nodal rhythm is excessively slow, angina or Stokes-Adams attacks may occur, and atropine may be of value. If nodal rhythm is associated with acute myocardial infarction, correction of any hypertension or heart failure may revert the rhythm to normal. If a reasonable possibility of digitalis toxicity exists, the digitalis preparation should be discontinued and, if necessary, potassium and magnesium should be administered carefully.

2. Re-entry Supraventricular Tachycardias

a. Pathophysiology of Re-entry

The main tachyarrhythmias clearly due to re-entry are those due to accessory bundles. The re-entry tachycardias tend to be paroxysmal. About 50% to 60% of patients with re-entry tachycardias have the paroxysms of re-entry sustained by circuits within the AV node, and about 20% to 30% have accessory bypass connections that are "hidden" during sinus rhythm. In 10% to 20% the circuit is unclear. In about half of the accessory bypass connections, the AV node participates as part of the circuit.

The electrophysiologic explanation for sustained re-entry within the AV node hypothesizes that there are two functionally different pathways creating a re-entry loop (Fig. 3.11). One pathway, termed the alpha pathway, has a slow conduction and a short refractory period, and the other pathway, called the beta pathway, has faster conduction and a longer refractory period. About 90% of sustained AV nodal re-entry appear to have the impulse propagated antegradely down the alpha (slow) pathway and retrogradely up the beta (fast) pathway. Because the atrial depolarization occurs soon after ventricular depolarization through the fast pathway, the ECG evidence of atrial depolarization frequently is hidden in the QRS complex or is visible just after the QRS complex. In patients

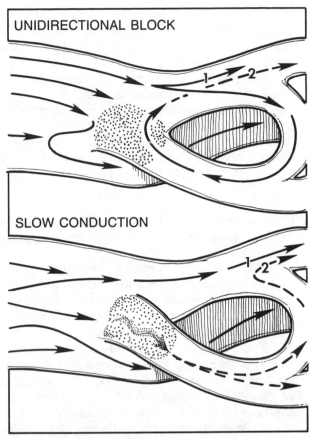

UNIDIRECTIONAL BLOCK

SLOW CONDUCTION

Figure 3.11 Disturbances in impulse conduction, re-enty phenomena. Unidirectional block: The conduction of an impulse travels down the open pathway and depolarizes the surrounding myocardium; it may find the previously blocked or refractory pathway excitable, thereby generating another wave of depolarization (broken arrow). Pathway of slow conduction; an impulse (solid arrows) traveling through an area of slow conduction may emerge to find the surrounding myocardium repolarized, and therefore capable of generating another wave of depolarization (broken arrows). (From Dolan, JT: Critical Care Nursing. FA Davis, Philadelphia, 1991, p 806, with permission.)

with concealed bypass connections, the re-entry circuit is formed by the normal AV node and infranodal conducting system, which propagate the impulse antegradely, and the bypass connection, which carries the signal retrogradely back into the atrium.

b. Diagnosis

Re-entry tachycardias are usually paroxysmal and tend to occur in individuals with no evidence of structural heart disease. They may, of course, also be seen with one of the pre-excitation syndromes. Occasionally they are seen with rheumatic heart disease, acute pericarditis, acute myocardial infarction, or even mitral valve prolapse. The symptoms generally consist of palpitations and/or light-headedness. A history of similar attacks beginning and ending abruptly may be very helpful. Even if the BP is normal, cardiac output is often reduced.

Re-entrant SVT can be differentiated from other narrow QRS tachycardias about 80% of the time on the surface ECG. The rate is usually 160 to 200 beats per minute, and if there is an alteration in the QRS complex, a bypass connection has been revealed. If the P wave cannot be seen, it is a re-entrant nodal tachycardia. If the P wave occurs after the QRS, it is a re-entrant tachycardia using a concealed bypass connection.

Of the patients with the Wolff-Parkinson-White (WPW) syndrome who develop tachycardia, 80% will have paroxysmal atrial tachycardia (PAT). In the WPW syndrome with PAT, if antegrade conduction proceeds down the normal pathway, the QRS configuration is normal. Under such circumstances, PAT due to the WPW syndrome will not be distinguishable from other types of PAT during the tachycardia. However, the ECG during normal sinus rhythm will generally give the diagnosis of WPW.

Re-entrant SVT can usually be converted by impeding conduction through one limb of the re-entry circuit. Maneuvers that increase vagal tone, by slowing conduction through the AV node and prolonging its refractory period, will tend to break the circuit. Initially, vagal stimulation often causes a slowing of the ventricular rate, followed by a sudden termination of the SVT and resumption of sinus rhythm. Vagal stimulation with other types of SVT may also result in slower ventricular rates, but the SVT continues.

AXIOM

Vagal maneuvers should not be attempted in patients with digitalis toxicity because they may cause ventricular fibrillation which may be difficult to correct.

The most frequent vagal-stimulating maneuvers include:

1. The Valsalva maneuver, which involves bearing down with a closed glottis after a deep breath. This should be done quite strenuously for at least 10 seconds. This may be the simplest therapeutic maneuver and should be repeated if necessary.

2. Carotid sinus massage (CSM), in which one attempts to massage the carotid sinus against the transverse processes of the cervical vertebrae. CSM must be done very carefully, especially in someone with possible cerebrovascular disease. It should be done for only 10 seconds at a time, and should be attempted first on the side of the nondominant cerebral hemisphere.

3. Facial immersion in cold water (diving reflex). This is usually done for at least 30 seconds and may be especially helpful in infants. The duration of time that the breath is held is more critical than the temperature of the water.

4. Tickling the back of the throat. This is considered by some physicians to be the simplest and most effective technique.

5. Pressing on the eyeballs. This can damage the eyes, and its use is generally discouraged now.

AXIOM

Carotid sinus massage should never be done simultaneously on both sides.

CSM should be viewed as a possible risky procedure. It may cause a prolonged AV block in patients who have AV node disease or are on digitalis. CSM in patients with carotid artery stenosis may cause cerebral ischemia or infarction, especially if done too vigorously.

c. Treatment

If the patient has angina or any hemodynamic instability such as hypotension, heart failure, or evidence of decreased cerebral perfusion (seizures, coma, confusion, etc.), the SVT is best treated by immediate synchronized cardioversion. If the patient has been taking a digitalis preparation, one should start with 10 joules (watt-sec) and increase by 10 joules each time if additional shocks are necessary. In other patients, one can begin with 50 joules. Cardioversion can release digitalis into the blood from various storage sites.

AXIOM

Synchronized cardioversion should be avoided or is performed with less energy in patients who are on digitalis preparations.

If the patient is stable, one can try the various vagal maneuvers. If the re-entrant SVT in a stable patient is resistant to the vagal maneuvers or is rapidly recurrent, there are several drugs that can be helpful.

1. Verapamil is the drug of choice if there is no abnormal conduction pathway. One can give 0.075 to 0.15 mg/kg (5 to 10 mg in adults) IV over 30 to 60 seconds with a repeat dose in 30 minutes if necessary. Studies have found that more than 90% of adults with re-entrant SVT will respond within 1 to 2 minutes to verapamil.

2. Edrophonium can be used to increase parasympathetic tone. A 1.0-mg IV test dose is given. If there are no adverse reactions in the next 3 to 5 minutes, one can give 5 to 10 mg IV over 60 seconds.

3. Vasoconstrictors can be used to enhance vagal tone by pharmacologically elevating blood pressure. Agents, such as epinephrine, that have beta-adrenergic activity should not be used. This method can be combined with carotid sinus massage. Blood pressure should be monitored frequently, and diastolic and systolic pressures should not be allowed to exceed 120 mm Hg or 180 mm Hg, respectively. This method should not be used if hypertension is already present. The vasoconstrictors used most frequently include:

  a. Metaraminol (200 mg/500 ml D_5W) or norepinephrine (4 mg/500 ml D_5W) at rates of 1 to 2 ml/min and increased slowly until the rhythm converts or the blood pressure limits are reached.

  b. Methoxamine or phenylephrine 0.5 to 1.0 mg IV over 2 to 3 minutes with repeat doses are required.

4. Propranolol 0.5 to 1.0 mg IV slowly over 60 seconds and repeated every 5 minutes until the rhythm converts or the total IV dose reaches 0.1 mg/kg. Historically, propranolol has about a 50% success rate in converting re-entrant SVT.

AXIOM

Beta-blocking drugs should not be given or should be given very cautiously if any heart failure or bronchospasm is present.

5. Digoxin 0.5 mg IV with repeat doses of 0.25 mg every 30 to 60 minutes until a response occurs or the total dose reaches 0.02 mg/kg. The chief drawback of digoxin is the long delay in the onset of its action and the potential hazards in patients with accessory (bypass) tracts.

3. Ectopic Supraventricular Tachycardia

The tachycardias associated with ectopic foci or increased automaticity include paroxysmal atrial tachycardia with block, nonparoxysmal junctional tachycardia, and multifocal atrial tachycardia.

a. Pathophysiology

Ectopic SVT usually originates in the atria but may begin anywhere above the bundle of His. It represents an atrial rate of 100 to 250 beats per minute (most commonly 140 to 200), with regular P waves, and often AV block. Ectopic SVT is most apt to be seen in patients with acute myocardial infarction, COPD, pneumonia, alcohol intoxication (holiday heart), and as a manifestation of digitalis toxicity. With digitalis toxicity, there is almost always AV block, and even though the arrhythmia is not paroxysmal, it is usually referred to as *PAT with block*.

b. Diagnosis

Clues to the existence of ectopic SVT include (1) presence of pre-existing cardiac disease, especially if treated with digoxin; (2) gradual (rather than abrupt) onset and disappearance of the arrhythmia; (3) presence of AV block; and (4) increased AV block and slowing of the ventricular rate in response to vagal maneuvers.

AXIOM

Any patient on digitalis who suddenly notices palpitations or a change in heart rhythm should be considered to have PAT with block until proven otherwise.

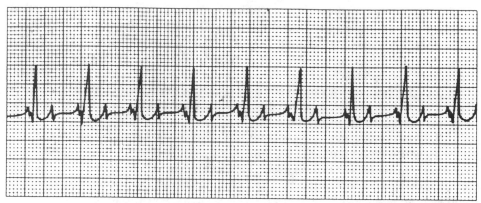

Figure 3.12 PAT with block.

The ventricular rate in PAT with block may be either fast or slow, depending upon the amount of AV block. Thus, clinical diagnosis may be extremely difficult. ECG diagnosis may also be a problem (Fig. 3.12). If there is a 2 : 1 block and a P wave is hidden in the QRS complex, it may even resemble normal sinus rhythm. If the atrial rate is very rapid, the ECG pattern may closely resemble atrial flutter; however, in atrial tachycardia with block, the atrial rate seldom exceeds 220 per minute, whereas atrial flutter is seldom less than 280 per minute.

Carotid sinus massage, by increasing the AV block and slowing the ventricular rate, may help the physician examine ventricular complexes on the ECG. Examination of II, III, and aVF may be particularly helpful.

Another type of ectopic supraventricular tachycardia is referred to as non-paraoxysmal AV junctional tachycardia or accelerated AV junctional rhythm (Fig. 3.13). It generally has a gradual onset and a ventricular rate of only 70 to 130 per minute. It is usually caused by digitalis toxicity or occasionally by a posterior or inferior myocardial infarction. When this arrhythmia is associated with an acute myocardial infarction, the mortality rate may be quite high. Since the ventricular rate is usually less than 130, rapid aggressive therapy is generally not required.

c. Treatment

The treatment of ectopic SVT can be divided into (1) ectopic SVT due to digitalis toxicity and (2) ectopic SVT not due to digitalis toxicity.

Ectopic SVT due to digitalis toxicity is treated by:
1. Discontinuing the digitalis.
2. Correcting hypokalemia as long as there is not a high-grade AV block

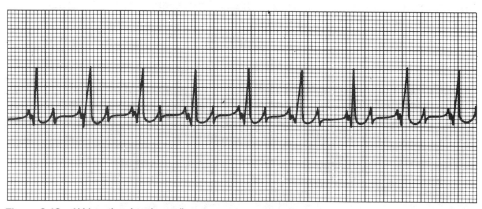

Figure 3.13 AV junctional tachycardia.

with a slow ventricular response. One can give 10 to 20, and occasionally (with great care) up to 40 mEq of potassium per hour IV with continuous ECG monitoring. If there is no or only a partial cardiac response to treating hypokalemia, one should try 1.0 to 2.0 g of MgSO$_4$ IV over the next 2 to 4 hours.

3. Phenytoin (Dilantin) can be infused intravenously at a rate less than 50 mg/min until either the desired response is achieved, the total dose reaches 15 to 18 mg/kg, or early signs of toxicity, such as nystagmus or ataxia, develop.

4. IV lidocaine may be effective.

5. Cardioversion is *not* effective and is potentially hazardous.

Ectopic SVT *not* due to digitalis toxicity is treated by:

1. Digoxin to control the ventricular response.

2. Quinidine or procainamide to reduce atrial ectopy once ventricular rate control has been achieved.

3. Cardioversion. This may be very effective, but one must be sure the patient is not in digoxin toxicity.

PITFALL

Use of cardioversion in a hemodynamically stable patient with possible digitalis toxicity.

4. Multifocal Atrial Tachycardia

Multifocal atrial tachycardia (MAT) is also known as chaotic atrial rhythm or wandering atrial pacemaker. The ECG characteristics are (1) two or more types of ectopic P waves, (2) varying PR intervals, (3) atrial rates or 90 to 250 beats per minute, and (4) frequent nonconducted ectopic P waves (Fig. 3.14). Because of the variation in the P-wave morphology, MAT may easily be confused with atrial flutter or fibrillation. Multifocal atrial tachycardia generally occurs in seriously ill, elderly patients with severe chronic lung disease, cor pulmonale, or pneumonia. Occasionally MAT may be a manifestation of digitalis intoxication.

Treatment is directed to the underlying disorder. Severe chronic lung disease should be treated aggressively along with correction of any hypoxemia, acidosis, or electrolyte imbalances that may be present. If serum theophylline or digoxin levels are elevated, they should be permitted to return to normal.

Although multifocal atrial tachycardia is usually quite resistant to drug treatment, it is often responsive to cardioversion. Of the various drugs, propranolol has usually been considered the drug of choice. Metoprolol also appears to be effective therapy for acute or chronic multifocal atrial tachycardia, and serious adverse effects are infrequent. Recent studies suggest that verapamil can safely reduce ventricular rate in many of these patients, and MgSO$_4$ 1.0 to 2.0 g IV over 5 to 15 minutes followed by 1 to 2 g/h to a total of 4 to 8 g can often abolish or reduce atrial ectopy and ventricular rates.

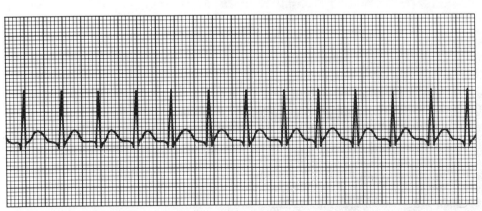

Figure 3.14 Multifocal atrial tachycardia.

5. Atrial Flutter

While most experimental evidence implicates re-entry as the mechanism of atrial flutter, clinical studies have been inconclusive and are consistent with either an ectopic focus or re-entry. Atrial flutter most commonly originates in a small localized region of the atria, usually the inferior right atrium. It is usually found only in patients with severe congestive heart failure, but also may be seen in association with chest pain or cerebrovascular symptoms (due to emboli).

The ECG itself is frequently diagnostic, as a typical "sawtooth" pattern seen best in I, II, and aVF, particularly if the atrial rate is 250 to 300 per minute (Fig. 3.15). Almost invariably, an AV block of some type (usually 2:1) is present, and the ventricular rate is usually about 140 to 160 per minute. However, if "improved" AV conduction suddenly allows all the atrial impulses to reach the ventricle, this will result in a severe ventricular tachycardia. This is most apt to occur in patients receiving quinidine without digitalis or in the WPW syndrome.

Carotid sinus massage may be helpful in making a diagnosis. This often increases the atrial rate slightly, but it may decrease AV conduction with temporary slowing of the ventricular rate (Fig. 3.16). The slowing of the ventricular rate often makes the typical sawtooth pattern become more obvious

The treatment of choice is now generally considered to be synchronized, direct-current cardioversion. If cardioversion is not used, rate control is achieved with digoxin, and then quinidine or procainamide can be used to slow or convert the arrhythmia chemically. If atrial flutter has persisted for only a few hours and the patient is in no distress, rapid digitalization over the next 24 hours may effect a conversion. When the ventricular rate has been controlled by digoxin but atrial flutter persists, a decision must be made either to push the digoxin to near toxic levels or to hold digoxin and try cardioversion.

Intravenous verapamil will convert atrial flutter into sinus rhythm about 30% of the time. Although it may convert the flutter into atrial fibrillation about 20% of the time, it will achieve ventricular rate control in about 90%. Intravenous flecainide will convert atrial flutter to sinus rhythm in about 40% of cases.

6. Atrial Fibrillation

a. Pathophysiology

In atrial fibrillation multiple areas of the atria are continuously contracting and recovering. This results in what appears to be a "quivering" of the atria with no effective contractions. Several theories have been proposed to explain its development, including the circus-movement theory, the ectopic focus theory, and the multiple re-entry theory. According to the circus-movement theory, a primary activation or impulse follows a circular path around the ostia of the two cavea, with irregular daughter waves given off erratically to depolarize the atria. According to the ectopic focus theory, one or more atrial sites initiate impulses at an extremely rapid rate. According to the multiple re-entry theory, an ectopic or sinus impulse occurs in a vulnerable period and causes flutter or fibrillation, which is perpetuated by the development of multiple re-entries and multiple

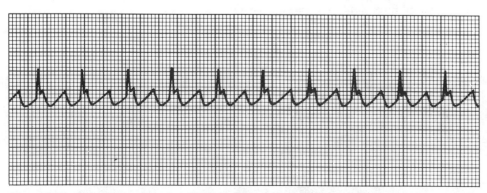

Figure 3.15 Atrial flutter with a 2:1 AV block. Note the sawtooth pattern.

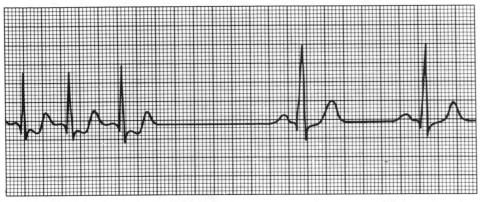

Figure 3.16 PAT response to carotid massage.

simultaneous circulating waves, each with its own "gap" and a "head" which is chasing its "tail."

b. Clinical Significance

Atrial fibrillation is usually persistent, chronic, and associated with cardiomyopathy or ischemic, hypertensive, or valvular heart disease. All these conditions can cause left atrial enlargement, a state that appears necessary for the maintenance of chronic atrial fibrillation. Occasionally, atrial fibrillation presents acutely following a myocardial infarction or cardiac surgery or in patients with the sick sinus (tachy-brady) syndrome.

In patients with decreased left ventricular function, the left atrial contraction at the end of diastole makes an important contribution to cardiac output, and the loss of effective left atrial contraction may precipitate heart failure. The stasis of blood in the atria in atrial fibrillation predisposes patients to the development of atrial thrombi, with the risk of subsequent pulmonary or systemic embolization. The incidence of embolism in chronic atrial fibrillation is about 30%, being somewhat higher in patients with mitral valvular or ischemic heart disease. Conversion from chronic atrial fibrillation to sinus rhythm carries a risk of 1% to 2% systemic embolization at the time of conversion regardless of which form of therapy is used to stop the fibrillation. Therefore, 2 weeks of anticoagulation are usually recommended prior to elective cardioversion. It also seem prudent to consider anticoagulation prior to conversion with antiarrhythmic drugs.

About 2% to 3% of patients with atrial fibrillation have no evidence of cardiac disease by history, physical examination, electrocardiogram, or chest radiograph, and such patients are said to have "lone atrial fibrillation." These patients are usually under the age of 60 years and have a lower risk of stroke than other patients with atrial fibrillation. Consequently, routine anticoagulation of such individuals may not be warranted.

c. Diagnosis

Atrial fibrillation is characterized by absent P waves and irregular oscillations of the baseline called *f* or fibrillation waves. The atrial rate is greater than 350 beats per minute. However, a variable amount of block is generally present so that even in untreated atrial fibrillation the ventricular rate seldom exceeds 150 to 170 per minute (Fig. 3.17). More rapid ventricular rates of 200 or more may be seen with the WPW syndrome or thyrotoxicosis.

If the ventricular rate is rapid, the QRS complex may be widened due to aberrant conduction because the rapidly firing atrial impulses find the conduction system of the ventricles in a relatively refractory state. Ventricular aberration may also occur with a long-short cycle sequence (Ashman's phenomenon) (Fig. 3.18). When atrial fibrillation occurs in the WPW syndrome, the QRS

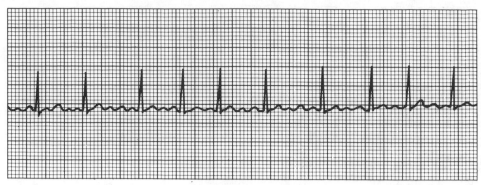

Figure 3.17 Atrial fibrillation.

complex is usually widened due to antegrade conduction along the aberrant pathway.

AXIOM

Any irregular irregularity of the heart rate and rhythm should be considered as due to atrial fibrillation until proven otherwise.

The rhythm of the ventricular contractions in patients with atrial fibrillation is extremely irregular. Because some ventricular contractions are feeble, a significant "pulse deficit" may exist between the apical heart rate and the palpable radial pulse rate.

If there is a problem with the diagnosis, carotid sinus massage increases the block at the AV node and slows the ventricular rate so that the underlying atrial rhythm may be much more obvious (Fig. 3.19).

d. Treatment

Whenever possible, atrial fibrillation should be controlled in order to (1) improve cardiac function, which may be reduced by 20% to 40% in some patients; (2) reduce the incidence of systemic emboli from clots forming in the left atrium; and (3) reduce the palpitations, which can be extremely bothersome to some patients. Treatment goals usually include controlling the underlying problem (particularly mitral valve disease) and slowing the ventricular rate to 70 to 80 per minute with digitalis.

If there is a rapid ventricular rate and the patient has hypotension, pulmonary edema, or chest pain, synchronized cardioversion should be attempted. However, if the ventricular rate is slow, no attempt should be made to revert the patient to normal sinus rhythm. If the patient is on digitalis, the digitalis should be discontinued and the ventricular rate watched closely to see if it rises.

Digitalis toxicity should be suspected with atrial fibrillation if the patient has (1) a slow ventricular rate (particularly less than 50 per minute), (2) a regular ventricular rate (implying some degree of AV block with an escape AV junctional pacemaker), or (3) frequent PVCs, especially ventricular bigeminy.

Pharmacologic control of the ventricular response during atrial flutter and atrial fibrillation in hemodynamically stable patients with the Wolff-Parkinson-

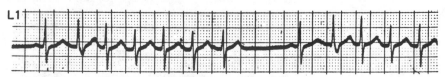

Figure 3.18 Ashman's phenomenon. (From Constant, J: Learning Electrocardiography, ed 3. Little, Brown & Co, Boston, 1987, p 486, with permission.)

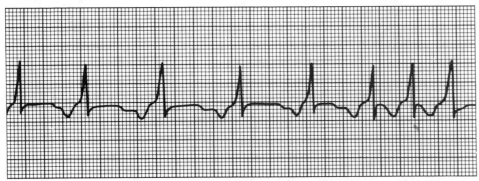

Figure 3.19 Atrial fibrillation. Carotid sinus massage increases the block at the AV node and slows the ventricular rate.

White syndrome requires depression of conduction and prolongation of refractoriness in the anomalous AV connection. Intravenous procainamide, 50 mg/min to a total dose of 10 to 20 mg/kg, followed by a constant infusion at 2 to 6 mg/min is the therapy of choice. Intravenous lidocaine treatment may also be effective in certain patients.

Medications that exert a depressive action on the AV node but not the anomalous AV connection may cause deleterious effects when ventricular pre-excitation is present. Intravenous digitalis therapy has a variable effect on the refractory period of anomalous AV connections and, in some cases, may actually shorten it and thereby accelerate the ventricular response. Beta-adrenergic blocking agents have little effect on conduction in the anomalous AV connection, while intravenous verapamil therapy may indirectly shorten the refractory period of the anomalous AV connection by a reflex sympathetic discharge in response to verapamil-induced hypotension. Intravenous verapamil has been reported to have provoked degeneration of atrial flutter and atrial fibrillation in the setting of ventricular pre-excitation into ventricular fibrillation.

PITFALL
Use of verapamil when atrial fibrillation may be associated with an anomalous AV connection.

Intravenous digitalis and verapamil should be considered contraindicated in the acute treatment of atrial flutter and atrial fibrillation associated with ventricular pre-excitation.

7. Ventricular Arrhythmias

Any cardiac impulse conducted from the atria is considered to be an ectopic ventricular beat. Since ventricular ectopic beats usually occur before sinus impulses would ordinarily reach the ventricle, they are also often referred to as premature ventricular contractions (PVCs) or ventricular premature beats (VPBs).

a. Ventricular Premature Beats (Premature Ventricular Contractions)

(1) Clinical Significance

VPBs are generally considered to be important because they may go on to cause ventricular tachycardia or ventricular fibrillation. However, VPBs are not uncommon, even in persons without evidence of heart disease. Nevertheless, VPBs are often seen in patients with ischemic heart disease and are nearly universal during the acute phase of myocardial infarction. VPBs are also common in digitalis toxicity and congestive cardiomyopathies and appear to be exacerbated by hypokalemia, alkalosis, hypoxia, and sympathomimetic agents.

Although available evidence suggests that repetitive VPBs (two or more in a row) increase the risk for sudden death in patients with coronary artery disease, the evidence for single or multiform VPBs is less convincing. Therefore, in the ambulatory setting, the decision to treat chronic VPBs involves assessing the patient for the extent of the ventricular ectopy, evidence of heart disease, and presence of symptoms to determine the likelihood that the PVCs may contribute to future morbidity. Some authors feel that most patients do not require specific antiarrhythmic therapy for single PVCs, regardless of how frequent or multiform.

In the setting of acute myocardial ischemia, the presence of VPBs may reflect the underlying electrical instability of the heart and indicate that the patient is a risk for primary ventricular fibrillation. It was previously thought that patients at risk for developing ventricular fibrillation had more serious degrees of VPBs (so-called warning arrhythmias), and that this would help select those patients who require extra monitoring or treatment. However, these warning arrhythmias are not always present before ventricular fibrillation.

In the setting of possible or definite acute myocardial ischemia, most physicians treat VPBs with intravenous lidocaine—not only to suppress ectopy, but also to prevent the occurrence of ventricular tachycardia or fibrillation. Some physicians also treat patients with a suspected acute myocardial infarction prophylactically with lidocaine prior to the detection of any ventricular ectopy. Depending on the underlying disease, the risk of subsequent ventricular fibrillation, and the degree of protection offered by treatment, it is likely that a large number of patients would have to receive prophylactic lidocaine treatment to prevent just one occurrence of ventricular fibrillation.

(2) Diagnosis

VPBs are characterized by a wide QRS complex (greater than 0.12 second), lack of preceding P wave, and an ST segment and T wave directed opposite to the major QRS deflection (Fig. 3.20). If the impulse from a VPB activates the atria, a P wave follows the QRS complex. Unless the rhythm is parasytolic, there is a constant coupling interval between the normal beat and the VPB, and the VPB is usually followed by a full compensatory pause. A ventricular fusion beat is a beat resulting from a simultaneously occurring sinus impulse and ventricular ectopic impulse. Its configuration is midway between the two.

PITFALL
Use of lidocaine to suppress ventricular ectopic beats when the basic ventricular rate is very slow.

(a) Escape beats

If the basic ventricular rate is less than 60 per minute, the ventricular ectopic beats may be an escape phenomenon and essential to life (Fig. 3.21). Under such circumstances, lidocaine is contraindicated; however, atropine or isoproterenol may help by increasing heart rate and thereby automatically suppressing the ectopic beats.

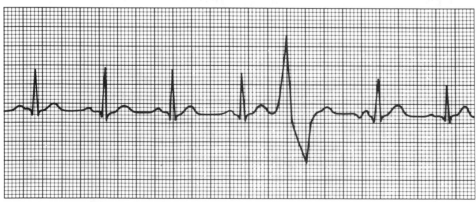

Figure 3.20 Ventricular ectopic beat.

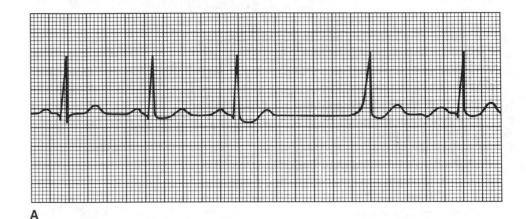

A

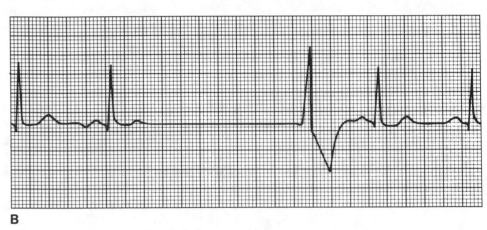

B

Figure 3.21 (*A*) Nodal and (*B*) ventricular escape beats.

(b) Interpolated Premature Ventricular Contractions	Another less frequent type of PVC is the interpolated beat that occurs between two consecutive normal sinus beats and does not interrupt the basic sinus rhythm. There is no compensatory pause, and this is truly an "extra" systole. The interpolated PVC usually occurs only if the sinus rate is relatively slow. With a rapid sinus rate, the ventricles and/or conducting system would be refractory to the first sinus impulse occurring after the premature beat.
(c) Premature Atrial Contraction with Aberrant Ventricular Conduction	If a premature atrial or AV nodal beat occurs soon after a preceding sinus beat, it may reach the bundle of His and its branches before they have completely recovered from the previous impulse. Since repolarization may not be perfectly uniform, some portions of the conducting system may handle the impulse normally while other areas may not. Consequently, the impulse may take an aberrant pathway through the ventricle, producing a bizarre, widened QRS complex. If a premature P wave can be seen in front of an abnormal QRS complex, the premature atrial impulse with aberrant ventricular conduction can be readily differentiated from the usual type of PVC (Fig. 3.22).

Differentiation between ectopic beats of ventricular origin and those of supraventricular origin but conducted aberrantly can be difficult, especially in sustained tachycardias with wide QRS complexes. Several guidelines might help in this distinction.

1. A preceding ectopic P wave is good evidence favoring aberrancy; however, coincidental atrial and ventricular ectopic beats or retrograde conduction can occur. AV dissociation suggests ventricular origin.

2. A fully compensatory pause after the beat in question is more likely after a ventricular beat, but exceptions do occur.

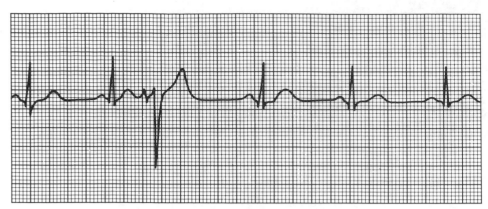

Figure 3.22 Premature atrial contraction with aberrant conduction.

3. Fusion beats are good evidence for ventricular origin, but exceptions do occur.

4. A varying bundle branch block pattern suggests aberrancy.

5. Coupling intervals are usually constant with ventricular ectopic beats, unless parasystole is present. Varying coupling intervals suggest aberrancy.

6. Carotid sinus massage will slow conduction through the AV node and may abolish re-entrant SVT and slow the ventricular response in other types of supraventricular tachyarrhythmias. Carotid sinus massage has essentially no effect on ventricular ectopy.

7. A QRS duration of longer than 0.14 second is usually found only in ventricular ectopy.

8. Aberration should be suspected if there is an RSR in V_1 or QRS in V_6.

(d) Parasystole

Parasystole may also be confused with VPBs. This is the occurrence of an independent cardiac pacemaker that is protected from the influence of the main pacemaker. A parasystolic pacemaker can arise anywhere in the heart, but it is most often located in the ventricles and is independent of the basic cardiac rhythm. Impulses arising from the main cardiac pacemaker do not influence the parasystolic focus (Fig. 3.23).

Diagnostic criteria of parasystole are (1) varying coupling intervals, (2) a constant interectopic beat interval, and (3) frequent fusion beats. Since the parasystolic and main pacemaker are firing independently, the interval between a normal beat and the parasystolic beat will vary, as opposed to fixed coupling intervals between a normal beat and a PVC. Unlike other ventricular arrhythmias, ventricular parasystole can sometimes be affected by carotid massage. Accelerated idioventricular rhythm is a form of parasystolic rhythm.

Ventricular parasystole is most often associated with coronary artery or hypertensive heart disease, acute myocardial infarction, or electrolyte imbalance. Parasystole is usually self-limited and is related to the underlying cardiac

V_1

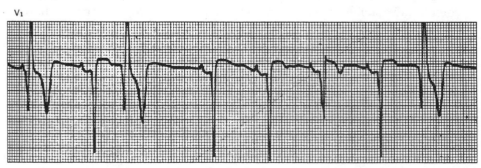

Figure 3.23 Parasystole.

disease. It is believed that the arrhythmia itself does not contribute to mortality or morbidity and may not require treatment.

(3) Treatment of Ventricular Premature Beats

Forney and Forney have recently emphasized that the majority of patients with VPBs are not in need of antiarrhythmic treatment. However, treatment should be considered for repetitive or early VPBs. Treatment of PVCs may involve a number of antiarrhythmic agents, but must also be directed at the underlying cardiac disease, which may include coronary insufficiency, hypoxia, heart failure, digitalis excess, epinephrine, caffeine, or amphetamines.

Ventricular ectopic beats associated with any of the following may be dangerous and should generally be treated quite aggressively.

1. The VPBs occur at, or just prior to, the peak of a T wave (R on T phenomenon).

2. There are more than 6 to 8 VPBs per minute.

3. The VPBs are multifocal.

4. A tachycardia is present.

5. The VPBs occur in bigeminy or trigeminy

6. The VPBs occur following an acute myocardial infarction.

If these criteria are present, lidocaine is given IV aggressively as two boluses of 1 mg/kg 5 minutes apart while an IV drip of 4 mg/min is started. If VPBs recur or continue, additional boluses (to a total of four or five) may be given. The lidocaine drip can be gradually tapered over the next 24 hours if no more VPBs occur. If there is an inadequate response to lidocaine, procainamide may be given. If digitalis toxicity is suspected, IV potassium chloride (KCl) should be given, possibly with magnesium and/or dilantin.

Although type-I antiarrhythmic agents, such as flecainide and encainide, have been shown to reduce the number of VPBs, the Cardiac Arrhythmia Suppression Trial (CAST) showed that the use of these agents to treat asymptomatic or minimally symptomatic arrhythmias in patients after myocardial infarction is associated with a substantial increase in the sudden-death rate and total mortality. However, beta blockers have consistently been shown to reduce mortality, despite the fact that they have little or no effect on VPBs.

It is important to emphasize that ventricular escape beats in the face of a ventricular bradycardia should not be treated with lidocaine. Atropine, isoproterenol, or a pacemaker should, however, be considered.

b. Accelerated Idioventricular Rhythm

Accelerated idioventricular rhythm (AIVR) is an ectopic rhythm of ventricular origin occurring at rates of 40 to 100 per minute. Even though AIVR is not a tachycardia, such terms as idioventricular tachycardia, nonparoxysmal ventricular tachycardia, or slow ventricular tachycardia have been applied to it.

The ECG characteristics of AIVR are (1) wide and regular QRS complexes, (2) rate between 40 and 100 (often close to the preceding sinus rate), (3) runs of short duration (usually only 3 to 30 beats), and (4) often beginning with a fusion beat (Fig. 3.24).

(1) Clinical Significance

AIVR most commonly occurs after an acute myocardial infarction, but it may also be seen in patients without heart disease. While there is some variable association with ventricular tachycardia, there is no apparent association with ventricular fibrillation. AIVR usually produces no symptoms itself. However, loss of atrial contraction may cause some fall in cardiac output.

(2) Treatment

1. Treatment is generally not necessary. Furthermore, AIVR may occasionally be the only functioning pacemaker, and suppression with lidocaine can lead to cardiac asystole.

2. If sustained AIVR produces symptoms due to a decrease in cardiac output, treatment with atrial pacing may be required.

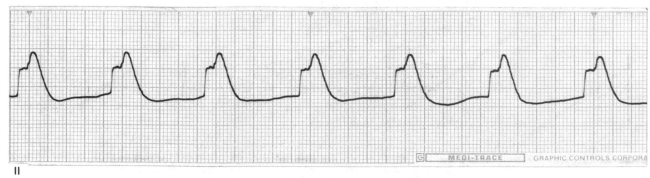

II

Figure 3.24 Accelerated idioventricular rhythm (AIVR). (From Brown, KR: Mastering Dysrhythmias. FA Davis, Philadelphia, 1988, p 126, with permission.)

c. Ashman's Phenomenon

Ashman's phenomenon is an aberrantly conducted beat that occurs shortly after a preceding long interbeat interval. Aberrant conduction occurs when the electrical impulse travels through myocardial cells instead of following the normal conduction pathway. Electrical conduction through the myocardial cells is much slower and results in a widened and sometimes bizarre QRS complex. Ashman's phenomenon can be difficult to identify and is easily misinterpreted as ventricular ectopy. Furthermore, runs of consecutive aberrant beats may mimic ventricular tachycardia and create a serious therapeutic dilemma.

Examination of V_1 will help differentiate aberrancy from ventricular ectopy. The arrhythmia should meet the following criteria if it is a supraventricular rhythm with aberrant ventricular conduction:

1. The initial deflection of the QRS complex is identical to the normal QRS complexes. This occurs because the conduction pathway is normal until the impulse reaches the bundle branches.

2. A "long-short" RR cycle will be present. The duration of the refractory period in the intraventricular conduction system is related to the heart rate. Increasing the RR interval (slower heart rate) prolongs the refractory period of the next beat. If the next beat is premature (short RR or faster heart rate) the chance of an intraventricular conduction delay (i.e., ventricular aberrancy) will be greater. When the irregular RR interval of atrial fibrillation suddenly lengthens, the refractory period of ventricles is also lengthened. If the following impulse is premature, aberrant conduction is likely to occur.

3. An RSR pattern in V_1 or MCL_1 will generally be present with an Ashman's beat. Normally, the right bundle branch has the longest refractory period of all the fascicles in the intraventricular conduction system. Therefore, premature supraventricular impulses are more likely to be blocked in this division, resulting in the RSR pattern characteristic of right bundle branch block. As a result of the irregularity of the rhythm, a prolonged RR interval that is immediately followed by another sinus beat may produce aberrant conduction. The left bundle branch will allow normal conduction to the left side of the heart, causing the appearance of a right bundle branch block pattern. Once the right bundle branch repolarizes normally, the patient's ECG will again reveal normal QRS morphology.

Treatment is not indicated for Ashman's phenomenon, but the underlying atrial fibrillation of other arrhythmia should be treated, The importance of Ashman's phenomenon is that its aberrantly conducted beats may be mistaken for ectopic ventricular activity. Misdiagnosis may influence the medical decision to withhold digoxin, which is usually needed if atrial fibrillation is present.

AXIOM

A patient with atrial fibrillation who develops what appears to be ventricular ectopy should have aberrant conduction (i.e., Ashman's phenomenon) ruled out before being treated with antiarrhythmic drugs for ectopy.

d. Ventricular Tachycardia

Ventricular tachycardia can be defined as any tachyarrhythmia that originates and is sustained in tissues below the bifurcation of the bundle of His. Operationally this is identified on the surface ECG as at least three wide QRS complexes in a row, occurring at a ventricular rate above 100 that usurps the underlying cardiac rhythm.

(1) Clinical Significance

Ventricular tachycardia is extremely dangerous because it may rapidly convert to ventricular fibrillation, particularly in the presence of ischemia, hypoxia, acidosis, or sympathomimetic drugs. Ventricular tachycardia rarely occurs in a normal heart, and over 70% of patients with this arrhythmia have significant ischemic heart disease. Although a ventricular rate of 150 to 200 per minute may cause only mild hemodynamic changes in a normal heart, ventricular tachycardia in patients with severe underlying heart disease can rapidly cause heart failure or shock.

(2) Diagnosis

The ECG in ventricular tachycardia shows widened (greater than 0.12 second), slurred QRS complexes with a slightly irregular rhythm at 150 to 200 per minute (Fig. 3.25). Varied configurations of the QRS complexes suggest multiple ectopic

Rate	Rhythm	Duration
Ventricular greater than 150	R-R regular	PR Interval absent
Atrial absent	P-P absent	QRS Complex widened and bizarre

Note: Sustained ventricular tachycardia is at risk to degenerate into ventricular fibrillation. It must be terminated without delay.

INTERVENTIONS:
- Assess vital signs, clinical status; document ECG strip.
- Determine patient's tolerance of dysrhythmia.
- Notify physician.
- Administer lidocaine bolus intravenously, and initiate lidocaine drip.
- Prepare for cardioversion.
- Monitor response to therapy.
- If unresponsive, call Code Blue and initiate CPR.

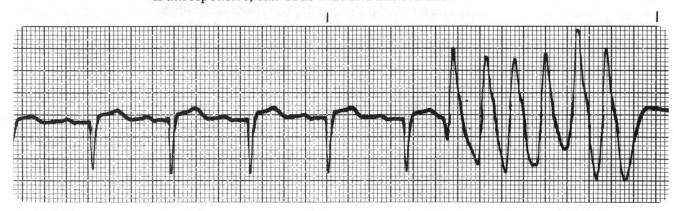

Lead MCL$_1$

Figure 3.25 Ventricular tachycardia. (From Dolan, JT: Critical Care Nursing. FA Davis, Philadelphia, 1991, p 812, with permission.)

foci and a much more dangerous condition. If sinus capture beats and/or ventricular fusion beats can be identified, the diagnosis is almost certain.

Ventricular flutter is probably not a distinct entity. It represents an extreme type of ventricular tachycardia that is about to convert to ventricular fibrillation within a few seconds. On the ECG, ventricular flutter is characterized by wide, regular, smooth ventricular waves at 150 to 300 per minute without recognizable P waves (Fig. 3.26).

(3) Treatment

If ventricular tachycardia causes hypotension, congestive failure, or loss of consciousness, direct-current cardioversion is the treatment of choice. At the same time, lidocaine is given in an IV bolus of 1.0 mg/kg (which is repeated in 5 minutes and then as often as needed, up to four or five times) while an IV drip of 4 mg/min is begun. If the patient is hemodynamically stable, lidocaine is given by itself. If the patient fails to respond rapidly to lidocaine and/or if cardioversion is not available or is not effective, procainamide in doses of 100 to 200 mg IV every 2 to 4 hours may also be attempted. If the ventricular tachycardia is still present, bretylium or amiodarone may be tried.

If ventricular tachycardia is due to digitalis toxicity, phenytoin 100 to 200 mg slowly by IV may convert the rhythm to normal in 15 to 20 minutes. In the rare patient with digitalis toxicity but an otherwise normally functioning myocardium, cautious administration of propranolol may be considered.

e. Torsade de Pointes

Torsade de pointes, first described by Desertenne in 1966, is a variant of ventricular tachycardia (VT) in which the QRS axis swings in polarity, producing a waxing and waning in the size of ventricular complexes (Fig. 3.27). The French term means *twisting of points*. It is an apt description of the ECG appearance. Available evidence indicates that this arrhythmia originates from a small area of ventricular myocardium and is generated by triggered automaticity. Torsade de pointes generally occurs at a ventricular rate of 200 to 240 per minute in nonsustained runs lasting 5 to 15 seconds. This form of ventricular tachycardia most often occurs in patients with serious myocardial disease who have prolonged and uneven ventricular repolarization, manifested as a prolonged QT interval. Drugs or toxins that prolong the QT interval can induce or aggravate this arrhythmia.

Despite its infrequency, much has been written about torsade de pointes because of its unusual nature, its occurrence with various forms of drug toxicity, and the fact that its treatment is so different from other varieties of VT. Sustained runs of torsade de pointes can be terminated with synchronized cardioversion, but because most occurrences of this arrhythmia are nonsustained, cardioversion is only rarely indicated. In addition, even if the arrhythmia is terminated and the underlying pathophysiology remains, recurrences are likely.

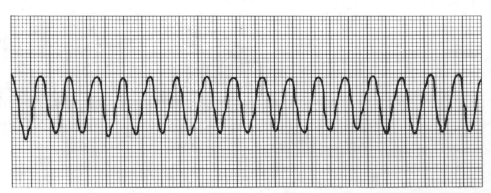

Figure 3.26 Ventricular flutter. (From Wilson, RF: Principles and Techniques of Critical Care, Vol 1. Upjohn, 1977, with permission.)

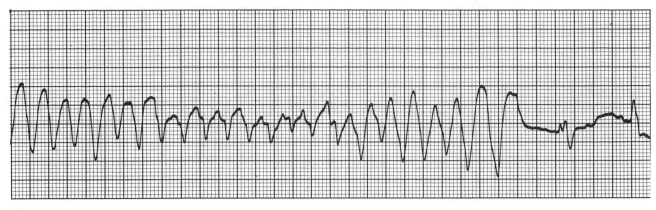

II

Figure 3.27 Torsade de pointes converting spontaneously to sinus rhythm. (From Brown, KR: Mastering Dysrhythmias. FA Davis, Philadelphia, 1988, p 124, with permission.)

AXIOM

Disease or drugs prolonging the QT interval increase the likelihood of causing torsade de pointes to start and persist.

The use of class Ia antiarrhythmics (such as quinidine, procainamide, or disopyramide) which prolong QRS duration, are usually ineffective and may aggravate torsade de pointes. Some of the antiarrhythmics that have been reported to suppress torsade de pointes include mexilitene, dilantin, bretylium, propranolol, verapamil, calcium gluconate, and atropine. However, no agent is reliably effective.

Other recommended treatment for torsade de pointes includes accelerating the heart rate (thereby shortening ventricular repolarization) with an isoproterenol infusion as an emergent but temporary solution, followed by a ventricular pacemaker for long-term control and prevention. The desired ventricular rate is 100 to 120. Overdrive pacing prevents torsade de pointes, allowing time for the physician to correct the underlying or contributing causes. Recent reports have shown that intravenous magnesium is often effective in abolishing torsade de pointes, and has few observed side effects.

f. Wide (QRS) Complex Tachycardia

Wide complex tachycardia can present a difficult therapeutic decision because it can be either VT or SVT with aberrancy. Consequently, the physician may make the wrong decision and institute treatment that is ineffective or harmful. Nevertheless, patients who are compromised by the rapid rate should be cardioverted. Because most sustained tachycardias are due to re-entry, this therapy will be effective for both.

For patients who are clinically stable, historical, clinical, and ECG factors can be used to make an educated guess differentiating VT from SVT with aberrancy (Table 3.1).

The response to carotid sinus massage may be helpful. Induction of an AV block usually allows a supraventricular arrhythmia to be better seen or terminated, but it generally has no effect on VT.

AXIOM

In elderly patients or those with known cardiac disease, wide complex tachycardia should generally be treated as ventricular tachycardia.

Unfortunately, historical, clinical, and electrocardiographic data are only guidelines to the diagnosis of a wide complex tachycardia, and the physician

Table 3.1

DIFFERENTIATION OF ABERRANT VENTRICULAR CONDUCTION FROM VENTRICULAR ECTOPY	*Characteristics Favoring Aberrant Ventricular Conduction*
	Right bundle-branch block with R′ > R in V_1
	Rate >170
	Initial QRS vector same as conducted QRS
	QRS duration <140 msec
	Normal axis
	Preceding P′
	Ashman's phenomenon
	Characteristics Favoring Ventricular Ectopy
	Left axis deviation
	QRS >140 msec
	Monophasic or diphasic in V_1
	Fusion or capture beats
	Rate <170
	AV dissociation
	R > R′ in V_1
	Concordant precordial pattern

must often decide a course of therapy without a definitive diagnosis. However, if the QRS complex is wide, the rhythm regular, the rate rapid, and the patient elderly or with known cardiac disease, wide QRS complex tachycardia is ventricular tachycardia at least 95% of the time. The best antiarrhythmic drugs to use in this situation are the class Ia antiarrhythmics (quinidine, procainamide, disopyramide), which affect the conducting system in a manner that is effective in both SVT and VT without producing harm.

PITFALL
Use of verapamil to treat wide complex tachycardia.

One must be particularly careful not to use verapamil in wide complex tachycardia because, in up to 40% of cases, it may accelerate the rate of ventricular tachycardia or produce a deterioration to ventricular fibrillation. Verapamil has been found to be useful in patients with wide complex tachycardia only where prior testing under controlled circumstances have demonstrated its effectiveness.

g. Ventricular Fibrillation

Ventricular fibrillation is an uncoordinated depolarization of ventricular muscle, resulting in abrupt cessation of effective blood flow (Fig. 3.28). This arrhythmia occurs only when the heart is severely damaged by ischemia, drugs (such as digitalis, quinidine, or procainamide in toxic doses), trauma, or contact with

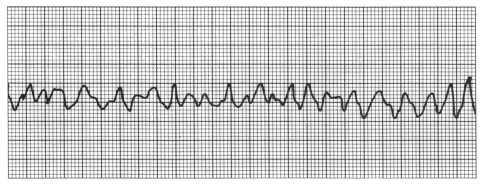

Figure 3.28 Ventricular fibrillation.

high-voltage electricity. Unless ventricular fibrillation is corrected immediately or unless an adequate cardiac output can be maintained with cardiac massage or cardiopulmonary bypass, ventricular fibrillation will be fatal in 3 to 5 minutes or less.

Occasionally, a sharp thump or punch directly over the precordium immediately after ventricular fibrillation has begun will convert the rhythm to normal. However, in any case with a cardiac arrest, electrical defibrillation should be attempted as soon as possible. While it may have little effect on asystole, it may be rapidly helpful with ventricular tachycardia or ventricular fibrillation

AXIOM
The quicker one attempts to electrically defibrillate a patient with cardiac arrest, the more favorable the outcome.

Sodium bicarbonate in an initial dose of 1.0 mEq/kg may be needed to combat the severe metabolic acidosis that may develop very rapidly following cessation of an effective cardiac output. However, in witnessed and rapidly treated cardiac arrests, bicarbonate administration should be based on arterial and mixed venous blood gas analyses.

If the ventricular fibrillation pattern is very weak, intravenous or intracardiac epinephrine in doses of 0.3 to 0.5 mg (3 to 5 ml of 1 : 10,000 solution), may help the heart develop a stronger fibrillation, which may be easier to convert electrically. If the rhythm converts to normal following electrical defibrillation and then reverts to ventricular fibrillation again, lidocaine should be given intravenously.

(8) Pre-excitation Syndromes

Pre-excitation occurs when, in relation to atrial events, all or part of the ventricular muscle is activated by the atrial impulses sooner than would be anticipated if the impulse reached the ventricles through the normal AV conduction system. A classification of the pre-excitation syndromes, based on their proposed anatomic connections, has been devised. Six separated pathways have been identified.

The AV bypass tract is the most frequently encountered type of pre-excitation and accounts for the WPW syndrome. The typical WPW-ECG pattern has a short PR interval (<0.12 second), a slurred upstroke of the QRS complex (delta wave), and a wide QRS complex (>0.12 second). This pattern results from the atrial impulse bypassing the normal delaying site (AV mode) to begin ventricular depolarization earlier than expected. The QRS complex abnormality is a fusion complex, a result of dual ventricular activation initiated by both the bypass trait and the normal AV conduction system.

James fibers are a continuation of the posterior internodal tract and connect the atrium and proximal His bundle. Atrial impulses can therefore completely bypass the AV mode to activate the ventricles. On ECG, this appears as a short PR interval, because the usual delay in the AV node is bypassed. The QRS complex appears normal because the James fibers insert directly into the infranodal conducting system and the ventricles are activated normally.

Mahaim bundles are composed of myogenic tissue, which originate from either the AV node, His bundle, or bundle branches, and insert into the ventricles in the septal region. Atrial impulses pass through the AV node normally but then bypass all or part of the infranodal conducting system to activate the ventricles. Ventricular activation then occurs from two sources. The initial depolarization starts at the ventricular insertion of the bypass tract and is spread slowly by cell-to-cell transmission of the impulse. Subsequent depolarization by way of the normal (faster) conducting system then overtakes the initial depolarization and activates the bulk of ventricular myocardium. On ECG this appears

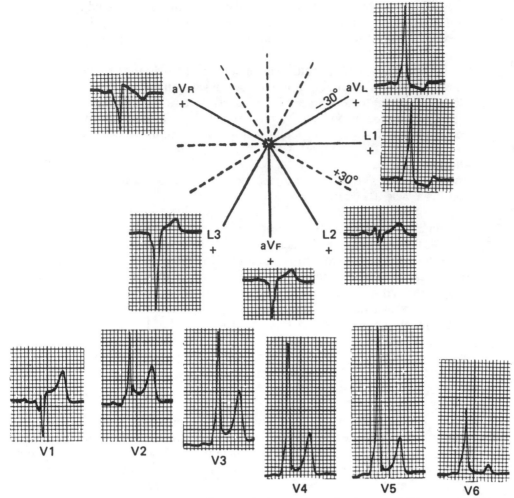

Figure 3.29 Accessory AV bundle type of pre-excitation, as shown by absence of PR segment, a delta wave, and a wide QRS. (From Constant, J: Learning Electrocardiography, ed 3. Little, Brown & Co, Boston, 1987, p 191, with permission.)

as a normal PR interval, and an initial distortion of ventricular depolarization (delta wave (Fig. 3.29).

Kent's bundles are composed of myogenic tissue and directly link the atria to the ventricles, completely bypassing the AV node and infranodal system. This is the most common form of pre-excitation and is the anatomic basis for the Wolff-Parkinson-White (WPW) syndrome. On ECG, this appears as a shortened PR interval and an initial distortion of ventricular activation (delta wave) (Fig. 3.30). If the bypass tract does not conduct an atrial impulse in the antegrade direction, the QRS complex is entirely normal. However, these concealed bypass tracts may also conduct retrograde impulses and thereby sustain a re-entrant SVT.

The WPW syndrome has been divided into types, depending on the direction of the initial delta wave on the surface ECG. This in turn is determined by where the bypass tract (bundle of Kent) inserts into the ventricles and which portion of the ventricles is activated first. However, accessory tracts can insert anywhere around the AV annulus.

Because there is altered depolarization, repolarization is often abnormal with changes in the ST segments and T waves. The ECG changes of WPW may mimic those seen with myocardial ischemia or infarction.

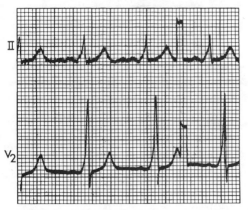

Figure 3.30 Wolff-Parkinson-White syndrome. (From Merch Manual, ed 15. Merck Sharp & Dohme, West Point, PA, 1987, p 475, with permission.)

(2) Clinical Significance

There is a high incidence of tachyarrhythmias in patients with AV bypass traits. These include atrial flutter, atrial fibrillation (10% to 20%), and paroxysmal re-entrant SVT (40% to 80%). The re-entrant SVT uses the normal AV conduction system as the antegrade limb and the bypass trait as the retrograde limb of the re-entrant circuit. Although less common, atrial fibrillation and flutter are potentially more life threatening since extremely rapid ventricular rates can result and precipitate ventricular tachycardia and/or fibrillation.

(3) Treatment

1. Re-entrant SVT in the WPW syndrome can be treated like other re-entrant SVT. Since the AV node is involved in the re-entry circuit, maneuvers or drugs (propranolol, digitalis) that slow conduction through the AV node tend to be effective.

2. Atrial flutter or fibrillation with a rapid ventricular response is best treated with cardioversion. As an alternative, agents that prolong the refractory period of the accessory tract—such as lidocaine or procainamide —can be used. In general, Dilantin, propranolol, or verapamil have a variable effect on accessory conduction and should not be used. Digitalis is contraindicated in atrial flutter or fibrillation with a bypass tract because it may shorten the refractory period and enhance conduction over the bypass tract.

AXIOM
Propranolol and digitalis can be of use in treating re-entrant SVT, but should be avoided in re-entrant atrial flutter or fibrillation.

h. Summary of Antiarrhythmia Therapy

In acute situations, it may be helpful to have a summary table of the more frequently used treatments for the various arrhythmias (Table 3.2).

B. DISORDERS OF CARDIAC CONDUCTION

1. Atrioventricular Conduction

The AV node is about $1 \times 2 \times 6$ mm and lies in the lower interatrial septum near its junction with the membranous interventricular septum. In about 90% of patients, the blood supply for the AV node comes from the posterior descending branch of the right coronary artery, and in about 10%, it comes from a posterior descending branch of the left circumflex artery. Interestingly, an area of vagal neuroreceptors (near the ostium of the coronary sinus) is only a few millimeters from the AV node, and thus the vagus nerve may be stimulated when the AV node is injured or ischemic. This may explain why ischemia of the AV node is often associated with an intense vagal discharge which can result in nausea, vomiting, bradycardia, or syncope. Disease or abnormalities of the AV node

Table 3.2

COMMON DYSRHYTHMIAS IN POSTOPERATIVE CARDIAC SURGICAL PATIENTS	Dysrhythmia	Treatment
	Ectopic Rhythms	
	Atrial premature contractions	1. Usually none required; but may indicate hypokalemia
	Ventricular premature contractions	1. None if <5–6 min, if unifocal, and if not close to T wave 2. Lidocaine 1.5 mg/kg bolus × 2, plus infusion begining at 4 mg/min 3. Overdrive pacing 4. Check electrolytes for hypokalemia
	Tachydysrhythmias Paroxysmal atrial tachycardia	1. Rapid atrial pacing 2. Propranolol 3. Increased vagal tone (carotid massage) 4. Cardioversion 5. Digoxin (but dysrhythmia may be precipitated by digitalis toxicity)
	Atrial flutter	1. Rapid atrial pacing 2. Beta blockade 3. Verapamil (not with WPW) 4. Cardioversion 5. Digoxin (not with WPW)
	Atrial fibrillation	1. Cardioversion (if acute and/or symptomatic) 2. Digoxin (not with WPW)
	Ventricular tachycardia	1. Lidocaine (if hemodynamically stable) 2. Cardioversion
	Ventricular fibrillation	1. Defibrillation 2. Cardiac arrest protocol 3. If refractory, procainamide or bretylium
	Bradydysrhythmias Sinus or nodal bradycardia (if symptomatic)	1. Atrial pacing when available 2. Atropine 3. Isoproterenol (rarely needed)
	Atrioventricular dissociation with slow ventricular response	1. Ventricular pacing (preferably AV sequential) 2. Atropine—rarely successful 3. Isoproterenol

usually slow AV conduction, but occasionally they accelerate it, as in the WPW syndrome.

AXIOM

Nausea, vomiting, and bradycardia may be due to vagal stimulation, possibly from posterior myocardial ischemia.

a. First-Degree Heart Block

When the PR interval is longer than normal, first-degree heart block is said to be present. The usual upper limit of normal for the PR interval in adults is 0.20 second but should be considered in terms of heart rate (Fig. 3.31). There are essentially no symptoms associated with this abnormality, but it may indicate the presence of significant underlying cardiac disease or drug toxicity, especially from digitalis. The PR intervals usually revert to normal with exercise or following atropine administration.

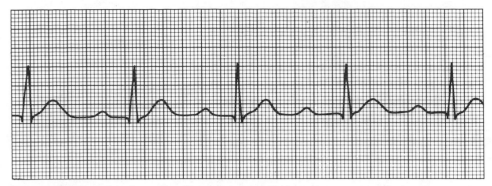

Figure 3.31 Normal rhythm with a first-degree heart block.

b. Second-Degree Heart Block

The two major types of second-degree heart block are the Mobitz type-I and the Mobitz type-II blocks. The Mobitz type-I block or Wenckebach phenomenon is characterized by a progressive lengthening of the PR interval for several successive beats until there is a P wave that is not followed by ventricular excitation (Fig. 3.32). Clinically, this problem may be recognized by dropped beats at relatively regular intervals. Underlying cardiac problems frequently associated with this arrhythmia include coronary artery disease, digitalis toxicity, rheumatic fever, and various viral infections.

The Mobitz type-II second-degree heart block is characterized by incomplete failure of AV conduction so that every second, third, or fourth atrial impulse is conducted to the ventricles (Fig. 3.33). This type of second-degree AV block usually represents a block in the His-Purkinje system below the AV node and is much more apt to progress to complete AV block than the Wenckebach phenomenon.

When second-degree heart block is due to digitalis or quinidine toxicity, these drugs should be withheld. If the atrial rate is rapid with a second-degree block, potassium may be contraindicated because it may relieve the AV block without slowing the atrial rate, thereby producing a very rapid ventricular rate. When second-degree heart block is due to ischemia, correction of any associated hypotension or heart failure may also correct the arrhythmia. If a Mobitz type-II block persists in spite of such therapy, a temporary transvenous pacemaker should be inserted.

c. Complete (Third-Degree) Heart Block

Failure of the AV node to conduct any atrial impulses to the ventricles is referred to as a complete AV block. It may be congenital in origin, but is more likely to be caused by ischemia, drugs, or trauma. Physical examination may reveal A waves in the neck veins unrelated to the pulse or heart sounds. Large cannon waves can also be detected in the neck veins when the atria contract while the

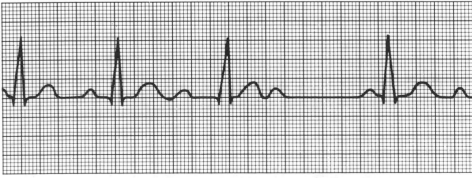

Figure 3.32 Mobitz type-1 second-degree heart block (Wenckebach phenomenon).

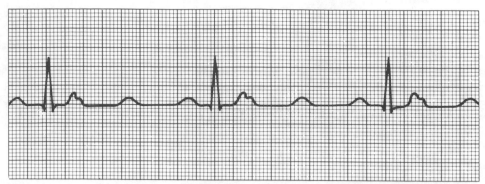

Figure 3.33 AV conduction with Mobitz type-II second-degree heart block.

AV valves are closed. On ECG, the P waves and QRS complexes are completely independent of each other. The heart rate is usually only 30 to 50 per minute and does not increase significantly with exercise (Fig. 3.34).

If a heart block is almost completely asymptomatic and is in the AV node, no treatment may be required. Symptoms of Stokes-Adams-Morgagni syndrome or congestive failure in a patient with a complete (third-degree) heart block or Mobitz type-II block below the AV node require insertion of a permanent transvenous demand pacemaker. Following an acute inferior myocardial infarction, a block in the AV node may be transient, and temporary pacing is often all that is required. However, if a third-degree block or a Mobitz type-II block persists for more than 3 or 4 weeks, a permanent pacemaker should be inserted.

d. AV Dissociation

The term AV dissociation should probably be reserved for instances in which the atria and ventricles are controlled by independent pacemakers, a retrograde AV block is present, the capacity for forward AV conduction is intact or only incompletely blocked, and the idioventricular rate is less than 150 per minute. This arrhythmia is usually transient, and if there is little or no AV block, no treatment is necessary. However, treatment of any underlying problem, particularly digitalis toxicity (the most frequent cause), is indicated.

2. Bundle-Branch Block

A bundle branch block is said to exist if conduction of the excitatory impulse from the AV node is delayed in a portion of the bundle of His or in the right or left bundle so that one ventricle is activated and contracts before the other. The most frequent causes are ischemia, hypertension, rheumatic disease, congenital abnormalities (especially septal defects), and aortic valvular disease. However, the bundle branch block itself rarely causes any symptoms.

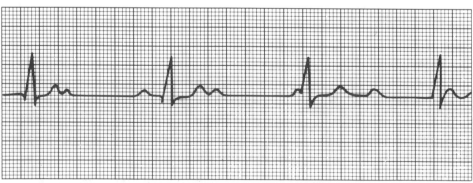

Figure 3.34 Complete AV dissociation with third-degree heart block.

The abnormal conduction of at least part of the impulse through the muscle mass (rather than the normal conducting system) distorts and widens the QRS complex. If the duration of the QRS complex is 0.10 to 0.12 second, an incomplete bundle branch block is said to exist. If the QRS complex is greater than 0.12 second, the bundle branch block is said to be complete.

a. Left Bundle-Branch Block

With complete LBBB, paradoxical splitting of the second heart sound may be heard during expiration. In leads aVL, V_5, and V_6 the ventricular deflections of greatest duration are upward, and the T waves are often inverted. The intrinsicoid deflection time (from onset of the QRS complex to the peak of the R wave) is of maximum duration in the left precordial leads (V_5 and V_6). In leads III, V_1, and V_2 the ventricular deflections are of the widest duration downward and the T waves are usually upright in V_1 through V_3 (Fig. 3.35). The biggest problem with LBBB is that it may mask the ECG changes of an acute myocardial infarction and, as a form of bifascicular block, it may be a harbinger of complete heart block.

AXIOM

In the presence of a LBBB, the ECG cannot be used to rule out an acute myocardial infarction.

b. Right Bundle-Branch Block

In a complete RBBB, ventricular deflections are of widest duration downward in lead I and upward in lead III. The intrinsicoid deflection is of maximum duration in the right precordial leads (V_1 and V_2), and the T waves are opposite in direction to the QRS deflection of greatest duration (Fig. 3.36). RBBB is usually asymptomatic; however, it may be associated with pulmonary hypertension or pulmonary emboli.

Incomplete RBBB is characterized by an Rr' of 0.10 to 0.12 seconds in V_1 and is normal in many individuals. However, a new incomplete RBBB may indicate acute right heart strain, as with a pulmonary embolus.

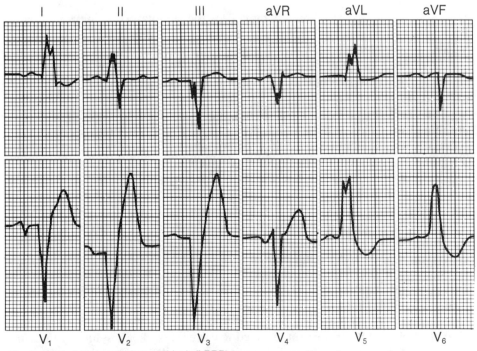

Figure 3.35 Left bundle branch block (LBBB).

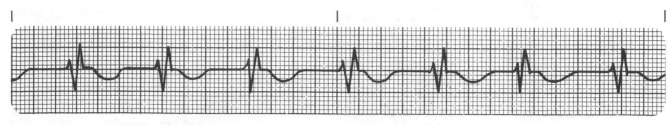

A Lead MCL₁

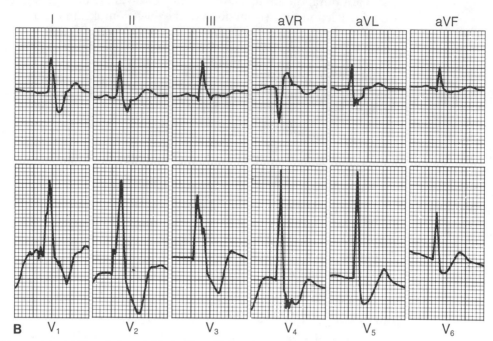

I	II	III	aVR	aVL	aVF

B V₁ V₂ V₃ V₄ V₅ V₆

Figure 3.36 (*A*) Incomplete right bundle branch block. (From Dolan, JT: Critical Care Nursing. FA Davis, Philadelphia, 1991, p 821, with permission.) (*B*) Complete right bundle branch block.

c. Left Ventricular Hemiblock

It is now recognized that the left branch of the bundle of His physiologically functions as a bifascicular system with a thin, elongated anterior division and a wider, shorter posterior division. However, there is also a central radiation or plexus of fibers to the midseptal area. Either the anterior or posterior divisions may be separately blocked as a result of myocardial infarction, fibrosis, or inflammation.

The term bifascicular block is now generally used to describe a RBBB combined with a left anterior of left posterior hemiblock, whereas a trifascicular block involves the right bundle and the anterior and posterior branches of the left bundle. Note that it is not quite a complete AV block because the central radiation of conducting fibers to the ventricles may still be intact.

(1) Left Anterior Hemiblock

Left anterior hemiblock (LAH) is much more common than left posterior hemiblock (LPH) and more easily identified. It should be suspected whenever the frontal plane axis is negative more than −30°. The QRS duration is lengthened only slightly and averages about 0.10 to 0.12 second (Fig. 3.37).

(2) Left Posterior Hemiblock

Left posterior hemiblock (LPH) generally indicates more extensive injury and is more difficult to detect than LAH. It occurs most often with posterior (inferior) myocardial infarctions, in which case the abnormal Q waves in leads II, III, and aVF are followed by prominent, delayed R waves (Fig. 3.38). While an uncomplicated posterior myocardial infarction tends to shift the frontal plane axis to the left, if LPH is present, the frontal plane axis is shifted to the right.

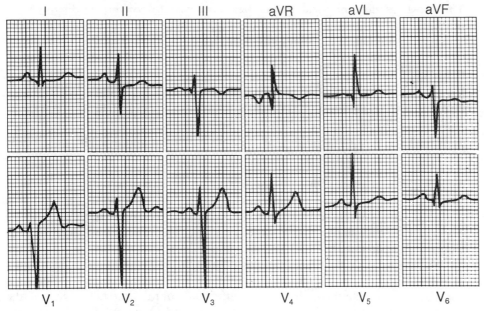

Figure 3.37 Left anterior hemiblock (LAH).

V. TREATMENT: GENERAL CONSIDER- ATIONS

The first step in evaluation of the patient with an arrhythmia should be a search for reversible causes such as hypoxia, myocardial ischemia, abnormal intracardiac pressures, and acid-base or electrolyte abnormalities. However, in many situations antiarrhythmic drugs will be required as temporary measures to permit stabilization of a patient's rhythm until the reversible factors may be normalized. Antiarrhythmic drugs may also be required continuously in patients whose underlying cardiac disease makes them chronically susceptible to arrhythmias.

The therapeutic modalities available for treating various arrhythmias include physical maneuvers, electrical equipment for pacing or cardioversion, and drugs.

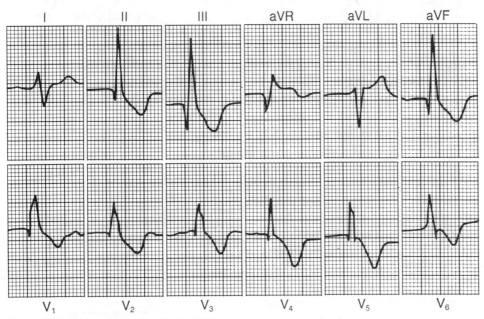

Figure 3.38 Left posterior hemiblock (LPH).

A. PHYSICAL MANEUVERS

The most frequent physical maneuvers employed to convert or diagnose arrhythmias are designed to stimulate the vagus nerve. This may be done with the Valsalva maneuver or carotid sinus massage.

PITFALL
It is dangerous to have a patient perform a Valsalva maneuver without first ruling out coronary artery disease, cerebrovascular disease, or hypovolemia.

1. Responses to Physical Maneuvers

The responses to vagal stimulation may have both diagnostic and therapeutic value (Table 3.3).

B. ARTIFICIAL CARDIAC PACEMAKERS

1. Components and Positioning

Artificial or exogenous cardiac pacemakers have two components; a power source (battery with pulse generator) and one or more electrodes inserted into the heart (transvenous, transthoracic, or epicardial). The pulse generator can be designated to operate in either a fixed-rate mode (syncronous or competitive) or a demand mode (synchronous or noncompetitive).

In the fixed-rate mode, the pulse generator produces an electrical signal at a predetermined rate regardless of the patient's own intrinsic cardiac rate. As a consequence, serious arrhythmias or ventricular fibrillation may occur if the pacemaker discharges during the vulnerable period (T wave). For this reason, fixed-rate pacing is rarely done now. In the demand mode, the pulse generator has a sensing circuit that detects spontaneous cardiac activity and will discharge only if no cardiac depolarization occurs after a preset interval. Demand pacemakers may have two response modes, either inhibited or triggered. In the inhibited response mode (most commonly used), the pulse generator is inhibited by the sensed cardiac activity and does not generate an impulse. In the triggered response mode, the pacemaker detects the patient's intrinsic cardiac activity and then discharges during the absolute refractory period.

A three-letter code system is used for pacemaker designation (Table 3.4). The most common type of pacemaker used—a ventricular demand inhibited-response pacemaker—would be designated as VVI. Atrioventricular demand inhibited-response pacemakers are designated as DDI.

Permanent pacemakers are powered by mercury-zinc or lithium batteries, which have approximate lifetimes of 5 to 6 years or 8 to 12 years, respectively. Most units are preset for rates around 70 per minute with a pacing interval of 0.84 second. The demand pacemaker has a built-in refractory period (0.2 to 0.4 second) during which it will not sense; this prevents it from being inhibited by its own stimulus. Most demand pacemakers have a magnetic switch that temporarily converts the pulse generator from the demand mode to the fixed-rate mode when a magnet is held over the unit. In this way the pacing rate can be quickly determined. However, the magnet should be applied for only short periods to avoid initiating tachyarrhythmias. In the newer programmable pacemakers, the rate and stimulus strength can be reset by noninvasive means.

Table 3.3

RESPONSE OF DYSRHYTHMIAS TO VAGAL MANEUVERS		
	Sinus tachycardia	Slows gradually, returns to intrinsic rate when maneuver is ended
	Ectopic atrial tachycardia	Stepwise decrease in AV conduction; may develop 2:1 or 3:1 conduction block
	Paroxysmal atrial tachycardia	No response or a sudden conversion to sinus rhythm
	Atrial flutter	Decrease in AV conduction; may go from 2:1 to 3:1 or 4:1 conduction block
	Atrial fibrillation	Gradual decrease in ventricular rate, returns to original rate after termination of maneuver
	Multifocal atrial tachycardia	No response or may cause some P waves to be nonconducted
	Ventricular tachycardia	No response

Table 3.4

CODING SYSTEM FOR PERMANENT PACEMAKERS	First Letter Chamber Paced	Second Letter Chamber Sensed	Third Letter Mode of Response
		A = atrium V = ventricle D = double (both)	I = inhibited T = triggered O = not applicable

Temporary pacemakers are powered by 9-V radio-type batteries. These pacemakers have settings for the mode (fixed or demand), rate (40 to 140), and stimulus strength (0.2 to 20 mA). During emergency pacing, initial setting should be in the demand mode with a rate around 70 and stimulus strength around 3.0 mA. The negative terminal should be connected to the distal electrode.

The pacing electrode may be either unipolar or bipolar. The unipolar setup has the negative electrode within the heart and the positive electrode in the chest wall. Permanent pacemakers using the unipolar setup have the positive electrode on their surface covering, while temporary pacemakers use a needle implanted in the skin of the anterior thorax. The bipolar setup has both electrodes within a few millimeters of each other, and both lie within the heart.

The most frequent electrode placement is into the apex of the right ventricle using a transvenous approach. The catheters used depend on the clinical situation. Rigid or semirigid catheters (6F or 7F) are inserted through a venous puncture or cutdown and usually require fluoroscopy for correct placement. Semifloating (3F and 4F) or flexible balloon-tipped catheters (3F or 5F) can be introduced and directed into the right ventricle without fluoroscopy using blood flow. However, flexible catheters can become dislodged quite easily by patient or cardiac movement and are usually replaced with semirigid catheters within 24 hours.

Transthoracic electrodes can be inserted into the anterior wall of the right ventricle through a left parasternal or subxiphoid puncture. They are used in cardiac resuscitation when rapid placement is essential. A major disadvantage of transthoracic electrodes is that they can become dislodged with closed-chest compression. In addition, coronary artery laceration or pericardial tamponade may occur. While electrical capture may be obtained in an occasional patient, it is rare to produce effective cardiac contractions with transthoracic pacing.

2. Indications for Emergency Pacing

Emergency cardiac pacing is indicated either therapeutically (for symptomatic bradyarrhythmias) or prophylactically (for conduction defects which have a high risk of developing sudden complete heart block or asystole) (Table 3.5).

a. Preventing Arrhythmias

Electrical pacing of the heart may be useful in the prevention or termination of many arrhythmias. The earliest uses of pacing were to prevent arrhythmias that tend to occur during bradycardia. Some arrhythmias are triggered by late diastolic premature beats. In bigeminal rhythms, the long pause after the premature beat can prolong repolarization after the subsequent normal beat and lead to an "R-on-T" phenomenon. In these two instances, overdrive pacing at faster rates may prove effective in preventing arrhythmias. In patients having a relative bradycardia associated with hemodynamic compromise that causes a secondary arrhythmia, pacing (atrial, ventricular, or dual-chamber) may help prevent further episodes. Unfortunately, overdrive pacing by itself is only occasionally successful for the long-term management of arrhythmias.

Most authors would recommend prophylactic placement of a pacemaker in any patient with acute myocardial infarction who has a new bifascicular or

Table 3.5

INDICATIONS FOR TEMPORARY CARDIAC PACING	
	1. Symptomatic bradyarrhythmias
	Sick sinus syndrome
	Bradycardia-tachycardia syndrome
	Complete heart block
	Carotid sinus hypersensitivity
	Other miscellaneous bradyarrhythmias
	2. Prophylactic pacing
	Mobitz II second-degree AV block
	After cardiac surgery
	Right heart catheterization with left bundle-branch block
	3. During acute myocardial infarction
	Symptomatic bradycardia
	Type-II second-degree AV block
	Third-degree AV block
	New bifascicular block
	New right or left bundle-branch block with anterior myocardial infarction
	4. Tachycardias
	Atrial flutter
	Torsade de pointes
	Other miscellaneous tachyarrhythmias

trifascicular block. Second-degree Mobitz II and third-degree (Mobitz III) AV blocks are also indications for pacemaker insertion. Despite successful pacing, patients with acute myocardial infarction and serious conduction blocks tend to have extensive left ventricular damage and a high mortality rate from pump failure.

The automatic internal cardioverter defibrillator (AICD) was approved for general use in the United States in 1986. this fully implantable device continually senses the heart's rhythm and is set to deliver shocks from internal electrodes in response to rapid or disorganized ventricular rhythms.

b. Treating Arrhythmias

One of the arrhythmias treated best with overdrive pacing is atrial flutter. The delivery of bursts of atrial stimuli at cycle lengths shorter than the atrial cycle lengths results in a change in the flutter wave on the ECG. In most cases this will either terminate the flutter or accelerate it to atrial fibrillation. Even if atrial fibrillation is produced, it is often easier to medically control the ventricular rate with atrial fibrillation than with atrial flutter. Re-entrant supraventricular tachycardias may also be terminated by overdrive pacing. Atrial fibrillation, multifocal atrial tachycardia, and automatic atrial or junctional tachycardias do not usually respond.

Direct-current countershock is the treatment of choice for arrhythmias that (1) are associated with hemodynamic collapse or with severe angina, (2) occur in patients with severe coronary artery disease, or (3) are resistant to other forms of treatment. When used to treat supraventricular arrhythmias or a well-tolerated ventricular tachycardia, the DC countershock delivery should be synchronized with the peak of the QRS complex to avoid precipitating ventricular fibrillation by delivering the shock during the T wave.

AXIOM

Digitalis toxicity should be excluded, if possible, prior to elective cardioversion since cardioversion releases tissue stores of digitalis into the blood. The resulting increased digitalis toxicity may lead to irreversible ventricular fibrillation.

Although some controversy still exists, there is now more or less general agreement on the situations in which a pacemaker is (1) definitely indicated, (2) probably indicated, or (3) not indicated.

Category I: Diagnoses definitely indicating implantation:

1. Acquired complete heart block with symptomatic bradycardia (congestive heart failure, ventricular ectopic activity, or low cardiac output)

2. Mobitz type-II second-degree atrioventricular block

3. Persistent bradycardia with a maximum RR interval of more than 3 seconds or a minimum heart rate below 40 beats per minute

4. Sinus node dysfunction with:
   a. Correlation of symptoms with arrhythmia
   b. A maximum RR interval of more than 3 seconds
   c. A minimum heart rate below 40 beats per minute

5. Tachycardia-bradycardia syndrome, with episodes of paroxysmal atrial fibrillation, atrial flutter, or supraventricular tachycardia, followed by a pause on termination lasting more than 3 seconds

6. Transient or persistent Mobitz II second-degree atrioventricular block or complete heart block during an acute myocardial infarction, except for atrioventricular nodal block with an inferior myocardial infarction

7. Postoperative Mobitz II second-degree atrioventricular block or complete heart block persisting longer than 5 days

8. Symptomatic bradycardia with a maximum RR interval of more than 3 seconds or a minimum heart rate below 40 beats per minute during drug therapy

9. Marked infranodal conduction disturbance (split His potentials, HV>90 msec, or prolongation of HV to >90 msec by pacing or procainamide administration)

Category II: Diagnoses possibly indicating implantation:

1. Symptomatic or persistent bradycardia without a documented heart rate consistently below 40 beats per minute or an RR interval of more than 3 seconds

2. Symptomatic tachyarrhythmias

3. Syncope of undetermined cause

4. Symptomatic bifascicular or trifascicular block

5. Congenital complete heart block

6. Transient atrioventricular block after operation or during infarction, with possible infranodal conduction disturbance

7. Symptomatic bradycardia or high-grade atrioventricular block associated with an intercurrent toxic or metabolic condition

Category III: Diagnoses in which pacemakers are usually inappropriate:

1. Bradycardia, in which the longest RR interval is less than 3 seconds and the minimum heart rate above 40 beats per minute, with no symptoms or no correlation of symptoms with arrhythmia

2. Asymptomatic sinoatrial node dysfunction, in which the longest RR interval is less than 3 seconds and the minimum heart rate above 40 beats per minute

3. Asymptomatic isolated bundle branch block or bifascicular block with normal infranodal conduction

4. Asymptomatic first-degree or Mobitz I second-degree atrioventricular block

5. Drug-induced bradyarrhythmia if the drug is unnecessary

6. Overdrive suppression of ventricular ectopic activity, except torsade de pointes

7. Transient atrioventricular block during operation or catheterization

3. Pacemaker Malfunction

AXIOM

Early pacemaker dysfunction is usually due to improper initial electrode placement or loss of an initially correct position.

Pacemaker malfunction can result from a failure to properly sense the intrinsic cardiac rhythm, a failure to effectively pace, or both. While the problem can be in the pulse generator, most acute pacemaker malfunctions are due to problems with the electrodes.

Failure to sense may occur when the voltage of the patient's own intrinsic QRS complex is too low to be detected by the sensing circuit of the pacemaker. Changing from a bipolar to unipolar setup (if possible) may help the pacemaker sense the intrinsic cardiac activity. However, unipolar electrodes are more sensitive to electric interference from muscle activity or external electric equipment. Such interference can inhibit the pacemaker and suppress impulse formation. A failure to sense may cause the pacemaker to discharge during the T wave and trigger serious arrhythmias.

Failure to pace may occur when tissue reaction around the electrode makes the myocardium insensitive to the electric discharge generated by the pacemaker. It is common for the pacing threshold to increase during the first few weeks after insertion, but further rises are infrequent.

Failure both to sense and pace may be due to battery exhaustion, fracture of the wires in the catheter, or displacement of the electrodes. Battery exhaustion is indicated when the pacing rate slowly decreases.

AXIOM

Greater than 10% change from the initial rate in a pacemaker is usually an urgent indication for battery replacement.

Catheter wire fracture may cause either sustained or intermittent interruption in electrical conductivity. Sudden onset of symptoms and/or bradyarrhythmias suggests catheter fracture. Catheter fractures are rarely seen on routine chest radiographs. The transvenous electrode is usually positioned in the right ventricular apex, and has a characteristic appearance on the chest x-ray and ECG. Displacement should be suggested whenever changes on the radiographs or ECG are noted.

C. ANTIARRHYTHMIC DRUGS

1. Electrophysiology

The interior of a resting cell is negatively charged compared to its exterior. This electrical difference, called the resting membrane potential, ranges from about -60 to -100 mV, depending on the type of cell and averages about -90 mV. The electrical gradient across the cell membrane is determined largely by the high concentration of sodium outside the cell. This ionic gradient is maintained by a Na-K ATPase pump that actively pumps out any excess sodium that might otherwise get inside the cell.

When an excitable cell such as a Purkinje fiber is stimulated, an electrical current or action potential is developed. The cellular action potential is divided into five phases (Fig. 3.39). In phase 0, the cell is stimulated and the permeability of the cell membrane to sodium increases. Sodium rapidly enters the cell, reversing the electrical charge across the cell membrane and causing depolarization. The next phase, known as *repolarization*, is characterized by changes in the conduction of sodium, potassium, and calcium across the cell membrane and is represented by phases 1, 2, and 3. Phase 4 is the resting potential.

2. Classification of Antiarrhythmic Drugs

Antiarrhythmic drugs exert their effects by means of interactions with ion channels. These drugs usually have a high affinity for open or inactivated channels, but low affinity for channels in the resting state. When channels are in the drug-bound state, conductance of the ion regulated by that channel is inhibited.

Several phenomena observed to be associated with antiarrhythmic drugs may be explained using a modulated receptor hypothesis. At faster rates, myocardial and conducting cells spend less time in the resting or drug-insensitive

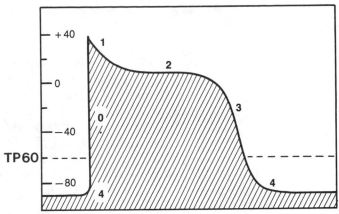

Figure 3.39 Phases of the action potential. TP threshold potential. (Modified from Dolan, JT: Critical Care Nursing, FA Davis, Philadelphia, 1991, p 734, with permission.)

state. Consequently, antiarrhythmic drugs will typically produce greater effects at faster rates. This phenomenon is called use or frequency dependence. The increased activity of many drugs on damaged cells is explained by the fact that loss of resting potential results in many inactivated channels and these also tend to have an increased sensitivity to drugs.

Antiarrhythmic drugs in the course of their activity affect the action potential in several ways. They can alter the rate of repolarization by changing the slope of phase 2 or phase 3, they can alter the threshold, or they can alter the slope of phase 4 so that it takes a longer or shorter time to reach threshold. Based on these changes, antiarrhythmic drugs can be divided into four main groups.

Class I agents are local anesthetic agents that are membrane stabilizers and have as their predominant effect a depression of sodium conductance during phase 0 of the action potential. These agents are further divided into three subclasses based on their effects on effective refractory period (ERP), action potential duration (APD), and the duration of the QRS.

Class II drugs are beta-receptor blockers. Class III agents include drugs that prolong repolarization. Class IV drugs include the calcium-channel blockers.

The dosages for the most frequent antiarrhythmic drugs are listed in Table 3.6.

Table 3.6

ABBREVIATED DOSAGE SCHEDULE FOR ANTIARRHYTHMIC DRUGS	Lidocaine: 1 mg/kg IV bolus. Repeat if necessary to maximal total dose of 4.5 mg/kg. Follow with infusion at 1–5 mg/min.
	Procainamide: 100 mg IV bolus at 25–50 mg/min: repeat in 5 min until arrhythmia is abolished, signs of QRS or QT prolongation appear, or a total dose of 1 g has been given.
	Quinidine: 300–400 mg p.o.q. 6 h.
	Propranolol: urgent situation 0.5–1.0 mg IV bolus not to exceed 1 mg/min. Repeat dose in 2–5 min. Nonurgent situation 10–20 mg p.o.q. 4–6 h, to 80 mg p.o.q. 6 h.
	Phenytoin: Cardiac arrhythmias: 100 mg IV over 5 min. Repeat dose in 5–15 min to total dose of 500–600 mg. Status epilepticus: 800–1000 mg may be necessary.
	Bretylium: 5 mg/kg IV bolus, followed by 5 mg/kg IM q. 6–8 h.
	Magnesium: Arrhythmias: 10–15 ml 20% $MgSO_4$ solution IV over 1 min followed by 4–6 h infusion of 500 ml of 2% $MgSO_4$ in D_5W (method of Iseri). Hypomagnesemia: 1 ml 20% $MgSO_4$ IM.

3. Specific Antiarrhythmic Drugs

The main class Ia agents are procainamide, quinidine, and disopyramide.

a. Class Ia Agents

(1) Procainamide (Pronestyl)

(a) Action

Procainamide depresses fast channel sodium conductance. It slows the rate of rise of the action potential (phase 0) and increases the action potential duration. It also elevates the threshold of ventricular muscle to electrical stimulation. It reduces automaticity by prolonging repolarization and the refractory period of cardiac muscle, thereby decreasing the slope of phase 4. It can directly depress myocardial conduction in normal and abnormal tissue as well as suppress ectopic or re-entrant foci. In contrast to quinidine (the other important class Ia agent), it has little effect on AV nodal conduction. Its active metabolite, N-acetylprocainamide (NAPA), is also an antiarrhythmic agent, but it has class III actions.

(b) Indications

Procainamide is generally used for ventricular arrhythmias that are resistant to lidocaine and attempted defibrillation. However, it can be very effective in SVT not responding to adenosine or esmolol. It is particularly effective in treating re-entrant and ectopic supraventricular arrhythmias, although it is not the drug of choice. It is, however, favored for the treatment of atrial flutter-fibrillation in the WPW syndrome.

Procainamide is contraindicated in patients (1) with second- or third-degree AV conduction defects, (2) sensitivity to amide anesthetics, (3) long QT syndrome, (4) history of torsade de pointes, or (5) hypokalemia.

(c) Dose

Procainamide is usually given IV in 100-mg boluses at 25 to 50 mg/min. This 100-mg dose may be repeated every 5 minutes until the arrhythmia is converted, hypotension develops, QRS and QT prolongation (50% or more) develops, or a total dose of 1 g has been given. Many physicians continue to give procainamide until the arrhythmia is corrected or until ECG effects are apparent. In renal failure, the dose must be reduced.

(d) Adverse effects

The most serious side effects of procainamide are its cardiovascular depressant effects, which are dose related. Consequently, the ECG and BP must be continuously monitored during procainamide administration, particularly following an acute myocardial infarction. At toxic doses, prolongation of the QRS and QT interval may be followed by progressive impairment of AV conduction, and finally by ventricular fibrillation. Hypotension can occur if the dose is excessive or if the drug is given too rapidly.

AXIOM

Procainamide is generally only used for acute problems because many side effects occur with prolonged use.

Chronic procainamide therapy can result in drug fever, eosinophilia, agranulocytosis, or a lupus erythematosuslike syndrome. Since this lupus syndrome may develop in up to 60% of the patients using procainamide chronically, it is seldom used except for acute problems in hospitalized patients.

(2) Quinidine

(a) Action

Quinidine, like procainamide, acts through depression of fast-channel sodium conductance. Quinidine prolongs APD and ERP and thereby depresses SA and ectopic pacemakers. It has mixed effects on AV nodal conduction. If AV conduction is normal, the vagolytic action of quinidine causes a reduction in the refractory period of the AV junction and may facilitate AV conduction. If AV conduction is depressed, quinidine may depress it further. Accessory pathways also display slowed conduction and prolonged refractoriness.

(b) Indications

Because quinidine can suppress ectopic atrial contractions and re-entry, it is very useful for the management of supraventricular tachyarrhythmias. It is also used for the conversion of atrial flutter or fibrillation to normal sinus rhythm.

PITFALL
If quinidine is used to treat atrial flutter of fibrillation without first giving digitalis, it may decrease the degree of AV block and cause the development of a dangerous, very rapid ventricular response.

Quinidine can also be used for the treatment of PVCs or recurrent ventricular tachycardia (VT). However, it should not be given in the presence of second- or third-degree AV conduction disturbances, prolonged QT syndrome, hypokalemia, or a history or torsade de pointes.

(c) Dose

Hypersensitivity or idiosyncratic reactions occasionally occur with quinidine. Consequently, when it is used orally, a test dose of 100 to 200 mg should be administered and the patient watched carefully over the next 4 to 6 hours. The usual oral dose of 300 mg every 6 hours will generally provide therapeutic serum levels of 3 to 6 mg/liter in 24 to 48 hours. Careful ECG monitoring is necessary, and quinidine blood levels should be obtained to guide treatment.

In urgent situations, quinidine gluconate can be administered IV in a dose of 200 mg. This dose may be repeated once or twice cautiously. The peak effect is not evident for about 1 hour.

AXIOM
The IV administration of quinidine can be extremely dangerous because it can cause severe hypotension or cardiac standstill.

Since quinidine is primarily metabolized by the liver, the dose must be reduced if there is liver failure. Quinidine metabolism is accelerated if it is given with agents, such a rifampin, phenytoin, or phenobarbital, which induce oxidative enzymes in hepatic microsomes.

PITFALL
Failure to adjust quinidine dosage for liver failure or for drugs that accelerate its metabolism may result in dangerous overdosing or underdosing.

(d) Adverse effects

Idiosyncratic reactions including urticaria, fever, and/or maculopapular eruptions, occur in up to 15% of patients receiving quinidine. Hemolytic anemia occasionally develops. Gastrointestinal symptoms, particularly nausea and diarrhea, occur in up to a third of patients. These symptoms can be controlled by lowering the dose using antispasmodics, or shifting to the IM route. Quinidine also decreases renal and nonrenal clearance of digoxin. Consequently, the dose of simultaneously given digoxin will often have to be reduced.

Cinchonism is a syndrome common to all cinhona alkaloids and includes vomiting, tinnitus, vertigo, and visual disturbances. Prolongation of the QT interval and ST-T wave depression are frequent and usually indicate only that therapeutic levels have been achieved.

Widening of the QRS complex to 0.16 second, or more than 50% greater than control, is a sign of toxicity and an indication to stop the drug. Other toxic effects include SA and AV block, PVCs, ventricular tachycardia, and ventricular fibrillation.

(3) Disopyramide

(a) Action

The direct electrophysiologic effects of disopyramide are similar to those of quinidine and procainamide. It depresses the rate of phase 0 depolarization, prolongs the duration of the action potential, and increases the ERP of atrial and

167

ventricular muscle. In Purkinje fibers, conduction velocity is delayed and the slope of spontaneous diastolic depolarization is decreased.

Disopyramide has significant anticholinergic properties and these tend to cancel out a direct depressant effect on atrioventricular conduction. Although disopyramide has little effect on the sinus node of normal individuals, it may produce marked sinus node depression in patients who already have some sinus node dysfunction. Disopyramide prolongs the HV interval, and in rare patients, it may precipitate AV block. During routine clinical usage, disopyramide at usual concentrations produces little change in the PR interval, and given orally, it causes little or no prolongation of the QRS. However, it may cause a moderate prolongation of the QT interval.

(b) Pharmacokinetics

Disopyramide may be administered either orally or intravenously, but only the oral preparation is currently available for use in the United States. The drug is well absorbed orally and reaches a peak serum concentration approximately 1 to 2 hours after ingestion. Real excretion of unchanged drug is the major mode of elimination. Elimination is prolonged in renal failure, and doses must be adjusted according to serum concentrations.

(c) Hemodynamic effects

Disopyramide has negative inotropic effects that can complicate its use in patients with congestive heart failure. It has been reported to lower cardiac output, raise systemic vascular resistance, and depress left ventricular function.

(d) Side effects

Disopyramide has potent anticholinergic effects, which include dry mouth, urinary hesitancy, and constipation. Acute urinary retention may occur in patients with prostate enlargement or diabetes mellitus. The drug may also precipitate acute glaucoma. Rare cases of hepatitis developing during its use have been reported.

(e) Dosage and administration

The usual loading dose is 300 mg orally, with subsequent doses of 100 to 200 mg every 6 or 8 hours. The interval between doses should be decreased in the presence of renal failure.

b. **Class Ib Agents**

(1) Lidocaine (Xylocaine)

(a) Action

Lidocaine is a local anesthetic of the amide type. It is only a moderately potent sodium-channel inhibitor. It also acts to shorten APD, increase potassium conductance, and suppress automaticity. It has minimal effect on the duration of the QRS complex or PR or QT intervals; however, in injured tissues, lidocaine enhances conduction at the Purkinje-myocardial cell junction and shortens the duration of the action potential. It also increases the threshold to ventricular fibrillation. It is effective in re-entrant rhythms because it enhances conduction and lessens the discrepancy between the refractory periods of normal and dysfunctional tissue.

(b) Indications

The most frequent indication for giving lidocaine is ventricular premature beats, which are frequent (more than five per minute), close coupled, multifocal in origin, or occurring in short bursts of two or more in succession. However, ventricular ectopy of any degree of frequency, when myocardial ischemia is suspected, can also be promptly suppressed with lidocaine. Lidocaine is also indicated in ventricular tachycardia or ventricular fibrillation, especially if it is resistant to defibrillation.

Lidocaine is generally ineffective for supraventricular arrhythmias. However, it has been reported to be effective in the treatment of atrial flutter-fibrillation in the WPW syndrome because it depresses conduction over the accessory pathway.

(c) Dose

For PVCs, a dose of 1 to 1.5 mg/kg is given as an IV bolus. This can be repeated every 5 minutes, up to four or five times, if necessary. The total toxic dose is variable. In patients without liver disease or severe heart failure, the total dose should not exceed 5.0 mg/kg in any 30-minute period. In other patients, the toxic dose may be much lower.

Following two initial boluses of 1.0 to 1.5 mg/kg IV, patients resuscitated from ventricular tachyarrhythmias and those having recurrent PVCs should receive an IV infusion of lidocaine, 1 to 4 mg/min, usually starting at the higher doses and continuing the infusion for at least the next 24 hours. Continuous oscilloscope monitoring should be provided while the drug is being administered.

(d) Adverse effects

The adverse effects of lidocaine generally correlate with elevated plasma levels. Most toxic reactions involve the CNS and include dizziness, parasthesias, light-headedness, confusion, lethargy, or even coma. Seizures, which are usually responsive to diazepam, may also occur with excessive doses. With a given dose, plasma levels are higher in patients with liver disease or congestive heart failure. Adverse effects can occur in such patients with doses of as low as 1 mg/kg.

PITFALL
Failure to reduce the doses of lidocaine in patients with severe cardiac or liver failure may cause severe lidocaine toxicity.

Lidocaine in very large doses has been reported to depress conduction in patients with either high-degree SA or AV block or with fascicular block, and it is relatively contraindicated in these situations. It is also contraindicated in patients who are allergic to local anesthetics of the amide type. However, lidocaine may be given to persons who are allergic to procaine hydrochloride, since procaine, tetracaine, and benzocaine are paraminobenzoic esters and cross-reactivity between the two groups is not expected.

(2) Mexiletin

(a) Action

Mexiletin resembles lidocaine in chemical structure and local anesthetic properties. It has a direct membrane effect in vitro, typical of quinidinelike drugs. It decreases the upstroke velocity of the action potential, shortens action potential duration, slows conduction velocity, and results in membrane stabilization, indicative of a local anesthetic effect.

(b) Indications

Efficacy has been reported in 74% to 92% of patients when used orally or intravenously to treat ventricular arrhythmias associated with recent myocardial infarction, digitalis intoxication, or cardiac surgery. Minimal associated cardiac depression, reasonable efficacy, a regimen of only two or three doses daily, and a low incidence of serious side effects make mexiletin suitable for long-term management of ventricular arrhythmias. Evidence indicates that mexiletin can be used with relative safety in patients with acute myocardial infarction or cardiomyopathy. Such patients have an increased risk of serious ventricular arrhythmias and many other antiarrhythmic agents are contraindicated.

(c) Dose

Mexiletin is primarily metabolized by the liver. The usual oral dose is 200 to 400 mg administered every 6 or 8 hours. The intravenous dose is generally 200 mg over 3 to 5 minutes followed by 1.0 to 1.5 mg/min.

(d) Adverse effects

Noncardiac adverse effects, such as tremor, diplopia, and nausea, have been reported in 40% to 70% of patients, and serious reactions, including thrombocytopenia, in 17%. Unwanted cardiovascular effects, such as depression of sinus node, atrioventricular node, or myocardial function is uncommon, except in patients with pre-existing disease.

Isolated incidents of serious arrhythmogenesis have been observed with mexiletin therapy, but none have been recognized in patients with chronic stable ventricular arrhythmias or in patients who received prophylactic mexiletin ther-

169

apy after acute myocardial infarction. The incidence of arrhythmia aggravation when mexiletin is used to treat refractory ventricular arrhythmias is generally lower than that reported with other drugs.

(e) Contraindications

Mexiletin should be used with caution in patients with known hepatic disease, refractory tachyarrhythmias, epilepsy, or a history of psychosis.

(3) Tocainide

(a) Action

Tocainide is another class Ib compound structurally related to lidocaine that has similar electrophysiologic properties. Its chief advantage over lidocaine is its long elimination half-life and its ability to be taken orally. After intravenous infusion, the drug produces only minor changes in sinus rate or in the PR, QRS, or QT intervals. When given to some patients with ventricular tachycardia, tocainide may paradoxically shorten the tachycardia cycle length and cause degeneration to ventricular fibrillation.

(b) Indications

Tocainide can suppress ventricular premature beats in 40% to 70% of patients with stable, asymptomatic arrhythmias. The response rate to tocainide for patients with sustained ventricular tachycardia or ventricular fibrillation is much lower; however, like mexiletin, it should probably not be used as a single agent in therapy of sustained ventricular tachyarrhythmias. Tocainide has not been shown to be of significant benefit during acute myocardial infarction.

(c) Dose

The recommended initial dose is 400 mg every 8 hours, and this can be increased to 600 mg every 8 hours as needed. Tocainide is rapidly absorbed orally with almost 100% bioavailability. Peak serum levels are seen 1 to 2 hours after oral ingestion. The drug is eliminated both by hepatic metabolism and by renal filtration. The elimination half-life is between 10 and 15 hours. Antiarrhythmic effects are noted at plasma concentrations of 5 to 12 mg/liter.

(d) Adverse effects

Central nervous system toxicity is a frequent complication of tocainide therapy, with tremors, headache, visual disturbances, dizziness, and paresthesia observed frequently, even with plasma levels below 10 μg/ml. Nausea, vomiting, dyspepsia, and anorexia are seen in approximately 10% to 25% of patients. Other much less frequent adverse reactions include an allergic rash, leukopenia, and pulmonary fibrosis. It should not be given to patients with second- or third-degree heart block.

(4) Diphenylhydantoin (Dilantin) (Phenytoin)

(a) Action

Dilantin acts somewhat like other class Ib antiarrhythmics. It enhances conduction at the Purkinje-myocardial junction and shortens the duration of the action potential in injured tissues. It also raises the threshold for ventricular fibrillation.

(b) Indications

AXIOM
Phenytoin's main cardiac use is the treatment of arrhythmias due to digitalis toxicity.

Dilantin is used primarily for chronic treatment of epilepsy. However, it may also be effective in the management of atrial and ventricular tachyarrhythmias due to digitalis toxicity. It may also be used to abolish some ventricular arrhythmias, but it is much less effective than other drugs for this, especially if the arrhythmias are due to ischemic heart disease.

(c) Dose

For ventricular arrhythmias, 100 mg is given IV over 5 minutes. The dose may be repeated every 5 to 15 minutes, as needed, to a total of 500 to 600 mg. In some instances, a full antiseizure loading dose of 18 mg/kg may be required, but it should not be given faster than 50 mg/min. Dilantin should not be given intramuscularly because absorption is erratic and unreliable.

(d) Adverse effects

PITFALL
Administering Dilantin rapidly IV.

Dilantin should not be given faster than 50 mg/min. Hypotension, asystole, or ventricular fibrillation can be produced by the administration of large, rapid bolus doses of Dilantin. This may be at least partly due to the diluent propylene glycol. Other adverse effects include urticaria, purpura, maculopapular eruptions, and bradycardia. Sinoatrial or AV conduction disturbances may occur but are unusual if the Dilantin is administered slowly. Dilantin should be given with caution in the presence of nodal or infranodal conduction defects.

c. Class Ic Agents

(1) Encainide

(a) Action

Most class Ic drugs markedly reduce sodium-membrane conductance and phase 0 of the action potential, but they have relatively little effect on repolarization. In Purkinje fibers, encainide depresses V_{max} during phase 0 of the action potential, shortens action potential duration, prolongs the ERP relative to the APD, and decreases the rate of spontaneous phase 4 depolarization. Conduction velocity in Purkinje fibers is markedly reduced. Normal sinus node function and AV nodal conduction are only slightly affected by IV encainide, but the HV interval is markedly prolonged. During chronic therapy, accumulation of active metabolites may also cause prolongation of the AH interval. Consequently, during chronic therapy the ECG of patients will usually show a prolonged PR interval and a widened QRS.

(b) Indications

Encainide is an effective agent for suppressing ventricular premature beats and nonsustained ventricular tachycardia in patients without important structural heart disease. Results in patients with a history of sustained arrhythmias are less predictable.

Encainide may be useful in patients with supraventricular arrhythmias. If relatively high doses (150 to 200 mg/day) are used, encainide can markedly prolong the ERP of, or even block conduction in, accessory pathways. The role of encainide in patients with paroxysmal atrial flutter or fibrillation has not been thoroughly investigated.

(c) Dose

Encainide therapy is usually started at a dose of 25 mg three times daily and cautiously increased every 3 to 4 days as needed up to a maximum dose of 200 mg daily. Rapid loading should be avoided because of the risk of overshooting the desired effects and either adversely affecting AV conduction or producing proarrhythmic effects.

Encainide is rapidly and well absorbed after oral administration, but in about 92% of the North American population, extensive first-pass hepatic extraction and metabolism occur before the drug reaches the systemic circulation. In these patients most of the clinically apparent effects are produced by metabolites.

Approximately 8% of the North American population genetically lack the ability to metabolize encainide readily. In these patients much higher plasma concentrations of encainide are seen, and the parent compound is responsible for the antiarrhythmic activity.

(d) Adverse effects

Encainide causes dose-related side effects that limit therapy in about 25% of patients. The most common adverse reactions are dizziness, blurred vision, ataxia, tremor, headache, and gastrointestinal upset. The relationship between these side effects and the plasma concentrations of encainide and its major metabolites is unknown.

Encainide, like flecainide and other similarly acting drugs, has a potential for producing proarrhythmic effects without warning. In the most severe form, these arrhythmias are sustained ventricular tachycardia with unusually wide QRS complexes that may be resistant to cardioversion attempts.

171

In the Cardiac Arrhythmia Suppression Trials (CAST), encainide and flecainide had a higher risk of sudden cardiac deaths (4.5%) than the placebo (1.2%). The incidence of total deaths was also increased (7.7% vs. 3.0%).

AXIOM

Because the use of encainide and flecainide has been associated with an increased mortality, these agents should be restricted to symptomatic ventricular arrhythmias not responding to other, safer medications.

(2) Flecainide

(a) Actions

Flecainide as a class Ic agent is a potent inhibitor of fast sodium-channel activity and markedly depresses the upstroke of the action potential during phase 0. Conduction velocity in Purkinje fibers and both atrial and ventricular muscle is slowed. Normal sinus node automaticity is usually not changed, but Purkinje fiber automaticity is inhibited. Conduction velocity in the AV node is also decreased. During electrophysiologic studies, flecainide prolongs both the AH and HV intervals, prolongs or blocks conduction times in accessory pathways, and produces minor increases in atrial and ventricular refractoriness.

During chronic flecainide therapy, increases in the PR interval and QRS duration may be seen. Increases in QRS duration of more than 25% indicate toxic blood levels.

(b) Indications

Although increased mortality rates have been noted with its use, flecainide is still a reasonable choice in patients with normal ventricular function and symptomatic ventricular arrhythmias not responding to other safer agents. Although it may be used in patients with compromised ventricular function, careful monitoring is required.

(c) Dose

AXIOM

Since cardiac toxicity to flecainide is commonly seen during the first few days of therapy, rapid loading is not recommended.

In stable patients without congestive heart failure, the initial dose should be 100 mg twice daily, with increases up to 200 mg twice daily after steady-state plasma concentrations have been achieved. In patients with heart failure, 50 mg twice daily is a more appropriate initial dose, and dosage increases should be made with caution.

Up to 95% of an oral dose is bioavailable and is not affected by food or antacids. Little first-pass hepatic extraction occurs. The average elimination half-life is between 12 and 24 hours, but this may be prolonged in patients with congestive heart failure or renal insufficiency. Careful monitoring from patient to patient is required to maintain plasma concentrations within the desired range and to avoid toxicity.

(d) Adverse effects

In stable patients with normal ventricular function, minor extracardiac side effects including dizziness, dysgeusia, blurred vision, nausea, and headache may be seen. In contrast, patients with more serious cardiac disease are susceptible to several life-threatening forms of cardiac toxicity. Flecainide decreases left ventricular ejection fraction, cardiac output, and stroke work, and increases left and right ventricular filling pressures.

During chronic oral therapy, 5% to 15% of patients treated with flecainide will either develop new or worsening congestive heart failure. Flecainide has also been associated with a 10% to 15% incidence of worsened arrhythmias when given to patients with sustained ventricular tachycardia or cardiac arrest. This proarrhythmic effect often presents as a sustained ventricular tachycardia with very wide, poorly defined QRS complexes that may not support an adequate blood pressure. This rhythm may be resistant to attempts at DC cardioversion and may prove fatal despite immediate and appropriate resuscitation attempts. Complete AV block may also be seen if flecainide is used in patients with pre-existing AV conduction system disease.

As mentioned previously, the Cardiac Arrhythmia Suppression Trial (CAST) has shown that the use of encainide and flecainide to treat asymptomatic or minimally symptomatic ventricular arrhythmias in patients after myocardial infarction is associated with a substantial increase in the sudden-death rate and total mortality.

d. Class II Agents (Beta-Adrenergic Blockers)

(1) Propranolol

(a) Action

Propranolol, timolol, and metoprolol have quinidinelike effects resulting in prolongation of the action potential. In therapeutic doses, however, its major effect is its beta-adrenergic blocking activity, thereby decreasing heart rate and depressing myocardial contractility. Thus, it may be used to help relieve myocardial ischemia and hypertension.

(b) Indications

Because of its long duration of action this agent is only rarely used now for emergency treatment of arrhythmias. The arrhythmias treated most frequently by propranolol have been supraventricular and ventricular tachyarrhythmias. It has been helpful when other drugs have failed and if excess endogenous or exogenous catecholamines are present. It can convert paroxysmal supraventricular tachycardia to normal sinus rhythm, and it can decrease the ventricular response in atrial fibrillation. It is also useful in the management of paroxysmal atrial tachycardia in the WPW syndrome.

(c) Dose

For urgent situations, 0.5 to 1.0 mg is given slowly IV over 2 to 5 minutes. The dose may be repeated in 5 minutes if needed. Significant myocardial depression can occur if more than 2 mg is given IV. Therefore, doses in excess of this should be given with great caution. In nonurgent situations, a starting dose of about 20 mg orally every 4 to 6 hours is usually employed.

AXIOM
When possible, beta-adrenergic blocking agents should be avoided in patients with asthma, heart failure, or hypotension.

(d) Adverse effects

Adverse effects include nausea, vomiting, light-headedness, mental depression, bradycardia, hypotension, bronchospasm, and pulmonary edema. Propranolol should generally not be administered to patients with asthma. It is also contraindicated in severe sinus bradycardia, advanced SA and AV conduction abnormalities, and in congestive heart failure or cardiogenic shock, unless the shock is clearly due to a tachyarrhythmia.

(2) Esmolol

(a) Action

Esmolol (Brevibloc) is one of the newer drugs available to treat SVT, and it has largely replaced propranolol for treatment of acute supraventricular tachycardias. It is a short-acting beta blocker that is rapidly metabolized by esterases coating the surface of red blood cells (RBCs). Its pharmacologic half-life is about 9 minutes with a therapeutic half-life of around 2 minutes. This rapid onset and short duration of action allow the clinician to titrate the degree of beta blockade desired quite exactly.

(b) Indications

Indications for esmolol include virtually any type of noncompensatory supraventricular tachyarrhythmias. It is effective on accessory bundles, as well as the AV node, so that it will not paradoxically accelerate VT due to these accessory bundles. It converts atrial fibrillation or flutter to NSR more consistently than do the calcium-channel blockers. It is very cardioselective and can usually be given to patients with bronchospastic disease (asthma/COPD) with relatively little risk.

AXIOM

Probably the biggest advantage of esmolol is its extremely short half-life.

If a patient does develop a side effect to the esmolol (usually mild hypotension or bradycardia), one stops the infusion, and within a few minutes the drug is metabolized and the problem is corrected. Esmolol is the most reversible of any of the agents currently used to treat SVT. If the drug does not control the rate, its effects are gone within about 20 minutes. One can then use another agent without risk of cross-reactivity.

(c) Dose

A bolus dose must be given to saturate the RBC esterases in order to rapidly achieve a therapeutic level with infusion. Esmolol may be mixed in almost any crystalloid fluid at a concentration of 10 mg/ml. This is achieved by adding 1 ampule (2.5 g) to 250 ml or 2 ampules to 500 ml of fluid.

The bolus dose is 500 μg/kg IV over 60 seconds, and then an IV infusion is begun at 50 mg$\cdot$kg$^{-1}\cdot$min^{-1}. If that dose is ineffective, the patient is rebolused at 500 μg/kg over another 60 seconds, and the IV infusion is increased to 100 mg$\cdot$kg$^{-1}\cdot$min^{-1}. The IV infusion dose can be increased by 50 mg$\cdot$kg$^{-1}\cdot$min^{-1} every 10 to 15 minutes. The maximal dose is 300 mg$\cdot$kg$^{-1}\cdot$min^{-1} but there is usually nothing gained by doses over 200 mg$\cdot$kg$^{-1}\cdot$min^{-1}.

Once control of the SVT is achieved, the IV infusion is maintained for another 30 minutes and the dose is then reduced by half. The infusion can then be stopped completely after another 30 minutes.

(d) Side effects

The main side effects are similar to those seen with any beta blocker, that is, bradycardia and hypotension; however, bronchospasm is unusual.

e. Class III Agents

(1) Bretylium Tosylate

(a) Actions

Soon after administration of bretylium, norepinephrine is released from the presynaptic nerve endings of postganglionic adrenergic neurons. In the heart, this causes a transient increase in sinus rate, AV conduction, and ventricular automaticity.

Subsequently, bretylium accumulates in the nerve ending, depletes norepinephrine stores, inhibits norepinephrine release, and blocks reuptake of catecholamines. This prolongs the ventricular action potential duration and ERP without changing V_{max} and conduction velocity. In animal models, bretylium increases ventricular fibrillation threshold, particularly during myocardial ischemia. These latter effects require 3 to 6 hours to become apparent.

Severe hypertension may be seen initially after bretylium administration. However, with continued therapy, hypotension is commonly observed. The hypotension is aggravated by postural changes, but may persist even if the patient remains supine. The cardiac index is usually unchanged unless adverse effects are produced by the hypotension.

(b) Indications

Bretylium may be effective against ventricular tachycardia and ventricular fibrillation unresponsive to other agents. The immediate and delayed antiarrhythmic effects of bretylium appear to be mediated by different mechanisms. At present, bretylium's role is restricted primarily to short-term control of ventricular fibrillation. Unfortunately, since the chief clinical experience with bretylium has been in cardiac arrest and in the management of patients with multiple factors contributing to their arrhythmias, an objective analysis of bretylium's clinical efficacy is not possible. There are no convincing data that bretylium is effective for hemodynamically stable ventricular tachycardia, and the hypotension it causes can be harmful.

(c) Dose

The usual dose for a persistent ventricular fibrillation is 5 mg/kg as an IV bolus, followed by electrical defibrillation. If ventricular fibrillation persists, the dose can be increased to 10 mg/kg and repeated at 15- to 30-minute intervals until a total dose of 30 mg/kg is given. In refractory or recurrent ventricular tachycardia, 500 mg of bretylium tosylate can be diluted to 50 ml, and 5 to 10 mg/kg can then be injected IV over 8 to 10 minutes. Once the loading dose has been given, the drug can be administered as a continuous infusion at a rate of 1 to 2 mg/min.

(d) Adverse effects

PITFALL
Failure to consider the severe hypertension and then hypotension that may develop with bretylium.

As norepinephrine is released from nerve endings, a sharp, severe hypertension may occur. However, subsequent hypotension necessitating withdrawal of the drug or the institution of vasopressors is common. Bretylium may also increase infarct size by the initial release of catecholamines and/or later development of hypotension. Rapid intravenous infusion of bretylium frequently also causes nausea and vomiting. This may be ameliorated if the drug is given by slow infusion over 8 to 10 minutes. Chronic oral therapy with bretylium has also been associated with parotitis.

(2) Amiodarone

Amiodarone was initially developed as an antianginal agent, but it also has powerful antiarrhythmic effects in patients with both supraventricular and ventricular arrhythmias. However, its unusual pharmacokinetics profile and its potential for producing toxicity in many organ systems have limited its usefulness.

(a) Actions

Since amiodarone is virtually insoluble in aqueous media, few reports on its acute, electrophysiologic effects are available. During chronic amiodarone therapy, sinus node automaticity is decreased and AV nodal conduction velocity and refractoriness are depressed. His-Purkinje conduction intervals are increased, as are the effective and functional refractory periods of the atria and ventricles. In patients with accessory pathways, both antegrade and retrograde refractory periods are increased.

During chronic amiodarone therapy, the ECG usually shows a moderate sinus bradycardia, a slight prolongation of the PR interval, a prolongation of QRS complexes, and the appearance of prominent U waves, particularly in the midprecordial leads.

There seems to be little change in left ventricular ejection fraction or cardiac output during chronic oral therapy. Nevertheless, some patients may not tolerate the sinus bradycardia usually seen during therapy.

(b) Indications

Amiodarone is an extremely potent antiarrhythmic agent. Most studies have dealt primarily with patients who had previously failed one or more antiarrhythmic drug trials. Nevertheless, long-term efficacy rates of 75% to 90% in patients with supraventricular arrhythmias and 45% to 75% in patients with ventricular arrhythmias have commonly been achieved. Amiodarone is highly effective in patients with recurrent atrial flutter and with paroxysmal supraventricular tachycardia (PSVT) due to either AV nodal re-entry or re-entry involving an accessory AV pathway. Paroxysmal atrial fibrillation also responds in many cases.

In patients with sustained ventricular tachycardia, amiodarone will often either eliminate or decrease the frequency of episodes. The rate of the tachycardia, should it recur, is usually significantly slowed.

(c) Dose

Amiodarone has variable and unusual pharmacokinetics parameters, and elimination kinetics are complex. Loading doses of 800 to 1600 mg/day orally for 1 to 3 weeks with in-hospital monitoring may be required before a therapeutic response occurs. Once adequate arrhythmia control has been obtained, the dose is gradually reduced to 400 to 600 mg/day. Plasma levels decline very slowly after discontinuation of chronic therapy and detectable plasma concentrations may be present as long as 6 to 12 months after the last dose.

AXIOM

One should use amiodarone with great care and only for life-threatening arrhythmias because significant toxicity may occur at all clinically useful doses and over a wide range of plasma concentrations.

(d) Adverse effects

The most dangerous side effect associated with amiodarone therapy is the development of pulmonary infiltrates. This reaction has been reported in up to 10% to 20% of patients treated chronically with amiodarone and it may appear at any point during therapy. Patients with amiodarone pulmonary toxicity usually present with dyspnea and a nonproductive cough. Pyrexia may also occur. Arterial blood gases can show a marked hypoxemia with a low or normal Pco_2. Pulmonary function tests indicate a restrictive defect, and diffusion capacity is usually markedly reduced.

Almost all patients receiving amiodarone chronically develop corneal microdeposits. Although these are readily visible during a slit-lamp examination, they only rarely affect visual activity. However, approximately 10% of patients report visual blurring or halo vision.

Iodine-induced hypothyroidism or hyperthyroidism may be seen, with the incidence dependent on the dietary iodine content of the population studied. Amiodarone also inhibits conversion of T_4 and T_3. Supplementation with thyroxine will prevent clinical symptoms of hypothyroidism without affecting antiarrhythmic activity.

Dermatologic toxicity is common and may be present in two forms. Up to 50% of patients develop increased photosensitivity to ultraviolet light, and a smaller percentage of patients develop bluish-gray discoloration of sun-exposed skin due to accumulation of lipofuscin granules in dermal macrophages.

Neuromuscular toxicity is commonly seen during amiodarone therapy, particularly in older patients, and usually includes proximal muscle weakness, tremor, and peripheral neuropathy.

Liver function abnormalities may be detected in approximately one third of patients receiving amiodarone. The usual finding is a minor (<twofold) elevation of serum glutamic oxaloacetic transaminase (SGOT), and lactic dehydrogenase (LDH) that may be either persistent or transient.

Bradycardias due to either sinus node suppression or drug-induced AV block are frequently encountered during long-term amiodarone therapy. Because of the long period required for drug elimination, permanent pacing of these bradycardias is often required.

f. Class IV Agents (Calcium-Channel Blockers)

Verapamil is the prototype for agents that selectively affect calcium transport. These "calcium blockers" have been used for treating hypertension, variant and typical angina, hypertrophic myopathies, and various arrhythmias.

(1) Verapamil

(a) Actions

Verapamil depresses action potentials dependent on slow channel activity in normal conduction tissue, the sinus and AV nodes, and partially depolarized fibers. Conduction velocity in these cells is also selectively depressed. However, fibers in which the action potential is mediated by fast channel currents are relatively unaffected.

Verapamil may depress sinus node function, particularly in patients with sinus node disease. The refractory period for antegrade conduction over accessory bypass tracts may either show no effect or actually shorten, but the latter effect may be reflex mediated. The ECG may show slight prolongation of the PR interval, whereas the QRS and QT intervals usually remain unchanged.

Verapamil has marked negative inotropic effects and also relaxes vascular smooth muscle. In most patients, the decrease in blood pressure after IV verapamil is primarily due to peripheral vasodilation, but left ventricular end-diastolic pressure also increases, and the drug may precipitate congestive heart failure. However, in many patients with mild or moderate heart failure, particularly after an acute myocardial infarction, the improvement in afterload and attenuation of ischemia may more than compensate for verapamil's negative inotropic effects.

(b) Indications

Verapamil can terminate most episodes of re-entrant supraventricular tachycardia in which the AV node is involved in the re-entry loop. In atrial flutter or fibrillation, conduction through the AV node is delayed and a stable ventricular rate may be achieved. However, reflex adrenergic stimulation in response to hypotension seen after verapamil injection may blunt these effects in unstable patients.

Oral verapamil is useful in the chronic prophylaxis of recurrent paroxysmal supraventricular tachycardia. It also can provide a stable ventricular rate in selected patients with chronic atrial fibrillation.

PITFALL
Using verapamil to treat a tachycardia when an accessory pathway may be present.

(c) Dose

Verapamil may be administered either orally or intravenously. When administered orally (usually 80 mg three or four times a day), the drug is well absorbed but undergoes substantial first-pass hepatic degradation. The elimination half-life for verapamil is about 3 to 6 hours. Elimination is prolonged in cirrhosis and in conditions with decreased hepatic blood flow. Verapamil can be administered intravenously at a dose of 0.75 or 0.15 mg/kg (5 to 10 mg total). It is best given in small boluses of 0.5 to 1.0 mg injected into the side of a rapidly running IV line. Effects can sometimes be obtained with just 2.0 to 2.5 mg.

(d) Adverse effects

The principal extracardiac side effect reported with oral verapamil is constipation. Nausea, vomiting, vertigo, headache, and nervousness have also been reported. After intravenous administration, hypotension and bradycardia may occasionally be seen. There are anecdotal reports that giving IV calcium before the verapamil will present the hypotension occasionally caused by verapamil, but this has not been tested extensively. Ventricular asystole has been reported in patients who previously received IV beta-adrenergic blockers.

When given to patients with Wolff-Parkinson-White syndrome conducting antegradely over an accessory pathway, verapamil may speed antegrade conduction and increase ventricular rates to the point that an almost irreversible ventricular fibrillation may develop. If verapamil is given in doses > 10 mg, it could occasionally cause ventricular fibrillation, even without underlying WPW.

AXIOM
As a general rule, verapamil should not be given to a patient with a wide complex tachycardia of unknown mechanism.

g. Other Agents

(1) Adenosine

(a) Mechanism of action

Adenosine is an endogenous nucleoside that is an intermediate metabolite in many biochemical pathways. It also has a role in the regulation of many physiologic processes including coronary and systemic vascular tone, platelet function, and lipolysis in adipocytes. Adenosine inhibits sinus node automaticity and depresses AV nodal conduction and refractoriness. Adenosine produces a transient AV nodal block, which breaks re-entrant circuits within the AV node. It has no effect on anterograde conduction over accessory pathways in patients with Wolff-Parkinson-White syndrome.

Adenosine may prove to be valuable in determining the origin of broad complex tachycardia. An adenosine-induced AV block can slow the ventricular rate and reveal the unaffected atrial arrhythmias. Adenosine acts on supraventricular tachycardias (SVT) with aberrant conduction, while having no effect on ventricular tachycardia. Unlike verapamil, which may produce severe hemodynamic deterioration in patients with VT for several minutes, adenosine has relatively little effect on blood pressure, and if the BP does fall, it is usually very transient.

(b) Indications

Adenosine is indicated for the acute treatment of paroxysmal supraventricular tachycardias, including those associated with Wolff-Parkinson-White syndrome. The drug has also been used to assist in the diagnosis of broad complex tachycardias. Although some feel that it is contraindicated in atrial fibrillation, it can assist with the diagnosis by slowing the ventricular rate enough to see the arterial pattern. In a recent study by DiMarco and colleagues, adenosine was found to be as effective as verapamil for PSVT, with a more rapid onset of action.

(c) Pharmacokinetics

Adenosine must be administered quite rapidly through an IV line with a relatively large needle. If it is given slowly, it can be metabolized in the blood before it even reaches the heart. The usual initial dose is 6 mg IV rapidly. If there is no effect within 1 to 2 minutes, a dose of 12 mg may be given rapidly IV. If this dose is not effective within 2 minutes, another dose of 12 mg may be given rapidly IV.

Adenosine has a very rapid onset of activity and can terminate most supraventricular tachycardias within 20 to 30 seconds. It also will induce an AV nodal block rapidly in patients with arrhythmias not requiring AV nodal conduction. Adenosine's duration of action is very short, usually less than 10 seconds, due to its rapid cellular uptake and metabolism.

Adverse reactions to adenosine are common, but very brief. The most common adverse reactions associated with adenosine are flushing (20%), dyspena (20%), and chest pain (20%). Headache, nausea, coughing, and malaise also have been reported. These effects are transient, usually acting less than 1 minute. A slight rise in blood pressure may occur after conversion to sinus rhythm.

Other cardiovascular adverse effects include sinus bradycardia, sinus arrest, atrial fibrillation, and various degrees of AV block.

(d) Drug interaction

Adenosine should not be used in patients receiving methylxanthines. Adenosine should be used with caution in patients receiving dipyridamole, which potentiates its clinical effects, and initial doses of adenosine should not exceed 1.0 mg in such patients.

(2) Digitalis Preparations

(a) Actions

Digitalis binds to the enzyme Na-K ATPase and thereby inhibits sodium and potassium movement across the cell membrane. It increases myocardial contractility, decreases the rate of impulse conduction, and prolongs the functional refractory period of the AV node. However, it shortens the refractory period of atrial muscle. ECG changes produced by digitalis include depression of the ST segment and decrease in the height of the T waves.

(b) Indications

The greatest use of digitalis preparations, especially digoxin, is in decreasing AV conduction, thereby slowing the ventricular rate in patients with atrial tachyarrhythmias, especially atrial flutter and fibrillation. It also can be used to control a variety of arrhythmias due to, or associated with, congestive heart failure. Some physicians feel that there is no place for digoxin in the emergency treatment of arrhythmias, and it should probably not be given without first checking digoxin and potassium levels.

(c) Dose

Depending on the urgency of the situation, digoxin may be given intravenously or orally. The total digitalizing dose for IV digoxin is usually 1.0 to 1.5 mg given in divided doses over 24 hours followed by a daily maintenance dose of 0.25 mg.

(d) Adverse effects

Side effects of digitalis preparations are frequent, but they are usually due to excessive dosage or failure to reduce the maintenance dose in patients with renal impairment.

PITFALL
Failure to adequately monitor serum potassium and calcium levels in patients receiving digitalis preparations.

Digitalis toxicity is most apt to occur in patients with hypokalemia, hypercalcemia, or acute myocardial infarction, and immediately after cardioversion or cardiopulmonary bypass. Gastrointestinal symptoms, such as nausea, are more common with oral preparations.

Digitalis can cause a wide variety of cardiac arrhythmias including frequent PVCs (often with multifocal coupling), interference dissociation, PAT with block, nonparoxysmal nodal tachycardia, varying degrees of AV block (often Wenckebach phenomenon), atrial fibrillation or flutter, and ventricular tachycardia or fibrillation.

AXIOM
PAT with block should be considered due to digitalis toxicity until proven otherwise.

Treatment of digitalis-induced arrhythmias generally involves discontinuing the digitalis preparation, at least temporarily. Potassium and magnesium may be given to reduce the digitalis effect, but they should not be administered to patients with atrial tachycardia with a high-grade (3:1 or 4:1) AV block or complete heart block due to digitalis. Cardioversion should generally also not be used in this situation because it may cause severe tachyarrhythmias due to increased digitalis toxicity.

AXIOM
Cardioversion releases digitalis from tissue stores and increases the tendency to digitalis toxicity.

(3) Potassium

Potassium decreases the sensitivity of the heart to digitalis and, therefore, may be valuable in treating digitalis toxicity. It is usually administered in urgent situations in doses of 10 to 20 mEq in 50 ml of D_5W by intravenous piggyback (IVPB) to run over a period of an hour. It usually takes at least 40 to 50 mEq of potassium chloride to raise serum levels by 1.0 mEq/liter while ECG and serum potassium levels are closely monitored. Since alkalosis tends to lower serum potassium levels and acidosis tends to raise serum potassium levels, the patient's acid-base balance should be checked prior to and during therapy.

Potassium may also be given in a variety of oral preparations in doses of 20 to 30 mEq three or four times a day. This may be particularly important in patients receiving loop diuretics that tend to increase urinary potassium loss.

(4) Magnesium

Many arrhythmias due to, or associated with, hypokalemia may also be related to hypomagnesemia. Magnesium may occasionally correct ventricular arrhythmias refractory to all other agents, even when the serum magnesium level is normal.

179

Serum magnesium levels may be normal in spite of moderate-to-severe total body magnesium deficits.

For cardiac arrhythmias, the dose is 10 to 15 ml of a 20% magnesium sulfate solution given IV over 5 to 10 minutes. This should be followed by an IV infusion of 2% magnesium sulfate in 250 to 500 ml of D_5W over 4 to 6 hours. Serum magnesium levels should be followed closely and the infusion stopped if the level rises above 3.0 mEq/liter or if deep-tendon reflexes disappear.

If blood levels exceed 3 to 4 mEq/liter, hyporeflexia often develops. Consequently, deep-tendon reflexes should be checked frequently whenever concentrated $MgSO_4$ is given. At 6 to 8 mg/liter, hypotension may develop, and at 10 mEq/liter, muscular and respiratory paralysis and complete heart block may occur.

(5) Atropine Sulfate

Atropine increases pulse rate and myocardial contractility by its parasympatholytic effect. It is useful in treating sinus bradycardia that is accompanied by hypotension or frequent ventricular ectopic beats. Atropine also is useful if the rate is less than 50 beats per minute in the presence of high-degree AV block at the nodal level and in the presence of ventricular asystole.

The recommended dose of atropine sulfate is 0.5 to 1.0 mg given IV and repeated at 5-minute intervals to a total dose of 2.0 mg or until the desired rate is achieved.

PITFALL
Failure to recognize that 0.5 mg of atropine may paradoxically slow the heart rate by either a peripheral parasympathomimetic or a central vagal-stimulating action.

Because tachycardia can greatly increase myocardial oxygen requirements, atropine should be used cautiously in the presence of acute myocardial ischemia. Excessive rate acceleration in such settings may cause an acute myocardial infarction or increase its size. Ventricular fibrillation and tachycardia can also occur following IV atropine. Urine retention and glaucoma may be severely aggravated by atropine, and atropine is generally contraindicated in patients with prostatism or glaucoma.

(6) Isoproterenol

Isoproterenol is a powerful beta-adrenergic stimulator, which can greatly increase heart rate and myocardial contractility. It is most useful in patients with severe sinus bradycardia or AV conduction abnormalities, especially if hypotension is present and the bradycardia is refractory to atropine. In patients with a weak, slow heart, it can greatly increase heart rate, BP, and cardiac output.

The optimal dose is usually 1 to 2 μg/min, usually as an IV infusion of 2 mg in 500 ml D_5W at 0.25 to 0.5 ml/min. Occasionally doses as high as 30 μg/min may be required, but these higher doses can cause sudden, severe tachyarrhythmias.

PITFALL
Use of isoproterenol to treat an asymptomatic sinus bradycardia in a patient with an acute myocardial infarction.

Isoproterenol is generally contraindicated in patients with an acute myocardial infarction. It tends to increase myocardial oxygen demand more than it increases coronary blood flow and thus may increase myocardial ischemia. A possible exception is the patient with congestive heart failure or hypotension resulting from a severe sinus bradycardia or AV conduction disturbance.

D. CARDIOVERSION

Cardioversion has become a well-accepted technique for rapidly controlling a wide variety of tachyarrhythmias, particularly those causing severe cardiovascular symptoms and those unresponsive to standard drug therapy.

1. Indications

The main indication for cardioversion of an arrhythmia is an "unstable" patient characterized by (1) hypotension (systolic BP <90 mm Hg), (2) severe heart failure (e.g., pulmonary edema), (3) unremitting chest pain, or (4) evidence of cerebrovascular insufficiency (confusion, seizures, coma).

a. Atrial Fibrillation

The most frequent arrhythmia for which cardioversion is used is atrial fibrillation. Up to 50% of patients with this arrhythmia may be successfully converted to normal sinus rhythm with direct current shock, but only about 10% to 15% will remain in normal sinus rhythm 1 year after successful cardioversion. Consequently, if the patient has few or no symptoms, conversion to normal sinus rhythm will produce relatively little clinical improvement.

Patients with atrial fibrillation who are most apt to be successfully converted to normal sinus rhythm by direct-current shock have had atrial fibrillation for less than 2 years, are less than 50 years old, have normal-size hearts, normal mitral valves, and hypertension or thyrotoxicosis as the etiology of their heart disease. Clinical benefit is most apt to be noted with conversion to normal sinus rhythm if (1) the ventricular rate is difficult to control; (2) atrial fibrillation precipitates or causes increased heart failure, angina, or systemic emboli; and (3) uncontrolled palpitations occur.

Patients least likely to have atrial fibrillation converted to normal sinus rhythm include those with atrial fibrillation present for more than 3 years, those with uncorrected mitral valve disease or multiple valvular operations, and those with low-amplitude fibrillatory waves.

Maintenance of normal sinus rhythm after successful cardioversion can be extremely difficult. Quinidine 300 mg qid is often helpful. If 10 to 20 mg qid of propranolol is also given, less quinidine seems to be needed.

b. Supraventricular Tachycardias

Up to 70% of patients who have PAT with block, atrial tachycardia, AV junctional tachycardia, or undefined atrial tachycardias have responded successfully to cardioversion. When AV block is present, the main problem is identification and elimination of digitalis intoxication as the cause of the arrhythmia.

AXIOM

Failure of a patient with an AV block to respond to potassium and Dilantin suggests that the arrhythmia is not due to digitalis and may respond successfully to cardioversion.

Atrial or junctional tachycardias should be treated first with vagal maneuvers or antiarrhythmic drugs such as Dilantin. If these are unsuccessful, cardioversion with low-energy discharges is usually effective.

Supraventricular tachycardias associated with pre-excitation WPW syndrome are often refractory to drugs, but they are often successfully cardioverted.

c. Ventricular Tachycardia

Cardioversion may be life saving when ventricular tachycardia causing shock or heart failure does not respond rapidly to lidocaine. Relatively high energy shocks, however, may occasionally be required.

d. Atrial Flutter

Since cardioversion terminates atrial flutter so easily, it is the treatment of choice for this arrhythmia. Energy levels as low as 10 to 25 watt-sec are often successful, and can usually be applied without anesthesia.

e. Arrhythmias in Acute Myocardial Infarction

Although there seems to be some reluctance to use cardioversion in patients with an acute myocardial infarction, this procedure is generally the treatment of choice for arrhythmias causing hypotension or heart failure in such patients.

2. Technique

Since cardioversion greatly increases the sensitivity of the heart to digitalis, particularly if the patient converts to normal sinus rhythm, digoxin is withheld, if possible, for at least 24 hours prior to cardioversion. Longer-acting digitalis preparations are discontinued 48 hours prior to cardioversion.

Some physicians administer quinidine sulfate (300 mg every 6 hours) prior to cardioversion. This can reduce the incidence and severity of atrial and ventricular extrasystoles following the procedure and help maintain a normal sinus rhythm.

Preanesthetic medications may include 100 mg of pentobarbital and/or 5 to 10 mg of morphine given about 1 hour prior to cardioversion. Immediately before cardioversion, atropine 0.4 to 0.6 mg IV is often given to prevent post-conversion bradyarrhythmias due to the increased vagal tone caused by electric shock.

If large energy discharges are likely to be needed, the patient is sedated with rapid-acting agents, such as sodium methohexital, sodium thiopental, or diazepam. Even if only small amounts of energy may be required, an anesthetist should always be present to manage any airway problems that may develop.

During the period of anesthesia, synchronized shock is administered starting with energy levels as low as 10 to 20 watt-sec. Placing the electrodes in anteroposterior rather than anterolateral positions generally accomplishes cardioversion more frequently and with less current. If low-energy shocks fail, the energy is increased by 25 to 50 watt-sec increments until a maximum of 400 watt-sec has been reached.

The cardiac rhythm is observed very carefully immediately following each shock. Extrasystoles are not infrequent following direct-current cardioversion, and higher energy levels seem to increase ventricular irritability.

Lidocaine should be available to be administered in boluses of 1 mg/kg IV if ventricular extrasystoles appear. If the extrasystoles are not controlled, up to three more boluses of lidocaine can be given, followed by a drip of 1 to 4 mg/min. If the extrasystoles persist or increase in spite of the administration of lidocaine, procainamide should be given.

If bradycardia develops and persists for more than 20 seconds following a cardioversion shock, more intravenous atropine sulfate (0.5 mg) should be given. If the bradycardia persists, isoproterenol (0.2 mg in 200 ml fluid) at 1 to 2 ml/min may increase the rate to normal.

3. Complications of Cardioversion

Ventricular fibrillation may occur if an inadvertent unsynchronized shock is delivered during the vulnerable period of the cardiac cycle. However, if this occurs, a second shock almost invariably terminates the ventricular fibrillation.

Ventricular tachycardia or other ventricular arrhythmias occasionally will develop following cardioversion in patients receiving digitalis or quinidine. This may occur because the shock causes release of potassium from the myocardial cells or because stimulation of the autonomic nervous system releases catecholamines. Consequently, these drugs are stopped, whenever possible, prior to cardioversion. If this is not possible, lidocaine (1 to 2 mg/kg) and/or diphenylhydantoin (250 mg IV slowly over a 5-minute period) may help reduce ventricular irritability.

High-energy shocks may cause a significant increase in LDH and SGOT levels, but release of these enzymes is probably from the chest wall and not from the heart itself. Other complications occasionally reported after cardioversion include pulmonary edema, hypotension, and pulmonary or systemic emboli. In general, patients with a history of such emboli should be anticoagulated prior to cardioversion.

SUMMARY POINTS

1. An upright P wave in aVR indicates a junctional rhythm, misplaced leads, or dextrocardia.
2. Presence of abnormal Q waves should be considered evidence of a myocardial infarction until proven otherwise.
3. A wide complex tachycardia may be an early warning of ventricular fibrillation.
4. One should not give calcium to a stable patient with prolonged QT intervals without first checking potassium and ionized calcium levels. T-wave flattening followed by a U wave can look like a prolonged QT interval.
5. QT interval is prolonged by bradycardia, hypocalcemia, myocardial ischemia, and quinidine. QT interval is shortened by tachycardia, hypercalcemia, digitalis, propranolol, and phenytoin.
6. The most common causes of depressed ST segments are digitalis and myocardial ischemia.
7. U waves are usually due to hypokalemia and myocardial ischemia.
8. Left bundle branch block (LBBB) causes intense left axis deviation, and RBBB causes right axis deviation.
9. If the conduction of electrical impulses in the left ventricle do not go through the Purkinje system, the T wave is of opposite polarity to the QRS complex.
10. The two most common causes of tachyarrhythmias are the presence of ectopic foci and re-entry or circus movement. Conditions that facilitate the development of re-entry phenomena are (1) increased length of the pathway of conduction, (2) decreased velocity of conduction, and (3) shortened refractory period.
11. Ectopic foci are usually due to local muscle ischemia, overuse of stimulants, or excess catecholamine release.
12. With any arrhythmia, one must obtain a careful history for ingestion of stimulants or other potentially cardiostimulatory or depressive drugs, especially digitalis, thyroid extract, and amphetamines.
13. An overly sensitive carotid sinus can cause such an increase in vagal tone that hypotension and/or syncope can occur with mild neck pressure.
14. Correction of an asymptomatic bradycardia, especially in a patient who may have coronary artery disease, may cause a disastrous fall in cardiac output and blood pressure.
15. Symptomatic bradycardia is usually best treated initially by atropine (0.5 to 1.0 mg at a time, up to 2.0 mg). If the bradycardia recurs or is persistent isoproterenol and/or transvenous pacing are used.
16. Atrial tachycardias tend to be much more regular than sinus tachycardias (ST).
17. Carotid sinus massage (CSM) causes a slight temporary slowing of SVT, but either has no effect on atrial tachycardia or causes it to cease abruptly.
18. Atrial ectopic premature beats (PACs) are followed by an incomplete compensatory pause (unless the basic rate is rapid), while PVCs tend to have a full or complete compensatory pause.
19. Paroxysmal atrial tachycardia (PAT) is the most frequent paroxysmal tachycardia in children and young adults.
20. When an arrhythmia precipitates or causes shock or severe heart failure, immediate cardioversion is usually the treatment of choice.
21. Propranolol may be effective in terminating supraventricular tachycardias, particularly those associated with digitalis toxicity. However, because of its marked negative inotropic effects, it should generally be avoided in patients with congestive heart failure or severe bronchospasm.
22. An arrhythmia developing while a patient is on a digitalis preparation should be considered as due to that drug until proven otherwise.
23. PAT with block is usually due to digitalis toxicity.
24. PAT with block should be suspected in any digitalized patient who notes either a sudden change in heart rhythm or a sudden onset of palpitations.

25. Sick sinus syndrome is often manifested as intermittent runs of sinus bradycardia and tachycardia (tachy-brady syndrome).
26. If P waves are seen with the QRS complexes in supraventricular tachycardia, the rhythm is often referred to as an atrial tachycardia. If the P waves cannot be seen or occur after the QRS, the tachycardia is often called a junctional (nodal) tachycardia.
27. In the WPW syndrome with PAT, if autograde conduction proceeds down the normal pathway, the QRS configuration is normal.
28. Increased vagal tone tends to convert many re-entry SVTs. However, vagal maneuvers in patients on digitalis can convert an SVT to a ventricular fibrillation that may be very difficult to convert.
29. Synchronized cardioversion is performed with less energy in patients who are on digitalis preparations.
30. Ectopic SVT *not* due to digitalis toxicity is treated by (a) giving digoxin to control the ventricular response, then (b) quinidine or procainamide to reduce atrial ectopy, and then if needed (c) cardioversion, but being sure the patient is not in digitalis toxicity.
31. Treatment of multifocal atrial tachycardia involves (a) correction of the underlying problem, especially chronic lung disease; (b) propranolol of metoprolol, verapamil, and/or $MgSO_4$; (c) cardioversion as needed.
32. Carotid sinus massage tends to slow the ventricular rate in atrial flutter so that the typical sawtooth pattern is more easily seen.
33. Digitalis toxicity should be suspected in atrial fibrillation if the patient has (a) a slow ventricular rate (particularly less than 50 per minute; (b) a regular ventricular rate, implying some degree of AV block with an escape AV junctional pacemaker; or (c) frequent PVCs, especially ventricular bigeminy.
34. Use of cardioversion in a hemodynamically stable patient with possible digitalis toxicity can be disastrous.
35. Any irregular irregularity of the heart rate and rhythm should be considered as due to atrial fibrillation until proven otherwise.
36. Verapamil should not be used to treat atrial fibrillation if it may be associated with an anomalous AV connection.
37. If a patient with atrial fibrillation develops what appears to be ventricular ectopy, one should rule out aberrant conduction (i.e., Ashman's phenomenon) before treating with antiarrhythmic drugs.
38. Factors favoring a supraventricular beat conducted aberrantly (versus a ventricular ectopic beat) are preceding ectopic P wave, varying bundle branch block pattern, varying coupling intervals, response to carotid sinus massage, RSR in V, and/or QRS in V_6. Factors favoring ventricular ectopic beats are a full compensatory pause, fusion beats, constant coupling intervals, and/or a QRS longer than 0.14 second.
39. Parasystoles from an independent cardiac pacemaker can be differentiated from PVCs by varying coupling intervals, a constant interectopic beat interval, and/or frequent fusion beats.
40. Ventricular ectopic beats (PVCs) may be extremely dangerous and should be treated aggressively when (a) they occur at or just prior to the peak of a T wave, (b) several occur in a short time, (c) several occur in succession (especially if the ectopic rate increases from beat to beat), (d) they are multifocal, or (e) a tachycardia is present. However, if the basic ventricular rate is less than 60, ventricular ectopic beats may be an escape phenomenon and essential to life.
41. Ventricular tachycardia can be defined as at least three wide QRS complexes of ventricular origin occurring at a ventricular rate $\geq$ 100 per minute (usually 150 to 200 per minute).
42. As soon as ventricular tachycardia is recognized, lidocaine should be given in an IV bolus of 50 to 100 mg (which may be repeated as needed) and by IV drip at a rate of 1 to 4 mg/min.

43. Torsade de pointes is an unusual form of ventricular tachycardia in which the QRS axis swings in a sinusoidal pattern. Disease or drugs prolonging the QT interval increase the likelihood of its occurrence and persistence.

44. Use of verapamil to treat wide complex tachycardia can accelerate the rate of ventricular tachycardia or cause ventricular fibrillation in up to 40% of cases.

45. The quicker one attempts to convert ventricular fibrillation, the more successful the attempt will be.

46. Propranolol or digitalis can be used to treat SVT, but they should be avoided in re-entrant atrial flutter of fibrillation.

47. Potassium, often given to help correct arrhythmias due to digitalis toxicity, may be contraindicated in patients with a second-degree heart block.

48. Symptoms of Stokes-Adams-Morgagni syndrome or congestive failure in a patient with a complete (third-degree) heart block or Mobitz type-II block below the AV node require insertion of a pacemaker.

49. The biggest problem with a LBBB is that it may mask the ECG changes of an acute myocardial infarction. As a form of bifascicular block, it may be a harbinger of complete heart block.

50. Carotid sinus massage should not be employed if there is any evidence of cerebrovascular disease.

51. Left anterior hemiblock (LAH) should be suspected with a QRS of 0.10 to 0.12 second and a left axis deviation $> -30°$. LPH is suspected by prominent delayed R waves after abnormal Q waves in II, III, and aVF with right axis deviation.

52. Prophylactic cardiac pacing is indicated with acute myocardial infarction if there is a new bifascicular, trifascicular, Mobitz II, or Mobitz III heart block.

53. Lidocaine and diphenylhydantoin are metabolized by the liver; quinidine, procainamide, propranolol, and digitalis are excreted primarily by the kidney.

54. Digitalis toxicity should be excluded, if possible, prior to elective cardioversion of arrhythmias, since digitalis toxicity may lead to irreversible ventricular fibrillation after countershock.

55. Early pacemaker dysfunction is usually due to improper initial electrode placement or loss of an initially correct placement.

56. Procainamide is generally only used for acute problems because it has so many side effects when used chronically.

57. If quinidine is used to treat atrial flutter of fibrillation without first giving digitalis, it may decrease the degree of AV block and cause the development of a dangerous, very rapid ventricular response.

58. Because encainide and flecainide have been associated with an increased mortality rate, its use should be restricted to arrhythmias not responding to other safer medications.

59. Since cardiac toxicity to flecainide is commonly seen during the first few days of therapy, rapid loading is not recommended.

60. When possible, beta-adrenergic blocking agents should be avoided in patients with asthma, heart failure, or hypotension.

61. One should use amiodarone with great care and only for life-threatening arrhythmias because significant toxicity may occur at all clinically useful doses and over a wide range of plasma concentrations.

62. One should carefully monitor serum potassium and calcium levels in patients receiving digitalis preparations.

63. One should know that 0.5 mg of atropine may paradoxically slow the heart rate by either a peripheral parasympathomimetic or a central vagal-stimulating action.

64. Failure of a patient with an AV block to respond to potassium and Dilantin suggests that the arrhythmia is not due to digitalis and may respond successfully to cardioversion.

BIBLIOGRAPHY

1. Amsterdam, EA, et al: Systemic approach to the management of cardiac arrhythmias. Heart Lung 2:747, 1973.
2. Artucio, H and Pereira, M: Cardiac arrhythmias in critically ill patients: Epidemiologic study. Crit Care Med 18:12:1383, 1990.
3. Brown, KR and Jacobson, S: Mastering Dysrhythmias: A Problem-Solving Guide. 1988.
4. Das, G, Talmers, FN, and Weissler, AM: New observations on the effects of atropine on the sinoatrial and atrioventricular nodes in man. Am J Cardiol 36:281, 1975.
5. DiMarco, JP, et al: Adenosine for paroxysmal supraventricular tachycardia: Dose ranging and comparison with verapamil. Ann Intern Med 113:104, 1990.
6. DiMarco, JP, et al: Adenosine for paroxysmal supraventricular tachycardia. Circulation 68:1254, 1983.
7. Dimond, EG: Electrocardiography and Vectorcardiography. Little, Brown & Co, Boston, 1976.
8. Dolan, JT: Clinical management through the nursing process. Crit Care Nurs, FA Davis, Philadelphia, 1991.
9. Dolan, JT: Critical Care Nursing. FA Davis, Philadelphia, 1991.
10. Escher, DJW: Types of pacemakers and their complications. Circulation 47:1119, 1973.
11. Forney, PD and Forney, MA: Ventricular arrhythmias: Appropriate patient selection and treatment options. Hosp Formul 25:1076, 1990.
12. Gabbetta, M and Lipp, H: Coronary care: The understanding and treatment of atrial and ventricular dysrhythmias. Med Clin North Am 57:125, 1973.
13. Gallagher, JJ, et al: Surgical treatment of arrhythmias. Am J Cardiol 61:27A, 1988.
14. Greenspan, AM, et al: Incidence of unwarranted implantation of permanent cardiac pacemakers in a large medical population. N Engl J Med 318:158, 1988.
15. Guidelines for permanent cardiac pacemaker implantation. May 1984: A Report of the Joint American College of Cardiology/American Heart Association Task Force on Assessment of Cardiovascular Procedures (Subcommittee on Pacemaker Implantation). J Am Coll Cardiol 4434, May 1984.
16. Horwitz, S, et al: Electrocardiographic criteria for the diagnosis of left anterior fascicular block. Chest 68:317, 1975.
17. Hurst, JW and Myerburg, RJ: Introduction to Electrocardiography. McGraw-Hill, New York, 1973.
18. Josephson, ME and Seides, SF: Clinical Cardiac Electrophysiology: Techniques and Interpretations. Lea & Febiger, Philadelphia, 1979.
19. Kastor, JA: Pacemaker mania. N Engl J Med 318:182, 1988.
20. Constant, J: Learning Electrocardiography, ed 2. Little, Brown & Co, Boston, 1981.
21. Littman, D: Textbook of Electrocardiography. Harper & Row, New York, 1972.
22. Mandel, WJ, Laks, MM, and Obayashi, K: Atrioventricular nodal reentry in the Wolff-Parkinson-White syndrome. Chest 68:321, 1975.
23. Marriott, HJL: Practical Electrocardiography, ed 8. Williams & Wilkins, Baltimore, 1988.
24. Pinski, SL and Maloney, JD: Adenosine: A new drug for acute termination of supraventricular tachycardia. Cleve Clin J Med 57:383, 2990.
25. Rankin, AC, et al: Value and limitation of adenosine in the diagnosis and treatment of narrow and broad complex tachycardias. Br Heart J 62:195, 1989
26. Rosen, KM, Ehsani, A, and Rahimtoola, SH: Myocardial infarction complicated by conduction defect. Med Clin North Am 57:155, 1973.
27. Ruskin, JN: Cardiac arrhythmia suppression trial (CAST). New Engl J Med 321:386, 1989.
28. Venkataraman, K, Madia, JE, and Hood, WB: Indications for prophylactic preoperative insertion of pacemakers in patients with right bundle branch block and left anterior hemiblock. Chest 68:501, 1975.
29. Vohra, J: Beta-adrenergic blockade in arrhythmias of acute myocardial infarction. Heart Lung 2:662, 1973.
30. Wines, IM and Macari-Hinson, MM: Torsade de pointes: A critical care nurse's dilemma. Heart Lung 19:500, 1990.
31. Woosley, RL and Funck-Brentano, C: Overview of the clinical pharmacology of antiarrhythmic drugs. Am J Cardiol 61:61A, 1988.
32. Wright, KE and McIntosh, HD: Artificial pacemakers: Indications and management. Circulation 47:1108, 1973.

CHAPTER 4

Heart Failure

I. INTRODUCTION

A. INCIDENCE

Congestive heart failure is an increasing problem in the United States. The National Center for Health Care Statistics noted that the number of annual hospital discharges for congestive heart failure increased from 570,000 in 1970 to 1,557,000 in 1982. In 1981 there were more than 4 million office visits for heart failure. The prevalence of cardiac failure is in the order of 60 per 1000 population over the age of 65 years and rises to 100 per 1000 over the age of 75. In the Framingham study, age-specific rates for heart failure doubled at each decade, with the incidence in men exceeding that in women in all age groups.

The mortality for heart failure has failed to decline despite the decrease in deaths from ischemic heart disease and the improvements in control of hypertension. For patients who have severe congestive heart failure that is refractory to standard treatment, the average survival is less than 1 year.

AXIOM

Cardiac failure is often defined as an inability of the heart to pump enough blood to meet the metabolic demands of the body. However, it is usually diagnosed from evidence of pulmonary or systemic venous overload.

B. DEFINITIONS

The term cardiac failure may have vastly different meanings to clinicians and physiologists. To many clinicians, it refers to signs and symptoms related to venous hypertension, pulmonary congestion, and/or reduced cardiac output. However, cardiac output is not reduced in all instances of heart failure. In some patients with heart failure, the cardiac output is normal or even elevated, provided the venous return is high enough to offset the diminished strength of the heart.

AXIOM

From the physiologist's viewpoint, cardiac failure is often defined as a diminished work output of the heart in relation to its filling pressure.

The pumping ability or contractility of the heart may be defined by cardiac function curves, which correlate the stroke work of the heart (mean blood pressure multiplied by stroke volume) with the filling pressures of the heart. Under these circumstances, left heart failure is considered to be present if there is a low left ventricular stroke-work index (LVSWI) in the face of a high pulmonary artery wedge pressure (PAWP) (Fig. 4.1). Right heart failure would be reflected by a low right ventricular stroke-work index (RVSWI) and a high central venous pressure (CVP).

The terms right heart failure and left heart failure are sometimes used clinically to describe the two major types of signs and symptoms seen with cardiac failure. With *right* heart failure, the main signs and symptoms are pedal edema, hepatomegaly, and distended neck veins. With *left* heart failure, the

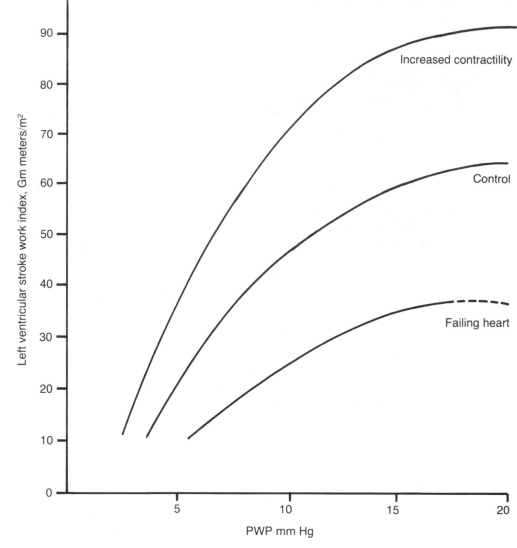

Figure 4.1 Contraction of the intact ventricle.

usual problems are pulmonary congestion with dyspnea, often with weakness or fatigue and light-headedness.

Since the left and right sides of the heart are two separate pumping systems, it is possible for one of the ventricles to fail independent of the other, at least transiently. The most frequent causes of heart failure, such as myocardial infarction, hypertension, or valvular heart disease, primarily affect only the left ventricle initially.

AXIOM
Right heart failure is usually due to left heart failure.

Isolated right heart failure due to chronic obstructive lung disease, acute pulmonary embolism, or right ventricular infarction is much less common than biventricular failure. When one side of the heart becomes weakened or fails, a sequence of events begins that eventually causes the opposite side to also fail. Thus, in most patients with heart failure, both chambers are involved to some degree.

The terms *backward* and *forward* heart failure (used infrequently now) attempted to differentiate between *symptoms* primarily related to venous congestion and symptoms primarily related to a decrease in cardiac output. In most patients, however, both problems are present, and one type of heart failure usually cannot be treated adequately without considering the other.

The terms *heart failure* and *congestive heart failure* are often used synonymously. Traditionally, heart failure referred to peripheral edema, distended neck veins, and hepatomegaly, whereas congestive heart failure referred to a more advanced degree of heart failure with signs and symptoms of overloading of the lungs, such as dyspnea and rales.

Systolic dysfunction of the heart is a more physiologic description of a heart that is unable to either eject adequate amounts of blood into the circulation or effectively empty itself. Diastolic dysfunction of the heart describes abnormal (excessive) filling of the ventricles resulting in increased filling pressures and pulmonary and/or systemic venous congestion.

C. RATE OF ONSET

Some degree of cardiac failure is present in many critically ill patients. Its rate of onset and severity are extremely variable. It may develop acutely (after an acute myocardial infarction, cardiac surgery, or cardiac arrest) or it may develop somewhat more slowly over a period of 24 to 48 hours or longer in patients with sepsis or shock of noncardiac origin. In many individuals cardiac failure develops gradually as a chronic process over a period of weeks, months, or years. If the process comes on slow enough, patients may be unaware of the problem until they begin to have dyspnea with moderate exertion.

II. ETIOLOGY

If a broad definition of cardiovascular failure is used (i.e., inadequate blood flow to meet the body's metabolic demands), three principal causes can be identified. These include primary cardiac failure, inadequate venous return, and circulatory overload (Table 4.1).

A. PRIMARY CARDIAC FAILURE

The primary or direct causes of inadequate heart function can be categorized into myocardial insufficiency, interference with diastolic filling, arrhythmias, and electrolyte and acid-base abnormalities.

1. Myocardial Insufficiency

Probably the single most frequent cause of inadequate cardiac function is myocardial infarction. The next most common cause is an excess pressure or volume load on the heart usually caused by pulmonary or systemic hypertension or cardiac valvular stenosis or insufficiency. Other direct causes of myocardial failure include cardiomyopathies and decreased efficiency of contraction due to ventricular aneurysms.

Table 4.1

CAUSES OF CARDIOVASCULAR FAILURE	1. Primary
	a. Cardiac changes
	Myocardial infarction, valve disorders, etc.
	Cardiomyopathy (alcoholic)
	Hypothyroidism
	b. Interference with diastolic filling (tamponade, constrictive pericarditis)
	c. Arrhythmias
	d. Electrolyte and acid-base abnormalities
	2. Inadequate venous return (hypovolemia, vasodilators, anesthesia, etc.)
	3. Circulatory overload
	a. Increased blood volume
	b. Increased venous return (high-output failure, AV fistulas, etc.)

2. Interference with Diastolic Filling

Pericardial tamponade and constrictive pericarditis interfere with cardiac function by limiting the diastolic filling of the ventricles. Acute pericardial tamponade can be caused by as little as 100 to 200 ml of pericardial fluid. If the pericardial fluid accumulates gradually, as with chronic uremic pericardial effusions, the pericardium has a chance to dilate, and over 1000 ml of pericardial fluid may be present without symptoms.

AXIOM

The most frequent cause of massive pericardial tamponade is chronic renal failure.

3. Arrhythmias

AXIOM

Although tachycardia up to 160 to 180 per minute usually improves cardiac output, if there is coronary artery disease, it severely limits myocardial blood flood.

Severe tachyarrhythmias reduce the time available for diastolic ventricular filling and coronary blood flow. However, severe bradycardias may drastically reduce cardiac output, particularly if there is any restriction of stroke volume. If the arrhythmia is confined to the atria in an otherwise normal heart, it seldom reduces cardiac output by more than 10% to 20% and, therefore, does not usually cause clinical heart failure. However, if mitral stenosis is present or if the heart is already failing, atrial fibrillation (by causing loss of the normal "booster-pump" function of the atria) can decrease cardiac output by 30% to 50% or more and greatly increase any tendency to congestive heart failure.

AXIOM

Atrial fibrillation should generally be prevented or rapidly corrected, especially in patients with severe mitral stenosis.

4. Electrolyte and Acid-Base Abnormalities

AXIOM

Potassium and calcium abnormalities should be prevented or rapidly corrected if there is any evidence of heart failure.

Severe hypokalemia or hypercalcemia tends to stop the heart in systole, whereas hyperkalemia or hypocalcemia tend to stop it in diastole.

AXIOM

Acidosis tends to depress cardiac contractility, but the increased catecholamine release it stimulates tends to override the depression unless the pH is less than 7.10.

Mild acidosis may improve cardiac action, but severe acidosis (pH less than 7.10) tends to reduce ejection fraction and cardiac output. Many patients with metabolic acidosis will have a compensatory respiratory alkalosis, and a $Paco_2$ of less than 20 mm Hg may also interfere with myocardial contractility and coronary blood flow.

B. HYPOVOLEMIA

Hypovolemia is a frequent cause of reduced cardiac output, especially after trauma or surgery. In addition, with severe prolonged shock, capillary permeability increases and fluid therapy may be relatively ineffective because of the tendency for fluid in the vascular space to "leak" into the interstitial fluid space. Venous return may also fall, in spite of a normal blood volume, if vascular capacity is increased by anesthetics, narcotics, or vasodilators.

It may be especially difficult to maintain an adequate intravascular volume in septic patients. The vasodilation and greatly increased capillary permeability associated with severe infection, particularly peritonitis, often increases fluid needs by more than 200 to 500 ml/h over and above measured losses. Because of increased capillary permeability, the lungs may appear to be overloaded with fluid even if the patient is hypovolemic.

AXIOM
Patients with sepsis may develop pulmonary edema in spite of reduced cardiac filling pressures.

Patients with hypertension not infrequently have a reduced blood volume. Consequently, these patients may easily develop sudden hypotension if vasodilators and diuretics are used to control the blood pressure (BP).

C. CIRCULATORY OVERLOAD

1. Increased Blood Volume

In healthy individuals, the difference in blood volume between hypovolemic shock and heart failure may exceed 3 to 4 liters. However, patients with pre-existing cardiac disease may go from hypovolemia to pulmonary edema with fluid infusions of as little as 500 to 1000 ml. Although fluid overloading may occur during the initial resuscitation from shock or trauma, it is more likely to occur during the fluid mobilization phase, which usually occurs 2 to 3 days after acute injury or surgery. If large volumes of fluid continue to be given or if urine output cannot keep pace with the shift of fluid from the interstitial space into the vascular space, hypertension and/or heart failure may result. Patients with renal or hepatic failure also often tend to accumulate water and have a tendency to develop heart failure.

If cardiac filling is increased by more than 30% to 50%, the cardiac muscle fibers may be stretched beyond their normal physiologic limits. This decreases the effectiveness of the heart as a pump and starts a vicious cycle of increasing fluid retention and cardiac failure.

2. High-Output Failure

Although the cardiac output may be high in patients with severe anemia, cirrhosis, arteriovenous fistulas, or thyrotoxicosis, the heart may have difficulty keeping up with the increased venous return. As a consequence, the filling pressures may be much higher than normal, producing a condition often referred to as high-output cardiac failure. The basic problem is not failure of the heart itself, but rather an overloading of the heart with too much venous return.

III. PHYSIOLOGIC CHANGES

The acute cardiovascular responses to a reduced BP or cardiac output are primarily due to an increased sympathetic nervous system activity.

A. RESERVE MECHANISMS

1. Acute (Cardiovascular) Changes

a. Baroreceptor Reflexes

Whenever cardiac output or blood pressure fall, a number of acute circulatory reflexes or responses become active in an attempt to restore blood pressure and flow to normal (Fig. 4.2). The best known of the acute circulatory reflexes involved in heart failure is the baroreceptor reflex. This is activated by reduction in arterial blood pressure, primarily by reducing stimulation of the baroreceptors in the carotid sinus. Normally the carotid sinus is stimulated by a rise in BP, which then inhibits the vasomotor center and causes a lowering of BP to more normal levels. With hypotension, the normal inhibition of the vasomotor center by the carotid sinus is removed. If systolic pressure falls to very low levels (below 60 mm Hg), the nervous system ischemic (baroreceptor) reflex will also be activated, with a rapid and powerful stimulation of the sympathetic nervous system. At the same time, the parasympathetic system is reciprocally inhibited.

In chronic heart failure, the ability of atrial and arterial baroreceptors to suppress sympathetic activity and reduce the release of vasopressin and catecholamines is impaired. Left atrial receptors are no longer appropriately activated by the increase in atrial pressure that follows volume expansion. The cause of this abnormal baroreceptor sensitivity may be related to changes in atrial and arterial compliance as well as to disruption and fragmentation of receptor endings. This baroreflex dysfunction greatly impairs the ability of the circulation to limit the release of vasoconstrictor neurohormones, even after the threat to cerebral perfusion has subsided. Consequently, most patients with heart failure demon-

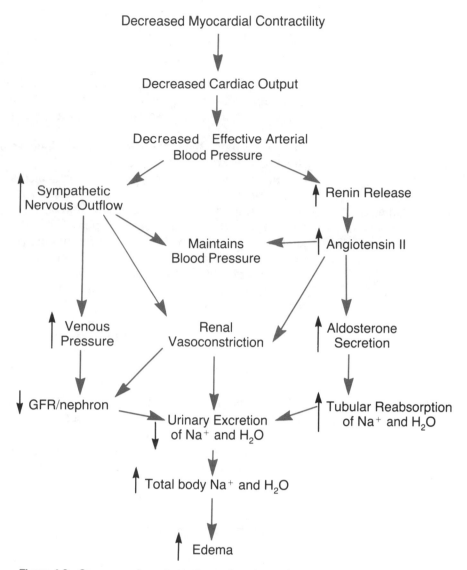

Decreased Myocardial Contractility

Decreased Cardiac Output

Decreased Effective Arterial Blood Pressure

↑ Sympathetic Nervous Outflow

↑ Renin Release

Maintains Blood Pressure

↑ Angiotensin II

↑ Venous Pressure

Renal Vasoconstriction

↑ Aldosterone Secretion

↓ GFR/nephron

Urinary Excretion of Na^+ and H_2O

↑ Tubular Reabsorption of Na^+ and H_2O

↑ Total body Na^+ and H_2O

↑ Edema

Figure 4.2 Sequence of events leading to the edema of congestive heart failure.

strate an increased activation of the sympathetic nervous system with elevated plasma norepinephrine levels, even at rest.

b. Cardiac Effects

Sympathetic stimulation of adrenergic receptors in the heart can greatly increase the force of myocardial contraction. Even a damaged myocardium usually responds to some extent to increased sympathetic stimulation. If a portion of the myocardium is damaged but not dead, sympathetic stimulation will usually also strengthen the contraction of the abnormal myocardium. If less than 40% of the ventricular myocardium is nonfunctional due to infarction, the normal muscle may compensate adequately for the nonfunctional muscle.

The chronic failing heart often lacks adequate stores of norepinephrine because of defective local catecholamine synthesis and storage. Consequently, the heart muscle may have to depend on epinephrine and norepinephrine released from the adrenal medulla and peripheral nerve endings for much of its adrenergic stimulation.

Interestingly, despite high circulating levels of catecholamines, the heart rate may not be greatly elevated in patients with chronic heart failure. Such observations suggest that some adaptation to prolonged sympathetic stimulation occurs. Consequently, the ability of the failing heart to respond to catecholamines becomes increasingly attenuated. This reduced responsiveness is not related to a defect in myocardial contractile elements since the failing myocardium usually responds normally to digitalis and calcium. The problem appears to be related to a specific intracellular deficiency of cyclic adenosine monophosphate (CAMP) in the failing heart.

AXIOM
Continuing heart failure is characterized by down-regulation of beta-adrenergic receptors.

The cause of the intracellular myocardial deficiency of cyclic AMP in chronic heart failure is most likely related to defects in the beta-adrenergic pathway. The failing myocardium becomes depleted of catecholamines, possibly because of defects in the synthesis and uptake of norepinephrine. In addition, the density of beta-adrenergic receptors is markedly decreased in failing human hearts, and this receptor loss is accompanied by a proportional decrease in the activity of adenylate cyclase and agonist-stimulated muscle contraction. A similar reduction in beta-receptor density and catecholamine responsiveness has been observed in the peripheral lymphocytes of patients with heart failure, and consequently, lymphocytes can be used to assess changes in adrenergic responsiveness in heart failure. In the ventricular myocardium, this beta-receptor down-regulation appears to be selective so that quite specific $beta_1$ agonists can no longer mediate a full positive inotropic response. In contrast, selective $beta_2$ agonists tend to retain full inotropic activity in patients with heart failure. Consequently, $beta_2$ receptors may serve an important supportive role in the failing myocardium.

In lymphocytes of patients with heart failure, there is a reduction in the amount of stimulatory G protein (G_s) that promotes cyclase activation. A similar reduction in G_s has also been noted in the ventricular myocardium of dogs in heart failure. Studies in failing human hearts have produced conflicting results, with some studies reporting decreased concentrations of G_s and impaired G_s function and others noting normal G_s function but an increase in inhibitory G protein (G_i). Thus, there seems to be some agreement that the $G_s : G_i$ ratio is reduced in heart failure and that this may contribute to the resistance seen to endogenous and exogenous catecholamines.

c. Vascular Effects

Sympathetic stimulation through alpha-adrenergic receptors increases the muscular tone of most blood vessels in the body. Arteriolar vasoconstriction tends to raise the blood pressure and shift blood toward vital organs, especially the heart and brain. The associated increase in venous tone reduces vascular capacity, thereby increasing venous return, which in turn can help return cardiac back up toward normal.

d. Increased Oxygen Extraction

With increased vasoconstriction and decreased perfusion, tissues are forced to extract more oxygen from the blood. Under normal circumstances, the body extracts about 25% of the oxygen available in the blood. However, when blood flow is greatly reduced, noncardiac tissues may extract more than 40% to 50% of the oxygen present. If the amount of oxygen taken up by the tissue is still inadequate, the arterioles must dilate to provide increased blood flow. If this is still inadequate, the tissues will be forced into anaerobic metabolism with development of a progressive lactic acidosis.

2. Subacute Compensatory Changes

The main change in subacute heart failure is increased salt and water retention.

a. Retention of Sodium and Water

The subacute compensatory changes in heart failure consist of an increase in blood volume and interstitial fluid due to retention of salt and water by the kidneys. The cycle usually begins with a reduced cardiac output, which, in turn, results in renal vasoconstriction with a reduction in glomerular filtration and urine output. In addition, if renal blood flow is decreased, it is diverted from the outer renal cortex to the inner (juxtamedullary) renal cortex, where there are less glomeruli. This also reduces glomerular filtrate. In addition, the juxtamedullary glomeruli have long loops of Henle; consequently, absorption of water and sodium is increased, producing a further reduction in urine output. Thus, in heart failure, the urine tends to be more concentrated (particularly in relation to nitrogen compounds, such as urea and creatinine) but usually has a low (less than 10 to 20 mEq/liter) sodium concentration.

Increased sympathetic tone, decreased renal arterial perfusion, and decreased sodium concentrations in the distal tubules all can activate the juxtaglomerular apparatus (JGA), which releases renin. The renin then cleaves angiotensin I from an alpha$_2$ globulin, and angiotensin-converting enzyme (ACE) converts angiotensin I to angiotensin II. Angiotensin II is a potent vasoconstrictor, especially on the renal afferent arterioles, and it stimulates the adrenal cortex to release aldosterone. Aldosterone causes even more sodium and water retention.

If blood flow to the brain or filling of the atria is reduced, increased amounts of antidiuretic hormone (ADH) are released from the posterior pituitary. The ADH causes increased absorption of water in the distal and collecting tubules, further expanding the extracellular fluid (ECF) and reducing urinary output.

As a result of these mechanisms, fluid retention in moderate cardiac failure may increase the blood volume by 5% to 15% or more. The increased venous return and diastolic filling of the heart may restore cardiac output to relatively normal levels. In severe cardiac failure, however, the salt and water retention may increase blood volume and venous return by 30% to 50% or more. Consequently, myocardial muscle fibers may be stretched beyond their normal physiologic limits, and cardiac output may fall.

AXIOM
Increasing hyponatremia may be an important indicator of impaired cardiac function.

b. Increased Erythropoiesis

Another cause of increased blood volume in patients with cardiac failure is increased production of red blood cells. Whenever oxygen delivery to the tissues is impaired, the bone marrow is stimulated to increase its erythropoietic activity, resulting in an increase in red blood cell volume. However, as the hematocrit rises, particularly above 55%, the resultant increased viscosity tends to increase cardiac work and decrease cardiac output, thereby aggravating the tendency to cardiac failure.

3. Chronic Compensatory Changes

In chronic heart failure there is cardiac hypertrophy and various changes to try to improve local organ blood flow and to reduce excessive accumulation of salt and water.

a. Myocardial Hypertrophy

The principal chronic hemodynamic adjustment to heart failure is hypertrophy of the ventricular myocardium. The rapidity and extent to which the myocardium will hypertrophy will vary with the acuteness of the problem and the type of overload with which the heart must contend. An acute overload (as may develop with acute mitral insufficiency secondary to a rupture of a papillary muscle) is usually tolerated very poorly. However, if the same degree of mitral insufficiency develops slowly over a period of months or years, the changes may be tolerated rather well for quite some time. In general, volume overloads (such as those resulting from aortic insufficiency) are tolerated better than pressure overloads (as may occur with aortic stenosis). Gradually increasing pressure overloads tend to cause hypertrophy. Cardiac dilatation will usually not occur until relatively late, after rather severe failure has developed.

Although myocardial hypertrophy may be an important compensatory mechanism, it makes the heart more susceptible to ischemia. Blood flow to the endocardium through long, narrow transmyocardial arterioles in thickened heart muscle falls very rapidly when diastolic aortic pressure decreases.

Katz in a recent review of the cardiomyopathy of overload has pointed out that the cells of the hypertrophied failing heart are not normal. The synthesis of the myosin heavy chains, which determine myosin adenosine triphosphatase (ATPase) activity (a measure of the rate of energy liberation by myosin in vitro) and muscle-shortening velocity (a measure of the rate of energy use by myosin in vivo), is altered by chronic hemodynamic overloading and heart failure. These changes are associated with an increased tendency to arrhythmias, slowed relaxation, and desensitization to sympathetic neurotransmitters. The decreased response to adrenergic stimulation is due to decreased numbers of beta-adrenergic receptor molecules and altered guanine nucleotide-binding proteins, also known as G proteins.

b. Increased Prostaglandin Production

Experimental studies have shown that renal and cardiac hypoperfusion release prostacyclin (PGI_2) and PGE_2, whose vasodilator properties help preserve renal and coronary blood flow. Recent clinical studies have confirmed these findings by showing that the plasma levels of the metabolites of PGI_2 and PGE_2 in patients with severe heart failure were 3 to 10 times higher than normal.

In the final phases of heart failure, there is increasing release of both renin and prostaglandins by the kidney. Both hormones interact to preserve glomerular filtration rate, despite the marked decrease in cardiac output and renal perfusion. Renal perfusion may become so severely compromised at this stage that atrial natriuretic peptide (ANP) may no longer be able to exert important renal effects. Consequently, prostaglandin may increasingly assume the role of antagonizing the intrarenal effects of the systemic vasoconstrictor hormones. Unlike the atrial peptide, however, prostaglandin increases (rather than decreases) the release of renin from the juxtaglomerular cells, and thus may lead to further activation of endogenous vasoconstrictor systems. The critical reduction in renal blood flow seen in the final phases of chronic heart failure may explain why hyponatremia—an important clinical indicator of severe renal hypoperfusion—has prognostic significance in patients with this disorder.

PITFALL
Use of prostaglandin synthesis inhibitors in patients with severe heart failure and hyponatremia.

With severe heart failure and hyponatremia, indomethacin (a prostaglandin synthesis inhibitor) can cause significant decreases in cardiac index and increases in pulmonary artery wedge pressure (PAWP). Patients with normal serum sodium levels usually have no significant hemodynamic change after indomethacin. Thus, the vasodilator effects of the prostaglandin may be an important compensatory mechanism in severe heart failure complicated by hyponatremia.

c. Atrial Natriuretic Factor

Considerable attention has been given recently to atrial natriuretic factor (ANF), a substance released by atrial cells in response to elevated filling pressures. This substance promotes sodium excretion by the kidneys and may be thought of as an endogenous natriuretic released in response to congestive heart failure or any other conditions elevating atrial pressure.

ANF also exerts potent, direct vasodilator actions by its ability to increase intracellular cyclic guanosine monophosphate (CGMP) and to antagonize the actions of most endogenous vasoconstrictors. Under experimental conditions, ANF inhibits not only the release of norepinephrine from nerve terminals, but also its effects on systemic vessels. It also enhances baroreceptor sensitivity and thereby reduces central activation of the sympathetic nervous system. ANF suppresses the formation of renin and opposes the actions of angiotensin II, including its vasoconstrictor actions and its ability to stimulate thirst and aldosterone secretion. ANF also inhibits the release of vasopressin and its vasoconstrictor effects on systemic vessels and its antidiuretic effects on the collecting ducts.

All of these observations suggest that ANF is a versatile neurohormonal antagonist to many of the physiologic changes occurring in heart failure. This antagonism not only may reduce cardiac distension but may also decrease the adverse effects of endogenous vasoconstrictors on the kidneys. This may explain why renal function is less impaired in subjects with cardiac failure than in subjects with hypovolemia, even when the cardiac output is reduced to the same degree.

Unfortunately many of these studies have been performed using doses of ANF that are far greater than those likely to be seen under clinical conditions. Roach and associates, for example, recently reported that pathophysiologic levels of ANF do not alter reflex sympathetic control in the vascular system. Obviously more work in this area is required.

AXIOM
Positive end-expiratory pressure (PEEP), which decreases the distension of the atria in heart failure, can significantly reduce ANF production, causing even more fluid retention.

B. ORGAN CHANGES IN HEART FAILURE

AXIOM
Myocardial oxygen consumption increases in heart failure, but coronary blood flow tends to fall.

1. Heart

In ventricular failure, the myocardium fails to contract with sufficient force to empty the ventricle properly, and end-diastolic volume and fiber length tend to increase. As a result, each ventricular fiber does not have to shorten as much to eject a given volume of blood. This might seem to be advantageous; however, according to the law of Laplace ($T = PR/2h$), as the ventricle dilates and its radius (R) increases, each fiber must develop more tension (T) at a given intraventricular pressure (P) to eject blood from the heart. This can result in a substantial increase in myocardial oxygen requirements. However, the reduced cardiac output, tachycardia, and high left ventricular diastolic pressures reduce coronary blood flow.

The increased tension required to develop a given pressure results in a decreased rate of myocardial fiber shortening, and consequently the pre-ejection phase of systole is prolonged. In addition, excessive dilation may make contraction of the ventricle less coordinated and less effective.

2. Lungs

AXIOM
One of the most sensitive indicators of increasing cardiac failure is a drop in the arterial PO_2.

In cardiac failure, the vital capacity and functional residual capacity in the lungs are decreased because of increased blood in the pulmonary vessels and increased fluid in the pulmonary interstitial space. Increased fluid and congestion in the lungs also make the lungs stiffer, increasing the work of breathing and the tendency toward atelectasis. If fluid accumulates in the alveoli, the protein present can inactivate surfactant, further increasing the tendency to atelectasis. If pleural effusions develop, there is even further impairment of ventilation.

The forces involved in the translocation of water into the lungs and other tissues in heart failure were defined by Starling in 1896. These have been described by the formula:

$$Q_f = K_t A \left[(P_c - P_i) - (\sigma_c - \sigma_i) \right].$$

Q_f is the net flow of water across a capillary, K_t is the filtration coefficient which defines the fluid conductance across a capillary membrane. A is the cross-sectional area of the involved capillaries. Sigma (σ) is the reflection coefficient which defines the effectiveness of the membrane in preventing protein leakage from the capillary. If none of the protein can move across the membrane, the reflection coefficient is 1.0. If capillary permeability is greatly increased, as in sepsis, it may approach zero. P_c and P_i are the hydrostatic pressures in the capillary and interstitial spaces, respectively, and σ_c and σ_i are the osmotic pressures in the capillaries and interstitial water. In the lungs, only two of these forces, P_c and σ_c, can be readily measured as PAWP and plasma colloid osmotic pressure (COP).

Assuming a normal plasma COP of 22 to 25 mm Hg and a normal PAWP of 6 to 15 mm Hg, the COP-PAWP gradient ranges from 7 to 19 (average 16) mm Hg. This favors fluid remaining inside the pulmonary capillaries. When the COP-PAWP is reduced by either elevation of PAWP or reduction of COP, increased fluid flux into the pulmonary extravascular space may occur. Some studies have indicated that critically ill patients with heart failure, with a COP-PAWP gradient of less than +4 mm Hg tend to develop pulmonary edema as determined by chest x-ray changes. However, most investigators have found a poor correlation between the COP-PAWP gradient and either the amount of extravascular lung water (EVLW) or the amount of shunting (Q_s/Q_t) in the lungs.

3. Liver, Spleen, and Intestines

The increased right atrial pressure present in heart failure tends to reduce venous return from the splanchnic circulation and to produce increasing congestion in the liver, spleen, and intestines. If cardiac failure is severe and persistent, the reduction in liver blood flow caused by the severe congestion may impair liver function. Eventually, the liver may become fibrotic, developing what has been referred to as cardiac cirrhosis.

4. Kidneys

Cardiac failure decreases glomerular filtration and urinary output and can produce a prerenal azotemia with an elevated blood urea nitrogen (BUN). If cardiac failure is severe and persistent, some degree of oliguric renal failure may develop with a significant increase in both serum creatinine and BUN levels.

5. Endocrine Organs

The secretion of renin, ADH, and norepinephrine tends to increase during acute heart failure, but the secretion of these substances is often relatively normal in patients with stable chronic heart failure. After trauma or during sepsis or shock, these substances are usually present in much greater concentrations, and there is an increased tendency to heart failure.

IV. DIAGNOSIS

A. SYMPTOMS

1. Left Ventricular Failure

a. Dyspnea

Patients with left-sided heart failure classically complain of feeling "short of breath" (due to congestion of the lungs) and/or weakness and fatigue (due to an inadequate cardiac output). Dyspnea with mild exertion is often the first symptom of heart failure and is usually associated with an increased respiratory rate (tachypnea). Since dyspnea is largely a subjective sensation, it often correlates poorly with objective measurements.

The exact cause of dyspnea is unknown, but it appears to be related to increased interstitial edema and pulmonary congestion, which decrease lung compliance, increase the work of breathing, and tend to cause hypoxemia. In addition, interstitial edema in the vicinity of the pulmonary capillaries may stimulate juxtacapillary receptors (J receptors) thereby reflexly causing rapid, shallow breathing. The disproportion between the increased work required of the ventilatory muscles and their reduced blood flow may also cause some of the sensation of breathlessness.

b. Cough

In some patients, coughing with excitement or effort may be the first symptom of heart failure and may erroneously lead to the assumption that a pulmonary, rather than a cardiac, problem is present. In some instances, the sputum may appear bloody or rusty (because of the presence of hemosiderin-laden alveolar macrophages), further increasing the suspicion of a pulmonary lesion.

PITFALL
Assuming that an increasing cough is due to a primary pulmonary problem.

c. Orthopnea and Paroxysmal Nocturnal Dyspnea

AXIOM
The symptoms of heart failure in younger patients are often primarily pulmonary.

Orthopnea and paroxysmal nocturnal dyspnea (PND) are particularly interesting symptoms of left heart failure. When the patient with moderate to severe heart failure is in the upright position, blood tends to pool in the most dependent portions of the body rather than return to the heart. Because of increased systemic capillary pressure in dependent areas, as much as 15% of the intravascular water can leak into the tissue spaces of the legs, producing dependent pedal edema. When the patient lies down, however, the blood that was pooled in the legs can now return to the heart, causing increased congestion in the lungs. The edema fluid in the formerly dependent tissues now tends to gradually return to the bloodstream, causing even more congestion.

If shortness of breath occurs as soon as the patient lies down, the patient is said to have orthopnea. On the other hand, patients who are relatively comfortable when they first lie down but awaken suddenly with severe dyspnea several hours later are said to have PND. PND is often considered specific for left-sided heart failure, but it may occasionally also be seen in patients with severe emphysema. The mechanism causing PND is probably related not only to the gradual uptake of fluid from areas of peripheral edema but also to some reduction in cardiac output because of increased vagal tone during sleep.

d. Other Symptoms

Breathlessness, orthopnea, and PND are often the cardinal symptoms of left ventricular failure in "younger" patients. However, in elderly patients, confusion, restlessness, and fatigue are often more common. Many factors have been proposed to account for this apparently disproportionate systemic sensitivity to reduced cardiac output in the elderly. Possibilities include a relative lack of physical exercise or increased sensitivity of the central nervous system to hemodynamic changes.

e. Pulmonary Edema

Occasionally, acute severe left ventricular failure may develop rather suddenly, while the right ventricle is still functioning relatively well. The abrupt rise in pulmonary venous and capillary pressures can cause fluid to accumulate rapidly in pulmonary interstitial spaces and alveoli. As the fluid accumulates in the alveoli, clinical pulmonary edema develops, and frothy, pink-tinged sputum may begin to advance up the bronchioles into the trachea, impairing ventilation as well as gas exchange. Under such circumstances, very severe hypoxemia may develop rapidly.

2. Right Ventricular Failure

Failure of the right side of the heart characteristically causes systemic venous hypertension with increasing neck vein distension and peripheral edema. The congested liver may become swollen and painful and may occasionally simulate acute cholecystitis. Other symptoms that may develop (because of severe congestion of the intestines) include anorexia, nausea, vomiting, and abdominal distention. Weakness and fatigue, which are most often considered symptomatic of left heart failure, may also be prominent in isolated right heart failure.

AXIOM

Nausea, vomiting, and abdominal pain and distension in patients with heart failure can sometimes simulate an acute surgical abdomen.

B. PHYSICAL FINDINGS

1. Heart

Sinus tachycardia, although a very nonspecific sign, is almost invariably present with cardiovascular failure. Cardiac dilatation may occur rapidly, but muscle hypertrophy usually requires at least several weeks or months to develop; it is seldom found in acutely ill patients without pre-existing cardiac disease.

AXIOM

A gallop rhythm should be considered an early sign of left ventricular failure until proven otherwise.

A third heart sound during diastole is an important sign of left ventricular failure, but it is frequently overlooked by noncardiologists. The cadence produced by the fixed sequence of two normal heart sounds followed by the abnormal third heart sound can, especially when the heart is beating rapidly, produce a sound very much like that of a galloping horse, hence the term *gallop rhythm*.

PITFALL

Failure to listen closely for a third heart sound in all patients with cardiac or pulmonary symptoms.

In children and young adults, a third heart sound is often a normal finding, whereas a fourth heart sound is usually evidence of a ventricular abnormality. With advancing age, however, the significance of these auscultatory findings is altered. In persons over the age of 50, the detection of a fourth heart sound is less specific because it will also be found in some relatively healthy individuals. In contrast, a third heart sound in older subjects correlates well with ventricular dysfunction and is frequently present in cardiac failure.

PITFALL

Failure to appreciate that a fall in pulse pressure may be an important sign of increasing cardiac failure.

Unless heart failure is severe, the systemic blood pressure will often be elevated or at high normal levels. The return toward normal of an elevated blood pressure is often considered a good clinical sign, but sometimes it indicates increasing cardiovascular failure. A low pulse pressure, in particular, tends to suggest the presence of hypovolemia, aortic stenosis, tamponade, or severe cardiac failure.

2. Lungs

In early left ventricular failure, rales may be present only at the lung base, but as cardiac decompensation increases, rales usually become more generalized. At times, the rales of congestion may be difficult to differentiate from those of atelectasis, particularly in patients with trauma or severe sepsis who may not be able to clear their bronchial secretions properly.

AXIOM

"All that wheezes is not asthma." One must also exclude cardiac failure and obstructing lesions in bronchi.

Wheezing is usually considered to be due to bronchial asthma. However, it may also occur with cardiac failure (in the absence of pulmonary disease) because of swelling and congestion of the mucosa in the smaller bronchioles. Pleural effusions resulting from heart failure empirically occur slightly more frequently on the right, whereas a left hydrothorax may be slightly more suggestive of a pulmonary embolus.

3. Neck Veins

One of the most readily available signs of heart failure is distention of the deep jugular veins to at least 3.0 cm above the sternal notch when the patient is sitting up at a 45° angle. This may be a helpful sign, but it is much less accurate than direct readings of the central venous pressure (CVP) or pulmonary artery wedge pressure (PAWP).

4. Hepatomegaly

Enlargement of the liver and a positive hepatojugular reflux (pushing on the liver producing increased neck vein distention) are important corroborative signs of congestive heart failure.

5. Pedal Edema

Swelling of the feet and ankles is frequently caused by chronically increased venous pressure in the legs resulting from right heart failure. Such patients also often develop incompetence of the valves in the leg veins due to chronic distention.

In the bedridden patient with heart failure, the sacral area, rather than the feet and legs, is the dependent portion of the body. Consequently, this is the area that should be examined for edema.

PITFALLS
Failing to examine the presacral area for edema in bed-ridden patients.

C. RADIOLOGIC STUDIES

On the upright chest x-ray, fine transverse lines of increased density particularly near the costophrenic angles (Kerley B lines) in the lung bases, are often the first radiographic indication of increased lung water. Increased prominence and dilatation of the central lung markings are usually detected somewhat later on but usually before cardiac failure becomes clinically apparent. Accumulation of fluid in the interlobar fissures and blunting of the costophrenic angles by free pleural fluid is usually a relatively late sign, but it should also be looked for carefully, especially on the right.

An enlarged heart suggests a chronic underlying cardiac problem. If the cardiac silhouette is enlarging rapidly, chronic heart failure with a superimposed severe acute process is usually present. Patients with pure mitral stenosis usually maintain a relatively normal cardiac size until right heart failure begins to develop. Patients with chronic obstructive pulmonary disease (COPD) tend to have a relatively small cardiac silhouette because the diaphragms tend to flatten and move lower in the chest, giving the heart a more vertical position.

AXIOM
An enlarged cardiac silhouette in spite of moderate-to-severe COPD is usually evidence of rather advanced heart failure.

If surgical management of coronary artery disease is contemplated, or if valve replacement is required and coexistent ischemic heart disease is suspected, coronary angiography is indicated. Cardiac catheterization and ventriculography are the established means of assessing the hemodynamic consequences of both valvular heart disease and myocardial dysfunction, but sophisticated noninvasive techniques are being increasingly utilized for diagnosis.

Using M-mode and two-dimensional echocardiography, the majority of cardiac structural abnormalities can be recognized and the severity of stenotic valve lesions can be estimated by measurement of their cross-sectional area. With the additional use of Doppler ultrasound, the direction and velocity of blood flow can be determined, permitting a quantitative assessment of valve gradients. Initial experience suggested that Doppler aortic velocity measurements were unreliable in the elderly, but the systematic use of several ultrasonic views now permits high-quality flow-velocity recordings to be obtained from patients of all ages. Echocardiographic studies on healthy subjects have enabled the effects of age on cardiac structure and function to be defined, but a detailed investigation of elderly patients with cardiac failure has yet to be undertaken.

Noninvasive measurements of left ventricular ejection fraction can also be performed using radionuclide angiography or special pulmonary catheters. A recent survey of hospitalized patients aged over 75 years revealed that, of those with chronic biventricular failure, over half had left ventricular ejection fractions exceeding 40%. Although the mean ejection fraction of this group was significantly lower than that found in patients of a similar age who did not have clinical evidence of heart disease, these findings imply that ventricular systolic dysfunction is often not the only or main cause of cardiac failure in the elderly.

D. ELECTRO-CARDIOGRAPHIC FINDINGS

Electrocardiographic (ECG) findings do not indicate the presence or absence of congestive heart failure, per se. However, right or left ventricular hypertrophy tend to indicate a chronic strain, usually due to increased afterload. Evidence of ischemia, infarction, conduction disturbances, tachyarrhythmias, or bradyarrhythmias may also provide important clues to the etiology of heart failure. If symptoms are intermittent, 24-hour Holter (electrocardiographic) monitoring may reveal a paroxysmal arrhythmia.

E. FILLING PRESSURES

1. Central Venous Pressures

Although CVP is usually elevated to at least 12 to 16 cm H_2O in patients with heart failure, it may be normal (4 to 8 cm H_2O), at least temporarily, if the decompensation is primarily left sided. An occasional patient with acute left ventricular failure after a cardiac arrest or an acute myocardial infarction will develop pulmonary edema in spite of a CVP of less than 5.0 cm H_2O. On the other hand, patients with severe pulmonary disease or sepsis may have a CVP greater than 12 to 16 cm H_2O in spite of hypovolemia and a low PAWP.

2. Pulmonary Artery Wedge Pressure

Left heart failure is usually associated with a PAWP of at least 18 mm Hg, and as a general rule, a PAWP exceeding 18 mm Hg is associated with an increased pulmonary blood volume and interstitial lung water. With a PAWP exceeding 22 mm Hg, distended pulmonary veins may often be noted on chest x-ray and basilar rales are often heard. At a PAWP of 25 to 30 mm Hg, increasing amounts of fluid begin to accumulate in the alveoli. The increased lung water decreases lung compliance and functional residual capacity (FRC) and reduces the arterial Po_2. When the PAWP exceeds 30 to 35 mm Hg, clinical pulmonary edema with frothy sputum and severe rales throughout the lung is often present. If there is increased pulmonary capillary permeability due to sepsis or other problems, pulmonary edema can occur at much lower PAWP levels.

Within the past several years, bedside measurements of right ventricular (RV) ejection fraction (RVEF) by a thermodilution technique using a specially modified pulmonary artery catheter have become available. Reuse, Vincent, and Pinsky recently reported results of measuring right ventricular volumes during fluid challenge with 300 ml of 4.5% albumin in 41 ICU patients. In patients with a right ventricular end-diastolic volume index (RVEDVI) less than 140 ml/m², fluid tended to raise cardiac output. However, in the 20% (8/41) of patients with an RVEDVI > 140 ml/m², the fluid challenge tended to decrease the cardiac output. Thus, these measurements can help to recognize the patients with a maximally dilated right ventricle who are unlikely to benefit from fluid therapy.

F. CIRCULATION TIME

Patients with congestive heart failure usually have a prolonged circulation time. However, circulation time reflects not only cardiac function, but also the volume of blood in the pulmonary vascular bed and heart. Consequently, patients with acute heart failure caused by a recent myocardial infarction and a reduced central blood volume may occasionally have a normal circulation time. Patients with high-output cardiac failure often have a normal or shortened circulation time.

G. LABORATORY STUDIES

With acute heart failure, there is usually some hemodilution because of increased plasma water. With chronic heart failure, increased bone marrow production of red blood cells, as a compensatory response to the chronic hypoxemia, may cause Hb and Hct values to rise above normal, thereby increasing blood viscosity and afterload. In addition, increasing renal ischemia may result in a progressively rising BUN. Later, with further reduction in arterial inflow and increased venous congestion, a progressive renal and hepatic dysfunction may cause rising plasma creatinine and bilirubin levels. Chronic use of diuretics and a low-salt diet will tend to cause hyponatremia and hypokalemia, and these, in turn, may also increase the tendency to renal dysfunction.

The arterial Po_2 is generally an excellent and sensitive guide to the severity of left ventricular failure. A falling Pao_2 usually indicates that the heart failure is increasing, whereas a rising Pao_2 is often a sign of improvement. If left ventricular function appears to be good, but the arterial Po_2 is falling, one must be concerned about the possibility of recurrent pulmonary emboli, especially in older or bed-ridden individuals.

AXIOM
A relatively sudden fall in the arterial Po_2 in a patient with heart failure should make one look carefully for pulmonary emboli.

H. NONINVASIVE TECHNIQUES

A number of noninvasive techniques, such as echocardiography and systolic time intervals (using ECG, phonocardiography, and carotid pulsations) have been developed to evaluate the functional capabilities of the heart. Various radioisotope techniques now allow estimations of right and left ventricular end-systolic and end-diastolic volumes. Currently, these techniques are being perfected with improved instrumentation to demonstrate volume changes with time during the cardiac cycle. The ejection fraction (ratio of stroke volume to ventricular end-diastolic volume), which is determined angiographically, is normally about 0.55 to 0.70 for the left ventricle and 0.45 to 0.60 for the right ventricle. This measurement is being used increasingly to quantitate myocardial performance before and after coronary artery surgery. Changes in end-systolic and end-diastolic volumes provide much more accurate estimates of the functional capabilities of the right and left hearts than do the CVP and PAWP.

I. CARDIAC OUTPUT

Cardiac output is being measured with increasing frequency in intensive care units using thermodilution techniques. Although cardiac output often does not fall below normal until relatively late in heart failure, the heart's response to a fluid challenge may be extremely helpful in planning treatment. In many of these patients, the cardiac response is rather flat. Calculations of oxygen transport and oxygen consumption can provide particularly helpful information.

J. CARDIAC CATHETERIZATION

If the patient has progressive heart failure that is of unknown etiology and is not responding to standard treatment, cardiac catheterization may provide extremely useful diagnostic information, particularly if pressures and oxygen contents are studied in each chamber. Cardiac catheterization can also be used to detect lesions that might be corrected surgically.

K. TRANSVENOUS ENDOMYOCARDIAL BIOPSY

Transvenous endomyocardial biopsy has become an accepted technique for evaluating cardiac transplants for rejection. This technique may also provide useful clinical information in patients in whom the cause of the heart failure is unclear. The most frequent pathologic diagnoses obtained on biopsy under such circumstances have included myocarditis, vasculitis, and congestive cardiomegaly.

V. TREATMENT

Treatment of congestive heart failure is primarily concerned with removing precipitating factors, reducing the work load of the heart, increasing myocardial contractility, and correcting arrhythmias (Fig. 4.3).

A. REMOVING PRECIPITATING FACTORS

The treatment of a patient with congestive heart failure should include aggressive treatment of the underlying causes. This often may include careful control of hypertension and myocardial ischemia, both of which may result in loss of normally functioning contractile tissue. Weight loss may be an extremely effective means of reducing the cardiac work load. Stress-related, exertional, or other environmental factors that may place an increased burden on the failing heart should be assiduously avoided.

AXIOM

The increased catecholamine release associated with stress and anxiety may cause heart failure to continue in spite of all other therapy.

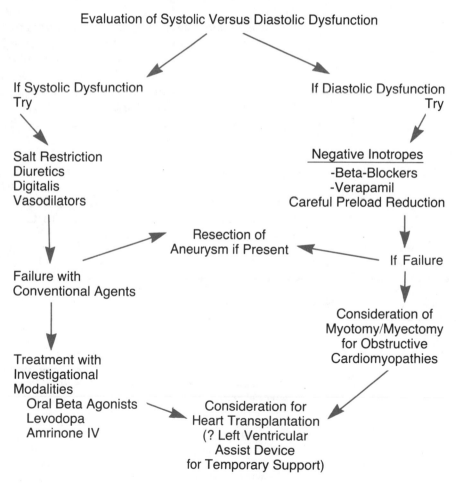

Figure 4.3 Treatment of congestive heart failure symptoms.

The physician should also be alert to the possibility that a patient with CHF may be taking a medication with myocardial depressive properties. Uncorrected valvular dysfunction or active systemic disease processes such as hemochromatosis, sarcoidosis, thyroid disease, or diabetes should be aggressively treated where possible. Careful monitoring of drug therapy for malignancy should be performed in order to avoid progressive myocardial dysfunction. Toxic agents such as tobacco or excessive alcohol or coffee should be avoided.

B. REDUCTION OF WORK LOAD

The work load on the heart can be diminished by reducing venous return (preload) (Table 4.2), by reducing the amount of vascular resistance against which the heart must pump (afterload), by decreasing cardiac contractility, and by decreasing the metabolic needs of the body.

1. Reduced Intake of Salt and Water

AXIOM

Moderate restriction of salt and water is often more successful than stricter regimens.

Restriction of water and salt can be a vital, nonpharmacologic means of reducing preload. Moderate salt restriction is very effective, but is often overlooked. A 2 to 4 g/d (34 to 68 mEq Na/d) salt diet is palatable, easily managed, does not require special foods, and will produce a significant reduction in salt intake to below that of the average American diet. Salt restriction to below 2.0 g/d is difficult to achieve as well as expensive because special diet foods are required. Fluid restriction may reduce plasma volume directly and also helps to correct the hyponatremia often observed in patients with congestive heart failure.

The hyponatremia of heart failure appears to be multifactorial in origin. An activated renin-angiotensin system plays a key role, and consequently therapy with captopril and furosemide may be very helpful. It is interesting that captopril treatment increases serum sodium only in hyponatremia heart failure patients (who also have the higher circulating renin activity levels). Since fluid restriction is poorly tolerated by many patients, and increased thirst is stimulated by accelerated angiotensin release, treatment of hyponatremia with a variety of drugs is often necessary.

2. Diuretics

A number of diuretics are available for treating heart failure. Thiazides are often recommended for the initial treatment of mild-to-moderate failure. However, there is little evidence that they are less prone to cause metabolic derangement than loop diuretics such as furosemide. In fact, thiazides may have a greater tendency to impair glucose tolerance and have been reported to occasionally

---

Table 4.2

METHODS OF PRELOAD REDUCTION	*Salt Restriction*
	Diuretic Therapy
	Thiazides
	Loop diuretics (furosemide, bumetamide, ethacrynic acid)
	Potassium-sparing agents (spironolactone, amiloride, triamterene)
	Fluid Removal by Phlebotomy, Hemodialysis, or Ultrafiltration
	Parenteral Vasodilators
	Nitroglycerine
	Nitroprusside
	Oral Vasodilators
	Nitrates (also effective in ointment or sublingual forms)
	Prazosin
	Captopril and enalapril
	Mechanical
	Surgical correction of regurgitant valvular lesions and shunts

cause severe hyponatremia. They are also ineffective when the glomerular filtration rate is less than 25 ml/min, and they may adversely affect renal function by causing vasoconstriction of afferent renal arterioles.

Furosemide (Lasix) is especially useful in the refractory edema of moderate-to-severe acute cardiac failure. The initial IV dose is generally 20 to 80 mg, depending on the urgency of the situation and the amount of fluid overload. The dose may then be increased until a satisfactory urinary output is obtained, or repeated until the fluid overload is adequately corrected. Interestingly, its rapid relief of pulmonary edema appears to be due to its ability to cause vasodilation and increase vascular capacity.

The margin of safety between fluid overload and hypovolemia in critically ill or injured patients may be very small, and many hypertensive patients are actually hypovolemic. If diuresis is excessive, patients with poorly functioning hearts may be pushed back and forth between hypovolemic shock and severe cardiac failure.

AXIOM
The most frequent cause of arrhythmias is hypokalemia due to excessive diuresis.

Severe electrolyte problems such as hypokalemia, hypomagnesemia, hypochloremia, and metabolic alkalosis may also develop during severe diuresis. These abnormalities may alter the cardiac response to digitalis and can precipitate dangerous arrhythmias. Hypovolemia may also cause azotemia and further activate the renin-angiotensin-aldosterone system.

Controversy persists about the routine use of potassium-sparing agents or potassium replacement in elderly patients requiring diuretic therapy. Hyperkalemia can occur relatively easily if the use of potassium-sparing agents is not carefully monitored, and potassium supplements may cause gastrointestinal side effects. The finding that chronic diuretic treatment does not always deplete total body potassium stores has led some authors to conclude that mild hypokalemia can be safely ignored unless the patient is receiving digoxin or has a tendency to arrhythmias. Nevertheless, extracellular potassium levels are a major determinant of the electrophysiologic properties of excitable tissues.

Many elderly patients with cardiac failure have underlying ischemic heart disease, and a dietary deficiency of protein and potassium is not unusual in such individuals. Thus, it may be argued that special steps should be taken to avoid hypokalemia and the associated increased risks of serious cardiac arrhythmias. However, it is important to avoid potassium-sparing diuretics if ACE (angiotensin-converting enzymes) inhibitors are also being given.

3. Tourniquet and Phlebotomy

Venous return can be reduced rapidly by elevating the head and chest and applying rotating tourniquets to the extremities. Phlebotomy is rarely used now. However, in desperate situations, removal of 50 to 100 ml of blood at 5- to 10-minute intervals up to a total 250 to 400 ml may help in the urgent management of acute pulmonary edema until previously administered drugs become effective. However, vital signs must be closely observed lest hypovolemia and hypotension develop.

4. Vasodilators

A wide variety of vasodilators are currently available for treating heart failure. These include nitrites and nitrates, alpha-adrenergic blockers, calcium blockers, ganglionic blockers, and other agents (Table 4.3). The hemodynamic effects of vasodilator drugs in severe left ventricular failure vary somewhat according to whether their predominant activity is on the arterial or venous circulation. Agents that are venoselective tend to reduce cardiac filling pressures (preload) more than vascular resistance (afterload) (Table 4.3).

When using the various vasodilators, it is essential not to let the blood

Table 4.3

VASODILATORS CLASSIFIED BY THEIR PRINCIPAL SITE OF ACTION	*Arterial Vasodilators Primarily*
	Hydralazine
	Minoxidil
	Arterial and Venous Vasodilators — "Balanced Vasodilators"
	Nitroprusside
	Phentolamine
	Prazosin
	Captopril
	Nifedipine
	Venous Vasodilators Primarily
	Nitrates (nitroglycerin, isosorbide dinitrate)

pressure drop too far. Farnett and colleagues recently reviewed 13 studies in which cardiovascular outcomes were stratified by the level of achieved diastolic BP in treated hypertensive patients. They found that diastolic BP levels below 85 mm Hg were associated with a significantly increased risk of adverse cardiac events.

5. Nitrates

a. Oral Nitrates

Nitrates dilate venous capacitance vessels and reduce ventricular size and central filling pressures. The resultant decreased ventricular wall tension is associated with a more favorable myocardial blood supply : demand ratio, and the decreased central filling pressure helps alleviate pulmonary congestion. Nitrates can be particularly useful in patients with predominant diastolic dysfunction, especially if it is due to ischemia. Indeed, correction of dyspnea alone by nitrates may improve exercise tolerance, even though cardiac output is not substantially improved.

(1) Nitroprusside

Sodium nitroprusside is an extremely potent, short-acting, vasodilator that relaxes vascular smooth muscle in both arteries and veins. Because of its potency, rapid onset, short duration of action, and remarkably linear dose-response relation, it is frequently used to manage acute severe heart failure and it has become the drug of choice for most hypertensive crises. However, with dissecting aneurysms, the increased dp/dt and reflex tachycardia caused by nitroprusside may be a problem; consequently, simultaneous use of a beta blocker is required.

AXIOM

Use of vasodilators in hypovolemic patients can be disastrous.

Sodium nitroprusside is considered a "balanced" vasodilator because it dilates both venous capacitance and arterial resistance vessels, thereby causing a decrease in both preload and afterload. In the patient with a normal blood volume, the venous pooling may cause a relative hypovolemia, and this, combined with a decreased afterload, can cause BP and cardiac output to fall abruptly. In contrast, when left ventricular function is severely impaired and preload is very high, the venous return will still be adequate following nitroprusside, and the concurrent drop in afterload will usually cause a rise in cardiac output. Pulmonary vascular resistance also falls during nitroprusside infusions, probably due to a direct effect on the pulmonary vascular bed. The dose of sodium nitroprusside required to produce a satisfactory reduction of afterload in cardiac failure varies from as little as 15 to as high as 400 μg/min (0.2 to 6.0 μg·kg^{-1}·min^{-1}), averaging approximately 50 μg/min (0.7 μg·kg^{-1}·min^{-1}).

Other than hypotension, the major side effects of nitroprusside are thiocyanate/cyanide toxicity and mild reductions in arterial oxygen tension due to nitroprusside-induced inhibition of the pulmonary vasoconstrictor response. Thiocyanate toxicity is manifested by confusion, hyperreflexia, and convulsions. Cyanide toxicity is first manifested by metabolic acidosis due to cyanide combining with cytochromes and inhibiting aerobic cellular metabolism. Thiocyanate or cyanide toxicity occurs almost exclusively in patients receiving high doses of nitroprusside for a prolonged period. Infusion rates of less than 3 $\mu g \cdot kg^{-1} \cdot min^{-1}$ for less than 72 hours are generally not associated with toxicity.

AXIOM

Nitroprusside should not be used in doses > 3.0 mg·kg⁻¹·min⁻¹ for more than 72 hours.

Some deaths during prolonged infusions of high doses of nitroprusside have been ascribed to cyanide toxicity. If discontinuation of the nitroprusside does not rapidly reverse metabolic acidosis and/or confusion which may be due to cyanide toxicity, one should consider using thiosulfate, sodium nitrate, or hydroxocobalamin to facilitate conversion of cyanide to thiocyanate. Monitoring blood thiocyanate levels can be used to follow toxicity in patients requiring infusions for longer than 2 to 3 days. Levels of thiocyanate below 10 mg/dl are usually considered safe.

Rapid discontinuation of a nitroprusside infusion can cause problems. These may include an increase in SVR, BP, and PAWP and a decrease in cardiac output.

(2) Nitroglycerin

In addition to its ability to dilate coronary arteries and relieve ischemic myocardial pain, nitroglycerin also dilates systemic arteries and veins, usually with a greater reduction in venous return than arterial resistance. Consequently, cardiac output may fall if the drug is administered to patients with only mild heart failure. However, in the presence of severe heart failure where an adequate preload will be maintained, the mild arterial dilating effect of nitroglycerin is usually enough to produce a substantial increase in cardiac output. Nitroglycerin also tends to reduce pulmonary arterial pressures, and this may be very helpful in patients with COPD or severe adult respiratory distress syndrome (ARDS). Intravenous nitroglycerin by slow infusion may be the vasodilator of choice if a high preload is the main problem and/or the patient has moderate-to-severe ischemic heart disease.

Intravenous nitroglycerin can be started in doses of 0.3 mg·kg⁻¹·min⁻¹ and gradually increased to about 3.0 $\mu g \cdot kg^{-1} \cdot min^{-1}$ as its hemodynamic effects become apparent. One of the main drawbacks to continued IV nitroglycerin therapy is the rapid development of tolerance. Consequently, intermittent therapy with IV nitroglycerin is often more effective and less apt to be associated with a loss of hemodynamic efficacy. Furthermore, it has been found that oral administration of N-acetylcysteine (Mucomyst) in doses of 200 mg/kg can at least partially reverse the tolerance that develops during continuous IV nitroglycerin therapy.

Sublingual nitroglycerin is used primarily to relieve angina pectoris, but it may also transiently help with CHF. However, a single sublingual dose usually lasts less than 20 minutes and generally causes a severe headache when it is first used.

(3) Isosorbide Dinitrate

Isosorbide dinitrate (ISDN) has been the most extensively studied longer-acting oral nitrate. A single dose can be effective for 4 to 6 hours. Doses of 20 mg may be sufficient for some patients, but many require 40, 60, or 80 mg, three or four times daily, to produce the desired pharmacologic effect. This agent may also be administered sublingually or chewed.

One study showed that a venous dilator such as ISDN may be preferable to arterial dilators for treating heart failure after an acute myocardial infarction. In another study, the drop in blood pressure with ISDN was similar to that seen with hydralazine, but there was less reflex sympathetic stimulation of the heart rate and a better reduction in myocardial oxygen consumption.

207

The principal concern in using nitrates in CHF is the development of tolerance, which occurs primarily in the arterial, rather than the venous, circulation. However, because improved exercise tolerance can often be maintained without a substantial increase in cardiac output in these patients, nitrate tolerance may not be as much of a problem in CHF as it is in angina. Given their relatively modest effects, nitrates are best used in combination with another vasodilator, such as hydralazine, that predominantly affects arterioles.

(4) Transdermal Nitroglycerin

Topical nitroglycerin applied to the anterior chest in an ointment form provides a more sustained effect that may last for 4 to 6 hours. However, the response to topical administration can be quite variable, and may be much less effective if used regularly in the long-term treatment of congestive heart failure. It has been postulated that due to interactions with membrane receptors, sustained levels of nitrates tend to be less effective than the peaks and valleys of serum levels associated with intermittent oral or sublingual preparations.

6. Alpha Blockers

a. Phentolamine

Phentolamine is considered one of the classical alpha-adrenergic blocking agents and causes blockade at both the postsynaptic (alpha$_1$) and presynaptic (alpha$_2$) receptors. Its potent vasodilator capabilities are secondary to both alpha-adrenergic blockade and a direct vasodilator effect on vascular smooth muscle.

Phentolamine can relax arteriolar and, to a lesser extent, venous smooth muscle and thus can increase cardiac output and reduce pulmonary and systemic venous pressures in patients with moderate or severe heart failure of all etiologies. The increased cardiac output and less-than-expected decreases in venous tone may be caused by an enhanced release of norepinephrine, which increases cardiac contractility and results in venous vasoconstriction. Although phentolamine is generally well tolerated in nonischemic cardiac failure, the tachycardia and norepinephrine release it causes can increase ischemia in patients with coronary artery disease.

Phentolamine is given as an intravenous infusion starting at 0.1 mg/min and increased slowly up to 2.0 mg/min as needed. Hemodynamic effects occur at 15 minutes after a bolus, usually peak by 30 minutes, and persist up to 60 minutes after the drug is stopped. The drug can be given orally in doses of 50 to 150 mg every 4 to 6 hours.

Because of the tachycardia that it can cause and its high cost, phentolamine is rarely used to treat heart failure. Other major side effects of phentolamine include vomiting, crampy abdominal pain, diarrhea, and rapid development of tolerance.

b. Prazosin

Prazosin is an oral selective alpha(postsynaptic)-adrenergic receptor antagonist that causes arteriolar and venous vasodilation by its receptor-blocking effects. In patients with heart failure, prazosin has balanced hemodynamic actions similar to those of nitroprusside, producing reductions in both systemic and pulmonary venous pressures. Cardiac output will tend to rise if an adequate preload is maintained.

Prazosin is well absorbed from the gastrointestinal tract and is given in doses of 1 to 10 mg every 6 to 8 hours. In many patients, the first dose of drug will produce orthostatic syncope. Some patients develop tachyphylaxis (decreased response with time) to the beneficial hemodynamic effects of this drug after only a few days of therapy. Consequently, prazosin is frequently not effective in the long-term therapy of congestive heart failure.

7. Calcium Blockers

Calcium-channel blocking agents interfere with muscular excitation-contraction coupling by reducing the movement of calcium into cells through the so-called slow channels. This results in peripheral and coronary artery vasodilation and a negative inotropic effect. However, the decreased contractility is often offset by a decreased left ventricular afterload, resulting in a favorable net effect on left ventricular function.

a. Nifedipine

Nifedipine has been widely used in the treatment of angina pectoris, and it may be of benefit in selected patients with heart failure. In patients with severe left ventricular failure, cardiac index tends to increase and systemic vascular resistance falls. Nevertheless, many clinicians are reluctant to use calcium-channel blockers in heart failure because the agents have a direct depressant effect on the myocardium. However, with nifedipine, the decrease in afterload is often more profound than the myocardial depressant effect, resulting in overall enhanced hemodynamics.

b. Verapamil

Verapamil has vasodilator properties, but its direct myocardial depressant effect is more profound, and this may seriously aggravate heart failure in patients with severe myocardial dysfunction. It may, however, be of value in treating tachyarrhythmias causing or contributing to the heart failure.

8. Arterial Vasodilators

a. Hydralazine

Hydralazine is a potent, direct dilator of vascular smooth muscle, especially in arterioles. Consequently, it primarily affects afterload (Table 4.4).

In patients with heart failure, hydralazine produces impressive increases in stroke volume by reducing arteriolar resistance. It has no effect or only a modest lowering effect on systemic venous or pulmonary venous pressures. For a given change in blood pressure, hydralazine increases cardiac output more than nitroprusside or nitrates. Hydralazine can also increase renal blood flow, thus promoting diuresis.

When using hydralazine in a critical care setting, intravenous administration is the most reliable route, but it must be given slowly and with constant hemodynamic monitoring to avoid hypotension. Administration should be started at 5 to 10 mg given by a slow intravenous drip over at least 20 to 30 minutes. The maximal effect occurs 25 to 45 minutes after injection, and the effect may last 4 to 24 hours. Subsequent doses of up to 20 mg can be administered intravenously every 6 hours. Given orally, the dosage is usually 25 to 100 mg every 6 hours with an onset of action at 60 minutes and peak effect at 2 to 3 hours.

A relatively small number of patients with heart failure develop tachycardia with hydralazine administration. This can exacerbate angina pectoris in patients with ischemic heart disease. Prolonged administration of hydralazine is associated with a lupuslike syndrome in 10% to 20% of patients, especially in those taking more than 400 mg daily.

Table 4.4

METHODS OF AFTERLOAD REDUCTION

Parenteral Vasodilators
  Nitroprusside*
Oral Vasodilators
  Prazosin*
  Captopril and enalapril*
  Nifedipine†
  Hydralazine†
  Minoxidil†
Mechanical
  Intra-aortic counterpulsation with balloon pumping
  Surgical correction of stenotic outflow valvular lesions

*Mixed arterial and venous dilating effects.
†Predominantly arterial dilating effects.

b. Minoxidil

Minoxidil is a potent, direct-acting, vascular smooth-muscle relaxant that acts primarily on the arterial bed. In doses of 5 to 20 mg orally, the drug produces beneficial hemodynamic effects similar to those seen with hydralazine. Side effects may include hirsutism and pericardial effusion. Because it may have fewer side effects than hydralazine, it has become the arterial vasodilator of choice for many physicians.

9. Angiotensin-Converting Enzyme Inhibitors

a. Captopril

Activation of the renin-angiotensin-aldosterone axis in congestive heart failure has several effects that may be deleterious. Increased angiotensin II and aldosterone production results in vasoconstriction and salt and water retention, which in turn result in increased preload and afterload.

Interruption of this system with ACE inhibitors, such as captopril, has several potentially beneficial hemodynamic effects. The primary mechanism of action is to reduce production of angiotensin II by competitive inhibition of the enzyme that converts angiotensin I into angiotensin II. Reduced levels of angiotensin II, in turn, promote vasodilation and lower aldosterone production. Captopril interferes with the action of angiotensin not only at peripheral vascular receptor sites, but also at central brain receptor sites, thus decreasing sympathetic outflow and reducing thirst. Furthermore, it may retard the breakdown of bradykinin, resulting in an increased tendency to vasodilation and increased production of prostaglandins.

Multiple clinical trials of oral forms of ACE inhibitors have shown both acute and chronic improvements in cardiac output, stroke-work index, and functional status along with lowered systemic and pulmonary vascular resistance and reduced ventricular filling pressures.

Captopril is available only in an oral preparation. Therapy is started with 25 mg every 6 hours and increased to a maximum daily dosage of 450 mg. Some investigators believe that much smaller doses should be used. They also believe that there is much less chance of hypotension developing if therapy is started at the lower doses and concurrent diuretic therapy is decreased as the captopril dose is increased. The duration of the hemodynamic effect is dose dependent, but the magnitude of the response is not. Tolerance to the drug has not developed in patients treated for up to 6 to 12 months. Maximal drug effectiveness is frequently obtained when an ACE inhibitor is used in combination with a diuretic such as furosemide.

Side effects with captopril include rash, hypotension, deterioration of renal function, and hyperkalemia. Therefore, potassium-sparing agents, such as spironolactone, should not be used concurrently. Development of sepsis while the patient is on an ACE inhibitor may result in extremely high rates of capillary leakage because ACE is important in inactivating bradykinin.

b. Enalapril

A consensus trial has concluded that the addition of enalapril, a newer ACE inhibitor, to other conventional therapy (including vasodilators) significantly reduces mortality in patients with New York Heart Association class IV heart failure but a relatively well-preserved blood pressure.

10. Ganglionic Blockers

a. Trimethaphan

Trimethaphan (Arfonad) is a short-acting ganglionic blocking agent which we used primarily for the treatment of hypertensive crises in the past. Its effect on venous capacitance vessels is usually greater than its arterial vasodilating effects. The inhibition of reflex sympathetic discharge by ganglionic blockage usually prevents an undesirable reflex tachycardia. However, the variability of the response to the drug and the occasional occurrence of severe orthostatic hypotension make its use somewhat difficult.

11. Oxygen

Since hypoxia can cause pulmonary artery vasoconstriction, giving oxygen can significantly reduce the afterload on the right ventricle. Severe hypoxia may also cause myocardial and peripheral tissue damage. Consequently, patients with congestive heart failure often benefit from the administration of sufficient oxygen to maintain an arterial Po_2 of at least 80 mm Hg.

AXIOM

One should be certain that a patient in heart failure has an SaO_2 of at least 90% and preferably 95%.

12. Beta Blockers

The calcium-channel blockers generally have negative inotropic properties. However, the beta blockers are much more powerful in this regard. Historically, the negative inotropic properties of the beta-adrenergic receptor antagonists were felt to preclude their use in patients with congestive heart failure. However, there are several beneficial effects these drugs may have, especially in patients with ischemic heart disease. The sympathetic autonomic system is activated early in the course of congestive heart failure. Initially, this adrenergic stimulation has useful results, including enhanced myocardial contractility, increased heart rate (which may preserve cardiac output), and peripheral vasoconstriction (which maintains systemic blood pressure). However, a chronic excess of circulating catecholamines may have direct toxic effects on the myocardium and may increase myocardial oxygen demands by elevating afterload, increasing heart rate, and enhancing the inotropic state. Beta blockers will counteract these effects, promote diastolic relaxation, and improve compliance.

Long-term studies such as the Beta Blocker Heart Attack Trial have shown no adverse effects of beta-blocker therapy in postmyocardial infarction patients with congestive heart failure. In fact there was often preservation or actual improvement of hemodynamic function with these medications, thereby lowering the risk of sudden death and overall mortality. Several smaller trials have also shown improvement in selected patients with chronic heart failure treated with beta blockers.

The reason for improved cardiac activity with beta blockers in selected patients in heart failure is not entirely clear. It is known, however, that long-term treatment with beta blockers is associated with up-regulation of beta receptors as well as improved catecholamine responsiveness.

It thus appears that selective reduction in myocardial responsiveness to catecholamines in chronic heart failure is a beneficial response that protects the failing ventricle from the deleterious effects of prolonged sympathetic stimulation. This may explain why therapeutic interventions that increase myocardial CAMP without a compensatory decrease in the activity of the beta-receptor pathway may produce adverse clinical effects in these patients.

13. Decreasing Metabolic Needs

The metabolic needs of the patient can be lowered by reducing apprehension, physical effort, and body temperature. Appropriate use of tranquilizers and sedatives in selected patients can be extremely helpful.

14. Mechanical and/or Surgical Support

Several surgical or mechanical means of treating the failing heart are available. The most common temporary mechanical treatment for the failing heart is intra-aortic balloon pumping (IABP). The main benefit of intra-aortic balloon pumping is improvement of coronary perfusion. There may also be some increase in cardiac output because of afterload reduction. Extracorporeal left ventricular assist devices, which can sustain a patient for a short time while awaiting definitive surgical therapy, are also available. However, their use is largely limited to major medical centers.

Surgical measures used to treat congestive heart failure include myocardial revascularization, defective valve replacement, closure of intracardiac shunts, and aneurysmectomy. At present, the use of mechanical artificial hearts for long-term treatment seems extremely limited due to poor short- and long-term results, multiple and often disabling complications, and the poor quality of life afforded to most of these patients. Cardiac transplantation, on the other hand, is increasingly successful and available and should be considered in younger individuals who have severe, unrelenting heart failure, but good function in all other organ systems.

C. INCREASING MYOCARDIAL CONTRACTILITY (TABLE 4.5)

1. Cardiac Glycosides

The mechanism by which cardiac glycosides, such as digitalis, increase myocardial contractility is not clear. However, it is thought that by inhibiting cell membrane sodium-potassium ATPase, sarcoplasmic reticulum and mitochondrial membranes are altered so that they release calcium more readily to the contractile elements. Although digitalis can have a vasoconstrictive effect on isolated vessels (with occasional mesenteric artery thrombosis in the elderly), its ability to increase cardiac output can reflexly reduce sympathetic tone, causing systemic vascular resistance to fall.

Digoxin is the only drug with positive inotropic properties that is commonly prescribed for elderly patients with cardiac failure. Controversy persists, however, regarding its benefit in the absence of atrial fibrillation. Withdrawal of digoxin rarely causes cardiac failure to deteriorate if sinus rhythm is maintained, implying that the routine use of this drug, with its narrow therapeutic range and numerous adverse side effects, can often be avoided in such patients. A possible explanation for the apparent lack of efficacy of digoxin in many patients is that not all patients with cardiac failure have markedly impaired ventricular systolic function.

The optimal digitalizing dose is quite variable, especially in critically ill or elderly patients, and occasionally half the usual dose may be adequate. The beneficial hemodynamic effects of digitalis can be obtained without any ECG changes. If ECG changes do occur, there is often some element of toxicity present.

Since the increased contractility produced by digitalis often increases myocardial oxygen requirements, it should be used with caution in patients with severe coronary artery disease. However, if cardiac dilatation due to heart failure is present, digitalis may decrease heart size enough to actually decrease myocardial oxygen consumption.

AXIOM

Any arrhythmia that develops in a patient receiving digitalis should be considered due to the digitalis until proven otherwise.

Table 4.5

METHODS OF IMPROVING CONTRACTILITY OF THE FAILING HEART	*Discontinue Agents with Negative Inotropic Effects (ethanol, anthracyclines, etc.)*
	 Oral Therapy
	    Digitalis preparations
	    Ibopamine (investigational dopaminelike drug)
	    Levodopa (investigational)
	 Intravenous Therapy
	    Beta-agonist agents (dobutamine, dopamine)
	    Amrinone
	    Epinephrine
	    Suproterenol
	 Mechanical
	    Change in pacemaker mode to allow atrioventricular synchrony
	    Left ventricular assist devices
	    Aneurysmectomy
	 Immunosuppression for Active Inflammatory Myocarditis (investigational)

One of the main drawbacks to digitalis preparations is the severe arrhythmias that can occur with digitalis toxicity. Paroxysmal atrial tachycardia (PAT) with varying AV block, is particularly due to digitalis. Consequently, before any digitalis is given to a patient in heart failure, it is important to determine if the patient is hypokalemic or hypercalcemic and if he or she has had any digitalis within the past 7 to 14 days. Furthermore, since digoxin is largely excreted by the kidneys, its maintenance dosage should be reduced if renal function is impaired.

AXIOM
Since digitalis tends to slow the conduction of impulses through the AV node and bundle of His, it should generally be avoided in patients with an AV block.

Other toxic effects of digitalis include anorexia, nausea, vomiting, and diarrhea. Abdominal pain and mesenteric venous occlusion may also rarely be caused by digitalis. Recently, severe digitalis intoxication has been successfully treated with digoxin-specific antibody fragments, which are developed in sheep and then isolated, purified, and fragmented.

2. Parenteral Beta Agonists

a. Dopamine

The hemodynamic effects of dopamine are extremely dose dependent. At 1 to 3 μg·kg^{-1}·min^{-1} it is primarily a splanchnic, and especially a renal, vasodilator. At 5 to 15 μg·kg^{-1}·min^{-1} it is primarily a positive inotropic agent. Although it has some peripheral vasoconstrictive effect, particularly at doses exceeding 20 to 30 μg·kg^{-1}·min^{-1}, and tends to raise blood pressure at most dosages, it is predominantly a positive inotropic agent. It is a relatively safe drug, except for an occasional tachyarrhythmia if the dose is increased too rapidly.

Dopamine is generally begun as a solution of 200 mg in 250 ml 5% G/W. The initial infusion rate is 5 to 10 microdrops per minute. This rate may be doubled every 3 to 5 minutes until an adequate response is obtained. At least part of the effect of dopamine is due to a release of endogenous myocardial catecholamines; consequently, it is less likely to be of benefit in chronic heart failure, which tends to be associated with depleted myocardial catecholamine stores.

b. Dobutamine

Dobutamine has cardiovascular effects somewhat similar to those of dopamine. However, it does not have the splanchnic vasodilating effect of dopamine, and it tends to cause systemic vasodilation rather than vasoconstriction and is less likely to increase heart rate and PAWP. Consequently, dobutamine in doses of 5 to 10 μg·kg^{-1}·min^{-1} is more likely to be used to treat cardiac failure when the cardiac output is low, systemic vascular resistance is increased, and the blood pressure is normal or increased. Dopamine, in contrast, is more apt to be used in septic shock when the blood pressure and systemic vascular resistance are reduced.

Recently, there has been increasing interest in pulsed inotropic therapy for long-term treatment of congestive heart failure. Several studies have shown significant improvement in the hemodynamic and metabolic parameters of heart failure patients treated with intermittent 72-hour infusions of dobutamine. Patients with systolic dysfunction have demonstrated significant symptomatic and hemodynamic benefit for as long as 2 months after a single treatment. Most studies suggest an initial titration of the dose, using data obtained through both invasive and noninvasive procedures. The infusion is usually started at 2.5 μg·kg^{-1}·min^{-1} and slowly titrated to doses in the 10 to 15 μg·kg^{-1}·min^{-1} range. Unfortunately, arrhythmias may develop with this type of therapy, and survival rates may actually be reduced.

c. Isoproterenol

AXIOM
Isoproterenol should probably be used only while the patient is bradycardic.

In patients with a slow, weak heart, such as may occur after valvular cardiac surgery, isoproterenol in doses of 1.0 to 2.0 μg/min may improve cardiac output without an excess increase in heart rate. It may be particularly helpful if pulmonary vascular resistance is increased in association with bronchospasm. However, if the pulse rate is greater than 120 per minute, isoproterenol tends to increase myocardial oxygen consumption much more than it increases coronary blood flow. This may be particularly detrimental in patients with coronary artery disease or pulmonary embolism.

d. Epinephrine

Epinephrine in doses of 1 to 2 μg/min may dramatically increase blood pressure and cardiac output in patients who have become unresponsive to dopamine and dobutamine. It can, however, cause significant tachycardias and ventricular arrhythmias. Tachyphylaxis may also develop fairly rapidly.

3. Phosphodiesterase Inhibitors

Amrinone is a bipyridine that, through its inhibition of phosphodiesterase fraction III, augments myocardial contractility and causes smooth-muscle relaxation. It can increase cardiac output and reduce filling pressures and systemic vascular resistance in patients with congestive heart failure. Heart rate and blood pressure usually do not change.

Indications for amrinone include (1) severe congestive heart failure that is refractory to conventional treatment with digoxin, diuretics, and oral vasodilators and that requires temporary inotropic support; and (2) acute heart failure associated with myocardial infarction (to reduce pulmonary vascular resistance and improve cardiac output).

Amrinone is given IV as a bolus followed by a maintenance infusion. A 0.75 to 1.5 mg/kg bolus is administered over 3 to 5 minutes, followed by an additional bolus of 0.75 mg/kg in 15 to 30 minutes if needed, and then a maintenance infusion of 5 to 10 μg$\cdot$kg$^{-1}\cdot$min^{-1}. A maximum dose of 10 mg every 24 hours is recommended. An alternative approach is to give 40 μg$\cdot$kg$^{-1}\cdot$min^{-1} for 1 hour, followed by 10 μg$\cdot$kg$^{-1}\cdot$min^{-1} as maintenance infusion.

Adverse effects of amrinone include nausea and vomiting (0.5% to 2.0%), thrombocytopenia (2.4%), hypotension (rare), fever (rare), and increase in ventricular dysrhythmogenicity. Although the oral preparation of amrinone has been studied, its multiple side effects, poor long-term efficacy, and possible increased mortality, particularly with severe congestive heart failure, have retarded its general use. Milrinone and enoximone are similar agents that may be released for oral treatment of chronic CHF.

In recent years there has been increasing search for potent, oral positive inotropic agents to treat chronic heart failure. This search has focused on drugs that inhibit cardiac phosphodiesterase activity, thereby increasing myocardial levels of cyclic AMP (cAMP) and enhancing the contractility of the failing ventricle. Milrinone, a bipyridine derivative, has been one of the most attractive of the phosphodiesterase inhibitors. Recently, DiBianco and associates reported on what may be the first well-controlled randomized trial of the long-term administration of milrinone compared to digoxin. Surprisingly, they found that digoxin improved left ventricular function and exercise tolerance better and had fewer side effects, including fewer ventricular arrhythmias.

4. Oral Adrenergic Agents

a. Prenalterol

Prenalterol is an adrenergic agonist that can be given IV or orally. It was hoped that it would be of benefit in the long-term treatment of heart failure. In one German study, prenalterol increased cardiac index and ejection fraction; however, with continued use, most of the beneficial effects disappeared after 3 to 6 months.

b. Pirbuterol

Pributerol, another orally active beta-adrenergic agonist, can raise cardiac index, stroke-work index, and ejection fraction, especially in patients with nonischemic cardiomyopathy and those with less severe heart failure. Its long-term effects, however, are still unknown.

c. Levodopa

Several other oral beta agonists are in the process of development and clinical testing. Levodopa is a naturally occurring catecholamine that is decarboxylated to form dopamine. It has been used experimentally in the treatment of congestive heart failure. Peak effects occur at about 1 hour, resulting in a sustained increase in cardiac index and a decrease in systemic vascular resistance. These responses can be attributed to activation of beta$_1$-adrenergic receptors by dopamine derived from levodopa. Unfortunately, its use has been associated with some significant side effects, including adverse hemodynamic effects and arrhythmias.

Murphy and Elliott, in a recent review of dopamine and dopamine-receptor agonists in cardiovascular therapy, noted that the novel DA$_1$-receptor agonist fenoldopam is claiming a role in the management of hypertension and heart failure and the preservation of renal function. DA$_2$-receptor agonists may have a role as potential antihypertensive agents.

d. Problems with Chronic Use of Beta-Adrenergic Agonists

Beta-adrenergic agonists have generally been unsuccessful in the treatment of heart failure. Although hemodynamic benefits may follow the administration of single doses of these drugs, long-term treatment is often accompanied by a reduction in beta-receptor density and loss of initial hemodynamic improvement. Consequently, these agents have not proved to be effective in placebo-controlled trials. Furthermore, abrupt withdrawal of these beta agonists after long-term treatment is not accompanied by worsening congestive heart failure. On the other hand, when attempts are made in patients with heart failure to stimulate the beta receptors and, at the same time, prevent the occurrence of receptor down-regulation (as with the intermittent use of intravenous dobutamine), serious arrhythmias may be observed and survival may be adversely affected.

5. Other Agents

a. Glucagon

AXIOM
Glucagon can be very helpful in supporting cardiac function in patients on (excess) beta blockers.

Glucagon is a polypeptide hormone that has positive inotropic and chronotropic actions. Glucagon's inotropic action is unaltered either by norepinephrine depletion or by alpha- or beta-adrenergic receptor blockade. Indeed, glucagon has been effective in restoring a stable cardiovascular state after beta-blocker overdose or toxicity in some patients.

Glucagon also promotes glycogenolysis in the liver and the development of hyperglycemia. It acts through specific receptors in the heart to increase contractility and heart rate. Evidence suggests that glucagon operates through adenyl cyclase to increase cAMP formation and thereby increase transcellular calcium flux. The usual dosage is 4 to 5 mg given directly IV followed by an IV infusion of 4 to 12 mg/h. Side effects may include severe hyperglycemia, as well as nausea and vomiting.

b. Thiamine

Chronic alcoholics occasionally develop severe myocardiopathy and cardiac failure which, like beriberi heart disease, may respond to large doses of thiamine (100 mg b.i.d. or t.i.d.).

6. Drug Combinations

The combination of vasodilators (such as nitroprusside or nitroglycerin) with inotropic agents (such as dopamine or dobutamine) may increase cardiac index much more than either agent alone. The PAWP and pulse rate may be much lower than with an inotropic agent alone. The combination of a vasodilator with furosemide can also produce better excretion of water and sodium than either agent alone.

The addition of hydralazine and isosorbide dinitrate to a therapeutic regimen of digoxin and diuretics can also have a favorable effect on left ventricular function and mortality. One study demonstrated a mortality reduction of 36% at 3 years in a group treated with hydralazine and isosorbide dinitrate compared with the results in patients taking only prazosin or a placebo.

D. CORRECTION OF ARRHYTHMIAS

Correcting arrhythmias is extremely important in patients with heart failure. Atrial tachycardia may respond to verapamil, quinidine, or cardioversion, and ventricular tachyarrhythmias may respond to intravenous lidocaine, procainamide, or cardioversion. Diphenylhydantoin (Dilantin) may help patients with tachyarrhythmias resulting from digitalis toxicity.

Beta-blocking agents such as propranolol are usually contraindicated in heart failure but may occasionally be helpful if the heart failure appears to be caused or significantly aggravated by an atrial tachyarrhythmia.

Patients with severe bradycardia, particularly if associated with a second- or third-degree heart block, may respond dramatically to atropine, isoproterenol, or a pacemaker.

E. ANTICOAGULATION

Deep venous thrombosis and pulmonary emboli are common in patients with congestive heart failure and may, in themselves, precipitate or aggravate cardiac failure.

AXIOM
The diagnosis of pulmonary emboli should be strongly considered in patients with recurrent heart failure of unknown etiology.

Although anticoagulant therapy probably has little or no effect on the incidence or severity of coronary artery thrombosis itself, it may significantly reduce venous thrombosis, pulmonary emboli, and systemic emboli from left atrial or left ventricular thrombi. In patients with an active thromboembolic process, 5000 units of heparin should be given rapidly IV as a loading dose of 5000 units, followed by 600 to 1200 units per hour by constant IV infusion, to maintain thrombin times or partial thromboplastin times (PTT) at 1.5 to 2 times normal. After the acute episode has subsided, Coumadin or other oral anticoagulants may be started and should generally be continued for at least 6 months. Coumadin may also be used prophylactically in patients who are at high risk of suffering an acute thromboembolic process.

F. TREATMENT OF ACUTE PULMONARY EDEMA

The emergency treatment of acute pulmonary edema involves many of the items discussed previously and should include:

1. Elevation of the patient's head and chest to an upright sitting position to improve ventilation and reduce venous return.

2. Oxygen by nasal catheter, mask, or intermittent positive-pressure breathing (IPPB). Positive-pressure ventilation with an endotracheal tube is indicated in the most severe cases and may help retard the development of alveolar fluid by increasing intra-alveolar pressure and reducing venous return. Alcohol in the nebulizing chamber reduces the stability of the bubbles in the pulmonary edema froth and may thereby improve ventilation.

3. Morphine sulfate, 5 to 15 mg, may be given IM or slowly IV, depending on the patient's blood pressure, with careful observation for respiratory depression or hypotension. However, morphine may be contraindicated in patients with pulmonary edema if the patient has (a) increased intracranial pressure, (b) severe pulmonary disease, or (c) severe lethargy or semicoma.

4. Furosemide, 40 mg IV, is given and repeated p.r.n. to obtain at least 200 to 500 ml of urine in the next hour.

5. Tourniquets can be applied to three extremities and rotated every 15 minutes to decrease venous return. Vasodilators and/or phlebotomy may also be used in particularly severe cases to reduce venous return. Vasodilators are most effective if the patient is hypertensive.

6. In the undigitalized patient, 0.5 to 1.0 mg digoxin may be given IV followed by additional increments of 0.25 mg every 4 to 6 hours three or four times as indicated. The dose must be adjusted if renal function and serum potassium or calcium levels are abnormal.

7. Cardioversion should be used if the patient has supraventricular or ventricular tachycardia that does not respond rapidly to the usual antiarrhythmic drugs. It is generally preferable to try cardioversion before a patient is given digitalis. If the patient has been digitalized, attempts at cardioversion may precipitate severe ventricular arrhythmias.

G. CARDIAC TRANSPLANTATION

The final frontier in the treatment of congestive heart failure is heart transplantation. The number of heart transplantation programs in the United States has greatly increased and 85% 2-year survival rates have been reported. However, the procedure is extremely costly and there continue to be problems with limited availability of donor organs, intensive frequent clinical follow-up, frequent invasive endomyocardial biopsies, and the morbidity of the immunosuppressive regimens. Nevertheless, results of this procedure are encouraging, and heart transplantation should be considered as an option for young, otherwise healthy patients with severe congestive heart failure which is refractory to all other forms of therapy.

SUMMARY POINTS

1. Cardiac failure is often defined as an inability of the heart to pump enough blood to meet the metabolic demands of the body. However, it is usually diagnosed from evidence of pulmonary or systemic venous overload.
2. From the physiologist's viewpoint, cardiac failure is often defined as a diminished work output of the heart in relation to its filling pressure.
3. Right heart failure is usually due to left heart failure.
4. The most frequent cause of a massive, relatively asymptomatic, pericardial tamponade is chronic renal failure.
5. Although tachycardia up to 160 to 180 per minute usually improves cardiac output, if there is coronary artery disease, it severely limits myocardial blood flow.
6. Atrial fibrillation should generally be prevented or rapidly corrected, especially in patients with severe mitral stenosis.
7. Potassium and calcium abnormalities should be prevented or rapidly corrected if there is any evidence of heart failure.
8. Acidosis tends to depress cardiac contractility, but the increased catecholamine release it stimulates tends to override the depression unless the pH is less than 7.10.
9. Patients with sepsis may develop pulmonary edema in spite of reduced cardiac filling pressures.
10. Continuing heart failure is characterized by down-regulation of beta-adrenergic receptors.
11. Increasing hyponatremia may be an important indicator of impaired cardiac function.
12. PEEP, which decreases the distension of the atria in heart failure, can significantly reduce ANF production, causing even more fluid retention.
13. Myocardial oxygen consumption increases in heart failure, but coronary blood flow tends to fall.

14. One of the most sensitive indicators of increasing cardiac failure is a drop in the arterial PO_2.
15. Increasing cough may be due to primary pulmonary or cardiac problems.
16. The symptoms of heart failure in younger patients are often primarily pulmonary.
17. Nausea and vomiting with abdominal pain and distension in patients with heart failure can sometimes simulate an acute surgical abdomen.
18. A gallop rhythm should be considered an early sign of left ventricular failure until proven otherwise.
19. A fall in pulse pressure may be an important sign of increasing cardiac failure.
20. "All that wheezes is not asthma." One must also exclude cardiac failure and obstructing lesions in bronchi.
21. One should examine the presacral area for edema in bed-ridden patients when looking for evidence of heart failure.
22. An enlarged cardiac silhouette in spite of moderate-to-severe COPD is usually evidence of rather advanced heart failure.
23. Moderate restriction of salt and water is often more successful than stricter regimens.
24. A relatively sudden fall in the arterial PO_2 in a patient with heart failure should make one look carefully for pulmonary emboli.
25. The increased catecholamine release associated with stress and anxiety may cause heart failure to continue in spite of all other therapy.
26. The work load on the heart can be diminished by reducing venous return (preload), by reducing the amount of vascular resistance against which the heart must pump (afterload), by decreasing cardiac contractility, and by decreasing the metabolic needs of the body.
27. The most frequent cause of arrhythmias is hypokalemia due to excessive diuresis.
28. Use of vasodilators in hypovolemic patients can cause an abrupt fall in BP and coronary blood flow.
29. Nitroprusside should not be used in doses > 3.0 mg $\cdot$ kg^{-1} $\cdot$ min^{-1} for more than 48 to 72 hours.
30. One should be certain that a patient in heart failure has an SaO_2 of at least 90% and preferably 95%.
31. Any arrhythmia that develops in a patient receiving digitalis should be considered due to the digitalis until proven otherwise.
32. Since digitalis tends to slow the conduction of impulses through the AV node and bundle of His, it should generally be avoided in patients with an AV block.
33. Isoproterenol should probably only be used in patients who are bradycardic.
34. Glucagon can be very helpful in supporting cardiac function in patients on beta blockers.
35. The diagnosis of pulmonary emboli should be strongly considered in patients with recurrent heart failure of unknown etiology.

BIBLIOGRAPHY

1. Awan, NA, et al: Hemodynamic actions of prenalterol in severe congestive heart failure due to chronic coronary disease. Am Heart J 101:158, 1981.
2. Beeson, PB and McDermott, W: Textbook of Medicine, ed 14, WB Saunders, Philadelphia, 1975.
3. Beregovich, J, et al: Dose-related hemodynamic and renal effects of dopamine in congestive heart failure. Am Heart J 87:550, 1974.
4. Bojar, RM, Rastegar, H, and Payne, DD: Methemoglobinemia from intravenous nitroglycerin: A word of caution. Ann Thorac Surg 43:332, 1987.
5. Bostrom, SL, et al: interaction of the antihypertensive drug felopidine with calmodulin. Nature 292:777, 1981.
6. Braunwald, E: Mechanism of action of calcium-channel blocking agents. N Engl J Med 307:1618, 1982.

7. Broder, MI: External counterpulsation in low cardiac output states. Surg Clin North Am 55:561, 1975.
8. Carleton, RA and Hauser, RG: The failing myocardium: II. Assisted circulation. Med Clin North Am 57:187, 1973.
9. Chernow, B and Lake, CR (eds): The Pharmacologic App. oach to the Critically Ill Patient, ed 2, Williams & Wilkins, Baltimore, 1988.
10. Civetta, JM, Taylor, RW, and Kirby, RR (eds): Critical Care, JB Lippincott, 1988.
11. Cleland, JGF, Gillen, G, and Dargie, HJ: The effects of fursemide and angiotensin-converting enzyme inhibitors and their combination on cardiac and renal haemodynamics in heart failure. Eur Heart J 9:132, 1988.
12. Cody, RJ, et al: Atrial natriuretic factor in normal subjects and heart failure patients: Plasma levels and renal, hormonal, and hemodynamic responses to peptide infusion. J Clin Invest 78:1362, 1986.
13. Cohn, JN: Inotropic therapy for heart failure (editorial). N Engl J Med 320:729, 1989.
14. Cohn, JN, et al: Neurohumoral control mechanisms in congestive heart failure. Am Heart J 102:509, 1981.
15. Cohn, L: Intra-aortic balloon counterpulsation in low cardiac output states. Surg Clin North Am 55:545, 1975.
16. DiBianco, R, et al: A comparison of oral milrinone, digoxin, and their combination in the treatment of patients with chronic heart failure. N Engl J Med 320:677, 1989.
17. Dzau, VJ, et al: Prostaglandin in severe congestive heart failure. N Engl J Med 310:347, 1984.
18. Dzau, VJ, et al: Relation of renin-angiotensin-aldosterone system to clinical state in congestive heart failure. Circulation 63:645, 1981.
19. Elkayam, U, et al: Acute hemodynamic effect of oral nifedipine in severe chronic congestive heart failure. Am J Cardiol 52:1041, 1983.
20. Erbel, R, et al: Hemodynamic effects of prenalterol in patients with ischemic heart disease and congestive cardiomyopathy. Circulation 66:361, 1982.
21. Farnett, L, et al: The J-curve phenomenon and the treatment of hypertension. JAMA 265:489, 1991.
22. Fennell, WH, et al: Propybutyldopamine hemodynamic effects in conscious dogs, normal human volunteers and patients with heart failure. Circulation 67:829, 1983.
23. Fleckenstein, A: Specific pharmacology of calcium in myocardium cardiac pacemakers and vascular smooth muscle. Annu Rev Pharmacol Toxicol 17:149, 1977.
24. Forrester, JS, deLuz, PL, and Chatterjee, K: Peripheral vasodilators in low cardiac output. Surg Clin North Am 55:531, 1975.
25. Francis, GS: Heart failure management: The impact of drug therapy on survival. Am Heart J 115:699, 1988.
26. Galvao, M: Role of angiotensin-converting enzyme inhibitors in congestive heart failure. Heart Lung 19:505, 1990.
27. Giles, TD: Defining the role of atrial natriuretic factor in health and disease. J Am Coll Cardiol 15:1331, 1990.
28. Goldberg, LI: Cardiovascular and renal actions of dopamine: Potential clinical applications. Pharmacol Rev 24:1, 1972.
29. Guyton, AC: Textbook of Medical Physiology, ed 4, WB Saunders, Philadelphia, 1971.
30. Guyton, AC and Jones, CE (eds): Physiology Series One: Cardiovascular Physiology. Butterworth & Co and University Park Press, Baltimore, 1974.
31. Harris, P: Congestive cardiac failure: Central role of the arterial blood pressure. Br Heart J 58:190, 1987.
32. Johnson, AK, et al: Plasma angiotensin II concentrations and experimentally induced thirst. Am J Physiol 240:R229, 1981.
33. Katz, AM: Cardiomyopathy of overload: A major determinant of prognosis in congestive heart failure. N Engl J Med 322:100, 1990.
34. Lambertz, H, Meyer, J, and Erbel, R: Long-term hemodynamic effects of prenalterol in patients with severe congestive heart failure. Circulation 69:298, 1984.
35. Langer, SZ: Presynaptic regulation of the release of catecholamines. Pharmacol Rev 32:337, 1980.
36. Leithe, ME, et al: Relationship between central hemodynamics and regional blood flow in normal subjects and in patients with congestive heart failure. Circulation 69:57, 1984.
37. Loeb, HS, et al: Beneficial effects of dopamine combined with intravenous nitroglycerin on hemodynamics in patients with severe left ventricular failure. Circulation 68:813, 1983.
38. Loeb, HS, Rahimtoola, SH, and Gunnar, RM: The failing myocardium: I: Drug management. Med Clin North Am 57:167, 1973.
39. Lundbrook, PA, et al: Acute hemodynamic responses to sublingual nifedipine dependence on left ventricular function. Circulation 65:489, 1982.
40. Majid, PA, Sharma, B, and Taylor, SH: Phentolamine for vasodilator treatment of severe heart failure. Lancet II:719, 1971.
41. Markham, RV, et al: Central and regional hemodynamic effects and nonhumoral consequences

of minoxidil in severe congestive heart failure and comparison to hydralazine and nitroprusside. Am J Cardiol 52:774, 1983.

42. Martiny, SS, Phelps, SJ, and Massey, KL: Treatment of severe digitalis intoxication with digoxin-specific antibody fragments: A clinical review. Crit Care Med 16:629, 1988.

43. Miller, RR, et al: Pharmacologic mechanisms for left ventricular unloading in clinical congestive heart failure: Differential effects of nitroprusside, phentolamine and nitroglycerin on cardiac function and peripheral circulation. Circ Res 39:127, 1976.

44. Moe, GW and Armstrong, PW: Recent advances in pharmacotherapy: Congestive heart failure. CMAJ 138:689, 1988.

45. Moulds, RFW, Jauernig, JA, and Shaw, JA: A comparison of the effects of hydralazine, diazoxide, sodium nitrite and sodium nitroprusside on human isolated arteries and veins. Br J Clin Pharmacol 1:57, 1981.

46. Murphy, MB and Elliott, WJ: Dopamine and dopamine receptor agonists in cardiovascular therapy. Crit Care Med 18:S14, 1990.

47. Myerburg, RJ, Kessler, KM, and Zaman, L: Pharmacologic approaches to management of arrhythmias in patients with cardiomyopathy and heart failure. Am Heart J 114:1273, 1987.

48. Needleman, P, et al: Cardiac and renal prostaglandin I_2 biosynthesis and biological effects in isolated perfused rabbit tissues. J Clin Invest 61:831, 1978.

49. Nelson, GIC, et al: Hemodynamic comparison of primary venous or arteriolar dilation and the subsequent effect of furosemide in left ventricular failure after acute myocardial infarction. Am J Cardiol 52:1035, 1983.

50. Ogilvie, RI: Effects of nitroglycerin in peripheral blood flow distribution and venous return. J Pharmacol Exp Ther 207:362, 1978.

51. Oliver, JA, et al: Participation of the prostaglandin in the control of renal blood flow during acute reduction of cardiac output in the dog. J Clin Invest 67:229, 1981.

52. Packer, M: Neurohormonal interactions and adaptations in congestive heart failure. Circulation 77(4):721, 1988.

53. Packer, M, et al: Prevention and reversal of nitrate tolerance in patients with congestive heart failure. N Engl J Med 317:799, 1987.

54. Pamelia, FX, et al: Acute and long term hemodynamic effects of oral pirbuterol in patients with chronic severe congestive heart failure: Randomized double-blind trial. Am Heart J 106:1369, 1983.

55. Parrillo, JE, et al: The results of transvenous endomyocardial biopsy can frequently be used to diagnose myocardial diseases in patients with idiopathic heart failure. Circulation 69:93, 1984.

56. Rackow, EC, Fein, A, and Siegel, J: The relationship of the colloid osmotic pulmonary artery wedge pressure gradient to pulmonary edema and mortality in critically ill patients. Chest 4:433, 1982.

57. Rajfer, SI and Goldbert, LI: Dopamine in the treatment of heart failure. Eur Heart J (Suppl 3) D:106, 1982.

58. Rajfer, SI, et al: Beneficial hemodynamic effects of oral levodopa in heart failure. N Engl J Med 310:1357, 1984.

59. Reuse, C, Vincent, JL, and Pinsky, MR: Measurements of right ventricular volumes during fluid challenge. Chest 98:1450, 1990.

60. Rieger, GAJ, Liebau, G, and Kochsiek, K: Antidiuretic hormone in congestive heart failure. Am J Med 72:49, 1982.

61. Roach, PJ, et al: Pathophysiologic levels of atrial natriuretic factor do not alter reflex sympathetic control: Direct evidence from microneurographic studies in humans. J Am Coll Cardiol 15:1318, 1990.

62. Robson, RH and Vishwanath, MC: Nifedipine and betablockade as a cause of cardiac failure. Br Med J 284:104, 1982.

63. Schatz, IJ and Wilson, RF: Cardiovascular failure following trauma. In Walt, AJ and Wilson, RF (eds): The Management of Trauma: Practice and Pitfalls. Lea & Febiger, Philadelphia, 1975.

64. Selzer, A: Changing aspects of the natural history of valvular aortic stenosis. N Engl J Med 317:91, 1987.

65. Shebuski, RJ and Aiken, JW: Angiotension II stimulation of renal prostaglandin synthesis elevates circulating prostacyclin in the dog. J Cardiovasc Pharmacol 2:667, 1980.

66. Starling, EH: On the absorption of fluids from the connective tissue spaces. J Physiol 18:312, 1896.

67. Tan, LB: Clinical and research implications of new concepts in the assessment of cardiac pumping performance in heart failure. Cardiovasc Res 21:615, 1987.

68. Timmis, AD, et al: Acute hemodynamic and metabolic effects of felodipine on congestive heart failure. Br Heart J 51:445, 1984.

69. Tweddel, AG, et al: Cardiovascular effects of prenalterol on rest and exercise hemodynamics in patients with chronic congestive heart failure. Br Heart J 102:548, 1981.

70. Vacek, JL, Emmot, WW, and Dunn, MI: New options in the management of congestive heart. Compr Ther 13(11):17, 1987.

71. Webb, SC and Impallomeni, MG: Cardiac failure in the elderly. Q J Med (New Series 64) 244:641, 1987.
72. Weissler, AM: Noninvasive methods for assessing left ventricular performance in man. Am J Cardiol 34:111, 1974.
73. Wientraub, M and Standish, R: Ibopamine: An orally active dopamine agonist. Hosp Formul 23:509, 1988.
74. Zaritsky, AL, Horowitz, M, and Chernow, B: Glucagon antagonism of calcium channel blocker-induced myocardial dysfunction. Crit Care Med 16:246, 1988.

CHAPTER 5

Shock

I. INTRODUCTION

Shock is a frequent occurrence in critically ill or injured patients. As a result of generalized or localized reductions in tissue perfusion, shock results in an inadequate delivery of oxygen and other nutrients to some or all tissues. Unfortunately, the process may not be recognized until the patient's general condition deteriorates so much that even the best treatment is apt to be unsuccessful.

AXIOM
Early diagnosis and rapid, aggressive therapy based on the trends and responses obtained from serial objective measurements offer the best chance for success in treating shock.

Death from hemorrhagic shock is unusual except with massive injuries to major structures or recurrent severe gastrointestinal bleeding in patients with impaired cardiopulmonary function. The duration and severity of shock are both critical. In a recent study of patients with abdominal venous injuries, the mortality rate was less than 15% if the shock was present for less than 15 minutes, but rose to 85% if the shock persisted for more than 30 minutes.

Septic shock is usually much more difficult to treat than hemorrhagic shock, especially if the primary infection is a pneumonia, peritonitis, or mediastinitis caused by aerobic Gram-negative rods. Gram-negative sepsis occurs in an estimated 70,000 to 140,000 patients in the United States annually and continues to be associated with a mortality rate of at least 40% to 70%.

Endotoxin, also known as lipopolysaccharide (LPS), initiates most of the physiologic and biochemical abnormalities that characterize septic shock. Endotoxin is a conglomerate molecule composed of both hydrophilic heteropolysaccharide as well as hydrophobic lipid, and has a molecular weight (MW) of nearly 1 million daltons. There are three major portions of the endotoxin complex: the outermost polysaccharide portion of the molecule is antigenic and has been termed the 0 antigen region. The so-called R core middle region is composed of both sugars and ketodeoxyoctanoate. The innermost section in the endotoxin complex is the lipid A region, which is thought to confer most, if not all, of the biological activity associated with endotoxin. Although endotoxin may itself cause host injury, it is the violent host inflammatory response that it initiates which triggers clearing of the invading microbe, but also results in host autoinjury through a variety of both cellular and humoral cascading events.

Although antibiotics may kill the invading microbe, they do not directly participate in clearance of endotoxin found on the bacterial cell wall. In fact, in some instances bacterial death may be associated with a Jarisch-Herxheimerlike reaction which probably emanates from a bolus of endotoxin released into the bloodstream.

Cardiogenic shock due to acute myocardial infarction continues to be a major cause of death. However, reopening of occluded coronary arteries in patients with evolving infarcts within 4 to 6 hours of the onset of pain with IV or intracoronary thrombolytic agents has improved survival substantially. Percutaneous transluminal coronary angioplasty (PTCA) and early coronary artery bypass grafting in selected individuals have also improved survival rates.

II. DEFINITION

AXIOM

Shock is usually associated with impaired tissue perfusion either in localized areas or in the body as a whole.

Shock may be defined in multiple ways, but basically it is a severe pathophysiologic syndrome associated with impaired cellular metabolism which in most instances is due to poor nutrient capillary perfusion. Since it includes a wide variety of problems, it is probably best thought of as a syndrome rather than a specific process. For many years, physicians tended to think of shock in rather simplistic mechanical terms and compared its complex pathophysiologic processes to simple "plumbing" problems, such as abnormalities in the pump, the pipes, or the fluid in the pipes. Such comparisons may be helpful in understanding hypovolemic and cardiogenic shock. It is increasingly apparent, however, that most patients with early septic shock and some patients with acute myocardial infarction (AMI) shock do not have the cold clammy skin, poor tissue perfusion, low cardiac output, and excessive vasoconstriction that were considered characteristic of all types of shock.

When the cardiac output is measured in patients with early septic shock, it is often found to be normal or increased, and total peripheral vascular resistance is frequently quite low. The skin, as might be expected in such a hemodynamic situation, is often warm and dry, and because the pulse pressure is often normal or increased, the peripheral pulses tend to be full and easily felt.

AXIOM

Septic shock may be associated with improper distribution of an overall increased cardiac output.

Many investigators feel that septic shock is a distributive problem with some vital areas having an impaired perfusion even though other areas and the body as a whole may have an increased blood flow. Others feel that the problem in sepsis is increased physiologic shunting resulting from abnormalities involving capillaries, cell membranes, and cell metabolism. For example, Duff and associates have shown that the uptake of xenon from peripheral muscle, which is accomplished through nutrient capillaries, correlates rather well with the increased cardiac output in septic patients. In addition, studies using radioactive microaggregates, which are too large to go through nutrient capillaries but can go through arteriovenous shunts, suggest that only a small portion of the increased cardiac output in sepsis goes through anatomic arteriovenous shunts. Another possibility is that even though blood may be going through nutrient capillaries in large quantities, the septic tissue cells may be unable to properly utilize the oxygen, glucose, and other materials brought to them.

III. CLASSIFICATION

From a relatively mechanistic point of view, shock may be classified into five categories: hypovolemic, cardiogenic, septic, neurogenic, and miscellaneous (Table 5.1).

Others have classified shock on a functional basis into hypovolemic, cardiogenic, obstructive, and distributive types. The obstructive type includes shock due to pulmonary emboli or pericardial tamponade. Sepsis is felt by some to be the most common type of distributive shock with maldistribution of blood flow,

Table 5.1

CLASSIFICATION OF SHOCK	A. Hypovolemic
	    Hemorrhage
	    Dehydration
	    Trauma (not always hypovolemia)
	B. Cardiogenic
	    Acute myocardial infarction
	    Pulmonary emboli, postcardiac
	      surgery, tamponade
	C. Septic
	    Hyperdynamic (early)
	    Hypodynamic (late)
		D. Neurogenic (rare) (*not head trauma*)
		    Sympathetic or spinal cord
		      damage
		    ?Fainting
		E. Miscellaneous
		    Hypoglycemia
		    Overdoses—especially
		      barbiturates

so that although cardiac output and flow to certain vascular beds is increased, other tissues may have an inadequate perfusion.

A. HYPOVOLEMIC SHOCK

Hypovolemic shock is caused by a decrease in the intravascular volume relative to the vascular capacity. In previously normal individuals, it is generally associated with a blood volume deficit of at least 25% and an even larger interstitial fluid deficit. This extracellular fluid (ECF) deficit may be caused by hemorrhage, vomiting, diarrhea, or any excessive loss of body fluid. Patients in hypovolemic shock almost invariably have a low cardiac output, increased systemic vascular resistance (SVR), increased heart rate, and decreased filling pressure in the right and left heart.

AXIOM
Shock following trauma is usually, but not always, due to hypovolemia.

Most patients with shock following trauma are hypovolemic, but other problems such as severe heart, lung, or brain damage may be present. Damaged tissue, in addition to sequestering large amounts of fluid, may release superoxide radicals and lysosomal enzymes, which can damage local and remote tissues and also release a variety of vasoactive substances that can alter cardiovascular, pulmonary, and metabolic function. Many patients with traumatic shock tend to have a normal or even high cardiac output, particularly if the associated hypovolemia has been corrected.

AXIOM
Although traumatic shock may occur without hypovolemia, inadequate administration of fluid is the most frequent cause for such shock to develop and persist.

B. CARDIOGENIC SHOCK

Cardiogenic shock is caused by impaired function of the heart as a pump. Patients with cardiogenic shock can be classified into six groups: acute left or right ventricular failure, acute mitral regurgitation, acute ventricular septal defect (VSD), acute pericardial tamponade, and acute pulmonary embolism. Most patients with cardiogenic shock have a low cardiac output with increased cardiac filling pressure, increased systemic vascular resistance, increased pulse rates, and a cool, clammy skin. Up to 20% to 30% of patients with acute myocardial infarction shock also have some hypovolemia due to prior vasoconstriction, diuretics, vomiting, or excessive sweating.

C. SEPTIC SHOCK

AXIOM
Early septic shock tends to be associated with systemic vasodilation and a normal or increased cardiac output.

Shock associated with severe sepsis is now generally divided into an early warm or hyperdynamic type (with abnormal or increased cardiac output) and a later cold or hypodynamic type (with a low cardiac output). Although many patients with early septic shock have a normal or increased cardiac output, probably due to peripheral vasodilation and a greatly increased beta-adrenergic activity, studies often reveal a reduced ejection fraction. Sepsis also impairs cell metabolism very early. Any maldistribution of blood flow or increased anatomic arteriovenous shunting will increase the tendency to impaired cell metabolism.

AXIOM

Septic patients with a low cardiac output may require very large quantities of fluid plus some inotropic support to maintain adequate tissue perfusion.

If sepsis continues, the increasing capillary leak may eventually cause enough hypovolemia to convert the process to hypodynamic septic shock. Even though continued severe sepsis is apt to further reduce right and left ventricular ejection fraction, most patients with hypodynamic septic shock can be converted, at least transiently, to hyperdynamic septic shock by administering adequate fluid.

D. NEUROGENIC SHOCK

Neurogenic shock is usually produced by damage to, or pharmacologic blockade of, the sympathetic nervous system, producing vasodilatation of arterioles and veins in the affected areas of the body with resulting hypotension and an increased vascular capacity. The increased vascular capacity can cause the patient to develop a relative hypovolemia. Thus, patients with neurogenic shock tend to have a low blood pressure, a relatively normal cardiac output, and greatly decreased systemic vascular resistance. Although a relative hypovolemia is present, damage to or blockade of the sympathetic nervous system results in warm, dry skin and a relatively normal pulse rate.

Neurogenic shock due to spinal anesthesia or trauma can usually be rapidly corrected by administering fluid or a vasopressor. Fainting after an emotional shock might also be considered a type of neurogenic shock, although any hypotension that results is usually mild and transient.

AXIOM

Brain injury does not cause hypotension until terminally when apnea occurs.

It must be emphasized that trauma to the brain itself almost never causes hypotension. In fact, damage to the brain usually causes an increased intracranial pressure which almost invariably produces a rise in the blood pressure. This will continue until there is failure of the respiratory and then vasomotor centers in the medulla. This is usually manifested first by apnea and later by hypotension. Shock in most patients with head trauma is caused by bleeding from an injury elsewhere in the body; however, the extent of blood loss from scalp lacerations coincident with head injury is often greatly underestimated.

AXIOM

Hypotension in the presence of respiratory effort is not due to head injury.

E. OTHER TYPES OF SHOCK

AXIOM

Shock in young individuals without apparent trauma or sepsis should be considered due to drugs, usually as an overdose, until proven otherwise.

One of the more important other types of shock is shock due to drug overdosage, particularly barbiturates. At normal doses, barbiturates cause only mild lethargy, but when they are used in higher doses, the resultant vasodilation can cause significant hypotension. After very large doses, respiration may be severely depressed (requiring ventilatory assistance). Correction of severe hypotension may require vasopressors and/or inotropic agents in addition to large amounts of fluid to fill the greatly increased vascular capacity.

An increased number of young individuals are being seen with acute severe neurologic or cardiopulmonary problems due to cocaine.

IV. DIAGNOSIS

AXIOM

Early diagnosis and treatment of shock greatly increases the chances of reversing the process before extensive deterioration of vital organ function has occurred.

The criteria most frequently used to diagnose shock are a systolic blood pressure less than 80 mm Hg or 90 mm Hg, severe oliguria, metabolic (lactic) acidosis, and clinical evidence of poor tissue perfusion (Table 5.2). If all of these signs are present, the diagnosis of shock is easy. However, these signs and symptoms may not be present in all types of shock, particularly in early sepsis.

A. BLOOD PRESSURE

The systemic arterial blood pressure consists of three parts: diastolic pressure, which correlates with the amount of arteriolar vasconstriction present; pulse pressure, which is primarily related to stroke volume and the rigidity of the aorta and its major branches; and systolic pressure, which is determined by a combination of these factors.

1. Pulse Pressure

AXIOM

Pulse-pressure changes reflect alterations in cardiac output much more accurately than systolic BP as shock is developing.

Pulse pressure is the most important pressure to monitor because it provides some indication of whether the stroke volume is increasing or decreasing. Although cardiac output and stoke volume tend to decrease with advancing age, pulse pressure tends to rise in the elderly because of increasing stiffness of the aorta and its larger branches.

There may be a poor correlation between stroke volume and pulse pressure when large groups of patients are averaged. However, in an individual patient, changes in pulse pressure often correlate quite well with changes in stroke volume. For example, if a patient's blood pressure changes from 120/80 to 110/90, the pulse pressure has fallen from 40 mm Hg to 20 mm Hg, and it is likely that the stroke volume has also decreased by about 50%.

2. Changes with Hemorrhage

AXIOM

Decreases in pulse pressure may occur because of tachycardia but are usually due to a decreased blood volume.

Table 5.2

SIGNS OF SHOCK		Early	Late
Blood pressure		Pulse pressure	Systolic pressure
Urine output		Urine volume	Urine volume
		Urine sodium concentration	
		Urine osmolality	
Acid-base changes		Respiratory alkalosis	Metabolic acidosis
Tissue perfusion		Restlessness	Cold, clammy skin
		Anxiety	Cloudy sensorium

In hypovolemic shock, major decreases in stroke volume and pulse pressure often occur long before there is any significant fall in the systolic pressure. Diastolic pressure often rises initially with hemorrhage because of sympathoadrenal stimulation, particularly if there is pain or tissue damage. However, since vasoconstriction can increase only to a certain maximum, continued blood loss will eventually result in a fall of both systolic and diastolic pressures.

In previously normal patients, the systolic pressure is often maintained relatively well until a blood-volume deficit of at least 25% has developed. In the average 70 kg man with a normal blood volume of 5000 ml, a rapid blood loss of 500 to 1000 ml may cause some decrease in the pulse pressure, but the systolic pressure often does not fall significantly until more than 1500 ml (30% of the normal blood volume) has been lost.

It is important to differentiate blood-volume *loss* from blood-volume *deficit*. If a patient lost 2000 ml of blood over a period of 1 hour, up to 1000 ml of extravascular fluid might move from the interstitial space into the vascular space to partially correct the hypovolemia; thus, the actual blood-volume deficit at the end of 1 hour might be only 1000 ml.

The severity of acute blood loss may be divided into four classes. In a previously normal 70 kg man, a class I blood loss is up to 750 ml or 15% of the expected blood volume (BV). A class II hemorrhage is 750 to 1500 ml (15% to 30% of the BV). A class III hemorrhage is 1500 to 2000 ml (30% to 40% of BV) and class IV is a greater loss. Class I and class II hemorrhages can usually be treated with crystalloid resuscitation alone, while classes III and IV hemorrhage generally require blood transfusions.

3. Unobtainable Cuff Blood Pressure

In patients with severe vasoconstriction and/or greatly reduced stroke volume, the vibrations produced as blood begins to flow past the main artery compressed by a blood pressure cuff may be too weak to produce Korotkoff sounds that are audible with an ordinary stethoscope (Fig. 5.1). Thus, there may be a large discrepancy between the central aortic pressure and the blood pressure obtained by the cuff technique.

PITFALL
Assuming that an unobtainable cuff BP is always extremely low.

An unobtainable cuff blood pressure usually results from a very low stroke volume and severe vasoconstriction. In the great majority of patients with an unobtainable blood pressure, the systolic blood pressure is less than 50 mm Hg; however, in up to 5% of patients, the intra-arterial pressure may actually be relatively normal or even high. Doppler-flow detectors can be very helpful in such patients by detecting vascular vibrations and providing fairly accurate systolic pressures long after Korotkoff sounds are no longer audible through an ordinary stethoscope.

4. Intra-Arterial Blood Pressure

If there is any difficulty obtaining a consistent and clear cuff blood pressure and if the patient's condition is not improving rapidly with therapy, an intra-arterial catheter should be inserted. In treating patients with shock, it is extremely important to be able to follow changes in blood pressure accurately and frequently.

The radial artery is generally the preferred for insertion of an intra-arterial catheter because of its accessibility. Complications of ischemia to the fingers or thumb are quite rare, particularly if (1) an Allen test reveals that the ulnar artery and palmar arch are patent, (2) the catheter is inserted percutaneously, and (3) it is removed in 48 to 72 hours. Not only can an intra-arterial line provide continuous blood pressure measurements, but it can also provide a ready source for obtaining frequent arterial blood gas samples.

The artery is occluded by the pressure of the cuff.

pressure = 140

Eddy currents distal to the compressed partially occluded vessel produce vibrations which cause noise (Korotkoff's sounds if the stroke volume is high enough)

pressure = 120

More open

pressure = 100

At the diastolic pressure the vessel is fully open; no eddy currents are produced and Korotkoff's sounds decrease or disappear.

pressure = 80

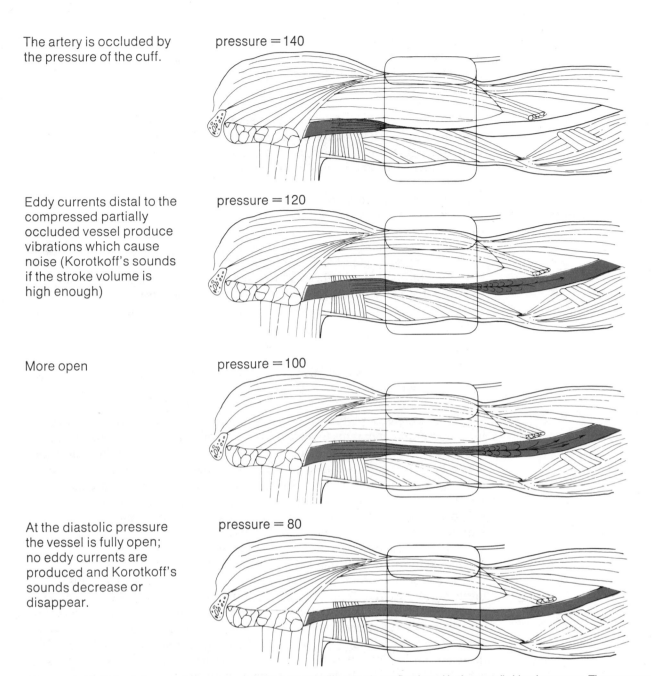

Figure 5.1 Cuff blood pressure. The pressure at which Korotkoff's sounds are first heard is the systolic blood pressure. The pressure at which Korotkoff's sounds disappear or greatly decrease in audibility is diastolic pressure. If excessive vasoconstriction exists above or below the cuff and/or stroke volume is severely decreased, then the flow is too weak to produce audible Korotkoff's sounds.

AXIOM
Systolic BP obtained from a radial artery catheter is usually higher than in the aorta.

The systolic pressure obtained through a radial artery line is usually at least 10 to 20 mm Hg higher than central aortic or cuff pressures. This discrepancy occurs because of the peripheral buildup of pressure waves proximal to small arteries. Nevertheless, mean BP determinations through a radial artery catheter are usually quite accurate. However, if there is excessive proximal vasconstriction, the mean radial artery pressure may be lower than the mean central aortic pressure.

Axillary artery catheters, although used in only a few centers, have a number of advantages over peripheral arterial catheters. Axillary artery catheters require less patient restraint, are less likely to occlude the cannulated vessel, and usually reflect central aortic pressures more accurately than peripheral catheters.

B. URINE OUTPUT

The kidney has been referred to as the *window of the viscera*, because renal perfusion, as reflected by the urine output, may be a rather accurate gauge of vital organ blood flow. Indeed, renal blood flow and urine output often fall long before other vital organ perfusion is significantly reduced.

1. Correlation with Cardiac Output

With any decrease in cardiac output or blood pressure, there is prompt renal artery and arteriolar vasoconstriction and a rapid reduction in renal blood flow. In addition, blood flow in the kidney is diverted toward the less numerous glomeruli in the juxtamedullary portion of the renal cortex. This results in a further decrease in glomerular filtrate, and since the juxtamedullary glomeruli have long loops of Henle, there is increased absorption of water and sodium. If the fall in blood pressure is gradual, urine sodium concentration will fall and the urine osmolality will rise before there is any significant change in the urine output.

AXIOM

A low urine sodium concentration is generally due to renal hypoperfusion, usually because of hypovolemia.

The decreased perfusion pressure in the renal arterioles stimulates the juxtaglomerular apparatus to secrete a protein called renin. Renin enzymatically converts an alpha$_2$ globulin in the blood to a decapeptide referred to as angiotensin I. This in turn is converted by angiotensin-converting enzyme (ACE) in the lung into angiotensin II. This very potent octapeptide can cause additional vasconstriction and also stimulates increased aldosterone release from the adrenal cortex. Aldosterone is a powerful mineralocorticoid hormone that causes the kidney to retain sodium, bicarbonate, and water. The four most important stimuli to aldosterone secretion are sympathetic stimulation, hypotension, decreased sodium in distal tubule fluid, and hyperkalemia.

The other important hormone that causes renal retention of water is antidiuretic hormone (ADH). The four main stimuli to the release of ADH, in order of their potency, are nausea, abdominal pain, hypovolemia, and hyperosmolality.

As a result of all these changes, the urine output may fall long before other signs of impaired tissue perfusion become evident. On the other hand, if the urine output is adequate without diuretics, it suggests that vital organ perfusion is probably adequate. However, in patients with sepsis or severe trauma, urine flow may be normal in spite of a renal blood flow as low as 25% of normal.

AXIOM

A low urine output usually reflects poor renal perfusion, but a normal urine output does not rule it out.

2. Urine Flow in Sepsis

Monitoring urine output is extremely helpful in detecting fluid deficits. Although sepsis usually causes a reduction in urine output, very occasionally severe sepsis can cause an inappropriate polyuria. The polyuria is termed inappropriate if urine output is much greater than normal in spite of an actual or relative hypovolemia. The polyuria may be particularly deceptive because many aspects of the clinical picture may suggest that the patient is overloaded with fluid. These patients tend to be edematous, they often have already been given large quantities of fluid, the central venous pressure (CVP) is elevated, rales can often be heard over much of the lungs, and the chest x-ray often shows evidence of increasing congestion or even early pulmonary edema. Under such circumstances, the polyuria may appear to be appropriate, and it is often assumed that the intravenous fluid intake can or should be drastically reduced. However, if the fluid intake is restricted without close continued observation of the patient, blood pressure and urine output may fall rather suddenly, and oliguric renal failure may develop.

AXIOM

In a septic patient with polyuria, a low urine sodium concentration should make one suspect an inappropriate polyuria.

If the polyuria is appropriate, urine sodium levels will tend to be high; however, with the inappropriate polyuria of sepsis, urine sodium concentrations will tend to fall and be less than 10 to 20 mEq/liter as the patient becomes hypovolemic.

3. Sodium Concentration and Osmolality of the Urine

AXIOM

A falling urine sodium concentration and rising osmolality suggest that the patient is becoming (more) hypovolemic.

If the urine sodium falls to less than 10 to 20 mEq/liter, the kidneys are usually functioning quite well but are probably not being perfused satisfactorily. A urine-to-serum osmolality ratio greater than 1.5 may also be a fairly reliable index of reduced renal perfusion. Although the reduced renal blood flow under such circumstance may occasionally be caused by renal artery stenosis or cardiac failure, in most instances it is due to hypovolemia.

C. ACID-BASE CHANGES

The characteristic acid-base abnormality in established shock is a lactic (metabolic) acidosis. However, early shock is often characterized by a respiratory alkalosis. Terminally, the patient may have a combined metabolic and respiratory acidosis.

1. Respiratory Alkalosis

AXIOM

An increasing respiratory alkalosis (falling $PaCO_2$) is an important sign that a patients' condition is deteriorating and should stimulate a search for hypoxemia, sepsis, hypovolemia, or pulmonary emboli.

Trauma, sepsis, and shock are usually powerful stimuli to ventilation. Therefore, arterial blood gas analyses in patients just beginning to go into shock generally reveal a low $PaCO_2$, a normal bicarbonate, and an elevated pH. This initial respiratory alkalosis is generally not a compensatory mechanism, but rather a nonspecific response to stress. If the effects of the trauma, shock, or sepsis are not rapidly corrected, however, and oxygen consumption falls below critical levels, metabolic acidosis ultimately develops, causing a further increase in hyperventilation. If the $PaCO_2$ is driven below 20 to 25 mm Hg, this severe hypocapnia may in itself cause some hemodynamic impairment.

Tachypnea is often a valuable sign that an otherwise stable patient may be deteriorating. Noticeable breathing is not normal, yet it may initially be interpreted as "good" ventilation. If breathing is clearly noticeable, the patient usually has a minute ventilation which is 1.5 to 2.0 times normal.

AXIOM

If a patient with shock or sepsis is not hyperventilating, one should suspect that the patient may be developing ventilatory failure.

2. Metabolic Alkalosis

Metabolic alkalosis may be found in many critically ill and injured patients, prior to their going into severe shock. Some of the more frequently recognized causes of metabolic alkalosis in an intensive care unit (ICU) include administration of large amounts of antacids to reduce gastric acidity, hypokalemia due to excessive diuresis and/or the use of corticosteroids, and metabolism of citrate (from blood transfusions) or lactate (from Ringer's lactate).

3. Metabolic Acidosis

AXIOM
Metabolic (lactic) acidosis often indicates a fairly advanced state of hypoperfusion or impaired cell metabolism.

Normal oxygen consumption (Vo_2) at rest is about 120 to 160 $ml \cdot min^{-1} \cdot m^{-2}$. As shock progresses, impaired cellular metabolism associated with a reduction in Vo_2 to below 100 $ml \cdot min^{-1} \cdot m^{-2}$ eventually results in the development of metabolic (lactic) acidosis. This first occurs intracellularly and then at the capillary and venous levels. A metabolic acidosis in arterial blood is a relatively late finding. Alterations in cell membrane potential and intracellular pH may occur long before changes are apparent in the arterial blood gas samples. Nevertheless, blood lactate determinations can be very helpful as an indicator of progress and prognosis.

In the early phases of metabolic acidosis, the acid-base abnormality can usually be corrected by improving tissue perfusion. Later, however, sodium bicarbonate may be necessary, particularly if the arterial pH falls below 7.10. If the metabolic acidosis continues to progress, the amount of bicarbonate needed for correction increases almost geometrically.

4. Combined Metabolic and Respiratory Acidosis

Ordinarily, the lungs excrete carbon dioxide easily. However, in the terminal stages of prolonged shock, the number of functional pulmonary capillaries can be so critically reduced that it may be impossible for the patient to eliminate carbon dioxide properly in spite of a minute ventilation that is two to three times normal. If a combined metabolic and respiratory acidosis is allowed to develop, the chances for ultimate survival are extremely poor. A rise in the venous Pco_2, with an increasing $P(a-v)co_2$ and pH falling below 7.30 to 7.35 usually indicates a severe reduction in perfusion of functional pulmonary tissue.

D. TISSUE PERFUSION

1. Pulse Pressure

PITFALL
Assuming that tissue perfusion is adequate because systolic BP is normal or increased.

With decreasing tissue perfusion, systolic BP may remain relatively normal in spite of significant decreases in cardiac output. Consequently, cardiac output determinations can be very helpful. Changes in stroke volume can be estimated to a certain extent by noting the changes in pulse pressure and the ease with which the peripheral pulses can be palpated. In individual patients, changes in pulse pressure often correlate with changes in stroke volume fairly well, and are usually a much better indication of blood flow than the systolic pressure.

2. Skin Changes

PITFALL
Assuming that tissue perfusion is adequate because the skin is warm.

If the patient has cold and clammy skin, the cardiac output is usually very low and total peripheral vascular resistance is high secondary to intense sympathoadrenal stimulation. However, many patients with early sepsis and occasional patients with AMI have warm, dry skin. In the septic patient, such vasodilatation may be at least partially due to vasoactive substances such as bradykinin. In AMI shock, lack of an appropriate amount of vasoconstriction may be due to abnormal or pathologic reflexes originating from the ischemic myocardium.

3. Mentation

AXIOM
Questioning the patient to establish mentation and cognitive function may provide early evidence of sepsis or hypovolemia.

A cloudy sensorium may be an important sign of poor tissue perfusion. It may also be the first sign that a patient is becoming septic. In alcoholic patients it may be difficult to differentiate between impending or mild delirium tremens and sepsis.

4. Arteriovenous Oxygen Difference

AXIOM
A fall in arteriovenous (a-v) O_2 differences may be an early sign of sepsis, while a rise in a-v O_2 differences often indicates a reduction in blood volume and/or cardiac output.

Trends in cardiac output may be indicated by changes in a-v oxygen differences or pulmonary artery (mixed venous) oxygen saturation. If the $C(a-v)O_2$ is greater than 6.0 vol % or if Svo_2 is less than 60%, tissue perfusion is probably impaired.

5. Urine

If urine output and urine sodium concentrations are falling and urine osmolarity is rising, it can generally be assumed that there is inadequate renal perfusion, usually due to hypovolemia.

V. PATHO-PHYSIOLOGY

A. EARLY SHOCK

1. Ventilation

In early shock, hyperventilation occurs, and the minute ventilation is increased to at least 1.5 to 2.0 times normal. Although tidal volume is often reduced, the respiratory rate is increased twofold to threefold. If a patient with increasing sepsis or early shock is not hyperventilating, something is wrong, and unless the condition is corrected, ventilatory failure is likely to develop.

AXIOM
The combination of shock and respiratory failure is highly lethal.

In spite of the hyperventilation that is characteristic of sepsis and shock, hypoxemia can develop rapidly because of pulmonary changes that are at least partially due to release of toxic oxygen radical from polymorphonuclear leukocytes (PMNs) in the lung and activation of the complement and coagulation systems by infected or ischemic tissue. The C4a and C5a fractions of complement, sometimes referred to as anaphylatoxins, leukotriene LTB_4, cause circulating PMNs to stick to pulmonary capillary endothelium.

PMN release of superoxide radicals may be particularly important in early lung damage. PMN lysosomal enzymes are also released, and these tend to cause more long-term injury. Fibrin and aggregated blood cells can cause additional problems by occluding pulmonary capillaries, thereby increasing pulmonary dead space.

AXIOM
Much of the tissue damage in shock may be due to increased production of oxygen-free radicals or lack of their endogenous scavengers.

There has been increasing interest in free radicals and their effects in shock. Under normal circumstances, most of the molecular oxygen in cells undergoes tetravalent reduction to water in the cytochrome oxidase system by the following equation:

$$O_2 + 4e^- + 4H^+ \longrightarrow 2\,H_2O.$$

However, under certain circumstances, univalent reduction can occur with transfer of only one electron (e^-), resulting in the release of highly reactive free radical intermediates. Under certain conditions, particularly reperfusion after a period of ischemia, the release of free radicals may overpower the natural protective mechanisms, resulting in rapid, extensive cellular damage.

A free radical is defined as any atom or molecule with one unpaired electron in its outer orbit. The conversion of molecular oxygen to toxic oxygen radicals occurs by single electron transfer by the mitochondrial or microsomal electron transport chain or through oxidant enzyme systems, such as xanthine oxidase, aldehyde oxidase, flavin dehydrogenase, amine oxidase, cyclo-oxygenase, and lipo-oxygenase. Normally hypoxanthine, which is one of the terminal metabolites of adenosine triphosphate (ATP), is converted to xanthine by xanthine dehydrogenase (XDH) by the following reaction:

$$\text{hypoxanthine} + \text{NAD} + H_2O \xrightarrow{\text{XDH}} \text{xanthine} + \text{NADH} + H^+.$$

However, in the presence of ischemia, xanthine oxidase (XO) is formed instead of xanthine dehydrogenase and the following reaction occurs:

$$\text{hypoxanthine} + 2O_2 + H_2O \xrightarrow{\text{XO}} \text{xanthine} + 2O_2^- + 2H^+.$$

These potentially cytotoxic substances include the superoxide radical (O_2^-), hydrogen peroxide (H_2O_2), and the hydroxyl radical (OH), which may be produced by the following reactions:

$$O_2 + e^- \longrightarrow O_2^-$$
$$O_2 + 2e^- + 2H^+ \longrightarrow H_2O_2$$
$$O_2 + H_2O_2 + H^+ \longrightarrow O_2 + H_2O + OH.$$

There are no physiologic defenses against excess generation of the hydroxyl radical; however, H_2O_2 may be converted directly to water by catalase or by reduced glutathione under the influence of glutathione peroxidase.

Since free radical scavengers, such as alpha-tocopherol (vitamin E) and phenylbutylnitrone, can prevent many of the hemodynamic and metabolic changes seen in endotoxemia, it would appear that free radicals are an important factor in the organ damage that develops in sepsis and ischemia.

2. Cardiac Stimulation

Stimulation of beta-adrenergic receptors results in a faster heart rate (chronotropic effect), an increased force of myocardial contraction (inotropic effect), vasodilation in skeletal muscle arteries, and venous constriction in many vascular beds. The net result of these stimuli is improved circulation to skeletal muscle and vital organs.

PITFALL

Assuming that absence of a severe tachycardia in an elderly patient with hypotension is evidence of a better prognosis.

Patients who fail to develop an appropriate tachycardia with shock or sepsis have a poor prognosis. Increasing the pulse rate to 100 to 110 per minute (using isoproterenol, atropine, or a temporary transvenous pacemaker) may significantly increase cardiac output in patients with a fixed stroke volume because of old age or cardiac disease.

Because of excessive beta-adrenergic stimulation, particularly in septic patients, tachyarrhythmias may develop before other signs of sepsis or shock become evident.

AXIOM
Sudden onset of an explained tachyarrhythmia should be considered due to sepsis or a pulmonary embolus until proven otherwise.

Elevated plasma catecholamine levels during shock tend to be directly related to the severity of the physiologic insult and can eventually lead to down-regulation of receptors with decreased responsiveness of the myocardium to hormonal stimulation. Myocardial dysfunction may also be due to reduced ability of myocardial cells to generate cyclic adenosine monophosphate (cAMP).

AXIOM
Assuming that cardiac performance in sepsis is satisfactory because the cardiac output is normal or high.

Although cardiac output may be higher than normal in early (warm) septic shock, there is increasing evidence that myocardial performance, as determined by left ventricular ejection fractions, is reduced in many of these patients. In fact, ECGs and echocardiograms suggesting the presence of an acute myocardial infarction should be cautiously interpreted in septic patients. Studies have shown that segmental myocardial abnormalities in sepsis may be due to reversible local factors. In addition, the systemic vasodilation of sepsis allows cardiac output to increase even if cardiac contractility is impaired.

Jardin and colleagues recently noted that 6 of 21 patients with septic shock had marked depressed left and right ventricular function with a cardiac index of 2.2 ± 0.8 liters·min^{-1}·m^{-2} and LVEF of $21 \pm 8\%$ in spite of a normal left ventricular end-diastolic volume. However, this sepsis-related cardiogenic shock was reversible within 24 to 48 hours by inotropic support.

In an accompanying editorial, Parillo noted that inadequate volume loading in the low left ventricular end-diastolic volume may have been related to inadequate volume loading. He emphasized that despite a normal or elevated cardiac index, myocardial performance is substantially depressed during septic shock syndromes in humans. Most patients compensate for this with increased heart rates and ventricular dilation to maintain an adequate stroke volume. Consequently, volume loading and inotropic support may both play a role in treatment.

3. Vasoconstriction

AXIOM
The initial vasoconstriction seen in hypovolemic shock is an important mechanism for maintaining perfusion of vital organs.

Catecholamine stimulation of the sympathetic nervous system's alpha-adrenergic receptors results in arterial vasoconstriction, particularly in tissues (such as the skin and kidneys) that are more resistant to hypoxia and ischemia. Initially this vasoconstriction is beneficial because it diverts blood to vital organs, such as the heart and the brain, which cannot tolerate an inadequate blood flow for more than a few minutes. In combination with the arteriolar vasoconstriction, vascular capacity is also substantially reduced because of narrowing of the larger veins. Since approximately 60% of the systemic blood volume is normally present in large (capacitance) veins, this reduction in vascular capacity is one of the most important compensatory mechanisms for tolerating blood volume deficits as high as 25% without severe hypotension.

PITFALL
Administration of narcotics to a septic or injured patient without first ensuring that the patient is not hypovolemic.

235

Patients who receive narcotics to relieve pain, especially after severe trauma, will occasionally have a sudden severe drop in blood pressure. In retrospect, it is usually clear that such patients were hypovolemic, but the blood pressure was being maintained at relatively normal levels prior to the narcotic by vasoconstriction of arteries and veins. Narcotics and other vasodilators not only inhibit arteriolar vasoconstriction, but may also increase vascular capacity by 1 or 2 liters or more, which can produce a sudden, severe relative hypovolemia. Before a narcotic is given to any patient with trauma or sepsis, it should be ascertained that the patient is not hypovolemic. In addition, one or two large intravenous lines should be in place for rapid infusion of blood or fluid if the blood pressure does begin to fall. If there is any question about the status of the patient's cardiovascular or respiratory system and if narcotics appear to be necessary, it is preferable to administer them intravenously in multiple small doses.

a. Peripheral Vascular Function

Recent clinical studies suggest that many patients in septic shock die as a result of peripheral vascular dysfunction rather than cardiac failure. Persistent, severe vasodilation is the major hemodynamic problem seen in many nonsurvivors who maintain a high cardiac index until shortly before death.

AXIOM
Death in advanced septic shock may be due to terminal cardiac or vascular failure.

From electrophysiologic studies of vascular smooth muscle (VSM) during hemorrhagic hypotension, Lombard and associates have drawn three conclusions: (1) transmembrane potential (Em) plays an important role in controlling the response of VSM to shock, (2) Em-dependent constriction of veins is a crucial factor in the compensatory response to hemorrhagic shock, and (3) failure of the adrenergic neuroeffector junctions in VSM is characteristic in the decompensatory phase of late hemorrhagic shock.

Some of the explanations for the abnormal adrenergic vascular function seen in sepsis include the following: (1) chronic sepsis down-regulates $alpha_1$-adrenergic receptors, (2) endotoxin depresses peripheral vascular adrenergic action, (3) endogenous opioids impair norepinephrine release, (4) endogenous prostanoids impair adrenergic function, and (5) numerous vascular mediators interfere with each other's actions. In septic shock one can find both vasoconstrictors (such as angiotensin, catecholamines, serotonin, PFG_2, and thromboxane A_2) and vasodilators (such as histamine, bradykinin, PGI_2, and endorphins). Therefore, in a late vasodilated state, a therapeutic vasoconstrictor may be totally ineffective. In addition, unlike hemorrhage or hypothermia in which the rise in plasma catecholamine levels is rapid, in sepsis the catecholamine response is often delayed.

AXIOM
Failure to respond to vasoconstrictors in advanced shock may be due to severe acidosis, excess quantities of endogenous vasodilators, or inadequate receptor response.

The relationship between catecholamines, angiotensin, and enkephalins is being increasingly studied. Catecholamines and angiotensin II stimulate secretion of one another, and blockade of both would appear to be necessary to completely prevent vasoconstriction in advanced shock. In addition, enkephalins are stored with catecholamines in adrenal chromaffin cells and may suppress cholinergic-dependent catecholamine release from the adrenal glands. Opiate antagonists, such as naloxone, might act either by blocking this suppression locally or by antagonizing central enkephalinergic inhibition.

Based on numerous observations on the processes involved in vasoconstriction, a new working model of the mechanism of alpha$_1$-adrenergic receptors in vascular smooth-muscle cells has been developed.

b. The Phosphatidyl-Inositol System

According to this model, binding of catecholamines to their various receptors can initiate either (1) opening of calcium channels (either receptor-operated or voltage-regulated) or (2) activation of a phosphoinositide-specific phospholipase C. Following opening of the calcium channels, intracellular Ca^{++} is increased, thereby activating a calcium/calmodulin-dependent protein kinase that mediates the phosphorylation of myosin light chains and ultimately causes vasoconstriction. It now appears that calcium channels mediate the tonic phase of contraction for alpha$_1$-receptors, while serotonin receptors (which have been activated by phospholipase C) mediate the phasic component.

After hydrolysis of polyphosphoinositides, the compound known as inositol 1,4,5-triphosphate (IP3) is released along with diacylglycerol (DAG). The IP3 mobilizes intracellular Ca^{++}, and DAG activates protein kinase C. The elevated intracellular Ca^{++} and activated protein kinase C acting in synergy mediate vasoconstriction by phosphorylation of myosin light chains. This model suggests that one might intervene in hypotensive states at a number of levels including the calcium channels, phospholipase C, and protein kinase C.

4. Fluid Shifts

AXIOM

Transcapillary refill of the vascular system is important in hypovolemia, but it may be totally inactive or reversed in sepsis.

Normally (Fig. 5.2) the net pressure pushing fluid out of the capillary at its arteriolar end (8.5 mm Hg) exceeds the net pressure pulling fluid in at its venous end (7.5 mm Hg) so that fluid tends to leave the capillary and enter the interstitial fluid space. The fluid entering the interstitial fluid space is then

Forces moving fluid out of arteriolar end of the capillary	mm Hg
1. Capillary hydrostatic pressure	25
2. Interstitial fluid pressure (minus)	7
3. Interstitial colloid osmotic pressure	4.5
	36.5
Forces moving fluid into the capillary	
4. Plasma colloid osmotic pressure	28
∴ Net force moving fluid out of the arterial end of the capillary	8.5
Forces moving fluid out of venous end of the capillary	
5. Capillary filtration pressure	9
6. Interstitial fluid pressure	7
7. Interstitial colloid osmotic pressure	4.5
	20.5
Forces moving fluid into the capillary	
8. Plasma colloid osmotic pressure	28
∴ Net force moving fluid into the capillary at the venous end	7.5
∴ Net force moving fluid out of the entire capillary = 8.5 − 7.5 = 1.0 mm Hg	

Figure 5.2 Fluid shifts.

eventually returned to the circulation through the lymphatic system. When hypovolemia develops, the filtration pressure at the arteriolar end of the capillaries falls, and fluid tends to move from the interstitial space into the vascular space. According to the Frank-Starling hypothesis, this fluid shift occurs largely because the colloid osmotic pressure is still relatively normal, but the filtration pressure at the arteriolar end of the capillaries is reduced as a result of both a decreased arterial blood pressure and an increased vasoconstriction of arterioles and precapillary sphincters.

After the interstitial space has become about 50% depleted and the plasma proteins are progressively diluted by transcapillary movement of interstitial fluid, the shift of fluid from the interstitial to the intravascular space decreases.

AXIOM
Malnourished individuals with low plasma glucose and protein levels tend to have impaired defenses against hypovolemia.

Failure to develop an appropriate hyperglycemia or failure to maintain proper levels of plasma proteins because of nutritional deprivation may greatly reduce transcapillary refill with hypovolemia. Because glucose crosses the tissue cell membrane poorly, hyperglycemia in the interstitial fluid spaces can osmotically pull fluid out of cells into the extracellular fluid space.

AXIOM
Septic patients can develop tissue edema rapidly, even when hypovolemic.

In sepsis, capillary permeability may be increased very early so that the colloid osmotic pressure is not as effective and the fluid shift is quickly reversed, so that fluid tends to "leak" into the interstitial fluid space. Consequently, septic patients often require much more fluid and become much more edematous than other patients with similar degrees of hypotension.

AXIOM
Any patient without obvious excess loss of fluid or blood who requires more than 200 ml of fluid per hour to maintain normal vital signs and urine output should be considered septic until proven otherwise.

5. Platelet Aggregation

Platelet activation and aggregation increase markedly in early sepsis and shock. This process can cause platelet deficiencies, and the aggregates can interfere with microcirculatory blood flow in vital organs. The platelet aggregates and the vasoactive substances they release may also form microemboli which can migrate to the lungs. This may be a contributory factor in the development of respiratory and other organ failure seen with persisting sepsis or shock.

6. Impaired Cell Metabolism

AXIOM
A progressive drop in the platelet count should make one very suspicious of sepsis or the development of disseminated intravascular coagulation (DIC).

As the shock process continues, there is increasing evidence of disturbed cell metabolism. Energy for the cell comes from a variety of sources. One of the most important sources in shock is the conversion of glucose to pyruvate. This process can occur anaerobically, but it results in the net formation of only two moles of adenosine triphosphate (ATP) from each mole of glucose.

Under normal aerobic conditions, pyruvate, when converted to acetyl-CoA, can enter the Krebs cycle to be broken down into carbon dioxide and hydrogen. The hydrogen ions then enter the electron transport system, where they combine with oxygen to form water, with the eventual release of 36 more moles of ATP from each mole of glucose. Thus, aerobic metabolism is almost 20 times as effective as anaerobic metabolism.

AXIOM
Elevated plasma lactate levels indicated inadequate cellular oxidative metabolism and inefficient utilization of energy sources.

When there is not enough oxygen present to combine with the hydrogens released by metabolism of pyruvate (as acetyl-CoA), the Krebs cycle grinds to a halt. The pyruvate is then converted to lactate with the formation of two more moles of ATP.

Adenosine triphosphate (ATP) synthesis and calcium transport rates in liver, kidney, and brain mitochondria decline rapidly during severe circulatory shock. The specific enzyme functions most affected by low flow states are ATP synthetase, adenine nucleotide translocase, and carrier-mediated calcium transport.

Mitochondrial oxidative phosphorylation, the mechanism by which the transfer of electrons along the respiratory chain is used to form high-energy phosphates, requires a continuous supply of oxygen and reducing equivalents. One of the first changes recorded in hemorrhagic shock is reduction of brain mitochondrial nicotinamide adenine dinucleotide (NAD) to NADH with an associated leakage of K^+ into the extracellular space. Another mitochondrial function, the takeup of Ca^{++} ions from the cytoplasm, is impaired by endotoxic and hemorrhagic shock. As shock continues, intracellular levels of K^+ and Mg^{++} decrease, and intracellular Na^+, Cl^-, Ca^{++}, and water increase.

AXIOM
Impaired cellular function may be manifested by a progressive decrease in plasma levels of sodium and ionized calcium.

By virtue of its mass, skeletal muscle is often the major consumer of glucose in the body. Under normal aerobic conditions, it oxidizes fatty acids and most of the glucose to carbon dioxide and water; only a small portion of the glucose is metabolized anaerobically to pyruvate and lactate. However, if lactate levels rise and adequate oxygen becomes available, red skeletal muscle (especially the heart), preferentially oxidizes lactate instead of the fatty acids and glucose, which are normally its major oxidative substrates. Thus, under normal aerobic conditions, coronary sinus lactate levels are lower than arterial levels.

AXIOM
Increased coronary sinus lactate is relatively reliable evidence of myocardial ischemia.

Ischemia must usually be rather severe and prolonged before there is almost complete loss of high-energy phosphates from muscle. Initially, creatinine phosphate is progressively depleted, and ATP depletion occurs only after creatinine phosphate stores are virtually exhausted. In experimental animals, it can take up to 2 hours of total ischemia before muscle glycogen stores are depleted and high levels of lactate accumulate intracellularly.

AXIOM
Rising arterial lactate levels, especially above 8.0 mmol/liter, generally indicate a poor prognosis.

There is a strong belief by many investigators that plasma lactate levels have great prognostic value in shock. However, others feel that although high blood lactate levels in hypovolemic or cardiogenic shock tend to be associated with increased mortality rates, whole blood lactate concentrations at the onset of resuscitation in septic shock in some studies have been similar in both survivors and nonsurvivors, and one may be able to predict outcome only from serial measurements of lactate.

In one study, however, lactate measurements were less valuable in estimating prognosis than serial measurement of simple hemodynamic variables such as BP and pulse rate. Furthermore, arterial lactate and acid-base changes often do not accurately reflect metabolic changes of shock at the tissue level. Significant changes in muscle membrane potential and tissue pH may occur long before there is any change in arterial lactate or bicarbonate concentrations.

7. Complement Activation

AXIOM

Some complement activation may be important in host defense, but excess or prolonged complement activation can be very damaging to tissues.

The classical complement pathway, in which C1, C4, C2, and finally C3 are serially activated, is typically initiated by antigen-antibody complexes. The alternative pathway, which if often initiated by endotoxin, bypasses these early components and directly activates factors D and B and then C3. In a study of 42 patients with septic shock, low levels of C3 correlated with low levels of both C4 and factor B in patients in shock for more than 4 hours. This indicates activation and consumption of factors from both complement pathways, and tends to be associated with a poor prognosis. However, in shock of less than 4 hours' duration, C3 and factor B levels were reduced, but C4 levels were normal, suggesting that only the alternative pathway was activated early.

B. LATE SHOCK

1. Lysosomal Breakdown

If shock is allowed to persist into its later stages, progressive deterioration in cellular and organ function is seen. Much of this dysfunction may be due to lysosomal enzymes and toxic oxygen radicals. The intracellular vacuoles called lysosomes are particularly prominent in phagocytes. These are occasionally referred to as *intracellular stomachs* because bacteria or particles taken in by the phagocytes are "digested" or broken down by these lysosomes. The limiting lipoprotein membrane that surrounds lysosomes can break down rapidly in shock, sepsis, or trauma, resulting in a release of toxic free oxygen radicals and powerful hydrolytic enzymes into the cell and then into the bloodstream. The free radicals can destroy any compounds they encounter. The proteolytic enzymes from the lysosomes can convert inactive kininogens (vasoactive polypeptides combined with alpha$_2$ globulins) into active kinins by enzymatically splitting off the protein.

In a recent report, Tanaka and associates found that the levels of granulocyte elastase (GE) and alpha$_1$-protease inhibitors were elevated in both hemorrhagic and septic shock. These levels fell in resuscitated hemorrhagic shock patients, but were persistently elevated in the patients with septic shock. The authors felt that increased GE activity in local tissues, such as lung alveoli, may be responsible for the multiple-organ failure of sepsis.

2. Vasoactive Polypeptides

The two most important vasoactive polypeptides in shock are bradykinin and myocardial depressant factor. Bradykinin is one of the most potent vasodilators known to man. This vasodilator causes much of the skin flushing that occurs with alcoholism, sepsis, pancreatitis, and the carcinoid syndrome. Bradykinin also greatly increases capillary and small vein permeability and may be a major factor in the formation of the edema that develops in sepsis and prolonged shock. Bradykinin is metabolized, at least partially, by the angiotension-converting enzyme (ACE).

AXIOM

Patients on ACE inhibitors may have especially severe edema or hypotension if they develop shock or sepsis.

Myocardial depressant factor (MDF) comes primarily from an ischemic pancreas. It can cause severe splanchnic vasoconstriction and depression of myocardial contractility. Although some investigators initially felt that MDF was a chemical artifact, our previous bioassays on blood from patients with shock, sepsis, or pancreatitis indicated the presence of multiple vasoactive substances, some of which had marked effects on contraction or dilation of ox carotid strips suspended in a physiological solution.

3. Induced Histamine

Additional microcirculatory changes can be caused by induced histamine that is produced at the cellular level in response to many types of injury. This "induced" histamine, unlike the "preformed" histamine that is stored in mast cells, is difficult to measure and is not inhibited or blocked by the antihistamines used to treat allergic reactions. During severe hemorrhagic shock in dogs, the presence of increased amounts of induced histamine has been inferred from the increased levels of histidine decarboxylase (which converts inactive histidine to histamine) that are found.

More recently, increased local histamine levels have been demonstrated in liver, lungs, spleen, left atrium, left ventricle, and various blood vessel walls. In severe advanced shock, the histamine-to-norepinephrine ratio may be particularly increased in the left ventricle and blood vessels walls. It is postulated that this histamine, acting as a strong vasodilator, may moderate the excessive vasoconstriction due to norepinephrine in severe hemorrhagic shock and may represent a positive factor for survival. However, increased amounts of induced histamine in sepsis may contribute to excessive vasodilation.

4. Prostaglandins and Leukotrienes

Prostaglandins and leukotrienes are synthesized by arachidonic acid through the cycloxygenase and lipoxygenase pathways, respectively. The prostaglandins and leukotrienes are generated primarily by macrophages, neutrophils, platelets, and mast cells. These substances have a wide range of pharmacological effects on the cardiovascular system. Prostaglandins of the E and F groups exert directly opposing physiologic actions on the microcirculation (vasodilation vs. vasoconstriction), and the eventual reaction depends on the ratio of the concentrations of these metabolites to each other. The ratio of thromboxane to prostacyclin levels in organs such as the heart and lung are particularly important for determining local capillary blood flow. Because the ratios of these substances may be so variable, early pharmacologic attempts with indomethacin and aspirin to block the adverse effects of the prostaglandins in shock have provided widely differing results. More selective blocking agents may help clarify this situation.

Leukotrienes contribute to many of the changes seen in inflammation, including chemotaxis (5-HETE and LTB_4), vasoconstriction (LTC_4), broncho-constriction (LTD_4), and increased vascular permeability (LTE_4). The slow reacting substance of anaphylaxis (SRS-A) is now recognized as a group of acidic lipopeptides (leukotrienes) of the C, D, and E classes. There are no clinically selective useful inhibitors of the lipo-oxygenase pathways. However, since glucocorticoids inhibit the common arachidonate phospholipase A_2, they block both the cyclo-oxygenase and lipo-oxygenase pathways.

5. Endorphins

Following stress, adrenocorticotrophic hormone (ACTH) and beta-endorphin (derived from the same precursor as ACTH) molecules are released in equimolar quantities from the anterior pituitary in response to corticotrophin-releasing factors (CRF). Although many of the hemodynamic effects attributed to beta endorphins were thought to be mediated centrally, it has been shown that adrenalectomy can block the pressor response to naloxone.

Since the original report of Holaday and Faden in 1978, there has been a great deal of work on the role of endorphins in shock. Continuing studies support the theory that beta endorphins mediate many of the hemodynamic changes in shock. Interestingly, there is some work that suggests that another endogenous opiate, metenkephalin, may be even more important than beta endorphins in shock.

6. Serotonin

Although serotonin is generally felt to cause vasoconstriction, bronchoconstriction, and platelet aggregation, it is an amphibaric substance and therefore has varying effects on vascular smooth muscle depending on the vessels being tested and their underlying contractile state. It may also desensitize blood vessels to norepinephrine and thereby reduce their vascular responsiveness. Furthermore, serotonin tends to increase blood levels of beta endorphins which oppose the vascular constriction caused by norepinephrine.

7. Hormones

AXIOM
The hormonal response in shock appears to be designed to increase blood levels of glucose and raise cardiac output to facilitate "fight or flight."

During shock, blood levels of catecholamines, glucagon, cortisol, and growth hormone rise, while insulin levels tend to be relatively low. Indeed, infusion of the three "counter-regulatory hormones" (epinephrine, glucagon, and cortisol) are able to produce a catabolic response very similar to that seen with severe injury and other stress.

Recently there has been increased attention paid to the role of the thyroid gland in sepsis and shock. Some researchers feel that thyroidectomy increases the release of thyrotropin-releasing hormone (TRH) from the pituitary, thereby improving the hemodynamic response to shock. However, hypothyroidism increases susceptibility to experimental sepsis. In addition, T_3 (3,5,3′-triiodothyronine) has been reported to be of benefit in experimental hemorrhagic shock by increasing systemic vascular resistance and decreasing pulmonary vasoconstriction.

8. Fluid Shifts

In late shock, fluid tends to leave the vascular system because of increasing capillary permeability and impaired cell membrane function. This can cause significant hypovolemia regardless of the etiology of the shock. The so-called sodium pump, which maintains low sodium concentrations (10 to 12 mEq/liter) inside the cell, in spite of a sodium concentration of 135 to 142 mEq/liter in the extracellular fluid, depends on active (energy-mediated) cellular metabolism. In damaged or ischemic cells, sodium begins to diffuse into the cells. At the same time, potassium, which normally has a concentration of about 120 to 150 mEq/liter inside cells, diffuses out into the extracellular fluid, where its normal concentration is only 3.5 to 5.0 mEq/liter. Since water tends to follow the sodium, which diffuses faster, the cells begin to swell, pulling in fluid from the extracellular fluid space, which is thereby depleted.

AXIOM
As shock progresses there is an increasing tendency to hypovolemia.

As shock or sepsis progresses, the endothelial cells of capillaries and small veins begin to swell and separate, leaving progressively enlarging intercellular capillary spaces. Fluid can then escape at an increasingly rapid rate through the capillaries and small veins into the interstitial space. As the spaces between the abnormal endothelial cells progressively widen, increasingly larger particles, including protein molecules and eventually even red blood cells, can also pass through the capillary wall into the interstitial fluid space. This increasing capillary leak, plus the increasing intracellular edema, may result in fluid leaving the circulation at rates exceeding 200 ml/h.

AXIOM

Progressively increasing fluid needs far above measured losses may be an important early sign of sepsis.

9. Calcium

In sepsis or shock, inadequate cell metabolism will allow movement of free ionized calcium (Ca^{++}) from the extracellular fluid space, where its concentration normally is about 1.05 to 1.20 mmol/liter (10^{-3} mol) into the cellular cytoplasm, where its concentration can be as low as 10^{-7} mol. This 10,000:1 gradient for Ca^{++} across the cell membrane can be maintained only if adequate cellular ATP is available.

Increased free Ca^{++} in the cytoplasm sets off a number of deleterious reactions resulting in a progressive impairment of cellular and cardiovascular function. As the mitochondria take up the increased cytosolic calcium, their production of ATP drops.

AXIOM

Falling ionized calcium levels in blood are often a sign of increasing impairment of cell function.

10. Further Impairment of Organ Function

a. Lung

The pulmonary capillary endothelium becomes increasingly damaged in prolonged sepsis or shock, resulting in more severe interstitial edema and congestive atelectasis, which are reflected by rising alveolar-arterial oxygen differences and increasing shunting (Qs/Qt). Physiologic dead space may also increase from a normal of 0.3 to levels exceeding 0.6, so that terminally the patient may become hypercarbic in spite of a minute ventilation that is more than two to three times normal.

b. Liver

Until recently there have been few measurements of hepatic blood flow in clinical shock. In one study of six patients with shock, calculated effective liver blood flow (as determined by galactose clearance studies in peripheral blood) was reduced to less than a third of normal. In addition, the systemic clearance of morphine was reduced by more than 50%. However, Dahn and coworkers have shown, using hepatic vein studies, that sepsis actually increases total hepatic blood flow.

Not only are metabolic functions of the liver profoundly impaired in severe shock or sepsis, but there is usually also concurrent impairment of the hepatic reticuloendothelial system (RES). The liver contains about 90% of the body's RES phagocytes, and the hepatocytes may also be involved in the removal of a number of toxic substances absorbed from the intestine during shock. Failure of the liver to handle these substances can, in turn, cause progressive impairment of cardiovascular and other organ function.

AXIOM

Hepatic dysfunction in late shock has dire consequences on metabolism and host defenses.

c. Bowel

The cause of a continued septic picture in patients who have had prolonged sepsis with no apparent site of infection has been the subject of much discussion. Deitch and others have presented data suggesting that movement or "translocation" of bacteria and various bacterial products through intestinal mucosa into intestinal lymphatics and the portal vein occurs under a variety of circumstances. This may be an important cause of a sepsislike picture, particularly in chronic ICU patients, in the absence of any apparent site of infection even at autopsy.

Such findings were described as a nonbacteremic clinical sepsis by Meakins and associates. They found that the classic presentation of sepsis, characterized by a hyperdynamic cardiovascular response, was uncommon in their ICU patients. Instead, most of their septic patients had multiple-organ failure (MOF) with hypoxemia, hyperbilirubinemia, gastric bleeding, renal failure, thrombocytopenia, abnormal mentation, and transient hypotension. Since only 22 of their 42 patients with clinical sepsis had positive blood cultures, there was concern that the gut might be the "motor" or cause of the septic picture.

Although bacterial translocation is an attractive hypothesis to explain many of the findings in ICU patients with multiple-organ failure, negative blood cultures are not unusual in patients with demonstrated foci of infection, especially if they are on antibiotics. Furthermore, in at least one study of patients who seemed to have nonbacteremic clinical sepsis, careful autopsies often revealed clinically unsuspected septic foci in the lungs.

d. Brain

Brain ischemia for as little as 2 to 3 minutes can result in (1) abnormal potassium and calcium ion homeostasis, (2) altered phospholipids, prostaglandin, and leukotriene metabolism, and (3) production of oxygen-free radicals. It has been suggested that, to prevent these changes during shock, various cerebral arterioles dilate so as to redistribute blood flow within the brain to areas necessary for the immediate survival of the animal.

e. Kidney

Even if urine output is restored to fairly normal levels after shock or sepsis, renal plasma flow can be very low and creatinine clearance and free water clearance tend to become progressively impaired. Interestingly, serum creatinine levels may not adequately reflect the degree of renal impairment because creatinine excretion after shock or during sepsis often falls from a normal of 1400 to 1800 mg/d to less than 300 to 600 mg/d. If creatinine excretion is markedly reduced, there is much less correlation of serum creatinine levels and creatinine clearance by the kidneys.

AXIOM
In advanced sepsis and shock there is often a poor correlation between serum creatinine levels and other measures of renal function.

11. Intravascular Coagulation

As vasoactive substances and acid metabolites accumulate in the progressively stagnant capillaries of shock, there is increasing red cell aggregation and a tendency to intravascular clotting. Because platelets, fibrinogen, factor V, factor VIII, and prothrombin are "consumed" by intravascular coagulation, this process in its advanced stages is often referred to as disseminated intravascular coagulation (DIC) or "consumption coagulopathy."

Concentrations of the various clotting factors may be extremely variable in critically ill and injured patients. Serial clotting studies are important in these patients, because they will often demonstrate significant trends long before other laboratory values become severely abnormal or before the clinical picture characteristic of DIC develops.

AXIOM
By the time DIC is clinically reflected in troublesome bleeding from needle puncture sites and mucosal surfaces, the concentrations of clotting factors are very low, and the problem is extremely difficult to correct.

In patients with traumatic shock, the tendency to consumption coagulopathy is further aggravated by (1) thromboplastin-rich materials entering the blood stream due to the injury, and (2) dilution of platelets and coagulation factors by infusion of large quantities of crystalloids and old bank blood. The importance of the initial shock in causing coagulation changes is reflected by a report on 180 patients with major trauma who eventually died. Almost all (97%) of these patients had coagulation abnormalities, and 60% had full-blown DIC before blood or crystalloid was infused. In fact, 12 of the 180 patients could not be cross-matched due to inability of their blood to clot in the test tube.

Suffredini, Harpel, and Parrillo described in detail the changes in the fibrinolytic system after a single dose of endotoxin that produced many of the abnormalities seen in early clinical sepsis. There was an initial rapid release of TPA. This was followed by an early increase in plasminogen activation and alpha$_2$-plasmin inhibitor-plasmin complexes which reached a maximum at 2 and 3 hours, and decreased by 3 and 5 hours. The decrease in fibrinolytic activity was due in part to the appearance of plasminogen-activator inhibitor-1 activity at 3 to 5 hours. In contrast, alpha$_1$-antitrypsin-elastase complexes (which reflect neutrophil activation) and von Willebrand factor antigen (a marker for endothelial cell stimulation) became significantly elevated at 3 hours and remained elevated for 24 hours after endotoxin.

Thus, endothelial cell abnormalities due to endotoxin infusion could cause increased blood levels of TPA and von Willebrand factor. Since hypotension, DIC, and neutrophil activation are all triggered by the interaction of factor XII with plasma kininogens and prekallikrein, the use of inhibitors of the contact activation system may be of therapeutic value.

12. Toxins

Of various clinical problems felt to be due to bacterial toxins, one of the most widely described is the toxic shock syndrome (TSS). TSS was first recognized in 1978 and is characterized by (1) fever, (2) a diffuse macular erythematous rash, (3) hypotension, (4) multisystem organ failure, and (5) desquamation of the palms and soles 1 to 2 weeks after onset of the fever. In 1980, TSS was noted to be causally related to tampon use during menstruation; however, an increasing incidence of surgical nonmenstrual TSS has been noted.

Over 90% of *Staphylococcus aureus* isolated from menstrual TSS patients produce an antigen referred to as toxic shock syndrome toxin-1 (TSST-1); however, it is only found in 25% of patients who have *S. aureus* but do not have TSS. TSST-1 is a protein with a molecular weight of 22,000 d. On a weight-for-weight basis it is 500 to 1000 times more active in inducing interleukin-1 (IL-1), the human endogenous pyrogen, from macrophages than the endotoxin of Gram-negative bacteria.

TSST-1 is also capable of suppressing a number of immune responses. For example, patients with TSS have lower levels of antibody to staphylococcal enterotoxins A, B, and C than do controls. Interestingly, many patients with TSS develop repeat infections; however, no patient who has developed antibodies to TSST-1 has had a recurrence of the syndrome.

AXIOM
Relatively mild postsurgical infections can cause severe toxic shock syndrome.

Although many physicians tend to think of TSS as primarily a menstrual or gynecological problem, TSS has also been seen with a wide variety of staphylococcal infections from other sites. The overall incidence of nonmenstrual TSS is lower (about 15% to 20% of all TSS). However, nonmenstrual TSS tends to be more serious and has a higher death rate (13% vs. 2%).

Almost all *S. aureus* from women with menstrual-related TSS produce TSST-1; however, many nonmenstrual isolates do not. Nevertheless, nonmenstrual TSST-1 negative isolates all produce at least one enterotoxin, suggesting that enterotoxin may also serve as a TSS toxin.

C. MONONUCLEAR RESPONSES

1. Inhibition by Trauma

Lymphocytes from trauma patients do not proliferate nearly as well as controls in response to mitogen stimulation. This depression appears to be due to generation of serum inhibitory factors. Reversal of the normal helper/suppressor T cell ratio, as determined by the ratio of monoclonal antibodies OKT-4 and OKT-8, respectively, can also occur after multiple trauma and severe burns, even in the absence of infection. This trauma-induced depression in lymphocyte function is postulated to contribute to the high incidence of infection seen after many types of trauma. In a study of septic patients developing multiple-organ failure, the peripheral total lymphocyte count, T-lymphocyte count, and response to phytohemagglutinin (PHA) and concanavalin A (ConA) were decreased in all patients. OKT-3 and immunoglobulin levels fell only in nonsurvivors.

2. Interleukin-2

Interleukin-2 (IL-2), a T-cell-produced factor, is required for (1) proliferation of T lymphocytes in response to mitogen and antigens, (2) generation of cytolytic T cells, and (3) T cell modulation of humoral responses. Both severe burns and multiple trauma have been shown to reduce the production of IL-2 by peripheral blood mononuclear cells. Anesthetized hemorrhage without any tissue injury also produces a profound suppression in IL-2 production by peripheral blood T lymphocytes. The depression in IL-2 generation is greatest 2 hours after hemorrhage and then gradually disappears over the next 48 hours.

3. Endotoxin

Many of the deleterious effects of clinical Gram-negative sepsis can be produced in animals by the administration of endotoxin, which is the lipopolysaccharide component of bacterial cell walls. However, examining animals genetically resistant or hyporesponsive to endotoxin has suggested that many of the pathophysiologic changes induced by endotoxin are mediated through factors (monokines) secreted by macrophages.

Another type of endotoxin hyporesponsiveness is due to prior exposure to endotoxin and has been designated endotoxin tolerance. Such tolerance is transient, shows no antigen O specificity, and is not associated with antibody production. When challenged with endotoxin, tolerant animals produce less monokines, lysosomal enzymes, and arachidonic acid metabolites than nontolerant control animals.

Although bacterial endotoxin is highly toxic to most mammals, endotoxin does not appear to injure host tissues directly, but rather through the action of endogenous mediators from various cells of hematopoietic origin, especially macrophages.

4. Tumor Necrosis Factor (Cachetin)

Cachetin is also known as tumor neurosis factor (TNF). This protein is produced in large quantities by endotoxin-activated macrophages and has been implicated as an important mediator of the lethal effects of endotoxin. Recombinant cachetin (formed by yeast with an artificial gene), when given to unanesthetized rats, can produce almost all of the hemodynamic, metabolic, and pathologic changes characteristic of endotoxin shock. Tracey and colleagues have also found that antibodies against TNF can prevent septic shock during lethal bacteremia. Interestingly, if an animal cannot make TNF, it does not show the typical signs of sepsis, but is much more likely to die.

A recent study of 86 patients in shock (74 with sepsis) by Marks and associates demonstrates that TNF is present in a significantly greater number of patients with septic shock (27/74 = 36%) than in patients with shock due to other causes (1/12 = 8%). They also showed that TNF is present in septic shock regardless of whether the bacteria are Gram-positive or Gram-negative. TNF is present early in the course of septic shock, and the presence of TNF is associated with a higher incidence of adult respiratory distress syndrome (ARDS) (55% vs. 26%) and mortality (81% vs. 43%). They also found that TNF levels were highest upon admission to the study. The levels then rapidly declined over the next 12 to

24 hours. Because of this rapid decline, attempting to measure TNF has limited value for prospectively identifying septic shock patients at risk for developing ARDS or dying.

AXIOM
Some TNF appears to be an important aspect of the host response to infection, but excess TNF may be very deleterious.

5. Fibronectin, Antithrombin, and Prekallikrein

Blood-borne particles, including tissue debris, fibrin clots, and bacteria, are removed from the circulation by cells of the mononuclear phagocyte system (MPS). Plasma fibronectin is a integral component of the MPS, in which it functions as "the third opsonin," with the first two opsonins being immunoglobulins and complement. All of these opsonins can bind to bacteria or circulating particulate matter to facilitate their clearance by phagocytes. One consequence of hemorrhagic shock, nutritional deprivation, or traumatic injury is a suppression of the mononuclear phagocyte system. This results in reduced clearance of potentially damaging particles from the blood, thereby increasing the risk of sepsis, organ failure, and death.

Plasma fibronectin levels fall in sepsis because of decreased synthesis and more rapid clearance from the circulation. In preliminary attempts to raise fibronectin levels with infusions of cryoprecipitate (which is rich in fibronectin) into septic burn and trauma patients, Saba found a significant reduction in multiple organ failure and mortality. However, later work by other investigators has not substantiated these findings.

AXIOM
Low antithrombin, prekallikrein, and fibronectin levels indicate an increased likelihood of sepsis.

Plasma levels of antithrombin (AT), prekallikrein (PK), and fibronectin (FN) are consumed when the coagulation and kallikrein cascades are stimulated by bacteria. Wilson and associates found that severe decreases in the plasma levels of AT, PK, and/or FN during the first 24 to 48 hours after trauma reliably predicted later sepsis in surgery patients before it became clinically apparent. Indeed, FN, PK, and AT levels in septic patients fell to significantly lower levels than in those without sepsis, and those with sepsis who died had lower levels than septic patients who lived.

Patients who enjoyed an uneventful recovery following major trauma had only moderately reduced AT, PK, and FN levels, and these returned to normal within 3 to 4 days. If AT, PK, and FN levels were extremely low and remained below 60% of normal for more than 6 days, the patients almost invariably developed septic complications.

VI. MONITORING

Close observations for trends help to identify patients who are beginning to go into shock. However, since there often is not enough equipment or personnel to monitor every patient closely, the exercise of clinical judgment is necessary.

Patients who may go in shock should have almost continuous monitoring of the following:
1. Blood pressure (using an intra-arterial line if necessary)
2. Heart rate and rhythm (cardioscope)
3. Respiratory rate, also noting depth and effort
4. CVP (and PAWP in selected cases)
5. Urine output (ml/h)
6. Serial arterial blood gases and electrolytes

Monitoring of cardiac output can be extremely important. This not only allows estimation of cardiac contractility but also allows one to calculate oxygen transport (Do_2) and oxygen consumption (Vo_2). The Do_2 and Vo_2 are probably the best parameters for evaluating the adequacy of resuscitation of patients who are, or may be, developing shock.

Currently, cardiac output is measured primarily by thermodilution technique. This technique is reasonably acute at normal values but is much less accurate with values much higher or lower than normal. One of the main problems with this technique is that it can be performed only intermittently.

There has continued to be interest in noninvasive techniques for continuous monitoring of cardiac output. Thoracic electrical bioimpedance (TEB) is currently the only noninvasive method for determination of cardiac output which can measure on-line cardiac performance with little technical effort. Many studies have compared TEB with standard methods, such as thermodilution (TD). The majority of authors conclude that TEB reliably estimates SV and cardiac output. Even critics of TEB admit that TEB accurately reflects trends even if there is a weak correlation with absolute cardiac output values. There has also been concern that positive end-expiratory pressure (PEEP) might affect the accuracy of TEB cardiac outputs.

In a recent study by Castor and associates in six patients undergoing neurosurgical interventions, TEB cardiac output measurements were compared during zero end-expiratory pressure (ZEEP) (r = 0.93) and during PEEP (r = 0.91). However, during normal or decreased cardiac output, TEB overestimated cardiac output compared with TD, whereas TEB underestimated cardiac output compared with TD during increased cardiac output, especially during PEEP.

Wherever possible, these numbers should be graphed. Rapid scanning of columns of numbers does not facilitate appreciation of subtle trends. However, graphic recordings of vital signs, particularly the pulse pressure, can be extremely helpful in this regard.

AXIOM

Isolated measurements are of much less value than serial determinations to demonstrate trends in the patient's condition and response to treatment.

VII. TREATMENT

A. PRIMARY PROCESS

Although it is sometimes necessary to treat patients who are in shock without knowing the initial or primary cause of the problem, a strong effort should always be made to establish an accurate etiologic diagnosis as soon as possible. Left uncorrected for more than a few hours, problems such as intra-abdominal abscesses, necrotic bowel, torn spleen, or ruptured ectopic pregnancy can carry an extremely high mortality rate, regardless of how well the cardiovascular, respiratory, and metabolic changes are managed (Table 5.3).

B. RESUSCITATION

1. Ventilation and Oxygen

a. Need for Increased Ventilation

AXIOM

A patient in shock who is not hyperventilating somewhat is more likely to develop respiratory failure.

Patients with severe sepsis or shock typically have a minute ventilation of more than double normal. In such patients, a "normal" minute ventilation of 6 liters is usually inadequate. If the patient has severe sepsis or shock and is not hyperventilating, one must suspect a significant ventilatory problem and provide early ventilatory assistance.

The $Paco_2$ in early to moderate shock is usually 25 to 35 mm Hg. If the $Paco_2$ is greater than 45 to 50 mm Hg and the pH is less than 7.35, the patient should be intubated and ventilation mechanically assisted. However, in the occasional patient who has severe chronic obstructive pulmonary disease (COPD) with CO_2 retention, the Pco_2 should not be reduced by more than 5

Table 5.3

AN OUTLINE OF THE TREATMENT OF SHOCK	A. Correction of primary problems (stop bleeding, drain pus, etc.)
	B. Resuscitation
	   1. Intubation and positive-pressure ventilation if there is a possibility of inadequate tidal volume or minute ventilation.
	   2. Oxygen, if PaO_2 is less than 80 mm Hg.
	   3. Fluids to correct hypovolemia without overloading—PAWP is important if there is acute myocardial infarction, sepsis, or respiratory failure.
	   4. Inotropic agents:
	     Dopamine—to raise BP and cardiac output.
	     Dobutamine—to raise cardiac output if BP is adequate.
	     Epinephrine—if dopamine and dobutamine are ineffective.
	     Isoproterenol—if pulse rate is less than 100.
	     Glucagon—occasionally helps if beta blockers were given.
	   5. Correction of acid-base and electrolyte abnormalities.
	   6. Corticosteroids—small doses if adrenal insufficiency is present.
	   7. Vasopressors*—norepinephrine plus phentolamine—to raise blood pressure, especially in patients with vascular disease.
	   8. Vasodilators*—for severe vasoconstriction and low cardiac output but a reasonable BP.
	   9. Diuretics—as needed to get a urine output of at least 0.5 ml·kg^{-1}·h^{-1}.
	  10. IABP—for persisting cardiogenic shock.

*Combined with inotropic agents as needed.
BP = blood pressure; IABP = intra-aortic balloon pumping; PAWP = pulmonary artery wedge pressure.

mm Hg/h. Other common clinical and blood gas parameters for initiating mechanical ventilation in shock are listed in Table 5.4.

b. Oxygen

Even if ventilation is adequate, virtually all patients in shock benefit from the administration of some oxygen. Oxygenation in the lungs can become impaired very quickly and, if cardiac output is decreased, tissue oxygenation may be totally inadequate. Consequently, virtually all patients in shock should be given oxygen during the initial 4 to 6 hours of resuscitation to maintain an arterial Po_2 of at least 80 mm Hg (oxyhemoglobin saturation of 95%). At this stage, providing sufficient oxygen to the tissues is the primary concern; oxygen toxicity is a very secondary consideration.

AXIOM

In patients with sepsis or shock, oxygen delivery (DO_2) should be increased until oxygen consumption (VO_2) no longer rises or is significantly above normal.

2. Fluids

In the recently injured patient in obvious hypovolemic shock, 3 liters of a balanced electrolyte solution is given over 10 to 15 minutes. If the blood pressure does not return to normal after such aggressive fluid resuscitation, type-specific blood and additional balanced electrolyte should be administered rapidly. Since

Table 5.4

INDICATIONS FOR ENDOTRACHEAL INTUBATION AND VENTILATORY ASSISTANCE IN PATIENTS IN SHOCK	1. Minute ventilation less than 9–12 liter/min (or > 18 liter/min) 2. Tidal volume less than 4 to 5 ml/kg 3. Vital capacity less than 10 ml/kg 4. $PaCO_2$ greater than 45 mm Hg if a metabolic acidosis is present or $PaCO_2$ greater than 50 to 55 mm Hg with normal bicarbonate 5. PaO_2 less than 80 mm Hg on 40% oxygen or PaO_2 less than 200 mm Hg on 100% oxygen 6. Respiratory rate greater than 30–35 per minute 7. Excessive ventilatory effort

the patient is probably losing blood rapidly, possibly from internal injuries, emergency surgical control of the bleeding should be considered.

AXIOM

The simplest and most effective treatment for most shock, particularly after trauma or surgery, is early and aggressive administration of fluids.

a. **Types of Fluids**

(1) Isotonic Crystalloids

The terms *crystalloid* and *colloid* were coined by Thomas Graham in 1861 and refer respectively to solute particles that will or will not pass through semipermeable membranes and are smaller or larger than an arbitrarily determined particle weight, usually taken as 10,000 d. The crystalloids generally used in resuscitation are solutions that are isotonic with plasma, contain sodium as their major osmotically active particle, and have no particles with molecular weight (MW) greater than 10,000.

Ringer's lactate and normal (0.9%) saline are the crystalloids used most frequently in resuscitation. Each liter of Ringer's lactate contains 130 mEq sodium, 109 mEq chloride, 28 mEq of lactate, 4 mEq potassium, and 3 mEq calcium. The calcium present may cause bank blood to clot in the tubing if it is given in the IV line. The lactate present in Ringer's lactate solution does not usually increase the lactic acidemia of shock unless the patient has severe liver dysfunction. Half (14 mEq) of the lactate is L-lactate and can undergo hepatic metabolism to bicarbonate. The other 14 mEq is R-lactate which is excreted unchanged in the urine.

Normal (0.9%) saline contains 154 mEq/liter each of sodium and chloride. The theoretical concern that large volumes of normal saline can produce a hyperchloremic acidosis is not generally a problem clinically. In fact, normal saline is preferred over Ringer's lactate in patients with severe liver disease, hypercalcemia, hyperkalemia, or hyponatremia.

Crystalloids are inexpensive, readily available, easily stored, reaction free, and can quickly correct most extracellular volume deficits. However, only 20% to 33% of these solutions remain in the circulation after 1 hour. Because so much of the crystalloid administered is sequestered in the interstitial fluid space, some peripheral edema is often seen in patients receiving more than 10 to 15 liters of these solutions in 24 hours. Pulmonary edema may also occur if tissue damage or severe sepsis is also present.

b. **Colloids**

(1) Albumin

Human serum albumin can be very effective in rapidly restoring blood volume, particularly if albumin levels are <2.0 to 2.5 g/dl. Albumin is clinically available as 5% or 25% solutions in isotonic saline. One gram of albumin binds about 18 ml of water by its oncotic activity, so that when 100 ml of a 25% albumin solution (25 g albumin) is infused, an increase in the intravascular volume to a final volume of about 450 ml occurs over the next 30 to 60 minutes. However, administered albumin rapidly distributes itself throughout the extracellular space, and its plasma half-life is usually less than 12 to 16 hours. The normal disappearance rate of iodine 131 tagged albumin from the circulation is 6% to 8% per hour. In shock or sepsis, the disappearance rate often exceeds 20% to 30%.

There is great controversy about the value of albumin in the treatment of shock. Shoemaker and others have found it to be a valuable, rapid plasma expander, while Lucas and associates have found many problems with its use, including increased organ failure and decreased coagulation proteins and immunoglobulins. Recently, Emerson reviewed some of the features of albumin that might make it of some efficacy during resuscitation of critically ill patients. These include (1) scavenging free radicals to limit lipid peroxidation, (2) binding to various toxic products such as lysosomal enzymes and free fatty acids, (3) inhibition of pathologic platelet activation, (4) enhanced inhibition of factor Xa by antithrombin III, and (5) maintenance of normal microvascular permeability to protein.

Albumin costs more than other plasma expanders and is at least 30 times as expensive as the amount of crystalloid needed to produce an equivalent expansion of blood volume. Some investigators feel that the increased pulmonary capillary permeability in sepsis allows more albumin to enter the interstitial fluid space, contributing to the formation of increased extravascular lung water.

Although there is no hepatitis risk with albumin, large quantities of albumin can reduce plasma concentrations of immunoglobulins and various coagulation proteins, possibly by interfering with their production.

AXIOM
Although plasma albumin levels are often very low in sepsis and shock, administration of albumin usually produces only transient benefits and can cause many complications if given in excess.

(2) Dextran

Dextran is a large glucose polymer which is available in two commercial preparations having an average molecular weight of 40,000 (dextran 40) or 70,000 (dextran 70). A 500 ml bolus of dextran 40 produces an intravascular volume expansion of 750 ml at 1 hour and 1050 ml at 2 hours. The smaller dextran molecules are rapidly lost through the kidney. The remaining molecules equilibrate with the entire ECF. Particles of MW >80,000 are taken up by the reticuloendothelial system (RES) and are eventually metabolized to carbon dioxide and water.

Dextran 40 improves blood flow in capillaries by decreasing viscosity and reducing aggregation of blood cells. In experimental animals hydroxyethyl starch (HES) and dextran 40 or dextran 70 produce more volume expansion than albumin, but dextran 70 produces higher pulmonary pressures, transiently higher colloid osmotic pressure (COP), lower cardiac output, and greater pulmonary edema. The increased pulmonary edema with dextran may be due to a combination of factors, including high pulmonary microvascular pressure and increased transvascular escape of dextran and endogenous macromolecules (because of a dextran effect on capillary permeability).

PITFALL
Administration of dextran 40 to patients with large open wounds can cause increased blood loss.

Dextran increases the likelihood of oozing from raw surfaces by (1) reducing platelet adherence and degranulation; (2) decreasing activation of clotting mechanisms; and (3) polymerizing with fibrin monomers, producing a less stable clot. To avoid excessive bleeding, the total dosage should be less than $1.5 \text{ g} \cdot \text{kg}^{-1} \cdot \text{d}^{-1}$ of D 40 and $2.0 \text{ g} \cdot \text{kg}^{-1} \cdot \text{d}^{-1}$ of D 70.

PITFALL
Relying on a urine output of 0.5 to 1.0 $\text{ml} \cdot \text{kg}^{-1} \cdot \text{h}^{-1}$ to indicate adequate renal perfusion after a patient has received a large bolus of dextran 40.

Since small dextran molecules can produce an almost immediate osmotic diuresis, urine output may not be a good guide to the adequacy of the resuscitation after such therapy. Furthermore, dextran-induced renal failure may occur because of precipitation of dextran in the tubules, especially in the presence of unrecognized hypovolemia.

The incidence of anaphylactoid reactions to dextran may be as high as 1% to 5.3%, but bronchospasm, shock, and death are uncommon. Allergic reactions, such as urticaria, rash, and nausea, usually occur within a half hour of the infusion beginning.

PITFALL

Not notifying the laboratory attempting to perform a type and cross-match when a patient has received dextran.

Dextran can interfere with the cross-matching of blood by reducing the tendency for red blood cells (RBCs) to aggregate. Consequently, blood should be drawn for type and cross-match prior to dextran infusions. If dextran has already been given, the RBCs should be washed prior to testing.

(3) Hydroxyethyl Starch (Hetastarch)

Hydroxyethyl starch (HES) (hetastarch) is a synthetic molecule with an average molecular weight of 69,000 and a range of 10,000 to 1,000,000. It is available as a 6% solution in normal saline. Infusions of hetastarch increase intravascular volume by an amount equal to or greater than the volume infused for at least 3 hours. Excretion is relatively slow, and 46% of an administered dose is excreted in the urine by 2 days and 64% by 8 days.

PITFALL

Administration of large amounts of hetastarch to patients who are bleeding or have a coagulopathy.

There has been some concern about the tendency of HES to prolong prothrombin and partial thromboplastin times and cause transient slight decreases in platelet count and clot tensile strength. However, there appears to be no significant increase in clinical bleeding in most patients if less than 1500 ml is given daily.

Serum amylase levels rise to about double normal values for up to 5 days after hetastarch administration. This occurs because amylase complexes with the hetastarch creating macroamylase particles that are only excreted slowly in the urine.

Hetastarch costs about one fourth as much as an equivalent amount of 5% albumin. Although hetastarch costs more than dextran, it has fewer side effects and is less likely to cause an anaphylactoid reaction.

(4) Fresh-Frozen Plasma

Fresh-frozen plasma (FFP) is prepared from whole blood by separating and freezing the plasma within 6 hours of phlebotomy. It may be stored for up to 1 year at −18°C. The labile clotting factors (V and VIII) deteriorate to a minimal extent during such storage. FFP takes 20 to 40 minutes to thaw and must be given through a filter. FFP has no functional platelets, but if used within 2 hours of thawing, it contains normal levels of all the other coagulation factors. However, delay of infusion for more than 2 hours rapidly decreases coagulation factor activity, especially for factor VII.

FFP exposes the recipient to the risks of hepatitis, AIDS, and other transfusion-transmitted diseases and should be used only to treat multiple-coagulation defects or antithrombin deficiency. Compatibility testing is not required, but ABO compatibility is advisable.

AXIOM

FFP should generally be used only to treat coagulopathies confirmed by appropriate laboratory tests.

c. Crystalloids versus Colloids

AXIOM

Successful resuscitation from hypovolemic shock is dependent more on the rapidity with which the plasma and ECF volumes are restored than the composition of the fluid used.

Controversies over the selection of the type of fluid for resuscitation (colloid versus crystalloid) center mainly on issues relating to philosophy, side effects, and economics. Proponents of colloids argue that (1) replacement with colloid is more rapidly effective in restoring circulating blood volume; (2) crystalloids reduce colloid osmotic pressure, thus favoring the development of pulmonary edema; (3) crystalloids, because they rapidly equilibrate with extracellular fluid (ECF), must be infused in amounts exceeding estimated losses by at least three to four times. In one study of critically ill patients, 1000 ml of crystalloid solution increased plasma volume by only 194 ml, whereas 500 ml of 5% albumin increased plasma volume by 700 ml.

In another study favoring colloid administration, 31 patients admitted with systolic blood pressure less than 70 mm Hg following trauma were prospectively randomized by odd and even dates to receive either (1) 6% dextran 70 (1.0 to 1.5 liters) plus as much Ringer's acetate (average 2 to 3 liters) and blood (average 5 units) as needed to maintain a systolic BP >100 mm Hg, or (2) as much Ringer's acetate (average 5 to 8 liters) and blood (average 5 units) as needed to obtain similar goals. No ARDS developed in the dextran 70 group, whereas it occurred in 5/17 (29%) of the Ringer's acetate group. Later fluid challenges with 500 ml of dextran 70 raised cardiac index (CI) by 29% ± 3% whereas 2.0 liters of Ringer's acetate raised CI by only 15% ± 5%.

Nevertheless, since the classic studies of Shires, there have been a multitude of studies showing that crystalloids are as good as colloids in resuscitation; are much less expensive; and have no risk of anaphylactoid shock, increased bleeding tendency, or transmitted diseases. Although it may take a bit longer to restore normal blood pressures with crystalloids and there may be a greater tendency to peripheral edema, overall they seem to be almost as effective and significantly safer than colloids. Lucas and associates, in a number of studies, have shown that large amounts of albumin can cause increased pulmonary, cardiac, and renal failure and decrease the production of immunoglobulins and various coagulation factors.

Massive albumin resuscitation of hemorrhagic shock over several days may have adverse effects on coagulation, immunoglobulin activity, cardiopulmonary function, and extravascular flux of nonalbumin protein; however, FFP resuscitation in moderation apparently does not. Furthermore, Shoemaker and co-workers have shown greatly improved results using albumin to resuscitate critically ill and injured patients.

AXIOM
Although albumin is expensive, if it reduces an ICU stay by 1 day, even large quantities will more than pay for themselves.

d. Hypertonic Saline Solutions

Hypertonic saline solutions (HSS) (1000 to 2500 mOsm/liter), have been shown to produce better outcomes than normal saline solution (NSS) (300 mOsm/liter), in a wide variety of situations. The decreased edema (interstitial fluid) that might occur in the heart, gastrointestinal tract, skin, and brain with HSS may also improve function and healing in those organs and decrease the risk of infection.

In addition to pulling intracellular fluid into the extracellular space, hypertonic saline tends to be a vasodilator and may exert direct inotropic actions on the myocardium. HSS also attenuates the ACTH, cortisol, aldosterone, and angiotensin II response to trauma and shock. Interestingly, it has been found in some studies that, if HSS is infused into dogs with hemorrhagic shock, denervation of the lungs may abolish the beneficial effects of HSS without affecting the changes in plasma osmolarity. Consequently, some of the hemodynamic benefits of HSS may be due to pulmonary osmoreceptors that stimulate CNS vasomotor centers by way of the vagus nerves.

In patients with head trauma and sepsis, it may be advantageous to use HSS to keep the ICP as low as possible. In a study in dogs, Ringer's lactate (RL) (274 mOsm/liter) raised ICP 55% more than HSS (2500 mOsm/liter). However, because of hemodilution, cerebral oxygen delivery (CDo_2) was reduced more by HSS (33%) than by Ringer's lactate (28%).

HSS may be more effective than isotonic crystalloids for increasing mean arterial pressure and decreasing third-space losses in selected hypotensive patients who may require large volumes of fluid, particularly if excess peripheral or central edema would be detrimental. A combination of 7.5% HSS (2400 mOsm/liter) with 6% to 12% dextran 70 might be particularly effective in such circumstances.

The main problems with HSS include a tendency to severe hypernatremia, which can cause fever and various hyperosmolarity problems and a tendency to vasodilation so that higher blood volumes may be needed to attain certain blood pressures. As a general rule, HSS is discontinued if serum sodium levels exceed 160 to 165 mEq/liter. This degree of hypernatremia has been reported by Mattar and colleagues and Krauz and associates as having a significant mortality.

AXIOM

HSS may reduce tissue edema in patients who would otherwise require large quantities of resuscitation fluid. However, the tendency to hypernatremia and vasodilation may be a problem.

Another problem that has surfaced with HSS, especially if combined with dextran, is an increased tendency to bleeding. At least one mechanism for this is the ability of hypertonic saline to vasodilate blood vessels. This could allow bleeding to be more severe by preventing the normal vasoconstrictive response to vascular injury. However, it is also possible that hypertonic saline may have anticoagulant effects on plasma clotting factors and platelet reactions.

Reed and associates determined that significant deteriorations in plasma clotting times and platelet aggregation developed when 10% or more of the normal plasma was replaced by HSS without dextran. This anticoagulant effect would probably be more pronounced if clotting factors and platelets are already reduced by shock, tissue damage, or hemodilution with other fluids.

In a recent study Maningas and colleagues found that prehospital administration of 250 ml of 7.5% NaCl in 6% dextran 70 or the isotonic crystalloid plasmalyte A to hypotensive victims of penetrating trauma with a BP < 90 mm Hg could be done safely. However, they did not show the survival advantage previously demonstrated by Holcroft and associates. Flint, in an accompanying editorial, questioned whether the immediate sharp rise in BP might predispose patients to recurrent bleeding. He also wondered if there might be late complications due to the hyperosmolarity.

The hypertonic (7.5%) saline-dextran 70 formulation appears promising for resuscitation of trauma patients, particularly in the prehospital setting. However, there have been some concerns that these solutions could cause several complications. For example, a rapid increase in plasma osmolality or sodium concentration in a chronically debilitated patient with pre-existing hyponatremia could produce central pontine myelinolysis. Rapid expansion of the plasma volume without concomitant potassium replacement could produce hypokalemia, which could cause an arrhythmia. Increased plasma chloride concentrations could produce metabolic acidemia that could compromise cardiac function or cause arrhythmias. Rapid re-establishment of blood volume and blood pressure combined with hyperosmolar shrinkage of an injured brain could precipitate intracranial hemorrhage and potentiate nontamponaded bleeding, like that caused by penetrating injuries or by injuries to the spleen or to the intraperitoneal portion of the liver.

Recently, Vassar, Perry, and Holcroft evaluated the potential side effects of rapidly infusing 250 ml of either 7.5% sodium chloride or 7.5% sodium chloride with 6% dextran 70 using Ringer's lactate as the control to 106 critically injured patients in two prospective double-blinded emergency department trials. Eight patients had a significant hyperchloremic acidemia in association with infusion of the hypertonic solutions, but all eight were moribund before infusion and many factors other than hyperchloremia could have contributed to their acidemia. Other blood chemistry changes that might have been associated with the hypertonic solutions, such as hyperosmolality or hypernatremia, were made insignificant by other factors, such as high blood alcohol levels or concomitant administration of sodium bicarbonate. There were no cases of central pontine myelinolysis; bleeding was not potentiated. There was no difficulty with cross-matching of blood, and no anaphylactoid reactions occurred. Thus, in a setting of limited volume resuscitation, hypertonic (7.5%) saline solutions are likely to have a favorable risk-to-benefit ratio.

e. Blood Transfusions

Almost all blood transfusions today are packed RBCs. A unit of packed RBCs has a volume of approximately 250 ml with a hematocrit between 60% and 80% so that each unit of blood has only 40 to 50 ml of plasma. To restore clotting factors, FFP must usually be given.

A hematocrit of 20% to 25% usually provides adequate oxygen delivery if cardiopulmonary function is normal. However, in critically ill or injured patients, a hematocrit of at least 30% to 35% may be preferred. In fact our survival rates tend to be best when the patient maintains a hematocrit of 35% to 40%. Indeed, D'Orio and associates studied variables affecting prognosis in patients with septic shock and found that an increased hematocrit was one of the significant variables separating those who survived from those who died. On admission to the ICU these hematocrits were 46% $\pm$ 3% and 39% $\pm$ 4%, respectively. However, in a recent report by Dietrich and colleagues on critically ill volume-resuscitated nonsurgical patients, raising the hemaglobin from 8.3 $\pm$ 0.2 gm/dl to 10.5 $\pm$ 0.2 gm/dl raised Do_2 from 410 $\pm$ 22 ml$\cdot$min$^{-1}\cdot$m^{-2} to 525 $\pm$ 29 ml$\cdot$min$^{-1}\cdot$m^{-2} but did not increase Vo_2 (120 $\pm$ 7 ml$\cdot$min$^{-1}\cdot$m^{-2} to 118 $\pm$ 6 ml$\cdot$min$^{-1}\cdot$m^{-2} or reduce lactate (4.1 $\pm$ 0.2 mm/liter to 4.1 $\pm$ 1.0 mm/liter).

(1) Typing and Crossing of Blood

The "safest" type of blood to administer is that which has been fully cross-matched. A full cross-match takes 30 to 45 minutes to perform; therefore, in an emergency, one may use O-negative or type-specific uncross-matched blood. However, because the plasma of O-negative blood contains anti-A and anti-B antibodies, significant minor transfusion reactions can occur if large volumes of this type of blood are infused. In addition, if more than 4 units of O-negative blood are administered to a patient with a different blood type, subsequent cross-matching may be complicated.

Blood of the recipient's type (i.e., type-specific blood) that has not been cross-matched can be administered safely and can usually be released for transfusion within 10 to 15 minutes.

(2) Complications of Transfusion

(a) Allergic and incompatibility reactions

The most frequent type of transfusion reaction, occurring in 2% to 10% of blood transfusions, is nonhemolytic fever. Urticaria, hives, or asthma also occasionally occur. Such reactions are usually thought to be related to an allergy by the recipient to leukocytes or proteins in the donor plasma. The incidence of these reactions may be reduced by the use of packed or washed RBCs or special filters for the removal of leukocytes.

Major hemolytic transfusion reactions occur from the interaction of preformed antibodies in the plasma of the recipient with antigens in the red cells of the donor. These reactions are usually due to clerical errors, allowing administration of blood to the wrong patient.

(b) Decreased ATP and 2,3-DPG

Anticoagulant preservative solutions and refrigeration increase plasma-free hemoglobin and potassium concentrations and reduce red blood cell viability and their concentrations of ATP and 2,3-diphosphoglyceric acid (DPG). Low levels of ATP result in decreased RBC deformability, thereby interfering with capillary blood flow. Low levels of 2,3-DPG shift the oxyhemoglobin dissociation curve to the left, thereby reducing the Po_2 and oxygen availability to the tissues.

AXIOM

The reduced 2,3-DPG in transfused blood after massive transfusions may result in good oxygen delivery but reduced oxygen consumption.

(3) Coagulation Changes in Stored Blood

Within 24 hours, most platelets in stored blood have disappeared and any platelets that still remain are nonfunctional. By day 14, approximately 25% of factor VIII and 60% of factor V are lost, even with the newer blood preservatives. Although one study showed that 45% of patients receiving 20 or more units of blood in 24 hours had partial thromboplastin times (PTTs) more than double normal, thrombocytopenia is the most important defect causing excessive bleeding following massive blood transfusions.

(a) Potassium changes

During storage, potassium levels in the plasma of bank blood may rise by up to 1.0 mEq/liter per day. However, in one of our studies, only 7% of patients receiving more than 10 units of blood developed a serum potassium level greater than 5.0, whereas up to 38% developed hypokalemia (K < 3.5 mEg/liter).

(b) Hypocalcemia

Ionized calcium levels in plasma can fall rapidly during shock because of increased movement of calcium into the cytoplasm of cells that have impaired metabolism. In addition, the citrate in bank blood binds divalent cations, such as calcium, further reducing plasma levels of ionized calcium and magnesium. Plasma ionized calcium levels below 0.7 mmol/liter (1.4 mEq/liter) may produce prolongation of the QT interval and impaired myocardial contractility.

AXIOM

Calcium is not usually given to patients receiving transfusions unless the rate of administration is rapid (less than one unit every 5 minutes) and the patient has persistent shock or heart failure.

(c) Citrate toxicity

In shock patients receiving massive transfusions, plasma citrate levels may reach 60 to 100 mg/dl, causing further falls in ionized calcium levels. Citrate may also have a separate direct depressant effect on the myocardium. The presence of hepatic dysfunction or hypothermia increases the likelihood of citrate toxicity.

(d) Hypothermia

Hypothermia often occurs during massive transfusions to patients in persistent shock, especially during surgery, no matter how much effort is made to prevent it. Once the major bleeding is controlled with packs or clamps, every effort should be made to warm the patient to at least 35°C before proceeding with the completion of the surgical procedure. Core temperatures less than 32°C in massive transfusion patients have been associated with mortality rates exceeding 85%.

(e) Blood-transmitted diseases

Viral hepatitis, usually of the non-A non-B (HVC) type, is the major infectious complication of blood transfusions. The risk is 0.5% to 1.5% per unit of blood product and it affects 7% to 12% of all recipients. The risk of AIDS is now greatly reduced to about 1:250,000 units of blood products. However, non-A and non-B hepatitis is still a risk in patients requiring multiple transfusions.

(4) Autologous Transfusions (Autotransfusion)

Autotransfusion involves the collection and then reinfusion of the patient's own shed blood during surgery or after trauma. Autotransfusion blood can be available for administration without the delay of a complete cross-match, and it is free of the risk of transmitted disease (such as hepatitis and AIDS) and hemolytic, febrile, or allergic reactions. However, administration of large volumes of autotransfused blood may cause thrombocytopenia, decreases in coagulation factors, and heparinization of the patient despite washing of the RBCs. In patients with extensive tissue damage or prolonged shock, autotransfused blood increases the tendency to disseminated intravascular coagulation and activation of fibrinolytic mechanisms. In such individuals, one should probably not autotransfuse more than 4 to 6 units of blood. Patients being autotransfused should have serial coagulation studies (platelet count, bleeding time, PT, PIT, and fibrinolytic activity).

AXIOM
Large quantities of autotransfused blood increase the risk of coagulopathies.

(5) Artificial Blood

The two main types of artificial hemoglobin solutions that have been studied are stroma-free hemoglobin (SFH) and fluorocarbons. The main problem with SFH has been its very high oxygen affinity. Although much oxygen is delivered to the tissues, very little is actually given up. However, recently developed products, including polymerized pyridoxalated hemoglobin (SFH-PLP) with a P_{50} (Po_2 at an oxyhemoglobin saturation of 50%) of 20 mm Hg (normal = 26.2 mm Hg), appear to have overcome this.

Fluosol-DA 20% (Fluosol) has been used in research studies to treat life-threatening blood loss in patients who have refused blood products for religious reasons. However, a number of patients treated with this agent have developed severe complications, including fever, leukocytosis, diffuse pulmonary infiltrates, and hypoxemia. As a consequence, it has been withdrawn from the U.S. market.

f. Amounts of Fluid

The amount of fluid to be given in shock is determined by multiple factors, including BP, pulse rate, urinary output, and skin perfusion. One must also search for rales or distended neck veins that might indicate fluid overload. The response of the CVP to a fluid load can be very helpful in estimating further fluid requirements. However, if the amount of fluid given seems excessive or if the patient has severe sepsis or respiratory failure, a PAWP catheter should be inserted to help monitor cardiovascular function.

(1) Central Venous Pressure Determination

Many factors affect the CVP level, particularly blood volume, right heart contractility, the amount of systemic arterial and venous constriction, and the resistance to blood flow in the lungs. Therefore, when monitoring the CVP, the response to a fluid load is much more important than the actual CVP level. Nevertheless, some physicians still say that if the CVP is above 12 or 15 cm H_2O, fluid administration should be stopped because the patient is probably overloaded.

The CVP in critically ill patients is extremely variable and frequently correlates poorly with blood volume and fluid needs (Fig. 5.3). We have seen a number of patients, particularly those with severe sepsis or respiratory failure, who had a CVP above 20 cm H_2O, but had a relatively low PAWP, and responded to a fluid challenge with increased cardiac output and improved tissue perfusion and little or no change in the CVP. In such instances, the high CVP is probably due to an increased pulmonary vascular resistance.

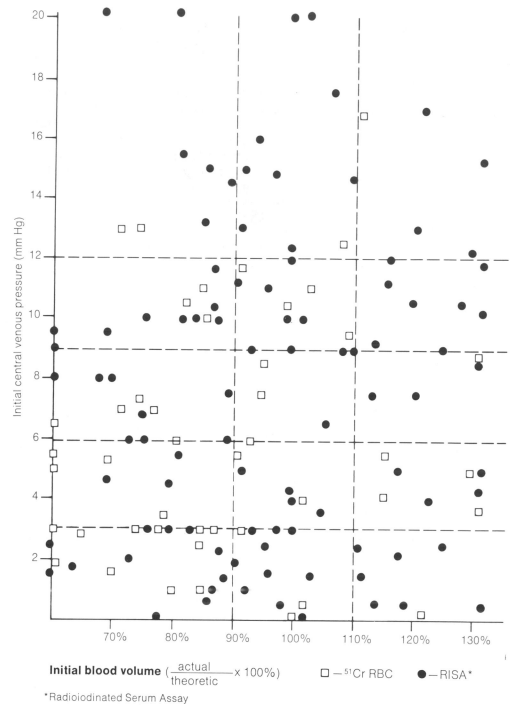

Initial central venous pressure (mm Hg)

Initial blood volume ($\frac{\text{actual}}{\text{theoretic}}$ x 100%)   □ — ⁵¹Cr RBC   ● — RISA*

*Radioiodinated Serum Assay

Figure 5.3 Relationship between initial central venous pressure and blood volume.

PITFALL
Relying on a CVP to determine fluid needs, particularly in a patient with ARDS or pulmonary disease.

The use of high tidal volumes and large amounts of positive end-expiratory pressure (PEEP) may increase the PAWP, and especially the CVP, by 5 to 10 cm H_2O or more. This must be taken into account if the patient cannot be taken off the respirator while the CVP or PAWP is being measured.

AXIOM

If more than 10 cm H₂O PEEP is used, a third of the PEEP pressure may be subtracted from the PAWP to obtain a "true" PAWP.

The CVP and PAWP may also be deceptively high if the patient is receiving large doses of vasopressor drugs. The arterial vasoconstriction caused by vasopressors increases the resistance against which the heart must pump, thereby tending to reduce cardiac output. Increased venous constriction also reduces vascular capacity, thereby increasing venous return to the heart.

If the patient's fluid status is in doubt, a fluid challenge of isotonic crystalloid (3 ml/kg) can be given over a period of 10 minutes. If the CVP rises more than 5.0 cm H₂O, fluids should be stopped until the CVP returns to within 2.0 cm H₂O of baseline. One or two other intravenous lines should be available for fluid administration so that the CVP can be monitored continuously. Water manometers tend to provide a CVP reading midway between the mean and peak CVP that is evident on transducer waveform monitoring.

AXIOM

If there are wide swings in CVP with positive-pressure ventilation, the water manometer will tend to provide deceptively high readings.

(2) Pulmonary Artery Wedge Pressure Determinations

In most instances the function of the right and left ventricles is quite similar. Consequently, changes in the filling pressures in the right heart normally correlate fairly well with changes in the filling pressures of the left heart. However, in a number of instances, the CVP and PAWP may be quite disparate. For example, an acute myocardial infarction may transiently produce an isolated acute left ventricular failure with a low CVP and high PAWP. Such patients may develop pulmonary edema with a CVP that was initially less than 5.0 cm H₂O. It is important to note this possibility because hypotensive patients with a very low CVP are often given large quantities of fluid rapidly without considering the possibility of an isolated left ventricular failure. The other extreme, however, is much more likely. In other words, the CVP is likely to be elevated in patients with hypovolemia if they are septic or have pulmonary disease.

AXIOM

Many patients with sepsis or acute respiratory failure have impaired pulmonary blood flow and a high CVP in spite of hypovolemia and a low PAWP.

Although there has been some concern about overuse and abuse of PAWP monitoring, it can be extremely helpful in monitoring critically ill patients, particularly those with severe pulmonary problems and those not responding favorably to standard fluid therapy. The ability of clinicians to predict whether pulmonary artery pressure, PAWP, and cardiac output are low, normal, or high in ICU patients is usually only about 40% to 50% accurate.

PAWP and cardiac output are particularly helpful in monitoring (1) patients with suspected cardiopulmonary disorders; (2) clinically unclear volume status in hypotensive patients; (3) afterload reduction in patients with impaired myocardial function; (4) treatment of shock in patients with acute myocardial infarction, sepsis, or ARDS; and (5) differentiation of cardiac and noncardiac causes of diffuse pulmonary infiltrates.

Maintenance of optimal ventricular filling intraoperatively and postoperatively may be of help in reducing postoperative complications. In high-risk surgical patients, Vinod Puri noted that intraoperative and postoperative maintenance of the PAWP within 4 mm Hg of the optimal value determined with Starling's curve preoperatively was associated with a complication rate of only 14%. In contrast, in patients in whom the PAWP was allowed to fall intraoperatively or postoperatively more than 4 mm Hg below the optimal value, the complication rate was 79% (15/19). The optimal PAWP on Starling's curve is determined by progressively raising the PAWP from normal to that level at which the cardiac output reaches a maximum without an abrupt rise in the PAWP.

We have found that errors in measuring pulmonary artery wedge pressure (PAWP) may occur in more than 15% of patients on digital monitors. Pressures taken off the waveforms are more accurate, particularly if there are wide swings in ventilatory pressures (Fig. 5.4).

PITFALL

Accepting a PAWP if it is recorded as higher than the pulmonary artery diastolic pressure (PADP).

One must always suspect the accuracy of a PAWP reading if it is higher than the PADP. This is most apt to occur if the tip of the PAWP catheter is in a portion of the lung where the alveolar pressure exceeds pulmonary venous pressure during at least part of the ventilatory cycle.

Even when PAWP is accurately measured, variances in left ventricular compliance may result in a poor correlation between PAWP and left ventricular end-diastolic volume (LVEDV) as measured by radionuclide angiography.

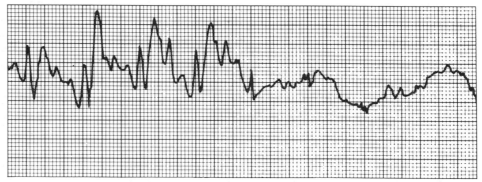

The shift from pulmonary artery pressure to PWP occurs when the balloon is inflated and the pulmonary artery is occluded proximal to the catheter tip.

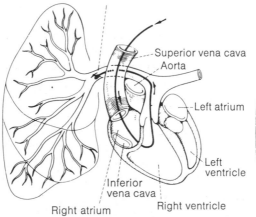

The Swan-Ganz catheter resting in the right pulmonary artery. The arrow in the superior vena cava shows where an ordinary CVP catheter terminates.

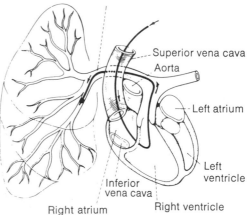

The Swan-Ganz catheter is advanced to a branch of the pulmonary artery, and the balloon is inflated.

Figure 5.4 Use of the Swan-Ganz catheter.

3. Continuous Measurement of Mixed Venous Oxygen Saturation

Continuous measurement of oxygen saturation in mixed venous blood (Svo_2) in the pulmonary arteries is now possible using flow-directed triple-lumen pulmonary artery catheters which incorporate fiberoptic filaments (Oximetrix, Incorporated, Mountain View, California). A decrease of 5% or more in Svo_2 may provide an early warning of deteriorating cardiopulmonary function, and an Svo_2 of less than 60% should make one suspect either impaired oxygen delivery (Do_2) to tissues or an increased oxygen consumption (Vo_2). Although occasional reports indicate no advantage to continuous Svo_2 monitoring in critically ill patients, we have seen numerous examples in which it provided early important information that significantly altered therapy.

a. Transcutaneous Oxygen Monitoring

Several noninvasive transcutaneous techniques for measuring O_2 and CO_2 have been studied by a number of investigators. Correlation with arterial blood gases in normodynamic or hyperdynamic critically ill patients is relatively good. However, if there is impaired perfusion to the area monitored, the correlation with ABG may be very poor.

The use of pulmonary oximetry as a type of transcutaneous monitoring of oxygen saturation and pulse amplitude in the fingers or toes can provide early warning of pulmonary or cardiovascular deterioration before it is clinically apparent. Such devices are now almost "standard-of-care" in the OR, PAR, and ICU.

Measurement of conjunctival oxygen tension ($Pcjo_2$) can also help provide early warning of inadequate tissue perfusion or blood gas changes. In one report, a $Pcjo_2:Pao_2$ ratio of 0.57 or less detected a measured blood volume of less than 85% of normal in 8 of 8 hypovolemic but normotensive patients. $Pcjo_2$ and transcutaneous oxygen tensions ($Ptco_2$) can also readily detect decreases in oxygen transport. To a certain extent, conjunctival Po_2 may also reflect O_2 delivery to the brain because the ophthalmic artery is the first branch of the internal carotid artery.

4. Cardiac Output

Restoration of normal or greater than normal cardiac output and tissue perfusion is important in the management of shock. Although measurement of cardiac index (cardiac output per square meter of body surface area) is difficult in the emergency department, it should be measured in ICUs and in critically ill patients in the OR.

In general, fluid should be given rapidly to shock patients as long as cardiac output is rising and there is little or no increase in filling pressures. Even when cardiac output is higher than normal, certain tissues, especially the intestines and liver, may still not have adequate perfusion. In one study, traumatized baboons that were resuscitated to their pretrauma mean arterial BP or left atrial pressure (LAP), still had blood volumes that were often only 70% to 80% of baseline. In addition, blood flow to the large and small intestine, stomach, spleen, kidney, and liver remained significantly lower than control values for at least 18 hours after resuscitation.

5. Oxygen Consumption

AXIOM

The best single guide to the resuscitation of severe shock is the oxygen consumption index (VO_2/m^2).

In critically ill or injured patients, Vo_2/m^2 should be increased to at least normal levels (120 to 160 $ml \cdot min^{-1} \cdot m^{-2}$). After resuscitation from shock, the Vo_2 will usually have to be at least 50% above normal to repay the O_2 debt that developed while the tissues were inadequately perfused. The oxygen debt is due not only to the anaerobic metabolism that occurred while blood flow was inadequate but also hypermetabolism caused by increased release of catecholamines, glucagon, and corticosteroids.

In many shock studies, returning the LAP to normal provided adequate blood pressure restoration. Even after large quantities of fluid are given to return the LAP and systemic BP to baseline values, blood volume and splanchnic blood flow usually remain lower than control for at least 12 to 18 hours. However, if one increases O_2 delivery (Do_2) until O_2 consumption (Vo_2) no longer rises, resuscitation is usually complete.

Shoemaker has repeatedly shown that using pulmonary artery catheter monitoring to raise cardiac index (in surgical patients) to 4.5 $liters \cdot min^{-1} \cdot m^{-2}$, oxygen delivery to greater than 600 $ml \cdot min^{-1} \cdot m^{-2}$ and oxygen consumption to greater than 170 $ml \cdot min^{-1} \cdot m^{-2}$ will significantly reduce morbidity and mortality. Most recently, he has also shown that such a protocol reduces the cumulative oxygen debt and incidence of organ failure.

6. Blood Volume Determinations

Blood volume determinations as guides to the rate or amount of fluid administration are seldom measured except during research studies, and they can be very deceptive. Blood volume normally varies widely from patient to patient. One standard deviation for blood volume in normal individuals averages about 10%. Furthermore, the actual blood volume is not nearly as important as its dynamic relationship with vascular capacity.

Vascular capacity can change rapidly with vasoconstriction or vasodilation. For example, vascular capacity may be reduced up to 25% by vasoconstriction. With vasodilation, vascular capacity may be increased by 50% or more. Blood volume determinations with radioiodinated serum albumin (RISA) are particularly deceptive in shock because the normal RISA disappearance rate of 6.0% to 8.0% per hour may rise to exceed 30% to 35% per hour in patients with shock or severe sepsis. A method using serial sampling every 10 minutes, however, may provide more accurate and consistent results than "one-shot" techniques.

a. Rapid Fluid Administration Sets

A "rapid solution administration set" utilizing a 40 micron screen blood transfusion filter, a heat exchanger, and 8.5 French IV catheter has been developed and is capable of infusing 37°C fluid at up to 1600 ml/min. Another similar device, called the Infuser, is a pressure chamber for rapid fluid administration. Routine use of such equipment may be life saving with certain types of trauma or surgery.

7. Myocardial Support

a. Digoxin

Digoxin is used rarely in the management of acute severe heart failure in shock because of (1) the difficulty and time delay in obtaining optimal tissue levels, (2) frequent prolonged side effects, and (3) relatively minor inotropic effects. However, it can be very helpful in patients with a dilated failing heart or atrial fibrillation. It may also increase vascular responsiveness to both norepinephrine and angiotensin, thereby helping to correct the intractable vasodilation seen in some septic patients.

The amount of digoxin needed in shock patients can vary greatly. Although an ECG response is generally not a good criterion for regulating dosage, it may be the only means to obtain some reasonable idea of the digoxin effect. Patients who are elderly or in shock may be adequately digitalized or may even develop digitalis toxicity with half the usual dosage.

b. Dopamine

Dopamine in doses of 0.5 to 2.0 μg·kg^{-1}·min^{-1} affects dopaminergic receptors primarily, thereby dilating renal and splanchnic vessels and increasing renal blood flow, urine output, and urine sodium excretion. At 2.0 to 4.0 μg·kg^{-1}·min^{-1}, beta receptors are also stimulated, resulting in an increased cardiac output and a variable tendency to tachycardia.

AXIOM

Dopamine is generally the inotropic agent of choice in patients with hypotension and a low cardiac output.

In doses of 5 to 15 μg·kg^{-1}·min^{-2}, dopamine acts primarily as a positive inotrope. At doses exceeding 20 to 30 μg·kg^{-1}·min^{-1}, it can cause increasing vasoconstriction.

However, in some septic patients the vasoconstrictor effect may not be apparent even at doses exceeding 50 μg·kg^{-1}·min^{-1}. In choosing between dopamine and another catecholamine, the decision is less dependent on the pharmaceutical characteristics of the agent(s) than it is on the clinical circumstances of the patients. In vasodilated septic patients with hypotension and oliguria, dopamine is probably the inotrope of choice. The most frequent problem with dopamine under such circumstances is tachycardia. Occasionally it may be difficult to wean patients from dopamine because they have become catecholamine depleted.

c. Dobutamine

AXIOM

Dobutamine is generally the inotrope of choice in patients with a low cardiac output and a normal or increased BP.

Dobutamine in doses of 5 to 20 μg·kg^{-1}·min^{-1} has a positive inotropic effect plus some vasodilator properties. It is particularly helpful in acute myocardial infarction shock characterized by a low cardiac output, normal BP, and high systemic vascular resistance. Dobutamine may also be a good agent for treating shock due to massive pulmonary embolism. As a rule, dobutamine causes less of an increase in heart rate, PA pressure, and PAWP than dopamine. Shoemaker has found it to be especially helpful for increasing oxygen delivery in critically ill postoperative patients.

Vincent, Roman, and Kahn recently noted that adding 5 μg·kg^{-1}·min^{-1} of dobutamine to a standard septic shock treatment protocol raised cardiac output, oxygen delivery, and oxygen consumption (137 ± 42 ml·min^{-1}·m^{-2} to 162 ± 66 ml·min^{-1}·m^{-2}). BP also rose in 12 of 18 patients.

d. Dopamine Plus Dobutamine

We frequently use combinations of dopamine (5 to 10 μg·kg^{-1}·min^{-2}) and dobutamine (5 to 15 μg·kg^{-1}·min^{-2}) to improve myocardial function in elderly patients. This combination has worked so well in many of these patients that we sometimes refer to it as "vitamin D." So far we have seen no problems with our inotropic vitamin D unless the patient already has a tendency to tachycardia.

e. Amrinone

Amrinone (Inocor) is a relatively new inotropic agent. Its mode of action is not completely understood but is probably associated with an inhibition of phosphodiesterase (the substance that breaks down cyclic adenosine monophosphate). Consequently, amrinone can potentiate the actions of various adrenergic agents. Since it is not inhibited by beta-blocking agents, it can be useful in patients receiving these agents up to the time of coronary artery bypass surgery. Amrinone can also be a good vasodilator, especially in the lungs, and because of this property it is being used increasingly in ICU patients with pulmonary hypertension, especially after cardiac surgery. One problem with amrinone, however, is that of having to use a loading dose (0.75 mg/kg) and then a maintenance dose (5 to 10 $\mu g \cdot kg^{-1} \cdot min^{-1}$). It also has a long half-life (3.6 to 5.8 hours) which can be a problem at times, especially if side effects develop.

f. Epinephrine

Epinephrine in doses of 1 to 5 $\mu g/min$ is used by some physicians when it is felt that a stronger combination of an inotropic agent and vasoconstrictor might be of benefit. However, dopamine tends to produce a somewhat more uniform response and a better rise in cardiac output, with much less tendency to tachyarrhythmias.

g. Isoproterenol

PITFALL
Using isoproterenol in patients with tachycardia, acute myocardial infarction, or pulmonary embolus.

In the unusual shock patient who has a slow pulse rate, isoproterenol in doses of 1 to 2 $\mu g/min$ may dramatically improve cardiac output. However, if the heart rate exceeds 100 per minute, isoproterenol can increase myocardial O_2 consumption (MVo_2) much more than it increases coronary blood flow. It can also cause dangerous tachyarrhythmias. For these reasons, isoproterenol should generally not be given to patients with an acute myocardial infarction or pulmonary embolus.

h. Glucagon

Glucagon can be an effective inotropic and chronotropic agent in patients with heart failure or cariogenic shock. In about 20% to 30% of the patients in whom relatively large doses (4 mg bolus and then 10 mg/h by constant intravenous infusion) are used, it has produced some improvement, although often only temporarily.

Glucagon should be reconstituted hourly, as it rapidly loses its potency at room temperature. Since this agent acts at least partially by stimulating adenyl cyclase activity and thereby increasing cAMP production in the myocardium, its effectiveness may be increased by the simultaneous administration of aminophylline, which inhibits phosphodiesterase, the enzyme that converts cAMP into inactive 5-cAMP. Glucagon's cardiovascular actions are calcium dependent and require adequate ionized calcium levels.

PITFALL
Failure to consider the use of glucagon in patients who are on beta blockers and have developed shock or acute heart failure.

Glucagon may be particularly helpful in the treatment of shock in patients taking beta blockers because its effectiveness is based on an entirely different mechanism of action. However, it can cause nausea, vomiting, and hyperglycemia.

i. Calcium

Administration of calcium to hypocalcemic patients with shock or sepsis may improve myocardial function for 30 to 45 minutes. However, if tissue perfusion and cell function have not been restored to normal, much of the calcium that was administered will move into the myocardium and vascular smooth muscle. Furthermore, if cell metabolism is still impaired, the additional calcium entering the cytoplasm will move into the mitochondria, where it will further interfere with ATP production.

Calcium should probably be given only to patients in persistent shock or heart failure if they are receiving massive blood transfusions rapidly or the patient has been on beta-adrenergic blockers and calcium-channel blockers.

In experimental hemorrhagic shock in dogs, some of whom had parathyroidectomy, calcium supplementation, plus an intact calcium-parathyroid axis seems to enhance the resuscitation effort. In one study of dogs with ligation of coronary arteries, the molecular fragment 1-34 of synthetic bovine parathyroid hormone exerted a tissue-sparing effect on myocardium, restored left ventricular function, and prevented the development of shock.

In hypotensive and bradycardic individuals taking beta blockers and slow-channel calcium blockers, IV calcium chloride may produce an immediate and dramatic beneficial hemodynamic response. Patients who have been on beta blockers or who have pre-existing myocardial dysfunction are especially likely to develop myocardial dysfunction during rapid transfusion with citrated blood. Hypocalcemia may sometimes be picked up early on a cardioscope by noting QT prolongation.

j. Glucose-Insulin-Potassium

An occasional patient who is unresponsive to inotropes and vasoconstrictors will respond, at least transiently, to "polarizing" solutions containing increased quantities of glucose, insulin, and potassium. The usual solution is a liter of 10% to 20% glucose containing 20 to 40 units of insulin and 40 to 80 mEq of potassium chloride given over 4 to 6 hours. Experimental studies suggest that GIK solutions may improve myocardial blood flow and metabolism. They have also been shown to reduce the incidence of arrhythmias clinically in acute anterior myocardial infarctions.

AXIOM

Glucose-insulin-potassium solutions may be of value in some arrhythmia-prone individuals.

8. Cardiac Pacing

Cardiac pacing for heart block or severe bradycardia in patients with a fixed low stroke volume can be extremely helpful, particularly if atropine or isoproterenol are not effective. Overdrive pacing may also improve cardiac output in some patients with tachyarrhythmias.

Cardiac pacing may also be helpful in some patients with right ventricular infarction. The syndrome of right heart failure, low cardiac output, and hypotension following right ventricular infarction is seen in 3% to 8% of all acute myocardial infarctions. Some of the patients will have the Beck I triad (hypotension, distended neck veins, and muffled heart tones) and will be suspected of having pericardial tamponade. Heart block and bradyarrhythmias are common in these patients, and AV sequential pacing may be needed to increase cardiac output and blood pressures.

Recently, there has been increasing interest in an arrhythmia known as torsade de pointes. Although it is often mistakenly diagnosed as ventricular tachycardia, it is characterized by spontaneously terminating runs of a fast polymorphic tachycardia with "twisting" of the QRS axis and prolongation of the QT interval. It usually occurs secondary to antiarrhythmics, especially type I agents such as quinidine on procainamide. Treatment consists of withholding those antiarrhythmic drugs and correcting any hypokalemia. Although IV $MgSO_4$ is now considered to be the drug of choice by many physicians, transvenous pacing sometimes will be more effective.

9. Optimizing Oxygen Delivery

AXIOM

Probably the ideal way to ensure that tissue perfusion is optimal is to increase oxygen delivery until oxygen consumption is well above normal and not flow dependent.

It is becoming increasingly clear that oxygen delivery (Do_2) should be high enough in critically ill patients so that the oxygen consumption (Vo_2) is greater than the basal normal of 120 to 160 $ml \cdot min^{-1} \cdot m^{-2}$. In other words, Do_2 should be increased (by raising cardiac output, hemoglobin levels, and arterial oxygen saturation) until the Vo_2 is well above normal or until there are no further increases in Vo_2 with increased Do_2.

Another technique is to attempt to achieve a set of optimal goals. Optimal goals suggested by Shoemaker have included a cardiac index more than $4.5 \cdot min^{-1} \cdot m^{-2}$, blood volume 500 ml more than normal, Do_2 of more than 600 $ml \cdot min^{-1} \cdot m^{-2}$, and Vo_2 of more than 170 $ml \cdot min^{-1} \cdot m^{-2}$. Utilizing this approach, Shoemaker was able to reduce the mortality in high-risk postoperative ICU patients from 35% (using "normal" values as the goal) to 13% (using "optimal" values as the goal).

In another study by Shoemaker, a three-leg prospective clinical study was established to further determine if optimizing PAWP, Do_2, and Vo_2 was of value. High-risk postoperative patients were randomized to be treated and monitored with (1) a CVP catheter, (2) a pulmonary artery catheter with normal values as the goal, or (3) a pulmonary artery catheter with optimal values as the goal of therapy. The results of this study showed no statistically significant difference between the mortality of patients managed with CVP catheter (23%) and those managed with a pulmonary artery catheter using normal values as the therapeutic goals (34%). However, use of the pulmonary artery catheter with optimal goals led to a significantly reduced (4%) mortality. In addition, the patients managed with a PA catheter and optimal goals developed less ARDS, renal failure, and sepsis than the other two groups.

These data are consistent with the concept that, in many critically ill patients, the Do_2 may be normal but may not be adequate to meet the increased metabolic requirements caused by trauma or sepsis. The longer unrecognized tissue hypoxia persists, the more likely the patient is to develop complications, some of which may be lethal.

We have noted that septic patients who have Vo_2 which is persistently less than 100 $ml \cdot min^{-1} \cdot m^{-2}$ have a mortality rate that approaches 100%. However, raising the Do_2 above normal limits (500 to 700 $ml \cdot min^{-1} \cdot m^{-2}$) does not always raise the Vo_2 above the normal of 120 to 160 $ml \cdot min^{-1} \cdot m^{-2}$. In one study in which oxygen delivery (Do_2) was progressively increased in critically ill septic patients, Vo_2 could be driven beyond normal only in patients who had lactic acidosis.

10. Pneumatic Antishock Garment

Since 1956, when Gardner reintroduced Crile's concept of external counterpressure to combat hypovolemia, MAST (military antishock trousers), another form of pneumatic antishock garment (PASG), became very popular with ambulance personnel and emergency physicians for treating shock in the field and during transport. Numerous studies have been performed to determine its hemodynamic effects. Although some of its advocates have felt that PASG raises BP by autotransfusing blood from the lower body to the central circulation, it now seems clear that PASG raises BP primarily by increasing afterload. This may cause CVP and PAWP to rise, but cardiac output tends to be unchanged or even fall. In addition, in one study, PASG reduced vital capacity by an average of 14%. This may be an important consideration in patients with marginal pulmonary function.

AXIOM

PASG may be helpful in prolonged ambulance transport of patients in shock, but it can also impair cardiac and pulmonary function.

In a recent prospective randomized study in Houston, Texas, 352 trauma victims with prehospital systolic blood pressures of less than 90 mm Hg were randomized on an alternate-day basis to receive treatment with military anti-shock trousers MAST (163 patients) or "No-MAST" (189 patients). In those patients with prehospital transport times of 30 minutes or less, MAST provided no advantage with regard to survival, length of hospital stay, or reduced hospital costs. Nevertheless, such devices may reduce loss of blood or fluid into the pelvis or lower extremities of patients with severe fractures or trauma in those areas. Prolonged application, however, increases the risk of compartment syndrome in the lower extremities.

11. Acid-Base Therapy

Most acid-base problems in shock will improve spontaneously if adequate ventilation and tissue perfusion are provided. However, if severe metabolic acidosis with a pH less than 7.10 persists in spite of optimal fluid loading and inotropic drugs, it may be wise to give enough bicarbonate to raise the pH to 7.20 to 7.25. If hyperventilation is used to raise the pH, one should not reduce the Pco_2 below 25 mm Hg because of the possible advance effects severe hypocarbia might have on the cerebral circulation. One must also be careful not to produce an overshoot alkalosis because it can markedly reduce the Po_2, O_2 availability, and ionized calcium and magnesium levels.

AXIOM

In shock, bicarbonate should probably be used only to partially correct severe acidosis that has not been responsive to fluids and inotropes.

The total bicarbonate deficit can generally be calculated by considering the bicarbonate space in man to be equal to 30% to 50% of the body weight, with the larger figure being applicable to base deficits greater than 15 mEq/liter. Thus, a base deficit of 10 mEq/liter in a 70 kg man can generally be corrected with about 210 mEq of bicarbonate. If the base deficit in the same patient were 18 mEq/liter, however, it might take 630 mEq or more of bicarbonate to correct the deficit. Only half the base deficit should be corrected at a time and generally at a rate not exceeding 3 to 5 mEq of bicarbonate per minute.

12. Steroids

The use of massive doses of steroids in shock and sepsis has largely been discontinued because of two large multi-institutional prospective studies. However, subclinical adrenal insufficiency may be present in 5% to 15% of critically ill patients. Consequently, patients with shock that is unresponsive to fluid loading and inotropic agents should probably be given at least 200 mg of hydrocortisone by rapid IV injection. If the patient responds, 50 to 100 mg of hydrocortisone can then be given every 6 to 8 hours as needed.

AXIOM

The only proven benefit of steroids in the treatment of shock is in individuals with adrenal insufficiency.

Experimentally, adrenocortical-like steroids in "massive" doses equivalent to 150 mg of hydrocortisone per kilogram of body weight were thought to be helpful in shock by (1) preventing uncoupling of mitochondrial electron transport and oxidative phosphorylation, (2) reducing lysosomal fragility and capillary membrane permeability, (3) improving cardiovascular function, and (4) reducing excessive activation of complement. More recently steroids have also been shown to block transcription and mobilization of tumor necrosis factor messenger RNA in macrophages. Thus, if given early enough, steroids could prevent irritation of the septic shock cascade. Hinshaw, Beller-Todd, and Archer have shown repeatedly that baboons can achieve a 100% survival in spite of an LD_{100} infusion of live *Escherichia coli* by early administration of appropriate antibiotics plus massive steroids.

PITFALL
Failure to consider the possibility of a subclinical adrenal insufficiency in patients with persistent hypotension in spite of adequate fluid loading, inotropes, and oxygen.

In the largest prospective randomized double-blind study performed at a single institution with pharmacologic doses of corticosteroid in septic shock, Schumer found that patients treated with a placebo had a mortality rate of 43% while those treated with steroids, usually less than 2 hours from the onset of shock, had a mortality rate of only 14%.

Sprung and associates performed a more recent double-blind prospective randomized study on 59 medical patients with septic shock. The patients were given either dexamethasone (6 mg/kg), methylprednisolone sodium succinate (30 mg/kg), or a placebo every 4 hours as needed. These patients were treated an average of 17 ± 5 hours after the onset of shock. Of those treated within 4 hours of the onset of the shock, reversal of the shock occurred in 73% (8/11) of those given steroids as compared to 20% (1/5) in controls. This difference was statistically significant ($P < 0.05$).

Two large multi-institutional prospective double-blind studies on the use of massive steroids in sepsis and septic shock have also been completed and suggest that there is little place for massive steroids in the treatment of sepsis or septic shock. Although a favorable response in patients with Gram-negative sepsis was found in one of the studies and was almost significant, the results with Gram-positive organisms was poor. Other steroid problems included an increased tendency to ARDS and increased mortality rates in patients with elevated serum creatinine levels.

13. Vasopressors

Vasopressors should be considered potentially lethal drugs. They should probably be given only as a temporary measure when there appears to be no other rapidly effective method of restoring an adequate coronary or cerebral blood flow in patients with severe coronary or cerebral vascular disease. They should generally be administered only after an adequate trial with ventilation, oxygen, fluids, acid-base correction, and inotropic agents. Dopamine, particularly if doses greater than 20 to 30 $\mu g \cdot kg^{-1} \cdot min^{-1}$ are used, can raise the BP quite adequately in about 80% to 90% of patients who require drugs to correct their hypotension. Thus, only a relatively small number of patients with shock require vasopressors, such as metaraminol or norepinephrine.

PITFALL
Administration of large doses of vasopressors to hypotensive patients who are still hypovolemic.

Administration of large amounts of norepinephrine to hypovolemic animals can cause complete arteriolar occlusion with resultant tissue necrosis and death of the animal. As a consequence, vasoconstrictor drugs should not be given to hypovolemic patients except very transiently to maintain perfusion in older patients while other treatment is being initiated.

The choice of vasopressors may be extremely important. Agents such as phenylephrine and methoxamine, which have only a peripheral vasoconstriction effect, can effectively raise blood pressure, but at the same time they can also cause severe reductions in cardiac output and tissue perfusion. Norepinephrine and metaraminol, which are predominantly vasoconstrictors but also have some cardiac effect, generally cause less of a drop in cardiac output than the pure vasopressors. With norepinephrine, doses less than 1 to 2 μg/min cause less vasoconstriction and more of a positive inotropic effect than larger doses.

Our current favorite vasopressor in appropriate patients is dopamine in large doses (20 to 60 μg$\cdot$kg$^{-1}\cdot$min^{-1}). If this is ineffective, we may use four ampules (16 mg) of norepinephrine and two ampules (10 mg) of phentolamine in 500 ml of D$_5$W. Phentolamine (Regitine) in this dosage may prevent excessive vasoconstriction, but it does not significantly reduce BP. Furthermore, if the norepinephrine should extravasate into tissues around the IV catheter, the phentolamine prevents the local necrosis that can be caused by the excessive vasoconstrictive effect of the norepinephrine. In instances when the patient already seems excessively vasoconstricted, the concentration of phentolamine may be increased to two ampules for each ampule of norepinephrine. Low doses (1 to 2 μg/min) of norepinephrine combined with moderate doses (5 to 15 μg$\cdot$kg$^{-1}\cdot$min^{-1}) of dopamine may also be of value in septic shock.

In patients with significant coronary artery disease, raising the mean blood pressure to 80 mm Hg may increase coronary blood flow more than it increases myocardial oxygen demands, and cardiac output may rise. However, higher blood pressures are apt to increase myocardial oxygen demand (Mvo$_2$) more than myocardial oxygen delivery (MDo$_2$) and may be very deleterious. Furthermore, there is no clinical evidence that vasopressors such as dopamine or norepinephrine increase survival of patients with circulatory shock.

14. Naloxone

ACTH and beta endorphins are derived from a common precursor (pro-opiocortin) and are secreted in equimolar amounts in response to stress at the hypothalamic level. Holaday and Faden in 1978 first reported that naloxone blocked the hypotension caused by endotoxin administration in rats. In canine endotoxin shock, naloxone attenuates the hypotension, reduces hemoconcentration and acidosis, prevents hypoglycemia, and increases survival. Cardiac output and left ventricular dp/dt may also improve.

In general, naloxone has been found to be beneficial in a wide variety of experimental shock models, especially if large doses are given before systemic deterioration is present. However, it has minimal, if any, hemodynamic effect in normal animals.

The majority of studies have related the overall beneficial effects of naloxone to a central (CNS) mechanism of action. However, both adrenalectomy and selective adrenal demedullation (with adrenal cortical function remaining intact) in rats not only enhance sensitivity to endotoxin, but also prevent the normal pressor response to naloxone during endotoxin shock. Thus, endogenous opiates appear to inhibit central autonomic sites that regulate the release of pressor substrates from the adrenal medulla.

Relatively few studies have evaluated the effects of naloxone on hypotension in humans. Peters and associates gave naloxone (0.4 to 1.2 mg) to 13 patients with prolonged hypotension secondary to sepsis. In eight of nine patients not taking corticosteroids there was a rapid (less than 5 minutes) increase in blood pressure which then returned to baseline over 30 to 60 minutes. Patients on prior corticosteroid therapy had no response to naloxone.

Rock and colleagues reported on the use of naloxone in 12 patients who were in septic shock for more than 12 hours and who were being treated with dopamine or norepinephrine. The dose of naloxone was begun at 0.1 mg/kg and doubled every 15 minutes up to 1.6 mg/kg or until there was a BP rise. Only 4 of the 12 patients had a rise in BP of at least 10 to 15 mm Hg for 15 or more minutes. Moreover, 11 of the 12 patients died, and four patients had severe reactions, including congestive heart failure or seizures.

DeMaria and McCabe, Seidel, and Jagger performed a prospective randomized double-blind study on 23 patients using 0.4 to 1.2 mg naloxone IV or a placebo. There were no hemodynamic differences between the two groups, and the mortality rates were 67% (6/9) and 77% (10/13), respectively. The average rise in BP was 13% for naloxone and 11% for the placebo.

Unpublished studies conducted at Wayne State University by Antonenko and Martin showed that naloxone could increase BP and cardiac output in most patients in advanced septic shock, but there were no survivors. Furthermore, many of the patients became very restless and difficult to manage after receiving naloxone.

In a recent study of 13 patients in septic shock, Hackshaw, Parker, and Roberts found no overall effect of naloxone (0.03 mg/kg IV push followed by a constant infusion of $0.2 \text{ mg} \cdot \text{kg}^{-1} \cdot \text{h}^{-1}$) on survival in spite of a significant rise in BP.

AXIOM
Naloxone may raise BP, but otherwise it is of little or no benefit in advanced shock in humans.

15. Thyrotropin-Releasing Hormone

Thyrotropin-releasing hormone (TRH) has been found to improve cardiovascular function and survival in experimental hemorrhagic and endotoxic shock. In contrast to naloxone, TRH does not bind to opiate receptors or alter the analgesic properties of various drugs. However, it does antagonize many of the other biological effects of endorphins. TRH may be of particular benefit if an antiendorphin is to be used in settings where adequate pain control is also important.

TRH, in a dose-related fashion, increases MAP, heart rate, and respiratory rate in experimental shock, and survival is also improved. TRH, like naloxone, appears to function largely through CNS effector sites and is dependent on an intact sympathetic-adrenal complex. However, TRH is more efficacious and appears to have more direct peripheral effects than naloxone. The effects of TRH also appear to be independent of its pituitary-thyroid regulatory function.

16. Vasodilators

If the patient shows evidence of excessive vasoconstriction and poor tissue perfusion in spite of all other therapy and blood pressure is normal or high, a vasodilator may greatly improve tissue perfusion.

PITFALL
Using a vasodilator to improve perfusion in shock without first ensuring that the patient is not hypovolemic.

Vasodilators should not be used in patients who are hypovolemic. Vasodilators may increase vascular capacity by 2 to 3 liters, making an even greater discrepancy between vascular capacity and intravascular volume in hypovolemic patients. This can cause sudden severe hypotension. Even if the patient has a normal blood volume, vasodilators will often cause the blood pressure to fall by at least 5 to 10 mm Hg. If the patient is already hypotensive, such a drop in blood pressure may jeopardize coronary and cerebral blood flow, particularly if these vessels have a 70% to 80% occlusion that makes flow through them pressure dependent.

AXIOM
To use a vasodilator effectively, one should have PAWP and arterial catheters in place. One should also be prepared to give fluid rapidly if the BP falls significantly as the vasodilator is started.

Nitroprusside in doses of 0.3 to 3.0 $\mu g \cdot kg^{-1} \cdot min^{-1}$ tends to reduce afterload more than preload, thereby increasing cardiac output. In contrast, nitroglycerin in similar doses primarily reduces preload and dilates coronary arteries. In addition to causing occasional sudden drops in BP, large doses (>3 to 5 $\mu g \cdot kg^{-1} \cdot min^{-1}$) of nitroprusside given for more than 36 to 48 hours may result in toxic levels of thiocyanate.

Other agents that can decrease total peripheral vascular resistance include prostacyclin, ATP-MgCl$_2$, narcotics, sedatives, and glucose-insulin-potassium solutions.

17. Nonsteroidal Anti-inflammatory Drugs

During shock and sepsis there is a greatly increased conversion of membrane phospholipids to arachidonic acid. Increased quantities of and/or abnormal relationships between these arachidonic acid metabolites may be responsible for many of the changes seen in both experimental endotoxic and clinical septic shock.

A number of prostaglandin inhibitors (including aspirin, indomethacin, ibuprofen, and imidazole) have been beneficial in experimental shock, especially when used as pretreatment. However, clinical benefit in proper trials is still to be demonstrated.

18. Diuretics

If the patient does not have an adequate urine output after all the extracellular volume has been restored, and if BP and cardiac output have been optimized as much as possible, diuretics should be tried. Patients with severe sepsis or trauma who develop oliguric renal failure and require dialysis almost always die. In contrast, 40% to 60% of the patients who develop nonoliguric renal failure will survive.

AXIOM

It is very important to maintain a urine output of at least 0.5 to 1.0 ml·kg^{-1}·h^{-1}, using fluids rather than diuretics whenever possible.

The most effective method for obtaining a satisfactory urine output is to administer adequate fluids. If there is absolutely no urine output, one must be alert for a mechanical problem, such as obstruction of a Foley catheter or the ureters.

As an initial diuretic effort, 12.5 to 25.0 g of mannitol may be given intravenously over a period of 10 to 15 minutes followed by an infusion of 6.25 to 12.5 g/h. Dopamine in doses of 1 to 3 $\mu g \cdot kg^{-1} \cdot min^{-1}$ may also help promote a diuresis.

If there is still oliguria, 20 to 80 mg of furosemide may be given every 4 to 8 hours as needed to maintain a urine output of at least 0.5 ml·kg^{-1}·h^{-1}. If there is not a rapid response, the dose of furosemide may be doubled every 15 to 30 minutes until a 500 to 1000 mg dose is used.

If oliguria persists in spite of all these drugs, the patient is in renal failure and should be treated accordingly. Such a situation, however, makes the treatment of shock extremely difficult. Under such circumstances one should consider the use of slow continuous ultrafiltration (SCUF) to remove excess water and to control the potassium levels and uremia. The usual forms of hemodialysis are not tolerated in shock patients.

19. Antibiotics

Patients with prolonged shock have a greatly decreased resistance to infection. The mucosal barrier in the intestine may become increasingly permeable to bacteria and bacterial products. The reticuloendothelial system, particularly in the poorly perfused liver, will be less effective at sequestering and combating these agents. Consequently, in shock patients, antibiotics should be started at the earliest indication of any infection or contamination, but only after appropriate smears and cultures have been obtained.

271

The choice of antibiotics will depend upon past experience with the antibiotic sensitivities of the organisms most likely to be involved in a particular hospital. For infections involving the peritoneal cavity following disease or trauma to the distal small bowel or colon, it is wise to use a combination of antibiotics to cover Gram-negative aerobes, such as *E. coli*, and anaerobes, particularly *Bacteroides fragilis*. Need for coverage of enterococci will vary with the experience at that hospital.

20. Enhancing Host Defenses

a. E. coli *Antisera and Vaccines*

In infections with Gram-negative bacteria, certain cell-wall components contribute to the development of bacteremic shock. The outermost layer of the cell wall of Gram-negative bacteria is a polysaccharide referred to as O or somatic antigen. This chain of repeating olgiosaccharide units is unique for each serotype of Gram-negative organism, and it is responsible for the smooth appearance of the colonies when grown on culture media. The colonies of mutant organisms that lack the O antigen and show only core polysaccharide on their surface appear rough (R) on culture. Core polysaccharide is attached through 2-keto-3-deoxyoctulosonate (KDO) to a lipid moiety, called lipid A.

The KDO-lipid A segment appears to be immunologically identical in almost all aerobic Gram-negative bacteria studied. Together, the three component layers—O antigen, R-core antigen, and lipid A—make up endotoxin, which is also called lipopolysaccharide (LPS). Although the term endotoxin was originally chosen because it was thought that this toxic bacterial component was an integral part of the bacterial cell wall, it has since been noted that endotoxin can exist in a free state, can be released by bacteria growing in culture, and retains its biologic activity after extraction from bacteria.

Studies with the J5 mutant of *E. coli* 0111:B4, a mutant unable to incorporate exogenous galactose into its outer polysaccharide layer, indicate that antibodies to core lipopolysaccharides (R-core antigen plus lipid A) can be cross-protective. In a study reported by Ziegler and associates, antiserum to core lipopolysaccharide was randomly given to 103 to 212 patients with Gram-negative infections. The mortality rate of the control group was 39% compared to 22% in the antiserum group. Its effect in those with shock was even greater, with mortality rates of 77% in controls and 44% in the antiserum group.

In another prospective randomized study, Lachman, Pitsoe, and Gaffin used freeze-dried human plasma which was rich in antilipopolysaccharide (anti-LPS) IgG to treat septic shock in OB-GYN patients. The mortality was 47% (9/19) in conventionally treated patients and 7% (1/14) with anti-LPS. Anti-LPS also caused mean arterial blood pressure rise from 45 ± 8 mm Hg to 69 ± 9 mm Hg within 75 minutes of administration.

Interestingly, another study by Aitchison et al showed markedly different results. In a randomized double-blind trial of human antilipopolysaccharide-specific globulin versus placebo in the treatment of severe septic shock, the hospital mortality rate was 53% (9/17) in the treated group and 59% (10/17) in the control group. Measurement of serum endotoxin and anti-LPS levels at the time of admission to the study and 24 hours later revealed no significant difference between controls and treated patients.

Baumgartner and colleagues in 1985 reported on the prophylactic effect of J5 immune plasma in surgical patients at high risk for postoperative infections. Results demonstrated that the prophylactic administration of J5 immune plasma to high-risk surgical patients reduced the frequency of Gram-negative septic shock. Although prophylaxis did not lower the infection rate, it did prevent serious consequences of Gram-negative infections and thus improved the overall prognosis.

b. *Monoclonal Antibodies*

Difficulty in preparation, lack of homogeneity, and risks associated with administration of antiserum lead to the concept of developing immunotherapy based on monoclonal antibody (MAB) technology. Dunn and associates experimentally produced MABs directed against certain common antigens on core LPS. They found that anti-J5 MABs significantly protected mice from three bacterial challenges, two of which represented organisms that were sterotypically distinct from *E. coli* J5. Antonacci and colleagues found that MABs were effective in significantly decreasing mortality rates in mice given an LD_{60} to LD_{70} dose of Gram-negative bacteria. An increasing number of studies suggest that monoclonal and polyclonal antibodies to endotoxin can significantly improve survival rates in severe sepsis and/or septic shock.

Teng and associates developed a cell line, A6H4C5, which produced a human monoclonal antibody (HA-1A) that cross-reacted with endotoxins from a large number of unrelated species of Gram-negative bacteria. The administration of the MAB protected rabbits against the endotoxin-induced dermal Shwartzman reaction, and also protected mice against lethal Gram-negative bacteremia.

In a phase I trial, Fisher and colleagues evaluated the safety, pharmacokinetics, and immunogenicity of HA-1A, in septic patients. Thirty-four patients received either 25 mg, 100 mg, or 250 mg of HA-1A as a single intravenous infusion over 15 minutes. Clinical monitoring for evaluation of safety was carried out through 14 to 21 days after infusion. The mean serum concentration at 1 hour following a 100 mg dose of HA-1A was 33.2 μg/ml with a mean half-life of 15.9 hours. There were no reports of adverse or allergic reactions thought to be related to the HA-1A infusion, and there was no evidence of an antibody response to HA-1A during the study period.

Ziegler and associates evaluated the efficacy and safety of HA-1A in Gram-negative bacteremia and sepsis. The clinical trial was a prospective, placebo-controlled, double-blind study of 543 patients with suspected Gram-negative sepsis of which 200 patients were diagnosed with Gram-negative bacteremia and sepsis. Patients received either a 100 mg single dose of HA-1A or a placebo and were evaluated for a 28-day study period. Mortality was statistically significantly reduced from 49% on placebo to 30% on HA-1A in patients with Gram-negative bacteremia. In addition, mortality was significantly reduced from 57% on placebo to 33% on HA-1A in patients with Gram-negative bacteremia and shock.

21. Other Agents

a. Cimetidine

Hansbrough and associates have shown that treatment with the histamine$_2$ blocker cimetidine, prevents burn-induced suppression of delayed hypersensitivity. In a more recent study, cimetidine prevented postburn depression of both delayed cutaneous hypersensitivity and T-helper cell/T-suppressor cell ratios. However, it failed to restore ConA responses. The value of this agent in improving host defenses clinically has still not been clarified.

b. Antithrombin

Varying amounts of intravascular coagulation develop in many patients with severe persistent shock, particularly if the patient is septic. Only a small percentage, however, develop the full-blown clinical syndrome of disseminated intravascular coagulation (DIC). Although there is some controversy regarding the value of heparin for the treatment of DIC, if serial coagulation studies reveal a progressive reduction in the platelet count and the concentrations of factor V, factor VIII, fibrinogen, and prothrombin, and if there is no evidence of fibrinolysis (i.e., fibrin split products are not elevated), heparin therapy may be of value. Most DIC is associated with increased fibrin split products and consequently, therapy is directed at controlling the primary process and restoring adequate clotting factors, usually by administering FFP.

Recent studies with antithrombin have shown that antithrombin levels drop rapidly in sepsis and shock. Low antithrombin levels probably increase the tendency to subclinical DIC and multiple organic failure.

c. Pentoxifylline

Recently there has been increased interest in using pentoxifylline (PTF) to treat septic shock. This methylxanthine derivative has been used to improve peripheral circulation in atherosclerotic vascular disease. Waxman noted in an editorial that PTF increases RBC deformability, and therefore improves blood flow through a constricted microcirculation. Thus, it might also improve oxygen delivery through the altered microcirculation of sepsis. PTF increases prostacyclin release, and this may also reverse some of the microcirculatory flow disturbances of sepsis. In addition, PTF has been shown to have a variety of effects on PMN leukocytes, including decreasing adhesiveness of activated PMN leukocytes to the endothelium, and possibly decreased release of lysosomal enzymes and superoxide radicals.

Activated PMNs adhering to the endothelium in a constricted capillary can completely occlude RBC flow through that capillary. Thus, decreasing PMN leukocyte adhesiveness could improve tissue oxygenation. In addition, activation and endothelial adherence of PMN leukocytes are initial steps toward lysosomal and superoxide radical release at the endothelial level. Because these effects may be central to the autodestructive inflammatory process of sepsis, inhibition of PMN leukocyte adhesiveness by PTF might be of therapeutic benefit. Most recently, PTF has been shown by Streiter, Remick, and Ward also to inhibit production of the tumor necrosis factor (TNF).

Tighe and associates demonstrated that pretreatment with PTF in a pig peritonitis model ameliorated the hemodynamic changes usually seen during the onset of sepsis, most particularly the decrease of wedge pressure and increase of systemic and pulmonary vascular resistance. These hemodynamic changes were associated with other beneficial changes including decreased neutrophil adhesiveness, less capillary occlusion, less leukostasis, and less endothelial disruption.

Sullivan and colleagues and Lilly and associates have demonstrated that PTF prevents the lung injury induced by TNF in animals, not only by inhibiting TNF production, but also by reducing the activation of PMNs induced by TNF, interleukin-1, and perhaps interleukin-2. Heath and coworkers showed that PTF can also provide considerable protection against leukostasis and lung damage in rabbits with severe fecal peritonitis.

22. Removal of Endotoxin from Plasma by Adsorption

Recently Bysani and associates have reported successful detoxification of plasma by extracorporeal clearance of endotoxin using a variety of specific and nonspecific adsorbants. After the plasma has been "detoxified," injection into mice is much less lethal than nonadsorbed plasma. Similar beneficial results were obtained with septic shock in dogs using polymyxin B immobilized fibers.

23. Correcting Hypothermia

AXIOM

Hypothermia, particularly below 32°C, must be prevented in patients, particularly those with shock and massive transfusions.

During prolonged surgery, particularly for traumatic shock due to injuries in the chest and abdomen, severe hypothermia may develop. This may not only increase the incidence of arrhythmias but also reduce myocardial function and vascular reactivity to vasoactive agents. The mortality rate in our massive transfusion patients who developed a core temperature $<32°C$ was 85%.

Experimental studies suggested that hypotensive patients with a core temperature below 29°C may benefit from exogenous catecholamines, especially if they are responding poorly to fluids.

24. Correcting Disseminated Intravascular Coagulation

The diagnosis of DIC in shock patients can be difficult at times. Carr, McKinney, and McDonagh reviewed the role of D-dimers in assisting with this problem. Several MABs that can recognize the unique fibrin degradation fragment D-dimer (DD) have become available for routine laboratory use. D-dimers and high molecular weight (HMW) complexes are generated with plasmin lysis of cross-linked fibrin clots. In contrast to fragments X, Y, D, and E, which are generated by the lysis of fibrinogen and non-cross-linked fibrin, the presence of fragment DD (D-dimers) documents that both thrombin generation (causing cross-linking of fibrin clot through thrombin activation of factor XIII) and plasmin generation (causing fibrinolysis) have occurred. Detection of D-dimers, therefore, offers a unique advantage over other laboratory tests for diagnosing DIC because it addresses both dimensions of DIC.

If DIC is diagnosed, treatment is mainly directed at correcting the primary process, including improving tissue perfusion. Restoration of clotting factors with platelet concentrates and fresh-frozen plasma is also important. In the past, heparin was also given to reduce the ongoing intravascular clotting. Now it is generally considered safer to avoid the increasing hemorrhage that might occur with heparin administration to a patient who is already bleeding excessively.

a. Mechanical Support

Intra-aortic balloon pumping (IABP) has been of greatest use in treating acute myocardial infarction shock and severe myocardial dysfunction after cardiac surgery. It may also be useful in any type of shock which has a major component of myocardial dysfunction. By deflating a 27 to 35 ml balloon in the descending aorta as the aortic valve is opening, systolic pressure, systolic time, and heart size tend to decrease. The resulting decrease in systolic tension-time index can greatly reduce myocardial oxygen consumption. By inflating the balloon at the beginning of diastole, diastolic aortic pressures increase, thereby improving myocardial blood flow (Fig. 5.5).

AXIOM

In patients with shock following cardiac surgery or an acute myocardial infarction shock, IABP can often raise BP and cardiac output, and reverse myocardial ischemia.

In an occasional patient with severe right heart failure, an intra-aortic balloon pump (IABP) has been inserted into the main pulmonary artery in an attempt to improve right ventricular output. Membrane oxygenators have also been used for acute right heart failure, but these are also only occasionally successful in adults.

If the cardiogenic shock is refractory to the IABP, one may try to support the circulation of selected individuals with arteriovenous extracorporeal membrane oxygenation (ECMO). Reedy and associates reported their experience with 38 patients supported with ECMO at St. Louis University Medical Center. Nine (24%) were long-term survivors. Their results indicate that resuscitative ECMO is useful for 12 to 24 hours and is best applied to (1) patients less than 60 years of age, (2) patients with acute events (such as a failed PTCA amenable to surgical correction), and (3) candidates for cardiac transplantation who could be switched to more sophisticated devices within 12 to 24 hours.

VIII. REVERSIBLE CAUSES OF SO-CALLED IRREVERSIBLE SHOCK

Frequently shock may be so severe and so unresponsive to standard therapy that the process appears irreversible. Under such circumstances the patient should be re-evaluated to determine whether some reversible causes of the persistent shock have been overlooked. Following are some of the more frequent, treatable causes of persistent shock:

1. Inadequate fluid administration
2. Inadequate ventilation or oxygen
3. Pneumothorax or hydrothorax
4. Pulmonary emboli
5. Pericardial tamponade

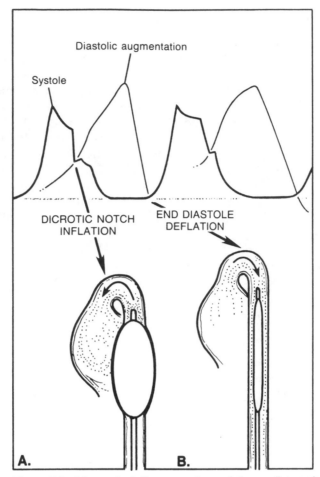

Figure 5.5 Intra-aortic balloon pumping and the cardiac cycle reflecting systole and diastole. Balloon inflation and deflation is depicted with inflation occurring at the dicrotic notch, and deflation occurring just prior to the next upstroke of the systolic wave. Diastolic augmentation reflects the increase in aortic pressures afforded by an inflated balloon during left ventricular diastole thereby increasing coronary artery perfusion pressures.

6. Inadequately treated sepsis
7. Adrenal insufficiency
8. Hypothermia
9. Hypocalcemia

SUMMARY POINTS

1. Early diagnosis and rapid, aggressive therapy based on the trends and responses obtained from serial objective measurements offer the best chance for success in treating shock.
2. Shock is usually associated with impaired tissue perfusion either in localized areas or in the body as a whole.
3. Shock following trauma is usually, but not always, due to hypovolemia.
4. Early septic shock tends to be associated with systemic vasodilation and a normal or increased cardiac output.
5. Septic patients with a low cardiac output may require very large quantities of fluid plus some inotropic support to maintain adequate tissue perfusion.
6. Brain injury does not cause hypotension until terminally, when apnea occurs.

7. "Warm" shock in young individuals without apparent trauma or sepsis should be considered due to drugs, usually as an overdose, until proven otherwise.

8. Early diagnosis and treatment of shock greatly increases the chances of reversing the process before extensive deterioration of vital organ function has occurred.

9. Changes in pulse pressure reflect alterations in cardiac output much more accurately than systolic BP does.

10. Decreased falls in pulse pressure may occur because of tachycardia, but they are usually due to a decreased blood volume or cardiac failure.

11. One should not always assume that an unobtainable cuff BP is extremely low.

12. Systolic BP obtained from a radial artery catheter is usually 10 to 20 mm Hg higher than in the aorta.

13. A low urine sodium concentration is usually due to hypovolemia.

14. A low urine output usually reflects hypovolemia, but a normal urine output does not rule it out.

15. In a septic patient with polyuria, a low urine sodium concentration should make one suspect an inappropriate polyuria.

16. A falling urine sodium concentration and rising osmolality suggest that the patient is becoming (more) hypovolemic.

17. An increasing respiratory alkalosis is an important sign that a patient's condition is deteriorating and should stimulate a search for hypoxemia, sepsis, hypovolemia, or pulmonary emboli.

18. If a patient with shock or sepsis is not hyperventilating, one should suspect that the patient may be developing ventilatory failure.

19. Metabolic (lactic) acidosis often indicates a fairly advanced state of hypoperfusion or impaired cell metabolism.

20. One should not assume that tissue perfusion is adequate because systolic BP is normal or increased.

21. One should not assume that tissue perfusion is adequate because the skin is warm.

22. Checking a patient's orientation and cognitive function may provide early evidence of sepsis or hypovolemia.

23. A fall in a-v oxygen differences may be an early sign of sepsis, while a rise in a-v oxygen differences often indicates a reduction in blood volume and/or cardiac output.

24. The combination of shock and respiratory failure is highly lethal.

25. Much of the tissue damage in shock may be due to increased production of oxygen-free radicals or lack of their endogenous scavengers.

26. Absence of tachycardia in an elderly patient with hypotension is usually evidence of a poor prognosis.

27. Sudden onset of an explained tachyarrhythmia should be considered due to sepsis or a pulmonary embolus until proven otherwise.

28. The initial vasoconstriction seen in hypovolemic shock is an important mechanism for maintaining perfusion of vital organs.

29. One should not administer narcotics to a septic or injured patient without first ensuring that the patient is not hypovolemic.

30. Continued hypotension in advanced septic shock may be due to continuing hypovolemia or cardiac or peripheral vascular failure.

31. Failure to respond to vasoconstrictors in advanced shock may be due to severe acidosis, excess quantities of endogenous vasodilators, or an inadequate adrenergic receptor response.

32. Transcapillary refill of the vascular system is important in hypovolemia, but it may be totally inactive or reversed in sepsis.

33. Malnourished individuals with low plasma glucose and protein levels tend to have an impaired response to hypovolemia.
34. Septic patients can develop tissue edema rapidly, even when hypovolemic.
35. Any patient without obvious excess loss of fluid or blood who requires more than 200 ml of fluid per hour to maintain normal vital signs and urine output should be considered septic until proven otherwise.
36. A progressive drop in the platelet count should make one very suspicious of sepsis or the development of DIC.
37. Impaired cellular function may be manifested by a progressive decrease in plasma levels of sodium and ionized calcium.
38. Increased coronary sinus lactate is relatively reliable evidence of myocardial ischemia.
39. Rising arterial lactate levels in shock generally indicate a poor prognosis.
40. Some complement activation may be important in host defense, but excess or prolonged complement activation can be very damaging to tissues.
41. Patients on ACE inhibitors may have especially severe edema or hypotension if they become septic because of decreased bradykinin breakdown.
42. The hormonal response in shock appears to be designed to increase blood levels of glucose and raise cardiac output to facilitate "fight or flight."
43. As shock progresses, the patient has an increasing tendency to hypovolemia.
44. Progressively increasing fluid needs, far above measured losses, may be an important early sign of sepsis.
45. Falling ionized calcium levels in blood are often a sign of increasing impairment of cell function.
46. Hepatic dysfunction in late shock has dire consequences on metabolism (because of hepatocyte failure) and host defenses (because of failure of hepatic phagocytes).
47. In advanced sepsis and shock, there is often a poor correlation between serum creatinine levels and other monitors of renal function.
48. By the time DIC is clinically reflected in troublesome bleeding from needle puncture sites and mucosal surfaces, the concentrations of clotting factors are very low, and the problem is extremely difficult to correct.
49. Relatively mild postsurgical infections can cause severe toxic shock syndrome.
50. Some TNF appears to be an important aspect of the host response to infection, but excess TNF may be very deleterious.
51. Low antithrombin, prekallikrein, and fibronectin levels indicate an increased tendency to develop sepsis.
52. It must be emphasized repeatedly that isolated measurements are of much less value than serial determination to demonstrate trends in the patient's condition and his or her response to treatment.
53. A patient in shock who is not hyperventilating is more likely to develop respiratory failure.
54. In patients with sepsis or shock, oxygen delivery (DO_2) should be increased until oxygen consumption (VO_2) no longer rises or is significantly above normal.
55. By far the simplest and most effective treatment for most shock, particularly after trauma or surgery, is early and aggressive administration of fluid.
56. Although plasma albumin levels are often very low in sepsis and shock, administration of albumin usually produces only transient benefits and can cause many complications if given in excess.
57. Administration of large amounts of dextran 40 to patients can cause increased blood loss from large open wounds.
58. One should not rely on a urine output of 0.5 to 1.0 $ml \cdot kg^{-1} \cdot h^{-1}$ to indicate

adequate renal perfusion after a patient has received a large bolus of dextran 40.

59. One should notify the laboratory when performing a type and cross-match on a patient who has received dextran.

60. One should not administer large amounts of hetastarch to patients who are bleeding or have a coagulopathy.

61. FFP should generally be used only to treat coagulopathies confirmed by appropriate laboratory tests.

62. Successful resuscitation from hypovolemic shock is dependent more on the rapidity with which the plasma and ECF volumes are restored rather than the composition of the fluid used.

63. Although albumin is expensive, if it reduces an ICU stay by 1 day, even large quantities more than pay for themselves.

64. Hypertonic saline solutions may reduce tissue edema in patients who would otherwise require large quantities of resuscitation fluid. However, the tendency to hypernatremia and vasodilation may be a problem.

65. The reduced 2,3-DPG after massive transfusions of old bank blood may result in good oxygen delivery but reduced oxygen availability and consumption.

66. Calcium is not usually given to patients receiving transfusions unless the rate of administration is rapid (more than one unit every 5 minutes) and the patient has persistent shock or heart failure.

67. The use of autotransfused blood has many benefits, but in patients requiring massive transfusions, it may contribute significantly to the development of a severe coagulopathy.

68. One should not rely on isolated CVP levels to indicate fluid needs.

69. One should not rely on a CVP to determine fluid needs in a patient with ARDS or pulmonary disease.

70. If there are wide swings in CVP with positive-pressure ventilation, the water manometer will tend to provide deceptively high readings.

71. Many patients with sepsis or acute respiratory failure have impaired pulmonary blood flow and a high CVP in spite of hypovolemia and a low PAWP.

72. A PAWP that is higher than the PADP is inaccurate and usually reflects malposition of the tip of the PA catheter.

73. The responses of the BP, SV, and PAWP to fluid challenges are far more informative than absolute levels.

74. Continuous monitoring of pulmonary artery oxygen saturations (SvO_2) may provide early warning of important changes in cardiovascular or pulmonary function.

75. In critically ill patients, a cardiac output greater than normal is probably needed to adequately perfuse vital organs, especially the liver.

76. The best single guide to the resuscitation of severe shock is the oxygen consumption index (VO_2/m^2).

77. Dopamine is generally the inotropic agent of choice in patients with hypotension and a low cardiac output.

78. Dobutamine is generally the inotrope of choice in patients with a low cardiac output and a normal or increased BP.

79. One should not use isoproterenol in patients with tachycardia, acute myocardial infarction, or pulmonary embolus.

80. One should consider the use of glucagon in patients who are on beta blockers and have developed shock or acute heart failure.

81. Calcium should probably only be given to patients in persistent shock or heart failure if they are receiving massive blood transfusions rapidly or the patient has been on beta-adrenergic blockers or calcium-channel blockers.

82. Glucose-insulin-potassium solutions may be of value in preventing arrhythmias in individuals with acute myocardial infarction shock.

83. Probably the ideal way to ensure that tissue perfusion is optimal is to increase oxygen delivery until oxygen consumption is well above normal and not flow dependent.

84. PASGs may be helpful in prolonged ambulance transport of patients in shock, but they can impair cardiac and pulmonary function and may cause compartment syndromes.

85. In shock patients bicarbonate should probably be used only to partially correct severe acidosis not responsive to fluids and inotropes.

86. The only proven benefit of steroids in the treatment of shock is treatment of adrenal insufficiency.

87. One should consider the possibility of a subclinical adrenal insufficiency in patients with persistent hypotension in spite of adequate fluid loading, inotropes, and oxygen.

88. One should not administer large doses of vasopressors to hypotensive patients who are still hypovolemic.

89. Naloxone may raise BP, but otherwise it is of little or no benefit in advanced shock in humans.

90. One should not use vasodilators to improve perfusion in shock without first ensuring that the patient is not hypovolemic.

91. To use a vasodilator effectively, one should have PAWP and arterial catheters in place. One should also be prepared to give fluid rapidly if the BP falls significantly as the vasodilator is started.

92. During and following resuscitation from shock, it is very important to maintain a urine output of at least 0.5 to 1.0 $ml \cdot kg^{-1} \cdot h^{-1}$, using fluids rather than diuretics whenever possible.

93. Hypothermia, particularly below 32°C, must be prevented, especially in patients with shock and massive transfusions.

94. In patients with shock following cardiac surgery or an acute myocardial infarction, IABP can often raise BP and cardiac output, and reverse myocardial ischemia.

BIBLIOGRAPHY

1. Abraham, E and Chang, YH: The effects of hemorrhage on mitogen-induced lymphocyte proliferation. Circ Shock 15:141, 1985.
2. Abraham, E, Oye, RK, and Smith, M: Detection of blood volume deficits through conjunctival oxygen tension monitoring. Crit Care Med 12:931, 1984.
3. Abraham, E and Regan, R: The effects of hemorrhage and trauma on interleukin-2 production. Arch Surg 120:1341, 1985.
4. Adeleye, GA, Furman, BL, and Parratt, JR: Possible involvement of opiate receptors in the response of conscious rats to Escherichia coli endotoxin: Protective effect of naloxone. Physiol Soc: 31P, April, 1981.
5. Aitchison, JM and Arbuckle, DD: Anti-endotoxin in the treatment of severe surgical septic shock: Results of a randomized double-blind trial. SAMJ 787, 1985.
6. Almqvist, PM, et al: Increased survival of endotoxin injected dogs treated with methyprednisolone, naloxone and ibuprofen. Circ Shock 14:129, 1984.
7. Antonacci, AC, et al: Development of monoclonal antibodies against virulent gram-negative bacteria: Efficacy in a septic mouse mode. Surg Forum 35:116, 1984
8. Bashour, TT, et al: Hypocalcemic acute myocardia failure secondary to rapid transfusion of citrated blood. Am Heart J 108:1040, 1984.
9. Baumgartner, JD, et al: Prevention of gram-negative shock and death in surgical patients by antibody to endotoxin core glycolipid. Lancet 2:59, 1985.
10. Beamer, KC and Vargish, T: Effect of methylprednisolone or naloxone's hemodynamic response in canine hypovolemic shock. Crit Care Med 14:115, 1986.
11. Bell, RC, et al: Multiple organ system failure and infection in adult respiratory distress syndrome. Ann Intern Med 99:293, 1983.
12. Bender, EM, et al: Prevention of post burn alterations in helper and suppressor T-lymphocytes by cimetidine. Surg Forum 35:156, 1984.
13. Bessey, PQ, et al: Combined hormone infusion simulates the metabolic response to injury. Ann Surg 200:264, 1984.

14. Bessler, H, et al: Effect of pentoxifylline on the phagocytic activity, cAMP levels and superoxide anion production by monocytes and polymorphonuclear cells. J Leukocyte Biol 40:747, 1986.

15. Bickell, WH, Shaftan, GW, and Mattox, KL: Intravenous fluid administration and uncontrolled hemorrhage. J Trauma 29:409, 1989.

16. Bone, RC and Jacobs, ER: Research on ibuprofen for sepsis and respiratory failure: Symposium on Motrin (ibuprofen), past, present and future. Am J Med 77:114, 1983.

17. Bonnet, F, et al: Naloxone therapy of human septic shock. Crit Care Med 13:972, 1985.

18. Boutros, AR and Lee, C: Value of continuous monitoring of mixed venous blood oxygen saturation in the management of critically ill patients. Crit Care Med 14:132, 1986.

19. Bronsveld, V, et al: Effects of glucose-insulin-potassium (GIK) on myocardial blood flow and metabolism in canine endotoxin shock. Circ Shock 13:325, 1984.

20. Bryan-Brown, CW, et al: The axillary artery catheter. Heart Lung 12:492, 1983.

21. Buckingham, JC: Hypothalamo-pituitary response to trauma. Br Med Bull 41:203, 1985.

22. Burchard, KW, Slotman, G, and Jed, E: Positive pressure respirations and pneumatic antishock garment application: Hemodynamic response. J Trauma 25:83, 1985.

23. Bysani, GK, et al: Detoxification of plasma containing lipopolysaccharide by adsorption. Crit Care Med 18:67, 1990.

24. Calvin, JE, Driedger, AA, and Sibbald, WJ: Does the pulmonary capillary wedge pressure predict left ventricular preload in critically ill patients? Crit Care Med 9:437, 1981.

25. Carr, JM, McKinney, M, and McDonagh, J: Diagnosis of disseminated intravascular coagulation. Am J Clin Pathol 91:280, 1989.

26. Castor, G, et al: Determination of cardiac output during positive end-expiratory pressure: Noninvasive electrical bioimpedance compared with standard thermodilution. Crit Care Med 18:544, 1990.

27. Chernow, B and Roth, BL: Pharmacologic manipulation of the peripheral vasculature in shock: Clinical and experimental approaches. Circ Shock 18:141, 1986.

28. Chernow, B, et al: Glucagon: Endocrine effects and calcium involvement in cardiovascular actions in dogs. Circ Shock 19:393, 1986.

29. Chu, DZJ, Nihioka, K, and Romsdahl, MM: Effect of tuftsin on post splenectomy sepsis. Surg Forum 35:162, 1984.

30. Connors, AF, Jr, McCaffree, DR, and Gray, BA: Evaluation of right-heart catheterization in the critically ill patient without acute myocardial infarction. N Engl J Med 308:263, 1983.

31. Cournand, A, et al: Studies of the circulation in clinical shock. Surgery 13:964, 1943.

32. Cowan, BN, et al: The relative prognostic value of lactate and hemodynamic measurements in early shock. Anesthesia 39:750, 1984.

33. Crass, BA and Bergdoll, MS: Toxin involvement in toxic shock. J Infect Dis 153:918, 1986.

34. Daily, EK: Use of hemodynamics to differentiate pathophysiologic causes of cariogenic shock. Crit Care Nurs Clin North Am 1(3):589, 1989.

35. Dawidson, I: Hypertonic saline for resuscitation: A word of caution. Crit Care Med 18:245, 1990.

35a. Deitch, EA, Maejima, K, Berg, R: Effect of oral antibiotics and bacterial overgrowth on the translocation of the GI-tract microflora in burned rats. J Trauma 25:385, 1985.

36. DeMaria, A, et al: Naloxone vs placebo in treatment of septic shock. Lancet i:1363, 1985.

37. DeMueles, JE: In vitro reversal of cardiac deterioration in septic shock with tetraethylammonium chloride. Arch Surg 121:65, 1986.

38. Denis, R, et al: The beneficial role of calcium supplementation during resuscitation from shock. J Trauma 25:594, 1985.

39. DePriest, JL: Septic shock: What to do until a breakthrough comes along. Postgrad Med 86:71, 1989.

40. Derrington, MC: The present status of blood filtration. Anesthesia 40:334, 1985.

41. Devennto, F: Hemoglobin solutions as oxygen delivery resuscitation fluids. Crit Care Med 10:238, 1982.

42. Dietrich, KA, et al: Cardiovascular and metabolic response to red blood cell transfusion in critically ill volume-resuscitated nonsurgical patients. Crit Care Med 18:940, 1990.

43. D'Orio, V, et al: Accuracy in early prediction of prognosis of patients with septic shock by analysis of simple indices: Prospective study. Crit Care Med 18:1339, 1990.

44. Ducey, JP, et al: A comparison of the cerebral and cardiovascular effects of complete resuscitation with isotonic and hypertonic saline, hetastarch, and whole blood following hemorrhage. J Trauma 29:1510, 1989.

44a. Duff, JH: The relationship between oxygen uptake and a toxic factor in septic shock. Adv Exp Med Biol 23:305, 1971.

45. Dunn, DL, Mach, PA, and Cerra, FB: Monoclonal antibodies protect against lethal effect of gram-negative bacterial sepsis. Surg Forum 34:142, 1983.

46. Dunn, R, et al: Diethyl-carbamazine, a leukotriene inhibitor, improves in-vitro microcirculatory flow during endotoxemia. Circ Shock 17:69, 1985.

47. Edwards, JD: Practical application of oxygen transport principles. Crit Care Med 18:S45, 1990.

48. Emerson, TE: Unique features of albumin: A brief review. Crit Care Med 17:690, 1989.
49. Feola, M, Gonzalez, H, and Canizaro, P: Vasoactive parathyroid hormone in the treatment of acute ischemic left ventricular failure and the prevention of cariogenic shock. Circ Shock 17:163, 1985.
50. Fisher, C, et al: Initial evaluation of human monoclonal anti-lipid-A antibody (HA-1A) in patients with sepsis syndrome. Crit Care Med 18:1311, 1990.
51. Flint, IM: (editorial comment) Am J Surg 157:533, 1989.
52. Fried, SJ, Satiani, B, and Zeep, P: Normothermic rapid volume replacement for hypovolemic shock: An in vivo and in vitro study utilizing a new technique. J Trauma 26:183, 1986.
53. Gaffney, FA and Thal, ER: Hemodynamic effects of medical antishock trousers (MAST garment). J Trauma 21:931, 1981.
54. Gilbert, EM, et al: The effect of fluid loading, blood transfusion, and catecholamine infusion on oxygen delivery and consumption in patients with sepsis. Am Rev Respir Dis 137:873, 1986.
55. Girotti, MJ, et al: Effect on cardiopulmonary changes of Gram-negative endotoxinemia in the sheep after type-specific, cross-reactive and non-specific immune stimulation. Circ Shock 18:171, 1986.
56. Goenen, M, et al: Amrinone in the management of low cardiac output after open heart surgery. Am J Cardiol 56:33B, 1985.
57. Gordfarb, RD: Cardiac dynamics following shock: Role of circulating cardiodepressant substances. Circ Shock 9:317, 1982.
58. Greenblatt, GM and Ward, CF: A new device for rapid fluid administration. Can J Emerg Med 4:197, 1986.
59. Groeger, JS, Carlon, GC, and Howland, WS: Naloxone in septic shock. Crit Care Med 11:650, 1983.
60. Groeneveld, ABJ, Bronsveld, W, and Thijs, LG: Hemodynamic determinants of mortality in human septic shock. Surgery 99:140, 1986.
61. Gross, D, et al: Quantitative measurements of bleeding following hypertonic saline therapy in "uncontrolled" hemorrhagic shock. J Trauma 29:79, 1989.
62. Gross, D, et al: Is hypertonic saline resuscitation safe in "uncontrolled" hemorrhagic shock? J Trauma 28:751, 1988.
63. Gump, FE, Price, JB, and Kinney, JM: Whole body and splanchnic blood flow and oxygen consumption measurements in patients with intraperitoneal infection. Ann Surg 67:577, 1970.
64. Guthrie, JP, Jr: Effects of digoxin on responsiveness of the pressor actions of angiotensin and norepinephrine in man. J Clin Endocrinol Metab 58:76, 1984.
65. Hackshaw, KV, Parker, GA, and Roberts, JW: Naloxone in septic shock. Crit Care Med 18:47, 1990.
66. Haljamae, H: Interstitial fluid response in shock and related problems. In Ships, GT (ed): Clinical Surgery International. Churchill Livingston, New York, 1984, p 44.
67. Halushka, PV, Cook, JA, and Wise, WC: Beneficial effects of UK27248, a thromboxane synthetase inhibitor, in experimental endotoxic shock in the rat. Br J Clin Pharmacol 15:133S, 1983.
68. Halushka, PV, Wise, WC, and Cook, JA: Studies on the beneficial effects of aspirin in endotoxin shock: Aspirin Symposium. Am J Med 77:91, 1983.
69. Hansbrough, JF, et al: Post burn immunosuppression in an animal model: Monocyte dysfunction induced by burned tissue. Surg 93:415, 1983.
70. Harke, H, et al: The influence of different plasma substitutes on blood clotting and platelet function during and after operations. Anaesthesist 25:366, 1976.
71. Haupt, MT, Gilbert, EM, and Carlson, RW: Fluid loading increases oxygen consumption in septic patients with lactic acidosis. Am Rev Resp Dis 131:912, 1985.
72. Heath, MF, et al: Relevance of serum phospholipase A_2 assays to the assessment of septic shock. Crit Care Med 18:766, 1990.
73. Henry, M, Kay, MM, and Viccellio, P: Cariogenic shock associated with calcium channel and beta blockers: Reversal with intravenous calcium chloride. Am J Emerg Med 3:334, 1985.
74. Hinder, RA and Stein, HJ: Oxygen-derived free radicals. Arch Surg 126:104, 1991.
75. Hinshaw, LB, Beller-Todd, BK, and Archer, LT: Current management of the septic shock patient: Experimental basis for treatment. Circ Shock 9:543, 1982.
76. Holaday, JW: Commentary: Cardiovascular consequences of endogenous opiate antagonism. Biochem Pharmacol 32:573, 1983.
77. Holaday, JW, et al: Adrenalectomy blocks pressor responses to naloxone in endotoxic shock. Evidence for sympathomedullary involvement. Circ Shock 11:201, 1983.
78. Holcroft, JW, et al: 3% NaCl and 7.5% NaCl/dextran 70 in the resuscitation of severely injured patients. Ann Surg 206:279, 1987.
79. Holaday, JW and Faden, AI: Naloxone reversal of endotoxia hypotension suggests role of endorphins in shock. Nature 275:450, 1978.

80. Hughes, GS: Naloxone in methylprednisolone sodium succinate enhance sympathomedullary discharge in patients with septic shock. Life Sci 35:2319, 1984.

81. Hunninghake, G, Gadek, J, and Crystal, R: Mechanism by which cigarette smoke attracts polymorphonuclear leukocytes to lung. Chest 77:273, 1980.

82. Jardin, F, et al: Sepsis-related cardiogenic shock. Crit Care Med 18:1055, 1990.

83. Jardin, F, et al: Dobutamine: A hemodynamic evaluation in pulmonary embolism shock. Crit Care Med 9:329, 1981.

84. Kapin, MA, et al: The cerebral circulatory response during canine anaphylactic shock. Circ Shock 20:115, 1986.

85. King, EG and Chin, WDN: Shock: An overview of pathophysiology and general treatment goals. Crit Care Clin 1:547, 1985.

86. Krauz, MM, et al: Hypertonic saline treatment increases bleeding and mortality in "uncontrolled" hemorrhagic shock. Circ Shock 24:244, 1988.

87. Kumakura, K, Karoum, F, and Guidotti, A: Modulation of nicotinic receptors by opiate receptor antagonists in cultured adrenal chronaffin cells. Nature 283:489, 1980.

88. Lachman, E, Pitsoe, SB, and Gaffin, SL: Anti-lipopolysaccharide immunotherapy in management of septic shock of obstetric and gynecological origin. Lancet 1: 981, 1983.

89. Ledingham, IM and Ramsey, G: Hypovolemic shock. Br J Anaesth 58:169, 1986.

90. Lee, JC and Lum, BKB: Protective action of calcium entry blockers in endotoxin shock. Circ Shock 18:193, 1986.

91. Lefer, AM: Eicosanoids as mediators of ischemia and shock. Fed Proc 44:275, 1985.

92. Lefer, AM: Blood-borne humoral factors in the pathophysiology of circulatory shock. Circ Res 32:129, 1973.

93. Lefer, AM, Tabas, J, and Smith, EF: Salutary effects of prostacyclin in endotoxic shock. Pharmacology 21:206, 1980.

94. Livingston, DH, et al: The effect of tumor necrosis factor-alpha and interferon-gamma on neutrophil function. J Surg Res 46:322, 1989.

95. Lombard, JH, et al: Vascular smooth muscle transmembrane potentials during hypotensive stress. Circ Shock 18:131, 1986.

96. Long, JB, et al: Effects of naloxone and thyrotropin releasing hormone on plasma catecholamines, corticosterone and arterial pressure in normal and endotoxemic rats. Circ Shock 18:1, 1986.

97. Love, JC, et al: Reversibility of hypotension and shock by atrial or atrioventricular pacing in patients with right ventricular infarction. Am Heart J 108:5, 1984.

98. Lucas, CE, et al: Effect of fresh frozen plasma resuscitation on cardiopulmonary function and serum protein flux. Arch Surg 121:559, 1986.

99. MacNab, MSP, et al: Profound reduction in morphine clearance and liver blood flow in shock. Crit Care Med 12:366, 1986.

100. Majno, G, Shea, SM, and Leventhal, M: Endothelial contraction induced by histamine-type mediators: An electron microscopic study. J Cell Biol 42:647, 1969.

101. Maningas, PA, et al: Hypertonic saline-dextran solutions for the prehospital management of traumatic hypotension. Am J Surg 157:528, 1989.

102. Marks, JD, et al: Plasma tumor necrosis in patients with septic shock: Mortality rate, incidence of adult respiratory distress syndrome, and effects of methyprednisolone administration. Am Rev Respir Dis 141:94, 1990.

103. Martin, DJ, et al: Fresh frozen plasma supplement massive red blood cell transfusion. Ann Surg 202:505, 1985.

104. Mattar, JA, Weil, MH, and Shubin, H: A study of hyperosmolal state in critically ill. Crit Med Care 6:293, 1973.

105. Mattar, JA, et al: Cardiac arrest in the critically ill. II. Hyperosmolal states following cardiac arrest. Am J Med 36:162, 1974.

106. Mattox, KL, et al: Prospective randomized evaluation of antishock MAST in post-traumatic hypotension. J Trauma 26:779, 1986.

107. Mazzoni, MC, et al: Capillary narrowing in hemorrhagic shock is rectified by infusion of 7.5% NaCl/6% dextran 70. Circ Shock 27:348, 1989.

108. McCabe, JB, Seidel, DR, and Jagger, JA: Antishock-trousers inflation and pulmonary vital capacity. Ann Emerg Med 12:290, 1983.

109. McIntosh, TK, et al: Endorphins in primate hemorrhagic shock: Beneficial actions of opiate antagonists. J Surg Res 40:265, 1986.

110. McKechnie, K, Furman, BL, and Parratt, JR: Modification by oxygen free radical scavengers of the metabolic and cardiovascular effects of endotoxin infusion in conscious rats. Circ Shock 19:429, 1986.

111. McNamara, JD, et al: Resuscitation from hemorrhagic shock. J Trauma 23:552, 1983.

112. Meakins, JL, et al: The surgical intensive care unit: Current concepts in infection. Surg Clin North Am 60:117, 1980.

113. Mela-Riker, L and Tavaroli, H: Mitochondrial function in shock. Am J Emerg Med 2:2, 1983.

114. Michie, HR, et al: Detection of circulating tumor necrosis factor after endotoxin administration. N Engl J Med 318:481, 1988.

115. Mihm, FG and Halperin, BD: Noninvasive detection of profound arterial desaturations using a pulse oximetry device. Anesthesiology 62:85, 1986.

116. Millawah, HA: The relationship between hepatic and cardiac function during hemorrhagic shock in dogs. Ann Surg 51:537, 1985.

117. Moley, JF, et al: Hypothyroidism abolishes the hyperdynamic phases and increases the susceptibility to sepsis. J Surg Res 36:265, 1984.

118. Morris, AH, Chapman, RH, and Gardner, RM: Frequency of wedge pressure errors in the ICU. Crit Care Med 13:705, 1985.

119. Morrison, DC and Ryan, JL: Endotoxins and disease mechanism. Annu Rev Med 38:417, 1987.

120. Mudig, J: Effectiveness of dextran-70 versus Ringer's acetate in traumatic shock and adult respiratory distress syndrome. Crit Care Med 14:454, 1986.

121. Murphy, MB and Elliott, WJ: Dopamine and dopamine receptor agonists in cardiovascular therapy. Crit Care Med 18:S14, 1990.

122. Nagy, S, et al: Histamine levels changes in the plasma and tissues in hemorrhagic shock. Circ Shock 18:235, 1986.

123. Nishijima, MK, et al: Serial changes in cellular immunity of septic patients with multiple system organ failure. Crit Care Med 14:87, 1986.

124. Oettinger, WKE, et al: Endogenous prostaglandin F_2 in the hyperdynamic state of severe sepsis in man. Br J Surg 70:237, 1983.

125. O'Mahony, JB, et al: Depression of cellular immunity after multiple trauma in the absence of sepsis. J Trauma 24:869, 1984.

126. Ordog, FJ and Wasserberger, J: Coagulation abnormalities in traumatic shock. Crit Care Med 14:519, 1986.

127. Parillo, JE: Myocardial depression during septic shock in humans. Crit Care Med 18:1183, 1990.

128. Parker, MM, et al: Profound but reversible myocardial depression in patients with septic shock. Ann Intern Med 100:483, 1984.

129. Parsonnet, J, Gillis, ZE, and Pier, GB: Induction of interleukin-1 strains of Staphlococcus aureus from patients with non-menstrual toxic shock syndrome. J Infect Dis 154:55, 1986.

130. Parsonnet, J, et al: Induction of human interleukin-1 by toxic shock syndrome toxin-1. J Infect Dis 151:514, 1985.

131. Petraglia, F, et al: Serotoninergic agonists increase plasma levels of beta-endorphin and beta-lipotropin in humans. J Clin Endocrinol Metab 59:1138, 1984.

132. Pearce, FJ, Connett, RJ, and Drucker, WR: Phase related changes in tissue energy reserves during hemorrhagic shock. J Surg Res 39:390, 1985.

133. Peitzman, AB, et al: Cellular function in liver and muscle during hemorrhagic shock in primates. Surg Gynecol Obstet 161:419, 1985.

134. Peters, WP, et al: Pressor effect of naloxone in septic shock. Lancet 1:529, 1981.

135. Pfeffer, MA, et al: Systemic hemodynamic effects of leukotrienes C_4 and D_4 in the rat. Am J Physiol 244:H628, 1983.

136. Piper, PJ: Pharmacology of leukotrienes. Br Med Bull 39:255, 1983.

137. Police, AM, Waxman, K, and Tominaga, G: Pulmonary complications after Flusol administration to patients with life-threatening blood loss. Crit Care Med 13:96, 1985.

138. Prough, DS, et al: Effects of hypertonic saline versus lactated Ringer's on cerebral oxygen transport during resuscitation from hemorrhagic shock. J Neurosurg 64:627, 1986.

139. Prough, DS, et al: Effects on cerebral hemodynamics of resuscitation from endotoxin shock with hypertonic saline versus lactated Ringer's solution. Crit Care Med 13:1040, 1985.

140. Puranapanda, V, et al: Erythrocyte deformability in canine septic shock and the efficacy of pentoxifylline and a leukotriene antagonist. Proc Soc Exp Biol Med 185:206, 1987.

141. Rackow, EC, Astiz, ME, and Weil, MH: Cellular oxygen metabolism during sepsis and shock: The relationship of oxygen consumption to oxygen delivery. JAMA 259:1989, 1988.

142. Rackow, EC, et al: Fluid resuscitation in circulatory shock. Crit Care Med 11:839, 1983.

143. Reed, RL, et al: Hypertonic saline alters plasma clotting times and platelet aggregation. Crit Care Med 31:8, 1991.

144. Reedy, JE, et al: Mechanical cardiopulmonary support for refractory cardiogenic shock. Heart Lung 19:514, 1990.

145. Regnier, B, Safrano, CJ, and Teisseire, B: Comparative hemodynamic effects of dopamine and dobutamine in septic shock. Intensive Care Med 5:115, 1979.

146. Roberts, N, et al: Right ventricular infarction with shock but without significant left ventricular infarction: A new clinical syndrome. Am Heart J 110:1047, 1985.

147. Rock, P, et al: Efficacy and safety of naloxone in septic shock. Crit Care Med 13:28, 1985.

148. Ruiz, CE, Weil, MH, and Carlson, RW: Treatment of circulatory shock with dopamine: Studies on survival. JAMA 242:165, 1979.

149. Sabe, TM, et al: Cryoprecipitate reversal of opsonic SB glycoprotein deficiency in septic surgical and trauma patients. Ann Surg 195:177, 1981.

150. Schlag, G and Redl, H: Macropology of the microvascular system in shock: Lung, liver and skeletal muscles. Crit Care Med 13:1045, 1985.
151. Schumer, W: Steroids in the treatment of clinical septic shock. Ann Surg 184:333, 1976.
152. Shatney, CH and Benner, C: Sequential serum complement (C₃) and immunoglobulin levels in shock/trauma patients developing acute fulminating systemic sepsis. Circ Shock 16:9, 1985.
153. Shepherd, RE, McDonough, KH, and Burns, AH: Mechanism of cardiac dysfunction in hearts from endotoxin-treated rats. Circ Shock 19:371, 1984.
154. Shibutani, K, et al: Critical level of oxygen delivery in anesthetized man. Crit Care Med 11:640, 1983.
155. Shigematsu, H, et al: Triiodothyronine improves survival in canine hemorrhagic shock. Circ Shock 16:61, 1985.
155a. Shires, GT, Williams, J, and Brown, F: Acute change in extracellular fluids associated with major surgical procedures. Ann Surg 154:803, 1961.
156. Shoemaker, WC, Appel, PL, and Bland, RD: Use of physiologic monitoring to predict outcome and to assist in clinical decisions in critically ill postoperative patients. Am J Surg 146:43, 1983.
157. Shoemaker, WC, Appel, PL, and Kram, HB: Tissue oxygen debt as a determinant of lethal and nonlethal postoperative organ failure. Crit Care Med 16:1117, 1988.
158. Shoemaker, MC, Trupin, I, and Goldberg, SV: Oxygen transport responses to colloids and crystalloids in critically ill surgical patients. Surg Gynecol Obstet 150:811, 1980.
159. Shoemaker, WC, et al: The efficacy of central venous and pulmonary artery catheters and therapy based upon them in reducing mortality and morbidity. Arch Surg 125:1322, 1990.
160. Shoemaker, WC, et al: Comparison of hemodynamic and oxygen transport effects on dopamine and dobutamine in critically ill surgical patients. Chest 96:120, 1989.
161. Shoemaker, WC, et al: Prospective trial of supranormal values of survivors as therapeutic goals in high risk surgical patients. Chest 94:1176, 1988.
162. Shoemaker, WC, et al: Comparison of two monitoring methods (central venous pressure vs pulmonary artery catheterization) and two protocols as therapeutic goals (normal values vs values of survivors) in a prospective randomized clinical trial of critically ill surgical patients (abstr). Crit Care Med 13:304, 1985.
163. Shoemaker, WC, et al: Effect of hemorrhagic shock on conjunctival and transcutaneous oxygen tensions in relation to hemodynamic and oxygen transport changes. Crit Care Med 12:949, 1984.
164. Sibbald, WJ, et al: Variations in adrenocortical responsiveness during severe bacterial infections: Unrecognized adrenocortical insufficiency in bacterial infections. Ann Surg 186:29, 1977.
165. Simmeson, NE, Simoneson, M, and Palade, GE: Permeability of intestinal capillaries: Pathways followed by dextrans and glycogens. J Cell Biol 53:365, 1972.
166. Singh, S, et al: Cardiorespiratory effects of volume overload with colloidal fluids in dogs. Crit Care Med 11:585, 1983.
167. Slotman, GJ, et al: Thromboxane, prostacyclin, and hemodynamic effects of graded bacteremic shock. Circ Shock 16:395, 1985.
168. Smith, GU, et al: A comparison of several hypertonic solutions for resuscitation of bled sheep. J Surg Res 39:517, 1985.
169. Sprung, CL, et al: Complement activation in septic shock patient. Crit Care Med 14:525, 1986.
170. Sprung, CL, et al: The effects of high-dose corticosteroids in patients with septic shock: A prospective controlled study. N Engl J Med 311:1137, 1984.
171. Stokes, CD, et al: Prediction of arterial blood gas by transcutaneous O₂ and CO₂ in critically ill hyperdynamic trauma patients. J Trauma 26:684, 1986.
172. Sterling, RP, et al: Early bypass grafting following intracoronary thrombolysis. J Thorac Cardiovasc Surg 87:487, 1984.
173. Strieter, RM, Remick, DG, and Ward, PA: Cellular and molecular regulation of tumor necrosis factor-alpha production by pentoxifylline. Biochem Biophys Res Commun 255:1230, 1988.
174. Suffredini, AF, Harpel, PC, and Parrillo, JE: Promotion and subsequent inhibition of plasminogen activation after administration of intravenous endotoxin to normal subjects. N Engl J Med 320:1165, 1989.
175. Sullivan, GW, et al: Inhibition of the inflammatory action of interleukin-1 and tumor necrosis factor (alpha) on neutrophil function by pentoxifylline. Infect Immun 56:1722, 1988.
176. Tanaka, H, et al: Role of granulocyte elastase in tissue injury in patients with septic shock complicated by multiple organ failure. Ann Surg 213:81, 1991.
177. Tempel, GE, et al: The improvement in endotoxin induced redistribution of organ blood blow by inhibition of thromboxane in prostagland synthesis. Adv Shock Res 7:209, 1982.
178. Teng, NH, et al: Protection against gram-negative bacteremia and endotoxemia with human monoclonal IgM antibodies. Proc Natl Acad Sci USA 82:1790, 1985.

179. Thomas, F, et al: Reversible segmental myocardial dysfunction in septic shock. Crit Med 14:587, 1986.

179a. Tighe, D, et al: Pretreatment with pentoxifylline improves the hemodynamic and histologic changes and decreases neutrophil adhesiveness in a pig fecal peritonitis model. Crit Care Med 18:184, 1990.

180. Todd, TX, Glenn, MFX, and Silver, E: A randomized trial of cryoprecipitate replacement of fibronectin deficiencies in the critically ill. Am Rev Respir Dis 129:A102, 1984.

181. Tounes, RN, et al: The role of lung intervention in the hemodynamic response to hypertonic saline solutions in hemorrhagic shock. Surgery 98:900, 1985.

182. Tracey, KJ, et al: Anti-cachectin/TNF monoclonal antibodies prevent septic shock during lethal bacteremia. Nature 330:662, 1987.

183. Tracy, VJ, et al: Shock and tissue injury induced by recombinant human cachetin. Science 2:470, 1986.

184. Tzivoni, D, Keren, A, and Cohen, AM: Magnesium therapy for torsade de pointes. Am J Cardiol 53:528, 1984.

185. Vassar, MJ, Perry, CA, and Holcroft, JW: Analysis of potential risks associated with 7.5% sodium chloride resuscitation of traumatic shock. Arch Surg 125:1310, 1990.

186. Vincent, JL, Roman, A, and Kahn, RJ: Dobutamine administration in septic shock: Addition to a standard protocol. Crit Care Med 18:689, 1990.

187. Waller, JL, et al: Clinical evaluation of new fiberoptic catheter oximeter during cardiac surgery. Anesth Analg 61:676, 1982.

188. Watson, JD, et al: Adrenal vein and systemic levels of catecholamines and metenkephalin-like immunoreactivity in canine endotoxic shock: Effects of naloxone administration. Circ Shock 13:47, 1984.

189. Waxman, K: Pentoxifylline in septic shock. Crit Care Med 18:243, 1990.

190. Weil, MH, Leavy, J, and Rackso, EC: Prognosis in shock. Anesthesia 41:80, 1986.

191. Weiss, SJ: Oxygen, ischemia and inflammation. Acta Physiol Scand (Suppl)548:9, 1986.

192. Weithmann, K: Reduced platelet aggregation by pentoxifylline stimulated prostacyclin release. J Vasc Dis 10:249, 1981.

193. White, CB, et al: The possible role of calcium blockers in cerebral resuscitation: A review of the literature and syntheses for future studies. Crit Care Med 11:202, 1983.

194. Wiencek, RG and Wilson, RF: Abdominal venous injuries. J Trauma 26:771, 1986.

195. Wilson, RF, et al: Antithrombin, prekallikrein, and fibronectin levels in surgical patients. Arch Surg 121:635, 1986.

196. Wise, WC, et al: Ibuprofen, methylprednisolone, and gentamicin as conjoint therapy in septic shock. Circ Shock 17:59, 1985.

197. Wisner, DH, Schuster, L, and Quinn, C: Hypertonic saline resuscitation of head injury: Effects on cerebral water content. J Trauma 30:75, 1990.

198. Yang, SC and Puri, VK: Role of preoperative hemodynamic monitoring in intraoperative fluid management. Am Surg 52:536, 1986.

199. Ziegler, EJ, et al: Treatment of gram-negative bacteremia and septic shock with HA-1A human monoclonal antibody against endotoxin. N Engl J Med 324:429, 1991.

200. Ziegler, EJ, et al: Treatment of gram-negative bacteremia and shock with human antiserum to a mutant Escherichia coli. N Engl J Med 307:1225, 1982.

201. Zimmerman, JL: Therapy for overwhelming sepsis: Clues of treating disease and not just the symptoms. Crit Care Med 18:118, 1990.

CHAPTER 6

Cardiopulmonary Resuscitation (CPR)

I. INTRODUCTION

It has been estimated that 200,000 to 600,000 persons in the United States die annually of cardiac arrest. Extensive research has been directed toward identifying the causes of this problem and determining its optimal treatment. The ideal solution would be to prevent the diseases that cause the cardiac arrest. Modest success has been obtained in the initial resuscitation of these victims, and increasing attention has been directed to treatment of out-of-hospital ventricular fibrillation.

Most cardiac arrests in the community are the result of ischemic heart disease. At least 40% of sudden deaths from ischemic heart disease occur during the first hour after a myocardial infarction, and the proportion is higher— around 60%—among middle-aged and younger men. Over 90% of these deaths occurring outside the hospital are due to ventricular fibrillation, a potentially reversible condition.

Cardiac arrests, particularly in young people, may be due to causes other than ischemic heart disease, such as acute asthma, drug overdose, electrocution, immersion, hypothermia, and so forth. In some circumstances, properly performed cardiopulmonary resuscitation can sustain life for up to an hour while treatment for the underlying condition is being provided. Prolonged resuscitation attempts are usually not appropriate, but they should be considered with cases of (1) drowning in cold water; (2) hypothermia; and (3) overdoses of hypnotic, narcotic, or sedative drugs.

Resuscitation should be started in all patients with sudden loss of consciousness and absent breathing and pulses. It is inappropriate, however, to attempt to resuscitate those patients whose lives are drawing naturally to a close because of irreversible disease.

The goal of CPR is to provide circulation of oxygenated blood to vital organs, especially the heart and brain, while restoring the heart to its precardiac arrest condition. One must halt the degenerative processes usually associated with severe ischemia and anoxia until spontaneous circulation is restored. A successful outcome is the discharge from the hospital of a functioning patient with an intact central nervous system.

AXIOM

CPR is not "successful" unless the patient is neurologically intact.

Cardiopulmonary resuscitation (CPR) is most apt to be effective if it is begun early and is coupled with specific therapeutic interventions. Most cardiopulmonary arrest is due to ventricular fibrillation, and early defibrillation offers the highest probability of success. External cardiac compression alone is inadequate to provide sufficient perfusion to vital organs and, therefore, cannot sustain life by itself, in most circumstances, for more than a few minutes. Many new techniques to increase cardiac output have been developed, but their value has not been established by randomized prospective clinical trials. The American Heart Association guidelines for CPR are still the basis for our current CPR regimen. The therapeutic interventions must be pursued systematically in an expeditious manner so that they key interventions are made within the first 5 minutes of arrest.

In spite of correct application of CPR, the incidence of successful resuscitation (leaving the hospital alive and neurologically intact) is only about 15%. For patients over the age of 70 years or with underlying diseases of cancer, sepsis, or acute stroke, the rate of successful resuscitation and ultimate survival is essentially nonexistent.

AXIOM

The single most accurate predictor of a successful outcome after a cardiac arrest is early electrical conversion of ventricular fibrillation.

Advanced cardiac life support (ACLS) includes (1) basic cardiac life support (BCLS), (2) use of special equipment and techniques, (3) cardiac monitoring and dysrhythmia recognition, (4) establishing IV infusion routes, and (5) treatment for suspected acute myocardial infarction.

II. BASIC CARDIAC LIFE SUPPORT

A. BASIC TECHNIQUES

1. Establishing Unresponsiveness

One shakes the patient and asks: "Are you all right?" "What's happening?" One also *quickly* looks for signs of breathing or chest-wall motion, feels for a carotid pulse, and listens to the chest for heart sounds.

2. Calling for Help

If the patient shows no signs of life, one should call for help, even if this requires that you leave the patient briefly.

3. Positioning the Victim

If the patient is not already supine, one should carefully turn the patient flat on his or her back. However, one must be aware of the possibility of regurgitation of gastric contents and be prepared to turn the head to the side and/or suction out the regurgitated material. If the patient's neck has been injured, it is preferable to "logroll" the entire patient to the side to prevent twisting of the neck.

AXIOM

Patients with a cardiac arrest tend to open their sphincters and have a greatly increased chance of regurgitating gastric contents into their upper airway.

4. Opening the Airway

If there is already evidence of vomitus or blood in the upper airway, one should turn the patient's head to the side (unless cervical spine injury is suspected), and clean out the mouth and pharynx. A tonsil sucker can be very helpful for clearing blood and secretions from the upper airway.

AXIOM

Prolapse of the tongue into the pharynx is the most frequent cause of upper airway obstruction in unconscious individuals.

Whenever a patient loses consciousness, the tongue tends to fall back and occlude the airway. Since the tongue is attached to the anterior mandible by the genioglossus muscle, the upper airway can be opened by using any one of several techniques to move the mandible forward. The techniques most frequently used are referred to as the head tilt-neck lift, head tilt-chin lift, or jaw thrust.

Frontispiece

CARDIOPULMONARY RESUSCITATION (CPR)

(Basic Life Support)

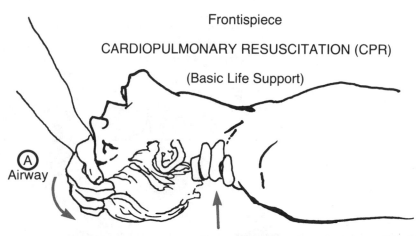

Airway

Figure 6.1 Head tilt–neck lift to open the upper airway. One way to open the airway of an unconscious individual is to lift up on the back of the neck with one hand and press down and back on the forehead with the other hand. This will tilt the jaw forward and hopefully open the airway by pulling the tongue out of the pharynx. This obviously cannot be performed safely on a trauma victim who may have a cervical spine injury. (JAMA, 227:1974.)

a. Head Tilt-Neck Lift (Fig. 6.1)

In patients without trauma, tilting the head back at the occipitocervical junction can be used to open the airway by moving the pharynx back from the tongue and mandible. One hand lifts up the neck close to the occiput while the other hand gently tilts the head backward by pressing on the forehead.

AXIOM

The head tilt cannot be used in trauma victims who may have a cervical spine injury.

b. Head Tilt-Chin Lift (Fig. 6.2)

This maneuver is often the most satisfactory for rescue breathing if the patient is wearing dentures. The head tilt-chin lift can also be used for unconscious patients who are breathing spontaneously. The thumb and index finger of one hand grasp the chin and lift it upward. The fingers should not press on the soft tissues under the chin because this will tend to push the tongue backward into the posterior pharynx. The chin is lifted so that the teeth are brought nearly together, but without completely closing the mouth. The victim's forehead is tilted back with the other hand.

c. Jaw Thrust (Fig. 6.3)

This is a relatively safe method for opening the airway of a victim with suspected neck injury. Nevertheless, in accident victims someone should stabilize the head

Frontispiece

CARDIOPULMONARY RESUSCITATION (CPR)

(Basic Life Support—Adult)

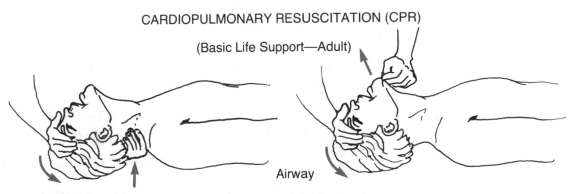

Airway

Figure 6.2 Head tilt–chin lift. Another method for opening the airway of an unconscious individual is to put one hand on the forehead to tilt the head down and back while pushing up the chin or lifting it with the other hand. (JAMA, 244:453, 1980.)

289

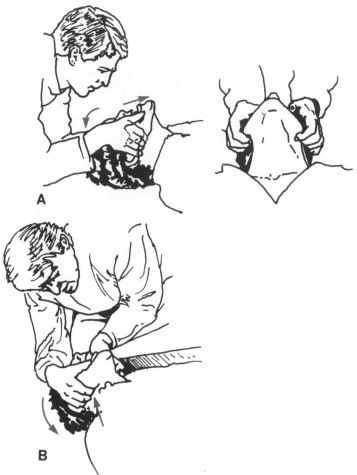

Figure 6.3 Jaw thrust. If the victim is unconscious and not breathing adequately with the backward head tilt or the chin lift, one can try the jaw thrust. To thrust the jaw forward, one grasps the ascending rami of the mandible in front of the ear lobes with the fingers of both hands and pulls forcibly upward (forward), displacing the mandible so that the lower teeth jut out in front of the upper teeth. The lower lip is retracted with the thumbs. It must be emphasized that one does not grasp the horizontal ramus of the mandible on each side because this will close the mouth rather than open it. (Safar, P and Bircher, NG: Cardiopulmonary cerebral resuscitation, 3d ed, WB Saunders, Philadelphia, 1988, p 23.)

while any maneuvers are made to open the airway or insert an endotracheal tube.

To perform the jaw thrust technique, the fingers of both hands are placed on the sides of the face near the angle of the mandible and the mandible is pushed upward and forward without disturbing the position of the cervical spine.

5. Establishing Breathlessness

While maintaining an open airway, one listens carefully over the victim's mouth and nose for air escaping during exhalation. One also looks closely to see if any chest-wall motion occurs that might indicate even some attempt at inspiration. If the patient is not breathing adequately within 5 seconds, rescue breathing should be begun.

6. Rescue Breathing

During rescue breathing one gently pinches the nostrils closed with the thumb and index finger of the hand that is pushing the forehead back to establish the airway. If the jaw thrust is used to open the airway, both hands are occupied, consequently the nares are occluded by placing the cheek tightly against them.

After taking a deep breath, the rescuer places his mouth around the outside of the victim's mouth, making a tight seal. Two quick breaths are given, allowing some lung deflation between breaths.

AXIOM

Whenever possible, one should use a pocket mask, rather than mouth-to-mouth breathing, to inflate the patient's lungs.

When interspersing breaths between cardiac compressions, one should make sure that the patient's chest rises with each breath that is delivered. After delivering each breath, the rescuer's head is turned toward the victim's chest to breathe in fresh air. Atmospheric air contains about 21% oxygen and a negligible amount of carbon dioxide (0.04%), while exhaled air contains 15% to 17% oxygen which should create an arterial Po_2 of about 60 to 70 mm Hg in a patient with otherwise normal lungs.

7. Establishing Absence of Pulses

After giving the two quick breaths and while still kneeling at the victim's side, one hand is placed on the patient's forehead to maintain correct head position and the other hand is used to palpate the carotid pulse. If a carotid pulse is present, but ventilation is absent, rescue breathing is continued at a rate of one breath every 5 seconds. The carotid pulse should be checked once a minute or after every 12 ventilations.

B. CLOSED-CHEST CARDIAC COMPRESSION

AXIOM

If a patient who is thought to have a cardiac arrest has a heart beat but has no effective blood flow, closed-chest cardiac compression should be started.

1. Procedure

If the patient does not have a carotid pulse, external cardiac compression should be started. The correct hand position for external cardiac compression in adults involves placing the heel of one hand one finger breadth above the lower edge of the sternum. The other hand is placed on top of the hand on the sternum. Both hands should be parallel to each other and perpendicular to the sternum. The fingers should be kept off the chest wall. The shoulders are positioned directly over the sternum so that the thrust of compression is straight down. The sternum is depressed 1.5 to 2.0 in with each compression. Optimal cardiac output is achieved if compression comprises 50% to 60% of the cycle. It is important to release the pressure on the sternum completely between compressions to allow the heart to fill maximally.

a. One-Rescuer CPR

If only one rescuer is present, CPR should be performed at 15 chest compressions per cycle at a rate of at least 90 to 100 compressions per minute (5 to 6 cycles per minute at 15 compressions per cycle). After completing one cycle of chest compressions, the rescuer moves the victim's head, the airway is opened, and two quick breaths are delivered before resuming chest compressions. The above cycle is repeated five to six times each minute with a check for the presence of a carotid pulse or spontaneous breathing after each cycle. If spontaneous ventilation and cardiac activity do not occur in the first 1 to 2 minutes, CPR is continued and a check for return of spontaneous breathing and pulse is made every 4 or 5 minutes.

b. Two-Rescuer CPR

When a second rescuer becomes available, he or she interposes rescue breathing during the upstroke of each fifth chest compression. In one of the newer techniques, the ventilation is provided during the cardiac compression. This may increase intrathoracic pressure and thereby increase cardiac output.

The individual ventilating the patient should feel for the carotid pulse frequently to assess the effectiveness of the chest compression. One should also check for the return of spontaneous breathing and pulses every 4 to 5 minutes.

c. Infants and Children

In children, one-rescuer CPR is used. The compression rate should be at least 100 beats per minute in infants, using a ratio of five compressions to one ventilation. Care should be taken to avoid extreme hyperextension of the neck in children, as this may close off the airway. The breaths delivered should not be excessive but should be of a volume sufficient to make the chest rise.

AXIOM
Since the heart of an infant or child is higher in the chest, external cardiac compression is applied to them over the midsternum.

The degree of sternal compression is much less in infants and children than in adults. In infants (less than 2 years of age), the midsternum is depressed only 0.50 to 0.75 inches, using only the tips of the index and middle fingers. For small children (2 to 8 years), the midsternum is depressed 1.0 to 1.5 inches, using the heel of one hand.

2. Effects of Hypothermia

The extreme levels of bradycardia, bradypnea, and peripheral vasoconstriction that often accompany profound hypothermia may complicate the accurate diagnosis of cardiopulmonary arrest in an unmonitored patient. Although CPR is indicated in the truly pulseless, apneic victim of hypothermia, chest compressions may convert a nonpalpable but adequately perfusing sinus bradycardia to ventricular fibrillation. This dilemma has led to disagreement among clinicians and hypothermic researchers about prehospital care protocols for severely hypothermic patients.

PITFALL
Pronouncing a cold patient dead before the hypothermia has been corrected to at least 32°C and preferably 35°C.

3. Improving Closed-Chest Cardiac Massage

Efforts to improve the results of closed-chest cardiac massage have included (1) abdominal binding or pneumatic antishock garment (PASG), (2) simultaneous compression-ventilation CPR (SCV-CPR), (3) pneumatic vest CPR (PV-CPR), (4) interposed abdominal compression CPR (IAC-CPR), and (5) faster compression rates.

a. Abdominal Binding of the Pneumatic Antishock Garment

Abdominal binding or inflation of a pneumatic antishock garment (PASG) was thought to increase the effectiveness of closed-chest cardiac massage by preventing the descent and eversion of the diaphragm. Abdominal binding tends to increase afterload, systolic blood pressure (BP), and carotid blood flow, but it did not improve myocardial perfusion and cardiac resuscitability. In addition, there was some concern about the possibility of an increased incidence of liver lacerations with this technique.

b. Simultaneous Compression-Ventilation CPR

Simultaneous compression-ventilation CPR (SCV-CPR) is a method of resuscitation designed to increase intrathoracic pressure through simultaneous chest compressions and ventilations at high airway pressures. Early studies demonstrated that simultaneous compression-ventilation CPR produced superior systolic, diastolic, and mean arterial pressures, carotid blood flow, and cardiac output. In addition, SCV-CPR has been shown to provide statistically significant increases in cerebral blood flow when compared with standard external CPR (SE-CPR) in selected animal models.

Simultaneous compression-ventilation CPR has been shown to increase coronary artery blood flow as compared with SE-CPR in some experimental studies, but not in others. Although Luce and associates found statistically significant increases in coronary perfusion pressure with SCV-CPR at high intrathoracic pressures as compared with low intrathoracic pressures, no SE-CPR controls were provided. To date, SCV-CPR has not produced myocardial blood flows greater than the 20 ml·min⁻¹·100 g⁻¹ which is thought to be necessary to maintain the viability of the fibrillating heart. Bircher and Safar studied SCV-CPR after 4 minutes of ventricular fibrillation and 30 minutes of CPR, demonstrating no superiority of SCV-CPR in resuscitability, survival, or neurologic deficit score at 24 hours in experimental animals when compared with SE-CPR.

In studies on 10 patients, Chandra and colleagues demonstrated significant increases in radial artery pressure and carotid blood flow with SCV-CPR. Martin and associates, however, could find no superiority of SCV-CPR over SE-CPR in coronary perfusion pressures in five patients undergoing CPR.

c. Pneumatic Vest SCV-CPR

Using a pneumatic vest to increase the effectiveness of SCV-CPR, Luce and coworkers and Halperin and associates in separate studies reported increased cerebral blood flow. Halperin and associates were also able to show an improved survival and neurologic outcome. However, the high pressures (380 mm Hg) used in the vest may be a problem.

d. Interposed Abdominal Compression CPR

The addition of interposed abdominal compressions to otherwise standard CPR has enhanced circulation in anesthetized dogs with ventricular fibrillation, primarily by increasing venous return to the heart. Limited clinical studies confirm that IAC-CPR can improve perfusion pressures in humans, and that complications of the technique are rare. However, no study has demonstrated that IAC-CPR improves either short- or long-term survival. Accordingly, the method remains experimental and cannot be recommended for basic life support or CPR at this time.

e. Faster Compression Rates

AXIOM
Faster rates of chest compression tend to increase BP and cardiac output.

Feneley and others have found that increasing the closed-chest massage rate from 60 to 120 per minute increased the incidence of successful defibrillation from 40% (6/13) to 92% (12/13). Maier and colleagues also found that the more rapid rate, particularly if combined with increased force, significantly increased myocardial blood flow.

f. Cardiopulmonary Bypass

Martin and his group have been working some time on the feasibility of using cardiopulmonary bypass (CPB) in animals and in selected patients who are unresponsive to standard CPR. Although it requires a skilled team to get these patients on CPB promptly, it quickly restores a normal cardiac output and seems to greatly improve the chances of a complete neurologic recovery.

4. How Does Chest Compression Generate Blood Flow?

a. Classic Concept

For a number of years it was thought that external cardiac compression squeezed the heart between the sternum and thoracic vertebrae and thereby forced blood out of the left ventricle into the aorta and out of the right ventricle into the lungs. Retrograde flow back into the heart was prevented by the cardiac valves. Total intrathoracic pressures were not considered to play any significant role, except perhaps for retarding venous return to the heart.

b. Cough CPR

One of the main reasons that investigators began to question the classic concept of how external CPR worked was the observation by Criley, Blaufuss, and Kissell that patients who developed ventricular fibrillation during cardiac catheterization could maintain themselves in a conscious state for up to 90 seconds by frequent forceful coughing. They also noted that forceful coughing could generate systolic pressures of 100 to 160 mm Hg. Increasing the amplitude of the cough increased the pressure generated, which in turn increased blood flow in a linear fashion. The effects of forceful coughing on BP caused investigators to feel that the total intrathoracic pressure might be a major factor in producing blood flow with closed chest CPR.

293

AXIOM

Forward blood flow with external cardiac massage is probably due primarily to changes in intrathoracic pressure rather than direct compression of the heart.

c. Pressure Gradients

In animal studies, no gradient has been found between the major arteries and veins in the chest during the compression phase of external CPR. In all instances, the pressures inside intrathoracic vessels were nearly equal to the intrathoracic pressures outside the vessels. However, in vessels outside the chest, there was a definite gradient between the major arteries and veins. Thus, the intrathoracic pressures developed during external CPR were transmitted to extrathoracic arteries, but not to extrathoracic veins.

Neimann and associates showed that the intrathoracic-to-extrathoracic venous pressure gradient in dogs is caused by venous valves at the thoracic inlet. Venous valves were identified by human anatomists in the 19th century. Their functional status in men was defined by Fisher and colleagues who studied thoracic inlet venous valves during cardiac catheterization and showed that these valves were competent and prevented the cephalad transmission of intrathoracic pressure and flow of blood at transvalvular pressures of >100 mm Hg.

Extrathoracic arterial pressures are similar to intrathoracic arterial pressures, but because of venous valves and possibly venous collapse, the intrathoracic venous pressure is significantly higher than extrathoracic venous pressure. Hence, a peripheral arterial-venous (a-v) pressure gradient is generated and results in the forward flow of blood. Thus, venous valves are key in developing the extrathoracic pressure gradient (which is essential for flow in any fluid-filled system) that is independent of the mechanism by which blood flow is primarily occurring.

AXIOM

Blood flow occurs during external chest compressions or coughing because of an extrathoracic a-v pressure gradient.

During closed-chest CPR, blood circulates because, although the increased intrathoracic pressure is transmitted equally to all intrathoracic structures, it is transmitted unequally to the extrathoracic arteries and veins. This creates an extrathoracic a-v pressure gradient that allows forward blood flow. After each compression, intrathoracic pressure falls to normal, and blood flows into the lungs as a result of an extrathoracic venous-to-intrapulmonary pressure gradient (Fig. 6.4).

Recent detailed hemodynamic studies in large dogs support the hypothesis that during CPR in humans, manipulation of intrathoracic pressure contributes substantially to the blood flow that occurs during prolonged resuscitation. This hypothesis is strengthened by their observation that abdominal compression with no sternal movement can produce BP values comparable with those generated by sternal displacement.

d. Other Techniques

The finding that blood flow during external chest compression may be due to increased intrathoracic pressure and the subsequent reporting of increased carotid blood flow with simultaneous ventilation and chest compression or with abdominal binding during CPR ignited a flurry of investigations into alternative approaches to CPR. A number of alterations of the conventional CPR technique resulted in improved hemodynamics. However, some of the proposed methods increased cerebral blood flow but decreased myocardial perfusion. Others improved systolic pressures but decreased vital organ blood flow. More important, most studies with survival as an end point failed to show a benefit when alternative approaches to CPR were used. Therefore, it is unlikely that there will be significant changes in the recommendations for the use of mechanical adjuncts during CPR.

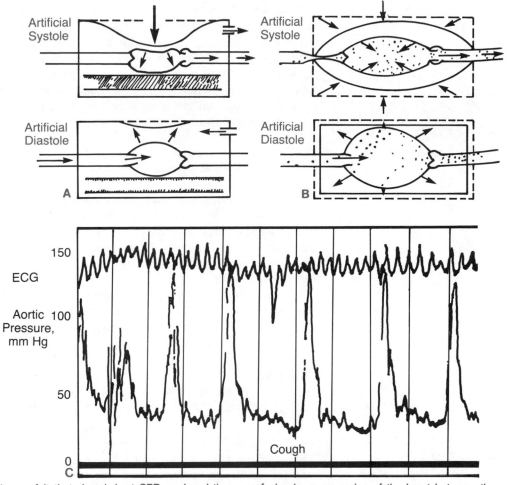

Figure 6.4 (*A*) Traditionally it was felt that closed-chest CPR produced tissue perfusion by compression of the heart between the sternum and the spine. According to this theory, as the heart is compressed, the cardiac valves prevent retrograde flow, and blood is forced out of the heart. Between compressions, chest resiliency generates a negative pressure and draws blood into the heart. This is called the "cardiac pump mechanism." (*B*) An alternate view, that of the "thoracic pump mechanism," holds that it is compression of the chest, not the heart, that propels blood during closed chest cardiac massage. According to this view, thoracic compression generates a positive intrathoracic pressure, which is vented by arterial outflow to peripheral tissues. The cardiac valves are irrelevant. Between compressions, chest resiliency generates a negative pressure and draws blood into the heart. (*C*) Cough-induced arterial pressure spikes during ventricular fibrillation. Criley has found that regular vigorous coughing in patients who developed ventricular fibrillation during cardiac catheterization was able to maintain reasonable tissue perfusion and consciousness for short periods of time. (Elefteriades, JA: Cardiopulmonary resuscitation. In AE Baue, et al: Glenn's Thoracic and Cardiovascular Surgery vol. 2. Appleton & Lange, Norwalk, 1991, pp 1530–1531.)

5. Complications of Basic CPR

PITFALL

Failing to detect gastric dilatation until the patient has regurgitated and aspirated.

a. Gastric Distention

In most adults, rescue breathing with a tidal volume of 800 to 1200 ml will be adequate to make the chest rise. However, rescue breathing using such large tidal volumes is also apt to cause gastric distention. Consequently, smaller tidal volumes are now recommended. Gastric distention not only restricts lung volume by elevating the diaphragm, but it may also induce vomiting.

AXIOM

Excessive ventilatory force applied through mouth-to-mouth or mask-to-mouth ventilation increases the risk of aspiration of gastric contents.

295

If gastric distention does occur, excessive airway pressure should be avoided during continued ventilatory attempts. However, attempting to relieve gastric distention by pressing on the victim's abdomen will usually cause vomiting with likely aspiration. If vomiting does occur, the patient's head should be turned to the side, the mouth wiped or suctioned clean, and CPR resumed. As soon as possible, during or after the CPR, an endotracheal tube should be inserted, and the tracheobronchial tree should be suctioned out and also bronchoscoped to remove material from the smaller bronchi.

b. Visceral Injury

PITFALL
Use of excessive force during external CPR in an effort to obtain a better pulse.

In one study, 21% of the patients with external cardiac compressions had at least one complication directly due to the CPR. Patients who were resuscitated on the wards were more likely to have complications than those treated in intensive care units. Incorrect hand position or the application of excessive force can cause severe injuries, including fractured ribs or sternum and lacerations of the spleen or liver.

It has been found that the Recording Resusci-Anne manikin is much stiffer than the human chest. This may cause rescuers to use more force than necessary on patients. Consequently, newer manikins with characteristics more like a human chest should be constructed.

AXIOM
Hypotension after apparently successful closed-chest massage may be due to an abdominal visceral injury caused by the chest compressions.

III. AIRWAY OBSTRUCTION

A. DIAGNOSIS

Cardiac arrest may be prevented in some patients by early recognition and treatment of foreign bodies causing airway obstruction. If a foreign body is in the airway but air exchange is adequate, the victim can often cough. However, there may be inspiratory wheezing between coughs, indicating that a partial airway obstruction is present. As long as there is good air exchange, the victim is encouraged to continue with spontaneous coughing and breathing. A child with partial airway obstruction and good air exchange should not be turned upside down because this may cause a foreign body below the glottis to become impacted against the vocal cords.

PITFALL
Failing to consider a foreign body in the airway of someone who is having trouble breathing.

With complete airway obstruction, the victim is unable to speak, breathe, or cough at all. If he is awake, he may clutch his neck as a universal distress signal. In the unconscious victim, airway obstruction may be diagnosed by noting a lack of air movement in spite of efforts to ventilate the patient.

B. TREATMENT

1. Usual Techniques

AXIOM
Poor air exchange (characterized by a weak, ineffective cough, inspiratory stridor, and respiratory distress) should be managed as if it were a complete airway obstruction.

Three maneuvers that have been recommended for relieving airway obstruction by a foreign body include (1) back blows, (2) manual thrusts, and (3) manual foreign-body removal. Back blows produce an instantaneous increase in intrathoracic and airway pressure, which may result in either partial or complete dislodgement of the foreign body. Manual thrusts produce a more sustained increase in airway pressure and may further assist in dislodging the foreign body. Combining these two techniques may be even more effective.

AXIOM
The abdominal thrust is probably the safest and most effective method for dislodging a foreign body in the upper airway.

a. Back Blows

The back blow technique is a series of four rapid, sharp blows delivered over the spine between the shoulder blades with the heel of the hand. They may be given with the victim standing, sitting, or lying, and should be applied forcefully and rapidly. Whenever possible, the victim's head should be lower than his or her chest to make use of gravity.

b. Thrusts or Squeezes

(1) Manual Thrusts

The manual thrust technique is designed to suddenly force air out of the lungs. There appears to be no substantial difference in air flow or pressure generated by the abdominal or chest thrust. The chest thrust is useful if the rescuer cannot fully wrap her or his arms around the victim's abdomen, or when direct abdominal pressure is likely to cause complications, as in advanced pregnancy.

If the victim is lying down, the head and neck should be positioned so that the upper airway is open. The rescuer can be positioned either astride or alongside the victim. It is preferable to be alongside the victim because the rescuer has more maneuverability. The heel of one hand is placed against the victim's abdomen between the xiphoid and the umbilicus. This hand is covered with the heel of the other hand. One then presses into the victim's abdomen with a quick upward thrust.

Victims can perform the maneuver on themselves by delivering a quick upward thrust to the abdomen with the fist or by leaning forward and compressing the abdomen over any firm object, such as the back of a chair or table.

(2) Abdominal Thrust (Squeeze)

If the victim is sitting or standing, the rescuer stands behind the victim and wraps his or her arms around the victim's waist. A fist is made with one hand and the thumb side of that fist is placed against the victim's abdomen between the xiphoid and the umbilicus. The free hand is placed around the fist, and four quick upward thrusts are delivered (Fig. 6.5).

(3) Chest Thrust (Squeeze)

When it is necessary to perform a chest thrust on a victim who is standing or sitting, the rescuer stands behind the victim, places her or his arms under the victim's axillae, and encircles her or his arms around the victim's chest. The thumb side of one fist is placed on the victim's midsternum. The fist is grasped with the other hand, and four forceful compressions are delivered (Fig. 6.6).

c. Manual Removal of a Foreign Body

PITFALL
Pushing a high foreign body further down into the airway while attempting to remove it.

If a foreign body is seen in the victim's mouth, it should be removed. However, blind probing for a foreign body may aggravate an airway obstruction. In infants and small children, an adult's probing finger may force a foreign body into the larynx and cause complete airway obstruction. Nevertheless, with careful technique, a large foreign body can sometimes be dislodged and removed manually if it is at or above the level of the epiglottis.

The methods for opening a victim's mouth to remove a foreign body are the tongue lift (Fig. 6.7) and the crossed-finger technique (Fig. 6.8). With the tongue lift, the victim's head is up or turned to the side, and the tongue and lower jaw are grasped between the thumb and fingers and lifted. This pulls the tongue out

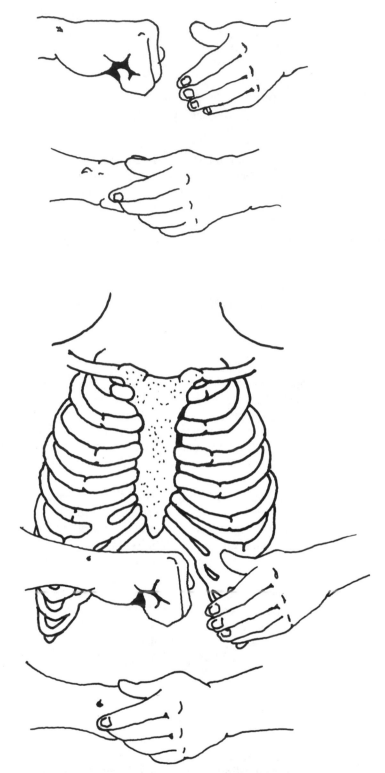

Figure 6.5 Abdominal thrust with victim standing or sitting. To perform an abdominal thrust on a conscious, choking patient, the rescuer stands behind the victim and wraps his arms around the victim's waist. He grasps his fist with the other hand and places the thumb side of his fist against the victim's abdomen, between the waist and the rib cage. He then presses his fist four times into the victim's abdomen with a quick inward and upward thrust. The rescuer's hands should never be placed on the xiphoid process of the sternum or on the lower margins of the rib cage. Use of the abdominal trust instead of the chest thrust in older victims might avoid fracture of brittle ribs. However, regurgitation of gastric contents can occur as a result of this maneuver. (JAMA 244:465, 1980.)

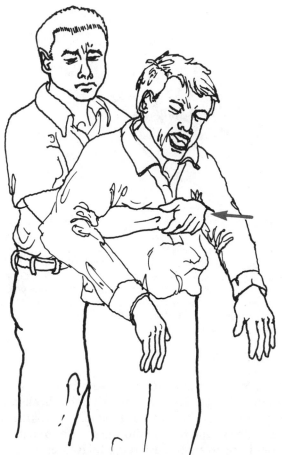

Figure 6.6 Chest thrust. This is an alternative technique to the abdominal thrust for relieving choking. The rescuer stands behind the victim, his arms directly under the victim's armpits, and encircles the victim's chest. He places the thumb side of his fist on the middle of the breastbone (sternum), taking care to avoid the xiphoid process and the margins of the rib cage. He then grasps his fist with his other hand and exerts four vigorous backward thrusts. Each thrust should be administered with the intent of relieving the obstruction without having to complete the full series. Whenever possible, the victim should be leaning forward to make the most effective use of gravity. (JAMA 244:465, 1980.)

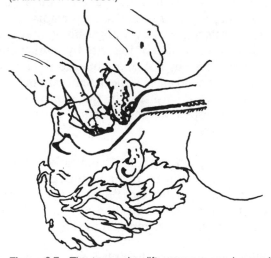

Figure 6.7 The tongue-jaw-lift maneuver can be used in patients with a fully relaxed jaw. The thumbs are inserted into the patient's mouth and throat. The tip of one thumb lifts the base of the tongue. The other fingers grasp the mandible at the chin and lift it up and anteriorly. (Safar, P and Bircher, NG: Cardiopulmonary cerebral resuscitation, 3d ed. WB Saunders, Philadelphia, 1988, p 26.)

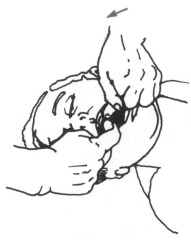

Figure 6.8 The crossed-finger maneuver is used to open the upper airway in patients with a moderately relaxed jaw. The rescuer is positioned at the top of the side of the patient's head. The index finger is inserted into the corner of the mouth and then pressed against the upper teeth to force the jaws apart. The thumb, crossed over the index finger, presses against the lower teeth. To leave ample room for instrumentation, the fingers are inserted into the far corner of the patient's mouth. (Safar, P and Bircher, NG: Cardiopulmonary cerebral resuscitation, 3d ed. WB Saunders, Philadelphia, 1988, p 26.)

of the posterior pharynx and away from the foreign body. The index finger is inserted along the inside of the victim's cheek and then moved around into the pharynx to the base of the tongue. A hooking action is used to dislodge the foreign body and slide it into the mouth so that it can be removed. One must be careful not to push the foreign body deeper into the airway. Once the foreign body comes within reach, it is removed. If the victim has dentures, they should also be removed.

2. Unconscious Patient

If the patient with an airway obstruction becomes unconscious, muscle tone tends to decrease, and this will occasionally loosen or dislodge the foreign body. If the foreign body remains in place, the airway should be opened and an attempt made to ventilate the patient with a quick breath. For airways that remain obstructed after several such attempts, rapidly delivered back blows and manual thrusts followed by a finger probe may succeed in clearing the airway. These maneuvers should be followed by another attempt to ventilate the patient. If the chest does not rise, the sequence should be repeated. External cardiac compression is of no value if the patient cannot be ventilated. If the foreign body becomes visible at any step in the sequence, it must be removed at once. Spontaneous respiratory and/or return of a pulse may occur once the foreign body is removed.

3. Infants and Small Children

The positioning and method of application of back blows and manual thrusts are slightly different in an infant or small child. Back blows should be applied to an infant with the victim face down on the rescuer's forearm and with the head and chest in a dependent position. If four back blows are ineffective, four firm sustained thrusts are delivered to the child's back between the shoulder blades.

4. Ancillary Procedures

a. Endoscopy

If facilities are available, direct laryngoscopy can be performed and the foreign body removed with forceps. Bronchoscopy, preferably of the rigid type, may be necessary to remove a foreign body that has lodged below the vocal cords.

b. Cricothyroidotomy (Coniotomy)

If the above maneuvers are unsuccessful, a cricothyroidotomy may be lifesaving. The technique can also be used to establish an airway when there is any intrinsic airway obstruction due to conditions such as laryngospasm, laryngeal edema, or tumor. For an adult, a cannula of at least 5 mm (inside diameter) should be inserted to ensure adequate air flow. In children under the age of 12 years, a 14- to 16-gauge needle cricothyroidotomy attached to intermittent wall oxygen is preferred. With a needle catheter cricothyroidotomy, however, carbon dioxide retention may be a problem.

c. Compressed-Air Insufflation

In some situations, adequate oxygen exchange can be maintained in an adult for 30 to 45 minutes by intermittent compressed-air insufflation through a 14-gauge intracatheter inserted into the cricothyroid membrane or upper trachea. The catheter is threaded 2 to 3 in down the trachea and is connected by extension tubing to a release valve, which may simply be a hole in the tubing that can be covered by a finger while insufflating the lung. This is connected by more tubing to a pressure adjustment valve on a source of compressed oxygen. If the lungs do not deflate when the insufflation pressure is released, expiration should be facilitated by compressing the chest. If the lungs still do not deflate, an alternate method of airway control is indicated.

d. Tracheostomy

PITFALL
Performing an unnecessary emergency tracheostomy.

Tracheostomy is generally performed as an elective procedure for long-term airway care with an endotracheal tube already in place. Occasionally, however, with a high upper tracheal obstruction or a traumatic cricotracheal separation, a tracheostomy may have to be performed as an emergency procedure.

IV. ADJUNCTIVE EQUIPMENT FOR CPR

Supplemental oxygen should be used as soon as it becomes available. Rescue breathing (exhaled-air ventilation) will deliver 15% to 17% oxygen to the patient, producing an alveolar oxygen tension of about 60 to 70 mm Hg under ideal circumstances. However, because of the low cardiac output with resultant very low venous oxygen levels and because of the increased intrapulmonary shunting associated with external chest compression, severe hypoxemia will generally be present unless supplemental oxygen is given.

A. ADJUNCTS FOR AIRWAY AND VENTILATION

1. Oxygen

2. Oropharyngeal (Oral) Airway

Oropharyngeal airways should be used whenever a bag-valve-mask system or manually cycled oxygen-powered resuscitator with mask is used on an unconscious patient. However, if the patient wakes up, the oral airway is apt to make the patient gag and/or vomit. As soon as appropriately trained individuals become available, the trachea should be intubated.

3. Esophageal Obturator Airway

The esophageal obturator airway (EOA) was developed by Don Michael in 1968. The device resembles an elongated endotracheal tube (ET), but is approximately 1.5 times the length of the standard ET. The distal end is occluded, and near the proximal end are numerous holes that will be located in the posterior pharynx and hypopharynx once the tube has been positioned. A face mask is attached to the most proximal end of the tube to prevent air from leaking out of the mouth. The device is passed blindly into the pharynx and esophagus, and then advanced until the mask is seated on the face. A balloon located near the distal end of the tube is inflated with approximately 30 to 35 ml of air to occlude the esophagus. Air is forced into the tube, and it exits through the holes in the proximal end of the tube lying in the pharynx and mouth. The air will then flow into the larynx and trachea. Proper positioning of the face mask and a good air-tight seal are essential for adequate ventilation. Proper placement of the device is confirmed by auscultation of breath sounds and visualization of chest-wall motion with each ventilation.

The esophageal gastric tube airway (EGTA) is a newer modification of the EOA. The distal tip of this tube is open, and there is a port on the face mask through which a tube can be passed to decompress the stomach. The lungs are ventilated through a separate port on the mask. The obvious advantage of this modification is that it permits passage of a nasogastric tube to decompress the stomach. However, the esophagus is still occluded to air or oxygen that is administered through the face mask.

Another variation of the EOA is a long tube, which is attached to a face mask with two ports. One port opens into the lumen of the tube, and the other port opens into the oropharynx. If the tube is passed into the esophagus, the patient is ventilated through the side port into the oropharynx. If the tube enters the trachea, direct ventilation through the tube can be accomplished.

The most recent alteration in this device is the development of an airway called the esophageal tracheal combitube (ETC). This is a double-lumen tube. One lumen resembles an endotracheal tube and the other resembles the EOA. There are two balloons on the airway: one on the distal end which can be inflated with 10 to 15 ml of air, and a proximal balloon that occludes the posterior pharynx when inflated with 100 ml of air. If the device is inserted into the esophagus, that portion of the tube is occluded and the opposite lumen is used to ventilate the patient.

Regardless of the device used, if the tube has been placed into the esophagus, endotracheal intubation should be performed as soon as possible, and the tube in the esophagus removed.

Following are advantages of the EOA over the endotracheal tube:

1. Minimal instruction is needed for its use.
2. Minimal skill and dexterity is required for its insertion.
3. It may be inserted blindly (vocal cord visualization not needed).
4. It is often performed more rapidly than endotracheal intubation.
5. No movement of the head or neck is necessary.

In a recent review by Pons, it was found that these "advantages" may be more perceived than real. In one report, the didactic training time for the EOA/EGTA was 3 hours versus 4.5 hours for endotracheal intubation (ETI) and the clinical practice times were 1 hour and 2.5 hours for EOA/EGTA and ETI, respectively. Another prehospital system documents that the training time for the EOA was 16 hours. The issues of skill, dexterity, and blind insertion are not as important as the ability and knowledge to recognize intubation of the wrong structure, regardless of which device is used.

Success rates for performing ETI or insertion of an EOA/EGTA reveal rather diverse results. Successful rates with ETI have ranged from 50% to 98%, although most studies indicate success rates between 88% and 97%. EOA/EGTA success rates are generally similar, with most reports showing 88% to 95% successful placement.

When used by well-trained individuals, complications occur rarely; however, a number of esophageal lacerations and ruptures have been reported, and even in experienced hands, the EOA may be inadvertently inserted into the trachea.

The esophageal obturator airway (EOA) has been in use for over 15 years and has been inserted in several million patients. However, its use is declining and it is rarely used in-hospital.

4. Endotracheal Intubation

As soon as practical, the trachea should be intubated by trained personnel. This isolates the airway, keeps it patent, prevents aspiration, and ensures the delivery of high concentrations of oxygen to the lungs. With a cuffed endotracheal tube, it is much easier to provide adequate ventilation, especially during CPR, than with bag-valve-mask techniques.

5. Mechanical Ventilation

Patients with a cardiac arrest are usually best ventilated by squeezing a bag; however, with prolonged CPR, a volume-cycled or time-cycled ventilator may be used. These ventilators have high instantaneous flow rates that can provide adequate ventilation, even during periods of increased intrathoracic pressure. Most can also function as inhalers for patients who are breathing spontaneously but require oxygen.

6. Suction Devices

Portable and installed suction equipment should be available for resuscitation emergencies. The portable unit should provide enough vacuum to remove copious, thick secretions or vomitus.

B. ADJUNCTS FOR CLOSED-CHEST MASSAGE

PITFALL
Attempting to give closed-chest cardiac massage while the patient is lying on a soft surface or bed.

1. Bedboard

CPR should be performed at the site where the victim is found. If the cardiac arrest occurs in a hospital bed, a bedboard should be placed beneath the patient's back so the patient will not bounce on the mattress. The bedboard should extend from the shoulders to the waist and across the full width of the bed. If the bedboard is not available, the patient should be gently moved to a stretcher or onto the floor.

2. Mechanical Chest Compressors

Mechanical devices that depress the sternum are usually not an adequate substitute for good manual external chest compression. However, they can be used as an adjunct by trained personnel to help with prolonged resuscitative efforts. Since the efficacy and safety of these devices have not been demonstrated in infants and children, their use should be limited to adults.

Simple, hinged, manually operated mechanical chest compressors can provide an adjustable stroke of 1.5 to 2 in and can be applied after only a brief interruption of the manual CPR. Advantages include relatively modest cost; ease of storage, transport, and assembly; light weight; and minimal possibility of mechanical breakdown. Problems related to their use include a tendency for the compressor head to shift position and for the tightening device to become loosened so that the plunger does not compress the chest adequately.

3. Pneumatic Antishock Garment

Central blood volume may be increased by elevation of the legs or by compression of legs and lower abdomen with a pneumatic antishock garment (PASG). PASGs have three compartments that allow for separate inflation of each lower extremity and the abdomen. Preliminary observations in animals suggest that, during cardiac arrest, blood pressure can be increased substantially while the garment is inflated. The pneumatic antishock garment has also been effective in treating hypovolemic shock from injuries to the lower extremities or pelvis. Much of the rise in BP with its use in trauma victims now appears to be due to an increased afterload, rather than an increased central blood volume.

PITFALL
If a PASG is inflated for too long a period, the chances of the patient developing a compartment syndrome are increased.

C. INTRA-AORTIC BALLOON PUMP

Another adjunct to circulation currently available is the intra-aortic balloon pump (IABP). Indications for using IABP include left ventricular power failure and severe persistent cardiogenic shock in spite of vasoactive drugs. Myocardial oxygen demand may be reduced and coronary blood flow increased dramatically with IABP.

303

V. INTERNAL (OPEN) CHEST CPR

A. EFFECTIVENESS

Open-chest CPR is a technique of resuscitation that has been employed in humans for many years and was the only means of cardiac massage until the early to mid-1960s, when closed-chest cardiac massage became increasingly popular. Nevertheless, many studies have shown that open-chest cardiac massage provides higher cardiac output and much more cerebral blood flow than closed-chest massage. Del Guercio found that closed-chest cardiac massage in patients produced only 20% of the control cardiac output while open cardiac massage resulted in a cardiac output that averaged more than 40% of control.

AXIOM

Open-chest cardiac massage provides much better coronary and cerebral blood flow than closed-chest compression.

Our own studies in the shock unit showed an average cardiac output of only 0.3 to 0.8 liter/min with closed-chest massage and cardiac outputs of 1.0 to 1.8 liters/min with open massage using the cardiogreen technique for measuring cardiac output. Furthermore, systolic BPs obtainable with closed-chest massage averaged only about 50 to 60 mm Hg whereas open massage would generally produce pressures at least 50% higher. Uniformly better results were obtained with open cardiac massage even though it was usually only started after 4 to 6 minutes had already been spent on closed-chest massage.

It has been shown that open-chest massage in dogs can produce a cardiac output that is 30% to 70% of control while closed massage produced a cardiac output of only 20% of control. Other benefits of open (vs. closed) cardiac massage have included significantly improved diastolic blood pressure, cerebral blood flow, and neurologic outcome. Significant clinical successes and a growing body of animal data have documented the superiority of open cardiac massage over standard closed-chest massage. However, except in trauma patients, the practice and teaching of open cardiac massage ceased almost entirely with the introduction of closed-chest massage in the 1960.

B. INDICATIONS

Emergency thoracotomy for open cardiac massage is now used almost entirely in cardiac arrests after trauma or cardiac surgery. Studies suggest that thoracotomy should continue to be the primary intervention in cardiac arrest secondary to penetrating trauma, particularly with chest injuries and if vital signs were present at the scene.

PITFALL

Use of closed-chest massage to resuscitate patients with cardiac arrest due to penetrating chest trauma.

Closed-chest CPR is usually of little value if the patient is hypovolemic or if pericardial tamponade is present. Indeed, with blunt trauma, closed-chest massage is very apt to aggravate the injuries.

Indications for emergency thoracotomy and open cardiac massage in non-traumatic arrests are less easy to define. However, it may be useful in any cardiac arrest where closed chest massage fails to result in successful resuscitation after several minutes. Conditions that may indicate a need for immediate institution of open cardiac massage include pericardial tamponade, massive pulmonary embolus, tension pneumothorax, chest-wall or vertebral abnormalities, air embolus, and third trimester of pregnancy.

C. CONTINUING QUESTIONS

Although there is ample evidence supporting the hemodynamic superiority of open cardiac massage over closed-chest massage, the closed technique remains a means of cardiopulmonary resuscitation that can be employed by lay persons as well as physicians both inside and outside the hospital. What remains to be defined is the appropriate role of open cardiac massage in the patients with nontraumatic cardiac arrest. Other specific questions are (1) What is the maximal period of total circulatory arrest that can be tolerated without causing severe central nervous system damage? (2) How long can standard CPR be performed after which open-chest CPR will no longer be efficacious? Randomized trials are needed to determine when open cardiac massage should be started if standard advanced cardiac life support does not result in prompt restoration of spontaneous circulation.

D. DIRECT MECHANICAL VENTRICULAR ASSISTANCE

Opening the chest and placing a mechanical compressing device directly on the heart can improve diastolic blood pressures and improve cardiac index for prolonged periods, even for days with normal outcome. McCabe found that direct mechanical ventricular assistance produced better diastolic pressures than CCM and OCCM (15 vs. 44 vs. 92 mm Hg) and better cardiac indices (19% vs. 59% vs. 86% of control). The clinical applicability of this device, however, is not clear.

VI. MONITORING

In addition to monitoring the patient clinically, one should also monitor his or her cardiovascular system and metabolic function as exactly and continuously as possible.

A. CLINICAL

The color and temperature of the skin may help indicate the adequacy of tissue perfusion. A warm, dry, pink skin tends to indicate a better perfusion than cold, mottled, cyanotic extremities. Reactive, medium-diameter pupils imply better perfusion than fixed dilated pupils. However, one must have a bright enough light to check for papillary responses.

AXIOM
The most common cause for nonreactive pupils is a weak flash light.

Pulses should be felt for at the wrist, groin, and in the neck. It is said that the following minimal systolic pressures are needed to feel the various pulses: carotid, 60 mm Hg; groin (femoral), 70 mm Hg; and wrist, 80 mm Hg. However, these numbers are not at all reliable, and it can be very difficult to differentiate the shaking of the body with each chest compression from the arterial pulse.

B. CARDIOSCOPE

Electrocardiographic monitoring should be established as soon as possible on all patients who have a suspected heart attack or sudden collapse. Most sudden deaths following acute myocardial infarction are caused by arrhythmias, especially ventricular fibrillation. The incidence of these arrhythmias is greatest immediately after myocardial damage or severe ischemia and for several hours thereafter.

C. ARTERIAL BLOOD GASES

PITFALL
Administering bicarbonate during CPR without first evaluating both arterial and mixed venous blood gases.

The amount of ventilation and bicarbonate provided during CPR should be guided by frequent arterial blood gas analyses rather than empiric rules. The arterial pH may be extremely variable during cardiac arrest, and giving sodium bicarbonate ($NaHCO_3$) to a patient who is already alkalemic may be disastrous. Furthermore, giving $NaHCO_3$ to a patient with a high mixed venous Pco_2 will only increase the tendency to a respiratory acidosis. An indwelling arterial line is preferable for ABG analysis because intermittent sticks might obtain venous rather than arterial blood.

D. ARTERIAL PRESSURE

If an intra-arterial pressure line can be inserted, usually by cut-down early in the CPR, it can help greatly in determining the effectiveness of the cardiac massage and need for more epinephrine for its alpha-vasoconstricting effect. Such a line can also be used for frequent ABG analysis.

E. CENTRAL VENOUS PRESSURE AND GASES

Knowing the central venous pressure (CVP) can be helpful in determining if further fluid should be given to improve blood pressure and coronary and cerebral perfusion. The differences between central venous and arterial pH and P_{CO_2} can also help determine the adequacy of overall blood flow. The greater the difference between arterial and central venous values, the poorer the overall cardiac output and blood flow to the lungs.

The central venous P_{CO_2} can be helpful in determining whether bicarbonate will improve an arterial metabolic acidosis. If the pH is <7.15 and the arterial and venous P_{CO_2} are both low, bicarbonate can be given. However, if the central venous or pulmonary artery P_{CO_2} is high, regardless of what the arterial P_{CO_2} is, bicarbonate is apt only to make the tissues develop an increasing respiratory acidosis.

The situation in which the arterial pH is relatively normal or even slightly alkalotic while the venous pH may be severely acidotic has been studied recently by von Planta and associates and further reviewed by Jaffe. The existence of an arterial-venous gradient across the coronary circulation due to anaerobic metabolism and the production of carbon dioxide and lactate is even greater than estimated from mixed venous blood.

Snyder and colleagues found that central venous oxygen tensions (P_{VO_2}) were a reliable predictor of poor short-term outcome after in-hospital cardiac arrest and resuscitation. Twelve of 14 survivors had an initial P_{VO_2} >37 mm Hg (4.9 kPa), whereas all 29 nonsurvivors had an initial P_{VO_2} <31 mm Hg (4.1 kPa). At 10 minutes, no survivors had a P_{VO_2} <41 mm Hg (5.5 kPa) and only four nonsurvivors had a P_{VO_2} >41 mm Hg (5.5 kPa).

F. END-TIDAL CARBON DIOXIDE

Some evidence suggests that the earliest sign of return of spontaneous circulation is a dramatic rise in end-tidal carbon dioxide (CO_2). Monitoring end-tidal carbon dioxide may also indicate appropriate times for interrupting CPR to evaluate ECGs, BP, and presence of palpable pulses. End-tidal carbon dioxide normally averages 3.0% to 3.5%. A sudden fall in end-tidal carbon dioxide after an apparently successful resuscitation generally indicates a sudden, severe fall in cardiac output.

PITFALL

Failure to monitor end-tidal carbon dioxide if it is available.

Weil and associates in 1985 reported that a $P_{ET}CO_2$ of ≥10 mm Hg (1.3 kPa) in animals was highly predictive of resuscitation and was achieved when coronary perfusion pressure exceeded 30 mm Hg (4.0 kPa). Barton and Callaham recently found that high $P_{ET}CO_2$ values reflect effective CPR through chest compression or a clinically undetectable perfusing cardiac rhythm. The patients who had a return of pulse had a $P_{ET}CO_2$ of 15 ± 1 mm Hg, whereas the 47 patients who did not have a return of pulse had a $P_{ET}CO_2$ of 4 ± 3 mm Hg. At the higher values, the $P_{ET}CO_2$ seems to correlate with improved pulmonary blood flow. There was, however, no overall correlation with Pa_{CO_2}.

AXIOM

$P_{ET}CO_2$ does not correlate with the likelihood of return of spontaneous circulation after high-dose epinephrine is administered.

VII. ESTABLISHING AND MAINTAINING IV INFUSION ROUTES

Following high-dose epinephrine (0.1 to 0.2 mg/kg), the correlation between a high $P_{ET}CO_2$ and increased return of spontaneous circulation is lost. Although high-dose epinephrine increases coronary cerebral perfusion pressure and the likelihood of a successful resuscitation, it also drops cardiac output and pulmonary blood flow so that $P_{ET}CO_2$ falls.

An essential part of ACLS is the early establishment of reliable IV route(s) for the administration of necessary drugs and fluids. Cannulation of either a peripheral or central vein is preferable to intracardiac injection. If an internal jugular or subclavian central venous line is in place when the arrest occurs, it should be used. If no vein is already cannulated at the time of arrest, cannulation of an antecubital vein should be the site of choice so as not to interrupt the CPR. The external jugular vein is another site for venous access that should be considered, both as a peripheral vein and for access to the central circulation.

Wrist or hand veins and distal saphenous veins in the legs are the least favorable sites for drug administration during cardiac arrest, as blood flow to the distal extremities is usually markedly diminished.

If a femoral vein is cannulated, advancing the catheter to a position above the diaphragm facilitates drug delivery. The intracardiac route is the last resort for injection of epinephrine if both IV and endotracheal routes are not available. Injection into the tracheobronchial tree can also be attempted, but absorption is erratic and the dose used may have to be increased 5- to 10-fold.

VIII. DRUGS USED IN ACLS

A. OXYGEN

In patients with cardiac arrest, 100% oxygen should be administered as soon as possible. Oxygen should also be administered to all patients with shock or airway obstruction.

B. IV FLUIDS

Expansion of circulating blood volume is a critical component of ACLS, particularly in patients who have sustained trauma or acute blood loss. In addition, up to 20% to 30% of patients with acute myocardial infarction shock may be hypovolemic and may benefit from volume expansion.

C. MORPHINE SULFATE

Morphine can be useful after an effective heart beat has been obtained. It can help to relieve acute pulmonary edema and the pain of acute myocardial infarction. In addition to its analgesic action, morphine increases venous capacitance and thereby decreases venous return. In patients with pulmonary edema, this can rapidly decrease pulmonary congestion. By reducing left ventricular end-diastolic pressure, systemic vascular resistance, and left ventricular afterload, myocardial oxygen consumption is also reduced.

Morphine is best given IV in doses of 2 to 3 mg every 5 to 30 minutes until the desired response is achieved. Although morphine can be a respiratory depressant, if it is given in multiple small IV increments, serious depression of ventilation is less likely. Hypotension after morphine is unusual, unless the patient is hypovolemic. Small intermittent doses will usually permit early recognition of any tendency to hypotension before serious consequences occur.

D. DRUGS USED FOR CONTROL OF HEART RATE AND RHYTHM

These include lidocaine, procainamide, bretylium, propranolol, atropine, and digitalis (see chapter on arrhythmias). Results from studies comparing the efficacy of lidocaine to bretylium in ventricular fibrillation are equivocal. However, because of bretylium's additional adverse hemodynamic side effects, lidocaine remains the drug of choice in treatment of ventricular tachyarrhythmias.

E. DRUGS USED TO IMPROVE BP AND BLOOD FLOW

These include dopamine, dobutamine, epinephrine, norepinephrine, metaraminol, nitroprusside, and nitroglycerin (see chapter on shock).

F. ALPHA-ADRENERGIC STIMULATION (VASOCONSTRIC-TION) AND CORONARY BLOOD FLOW

PITFALL

Failing to increase the amount of epinephrine given if a carotid or femoral pulse cannot be palpated during good external cardiac massage.

In their original report, Redding and Pearson recommended 0.1 mg/kg as the dose of epinephrine. For some reason, the ACLS guideline came out with a recommendation of only 0.5 to 1.0 mg (0.007 to 0.014 mg/kg) every 5 minutes. With that low dose, the aortic diastolic pressure seldom exceeds 8 to 10 mm Hg.

It has become increasingly apparent that the aortic diastolic right atrial pressure (ADRAP) gradient is extremely important in supplying adequate myocardial blood flow during cardiac massage. In both animals and man, a ADRAP gradient exceeding 15 to 17 mm Hg is essential for a return of spontaneous circulation. It has been repeatedly shown that increased alpha vasoconstriction to raise aortic diastolic BP is extremely important for providing adequate coronary blood flow. Closed-chest massage in dogs with standard doses of epinephrine (0.02 mg) generally produces an aortic diastolic blood pressure of less than 8 to 10 mm Hg. Doses of 0.2 mg/kg are much more likely to produce aortic blood pressures of at least 25 to 30 mm Hg which are usually needed for successful cardiac resuscitation.

Brown and colleagues in 1987 showed that epinephrine in very large doses of 200 μg/kg increased coronary blood flow almost 70 times more than standard doses of 0.02 mg/kg. The larger doses also improved subendocardial blood flow.

Interestingly, Martin and associates have shown that use of high-dose epinephrine was able to increase mean coronary perfusion pressure (CPP) a $\pm$ 12 mm Hg at a normal arterial pH (7.38 to 7.48) and 13 $\pm$ 11 mm Hg at an arterial pH <7.00, but with pHs above 7.42, the average increase in CPP was only 4 $\pm$ 6 mm Hg. Thus, the high-dose epinephrine worked well at normal or even severely acidotic pHs, but not in the face of alkalosis.

Goetling and coworkers recently reported improved survival of 40% (8/20) with high-dose epinephrine (0.2 mg/kg) versus 0% (0/20) with continued standard-dose epinephrine (0.01 mg/kg). The authors switched to the higher dose if two doses of 0.01 mg/kg given 5 minutes apart had not produced a hemodynamic response.

In patients, if one to two ampules (1 to 2 mg) of epinephrine do not restore an adequate BP within 3 to 4 minutes, it may be worthwhile to try doses 5 to 10 times as large over the next 5 to 10 minutes. Monitoring of intra-arterial BP might help greatly in making such decisions earlier. If there is a return of spontaneous circulation, an IV drip of epinephrine (four ampules = 4 mg) in 250 ml of D_5W to keep the systolic BP at 100 mm Hg or higher is essential.

Interestingly, if end-tidal carbon dioxide is monitored to follow the adequacy of the resuscitation, it will actually tend to go down with high-dose epinephrine. This occurs because, although aortic diastolic pressure and coronary perfusion pressure rise, cardiac output and blood flow through the lungs falls, reducing the end-tidal carbon dioxide. Thus, the end-tidal carbon dioxide is not helpful for following the adequacy of resuscitation after high-dose epinephrine.

G. ALPHA-ADRENERGIC STIMULATION (VASOCONSTRIC-TION) AND CEREBRAL BLOOD FLOW

Increased vasoconstriction due to large doses of epinephrine can greatly increase cerebral blood flow during closed-chest cardiac massage. In one study, epinephrine in doses of 200 μg/kg increased cerebral blood flow up to 43% of control while a 20 μg/kg dose provided cerebral blood flows that were only about 1% of control. Large doses of epinephrine also reduce external carotid blood flow to the facial structures and thereby further increase internal carotid blood flow to the brain.

H. ENDOTRACHEAL EPINEPHRINE

There has been some tendency to give epinephrine and some other agents endotracheally if an IV is not immediately available. Roberts found that the blood levels of epinephrine given endotracheally were only 10% of those given IV. Hornchen had similar findings and noted that 100 μg/kg given deeply endobrachially had an effect similar to that of 10 μg/kg given IV.

AXIOM

The dose of agents given endotracheally must usually be at least 5 to 10 times greater than those given IV

I. CORONARY VASODILATORS

Nitrites and nitrates can be used only to improve coronary or peripheral blood flow after an effective heart beat and adequate BP have been obtained. Sublingual nitroglycerin is readily absorbed and highly effective in angina pectoris, usually relieving the pain within 1 to 2 minutes. The therapeutic effect may last up to 30 minutes. Unfortunately, it causes a severe headache in many patients. If there is any hypovolemia, vasodilators can cause an abrupt drop in BP.

AXIOM

One must be very careful to not let the patient receiving vasodilators become hypovolemic.

J. SODIUM BICARBONATE

It has become evident that less sodium bicarbonate is needed than was previously assumed necessary during a cardiac arrest. If the pH is above 7.10 to 7.15, no bicarbonate is probably needed. Furthermore, by ensuring adequate alveolar ventilation, a major component of the acidosis that is present can usually be corrected. For each 10 mm Hg decrease in the arterial P_{CO_2}, the pH will rise 0.07 to 0.10. If alveolar ventilation is not adequate, administration of sodium bicarbonate can cause respiratory acidosis. Sodium bicarbonate is now generally recommended only after 10 minutes of cardiac massage and blood gas studies showing a severe metabolic acidosis. The initial dose of sodium bicarbonate is usually 1 mEq/kg followed by half this dose every 10 minutes as needed.

AXIOM

Sodium bicarbonate administration should be based primarily on arterial and mixed venous blood gas values.

Blood gas studies will often indicate that much higher or lower doses of bicarbonate, minute ventilation, or cardiac massage and epinephrine are required than would be expected clinically.

Considering the difficulty in obtaining serial ABGs on some patients, studies testing the predictability of central venous pH have been performed. One such study has shown that the central venous pH is a relatively good predictor of arterial pH in patients who have a pulse. All patients with a central venous pH $\geq$7.15 had an arterial pH $\geq$7.30, which is considered an acceptable end point for sodium bicarbonate therapy.

Sodium bicarbonate administration can cause a paradoxical cerebral acidosis because bicarbonate does not cross the blood-brain barrier, but the increased carbon dioxide that it produces does. If an alkalosis is suddenly induced by treatment, it can cause a variety of arrhythmias that may be partly due to a sudden decrease in ionized calcium. Bicarbonate can cause significant increases in serum osmolarity and sodium concentrations. It can also inactivate catecholamines when the two are given concomitantly in an IV.

K. DIURETICS

Furosemide (Lasix) and ethacrynic acid (Edecrin) are potent diuretic agents that inhibit the resorption of sodium in the proximal and distal tubules and in the loop of Henle. Furosemide also has a venodilating effect that may account for some of its prompt action in pulmonary edema. The onset of diuresis after IV administration usually commences within 5 minutes, reaches its peak within 30 minutes, and lasts for several hours. Furosemide or ethacrynic acid may be useful in the prevention or treatment of cerebral edema after cardiac arrest. For the treatment of pulmonary edema, furosemide in doses of 0.5 to 2.0 mg/kg should be injected slowly IV.

AXIOM

If diuretics produce an excessive urine output, one may have to administer additional fluids to prevent hypovolemic hypotension.

L. CORTICOSTEROIDS

For cerebral edema after cardiac arrest, methylprednisolone sodium succinate (50 to 100 mg), or dexamethasone sodium phosphate (10 to 20 mg) IV every 6 hours, has been recommended, but the effectiveness of corticosteroids under these circumstances is very controversial.

M. CALCIUM BLOCKERS

Within the past 5 to 10 years, there has been increasing interest in the role of calcium ions in a wide variety of pathologic cellular and organ changes following cardiac arrest. Recent data seem to implicate increased intracellular ionized calcium as a triggering element in a number of adverse reactions after shock, sepsis, trauma, and anoxia. Reports have also linked ionic calcium shifts to abnormalities in cellular metabolism, intracellular release of free fatty acids, production of oxidative free radicals, and the no-reflow phenomenon in the brain. All of these factors are implicated in neuronal injury after ischemic anoxia.

AXIOM

Calcium channel blockers may improve cerebral resuscitation but they can also increase the tendency to severe hypotension.

Movement of calcium into ischemic cerebral vascular smooth muscle cells may cause persistent cerebral vasoconstriction with resultant failure of cerebral reperfusion after strokes or cardiac arrest. Consequently, there has been increased interest in the use of calcium channel blockers for cerebral resuscitation. Calcium antagonists, such as flunarizine, verapamil, inimodipine, and $MgSO_4$ have been shown to protect cerebral cortical blood flow and cerebral oxygen consumption during reperfusion. Pioneer work by White and associates has demonstrated significantly improved early results with calcium channel blockers in several models of cerebral ischemic anoxia. Unfortunately, these calcium blockers also tend to cause vasodilation and a negative inotropic effect that may interfere with the cardiac resuscitation.

N. IRON CHELATING AGENTS

Use of a new class of drugs, the iron chelating agents, in advanced cardiac life support (ACLS) may prevent late deaths and brain damage following successfully cardiopulmonary resuscitation. It has been shown that free iron ions, liberated from bound intracellular stores during ischemia, catalyze initiation of free radical mediated reactions that propagate through membrane lipids and protein. Chelation of intracellular iron by deferoxamine, a commercially available drug that distributes to the intracellular space and has a great affinity for iron ions, may help prevent or reduce such reactions.

IX. CARDIAC ARREST AFTER AN ACUTE MYOCARDIAL INFARCTION

The mechanisms by which effective cardiac function can cease, especially after an acute myocardial infarction include ventricular tachycardia (5% to 10%), ventricular fibrillation (75% to 80%), asystole (10% to 20%), and electromechanical dissociation (5% to 15%).

Although a number of investigators (Cammins, Montgomery, Ritter and associates, Stueven and associates, and Sobel) have emphasized the value of bystander CPR, the main determinant of survival is how rapidly a reversible cardiac arrhythmia can be terminated with electrical defibrillation.

A. MANAGEMENT OF VENTRICULAR FIBRILLATION

AXIOM

The most important single factor determining if CPR will be successful is the rapidity with which ventricular fibrillation is converted to an effective rhythm by a defibrillator.

If ventricular fibrillation is identified in a patient who has been in cardiac arrest for less than 2 minutes, three successive defibrillation countershocks, increasing from 200 to 360 joules should be administered immediately, checking the cardioscope after each shock. If the patient has been in cardiac arrest for an undetermined period of time and has ventricular fibrillation, it is recommended by some that BCLS be performed for at least 2 minutes before an initial attempt at defibrillation is made. However, the time to defibrillation is the most important determination of eventual outcome, and an initial attempt at defibrillation before BCLS is given may be very worthwhile.

If a second series of countershocks is unsuccessful after 1 to 2 minutes of BCLS, it is recommended that one start an IV, give epinephrine, insert an endotracheal tube, and administer 100% oxygen. If severe metabolic acidosis (pH <7.10 to 7.15) is present, bicarbonate may be given. A third defibrillation attempt should then be made at settings that do not exceed 360 joules.

If a normal rhythm is obtained but the ventricular fibrillation recurs, the use of lidocaine, bretylium, or procainamide therapy may be helpful. In general, two IV lidocaine boluses of 70 to 100 mg are followed immediately by an infusion at 4 mg/min. If the patient's general condition is improved by good BCLS and ACLS, the energy required to defibrillate the heart may be substantially reduced. This has the advantage of minimizing electrical injury to the heart. Factors associated with an increased incidence of recurrent ventricular fibrillation include a history of congestive heart failure, prior myocardial infarction, low ejection function, and severe coronary artery disease.

B. VENTRICULAR TACHYCARDIA

Ventricular tachycardia with no effective blood flow is treated like ventricular fibrillation, but the results are usually much better.

C. MANAGEMENT OF VENTRICULAR ASYSTOLE

When ventricular asystole is present, a severe metabolic defect or extensive myocardial damage should be suspected, and the likelihood of a successful resuscitation is very low. High levels of parasympathetic tone can also (rarely) result in cessation of both supraventricular and ventricular pacemaker activity. In addition to beginning CPR, inserting an endotracheal tube for optimal ventilation, and starting an IV infusion, the following steps should be taken:

1. Epinephrine is given IV in progressively larger doses, as needed.
2. If a severe metabolic acidosis is present, sodium bicarbonate can be given.
3. If asystole persists, an IV infusion of epinephrine (at least 0.1 to 0.2 μg/min) may be started.
4. One should consider progressively increasing the dose of epinephrine if a palpable carotid pulse is not obtained with the cardiac massage.
5. In persistent asystole, a temporary transvenous pacemaker may, in rare instances, restore an effective ventricular rhythm.

**D. ELECTRO-
MECHANICAL
DISSOCIATION**

PITFALL
Failure to rule out hypovolemia tamponade, pneumothorax, or a pulmonary embolus in a patient who appears to have EMD.

In electromechanical dissociation, there is organized electrical activity on the ECG, but there are no effective myocardial contractions. Electromechanical dissociation carries a grave prognosis. However, it is important to recognize that pericardial tamponade may mimic EMD and is often readily treatable by pericardiocentesis. Myocardial rupture may also be confused with EMD, and an occasional case has been successfully treated with emergent surgical repair on cardiopulmonary bypass. Other problems such as hypovolemia, pulmonary embolus, and tension pneumothorax should also be ruled out.

The drugs recommended for electromechanical dissociation (EMD) in the 1980 *JAMA* guidelines include epinephrine, calcium chloride, and atropine. The effectiveness of epinephrine is felt to be due to its alpha-adrenergic (vasoconstrictor) properties; its beta-adrenergic activity may be a disadvantage. Calcium is now felt by many to be contraindicated, particularly because of its adverse effects on cerebral resuscitation reperfusion. Atropine may be useful if a slow, weak heart beat is obtained.

Paradis and others have noted that more than 40% of patients diagnosed as having EMD (because of no obtainable pulse or cuff BP in spite of fairly normal electrical complexes) actually have a significant pulse pressure when aortic pressure is monitored. These patients responded well to high-dose epinephrine and were much more likely to have a return of spontaneous circulation with vigorous resuscitation efforts.

**X. TERMINATION OF
BCLS OR ACLS**

CPR may be terminated when, despite adequate attempts (intubation, defibrillation, IV medications), intrinsic cardiac activity has not been achieved in 10 to 15 minutes in patients with asystole or severe bradyarrhythmias. CPR may also be discontinued in patients with other rhythms who have had CPR for more than 45 minutes without generation of any intrinsic cardiac activity. These criteria should not be used for victims of hypothermia before a core temperature of at least 32°C and preferably 35°C is achieved by active rewarming. Available data suggest that if these criteria are followed, many unproductive resuscitative efforts can be eliminated without jeopardizing potential survivors.

In patients with ventricular fibrillation or ventricular tachycardia, vigorous resuscitation is indicated. Patients with witnessed cardiac arrest who have had immediate CPR outside the hospital, but not definitive prehospital care, may benefit from ED CPR even if they have a bradyarrhythmia.

PITFALL
Stopping CPR early just because the patient has fixed-dilated pupils.

It is important to emphasize that fixed-dilated pupils do not necessarily indicate severe cerebral damage, and they do not indicate that CPR should be discontinued.

XI. RESULTS OF CPR

A. IN-HOSPITAL CPR

On the average, of the patients who have witnessed cardiac arrest in the hospital, about 40% to 50% will be at least temporarily resuscitated, but only about 10% to 20% will leave the hospital alive and fully functional. There are, however, a large number of factors that affect the results of CPR. The cause of the arrest is certainly a major factor. Prompt CPR and defibrillation where an electrical shock has caused a witnessed ventricular fibrillation in a young, previously healthy patient, should have an excellent result. CPR after an unwitnessed cardiac arrest in an elderly patient with chronic congestive heart failure and prior ischemic strokes will have dismal results.

B. TYPE OF ARRHYTHMIA

The type of arrhythmia causing the arrest is extremely important. In the few patients with ventricular tachycardia, one can expect an 80% to 90% incidence of success. With ventricular fibrillation, about 40% will be resuscitated and about 20% will leave the hospital in a fully functional state. With asystolic arrest, less than 3% to 5% will have a successful outcome.

C. OUT-OF-HOSPITAL CPR

With out-of-hospital cardiac arrests, the most important factor determining outcome is the total ischemic-anoxia time. Lund in 1976 in a study of 576 out-of-hospital cardiac arrests found that with less than 1 minute of anoxia, the survival rate was 61%, with 5 to 10 minutes of anoxia, it was 9%, and with more than 10 minutes of anoxia, the survival rate was 1%. If the patient got bystander CPR, the survival rate was 36%; without bystander CPR, the survival rate was 8%. Thompson in Seattle noted even better survival rates with bystander CPR (48%) than without bystander CPR (21%). However, Kowalski in Milwaukee noted by bystander CPR had no effect on resuscitability or survival in patients who were immediately defibrillated. Steuven and colleagues also found that bystander CPR made no real difference in survival: the main factor was how long the patient was anoxic before defibrillation was accomplished.

AXIOM

There is increasing evidence that prolonged closed-chest cardiac massage is of relatively little value in CPR. The time from cardiac arrest to electrical defibrillation is the critical factor.

XII. SUMMARY

The single most important factor in CPR producing a successful outcome (patient leaving the hospital alive with intact CNS function) is the speed with which ventricular fibrillation is converted to an effective rhythm with a cardiac defibrillator. During cardiac massage, very high doses of epinephrine (or other vasoconstrictors) can significantly increase coronary and cerebral blood flow and thereby improve the chances of a successful outcome. Open cardiac massage is more likely than closed-chest massage to produce good coronary and cerebral blood flow and should be considered in selected patients, especially young individuals with penetrating chest trauma.

SUMMARY POINTS

1. CPR is not "successful" unless the patient survives and is neurologically intact.
2. The most important single factor determining if CPR will be successful is the rapidity with which ventricular fibrillation is converted to an effective rhythm by a defibrillator.
3. Patients with a cardiac arrest tend to open their sphincters and have a greatly increased chance of regurgitating gastric contents into their upper airway and lungs.
4. Prolapse of the tongue into the pharynx is the most frequent cause of upper airway obstruction in unconscious individuals.
5. The head tilt cannot be used to open the upper airway in trauma victims who may have a cervical spine injury.
6. Whenever possible, one should use a pocket mask, rather than mouth-to-mouth breathing, to inflate the lungs of a patient with cardiac arrest.
7. If a patient who is thought to have a cardiac arrest has a heart beat but has

no effective blood flow, closed-chest cardiac compression should be started promptly.

8. External cardiac compression is given over the lower sternum in adults. However, since the heart of an infant or small child is higher in the chest, external cardiac compression is applied to them over the midsternum.

9. One should not pronounce a cold patient dead before hypothermia has been corrected to at least 32°C and preferably 35°C.

10. Chest compression at 80 to 100 times per minute tends to increase BP and cardiac output more than rates of only 60 to 80 per minute.

11. Forward blood flow with external cardiac massage is probably due to changes in intrathoracic pressure rather than direct compression of the heart.

12. Blood flow occurs during external chest compressions or coughing because of an extrathoracic a-v pressure gradient.

13. It is a clinical error not to detect gastric dilatation until the patient has regurgitated and aspirated.

14. Excessive ventilatory pressures applied through mouth-to-mouth or mask-to-mouth ventilation increase the risk of aspiration of gastric contents.

15. In an effort to obtain a better pulse, one should avoid use of excessive force during external CPR.

16. Hypotension after apparently successful closed-chest massage may occasionally be due to an abdominal visceral injury caused by the chest compressions.

17. If someone suddenly develops trouble breathing, especially while eating, one should rule out the possibility of a foreign body in the upper airway.

18. Poor air exchange (characterized by a weak, ineffective cough, inspiratory stridor, and respiratory distress) should be managed as if it were a complete airway obstruction.

19. The abdominal thrust is probably the safest and most effective method for dislodging a foreign body in the upper airway.

20. One must be careful to avoid pushing a high foreign body further down into the airway while attempting to remove it.

21. Emergency tracheostomy is rarely necessary.

22. One should not attempt to give closed-chest cardiac massage while the patient is lying on a soft surface or bed.

23. If a PASG is inflated for too long a period, the chances of the patient's developing a compartment syndrome are increased.

24. Open-chest cardiac massage provides much better coronary and cerebral blood flow than closed-chest compressions.

25. One should not use closed-chest massage to resuscitate patients with cardiac arrest due to penetrating chest trauma.

26. The most common cause for nonreactive pupils is a weak flashlight.

27. One should generally not administer bicarbonate during CPR without first evaluating both arterial and mixed venous blood gases.

28. End-tidal carbon dioxide can be used to monitor the effectiveness of cardiac massage.

29. PETCO$_2$ does not correlate with the likelihood of return of spontaneous circulation after high-dose epinephrine is administered.

30. One should increase the amount of epinephrine given if a carotid or femoral pulse cannot be palpated during what appears to be proper external cardiac massage.

31. The dose of drugs given endotracheally must usually be at least 5 to 10 times greater than those given IV.

32. One must be very careful to not let the patient receiving vasodilators become hypovolemic.

33. Sodium bicarbonate should be administered only according to arterial and mixed venous blood gases.

34. If diuretics produce an excessive urine output, one may have to administer additional fluids to prevent hypovolemic hypotension.

35. Calcium channel blockers may improve cerebral resuscitation but they can also increase the tendency to severe hypotension.

36. One should rule out hypovolemia, pericardial tamponade, pulmonary embolus, and pneumothorax in a patient who appears to have EMD.

37. One should not stop CPR just because the patient has fixed-dilated pupils.

38. There is increasing evidence that prolonged closed-chest cardiac massage is of relatively little value in CPR. The time from cardiac arrest to electrical defibrillation is the critical factor.

BIBLIOGRAPHY

1. Abramson, NS and BRCT I Study Group: Randomized clinical study of thiopental loading in comatose survivors of cardiac arrest. N Engl J Med 314:397, 1986.
2. Abramson, NS, et al: Lidoflazine administration to survivors of cardiac arrest. Ann Emerg Med 18:478, 1989.
3. Babbs, CF: Role of iron ions in the genesis of reperfusion injury following successful cardiopulmonary resuscitation: Preliminary data and a biochemical hypothesis. Ann Emerg Med 14:777, 1985.
4. Babbs, CF and Tacker, WA: Cardiopulmonary resuscitation with interposed abdominal compression. Circulation 74:IV37, 1986.
5. Babbs, CF, et al: CPR with simultaneous compression and ventilation at high airway pressure in four animal models. Crit Care Med 10:501, 1982.
6. Barton, C and Callaham, M: Lack of correlation between end-tidal carbon dioxide concentrations and $Paco_2$ in cardiac arrest. Crit Care Med 19:108, 1990.
7. Bellamy, RF, DeGuzman, LR, and Pedersen, DC: Coronary blood flow during cardiopulmonary resuscitation in swine. Circulation 69:174, 1984.
8. Bircher, N and Safar, P: Cerebral preservation during cardiopulmonary resuscitation. Crit Care Med 13:185, 1985
9. Bircher, N and Safar, P: Manual open-chest cardiopulmonary resuscitation. Ann Emerg Med 13:770, 1984.
10. Bircher, N and Safar, P: Open chest CPR: An old method whose time had returned. Am J Emerg Med 2:568, 1984.
11. Bishop, RL and Weisfeldt, ML: Sodium bicarbonate administration during cardiac arrest: Effect on arterial pH, Pco_2 and osmolality. JAMA 235:506, 1976.
12. Brown, CG, et al: The effect of graded doses of epinephrine on regional myocardial blood flow during cardiopulmonary resuscitation in swine. Circulation 75:491, 1987.
13. Brown, CG, et al: Comparative effect of graded doses of epinephrine on regional blood flow during CPR in a swine model. Ann Emerg Med 15:1138, 1986.
14. Chandra, NC, Rudikoff, M, and Weisfeldt, ML: Simultaneous chest compression and ventilation at high airway pressure during cardiopulmonary resuscitation. Lancet i:175, 1980.
15. Chandra, NC, et al: Observations of hemodynamics during human cardiopulmonary resuscitation. Crit Care Med 18:929, 1990.
16. Chandra, NC, et al: Augmentation of cardiac flow during cardiopulmonary resuscitation by ventilation at high airway pressure simultaneous with chest compression. Am J Cardiol 48:1053, 1981.
17. Chandra, ND et al: Contrasts between intrathoracic pressures during external chest compression and cardiac message. Crit Care Med 9:789, 1981.
18. Criley, JM, Blaufuss, AH, and Kiesell, GL: Cough-induced cardiac compression: Self-administered form of cardiopulmonary resuscitation. JAMA 236:1246, 1976.
19. Criley, JM, Blaufuss, AH, and Kiesell, GL: Self-administered cardiopulmonary resuscitation by cough-induced cardiac compression. Trans Am Clin Climatol Assoc 87:138, 1976.
20. Cummins, RO and Eisenberg, M: Pre-hospital cardiopulmonary resuscitation: Is it effective? JAMA 253:2408, 1985.
21. Cummins, RO, et al: Survival of out-of-hospital cardiac arrest with early initiation of cardiopulmonary resuscitation. JAMA 3:114, 1985.
22. Danne, PD, Finelli, F, and Champion, HR: Emergency bay thoracotomy. J Trauma 24:796, 1984.
23. Del Guercio, LR: A plea for open-chest CPR. Am J Emerg Med 2:565, 1984.
24. Don Micheal, TA, Lambert, EH, and Mehran, A: Mouth-to-lung airway for cardiac resuscitation. Lancet 2:1329, 1968.

25. Feneley, MP, et al: Influence of compression rate on initial success of resuscitation and 24 hour survival after prolonged manual cardiopulmonary resuscitation in dogs. Circulation 77:240, 1988.
26. Fisher, J, et al: Determinants and clinical significance of jugular venous valve competence. Circulation 65:188, 1982.
27. Frass, et al: The esophageal tracheal combitube: Preliminary results with a new airway for CPR. Ann Emerg Med 16:768, 1987.
28. Greene, HL: Sudden arrhythmic cardiac death: Mechanisms, resuscitation and classification: The Seattle Perspective. Am J Cardiol 65:4B, 1990.
29. Halperin, HR, et al: Vest inflation without simultaneous ventilation during cardiac arrest in dogs: Improved survival from prolonged cardiopulmonary resuscitation. Circulation 74:1407, 1986.
30. Hanashiro, PK, and Wilson, JR: Cardiopulmonary resuscitation. A current perspective. Med Clin North Am 70:729, 1986.
30a. Hornchen, U, et al: Endobronchial instillation of epinephrine during cardiopulmonary resuscitation. Crit Care Med 15:1037, 1987.
31. Jackson, RE, et al: Blood flow in the cerebral cortex during cardiac resuscitation in dogs. Ann Emerg Med 13:657, 1984.
32. Jacobs, IM and Berrizbeitia, LD: Prehospital trauma care. Emerg Med Clin North Am 2:717, 1984.
33. Jacobson, S: Current status of open chest procedures. Clin Emerg Med 2:121, 1983.
34. Jaffe, AS: New and old paradoxes: Acidosis and cardiopulmonary resuscitation. Circulation 80:1079, 1989.
35. Kern, KB, Sanders, AB, and Ewy, GA: Open-chest cardiac massage after closed-chest compression in a canine model: When to intervene. Resuscitation 15:51, 1987.
36. Kern, KB, et al: Dynamic changes in expired end-tidal carbon dioxide as a prognostic guide during CPR in dogs. Ann Emerg Med 17:392, 1988.
37. Kern, KB, et al: Comparison of mechanical techniques of cardiopulmonary resuscitation: Survival and neurologic outcome in dogs. Am J Emerg Med 5:190, 1987.
38. Koehler, RC, et al: Augmentation of cerebral perfusion of simultaneous chest compression and lung inflation with abdominal binding after cardiac arrest in dogs. Circulation 67:266, 1983.
38a. Kowalski, R, et al: Bystander CPR in prehospital coarse ventricular fibrillation. Ann Emerg Med 13:1016, 1984.
39. LeBlanc, R, et al: The effects of calcium antagonism on the epicerebral circulation in early vasospasm. Stroke 15:1017, 1984.
40. Levine, R, et al: Cardiopulmonary bypass cardiac arrest and prolonged closed-chest CPR in dogs. Ann Emerg Med 16:620, 1987.
41. Livesay, JJ, et al: Optimizing myocardial supply/demand balance with alpha-adrenergic drugs during cardiac resuscitation. J Thorac Cardiovasc Surg 76:244, 1978.
42. Luce, JM: The cardiovascular effects of mechanical ventilation and positive end-expiratory pressure. JAMA 252:807, 1984.
43. Luce, JM, Rizk, NA, and Niskanen, RA: Regional blood flow during cardiopulmonary resuscitation in dogs. Crit Care Med 12:258, 1984.
44. Luce, JM, et al: Regional blood flow during cardiopulmonary resuscitation in dogs using simultaneous and nonsimultaneous compression and ventilation. Circulation 67:258, 1983.
44a. Lund, I and Skulberg, A: Cardiopulmonary resuscitation by lay people. Lancet 2:702, 1976.
45. Maier, GW, et al: The physiology of external cardiac massage: High-impulse cardiopulmonary resuscitation. Circulation 70:86, 1984.
46. Marsden, AK: Basic life support: Guidelines for cardiopulmonary resuscitation. Br Med J 299, 1989.
47. Martin, GB, et al: Cardiopulmonary bypass versus CPR as treatment for prolonged cardiopulmonary arrest. Ann Emerg Med 16:628, 1987.
48. Martin, GB, et al: Aortic and right atrial pressures during standard and simultaneous ventilation and compression CPR in human beings. Ann Emerg Med 15:125, 1986.
49. Martin, GB, et al: Aortic and right atrial pressures during standard and simultaneous ventilation and compression CPR in human beings (abstr). Ann Emerg Med 14:497, 1985.
49a. McCabe, JB, et al: Direct mechanical ventricular assistance during ventricular fibrillation. Ann Emerg Med 12:739, 1983.
50. Michael, TA: The role of esophageal obturator airway in cardiopulmonary resuscitation. Circulation 74:134, 1986.
51. Montgomery, WH: The 1985 conference on standards and guidelines for cardiopulmonary resuscitation and emergency cardiac care. JAMA 255:2990, 1986
52. National Center for Health Statistics. Advance report: Final mortality statistics, 1981. Monthly Vital Stat Rep (Suppl DHHS) 33:4, 1981.
53. Niemann, JT, et al: Mechanical couth: Cardiopulmonary resuscitation during cardiac arrest in dogs. Am J Cardiol 55:199, 1985.
54. Niemann, JT, et al: Predictive indices of successful resuscitation after prolonged arrest and experimental cardiopulmonary resuscitation. Ann Emerg Med 14:521, 1985.

55. Niemann, JT, et al: Coronary perfusion pressure during experimental cardiopulmonary resuscitation. Ann Emerg Med 11:127, 1982.

56. Niemann, JT, et al: Pressure synchronized cineangiography during experimental cardiopulmonary resuscitation. Circulation 64:985, 1981.

57. Nowak, RM, et al: Selective venous hypercarbia during human CPR. Implications regarding blood flow. Ann Emerg Med 16:527, 1987.

58. Paradis, NA, et al: Central aortic pressure during human electromechanical dissociation: Identification of a subset with aortic pulse pressures (abstr). Ann Emerg Med 19:480, 1990.

59. Paradis, NA, et al: Coronary perfusion pressures during CPR are higher in patients with eventual return of spontaneous circulation. Ann Emerg Med 18:478, 1989.

60. Paradis, NA, et al: High-dose epinephrine and coronary perfusion pressure during cardiac arrest in human beings. Ann Emerg Med 18:478, 1989.

61. Paradis, NA, et al: Simultaneous aortic, jugular bulb, and right atrial pressures during cardiopulmonary resuscitation in humans: Insights into mechanisms. Circulation 80:361, 1989.

62. Pilcher, DB and DeMeules, JE: Esophageal perforation following use of esophageal airway. Chest 769:377, 1976.

63. Pons, PT: Esophageal obturator airway. Emerg Med Clin North Am 6:693, 1988.

64. Redding, JS: Abdominal compression in cardiopulmonary resuscitation. Anesth Analg 50:588, 1971.

65. Ritter, G, et al: The effect of bystander CPR on survival of out-of-hospital cardiac arrest victims. Am Heart J 110:932, 1985.

66. Rosenberg, JM, et al: The effect of CO_2 and non-CO_2 generating buffers on cerebral acidosis after cardiac arrest: A 31-P NMR study. Ann Emerg Med 18:341, 1989.

66a. Roberts, JR, Greenberg, MI, and Baskin, SI: Endotrachial epinephrine in cardiorespiratory collapse. JACEP 8:515, 1979.

67. Rosenthal, RE and Turbiak, TW: Open-chest cardiopulmonary resuscitation. Am J Emerg Med 4:248, 1986.

68. Sanders, AB, et al: End-tidal carbon dioxide monitoring during cardiopulmonary resuscitation. A prognostic indicator for survival. JAMA 262:1347, 1989.

69. Smith, JP, and Bodia, BI: Guidelines for discontinuing prehospital CPR in the emergency department: A review. Ann Emerg Med 14:1093, 1985.

70. Snyder, AB, et al: Predicting short-term outcome of cardiopulmonary resuscitation using central venous oxygen tension measurements. Crit Care Med 19:111, 1991.

71. Sobel, RM: Bystander cardiopulmonary resuscitation (CPR): The next decade. Ann Emerg Med 9:88, 1991.

72. Stajduhar, K, et al: Cerebral blood flow (CBF) and common carotid artery blood flow (CCABF) during open-chest cardiopulmonary resuscitation (OCCPR) in dogs. Anesthesiology (Suppl) 59:A117, 1983.

73. Steinman, AM: Cardiopulmonary resuscitation and hypothermia. Circulation 74:IV29, 1986.

74. Stueven, H, et al: Bystander/first responder CPR: Ten years experience in a paramedic system. Ann Emerg Med 15:707, 1986.

75. Swenson, RD, et al: Hemodynamics in humans during conventional and experimental cardiopulmonary resuscitation. Circulation 78:630, 1988.

76. Tsitlik, JE, et al: Elastic properties of the human chest during cardiopulmonary resuscitation. Crit Care Med 11:685, 1983.

77. von Planta, M, et al: Myocardial acidosis associated with CO_2 production during cardiac arrest and resuscitation. Circulation 80:684, 1989.

78. Weaver, WD, et al. Factors influencing survival after out-of-hospital cardiac arrest. J Am Coll Cardiol 7:752, 1986.

79. Weil, MH, et al: Difference in acid-base state between venous and arterial blood during cardiopulmonary resuscitation. N Engl J Med 315:153, 1986.

80. Weil, MH, et al: Cardiac output and end-tidal carbon dioxide. Crit Care Med 13:907, 1985.

81. White, BC, et al: Possible role of calcium blockers in cerebral resuscitation: A review of the literature and synthesis for future studies. Crit Care Med 11:202, 1983.

82. White, BC, et al: Effect of flunarizine on canine cerebral cortical blood flow and vascular resistance post-cardiac arrest. Ann Emerg Med 11:119, 1982.

83. Wiesfeldt, ML and Chandra, N: Physiology of cardiopulmonary resuscitation. Ann Rev Med 32:435, 1981.

CHAPTER 7

Stroke and Cerebral Resuscitation

I. STROKE

Stroke is a term used to indicate a variety of acute neurologic deficits resulting from ischemia or hemorrhage in a localized area of the brain. Stroke is by far the most common acute, nontraumatic brain problem and is the third leading cause of death in American adults.

More than 400,000 strokes occur in the United States every year, and nearly 150,000 of them are fatal. The elderly are especially at risk: the incidence of stroke more than doubles in each successive decade after age 55 years, with men suffering a 30% greater occurrence. Indeed, a stroke producing aphasia, paralysis, or even dementia is one of the most catastrophic conditions that can happen to an individual, and it can truly be a fate worse than death in its more severe manifestations. Somewhere between 54% and 85% of patients survive a first episode of stroke and remain at risk for future cerebrovascular complications. From 38% to 85% of survivors are still alive 5 years after the first cerebrovascular accident. This sizable population of elderly stroke survivors is at risk for many other problems, particularly pneumonia and acute respiratory failure. The economic impact of stroke syndromes is substantial, with medical, hospital, convalescent home care, and lost employment estimated to amount to approximately $14 billion per year in this country.

Patients who develop a stroke in the OR, especially during cardiovascular or neurosurgical procedures can be extremely difficult to manage, and may place a great burden on an ICU. Even in those patients who may survive, there is often the problem of quality of life thereafter, making the aggressiveness of the resuscitation sometimes come into question.

A. DIFFERENTIAL DIAGNOSIS

A wide variety of disorders may be misdiagnosed as a stroke. Isolated symptoms that are often seen with strokes but do not show other evidence of neurologic damage are seldom due to vascular disease. Thus, a patient with a sudden attack of vertigo is unlikely to have had a stroke. Similarly, isolated episodes of dysarthria, headache, double vision, confusion, delirium, memory loss, or coma can have multiple etiologies. However, a transient ischemic attack (TIA) or other vascular problem should be considered.

PITFALL
Attributing changes in mental status to cerebrovascular disease before metabolic, toxic, infectious, and neoplastic causes have been excluded.

AXIOM
The postictal state of epilepsy can be very difficult to differentiate from a stroke.

In a study of 821 consecutive patients admitted to a stroke unit, Norris and Hachinski noted that 13% had a disease other than stroke, and almost half of these misdiagnosed patients had seizures. The next largest group of mistaken diagnoses occurred in patients with drug intoxication, alcoholism, or metabolic abnormalities. Multiple sclerosis is a common cause of rapidly developing focal neurologic deficits, particularly in young patients. Focal mass lesions (such as cerebral tumors, abscesses, and subdural hematomas) may also present rather suddenly, simulating a stroke. Occasionally, encephalitis, hypoglycemia, and psychogenic symptoms can also be confused with stroke.

B. THE VASCULAR ANATOMY OF STROKES

1. Anterior (Carotid) Circulation

Hemiparesis, ranging from mild weakness to complete paralysis on one side of the body, is the hallmark of stroke. There is also often some degree of sensory loss in a distribution similar to the weakness. Most patients with such deficits have had a carotid distribution stroke, but hemiparesis and/or hemianesthesia does not always reliably differentiate carotid from vertebrobasilar ischemia.

AXIOM

The two symptoms of stroke that most accurately indicate carotid circulation involvement are aphasia and monocular blindness (Table 7.1).

Because the brainstem is more tightly compacted than the cerebral hemispheres, clinical syndromes due to an impaired posterior circulation are usually more complex. In brainstem stroke, bilateral neurologic signs are frequently present and cranial nerve and cerebellar abnormalities are often prominent (Table 7.2). Cranial nerve dysfunction (dysarthria, dysphagia, diplopia, dizziness), when seen in conjunction with hemiparesis or hemisensory loss, especially in a bilateral or crossed fashion, is usually a reliable indication of brainstem disease.

Deviation of the eyes may help localize a stroke. In hemispheric lesions, damage to the frontal lobe gaze centers causes the patient to look away from the hemiparetic side. With a brainstem stroke the patient also looks away from the hemiparetic side. However, with damage to the pontine gaze centers, the eyes look toward the hemiparetic side.

Weakness of just the lower part of the face on one side suggests damage in the cerebral hemispheres. A stroke affecting the brainstem will tend to paralyze the entire side of the face, including the forehead.

AXIOM

Most strokes (80%) involve the carotid artery system.

If there is doubt as to the origin of the lesion, it is probably in the carotid circulation, since it accounts for 80% of all strokes. The internal carotid and middle cerebral arteries are the major sites for atherosclerosis in the cerebrovascular system. In addition, most emboli from the carotid artery or the heart lodge

Table 7.1

CAROTID ISCHEMIA SYMPTOMS	*Symptoms of Carotid Ischemia*	*Frequency, %*
	Hemiparesis	65
	Hemisensory loss	60
	Monocular blindness	35
	Facial numbness	30
	Lower facial weakness	25
	Aphasia	20
	Headache	20
	Dysarthria	15
	Visual field loss	15

Table 7.2

VERTEBROBASILAR ISCHEMIA

Symptoms of Vertebrobasilar Ischemia	Frequency, %
Ataxia	50
Crossed or hemisensory loss	30
Vertigo	30
Crossed or hemiparesis	25
Dysarthria/dysphagia	25
Syncope or light-headedness	25
Headache	20
Deafness or tinnitus	10
Diplopia	10

in the middle cerebral artery. Brainstem strokes are generally due to hyaliniza-tion and thrombosis of small penetrating arterioles emerging directly from the vertebrobasilar arteries. Evaluation of a patient with carotid ischemia, therefore, usually focuses on atherosclerotic disease of the neck or cardiac sources of emboli.

Extensive evaluation of brainstem ischemia is seldom indicated because there is often little that can be done. However, brainstem strokes are usually small and have an excellent prognosis for full recovery, if the patient survives. Nevertheless, in the past 4 years, there has been increasing interest in surgery on the vertebral arteries to improve blood flow to the brainstem.

C. PATHOGENESIS OF STROKE

Vascular disease of the brain takes four major forms: thrombotic, embolic, lacunar, and hemorrhagic (Table 7.3).

Table 7.3

CHARACTERISTICS OF DIFFERENT TYPES OF STROKE

Type of Stroke	Onset	After TIAs, %	Seizure at Onset, %	Coma, %	Atrial Fibrillation, %	CT Scan	Other Features
Thrombotic	Stuttering, gradual	50	1	5	10	Ischemic infarction	Carotid bruit; stroke during sleep
Embolic	Sudden	10	10	1	35	Super-ficial (corti-cal) infarc-tion	Under-lying heart disease; periph-eral emboli
Lacunar	Gradual or sudden	30	0	0	5	Normal, or small, deep infarc-tion	Pure motor or pure sensory stroke
Hemorrhagic	Sudden	5	10	25	5	Hyper-dense mass	Nausea and vomit-ing; de-creased mental status

1. Thrombotic Strokes

Thrombotic strokes account for about 40% to 60% of all acute ischemic cerebrovascular problems. They are usually due to atherosclerotic stenosis of a large blood vessel, especially the internal carotid or middle cerebral artery. Because thrombotic occlusion tends to be a gradual process, the deficit it produces often has a slower onset than the other kinds of strokes and may present a stuttering or stepwise progression of symptoms over hours or days. Up to one half of all patients with thrombotic strokes report previous transient ischemic attacks (TIAs). About 40% of thrombolytic strokes occur at night, when the cardiac output and blood pressure are lower, and the patient who awakens in the morning with a new deficit has probably had a thrombotic stroke. Only 17% of embolic strokes occur at night, and they are less likely to cause a headache. Because atherosclerosis generally involves large vessels, the ischemia produced by thrombotic strokes tends to be large and the patients are often severely impaired.

AXIOM
Stuttering, slow, or nighttime strokes are usually thrombotic in origin.

2. Embolic Strokes

Emboli cause about 6% to 30% of all strokes. Embolic strokes arise from thrombi, platelets, cholesterol, fibrin, or other material breaking off from a diseased arterial wall or from the heart. Most strokes occurring in patients with atrial fibrillation or recent myocardial infarctions are embolic in origin. Patients with atrial fibrillation have a fivefold increased stroke risk compared with age-matched controls. Approximately 2.5% of patients with an acute myocardial infarction have an embolic stroke, and 15% of these patients will have a recurrent embolic stroke within 2 weeks. These patients also have often had peripheral emboli, such as renal infarcts or splinter hemorrhages in the conjunctiva and fingers.

Embolic strokes have an abrupt onset and the deficit tends to be maximal at the onset (80%) rather than progressive or stepwise. The emboli usually occlude distal cerebral cortical vessels and often cause major neurologic deficits, including aphasia, dense hemiparesis, and hemisensory loss. Global aphasia without hemiparesis, as well as isolated posterior cerebral artery syndromes, are usually cardioembolic in origin. The resultant defects often include seizures and aphasia if the dominant hemisphere is involved, and personality changes if the nondominant hemisphere is involved.

3. Lacunar Infarcts

Lacunar strokes represent approximately 20% of all strokes. The ischemic tissue is usually <1.0 cm in diameter and tends to occur where small perforating arterioles branch directly off large vessels. This distinctive anatomy occurs in the brainstem and the deep structures of the basal ganglia, thalamus, and internal capsule. The involved arterioles tend to become thickened and hyalinized and then thrombose, resulting in small local infarcts. Since they occur in deep subcortical regions of the brain, lacunar strokes tend to produce specific clinical deficits, the most common being hemiparesis without any sensory loss. A pure sensory stroke with no motor deficit is less common but may be seen. Although the functional deficits initially may be quite severe, the infarctions are usually small, and about 85% of the patients make a good recovery.

4. Hemorrhagic Strokes

Intracerebral hemorrhage accounts for about 10% of all strokes. The increased intracranial pressure (ICP) caused by sudden bleeding into the brain often causes headaches, nausea, vomiting, and altered consciousness.

AXIOM
The stroke patient who is lethargic or comatose has probably had an intracerebral hemorrhage.

Hemorrhages tend to occur in the same location as lacunae, deep within the brain in the region of the basal ganglia, internal capsule, and brainstem. Occasionally, intracerebral hematomas may appear following rupture of an aneurysm or arteriovenous malformation, and hypertension is much more common. The subcortical deficits are much more extensive than those seen with lacunae. Altered mental status, hemiplegia, hemisensory loss, and visual field defects are common. Although the initial mortality may exceed 50% to 70%, if the patient does survive, the residual deficits may be relatively mild.

D. CLINICAL EVALUATION OF STROKE

The history is the most reliable method of evaluating cerebrovascular disease. The neurologic or cardiac findings often only complement the history.

Surgery with a general anesthetic can greatly increase the risk of a stroke. The incidence of significant neurologic changes postoperatively in patients without a previous stroke is 0.2% to 0.7%, depending largely on the age of the patient. In patients with a prior stroke, the risk of recurrence during surgery is increased about 5- to 10-fold. Landercasper and associates recently noted a postoperative stroke rate of 2.9% in patients who had a past history of stroke. Maintenance of a normal or higher cardiac output and optimal oxygenation is essential in the OR, the postanesthetic recovery (PAR) room, and ICU. Use of anticoagulants may also be a risk. Landercasper and associates found that the most significant factors associated with perioperative strokes was the use of heparin preoperatively and systolic hypotension in the recovery room.

AXIOM
One should make great effort to avoid anticoagulants and hypotension in patients with a prior stoke, even if the event was very remote.

PITFALL
Failure to listen carefully for carotid or subclavian bruits in someone who has had a stroke.

Although examination of the carotid arteries is often unrewarding, it can be very helpful in detecting otherwise unsuspected vascular disease. However one cannot rely on the presence or absence of a bruit. No characteristic feature, including the volume, pitch, or duration of a carotid bruit, reliably indicates the degree of constriction of the vascular lumen. Carotid bruits are audible in some asymptomatic individuals who have no atherosclerosis and never suffer from cerebrovascular disease. It may also be absent in severely diseased vessels. Nevertheless, if a carotid bruit is detected, it should be investigated thoroughly.

PITFALL
Failure to perform a careful funduscopic examination on any patient who may have had a stroke.

Retinal vessels allow direct observation of arterial narrowing that may be due to hypertension or diabetes. Embolic strokes may be suspected because of embolic material in the retinal arteries. Cholesterol emboli often lodge in retinal artery bifurcations and are visible as shiny, refractile, orange-yellow crystals called Hollenhorst plaques. Retinal emboli composed of platelets and fibrin are grayish-white in color. Both kinds of emboli generally indicate the presence of carotid stenosis and ulceration.

PITFALL
Failure to completely evaluate the heart in a patient with a stroke.

Examination of the heart in a stroke patient should focus on detecting myocardial infarction, dysrhythmias, valve dysfunction, and bacterial endocarditis. The presence of heart disease is important because it greatly increases the morbidity and mortality from stroke. Up to 9% of patients with stroke have a concomitant myocardial infarction, which is often silent. One must, therefore, inquire carefully for chest pain, diaphoresis, nausea, dyspnea, or other symptoms of cardiac disease. Palpitations, dizziness, and light-headedness may be clues to dysrhythmias. The physician should also inquire about intravenous drug use and search for needle tracts, especially in younger patients and in individuals with endocarditis.

E. LABORATORY INVESTIGATION OF STROKE

Most patients with stroke have atherosclerotic or embolic cerebrovascular disease. Laboratory studies that may be of value in selected patients include a hematocrit, white blood cell count, blood cultures, and tests for sickle cells, syphilis, and vasculitis (such as sedimentation rate and antinuclear antibody). Metabolic encephalopathies can usually be detected by standard chemistry batteries including glucose, electrolytes, BUN, creatinine, and liver function tests.

An electrocardiogram (ECG) is necessary since myocardial infarction occurs frequently and is often clinically silent. Cardioscopic monitoring is important for detecting dysrhythmias early. CPK isoenzymes should be drawn every 8 hours times four. The chest radiograph may show cardiomegaly or other evidence of heart disease. Echocardiograms and Holter monitors are indicated if cardiac disease is suspected. An abnormal EEG may suggest a seizure rather than a stroke as the cause of focal neurologic symptoms.

F. RADIOGRAPHIC INVESTIGATION OF STROKE

Neuroradiographic imaging studies are the most useful procedures for evaluating stroke, and a CT scan of the head should be done on every stroke patient. Ischemic brain tissue gradually becomes hypodense (dark) on a CT scan.

PITFALL
Using an early "normal" CT scan of the brain to rule out an ischemic infarct.

CT scans obtained within the first 8 hours seldom demonstrate an ischemic infarct. They are usually positive by 24 hours, but it may be 2 or 3 days before an ischemic infarction becomes hypodense (dark) enough to be reliably detected.

PITFALL
Failure to obtain an early CT scan of the brain on patients who have neurologic changes that may be due to an intracranial lesion.

Free blood within the brain is hyperdense (white), and areas of bleeding can be detected immediately on a CT scan with almost 100% accuracy. Masses such as abscesses, brain tumors, and subdural hematomas, are reliably excluded by CT scanning, and CT scans can sometimes detect large arteriovenous malformations or aneurysms.

After 2 to 3 days, thrombotic infarcts are easily detected on a CT scan because of the large amount of ischemic brain tissue usually involved. Embolic strokes, causing smaller cortical lesions, are more difficult to detect. Lacunar strokes, which are often less than the 1.0 cm in diameter, usually cannot be demonstrated; however, more sophisticated CT scanners using thin-section slices may reveal many lacunar infarcts.

Because it can detect focal ischemia within hours, magnetic resonance imaging (MRI) is a much more sensitive test than a CT scan for early ischemic strokes. It is of special value in brainstem and posterior circulation strokes, since infarcts in that area are often obscured by adjacent bone and cannot be reliably detected on CT scans. Additional advantages of MRI are that it does not subject the patient to ionizing radiation and it does not require IV contrast. However, MRI does have some difficulty differentiating ischemic infarcts from hemorrhagic infarcts, abscesses, or neoplasms. The patient must also be more cooperative and remain motionless for a longer time than for a CT scan.

AXIOM
MRI should not be done on unstable or uncooperative patients.

G. MANAGEMENT OF THE STROKE PATIENT

AXIOM
Stroke patients often benefit from increased tissue oxygenation and a normal or slightly increased BP.

1. General Principles

Airway, breathing, and circulation should be supported, especially if the patient is comatose or unstable. After a stroke, most patients have a transient mild-moderate blood pressure elevation. Although this should be monitored carefully, intervention is seldom required unless the mean BP exceeds 140 mm Hg. In patients with ischemic stroke, it is generally preferable to let the BP stay slightly elevated rather than risk hypotension, which could enlarge the area of ischemia. Other support includes maintenance of adequate hydration, normal blood glucose levels, and electrolyte balance.

AXIOM
One should guard against aspiration of oral or gastric contents in the patient with strokes.

The leading cause of morbidity and mortality after a stroke is pneumonia, which is often due to aspiration. Patients should have their oral intake restricted until it is clear that they can swallow and cough well.

AXIOM
Fever after a stroke is often due to an infection, particularly pneumonia, or venous thrombosis.

Bedridden stroke patients are at high risk for deep venous thrombosis (DVT) with possible subsequent pulmonary emboli. Prophylaxis for DVT is controversial, but low-dose heparin therapy (5000 units subcutaneously b.i.d.) usually seems warranted, except in patients with bleeding. If heparin is contraindicated, pneumatic antiembolic stockings should be used to improve venous drainage in the legs.

AXIOM
Most patients admitted with a stroke have some underlying cardiac disease, and up to 9% have a concomitant myocardial infarction.

The myocardial ischemia in stroke patients is often unrecognized, and the patient should be examined carefully for any evidence of cardiac ischemia or dysfunction. Pre-existing heart disease, combined with the increased catecholamine release that often accompanies a stroke, probably accounts for the high incidence of dysrhythmias seen in these patients.

2. Treatment of the Stroke Itself

A great potential for recovery exists after most strokes, since many affected neurons are damaged rather than destroyed. Although there is no treatment, medical or surgical, that has been proven to alter the natural history of a completed stroke, there are some situations in which stroke victims require emergency or critical care.

STROKE AND CEREBRAL RESUSCITATION

325

a. Thrombotic Stroke

In addition to maintaining optimal blood flow and oxygenation of the brain, there is increasing use of antiplatelet therapy and thrombolytics. Barnaby, in a recent review, noted that antiplatelet therapy is increasingly recommended for completed thrombotic strokes in the form of aspirin 1 g per day, or 325 mg per day if there is gastrointestinal intolerance.

An exciting area of investigation is the use of thrombolytic therapy within 1 to 2 hours of a completed stroke. Early intra-arterial infusions have shown a high rate of recanalization and clinical improvement. There have been multicenter trials with tissue plasminogen activator (TPA) and single-chain urokinase plasminogen activator (SCU-PA) in patients with angiographically proven strokes.

In addition to these agents, another antithrombolytic drug, ancrod, a purified protein fraction of the venom of the Malayan pit viper, is undergoing multicenter trials. Ancrod has been used in Europe and Canada for treating peripheral vascular disease, deep-venous thrombosis, and, to a limited extent, stroke. Very preliminary evidence indicates that it may have fewer associated hemorrhage side effects than streptokinase or TPA.

(1) Stroke in Evolution

If the neurologic deficit is getting progressively worse, the patient is felt to have a "stroke in evolution" and heparin may be of some help. However, making an accurate diagnosis is essential, as tumors, subdural hematomas, infection, intoxication, and metabolic disturbances (hypoglycemia) have been known to mimic progressive stroke. A CT scan is mandatory to rule out intracerebral hemorrhage or hemorrhagic stroke. If the CT scan is negative for intracerebral hemorrhage, the patient is begun on IV heparin at about 1000 units per hour, with close monitoring of the prothrombin time (PT) and partial thromboplastin time (PTT). Many authorities do not give a 5000 unit loading dose of heparin because this might increase the likelihood of intracerebral hemorrhage. If the PTT exceeds 1.5 times normal, the dose should be reduced, but if the PTT is lower, the dose of heparin should probably not be increased. After a few days, warfarin therapy is started and adjusted to maintain the PT at about 1.5 times control. Heparin can then be stopped, and oral anticoagulation is then continued for at least 4 to 8 weeks.

AXIOM

Contraindications to anticoagulation include large cerebral infarctions, uncontrolled hypertension, or evidence of active bleeding.

(2) Increasing Intracranial Pressure

Some patients with a thrombotic stroke become much sicker due to development of increased intracranial pressure (ICP). Cytotoxic edema is common after a stroke and usually reaches a peak 3 to 5 days after the initial insult. As the brain tissue swells, the ICP can increase and cause further neurologic deficits. The first evidence of increased ICP is usually increasing lethargy progressing to stupor and coma.

AXIOM

Patients with coma may benefit from hyperventilation and diuretics.

Intubation and hyperventilation of the patient to a Pco_2 of 25 to 30 mm Hg causes cerebral vasoconstriction and can lower ICP rapidly. However, the mainstay of ICP reduction is diuretics (such as 40 to 80 mg of IV furosemide) and osmolar agents such as mannitol or glycerol. A dose of 100 g of mannitol can be administered intravenously as a bolus, and then 50 g can be given every 4 to 6 hours as needed. Giving the furosemide simultaneously may reduce the initial tendency to hypervolemia caused by mannitol alone.

High doses of steroids, 6 mg of dexamethasone every 4 hours, may be of some value. However, their use, except with rapidly growing brain tumors, is controversial, and they are usually not effective within the first few hours.

b. Embolic Stroke

Embolic cerebral infarction often occurs in the setting of continuing embolization from a cardiac source. Anticoagulation has been a mainstay of prophylactic treatment in high-risk groups for several years. Early anticoagulation reduces the chance of re-embolus to about one-third of the natural rate. However, concerns about early hemorrhagic transformation of an infarct and long-term complications of anticoagulation continue to be a concern. Recent studies suggest that CT should be obtained 48 hours after an embolic stroke to rule out hemorrhagic infarct. Anticoagulation with heparin can then be started in those patients who have relatively mild neurologic deficits. Patients with large infarcts tend to have the highest incidence of hemorrhagic complications with anticoagulation. In such patients, the CT scan can be repeated in 3 to 5 days. If no hemorrhagic transformation has occurred, heparin can then be started. Consideration should be given to obtaining a CT scan with contrast media, as enhancement can indicate the presence of small hemorrhage. An MRI would be of even greater value in ruling out hemorrhagic infarct. If hemorrhagic transformation is noted in very high-risk patients, acute anticoagulation can then be delayed for approximately 10 days. A lumbar puncture and cerebrospinal fluid examination offers no advantage over CT or MRI and is not necessary in the evaluation of embolic stroke. Once anticoagulation has been decided upon, heparin should be begun at an infusion rate of 1000 units per hour, with the goal of achieving a partial thromboplastin time (PTT) of 1.5 times the control value. Oral warfarin can be started after 3 to 4 days for chronic anticoagulation. Fibrinolytic therapy for acute embolic stroke is now undergoing study but is not currently indicated.

c. Lacunar Stroke

Occasionally, lacunar strokes can evolve or progress, but many authorities recommend against anticoagulating a lacunar stroke in evolution, since the risk of bleeding from one of the small perforating vessels may be greater than any potential benefit. These strokes are so small that edema is seldom a significant problem, and patients with lacunar strokes usually recover well, regardless of the severity of the initial deficit.

d. Intracerebral Hemorrhage

AXIOM
Controlling ICP is especially important in patients with hemorrhagic strokes.

The main danger from intracerebral hemorrhage lies in the increased ICP due to the amount of blood within the cranial cavity. This is the one setting after a stroke in which acute treatment of hypertension may be indicated in order to lower ICP. However, if the BP is allowed to drop too quickly, cerebral ischemia may result.

II. OTHER CEREBRO-VASCULAR SYNDROMES

A. TRANSIENT ISCHEMIC ATTACK

AXIOM
Patients with TIAs are at greatly increased risk of developing strokes.

TIAs are defined as acute thromboembolic neurologic deficits lasting no longer than 24 hours, with most events lasting only 10 minutes to 1 hour. TIAs are usually mild. Three general clinical types of TIA have been defined: (1) transient monocular blindness or amaurosis fugax, a sudden, painless dimness or loss of vision in one eye; (2) transient hemispheric attacks associated with focal motor and sensory symptoms, and, at times, language impairment; (3) vertebrobasilar TIAs which are most reliably diagnosed when "hard findings" such as diplopia, ataxia, or dysarthria are present. Unilateral weakness or sensory loss may also be present but are difficult to localize to the vertebrobasilar area.

A variant of these is crescendo TIA with recurrent cerebral hemisphere or monocular TIA lasting several minutes to a few hours and increasing in frequency to several attacks per day.

The diagnosis of TIA is made by obtaining a history of transient, but definite, focal findings that correlate well with carotid or vertebrobasilar territories. The incidence of strokes in patients suffering TIAs is 4 to 10 times greater than in the general population. The incidence of stroke is 5% to 6% per year, with the highest risk being in the first month after the initial TIA.

The term reversible ischemic neurologic deficit (RIND) has been applied to syndromes similar to TIAs, which last 24 to 96 hours and leave a minor neurologic deficit. Following a TIA or RIND with complete resolution of symptoms, subsequent CT or MRI has revealed a focal ischemic infarct in up to 25%. This has led to the designation of a third category, cerebral infarct with transient symptoms (CITS).

Treatment of TIAs is controversial. Only 20% to 30% of patients with TIAs have been found to have significant carotid disease. Carotid endarterectomy may be of benefit in certain selected patients. The ideal candidate is a symptomatic patient with little or no permanent deficit, who is in good general health, has a carotid artery stenosis of at least 50% to 60% or large ulcerated or hemorrhage plaque, has TIA symptoms in the specific carotid distribution, and has minimal other atherosclerotic manifestations.

Patients who are asymptomatic, have vertebrobasilar symptoms, casually detected lesions (such as asymptomatic carotid bruit), or lesions on the non-symptomatic side, or are about to undergo open heart or aortic surgery are not usually candidates for endarterectomy.

The therapeutic mainstay for TIAs includes antiplatelet and anticoagulation agents. A number of studies have demonstrated a significant reduction in TIAs (50%) and stroke risk (22%) in patients taking daily aspirin. No benefit has been demonstrated with dipyridamole (Persantin). Although doses of aspirin as small as 30 mg per day were thought to be efficacious in one study, the generally recommended dosage is 1 g per day (325 mg per day in those with gastrointestinal intolerance). In a recent randomized trial reported by Haas, Easton, and Adams, Ticlopidine (500 mg daily), another antiplatelet drug, was found to be somewhat more effective than ASA (1300 mg) in penetrating strokes in high-risk patients with TIAs, RIND, or prior minor strokes.

Anticoagulation with warfarin should be reserved for patients with TIAs caused by cardiac emboli or for those who do not respond to or cannot take aspirin. Warfarin probably should generally not be continued for longer than 6 months. After that period, the risk of complications from anticoagulation therapy exceeds the risk of cerebral infarction.

B. SUBARACHNOID HEMORRHAGE

1. Clinical Features

Subarachnoid hemorrhage is a true medical emergency in which prompt diagnosis is essential. Primary subarachnoid hemorrhage is responsible for approximately 10% of all stroke deaths. About 17% of patients with a ruptured intracranial aneurysm die before reaching the hospital, and one half of all these patients die during the initial hospital period. It is caused most commonly by bleeding from a saccular arterial aneurysm. Subarachnoid hemorrhage may occur at any age, but the peak incidence is the sixth decade, and there is a slight female predominance. Hypertension may contribute to rupture of an aneurysm, but this is not the sole cause of rupture. Normal blood pressure in an older patient with a hemorrhagic stroke should arouse suspicion of a ruptured aneurysm.

AXIOM

Sudden onset of the worst headache a patient ever had should be considered a leaking intracranial aneurysm until proven otherwise.

Sudden rupture of an intracerebral aneurysm frequently causes an abrupt, excruciating, well-localized headache, which is often described as the worst headache the patient has ever experienced. Irritation of the meninges by the intracranial blood may also cause nuchal rigidity and nausea and vomiting. Focal neurologic signs, such as hemiparesis or cranial nerve palsies, may occur, depending on the site of the ruptured blood vessel. The majority of these patients are initially alert and oriented, but up to 50% of patients become comatose immediately following a subarachnoid hemorrhage.

2. Diagnostic Evaluation

An ECG with rhythm strip and continuous cardioscopic monitoring is mandatory because the catecholamine surge and hypertension after subarachnoid hemorrhage often precipitate cardiac dysrhythmias. Bleeding parameters, including PT, PTT, platelet count, and bleeding time should also be measured. The syndrome of inappropriate antidiuretic hormone secretion (SIADH) may also develop after an intracranial bleed; consequently, fluid balance and serum electrolytes should also be checked carefully. In these patients a relatively mild hyponatremia (125 to 129 mEq/liter) may cause symptoms.

A CT scan without contrast enhancement detects the subarachnoid hemorrhage in approximately 75% to 90% of the patients. The CT scan can also often localize the site of the bleeding, and the aneurysm itself may occasionally be visualized. The CT scan may also rule out other CNS problems, or may show a large hematoma that would preclude a lumbar puncture.

AXIOM
The definitive test for subarachnoid hemorrhage is a lumbar puncture that reveals blood within the cerebrospinal fluid (CSF).

If the CT scan is equivocal or negative in a patient with a suspected subarachnoid hemorrhage, examination of the spinal fluid can be confirmatory. Lumbar puncture is usually safe provided there is no evidence of a high ICP and the CT scan does not show a focal mass of blood. If there is any question that blood in the CSF is due to a traumatic tap rather than a subarachnoid hemorrhage, the spinal fluid should be spun down in a centrifuge. Blood that is more than 2 hours old leaves a xanthochromic supernatant, confirming that blood was present before the lumbar puncture.

Although CT scanning and lumbar puncture can demonstrate blood in the subarachnoid space, angiography is necessary for precise localization and characterization of aneurysms or arteriovenous malformations. However, since angiography can cause or increase cerebral vasospasm, this test is usually deferred until just before surgery, so that any vasospasm present will not be aggravated unnecessarily. Patients with subarachnoid hemorrhage often deteriorate during the first few days following their initial bleed, usually because of cerebral arterial spasm. Consequently, the mortality for early surgery is high.

The continued high morbidity and mortality of patients with subarachnoid hemorrhage is principally due to rebleeding and the development of delayed cerebral ischemia due to cerebral arterial vasospasm. An estimated one third of patients will experience rebleeding, and one third ischemia, within 14 days of rupture if left untreated. Because of this danger, many neurosurgeons recommend early surgical intervention (within 72 hours) from aneurysm clipping and drainage of clot. With early intervention and newer microneurosurgical techniques 75% to 80% of patients admitted with grades I to III subarachnoid hemorrhage (with relatively mild deficits) in one series made a good neurologic recovery.

The administration of antifibrinolytic agents such as epsilon-aminocaproic acid and tranexamic acid have been given in a effort to retard clot lysis and prevent rebleeding, but these agents have been associated with an increased incidence of vasospasm with no reduction in overall morbidity or mortality.

One of the most promising modalities being used to prevent the effects of vasospasm is the calcium channel blocker nimodipine. Nimodipine is lipid soluble, enabling it to cross the blood-brain barrier more easily than its counterpart, nifedipine. Its mechanism of action is unknown; there is no significant difference in the degree of vasospasm in nimodipine and placebo-treated patients. It is speculated that nimodipine may have the effect of reducing intracellular influx of calcium, thus preventing the dramatic rise associated with ischemia, or that it may dilate small vessels not seen by angiography. Several studies have shown a dramatic reduction in delayed ischemic infarcts in patients when treated with nimodipine (60 mg orally every 4 hours) within 96 hours of presentation. Nimodipine seems especially effective in patients with large subarachnoid clots, as the degree of subsequent vasospasm and delayed infarct seems to correlate with the thickness of clot. The only significant complication reported with nimodipine was hypotension, which occurred in 6.5% of patients in one series.

3. Complications (Table 7.4)

AXIOM

Vasospasm and recurrent bleeding are the main dangers in an otherwise stable patient with intracerebral bleeding.

a. Rebleeding

Continued or recurrent bleeding from a cerebral aneurysm is often fatal, and up to 20% of these patients will rebleed, half within the first few days. Management to reduce the likelihood of recurrent bleeding includes bed rest, sedatives, a calm environment, and stool softeners.

Severe hypertension should be controlled as soon as possible. Antihypertensive medications, such as hydralazine and/or propranolol, are administered as needed. A combination of alpha- and beta-adrenergic blockers may be preferable. However, if the blood pressure is lowered too much, cerebral vasospasm may be induced or made worse. As a compromise, a pressure of about 140/90 is usually considered adequate. To prevent rebleeding, some physicians use antifibrinolytic agents such as epsilon-aminocaproic acid; however, its use is controversial.

b. Vasospasm

AXIOM

Early surgery or cerebral angiography may cause increased vasospasm.

Vasospasm usually begins about 3 days after the initial bleed and may persist for 2 to 3 weeks, rendering surgery impossible during that time (Table 7.5). The increasing vasospasm may be severe enough to cause a cerebral infarction, and this should be suspected if the patient develops new focal deficits. As mentioned earlier, some studies suggest that the calcium channel blocker, nimodipine may prevent or minimize vasospasm.

Table 7.4

COMPLICATIONS OF SUBARACHNOID HEMORRHAGE

Complication	Clinical Features	Diagnostic Tests	Therapy
Increased ICP	Decreased alertness	ICP monitor	Mannitol, steroids
Hydrocephalus	Decreased alertness	CT scan	Ventricular shunt
Vasospasm	Delayed focal deficit	Angiography	Maintain volume and BP
Recurrent hemorrhage	Worsening of deficits	CT scan and LP	Clip aneurysm
Seizures	Focal or generalized	EEG	Anticonvulsants
SIADH	Worsening of deficits	Serum and urine osmolarity	Fluid restriction

Table 7.5

CAUSES OF DETERIORATION AFTER SUBARACHNOID HEMORRHAGE	Time	Rebleed, %	Vasospasm, %	Hydrocephalus, %	Other, %
	1–6 days	60	20	5	15
	7–14 days	15	70	10	5
	15–21 days	5	80	10	5

c. Hydrocephalus

Hydrocephalus may be caused by blood blocking the resorptive pathways of the spinal fluid. In such instances early ventricular drainage by a shunt may be required.

d. Seizures

AXIOM
Great efforts should be made to prevent recurrent seizures after a stroke.

Seizures are usually best initially controlled with IV diazepam (Valium), and recurrences are best prevented by giving phenytoin (Dilantin), usually as a loading dose of 15 to 18 mg/kg and then at 300 to 400 mg per day. Some feel that a loading dose of Dilantin should be given as soon as a diagnosis of ruptured cerebral aneurysm is made.

e. Intracranial Hemorrhage

Intracerebral hemorrhage in the elderly is most often caused by chronic hypertension with its associated arteriopathy in the small arterioles that supply the basal ganglia, thalamus, and brainstem. Approximately 10% of all strokes are caused by intracerebral hemorrhage, and the majority of these cases occur between the ages of 55 and 75. Other causes include trauma, arteriovenous malformation, amyloid angiopathy, and coagulopathies. The most common locations, in order of frequency, are the putamen, thalamus, cerebral lobar areas, caudate nucleus, and cerebellum. The clinical picture is one of a gradual onset over minutes to hours and a focal neurologic deficit often accompanied by headache and vomiting.

Hemorrhage affecting the putamen often involves the adjacent internal capsule, producing contralateral hemiparesis, hemisensory deficit, and, frequently, hemianopsia. Thalamic hemorrhage commonly produces hemianesthesia more prominently than hemiparesis, along with impaired upward gaze. Significant hemorrhage into the pons is usually catastrophic, producing coma, quadriparesis, and a dramatic dysconjugate ocular mobility disorder. Lobar hemorrhages may produce unilateral hemiparesis and hemisensory deficits, and possible speech impairment. The CT scan reveals the lesion quite readily.

When considering therapy, hematomas can be divided into three groups:

1. Massive lesions producing profound neurologic deficits. Little can be done for these patients except for general supportive therapy.

2. Hematomas of 3 cm or greater with developing mass effect with mild-to-moderate neurologic deficit. This group of patients generally will benefit most from early surgical intervention.

3. Small hematomas (<3 cm in diameter) with associated relatively minor neurologic deficit. Most of these patients make an excellent spontaneous recovery, and therapy should consist of controlling hypertension and general supportive measures.

If the patient does exhibit signs of increasing intracranial pressure, controlled hyperventilation or mannitol therapy should be considered.

f. Cerebellar Hemorrhage

Cerebellar hemorrhage is most often caused by hypertension in the elderly and constitutes approximately 7% of all intracranial hemorrhages. Patients will often experience the abrupt onset of headache, vertigo, vomiting, and ataxia. A paralysis of conjugate gaze to one side can also be seen. No change in the level of consciousness is noted until a mass effect produces brainstem compression and coma. Rapid neurosurgical intervention is vital in patients exhibiting signs of an altered level of consciousness. Special views of the posterior fossa should be obtained. If MRI is available, a better radiologic evaluation of the cerebellar-brainstem area can be made to help determine if early surgical intervention is indicated.

III. BRAIN RESUSCITATION AFTER CPR

The goals of cerebral resuscitation after a period of severe global ischemia or anoxia are to (1) ameliorate CNS damage that has already occurred, (2) reverse ongoing mechanisms of injury, and (3) protect uninjured but endangered neurons. This may best be accomplished by aggressive establishment of optimal cardiopulmonary function, maintenance of vital organ oxygenation, and support of cerebral perfusion (Table 7.6).

A. IMMEDIATE CONCERNS

1. Intracranial Pressure

Intracranial pressure is not always elevated after ischemic or hypoxic insults. However, it may be increased in near drowning victims where it is a useful tool in predicting survival or death, but not residual brain damage. It is generally felt that ICP monitoring is an essential part of the management of patients who may have an elevated ICP, especially after a serious head injury. Monitoring of vital signs alone is inadequate to detect neurologic deterioration in patients with cerebral ischemia, especially if they are unresponsive.

2. Blood Pressure

AXIOM

One should make great efforts to keep a high normal CPP and low ICP in patients who have suffered cerebral ischemia.

Maintenance of arterial blood pressure in a high normal range is essential in the brain-injured patient. Inadequate perfusion pressure decreases the supply of nutrients and oxygen required for cerebral metabolic needs. Too high a blood pressure, on the other hand, increases cerebral blood volume (CBV) and may increase ICP. In head trauma, close monitoring of ICP and mean blood pressure (MBP) allows maintenance of adequate cerebral perfusion pressure (CPP) without compromising intracranial volume (ICV).

3. Central Venous Pressure

The CVP should be kept at normal or slightly lower levels, especially if there is any indication of an elevated ICP. However, if the CVP falls too low, blood pressure and cerebral blood flow may fall below ideal levels.

Table 7.6

GOALS OF CEREBRAL RESUSCITATION	*Maintain CNS Perfusion and Oxygenation* BP at normal or higher levels CVP and ICP as low as possible PaO_2 >80–100 mm Hg CPP >70–90 mm Hg
	Decrease Cerebral Metabolism Prevent seizures Barbiturates Prevent hyperthermia
	Prevent Chemical Damage to Brain Scavenge free radicals Desferoxamine Mannitol

---

B. CENTRAL NERVOUS SYSTEM PHYSIOLOGY AND PATHOPHYSIOLOGY

AXIOM

The brain needs an almost constant supply of oxygen, glucose, and other nutrients.

Unlike most other tissues, the brain has almost no storage capacity for oxygen or glucose and has only a slight capacity for anaerobic metabolism. Although the brain comprises only 2% of the body weight, it receives 15% to 20% of the cardiac output (750 to 1200 ml per minute). Neurotransmitter synthesis and maintenance of proper electrolyte concentrations across neuronal cell membranes require a great deal of energy. Energy consumption in the CNS is so high that, if circulation is cut off, an almost immediate cessation of neuronal function occurs. Within 4 to 6 minutes of almost complete global ischemia, all CNS high-energy phosphate compounds are consumed, leading to ion pump failure, loss of transmembrane electrical potential, and cellular edema. However, some neurons may recover limited activity even after 50 minutes of total ischemia.

Normal cerebral blood flow (CBF) averages 55 ml per 100 g tissue per minute, with white matter requiring somewhat less flow than gray matter. Cerebral perfusion pressure, derived by subtracting mean ICP from MBP, averages about 85 ± 15 mm Hg and is a relatively good indicator of CBF. Between mBPs of 55 and 150 mm Hg, CBF remains relatively constant in normal, supine subjects.

The intracranial contents include brain tissue (80% to 90%), blood in arteries (2% to 3%), blood in veins (3% to 6%), and cerebrospinal fluid (5% to 10%). If the brain progressively swells or there is intracranial bleeding, the amount of CSF present falls. As the ICP continues to rise, the amount of blood in cerebral veins and then arteries will also fall. If the ICP becomes high enough, there may be no cerebral perfusion.

Vasomotor control of cerebral arteries is determined primarily by $Paco_2$ and pH. Pao_2 plays a much less important role and affects cerebral vascular tone if it falls to less than 50 mm Hg. Hyperventilation-induced hypocapnia can causes a significant reduction of CBF and a resultant decrease in intracranial blood volume. Cerebral blood falls about 2% to 4% for each 1.0 mm Hg drop in the Pco_2.

1. Experimental Studies

In the absence of pharmacologic protection, the brain is the organ most sensitive to ischemic damage. It had long been thought that irreversible neuronal damage occurs after only 4 to 6 minutes of complete ischemia. However, there is increasing evidence that neurologic deficits following complete ischemia are not due to immediate neuronal death.

AXIOM

Brain death from transient ischemia is largely due to secondary processes rather than the initial insult.

In 1963, Ames and Guarian reported survival of retinal cells for more than 45 minutes in anoxic tissue baths. Hossmann and Kleiheus in 1973 found recovery of high-energy metabolism and action potential generation in cat cerebral neurons after 60 minutes of ischemic anoxia. Thus, ischemic-anoxic brain death may not occur in 4 to 6 minutes; however, the ischemic-anoxic episode apparently sets off a series of pathologic processes that eventually do lead to brain death.

2. Clinical Studies

a. After CPR

Although many observers have had great optimism about the results of CPR, the number of long-term survivors with normal cerebral function after cardiac arrest is quite low. Eisenberg, Copas, and Hallstrom, for example, reported in 1980 that only 6% of patients having an out-of-hospital cardiac arrest left the hospital alive. Furthermore, over 50% of those who survived had permanent severe neurologic disability. In another series, only one third of the survivors of CPR were able to return to their previous life style, and only 10% were without evidence of some intellectual impairment. On the other hand, if the heart were defibrillated within 4 to 6 minutes, 22% left the hospital alive and neurologic recovery was improved.

AXIOM
Early defibrillation is the best way to ensure recovery from a cardiac arrest with an intact CNS.

As the time from cardiac arrest to successful defibrillation begins to exceed 6 minutes, the outcome becomes progressively worse, even if CPR is begun immediately after the cardiac arrest. Closed-chest CPR, as it is currently done, does not adequately perfuse many tissues of the body, especially the brain. Cerebral blood flow (CBF) with closed-chest CPR in dogs is only 5% to 10% of normal. In addition, basic CPR usually does not produce an aortic diastolic pressure high enough to overcome coronary vascular resistance and adequately perfuse fibrillating hearts. In contrast, open-chest CPR with large epinephrine infusions may raise cerebral cortical blood flow (CCBF) to values greater than normal.

b. After Drowning

The neurologic outlook for near drowned individuals, especially children, is usually good, particularly in those who can develop spontaneous respiration soon after resuscitation. Although it had been thought in the past that an immersion time greater than 5 minutes was fatal, survival of small children has been reported after cold immersion times of 20 to 40 minutes.

IV. PATHOPHYSI-OLOGY OF ISCHEMIC-ANOXIC CELLULAR INJURY

A. CHANGES WITH TIME

About 15 seconds after complete cessation of cerebral blood flow, the brain's oxygen stores are totally depleted. By 5 minutes, the glucose and glycogen stores have been consumed so that even anaerobic glycolysis comes to a halt. Intracellular adenosine triphosphate (ATP) is also exhausted, and all energy requiring reactions cease. As soon as the plasma membrane sodium pump stops working, sodium, calcium, and water begin to enter the cell, causing increasing cellular edema. After about an hour of ischemic anoxia, frank necrosis of neurons becomes increasingly evident, as shown by vacuolization of mitochondria and breakdown of the plasma membrane.

B. CHANGES WITH SEVERITY OF ISCHEMIA

1. Clinical Changes

Progressive functional and metabolic disturbances increase with the severity of the ischemia. With perfusion rates above 30% of normal, neurons can maintain a fairly normal ATP content by using anaerobic glycolysis to make up for some of the compromised oxygen delivery. If oxygen and substrate delivery is then returned to normal, neuronal function is also brought rapidly back to normal.

AXIOM
Increasing lactate in cerebral venous blood is usually a sign of progressive cerebral damage.

Myocardial cells also maintain viability for prolonged periods if coronary blood flow is at least 30% of normal. However, if coronary blood flow falls to 15% to 30% of normal, glucose availability is limited and cellular ATP content rapidly declines. An increasing lactic acidemia progressively depresses anaerobic ATP production by inhibiting phosphofructokinase (PFK), the rate-limiting enzyme in glycolysis. Lactate begins to accumulate, and the lactate levels correlate rather well with irreversible injury in neurons and in the myocardium.

As severe cellular ischemic anoxia continues, protein and membrane degeneration occurs with release of lysosomal enzymes and superoxides. Lipid peroxidation of cell membranes may be particularly important. Eventually these changes result in irreversible cellular injury, even if normal blood flow is finally re-established. However, with absolute ischemia, all reactions rapidly stop, resulting in an "ischemic freeze," and the rate of cellular damage appears to be greatly decreased, at least for the next 30 to 60 minutes.

AXIOM
Complete ischemic anoxia may be better than a partial but inadequate blood flow.

Any precipitous fall in ATP content rapidly reduces the cell's ability to maintain ionic gradients across cell membranes with a resulting K^+ efflux and Na^+ influx. As sodium enters the cells and then the mitochondria, these structures absorb increasing amounts of water, causing cytotoxic edema and impaired function. If blood flow is completely arrested, these ion shifts are slower and there is relatively little change in the electrolyte content of the blood and interstitial fluid for some time. However, if a little blood flow persists, the fluid and electrolyte changes are usually much more severe and rapid.

2. Problems of Minimal Perfusion during Closed-Chest CPR

It is now clear that closed-chest CPR, especially if used for more than 6 to 8 minutes without restoring an adequate circulation, may be very deleterious to the brain. If CBF is only 10% of normal, there are massive increases in neuronal lactate and rapid development of irreversible mitochondrial injury. Continuous low oxygen delivery may also allow a number of other deleterious chemical reactions to occur. These include increased production of free radicals, increased movement of calcium into cells, and increased production of arachidonic acid metabolites, such as thromboxane and leukotrienes.

C. FAILURE OF CEREBRAL REPERFUSION (NO-REFLOW PHENOMENON)

AXIOM
Prolonged cerebral ischemia is followed by transient hyperfusion and then a progressive severe failure of reperfusion.

Restoration of cerebral perfusion after complete cessation of blood flow, if carried out within 5 to 10 minutes, results in an overall increase in cerebral blood flow, although some areas of hypoperfusion probably remain. This period of hyperfusion may last 5 to 15 minutes but is then followed by a rapid and progressive decrease in CBF to less than 30% to 50% of normal. This has been well confirmed in dogs where there is a progressive reduction of cortical CBF after a 20-minute cardiac arrest. This progressive failure of reperfusion may occur even if mean aortic pressure is maintained at 100 mm Hg following the cardiac arrest.

There appear to be several mechanisms for this progressive failure of reperfusion. Swelling of glial and endothelial cells together with red blood cell sludging and intravascular coagulation may contribute to the overall reduction in CBF. Normal carbon dioxide responses and CBF autoregulation are lost, and the ICP tends to rise as the tissues become more edematous. The finite space of the cranial vault becomes filled, and a critical point on the intracranial pressure-volume curve is reached where a small increase in volume (CSF, blood, or brain tissue) cause a significant increase in ICP.

Cerebrospinal fluid (CSF), which comprises only about 5% of the ICV, passes through the ventricles into the spinal subarachnoid space. Cerebral blood volume, compromises about 6% to 12% of the total intracranial volume (ICV), is affected by blood pressure, cerebral autoregulation, and vasomotor control. Because of the limited nature of the compensatory mechanisms that reduce CSF and CBF, the brunt of the pressure increase is taken by the intracranial neuronal tissue.

An extremely important factor in brain viability is the cerebral perfusion pressure (CPP), which is equal to the mean arterial blood pressure minus the ICP. The CPP must be maintained above 50 mm Hg. As ICP rises, cerebral perfusion pressure (CPP) falls. Swelling can become so great that CPP becomes inadequate. If cerebral blood flow (CBF) falls to less than 30% of normal and cannot be returned to normal, brain death is assured.

Global ischemia tends to produce edema that develops after recirculation, whereas focal ischemia can produce edema during the ischemic phase. Both cause cytotoxic edema, which is intracellular swelling due to cellular structural damage. Cerebral edema seen after trauma is predominately vasogenic and is caused by cerebral blood vessel injury. The resultant increase in vascular permeability causes additional fluid accumulation in the cerebral interstitial space. This phenomenon is commonly referred to as a breakdown of the blood-brain barrier. It is a major contributor to cerebral ischemia as ICP increases.

Another factor thought to contribute to the increased cerebral vascular resistance after ischemia is stiffening of RBCs due to a calcium influx. This results in a loss of deformability which is necessary for RBCs to squeeze through nutrient capillaries.

Although some investigators believe that an increased ICP and cerebral vascular resistance due to severe brain swelling are the main causes of the poor postresuscitation blood flow, recent studies indicate that intracranial pressures may not rise significantly for some time following the resuscitation. Intravascular clotting was also thought to play a role, but there is usually no evidence of fibrin deposition in cerebral vessels at autopsy.

D. REPERFUSION INJURY

During the period of progressive postischemic hypoperfusion, there is a concurrent cellular postischemic hypermetabolism. This causes an increasing discrepancy between blood supply and cellular demand. This may partially explain why cell damage due to ischemia seems to accelerate after reperfusion has begun. For example, the structure of ribosomes is maintained relatively well during 30 to 60 minutes of complete ischemia, but during reperfusion, the ribosomes rapidly degenerate so that, even if the cell survives, there is a prolonged severe disturbance of protein biosynthesis. Membrane-bound enzymes such as ATPase and cyclic nucleotide-related enzymes also rapidly lose their activity with reperfusion.

E. CALCIUM AND ISCHEMIC-ANOXIC INJURY

AXIOM

Movement of ionized calcium into cells appears to be a major factor in deterioration following ischemia-anoxia.

1. Calcium Entry into Ischemic Cells

Extracellular fluid normally has an ionized calcium concentration of 1.0 to 1.20 mmol/liter. This is equivalent to 10^{-3} molar. Katz and others have determined that cytoplasm has an ionized calcium content of only 10^{-7} molar. This 10,000 to 1 gradient across the cell membrane is maintained by mechanisms requiring active cell metabolism. As described by Filoteo et al, these include a low-affinity, slow-pumping carrier system and a high-affinity, rapid-pumping ATP-dependent mode induced by calcium-activated calmodulin. Carafoli described a third membrane calcium pump system which is an exchange mechanism that moves one calcium out of the cell in exchange for three sodium ions. Failure of these mechanisms disturbs the proper extracellular-intracellular distribution of calcium which is essential for proper function of cardiac, renal, and smooth-muscle cells. Loss of surface Ca^{++} also results in membrane degeneration and increased permeability to water and various ions.

Seisjo found that excess calcium entry into the cell activates proteases and phospholipases which can hydrolyze cell membranes and cause progressive loss of phospholipids and rapid liberation of free fatty acids (FFA) into the cytosol. The increased free-fatty acids in turn can act as detergents, damaging cell membranes and allowing further Ca^{++} and water entry into the cell. FFA also disrupt mitochondrial membranes, thereby reducing ATP synthesis. This loss of cell membrane function and reduced ATP synthesis then become part of a vicious cycle leading to irreversible cellular injury.

2. Mitochondrial Calcium Handling and ATP Formation

AXIOM

The inability of damaged cells to maintain an adequate cellular level of ATP following ischemia is a critical event leading to cell death.

Exposure of isolate mitochondria to calcium and metabolic substrates in vitro rapidly increases mitochondrial oxygen consumption and reduces ATP production. White and colleagues found that this is accompanied by leakage of protons out of the mitochondria and an uptake of calcium into the mitochondrial matrix. Thus, in the presence of increased calcium, the electrochemical gradient provided by the energy of oxidation in the Krebs cycle is used by mitochondria to take up the calcium rather than produce ATP.

3. Calcium-Activated Myofibrillar Contraction

a. Myocardium

In normal myocardium, transient increases in intracellular Ca^{++} initiate muscle contraction by releasing the troponin inhibition of actin and myosin cross-bridging. During anoxia and ischemia, failure to pump out calcium results in the development of sustained myofibrillar contracture, which increases diastolic resting tension and reduces cardiac output. Following reperfusion there is an even greater decrease in contractility and cardiac output. In addition, high myocardial Ca^{++} can trigger arrhythmias that may progress to ventricular fibrillation.

b. Vascular Smooth Muscle

Inadequate tissue perfusion following ischemic-anoxia may be further reduced by vascular smooth-muscle spasm caused by calcium influx. Once the actino-myosin complex is formed, high concentrations of Ca^{++} in vascular smooth-muscle cells hinder relaxation and increase vascular resistance.

4. Calcium and Arachidonic Acid Production

During ischemia, Ca^{++} influx into cells activates phospholipase A_2, which in turn causes a rise in arachidonic acid in the cytosol. During reoxygenation, arachidonic acid is metabolized or converted by cycloxygenase and lipoxygenase into a number of potentially cytotoxic compounds including thromboxane, endoperoxides, and leukotrienes. Thromboxane can cause platelet aggregation and severe vasospasm, thereby markedly reducing local blood flow. The leukotrienes and endoperoxides have free radical characteristics and can also cause vasoconstriction and cell damage.

F. FREE (SUPEROXIDE) RADICALS

Free radicals are extremely active oxygen derivatives with a single electron in their outer shell. All cells that have oxidative metabolism can produce free radicals as by-products, and under certain circumstances these free radicals can degrade membranes, proteins, and DNA, and thereby destroy the cell. Free radicals can also interfere with Ca^{++} uptake by the cardiac sarcoplasmic reticulum during reperfusion, thereby increasing Ca^{++} concentrations in the cytosol.

Three kinds of defense are normally available to control free radicals. These include (1) enzymes, such as catalase, peroxidase, and superoxide dismutase, which quickly react with free radicals to produce nontoxic compounds; (2) free radical scavengers, which include vitamins E and C and sulfur-containing amino acids and peptides; and (3) intact membranes, which provide a physical separation between normally occurring free radicals and sensitive biomolecules.

With reoxygenation after ischemia, increased damage by free radicals may occur for several reasons: (1) the activated arachidonic acid cascade produces increased amounts of intermediates with free radical characteristics, (2) degradation of high-energy phosphates leads to accumulation of xanthine which reacts with xanthine oxidase to produce free radicals, (3) damaged lipid membranes allow free radicals access to susceptible biomolecules, and (4) posthypoxic cells have decreased endogenous free radical scavengers such as superoxide dismutase and glutathione peroxidase. Thus, after ischemic anoxia, an increase in the production of free radicals and a decrease in the cellular defense mechanisms allow these agents to cause increasing cell damage. Consequently, a paradox develops following ischemic anoxia. The cells desperately need oxygen to survive, but oxygen also produces increased free radicals which can destroy the cell.

AXIOM
A little oxygen may be particularly damaging to ischemic cells because it may result in production of free radicals and little or no ATP.

V. TREATMENT

Therapy designed to improve cerebral resuscitation after a cardiac arrest includes maintaining adequate CNS perfusion, improving cerebral metabolism, and reducing cerebral metabolic demands. Platelet inhibitors and calcium blockers may also be useful.

A. MAINTENANCE OF ADEQUATE CEREBRAL PERFUSION

Cerebral perfusion is directly related to the cerebral perfusion pressure (CPP), which is equal to the mean arterial blood pressure (MBP) minus the intracranial pressure (ICP). In other words: CPP = MBP − ICP. CPP must be kept above 50 mm Hg, and preferably above 80 mm Hg, to prevent further brain damage.

1. Arterial Blood Pressure

As soon as possible after a cardiac arrest, one should obtain a systolic arterial BP of at least 90 to 100 mm Hg, and preferably 140 mm Hg. Cerebral blood flow should be at least 30% and preferably 100% of normal. This may be achieved best by rapid correction of hypovolemia and the use of inotropic and/or vasoconstrictor agents. Although one should not overload these patients with salt and water, it is important to rapidly correct hypoperfusion due to hypovolemia. Use of normovolemic hemodilution (to prevent RBC sludging and thereby increase capillary blood flow) may further reduce postanoxic brain damage.

During CPR one should attempt to maintain as high a cerebral blood flow as possible. In a study by Jackson and associates (1984) regional cerebral cortical blood flow (rCCBF) in 15 dogs was determined using the double thermistor dilution method during: (1) standard closed-chest massage (CCM), (2) CCM with epinephrine infusion at 30 $\mu g \cdot kg^{-1} \cdot min^{-1}$, and (3) open-chest cardiac massage (OCCM). As a percentage of prearrest flow values, the rCCBF was 9.8% with CCM, 35% with CCM plus epinephrine, and 156% with OCCM.

Although many studies describe carotid blood flows of less than 10% of normal during CCM, only a few have actually measured cerebral blood flow. The rCCBF of less than 10% during basic CCM is in good agreement with recent studies using radioactive microspheres as the perfusion marker. Thus, rCCBF during basic CCM is in a range that is apt to exacerbate neurologic injury rather than prevent or correct it. These findings offer some insight into the failure of prolonged basic cardiopulmonary resuscitation to consistently protect neurologic integrity.

The use of high-dose epinephrine to raise BP during CCM significantly improves rCCBF over that achieved with CCM alone. Although the dose of epinephrine used was considerably higher than that usually recommended clinically, its ability to improve rCCBF is encouraging.

Open-chest cardiac massage (OCCM) is far superior to CCM in maintaining diastolic pressure, cardiac output, and coronary and carotid blood flow. This technique is not associated with a general elevation of intrathoracic pressure. As a consequence it is less apt to produce the high central venous and intracranial pressures usually seen with CCM. Thus, OCCM may be the method of choice for prolonged resuscitative efforts, particularly for protecting the brain.

Rapid resuscitation of hypovolemia in patients requiring CPR is essential. Consequently, increased attention has been given to the use of colloids and hypertonic saline solution (HSS). HSS has been of particular interest because its use may be associated with much less edema in all tissues, including the brain. However, Ducey, Lamiell, and Gueller recently showed that restoration of mean arterial pressure (MAP) and cerebral perfusion pressure (CPP) after infusion of 7.5% hypertonic saline solution with 6% dextran (HSD) to treat severe hemorrhage in swine was poor. This apparently was related to the vasodilatory effects of HSD on the pulmonary and systemic circulations. Associated with the delay in restoration of CPP, there was suboptimal electrocortical brain recovery as reflected by somatosensory-evoked potentials.

2. Reducing Intracranial Pressure

a. Hyperventilation

(1) Hypocarbia

Hypocarbia causes cerebral arterial constriction. For each 1 mm Hg decrease in the P_{CO_2}, cerebral blood flow (CBF) falls by about 2% to 4%, and this will tend to reduce ICP. However, if the P_{CO_2} is reduced below 15 to 20 mm Hg, CBF may fall to dangerous levels (below 30% of normal). Because hypocarbia produces its greatest cerebral vasoconstriction in the most normal tissue, hypocarbia may actually increase flow to damaged areas of the brain, even though overall CBF may be reduced. A P_{CO_2} of 25 to 30 mm Hg represents a compromise that seems to provide a moderate reduction in ICP without a dangerous reduction in CBF.

Mackersie and Karagiones recently reported that end-tidal carbon dioxide tension can be reliably used to induce hypocapnia in head-injured patients. Although arterial blood gas analysis will always be necessary to establish the $P_{(a-ET)CO_2}$ gradient and confirm that the Pa_{CO_2} is low enough, it avoids the usual 15 to 20 minute delay in getting this information and leads to earlier, more accurate ventilator settings.

(2) Preventing Hypoxemia

High levels of P_{O_2} tend to cause some cerebral vasoconstriction. Since a low Pa_{O_2} can cause cerebral vasodilation and thereby increase ICP and reduce cerebral perfusion, the P_{O_2} following CPR should probably be kept at 80 to 100 mm Hg.

Demling and Riessen recently reviewed the etiology and management of pulmonary dysfunction after cerebral injury. More than two thirds of patients dying of intracranial hemorrhage have marked pulmonary congestion characteristic of neurogenic pulmonary edema. Even in the absence of pulmonary edema, patients with severe head trauma tend to have hypoxemia. The mechanisms for this are not clear, but their abnormal ventilating patters and hypermetabolism may play a role. In addition, there is a high incidence of pneumonia and pulmonary embolus, which may not always be clinically evident.

(3) Intrathoracic Pressure

Positive pressure ventilation will raise intrathoracic pressure and reduce venous return, thereby increasing ICP. As a consequence, the intrathoracic pressure should be kept at the minimum needed for maintaining the P_{CO_2} at about 25 to 30 mm Hg and the P_{O_2} at 80 to 100 mm Hg. It is probably best to avoid PEEP (if possible) and use faster ventilatory rates and lower tidal volumes to achieve the same minute ventilation. In addition, intermittent mandatory ventilation, which tends to cause a lower mean intrathoracic pressure, is probably preferable to assist-controlled (AC) ventilation.

(4) High-Frequency Ventilation

In ARDS, excellent oxygenation can be achieved in many patients with high-frequency ventilation (HFV) at lower mean airway pressures than those needed with standard low-frequency ventilation (LFV). Because there is a clear correlation between ICP and intrathoracic and jugular venous pressures, HFV may lower ICP and thereby increase brain perfusion. In addition, overall cardiac output may be improved if intrathoracic pressure falls and venous return increases.

Wide fluctuations of CBF during standard ventilator assistance causes more brain surface motion than during HFV. Some of this brain surface motion seems to be the result of changing arterial inflow due to variations of stroke volume and BP with each breath. Changing venous pressure also probably plays a role. Increased brain surface motion may cause increased capillary wall damage and lead to increased extravasation of fluid into the brain. The higher peak venous pressures occurring with standard ventilation may also impair CSF absorption. Both factors may be detrimental in patients with brain trauma.

AXIOM
Wide fluctuations in intrathoracic pressure with ventilatory assistance may further damage an injured brain.

(5) Reduced Effectiveness of Hypocarbia with Time

Because of bicarbonate ion shifts across the blood-brain barrier and renal compensation for respiratory alkalosis, the maximum beneficial effects of hyperventilation are thought to persist for only 48 to 72 hours, after which cerebral vasoconstriction is significantly diminished. Occasionally, additional hyperventilation to a lower $Paco_2$ may be useful, but such therapy should be accompanied by ICP monitoring to document any beneficial effect.

(6) Discontinuing Hyperventilation

When discontinuing hyperventilation, the $Paco_2$ should not be allowed to rise rapidly. A rapid elevation may cause cerebral vasodilation and a resultant increase in ICP.

b. Head Elevation

Elevation of the head may reduce ICP by improving jugular venous return. Each 5.4-in rise of the head above the level of the right atrium may reduce ICP by up to 10 mm Hg. If the mean arterial BP is kept constant, cerebral perfusion is correspondingly increased.

c. Central Venous Pressure

The CVP should be kept as low as possible while still maintaining a systolic BP of at least 90 to 100 mm Hg. As mentioned previously, unless the patient is hypovolemic, it is probably better to maintain BP with inotropes or vasoconstrictors, rather than with fluids. If the patient has a high CVP, it may be worthwhile to use a combination of inotropes, diuretics, and vasodilators.

d. Diuretics

(1) Osmotic Diuretics

Osmotic diuretics create an osmotic gradient between the brain and the blood, causing a shift of water from the brain tissue to the intravascular space and then to the kidneys for elimination. This water shift decreases brain volume and ICP. The dosage for mannitol is 0.5 to 1.5 g/kg over 10 to 20 minutes, followed by 0.25 to 0.50 g/kg every 4 to 8 hours. Ideally, osmotherapy is titrated through close monitoring of ICP and serum osmolarity, and it is usually beneficial for 48 to 72 hours.

Although osmotic diuretic agents have clinical usefulness, they also have potential drawbacks that can decrease their overall effectiveness. Mannitol, 10% glycerol, and urea, which are the most commonly used osmotic diuretics, must be given IV, usually in relatively large volumes. This can cause intravascular and CBV expansion which can increase ICP, at least transiently.

(2) Loop Diuretics

Furosemide is a rapid-acting vasodilator and loop diuretic. It may also reduce chloride ion shift into injured cells, thereby decreasing intracellular edema and ICP. In the patient who is at risk for congestive heart failure or pulmonary edema, furosemide, 0.5 to 1.0 mg/kg, given intravenously 15 minutes prior to mannitol, helps to avoid overhydration problems.

e. Corticosteroids

Corticosteroids given experimentally to animals with severe cerebral ischemia have a number of beneficial effects. They enhance free radical scavenging, stabilize cell membranes, prevent lysosomal activation and release of proteolytic enzymes, decrease CSF production, preserve the blood-brain barrier, and increase brain glucose availability. In addition, steroids reduce the drop in ATP formation that occurs in vitro when mitochondria are exposed to increased concentrations of calcium. Decadron may also block calcium-activated phospholipase A_2 and thereby decrease hydrolysis of cell membranes.

In spite of all these experimental and theoretical benefits, the only situation in which corticosteroids reduce ICP consistently is in patients with rapidly growing intracranial tumors, especially metastases. There is little or no evidence that steroids are of benefit in global anoxia-ischemia or head injury. In addition, steroids have a number of undesirable side effects, including an increased tendency to infection, stress gastritis, and hyperglycemia. This hyperglycemia increases the tendency to cerebral lactic acidosis and increases the ICP when vasogenic cerebral edema is present. Thus, steroids are probably not indicated in the treatment of traumatic and anoxic brain-injured patients.

f. Removal of Cerebrospinal Fluid

If the ICP rises above 20 mm Hg and remains elevated in spite of all other efforts to reduce it, one can consider drawing some CSF out through an intraventricular catheter. Removal of CSF through a lumbar tap increases the tendency for the brain to herniate through the tentorium cerebri or foramen magnum.

B. IMPROVING CEREBRAL METABOLISM

1. Adequate, but Not Excessive, Glucose

Under normal circumstances, the brain, particularly the neocortex, needs an almost constant supply of glucose to maintain adequate metabolism. After 1 to 2 weeks of starvation, however, the brain begins to use increasing amounts of keto acids for fuel. Although glucose levels are usually elevated in acute stress, liver glycogen stores may be rapidly depleted, with resultant hypoglycemia, particularly if there is significant pre-existing hepatic disease. Consequently, one should provide at least 100 to 150 g of glucose per day by IV infusion. However, raising blood glucose levels above 200 mg/dl may be detrimental because the hyperglycemia may increase cerebral lactate levels and cause a local acidosis.

2. Correcting Acidosis

Severe acidosis not only tends to dilate cerebral blood vessels and increase ICP, it also inhibits glycolysis and the Krebs cycle. However, giving large amounts of sodium bicarbonate to correct the acidosis may increase serum osmolarity and further increase ICP. In addition, if the cardiac output is low, bicarbonate administration can cause the Pco_2 in venous blood to rise rapidly. Consequently, it is better to correct the acidosis by improving perfusion and hyperventilating the patient. One should attempt to get the arterial pH up to at least 7.20 and preferably above 7.25. However, an overshoot alkalosis reduces the Pao_2 oxygen availability to tissue by 10% for each 0.10 pH rise.

3. Fructose Diphosphate

If there is difficulty correcting acidosis, a fructose-1,6-diphosphate infusion theoretically may be of value by bypassing the metabolic steps that require ATP and phosphofructokinase (which is greatly inhibited after ischemia or anoxia). In this manner, glycolysis can be maintained even in the presence of some cellular acidosis. The administration of fructose diphosphate during prolonged hemorrhagic shock in dogs has been shown to increase myocardial ATP production, and in one study it converted an irreversible shock model to 100% survival.

4. ATP-Magnesium Chloride

The severe depletion of ATP that occurs during a cardiac arrest may be partially corrected experimentally by an infusion of ATP with magnesium chloride ($MgCl_2$). Under normal circumstances, little or no ATP given IV gets into tissue cells. However, infusion of an ATP-$MgCl_2$ complex in experimental shock improves cellular ATP levels and increases survival to 80% in an otherwise "irreversible" hemorrhagic shock model. Infusion of ATP-$MgCl_2$ can also accelerate structural and functional recovery from postischemic renal and hepatic failure in animals. The mechanisms by which administration of ATP-MgCl$_2$ improves cellular ATP synthesis are still unclear, but plasma membrane stabilization, improved microcirculation, cytostructural stabilization, and increased ATP-membrane reactions that catalyze intracellular ATP production have all been suggested.

C. REDUCING CEREBRAL METABOLIC DEMANDS

1. Hypothermia

Hypothermia may help protect the brain not only during the ischemic-anoxic period but also later during reperfusion, when the brain would otherwise tend to become hypermetabolic. For each degree centigrade reduction in body temperature, metabolism drops by about 7% to 10%. Anecdotal cases of full recovery of near drowning victims with prolonged submersion in cold water tend to support the protective effects of hypothermia. Laboratory studies also document that hypothermia produces a decrease in the brain's inflammatory response to injury, decreased edema formation, and preservation of enzyme systems.

Nevertheless, the results of hypothermia in brain-injured patients are disappointing. The risks, with questionable benefits, make induced hypothermia a tenuous therapeutic modality for cerebral resuscitation.

AXIOM
With brain damage, hyperthermia is very deleterious, but hypothermia is of little or no proven value.

2. Barbiturates

For at least 20 years, barbiturates have been advocated enthusiastically as agents that can significantly reverse or modify the deleterious effects of both focal and global ischemia. Proposed mechanisms of action include decreased cerebral metabolism and oxygen demand, free radical scavenging, membrane stabilization, decreased ICP as a result of increased cerebral vascular resistance, redirection of CBF into ischemic regions, and blockage of calcium flux and autolytic pathways. However, the proposed benefits and mechanisms of action are controversial, and there is little agreement concerning barbiturate efficacy in cerebral resuscitation.

A recent multicenter, prospective, randomized study of sodium thiopental (30 mg/kg) administered to over 250 victims of cardiac arrest, concluded that there was no basis for the administration of thiopental as a means of cerebral protection or resuscitation in cardiac arrest victims. Half the patients were given enough sodium pentobarbital to produce electroencephalographic (EEG) burst suppression, and still no difference in outcome was noted. However, a significantly higher number sustained hypotension as a result of the barbiturate treatment. A retrospective study by Bohn and colleagues also showed that barbiturates, as a part of a combined protocol for near drowning victims, did not improve outcome.

In patients with intracranial hypertension due to acute brain injury, pentobarbital in loading doses of 4 to 7 mg/kg and maintenance doses of 1 to 4 mg/kg reduce heart rate and mean arterial BP by about 30%. Rectal temperature also falls 3°F to 4°F. The hypotension can be corrected by IV infusion of crystalloids or colloids. Consequently, the hemodynamic abnormalities seen after pentobarbital are probably largely due to an increase in venous capacitance with a relative hypovolemia and decreased barostatic reflexes, rather than just depression of myocardial function. Other problems include (1) respiratory depression, to the point of requiring mechanical ventilation; (2) increased risk of infection due to decreased white blood cell mobility; (3) patient immobility, with subsequent risk of a stasis-induced thromboembolic phenomenon; and (4) decubitus skin ulcers.

With high-dose barbiturate therapy, it can also be difficult to evaluate patients clinically or by EEG. However, when the EEG becomes isoelectric, somatosensory-evoked potentials (SSEP) can help determine if there is total brain damage or just barbiturate effect. In addition, the cortical SSEP responses have some prognostic value.

AXIOM
Although barbiturates can reduce a persistently elevated ICP, particularly in patients with brain trauma or focal ischemia, little solid clinical evidence supports their use in cerebral resuscitation.

3. Pancuronium (Pavulon)

Monkey experiments have suggested that paralysis with pancuronium (a curare-like drug) can be beneficial in cerebral resuscitation. This agent reduces oxygen demand, especially in restless subjects, and allows better control of extracranial organ failure. However, it can also cause respiratory depression and hypotension, which can be very deleterious.

4. Control of Seizure Activity

Seizures may occur in up to 30% of patients who have had a cardiac arrest. Seizure activity increases cerebral metabolic activity by as much as 300%. Such increased oxygen and metabolic substrate demand can tip the balance into the area of anaerobic metabolism with resulting permanent damage.

Clinical seizure activity may vary from subtle eyelid twitching to grand mal activity. Prophylactic seizure therapy is somewhat controversial, but any documented seizure activity after CPR should be quickly and aggressively treated with diazepam (5 mg IV), Dilantin loading (15 to 18 mg/kg IV over 30 to 60 minutes), and maintenance (300 mg daily) to prevent additional seizures.

Isenstein and Nasraway recently pointed out some of the potential hemodynamic problems with phenytoin infusion. They reported two patients with severe sepsis who developed hypotension while receiving Dilantin. They also noted that Dilantin is contraindicated in patients with a high degree of heart block or bradycardia.

AXIOM
Dilantin loading should be done very cautiously, if at all, in patients with severe sepsis, heart block, or bradycardia.

D. CALCIUM CHANNEL BLOCKERS

Ionic calcium (Ca^{++}) influx into injured cells contributes to the no-reflow phenomenon and a large number of metabolic derangements. When Ca^{++} moves into the cytosol, it activates phospholipase A_2, adenylate cyclase, and other enzymes that trigger increased production of free radicals, free fatty acids, and arachidonic acid metabolites.

E. CALCIUM BLOCKERS

1. Flunarizine

White and associates report that administration of calcium channel entry blockers can improve postischemic cerebral hypoperfusion and may protect against the development of early postischemic neurologic deficits. Following a 20-minute normothermic cardiac arrest, dogs maintained on cardiopulmonary bypass with a mean arterial pressure of 100 mg Hg had a cortical CBF of only 50% of normal. Similar dogs, treated with flunarizine, an experimental calcium blocker, after the 20-minute cardiac arrest had a normal cortical CBF on cardiopulmonary bypass.

In another more recent study by Newberg and colleagues flunarizine given after 10 minutes of global ischemia caused more harm than good. Cerebral blood flow, cerebral oxygen uptake, cerebral metabolites (including adenosine triphosphate and glucose), and the functional neurologic status at 48 hours, were similar in the treated and control animals. However, some of the flunarizine-treated animals developed severe pulmonary edema and died.

2. Lidoflazine

In a prospective blinded study by White and associates, animals treated with lidoflazine during resuscitation after a 15-minute cardiac arrest showed intact brainstem and beginning higher cortical function within 12 hours. Four of five dogs treated similarly but without this calcium blocker were functionally brain dead by this time.

In another study using lidoflazine after 10 minutes of cardiac arrest, cerebral recovery at 96 hours was significantly better in the lidoflazine-treated groups. In addition, cardiac output after arrest was significantly higher in the treated animals.

3. Nimodipine

In a study of monkeys subjected to 17 minutes of complete cerebral ischemia (produced by trimethaphan and neck cuff inflation), nimodipine significantly improved the neurologic outcome 96 hours after ischemia. The histopathologic and neurologic findings correlated significantly. A hypotensive response to bolus injection of the nimodipine was the only potentially adverse effect seen.

F. PROSTAGLANDIN INTERVENTIONS

The effects of prostaglandins on vascular tone are complex. Thromboxane causes vasoconstriction and platelet aggregation, while prostacyclin (PGI_2) produces vasodilation and decreased platelet aggregation. PGI_2 may also function as an endogenous Ca^{++} channel blocker during ischemia, and it has been shown to be a more potent stabilizer of lysosomes than steroids.

In animal models, infusion of PGI_2 during ischemia has helped protect the brain, heart, liver, and kidney. However, after severe ischemia and reperfusion, an uncontrolled surge of other prostaglandins and other compounds with free radical characteristics may result in ultimate cell death. Blockade of the cycloxygenase and lipoxygenase cascades in this situation may be protective.

Indomethacin decreases prostaglandin synthesis by inhibition of cycloxygenase activity. In some tissues it accomplishes this by phospholipase A_2 blockade. In high concentrations, it may also inhibit the lipoxygenase cascade. Protection of cerebral blood flow and improved neurologic recovery in dogs has been shown if indomethacin is infused shortly after the ischemic episode.

G. PLATELET INHIBITORS

Agents that prevent platelet aggregation may be of some value, particularly in reducing platelet aggregation in small vessels when there is acidosis and stasis. In this regard, aspirin, persantin, and indomethacin (by blocking the thromboxane effect) may be of particular benefit.

H. BLOCKAGE OF N-METHYL-D-ASPARTATE RECEPTORS

Cerebral ischemia and status epilepticus produce similar patterns of neuronal loss in the hippocampus. This suggests that enhanced calcium entry during either status epilepticus or the reperfusion phase after ischemia may explain selective neuronal vulnerability. Burst firing can be triggered in neurons at various sites by iontophoresis or aspartate acting on N-methyl-D-aspartate (NMDA)-preferring receptors. The excitatory effect of dicarboxylic amino acids at the postsynaptic receptor can be blocked by analogues of glutamate and aspartate such as 2-amino-7-phosphonoheptanoic acid (APH), a highly potent antagonist that is selective for NMDA receptors.

The effect of focally injecting APH into a hippocampus was examined in a rodent model in which bilateral carotid occlusion was combined with systemic hypotension to reduce forebrain blood flow to less than 5% of baseline. Occlusion for 30 minutes, followed by 2 hours of reperfusion, led to ischemic changes in pyramidal cells in both hippocampi. Microinfusion of APH into the dorsal hippocampus protected against ischemic damage to pyramidal, granule, and polymorphic cells.

These findings support the idea that excitatory synaptic activity and increased calcium entry contribute to selective neuronal vulnerability to ischemia. Pharmacologic blockage of excitatory receptors may help to reverse such changes.

I. COMBINATION THERAPY

The complex pathophysiology of postischemic encephalopathy includes reflow problems, hypotension, brain tissue acidosis, edema, membrane failure, impaired energy production, and hypermetabolism. Consequently, it was thought that multifacet therapy aimed at each of these postischemic changes might be helpful. In one study, complete global brain ischemia (GBI) was produced with a combination of trimethaphan-induced hypotension and neck cuff inflation to 1500 mm Hg. Control treatment of the postischemic animals consisted of normotension (MBP of at least 80 mm Hg), restored within 2 minutes postischemia, controlled ventilation for 24 hours with a $Paco_2$ of 25 mm Hg, normothermia, and phenytoin seizure prophylaxis beginning 20 hours postischemia. The 10 experimental animals received control treatment as well as hemodilution to a hematocrit of 25% within 4 minutes postischemia; hypertension to a MBP of 130 mm Hg for 5 minutes after hemodilution; hypothermia for 6 hours; and administration of pentobarbital (30 mg/kg) and dexamethasone (4 mg/kg) intravenously. Seven of ten animals in the treatment group, but only two of nine controls were either normal or awake with only some neurologic damage. The only brain death occurred in one control animal. Thus, a combination of hemodilution, hypertension, hypothermia, pentobarbital, and dexamethasone may help reduce postischemic brain damage.

J. OUTCOME

Jennett and coworkers from Glasgow, Scotland, and the Netherlands have devised a scoring system called the Glasgow Coma Scale (GCS), based on vocal response, eye movements, and motor response. Jennett's original data demonstrated that within the first 24 hours of injury, accurate predictions of outcome could be made in 44% of cases. This accuracy increased to 68% at 4 to 7 days. In patients with a GCS of three to four a week after injury, death or a persistent vegetative state is almost inevitable and further treatment may not be in the best interest of the patient, the patient's family, or society.

Predicting outcome reliably on patients who are in coma after a cardiac arrest is particularly difficult. However, in a study by Levy, absence of brainstem reflexes correlated with no meaningful recovery of neurologic function at 1 year. It must be emphasized that such data do not apply to children who may have full neurologic recovery in 10% to 15% of cases and who are initially flaccid and have fixed, dilated pupils after a cardiac arrest. This data should also not be applied to head trauma and infectious encephalopathies, which have a much better prognosis.

In another recent study of patients resuscitated after an out-of-hospital cardiac arrest, Bertini and associates found that patients who were conscious on admission had an in-hospital mortality rate of only 4%. Patients with an alteration of their state of consciousness on admission had an in-hospital mortality rate of 53%.

On admission, only the absence of spontaneous breathing was significantly predictive of an unfavorable outcome. The failure of response to painful stimulation and pupillary light reflex became significantly predictive of an unfavorable outcome only in the late in-hospital course. The time delay before onset of CPR was significantly longer in unconscious patients, but in this group no difference was observed between survivors and nonsurvivors. At discharge 3 of the 39 surviving patients showed severe neurologic impairment. The authors felt that their data indicated that, in patients with postanoxic coma, early clinical evidence of severe neurologic dysfunction is predictive of neither in-hospital death nor neurologic sequelae.

SUMMARY POINTS

1. One should not attribute changes in mental status to cerebrovascular disease until metabolic, toxic, infectious, and neoplastic causes have been excluded.

2. The postictal state of epilepsy can be very difficult to differentiate from a stroke.
3. The two symptoms with a stroke that most accurately indicate carotid circulation involvement are aphasia and monocular blindness.
4. Most (80%) strokes involve the carotid artery system.
5. Stuttering, slow, or nighttime strokes are usually thrombotic in origin.
6. The stroke patient who is lethargic or comatose has probably had an intracerebral hemorrhage.
7. One should listen carefully for carotid and subclavian bruits in all patients who have had a stroke.
8. One should perform a careful funduscopic examination on all patients who may have had a stroke.
9. One should completely evaluate the heart in all patients with a stroke.
10. One should obtain an early CT scan of the brain on patients who have neurologic changes that may be due to an intracranial lesion.
11. An MRI should not be done on unstable or uncooperative patients.
12. Stroke patients often benefit from increased tissue oxygenation and a normal or slightly increased BP.
13. One should guard against aspiration of oral or gastric contents in patients with strokes.
14. Fever after a stroke is often due to an infection, particularly pneumonia, or venous thrombosis.
15. Most patients admitted with a stroke have some underlying cardiac disease, and up to 9% have a concomitant myocardial infarction.
16. Contraindications to anticoagulation include large cerebral infarctions, uncontrolled hypertension, or evidence of active bleeding.
17. Patients with coma may benefit from hyperventilation and diuretics.
18. Controlling ICP is especially important in patients with hemorrhagic strokes.
19. Patients with TIAs are at greatly increased risk of developing strokes.
20. Sudden onset of the worst headache a patient ever had should be considered a leaking intracranial aneurysm until proven otherwise.
21. The definitive test for subarachnoid hemorrhage is a lumbar puncture that reveals blood within the cerebrospinal fluid (CSF).
22. Vasospasm and recurrent bleeding are the main dangers in an otherwise stable patient with intracerebral bleeding.
23. Early surgery or cerebral angiography may cause increased vasospasm.
24. Great efforts should be made to prevent recurrent seizures after a stroke.
25. One should make great efforts to keep a high normal CPP and low ICP in patients who have suffered cerebral ischemia.
26. The brain needs an almost constant supply of oxygen, glucose, and other nutrients.
27. Brain death from transient ischemia is largely due to secondary processes rather than the initial insult.
28. Early defibrillation is the best way to ensure recovery from a cardiac arrest with an intact CNS.
29. Increasing local lactate is usually a sign of progressive cerebral or cardiac damage.
30. Complete ischemic anoxia may be better than a partial but inadequate blood flow.
31. Prolonged cerebral ischemia is followed by transient hyperfusion and then a progressive severe failure or reperfusion.
32. Movement of ionized calcium into cells appears to be a major factor in deterioration following ischemia-anoxia.
33. The inability of damaged cells to maintain an adequate cellular level of ATP following ischemia is a critical event leading to cell death.

34. A little oxygen may be particularly damaging to ischemic cells because it may result in production of free radicals and little or no ATP.
35. Wide fluctuations in intrathoracic pressure with ventilatory assistance may further damage an injured brain.
36. With brain damage, hyperthermia is very deleterious, but hypothermia is of little or no proven value.
37. Although barbiturates can reduce a persistently elevated ICP, particularly in patients with brain trauma or focal ischemia, little solid clinical evidence supports their use in cerebral resuscitation.
38. Dilantin loading should be done very cautiously, if at all, in patients with severe sepsis, heart block, or bradycardia.

BIBLIOGRAPHY

1. Abramson, NA: Randomized clinical study of thiopental loading in comatose survivors of cardiac arrest. N Engl J Med 314:397, 1986.
2. Allen, GS, et al: Cerebral arterial spasm: A controlled trial of nimodipine in patients with subarachnoid hemorrhage. N Engl J Med 308:619, 1983.
3. Ames, A, III and Guarian, BS: Effects of glucose deprivation on function of isolated mammalian retina. J Neurophysiol 26:617, 1963.
4. Apstein, CS, et al: Graded global ischemia and reperfusion: Cardiac function and lactate metabolism. Circulation 55:864, 1977.
5. Aragno, R and Doni, MG: The exclusion of the cerebral circulation: Effect on the "in vivo" platelet aggregation. Thromb Res 9:319, 1976.
6. Auffant, RA, Shuptrine, JR, and Hotchkiss, RS: Effects of HFV vs IPPV on cerebral perfusion pressure and cardiopulmonary function. Anesthesiology 57:A88, 1982.
7. Babinskil, M and Albin, M: Effect of high frequency ventilation on ICP. Crit Care Med 9:159, 1981.
8. Barnaby, W: Stroke intervention. Emerg Med Clin North Am 8:267, 1990.
9. Barsan, W, et al: Identification and entry of the patient with acute cerebral infarction. Ann Emerg Med 17:1192, 1988.
10. Bassi, M and Bernelli-Zazzera, A: Ultrastructural cytoplasmic changes in liver cells after reversible and irreversible ischemia. Exp Mol Pathol 3:332, 1964.
11. Baue, AE, Chaudry, IH, and Wurth, MA: Cellular alterations with shock and ischemia. Angiology 25:31, 1974.
12. Bergner, L, et al: Evaluation of paramedic services for cardiac arrest. US Department of Health Services Research Report (HS 02456), December, 1981.
13. Bertini, G, et al: Prognostic significance of early clinical manifestations in postanoxic coma: A retrospective study of 58 patients resuscitated after prehospital cardiac arrest. Crit Care Med 17:627, 1989.
14. Bohn, DJ, et al: Influence of hypothermia, barbiturate therapy, and intracranial pressure monitoring on morbidity and mortality after near drowning. Crit Care Med 14:529, 1986.
15. Bragt, PC: Indomethacin inhibits in-vivo formation of the lipo-oxygenase product HETE during granulomatous inflammation in the rat. J Pharm Pharmacol 32:143, 1980.
16. Burst, JCM: Subarachnoid hemorrhage. In Rowland, LP (ed): Merrit's Textbook of Neurology, ed 8. Lea & Febiger, Philadelphia, 1989.
17. Brust, JCM: Transient ischemic attacks: Natural history and anticoagulation. Neurology 27:701, 1977.
18. Caplan, LR, Heir, D, and D'Cruz, I: Cerebral embolism in the Michael Reese Stroke Registry. Stroke 14:530, 1983.
19. Caplan, LR and Stein, RW: Stroke: A Clinical Approach. Butterworth & Co, Boston, 1986.
19a. Carafoli, E: Calcium-transporting systems of plasma membranes with special attention to their regulation. Adv Cyclic Nucleotide Protein Phosphorylation Res 17:543, 1984.
20. Chan, PH and Fishman, RA: Transient formation of superoxide radicals in polyunsaturated fatty acid induced brain swelling. J Med 298:659, 1978.
21. Chaudry, IH, Mohammed, SM, and Baue, AE: Effect of adenosine triphosphatemagnesium chloride administration in shock. Surgery 75:220, 1974.
22. Chiang, J, et al: Cerebral ischemia III: Vascular changes. Am J Pathol 52:455, 1968.
23. Clustin, WT, et al: Do calcium dependent ionic currents mediate ischemic ventricular fibrillation? Am J Cardiol 49:606, 1982.
24. Cooper, HK, Zalewska, T, and Hossman, KA: The effect of ischemia and recirculation on protein synthesis in the rat brain. J Neurochem 28:929, 1977.
25. Crowell, RM and Zervas, NT: Management of intracranial aneurysm. Med Clin North Am 63:695, 1979.

26. Daenen, W and Flameng, W: Myocardial protection by lidoflazine during one-hour normo-thermic global ischemia. Angiology 32:543, 1981.

27. Davis, DH and Sundt, TM: Relationship of cerebral blood flow to cardiac output, mean arterial pressure, blood volume, and a and b blockade in cats. J Neurosurg 52:745, 1980.

28. Dayton, WR and Schollmeyer, JV: Isolation from porcine cardiac muscle of a Ca^{++} activated protease that partially degrades myofibrils. J Mol Cell Cardiol 12:533, 1980.

29. Dearden, NM, et al: Effect of high-dose dexamethasone on outcome from severe head injury. J Neurosurg 64:81, 1986.

30. DeCree, J, et al: The rheological effects of cinnarizine and flunarizine in normal and patho-logical condition. Angiology 30:505, 1979.

31. DelMaestro, RF, et al: Free radicals as mediators of tissue injury. Acta Physiol Scand [Suppl] 492:43, 1980.

32. Del Zoppo, GJ, Ferbert, A, and Otis, S: Local intra-arterial fibrinolytic therapy in acute carotid territory stroke: A pilot study. Stroke 19:307, 1988.

33. Demling, R and Riessen, R: Pulmonary dysfunction after cerebral injury. Crit Care Med 18:768, 1990.

34. Dimant, J and Grob D: Electrocardiographic changes and myocardial damage in patients with acute cerebrovascular accidents. Stroke 8:448, 1977.

35. Ducey, JP, Lamiell, JM, and Gueller, GE: Cerebral electrophysiologic effects of resuscitation with hypertonic saline-dextran after hemorrhage. Crit Care Med 18:744, 1990.

36. Dusting, GL, Moncada, S, and Vane, JR: Prostacyclin in the enterogenous metabolite respon-sible for relaxation of the coronary arteries induced by arachidonic acid. Prostaglandins 13:3, 1977.

37. Earnest, MP, et al: Long term survival and neurologic status after resuscitation from out-of-hospital cardiac arrest. Neurology 30:1298, 1980.

38. Eisenberg, MS, Copas, MK, and Hallstrom, A: Management of out-of-hospital cardiac arrest: Failure of basic EMT service. JAMA 243:1049, 1980.

38a. Filoteo, AG, Gorski, JP, and Penniston, JT: The ATP-binding site of the erythrocyte mem-brane Ca2+ pump. Amino acid sequence of the fluorescein isothiocyanate-reactive region. J Biol Chem 262(14):6526.

39. Fisher, CM, Robertson, GH, and Ojemann, RG: Cerebral vasospasm with ruptured saccular aneurysm: The clinical manifestations. Neurosurgery 1:245, 1977.

40. Fishman, RA: Brain enema. N Engl J Med 293:706, 1975.

41. Flower, RJ: Drugs which inhibit prostaglandin biosynthesis. Pharmacol Rev 23:33, 1974.

42. Flower, RJ and Blackwell, GJ: Anti-inflammatory steroids induce biosynthesis of a phospho-lipase A_2 inhibitor which prevents prostaglandin generation. Nature 278:456, 1979.

43. Frank, JS, et al: Calcium depletion in rabbit myocardium, ultrastructure of the sarcolemma and correlation with calcium paradox. Circ Res 51:117, 1982.

44. Gadzinski, DS, et al: Alterations in canine cerebral cortical blood flow and vascular resistance post cardiac arrest. Ann Emerg Med 99:58, 1982.

45. Gaudet, RJ and Levine, L: Transient cerebral ischemic and brain prostaglandins. Biochem Biophys Res Commun 6:893, 1979.

46. Gisvold, SE, et al: Multifaceted therapy after global brain ischemia in monkeys. Stroke 15:803, 1984.

47. Grinwald, PM and Nayker, WG: Calcium entry in the calcium paradox. Cardiology 12:797, 1980.

48. Guarnieri, C, Flamigni, F, and Caldarera, CM: Role of oxygen in the cellular damage induced by re-oxygenation of the hypoxic heart. J Mol Cell Cardiol 12:797, 1980.

49. Hackel, DB, et al: Effects of verapamil on heart and circulation of hemorrhagic shock in dogs. Am J Physiol 241:H12, 1981.

50. Hallenbeck, JM and Furlow, TM: Prostaglandin I_2 and indomethacin prevent impairment of post-ischemic brain reperfusion in dogs. Stroke 19:629, 1979.

51. Hanley, MJ and Davidson, K: Prior mannitol and furosemide infusion in a model of ischemic acute renal failure. Am J Physiol 241:F556, 1981.

52. Harper, AM and Glas, HI: Effect of alterations in the arterial carbon dioxide tension on the blood flow through the cerebral cortex at normal and low arterial blood pressures. J Neurol Neurosurg Psychiatry 28:449, 1965.

53. Harris, RJ, et al: Changes in extracellular calcium activity in cerebral ischemia. J Cereb Blood Flow Metab 1:23, 1981.

54. Hart, RG and Easton, JD: Management of cervical bruits and carotid stenosis in preoperative patients. Stroke 14:290, 1983.

55. Hass, WK, Easton, JD, and Adams, HP: A randomized trial comparing ticlopidine hydro-chloride with aspirin for the prevention of stroke in high-risk patients. N Engl J Med 321:501, 1989.

56. Heffner, JE and Sahn, SA: Controlled hyperventilation in patients with intracranial hyperten-sion: Application and management. Arch Intern Med 143:765, 1983.

57. Hess, ML, Okab, E, and Kontos, HA: Proton and free oxygen radical interactions with calcium transport system of cardiac sarcoplasmic reticulum. J Mol Cell Cardiol 13:767, 1981.

58. Hoffmeister, F, Kaxda, S, and Krause, HP: Influence of nimodipine on the post ischemic changes of brain function. Acta Neurol Scand 60 [Supply] 72:538, 1979.

59. Hossmann, KA: Development of resolution of ischemic brain swelling. In Pappius, H and Fiendel, W (eds): Dynamic of Brain Edema. Springer-Verlag, Berlin, 1976, p 219.

60. Hossmann, KA and Kleiheus, P: Reversibility of ischemic brain damage. Arch Neurol 29:375, 1973.

61. Hossmann, V, Hossmann, KA, and Takagi, N: Effect of intravascular platelet aggregation on blood recirculation following prolonged ischemia of the cat brain. J Neurol 222:159, 1980.

62. Isenstein, D and Nasraway, SA: Hypotension during slow phenytoin infusion in severe sepsis. Crit Care Med 18:1036, 1990.

63. Jackson, RE, et al: Blood flow in the cerebral cortex during cardiac resuscitation in dogs. Ann Emerg Med 13:357, 1984.

64. Jacobsen, WK, et al: Correlations of spontaneous of neurologic damage in near-drowning. Crit Care Med 11:487, 1983.

65. Jenkins, LW, et al: Complete cerebral ischemia. An ultrastructural study. Acta Neuropathol (Berl) 48:113, 1979.

66. Jennet, B: Severe head injury: Prediction of outcome as a basis for management decisions. Int Anesthesiol Clin 17:133, 1979.

67. Jennet, B: Assessment of the severity of head injury. J Neurol Neurosurg Psychiatry 39:647, 1976.

68. Jennische, E, et al: Co-relation between tissue pH, cellular transmembrane potentials and cellular energy metabolism during shock and ischemia. J Mol Cell Cardiol 14:123, 1982.

69. Johnson, H: Effects of nifedipine on platelet function in-vitro and in-vivo. Thromb Res 21:523, 1981.

70. Jones, RN, et al: Effect of hypothermia on changes in high-energy phosphate production and utilization in total ischemia. J Mol Cell Cardiol 14:124, 1982.

71. Jugdett, BI, et al: Effect of indomethacin on collateral blood flow and infarct size in the conscious dog. Circulation 59:734, 1979.

72. Kaplan, L, Weiss, J, and Elsback, P: Low concentrations for indomethacin inhibit phospholipase A_2 of rabbit polymorphonuclear leukocytes. Proc Natl Acad Sci USA 75:2955, 1978.

73. Katz, AM and Messineao, FC: Lipid-membrane interactions and the pathogenesis of ischemic damage in the myocardium. Circ Res 48:1, 1981.

74. Katz, AM and Reuter, H: Cellular calcium and cardiac cell death. Am J Cardiol 44:188, 1979.

75. Landercasper, J, et al: Perioperative stroke risk in 173 consecutive patients with a past history of stroke. Arch Surg 125:986, 1990.

76. Lindsay, KW, et al: Evoked potentials in severe head injury analysis and relation to outcome. J Neurol Neurosurg Psychiatry 44:197, 1981.

77. Ljunggren, B, et al: Aneurysmal subarachnoid hemorrhage: Prevention of delayed ischemic dysfunction with intravenous nimodipine. Neurosurg Rev 10:255, 1987.

78. Lundar, T, Ganes, T, and Lindegaard, K: Induced barbiturate coma: Methods for evaluation of patients. Crit Care Med 11:559, 1983.

79. Mackersie, RC and Karagianes, TG: Use of end-tidal carbon dioxide tension for monitoring induced hypocapnia in head-injured patients. Crit Care Med 18:764, 1990.

80. Maiza, D, Theron, J, and Pelouza, GA: Local fibrinolytic therapy in ischemic carotid pathology. Ann Vasc Surg 2:206, 1989.

81. Markov, AK, et al: Irreversible hemorrhagic shock: Treatment and cardiac pathophysiology. Circ Shock 8:9, 1981.

82. Marshall, LF, Smith, RW, and Shapiro, HM: The outcome with aggressive treatment in severe head injuries, Part I: The significance of intracranial pressure monitoring. J Neurosurg 50:20, 1979.

83. McCarthy, ST: Low dose heparin as a prophylaxis against deep-vein thrombosis after acute stroke. Lancet 2:800, 1977.

84. Miller, VT and Hart, RG: Heparin anticoagulation in acute brain ischemia. Stroke 19:403, 1988.

85. Mohr, JP, et al: The Harvard cooperative stroke registry. Neurology 28:754, 1978.

86. Mohr, JP: Lacunes. Stroke 13:3, 1982.

87. Moncada, S, Higgs, EA, and Vane, JR: Human arteries and venous tissues generate prostacyclin: A potent inhibitor of platelet aggregation. Lancet 1:18, 1977.

88. Mori, E, et al: Intracarotid urokinase with thromboembolic occlusion of the middle cerebral artery. Stroke 7:802, 1988.

89. Myerburg, RJ, et al: Clinical, electrophysiologic and hemodynamic profiles of patients resuscitated from prehospital cardiac arrest. Am J Med 68:568, 1980.

90. Nemoto, EM, Hossmann, KA, and Cooper, HK: Post-ischemic hypermetabolism in cat brain. Stroke 12:666, 1981.

91. Newberg, LA, et al: Failure of flunarizine to improve cerebral blood flow or neurologic recovery in a canine model of complete cerebral ischemia. Stroke 15:666, 1984.
92. Nicholson, C: Measurement of extracellular ions in the brain. Trends in Neurosciences 3:216, 1980.
93. Niemann, JT, et al: Coronary perfusion pressure during experimental CPR. Ann Emerg Med 11:127, 1982.
94. Norris, JW and Hachinski, VC: Misdiagnosis of stroke. Lancet 1:328, 1982.
95. Nozick, JH, et al: The kidney and the calcium paradox. J Surg Res 11:60, 1971.
96. Nussbaum, E and Galant, SP: Intracranial pressure monitoring as a guide to prognosis in the nearly drowned, severely comatose child. J Pediatr 102:215, 1983.
97. Olinger, CP, et al: Use of ancrod in acute or progressive ischemic cerebral infarction. Ann Emerg Med 17:1208, 1988.
98. Patterson, AR: Brain resuscitation. In Civetta, J, Taylor, R, and Kirby, R (eds): Critical Care. JB Lippincott, Philadelphia, 1988, p 1261.
99. Petriek, KC, et al: Nimodipine treatment in poor-grade aneurysm patients: Results of a multicenter double-blind placebo controlled trial. J Neurosurg 68:505, 1988.
100. Piatt, JH and Schiff, SJ: High dose barbiturate therapy in neurosurgery and intensive care. Neurosurgery 15:427, 1984.
101. Przelomski, MM, et al: Fever in the wake of a stroke. Neurology 36:427, 1986.
102. Quandt, CM and de los Reyes, RA: Pharmacologic management of acute intracranial hypertension. Drug Intell Clin Pharm 18:105, 1984.
103. Rehncrona, S, Abdul-Rahman, A, and Siesji, BK: Local cerebral blood flow in the post-ischemia period. Acta Neurol Scand 72:294, 1979.
104. Rehncrona, S, Mela, L, and Siesjo, BK: Recovery of brain mitochondrial function in the rat after complete and incomplete cerebral ischemia. Stroke 10:437, 1979.
105. Rehncrona, S, Rosen, I, and Siesjo, BK: Brain lactic acidosis and cell damage: Biochemistry and neurophysiology. J Cereb Blood Flow Metab 1:297, 1981.
106. Rich, TL and Langer, GA: Calcium depletion in the rabbit myocardium: Calcium paradox protection by hypothermia and cation substitution. Circ Res 51:131, 1982.
107. Robbins, SL and Citran, RS (eds): Cell injury and cell death. In Pathologic Basis of Disease, ed 2. WB Saunders, Philadelphia, 1979, p 22.
108. Rokey, R, et al: Coronary artery disease in patients with cerebrovascular disease: A prospective study. Ann Neurol 1984: 16:50.
109. Rolak, LA: Cerebrovascular disease. In Joseph Civetta, J, Taylor, R, and Kirby, R (eds): Critical Care. JB Lippincott, Philadelphia, 1988, p 1217.
110. Ruigrok, TJC and Zimmerman, ANE: The effect of calcium on myocardial tissue damage and enzyme release. In Hearse, DJ and Leiris, JD (eds): Enzymes in Cardiology: Disease and Research. John Wiley & Sons, Chichester, 1979, p 399.
111. Safer, P: Amelioration of post-ischemic brain damage with barbiturates. Stroke 11:565, 1980.
112. Safar, P: Dynamic of brain resuscitation after ischemic-anoxia. Hosp Pract [OFF] 16:67, 1981.
113. Schanne, FA, et al: Calcium dependency of toxic cell death: A final common pathway. Science 206:700, 1979.
114. Schrier, RW: Acute renal failure. JAMA 247:2518, 1982.
115. Schwartz, JP, et al: Alterations of cyclic nucleotide-related enzymes and ATPase during unilateral ischemia and recirculation in gerbil cerebral cortex. J Neurochem 27:101, 1976.
116. Senter, HJ, Wolf, A, and Wagner, FC: Intracranial pressure in non-traumatic ischemic and hypoxic cerebral insults. J Neurosurg 54:489, 1981.
117. Shapiro, HM: Brain protection: Fact of infancy. In Shoemaker, W (ed): State of the Art, Vol 6. Society of Critical Care Medicine, Fullerton, CA, 1984.
118. Sherman, DG, et al: Antithrombotic therapy for cerebrovascular disorders. Chest 91:1405, 1989.
119. Siebke, H, et al: Survival after 40 minutes submersion without cerebral sequelae. Lancet 1:1275, 1975.
120. Siesjo, BK: Cerebral circulation and metabolism. J Neurosurg 60:883, 1984.
121. Simon, RP, et al: Blockade of N-methyl-D-asparate receptors may protect against ischemic damage in the brain. Science 226:850, 1984.
122. Smith, AL: Barbiturate protection in cerebral hypoxia. Anesthesiology 47:285, 1977.
123. Smolens, P and Stein, JH: Pathophysiology of acute renal failure. Am J Med 70:479, 1981.
124. Snyder, JV, et al: Global ischemia in dogs: Intracranial pressure, blood flow and metabolism. Stroke 6:21, 1975.
125. Sokoll, MD, Kassell, NF, and Davies, LR: Large dose thiopental anesthesia for intracranial aneurysm surgery. Neurosurgery 10:555, 1982.
126. Steen, PA, et al: Nimodipine improves cerebral blood flow and neurologic recovery after complete cerebral ischemia in the dog. J Cereb Blood Flow Metab 3:38, 1983.
127. Steen, PA, et al: Nimodipine improves outcome when given after complete cerebral ischemia in primates. Anesthesiology 62:406, 1985.

128. Todd, MM, Touland, SM, and Shapiro, HM: The effects of high frequently positive pressure ventilation on ICP and brain surface movement in cats. Anesthesiology 54:496, 1981.

129. Towart, R and Perzborn, E: Nimodipine inhibits carboxyclic thromboxzane-induced contractions of cerebral arteries. Eur J Pharmacol 69:213, 1981.

130. Traeger, SM, et al: Hemodynamic effects of pentobarbital therapy for intracranial hypertension. Crit Care Med 11:697, 1983.

131. Trunkey, DD, Holcroft, J, and Carpenter, MA: Calcium flux during hemorrhagic shock in baboons. J Trauma 16:633, 1976.

132. Vaagenes, P, et al: Amelioration of brain damage by lidoflazine after prolonged ventricular fibrillation cardiac arrest in dogs. Crit Care Med 12:846, 1984.

133. Van Reempts, J and Borgers, M: Brain protection: A histological assessment. J Cereb Blood Flow Metab (Suppl) 2:577, 1982.

134. Weglicki, WB, et al: Hydrolysis of myocardial lipids during acidosis and ischemia. In Dhalla, NS (ed): Recent Advances of Studies on Cardiac Structure and Metabolism. University Park Press, Baltimore, 1972, p 781.

135. Ward, JD, et al: Failure of prophylactic barbiturate coma in the treatment of severe head injury. J Neurosurg 62:383, 1985.

136. Weir, B: Antifibrinolytics in subarachnoid hemorrhage. Arch Neurol 44:116, 1987.

137. Weisman, S: Edema and congestion of the lungs resulting from intracranial hemorrhage. Surgery 6:722, 1939.

138. Weismann, DN: Altered renal hemodynamic and urinary prostaglandin response to acute hypoxemia after inhibition of prostaglandin synthesis in anesthetized dog. Circ Res 48:632, 1982.

139. White, BC, et al: Correction of canine cerebral cortical blood flow and vascular resistance after cardiac arrest using flunarizine, a calcium antagonist. Ann Emerg Med 22:118, 1982.

140. White, BC, Hoehner, PJ, and Wilson, RF: Mitochondrial O_2 use and ATP synthesis: Kinetic effects of Ca^{++} and HPO_4 modulated by glucocorticoid. Ann Emerg Med 9:369, 1980.

141. Yatsu, FM, et al: Anticoagulation of embolic strokes of cardiac origin: An update. Neurology 38:314, 1988.

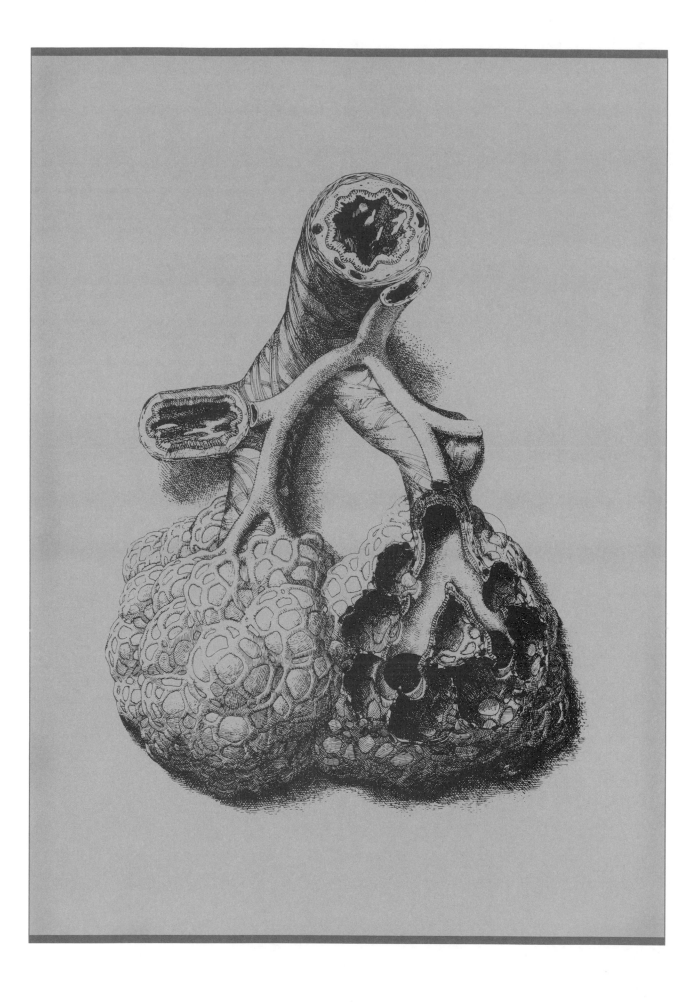

PART TWO

PULMONARY PHYSIOLOGY

CHAPTER 8

Pulmonary Physiology

I. FUNCTIONAL ANATOMY

The upper airway consists of the nose, mouth, pharynx, larynx, and cervical trachea (Fig. 8.1).

A. THE UPPER AIRWAY

1. Nose

The nose is lined by a vascular mucous membrane with ciliated columnar epithelium that warms and moistens the air and removes a certain amount of inhaled particulate matter. By the time air inhaled through the nose reaches the tracheal bifurcation, it is completely humidified and warmed to body temperature. Breathing through the mouth, because of nasal blockage or a greatly increased minute ventilation, may be very drying and irritating to the upper airway.

2. Pharynx

The pharynx is the common upper channel for both the respiratory and digestive tracts. Anatomically, it is divided into the nasopharynx, oropharynx, and laryngopharynx. The nasopharynx is superior to the soft palate, which helps to separate the oral cavity from the nasal cavity during the act of swallowing. The oropharynx extends down from the soft palate to the superior border of the epiglottis, which covers and protects the upper opening of the larynx during the act of swallowing. The hypopharynx is posterior and lateral to the larynx and extends from the upper border of the epiglottis to the lower border of the cricoid cartilage, where it becomes the esophagus. The pyriform sinuses are the lateral portions of the hypopharynx; foreign bodies are usually caught there if they do not enter the larynx or esophagus.

3. Larynx

The larynx extends from the epiglottis to the cricoid cartilage (at the level of the sixth cervical vertebra), where it connects with the trachea. One of its main functions is preventing entry of food and swallowed foreign bodies into the trachea. This is accomplished largely by the upward movement of the larynx and to a lesser extent by the downward motion of the flaplike epiglottis. Tight opposition of the vocal cords allows the patient to build up intrathoracic pressure just prior to coughing if any abnormal material enters the larynx or tracheobrachial tree.

AXIOM
Since a tracheostomy can limit upward motion of the larynx during swallowing, it may increase the tendency to aspiration of swallowed liquid or food.

The two important external laryngeal landmarks that are palpable are the thyroid cartilage, also known as Adam's apple, and the cricoid cartilage below it. The cricothyroid membrane stretches anteriorly between these two cartilages, is

Upper airway

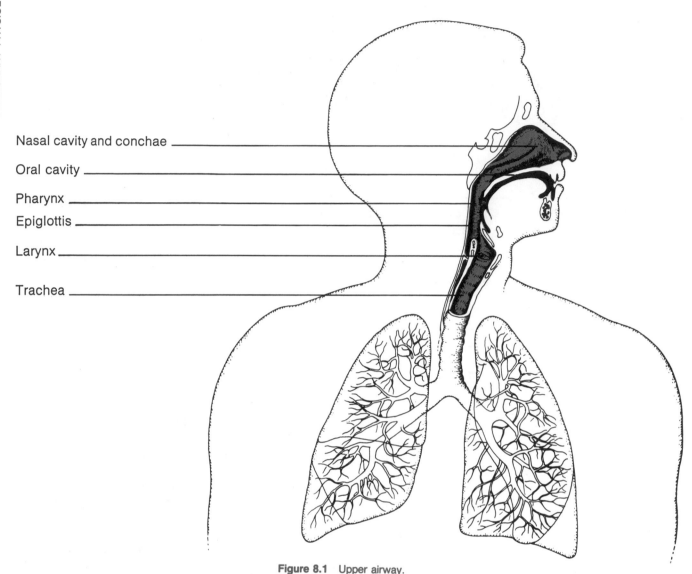

Nasal cavity and conchae

Oral cavity

Pharynx

Epiglottis

Larynx

Trachea

Figure 8.1 Upper airway.

quite thin, and is an excellent site for rapidly establishing an airway below the vocal cords. A cricothyroidotomy (coniotomy) in this area can generally be performed much more rapidly and safely than a tracheostomy.

AXIOM

A coniotomy is the preferred method for rapidly establishing an emergency airway if an endotracheal tube cannot be inserted.

Anatomically, the base of the tongue connects to the epiglottis. Anteriorly the tongue is attached to the mandible at the genoid tubercle by the genioglossus.

AXIOM

The most frequent cause of upper-airway obstruction in comatose patients is prolapse of the tongue into the posterior pharynx. Pulling the mandible forward is the best way to relieve this type of airway obstruction.

Speaking and singing are produced by vibration and movement of the vocal cords. The thinner, shorter, and tighter the vocal cords are, the higher the tone. Whispering does not require normal vocal cords and can be done even with severe laryngitis. Prolonged or forceful endotracheal intubation may damage the cords and result in speechlessness. If the patient has been intubated for more than a few days, he may be hoarse for several days or weeks following extubation.

AXIOM
The area between the vocal cords is the narrowest portion of the upper respiratory tract in an adult and is the most frequent site of upper-airway obstruction.

The recurrent laryngeal nerves, which control the vocal cords, may be damaged during thyroidectomy or parathyroidectomy. The left recurrent nerve curves around the ligamentum arteriosum and is vulnerable during surgery on the proximal descending thoracic aorta. The right recurrent laryngeal nerve curves around the proximal right subclavian artery. Damage to one recurrent laryngeal nerve usually only causes some hoarseness. Damage to both recurrent laryngeal nerves can cause the paralyzed vocal cords to come together in the midline and produce complete occlusion of the airway.

4. Trachea

The trachea is 10 to 12 cm long. It extends from the cricoid cartilage at the level of the sixth cervical vertebra down to the carina, where it bifurcates into the right and left mainstem bronchi at the level of the fifth thoracic vertebra. The inside diameter of the trachea, which is only 3 mm at birth, increases about 1 mm per year to the average adult diameter of 16 mm. Because of the small size of the upper airway in infants, laryngotracheobronchitis or inhalation of relatively small foreign bodies may rapidly cause severe respiratory difficulty. In adults, inspiratory stridor usually does not develop until the lumen of the larynx or the trachea is at least 70% to 80% obstructed.

AXIOM
Inspiratory stridor indicates a high-grade obstruction of the airway and is an indication for emergency endotracheal intubation or tracheostomy in the operating room.

The right mainstem bronchus is shorter, more vertically placed, and more directly in line with the trachea than the left. As a result, inhaled foreign bodies, aspirated oral secretions, or endotracheal tubes that go in too far tend to go down the right main bronchus. Up to 16% of endotracheal tubes may be in the right mainstem bronchus following resuscitation from a cardiac arrest.

Each of the 16 to 20 tracheal cartilages is an incomplete ring that spans the anterior two thirds of the trachea's circumference. Posteriorly, the tracheal wall is composed of a membrane containing fibrous and elastic tissue and smooth-muscle fibers. If the balloon on the end of an endotracheal or tracheostomy tube is inflated too much, the relatively immobile cartilages can quickly suffer pressure necrosis. The fibrous tissue that replaces the damaged cartilage tends to retract and narrow the tracheal lumen.

AXIOM
Allowing a slight air leak during inspiration helps to ensure that a balloon in the trachea is not overinflated.

Microscopically, the mucous membrane of the trachea is made up of pseudostratified, ciliated columnar epithelium interspersed with goblet cells. The cilia function in concert to move mucoid secretions upward along the trachea to the laryngeal opening. This process of mucociliary clearance, together with coughing, is responsible for removing most of the debris and inhaled particulate material that would otherwise accumulate in the lungs. However, the cilia are very sensitive, and smoking one cigarette can paralyze them for up to 20 to 30 minutes. Repeated smoking can cause replacement of this ciliated columnar epithelium with squamous epithelium.

When a tracheostomy is required because of airway problems, it is performed preferably through the second and third tracheal rings. In small children and infants, one must be especially careful to dissect directly on the trachea, because of the close proximity and friability of the pleura, which increases the risk of iatrogenic pneumothorax in children during a tracheostomy. Care must also be taken to make the tracheal incision high. If a tracheostomy is performed below the fourth or fifth tracheal ring, the risk of damage to the innominate artery by the tracheostomy tube or its balloon is increased.

AXIOM
Excessive pulsation of a tracheostomy tube is often due to increased pressure of the cuff or tip of the tube against the innominate artery.

The innominate artery crosses the trachea from left to right just below the center of the trachea. Unless a pulsating tracheostomy tube is pulled out somewhat and directed posteriorly, the tip or the balloon can cause erosion of the trachea and adjacent innominate artery.

B. CHEST WALL

1. Ribs

Functionally, the ribs may be divided into the first rib, the vertebral-sternal ribs, the vertebral-chondral ribs, and the floating ribs. The first rib is attached to the sternum very rigidly and moves only slightly during inspiration and expiration. The second to seventh ribs, also called the vertebral-sternal ribs, move about two axes simultaneously. Motion in one axis produces an increase in the anteroposterior diameter of the chest by a pump-handle motion. At the same time, these ribs also move in a bucket-handle fashion about the larger axes from their angles to the sternum, producing an increase primarily in the transverse diameter of the chest.

The eighth to tenth ribs, also called the vertebral-chondral ribs, move only in a bucket-handle fashion to increase the transverse diameter of the chest. As the diaphragm descends, movement of these ribs laterally also provides increased intra-abdominal space for displaced viscera. The ventral ends of the eleventh and twelfth ribs have no sternal or chondral attachments and are called floating ribs.

2. Diaphragm

At least 70% of the minute ventilation is normally due to the action of the diaphragm. Contraction of the muscles of the diaphragm during inspiration draws down its central tendon, increasing the volume of the thoracic cavity. At the same time the abdominal muscles usually relax and allow the upper abdomen to balloon out anteriorly. The costal fibers of the diaphragm also help to elevate the lower six ribs, thereby increasing the transverse diameter of the chest. The diaphragm, which is normally bowl shaped at rest, descends and flattens during inspiration to assume the shape of a saucer (Fig. 8.2). When, due to obstructive lung disease, the diaphragm is flattened or saucer-shaped following expiration, its function is severely limited.

During quiet expiration, the diaphragm rises back to its resting position, which is about the sixth intercostal space anteriorly. During forced expiration, contraction of the muscles in the abdominal wall increases intra-abdominal pressure and can force the diaphragm to rise as high as the third or fourth intercostal space anteriorly.

Each half of the diaphragm is supplied by a phrenic nerve which originates in the neck from the third to fifth cervical nerve roots. The intercostal muscles

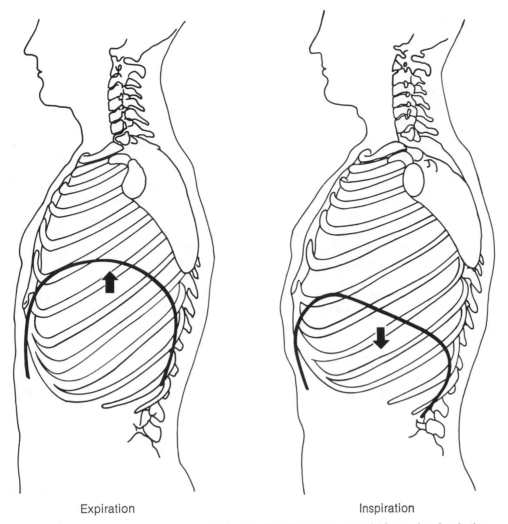

Expiration   Inspiration

Figure 8.2 The diaphragm on expiration and on inspiration.

between the ribs are supplied by corresponding intercostal nerves. Thus, an injury to the spinal cord at the level of C-6 will paralyze the lower intercostal muscles but will leave the diaphragm intact.

If the diaphragm is paralyzed because of injury to the phrenic nerves, it moves paradoxically while breathing; that is, upward with inspiration and downward with expiration. Impaired diaphragmatic function can also be seen in patients with large diaphragmatic hernias or ruptures following blunt trauma. Eventration of the diaphragm, due usually to chronic phrenic nerve paralysis, results in a thin, elevated diaphragm that may be difficult to differentiate from a ruptured diaphragm.

Adequate resting ventilation usually can be maintained by one hemidiaphragm or by the intercostal muscles alone. However, an increase in ventilatory requirements or the work of breathing can precipitate ventilatory insufficiency very rapidly in the presence of such impairment. The effectiveness of diaphragmatic contraction is altered by the degree of coordination with intercostal contraction, diaphragmatic position at the end of a normal quiet expiration, lung compliance, and intra-abdominal pressure. Neuromuscular diseases, phrenic nerve trauma, hypocalcemia, malnutrition, and various metabolic derangements can reduce diaphragmatic contractile strength, decreasing spontaneous ventilatory reserve and the ability to wean from mechanical ventilation.

Ventilatory muscle fatigue secondary to increased work of breathing is an important factor in respiratory failure.

AXIOM

As respiratory muscle fatigue progresses, ventilation tends to cease abruptly rather than gradually decline.

Aminophylline infusions and nutritional support may help improve diaphragmatic function in patients with critical illness or minimal ventilatory reserve.

3. Intercostal and Accessory Muscles of Respiration

The vertical chest cavity dimension is increased 1 to 4 cm during quiet tidal ventilation, but may exceed 8 cm during maximal inspiration. Contraction of the external intercostal muscles, which run from the lower, outer rib margins downward and forward to insert on the upper, outer margins of the ribs below, pulls the ribs upward and outward, increasing the anteroposterior chest cavity diameter. The accessory muscles of inspiration (scalenes, sternocleidomastoids, vertebral column extensors, anterolateral abdominal muscles, and pectoralis muscles) can also augment chest-wall expansion.

C. LUNGS

1. Bronchi

The right lung normally has three lobes (upper, middle, and lower) and the left has two lobes (upper and lower). In the average adult male, the right lung is larger, weighing about 600 to 650 g, and is responsible for 55% of the total ventilation. The left lung is smaller, weighing about 525 to 575 g, and accounts for 45% of the total ventilation. The weight of the lungs depends largely upon how much blood or fluid is present in lung tissue. In patients who die with severe congestive heart failure or acute respiratory failure, each lung will often weigh more than 1000 g.

Each lobar (secondary) bronchus divides into two to five segmental (tertiary) bronchi. Normally, there are ten (bronchopulmonary) segments in the right lung and eight in the left (Table 8.1).

2. Distal Bronchioles

As the bronchi proceed away from the hilum, they branch and become progressively smaller. Bronchioles less than 1.0 mm in diameter do not have cartilaginous rings and thus collapse quite readily during expiration. The terminal bronchioles are the smallest bronchioles that have no alveoli.

Closing volume refers to the amount of air still present in the lung at the time small bronchioles close during expiration. Closing volume is normally less than the functional residual capacity (FRC), which is the amount of air left in the lungs at the end of a normal quiet expiration.

AXIOM

If closing volume exceeds the functional residual capacity because of pulmonary disease, old age, pain, or the recumbent position, there is an increased tendency to atelectasis.

Table 8.1

BRONCHOPULMONARY SEGMENTS	Upper lobe	1. Apical 2. Posterior 3. Anterior	1. Apical-posterior 2. Anterior
	Middle lobe	4. Lateral 5. Medial	3. Superior lingular 4. Inferior lingular
	Lower lobe	6. Superior 7. Medial basal 8. Anterior basal 9. Lateral basal 10. Posterior basal	5. Superior 6. Anteriomedial basal 7. Lateral basal 8. Posterior basal

3. Acinus

The first order of bronchioles that have alveoli coming directly off their sides are referred to as respiratory bronchioles. The acinus, which is considered by many investigators to be the basic pulmonary unit, consists of a first-order respiratory bronchiole and two succeeding orders of smaller respiratory bronchioles, each with more alveoli in their walls. Each third-order respiratory bronchiole is followed by an alveolar duct, which is entirely alveolated. Each alveolar duct connects to an atrium, which is the entry to the main alveolar sacs (Fig. 8.3).

The portion of the lung with the respiratory bronchioles and alveoli comprise the respiratory zone (lung which is available for gas exchange). In the normal adult, this volume is about 3000 ml. With each inhaled breath, a tidal volume (about 500 ml) of inspired air moves through the conducting zone (i.e.,

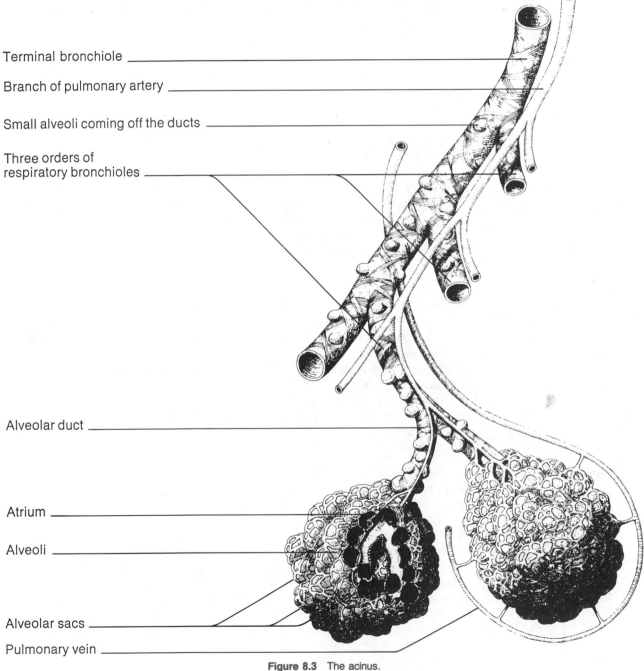

Terminal bronchiole

Branch of pulmonary artery

Small alveoli coming off the ducts

Three orders of respiratory bronchioles

Alveolar duct

Atrium

Alveoli

Alveolar sacs

Pulmonary vein

Figure 8.3 The acinus.

the dead space) to the respiratory zone (i.e., the blood-gas [alveolar-capillary] interface). Thus, only about 12% (350/3000) of the gas in the respiratory zone is changed with each breath.

Although the radius of each individual airway decreases with the 23 successive branchings of the bronchi, the total number of airways increases to a greater extent, resulting in an increase in the total airway cross-sectional area with each successive branching. Therefore, overall resistance to gas flow is normally highest in the larger airways and rapidly decreases as the airways' total cross-sectional area increases. Gas flow velocity also decreases in the smaller airways since the gas flows through a progressively larger cross-sectional area. In addition, the relatively higher flow rates in the large airways tend to cause some turbulence; however, in the smaller airways, velocity tends to slow and the flow becomes more laminar. This also contributes to lower resistance in the smaller airways.

The cross-sectional area of the alveolar ducts and alveoli is so large that gas movement is negligible and diffusion is the primary mechanism for gas exchange in these airspaces.

4. Blood Vessels

The lungs have a double arterial blood supply. The right and left pulmonary arteries and their branches bring venous blood from the right side of the heart to the pulmonary capillaries, where gas exchange with the alveoli is accomplished. The other (bronchial) arteries carry arterial blood to the supporting tissues of the lung, particularly the bronchi. There is usually one bronchial artery on the right and two on the left; their branches follow the bronchial tree down as far as the respiratory bronchioles.

A superior and inferior pulmonary vein carry oxygenated blood from the pulmonary capillaries in each lung to the left atrium. The bronchial venous drainage may go into the azygous and hemizygous systems or into the pulmonary veins. The bronchial venous blood, which enters the pulmonary veins, causes some desaturation of pulmonary venous blood. This accounts for a significant part of the normal physiologic shunt (pulmonary arteriovenous admixture) of 3% to 5% of the cardiac output.

D. MICROSCOPIC ANATOMY (FIG. 8.4)

1. Bronchioles

Microscopically, the bronchioles containing cartilage have much the same appearance as the trachea. Although the most distal bronchioles have fewer goblet cells, they have special cuboidal cells with many dense organelles believed to contain surfactant.

Broad longitudinal bands of elastin in the bronchioles are important in the normal elastic recoil of the lung. In the submucosal layer, two helical tracts of muscular fibers run in opposite directions to each other. Stimulation of this smooth muscle by histamine, serotonin, or local hypoxemia causes bronchoconstriction.

2. Alveoli

The 200 to 600 million alveoli in a normal lung have an average total alveolar surface area of 40 to 100 m². This surface area is directly related to body length and decreases by about 5% per decade after reaching a peak in young adults.

The epithelium of the alveoli is made up of two types of cells attached to a basement membrane. Most of a normal alveolus is lined by thin type I alveolar epithelial cells. The relatively small number of organelles in their cytoplasm reflects their relatively passive metabolic role in the lung. These cells are highly differentiated and when damaged cannot replicate. They are attached to a basement membrane, which in turn is separated by loose interstitial connective tissue from the capillary. The barrier to diffusion of alveolar gases normally consists of the alveolar cell wall, a basement membrane, loose interstitial connective tissue, and a capillary cell wall (Fig. 8.5). This "alveolar-capillary membrane" at its thinnest portion is usually only 0.2 μm wide, but it is considered to have an average thickness of about 0.6 μm.

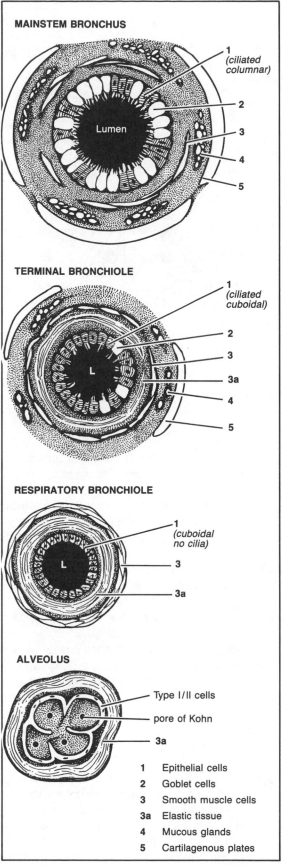

MAINSTEM BRONCHUS

1
(ciliated
columnar)

2

3

4

5

Lumen

TERMINAL BRONCHIOLE

1
(ciliated
cuboidal)

2

3

3a

4

5

L

RESPIRATORY BRONCHIOLE

1
(cuboidal
no cilia)

3

3a

L

ALVEOLUS

Type I/II cells

pore of Kohn

3a

1	Epithelial cells
2	Goblet cells
3	Smooth muscle cells
3a	Elastic tissue
4	Mucous glands
5	Cartilagenous plates

Figure 8.4 Microanatomy of airways in cross section at various points within the tracheobronchial tree, including the mainstem bronchus proximally, down to the alveolus, distally. (From Dolan, JT: Critical Care Nursing. FA Davis, Philadelphia, 1991, p. 555, with permission.)

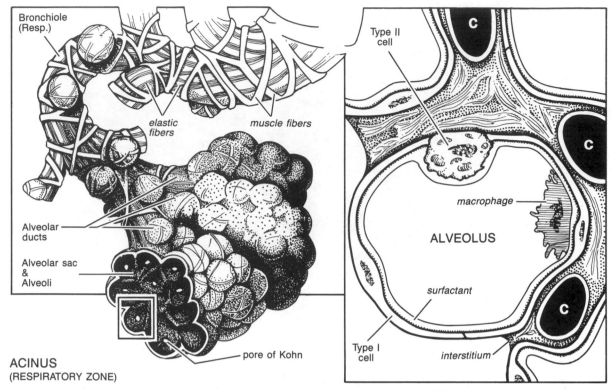

Bronchiole (Resp.)

elastic fibers

muscle fibers

Alveolar ducts

Alveolar sac & Alveoli

pore of Kohn

ACINUS (RESPIRATORY ZONE)

Type II cell

macrophage

ALVEOLUS

surfactant

Type I cell

interstitium

Figure 8.5 Ultrastructure of a pulmonary alveolus and capillaries. (From Dolan, JT: Critical Care Nursing. FA Davis, Philadelphia, 1991, p. 556, with permission.)

Type II alveolar cells are fewer in number. They are cuboidal in shape and have prominent organelles. The type II pneumocyte is usually found at the junction of the alveolar septae. These cuboidal cells are covered with microvilli. Surfactant is produced in the abundant cytoplasmic lamellar bodies and in the cytoplasmic microsomes of these cells. If the type I cells become damaged, as in ARDS, the type II cells usually multiply to fill in the gaps.

A third type of cell in the alveoli is the alveolar macrophage (dust cell). These phagocytes migrate from the capillaries to remove particles and foreign bodies in the alveoli. They then migrate either into the lymphatics or into the proximal bronchioles, where they are removed by the mucociliary clearance system. A proper sputum sample can be differentiated from saliva by the presence of these alveolar macrophages.

Pulmonary capillary endothelial cells are similar to endothelial cells found in other vascular beds. These cells produce and degrade prostaglandins, metabolize vasoactive amines, convert angiotensin I to angiotensin II, and produce, in part, coagulation factor VIII. Vasoactive agents synthesized by these cells may be partially responsible for regulation of ventilation and perfusion relationships. The endothelial cells are joined by loose intercellular junctions which are relatively permeable.

3. Blood Vessels

The pulmonary arteries and veins divide and become progressively smaller until they form the capillaries in the alveolar-capillary membranes (Fig. 8.6).

Two types of pulmonary capillaries are found within the alveolar matrix. The first passes through corner junctions where adjacent alveoli merge at a "triple point." These junctional capillaries probably do not participate in gas exchange, but are important for pulmonary fluid homeostasis. The other capillaries run within the alveolar septa separating adjacent airspaces. Suspensory collagen fibers attach to one side of these septal capillaries. An increase in lung

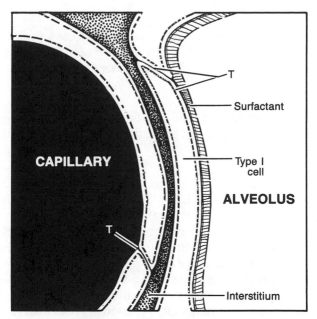

Figure 8.6 Ultrastructure of the alveolar-capillary membrane shown in cross section: pathway of diffusion. Diffusion of gases occurs through the various structural layers of the membrane including the fluid surfactant layer lining the alveolus, alveolar-epithelial type I cell, epithelial basement membrane, interstitial space, capillary basement membrane, capillary endothelial cell, and the red blood cell (not depicted). Tight junctions (*T*) are also depicted. (From Dolan, JT: Critical Care Nursing. FA Davis, Philadelphia, 1991, p. 566, with permission.)

volume with inspiration exerts traction on these suspensory fibers, causing the septal capillary to bulge outward into the airspace on one side of the septum. Approximately half of the capillaries in any septum will protrude into each contiguous airspace, thereby increasing the area of alveolar-capillary contact. Septal capillaries are thin where they bulge into the alveolus and are thick on the side that tends to stay in the septum. The thick portion is predominantly concerned with fluid and protein transfer between blood and the pulmonary interstitium. The thin portion is involved primarily in gas exchange.

The interstitial space between the alveoli and capillaries is generally thin, but it is thick around the larger arteries and veins. The perivascular interstitial space is the first area where excess interstitial fluid accumulates.

AXIOM
Early pulmonary edema will often produce a butterfly appearance on a chest x-ray because of the increased interstitial fluid around the segmental and subsegmental vessels extending out from the hilum.

II. PULMONARY FUNCTION

The four main processes related to gas exchange in the lungs include *ventilation* (movement of air in and out of the lungs), *distribution* of ventilated gases into the various lobes, segments, and lobules, *diffusion* of gases back and forth between the alveoli and plasma, and *perfusion* of blood through the pulmonary capillaries.

A. VENTILATION

Ventilation is a rhythmic act, brought about primarily by contraction of the diaphragm and intercostal muscles, which results in the movement of air or other gases into and out of the lungs.

AXIOM

The term *respiration* (often erroneously confused with the term *ventilation*) involves not only movement of gases in and out of the lung, but also all of the physiologic mechanisms involved in gas exchange, from inhalation of oxygen to its utilization at the cellular level.

Respiration may also be defined as all of the processes concerned with the exchange of oxygen and carbon dioxide between organisms (patients) and their environment.

1. Types of Ventilation

a. Minute Ventilation ($\dot{V}E$)

The minute ventilation is the total amount of new air or gas moved in and out of the airways and lungs each minute, and this is equal to the tidal volume multiplied by the respiratory rate. The normal tidal volume is about 500 ml (7 ml/kg) and the normal respiratory rate is 12 breaths per minute. Therefore, the normal minute ventilation averages about 6 liters/min. A person can live for only short periods of time with a minute ventilation as low as 1.5 liter and with a respiratory rate as low as two to four breaths per minute unless his metabolism is severely depressed, such as in deep hypothermia.

The respiratory rate occasionally rises to as high as 40 to 50 per minute, and the tidal volume can become almost as great as the vital capacity, which is about 4500 to 5000 ml in a young adult male. However, at rapid breathing rates (>30 per minute) individuals usually cannot sustain tidal volume greater than 50% of the normal vital capacity for more than a few minutes unless they are trained athletes.

b. Alveolar Ventilation ($\dot{V}A$)

The main function of the pulmonary ventilation is to continually renew the air or gases in the alveoli. The rate at which new air reaches these gas-exchange areas is called alveolar ventilation. During normal quiet ventilation, the tidal volume fills the tracheobronchial tree down as far as the terminal bronchioles, with only about 70% of the inspired air actually flowing all the way into the alveoli. The portion of each tidal volume (V_t) that never reaches the alveoli is referred to as anatomic dead space (V_d). In adults this is about 150 ml or 1.0 ml per pound of body weight. The ratio of V_d/V_t is normally 0.3. Alveoli that are not perfused are referred to as pathological dead space.

The new gas molecules move the last short distance from the terminal bronchioles into the alveoli by diffusion. Diffusion is caused by the kinetic motion of molecules with each gas molecule moving at high velocity between the other molecules. The velocity of movement of the molecules in the respiratory air is so great that the gases move the remaining distance to the alveoli in only a fraction of a second.

2. Control of Ventilation

a. Chemical Stimuli

The most important chemical stimuli to the respiratory center are hypercarbia, acidosis, and hypoxemia.

(1) Carbon Dioxide Changes

AXIOM

Increased carbon dioxide in the blood, through its effect on brain pH, is normally the most powerful stimulus to which the respiratory center is exposed. Relatively small increases in arterial PCO_2 may cause dramatic increases in minute ventilation.

In most people, the inhalation of 5% carbon dioxide will more than double the minute ventilation. This response takes longer than the circulation time from the lung to the brain and may persist for some time after the stimulus is withdrawn. For this reason, carbon dioxide probably does not act directly on the respiratory center, but rather through changes in the pH of the cerebrospinal fluid (CSF). Apparently, carbon dioxide diffuses freely into the CSF and then hydrogen ions are released by the following reaction:

$$H_2O + CO_2 \rightleftharpoons H_2CO_3 \rightleftharpoons H^+ + HCO_3^-.$$

Since CSF normally has almost no proteins and is poorly buffered, its pH changes rapidly with any alteration in its carbon dioxide concentration.

AXIOM

Persistently high arterial carbon dioxide concentrations, in the range of 60 to 70 mm Hg or higher, decreases the sensitivity of the respiratory center to carbon dioxide changes. Consequently, patients with chronic severe hypercarbia often must rely on hypoxemic stimulation of peripheral chemoreceptors to maintain adequate ventilation.

Ordinarily, the respiratory center responds to a decrease in the P_{CO_2} by decreasing the frequency and depth of ventilation. However, a paradox is often seen in patients with severe respiratory alkalosis who may have increasing hyperventilation until they pass out. The main determinant of cerebral blood flow is the arterial P_{CO_2}. Hypocarbia causes cerebral vasoconstriction and decreases cerebral blood flow by about 2% to 4% for each 1 mm Hg fall in P_{CO_2}. Thus, the patient who is hyperventilating and reduces his arterial P_{CO_2} (Pa_{CO_2}) to less than 15 to 20 mm Hg may experience such severe cerebral vasoconstriction that the brain becomes ischemic and develops a local metabolic acidosis. This acidosis then stimulates the respiratory center to produce even more hyperventilation.

AXIOM

A severe respiratory alkalosis may cause the respiratory control center to increase ventilation even more.

This cycle of increasing hyperventilation, respiratory alkalosis, and cerebral acidosis will tend to become progressively worse until it is interrupted in some manner. The simplest treatment is to have the patient rebreathe his expired air by breathing in and out of a paper bag. Expired air has a P_{CO_2} which is about 70% of the Pa_{CO_2}. After the patient's Pa_{CO_2} rises to a more normal range, the excessive cerebral vasoconstriction will relent and the cerebral metabolic acidosis will be corrected.

(2) pH Changes

Acidosis by itself, without any changes in the Pa_{CO_2}, can increase both respiratory rate and tidal volume. This is probably because of stimulation of the respiratory center and peripheral receptors. As mentioned earlier, most of the respiratory changes caused by the Pa_{CO_2} are probably related to its effect on the pH of the CSF.

Patients with ischemic brain damage often act as if they have a severe cerebral metabolic acidosis and may hyperventilate until arterial blood is quite alkalotic. Efforts to correct this respiratory alakalosis with large amounts of sedatives and/or increasing dead space are usually unsuccessful.

(3) Oxygen Changes

Hypoxia is a much weaker stimulus to ventilation than hypercarbia. Minute ventilation often does not increase significantly until the inhaled fraction of oxygen (F_{IO_2}) is decreased to 15% to 16% (at sea level).

AXIOM

Hypoxia indirectly stimulates the respiratory center through specific chemoreceptors in the carotid and aortic bodies.

Although the response to hypoxia is much weaker than the response to hypercarbia, the response to hypoxia persists until death. In some patients with severe chronic pulmonary disease, hypoxia is the main or only drive to ventilation. Consequently, administration of oxygen in volumes greater than 0.5 to 1.0 liters/min may result in removal of the hypoxic stimulus, thereby causing severe hypoventilation or apnea resulting in an increasing and sometimes lethal respiratory acidosis.

AXIOM

If oxygen is administered to a patient with severe chronic hypercarbia, the patient's ventilation must be watched very closely.

In anemia or carbon monoxide poisoning, the oxygen content of the blood may be greatly reduced with no appreciable change in Pao_2. Even though the tissues may be suffering severe oxygen lack, there may be little or no increase in ventilation until lactic acidosis due to impaired cell metabolism develops.

b. Reflex Stimuli

(1) From the Lungs

Moderate inflation of the lungs inhibits inspiration. This "inhibitoinspiratory reflex" is often considered to be the only stretch (Hering-Breuer) reflex. However, stretch reflexes also include an "excitatoinspiratory reflex" in which there is a stimulus to inspiration when the lungs become partially deflated. In addition, a "deep inspiration reflex" inflates the lungs even further if the lung becomes more than moderately inflated. This deep inspiration reflex may be an important factor in the sighing mechanism which periodically causes inflation of many of the alveoli that are not open during ordinary tidal volume ventilation.

(2) From Higher Centers in the Brain

A stressful emotion of any type, particularly fear or anger, increases ventilation. The vasomotor center is closely associated with the respiratory center in function. Consequently, any change that causes strong stimulation of the vasomotor center also tends to stimulate the respiratory center.

(3) From the Body

Sepsis is an extremely powerful stimulus to the respiratory center. Injection of endotoxin into the CSF is followed rapidly by a tremendous increase in the respiratory rate and minute volume, usually producing a relatively severe respiratory alkalosis.

AXIOM

Any hospitalized patient who begins to hyperventilate without obvious cause should be considered to have hypoxemia, sepsis, or a pulmonary embolus until proven otherwise.

3. Lung Volumes

A number of terms have been coined to describe the volume or capacity of the lungs at various phases of the inspiratory-expiratory cycle (Fig. 8.7). The spirogram formed by a maximal exhalation after a maximal inhalation is generally described in terms of four *capacities* and four *volumes*.

a. Definitions

TLC Total lung capacity represents the total volume of the lungs when they are maximally inflated. TLC can be divided into FVC and RV.
FVC Forced vital capacity is the volume of air that the patient can exhale after a maximum inspiration. It is a combination of inspiratory reserve volume, tidal volume, and expiratory reserve volume ($FVC = IRV + V_t + ERV$). It is also equal to the TLC minus the residual volume (RV).
RV Residual volume refers to the amount of gas remaining in the lung after a maximal exhalation.
V_t Tidal volume is the amount of air moved in and out of the lung during normal resting ventilation.

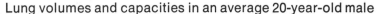

Lung volumes and capacities in an average 20-year-old male

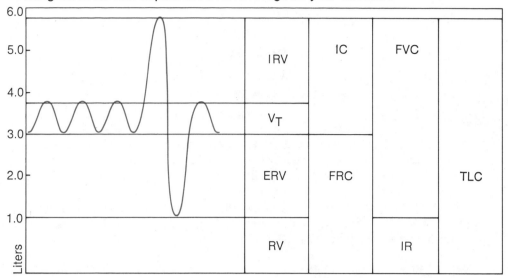

Spirometry in a normal patient. Normally at least 75% of the forced expiratory volume should be exhaled during the first second. The MMFR from 25% to 75% of the forced expiratory volume should be about 4.0 liters per second or about 240 liters per minute.

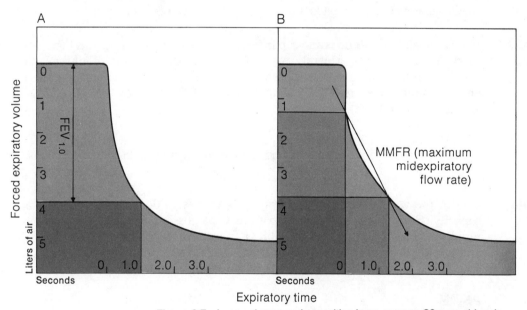

Figure 8.7 Lung volumes and capacities in an average 20-year-old male.

ERV Expiratory reserve volume is the amount of air that can be exhaled after a normal exhalation.

IRV Inspiratory reserve volume is the amount of air that can be inhaled after an inspiration of a normal tidal volume.

FRC Functional residual capacity, also called resting lung volume, consists of the ERV plus the RV. The FRC is the amount of air still present in the lungs after a normal exhalation.

IC Inspiratory capacity consists of V_t plus IRV. IC is the amount of air that can be inhaled after a normal exhalation.

369

The relationships of the various lung volumes or capacities can be expressed as follows:

$$TLC = VC + RV$$
$$VC = IRV + V_t$$
$$TLC = FRC + IC$$
$$FRC = ERV + RV$$
$$IC = IRV + V_t.$$

b. Normal Values

A seated, young adult who has a total lung capacity (TLC) of approximately 6.0 liters would typically have a residual volume (RV) of 1.2 to 1.5 liters, expiratory reserve volume (ERV) of 1.5 to 1.8 liters, a tidal volume (V_t) of 0.5 liters, and inspiratory reserve volume (IRV) of 2.5 liters (Table 8.2).

Other lung "capacities" in the same patient might consist of a vital capacity (VC) of 4.5 to 4.8 liters, and inspiratory capacity (IC) of 3.0 liters, and a functional residual capacity (FRC) of 3.0 liters (Table 8.3).

c. Changes with Age

With advancing age, TLC and FVC fall moderately and ERV and IC fall markedly. Thus, in patients who are 70 to 80 years old and apparently in good health, the TLC might be 4.2 liters, FVC 2.4 liters, RV 1.8 liters, ERV 0.8 liters, FRC 2.6 liters, and IC 1.6 liters.

AXIOM

If the FVC is more than 25% lower than expected for the patient's age, height, weight, and sex, the patient is said to have a restrictive pulmonary defect.

d. Changes in the Adult Respiratory Distress Syndrome

In ARDS, all lung volumes and capacities (particularly ERV, IRV, and FRC) are markedly reduced. In general, as the FRC falls, the amount of physiologic shunting in the lung increases. If ventilatory assistance with increasing positive end-expiratory pressure (PEEP) is applied, the FRC and Pao_2 tend to increase and the shunt (Qs/Qt) decreases.

AXIOM

In ARDS, the best correlation with increased shunting in the lung is the reduction in FRC.

e. Expiratory Flow Rate

One of the ways to determine airway resistance is to do a timed forced vital capacity (FVC). After taking as deep a breath as possible, the patient exhales as rapidly and deeply as possible (Fig. 8.8A). In most normal patients, at least 75%, and usually 85%, of the FVC will be exhaled in 1.0 sec. The $FEV_{1.0}$, depends on size, age, and sex, but in most healthy adults will be at least 3.0 liters.

AXIOM

If the $FEV_{1.0}$/FVC ratio is less than 75%, the patient is said to have an obstructive pulmonary defect.

Table 8.2

LUNG VOLUME CHANGES* WITH AGE AND ARDS		20 Years	70 Years	ARDS
	IRV	2.5	1.2	0.3
	VT	0.5	0.4	0.4
	ERV	1.8	0.8	0.3
	RV	1.2	1.8	1.5

*In liters.

Table 8.3

LUNG CAPACITY CHANGES* WITH AGE AND ARDS	20 Years	70 Years	ARDS
TLC	6.0	4.2	2.5
VC	4.8	2.4	1.0
IC	3.0	1.6	0.7
FRC	3.0	2.6	1.8

*In liters.

An $FEV_{1.0}/FVC$ ratio of 50% to 60% is said to be a moderate defect. If the $FEV_{1.0}$ is less than 50%, even with bronchodilator therapy, there is a major risk to any thoracic surgery.

The actual value of the $FEV_{1.0}$ also has some importance. In general, a patient should have an $FEV_{1.0}$ of at least 1.5 liters before having any thoracic surgery. If the $FEV_{1.0}$ is less than 0.8 liters following surgery, the risk of severe complications and/or the possibility that a patient will be a respiratory cripple are very high.

Using the timed FVC, one can also determine the maximum midexpiratory flow rate (MMEFR) from 25% to 75% of the FVC. Normally, this is about 4.0 liters/sec or 160 liters/min (Fig. 8.8).

The maximum expiratory flow rate from the first 200 ml of FVC to the 1200-ml mark can also be determined. Normally, this will be at least 8 liters/sec or 480 liters/min.

One can also use the $FEV_{1.0}$ to estimate the patient's maximum breathing capacity (MBC), which is also known as the patient's maximum voluntary ventilation (MVV). This is determined by having the patient breathe as deeply

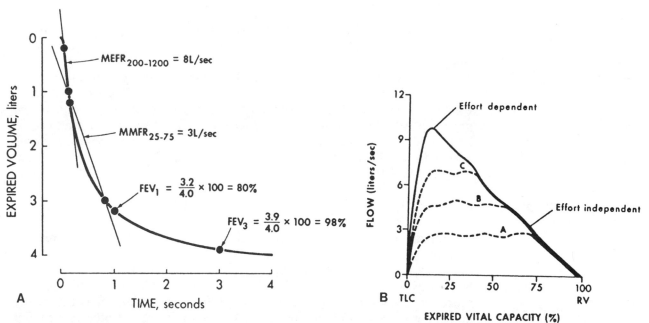

Figure 8.8 (A) Schematic representation of a normal forced vital capacity (FVC) maneuver (expired volume against time, heavy line) and the derivation of several variables commonly used to evaluate airway obstruction. (B) Expiratory flow-volume curves demonstrating the effect of varying degrees of effort: dashed lines A, B, and C represent increasing effort; solid center line represents maximal effort. The early effort-dependent and later effort-independent segments are shown. TLC = total lung capacity; RV = residual volume. (From Smith, LH and Thier, SO: Pathophysiology.WB Saunders, Philadelphia, 1981, p. 192, with permission.)

and rapidly as possible for 5 to 10 seconds and then multiplying the result by 6 or 12 to determine how much air could have been ventilated in 1 minute. The average normal for adult males is approximately equal to their age minus 25 in liters per minute. Thus, a 72-year-old man should have an MBC of about $200 - 72 = 128$ liters/min. In the absence of an obstructive defect, the MBC is equal to the $FEV_{1.0}$ multiplied by 40. Thus, the 40-year-old man should have an $FEV_{1.0}$ of about $128 - 40 = 3.2$ liters.

Another way of determining airway resistance is to plot flow during a FVC maneuver against expiratory volume, creating a maximal expiratory flow-volume curve. From this curve, peak flow and maximal flow rate at any given lung volume usually 50% ($Vmax_{50}$) or 75% ($Vmax_{75}$) of maximum can be determined and reported as a percentage of the predicted value for a normal subject of the same age, sex, and height.

The flow volume curve also can be used to demonstrate the effect of expiratory effort on flow rates. The family of curves formed by progressively increasing expiratory effort (Fig. 8.8B) demonstrates that increasing expiratory effort causes progressively higher peak flows early in expiration, but despite increasing effort, flow rates late in expiration remain unchanged.

A corollary of these observations is the fact that airflow resistance in the central "large" airways is largely effort dependent. On the other hand, measurements performed at lower lung volumes, toward the end of expiration, indicate that air flow in peripheral or "small" airways tends to be independent of effort.

AXIOM
Air flow in the small airways is largely effort dependent, particularly toward the end of forced vital capacity.

Of the various indices of airway resistance that can be derived from the dynamic recording of FVC, perhaps the one concerning most of the small airways is the maximal midexpiratory flow rate ($MMFR_{25-75}$), because it is less effort dependent than other parameters and reflects the behavior of small as well as large airways.

4. Dead Space

a. Anatomic and Pathologic Dead Space

The volume of the airways up to the gas exchange areas is called the anatomic dead space. On occasion, however, some of the alveoli are not functional because of a lack of blood flow to their pulmonary capillaries. From a functional point of view, these alveoli without capillary perfusion can be considered to be pathologic dead space. When the alveolar (pathologic) dead space is included, the total dead space is often called the physiologic (total) dead space. In the normal person, the anatomic and the physiologic dead spaces are nearly equal because all alveoli are functional. However, in persons with poorly perfused alveoli, the dead space/tidal volume ratio V_d/V_t) may rise from a normal of 0.30 to exceed 0.60 to 0.65.

b. Changes with Varying Tidal Volumes

Since dead space remains relatively constant, different tidal volumes can produce great changes in alveolar ventilation, even when the total minute ventilation remains constant. For example, if minute ventilation is 8 liters/min, respiratory rate is 16 per minute, tidal volume is 500 ml, and dead space is 150 ml per breath, alveolar ventilation will be 350 ml $\times$ 16 or 5.6 liters/min. On the other hand, if tidal volume is 200 ml and respiratory rate 40 per minute, the dead space per breath will generally fall to about 100 ml per breath, and consequently alveolar ventilation will only be about 4.0 liters/min. At the other extreme, if tidal volume is 1000 ml and the respiratory rate is 8 per minute, the dead space will probably increase to about 200 ml, but alveolar ventilation will increase to approximately 6.4 liters/min.

c. Shape of the Inspired Air Front

If the movement of inspired air through the conducting airways had a square front, and if the tidal volume were exactly equal to the anatomic dead space, there would theoretically be no effective alveolar ventilation with low tidal volumes. However, the front of the inspired air movement is wedge shaped, and there is facilitated diffusion past the terminal bronchioles so that, even when tidal volume is much less than the anatomic dead space, there is still some alveolar ventilation.

It has been noted that when a dog pants at very high respiratory rates, his tidal volume is less than his anatomic dead space, yet obviously the dog exchanges oxygen and carbon dioxide adequately. This helped stimulate interest in high-frequency ventilation which uses respiratory rates of 50 to 600 per minute and depends upon facilitated diffusion for alveolar gas exchange.

d. Determining Dead Space

The dead space/tidal volume ratio (V_d/V_t) can be calculated from the alveolar (end-tidal) $PACO_2$ and average expired PCO_2 ($PECO_2$) by the following formula:

$$V_d/V_t = \frac{PACO_2 - PECO_2}{PACO_2}.$$

Normally, the arterial PCO_2 is about 40 mm Hg and the average expired PCO_2 ($PECO_2$) about 28 mm Hg, making the ratio of total or physiologic dead space to tidal volume approximately 0.3. Example:

$$V_d/V_t = \frac{PaCO_2 - PECO_2}{PaCO_2} = \frac{40 - 28}{40} = \frac{12}{40} = 0.3.$$

Normally, there is little or no alveolar (pathologic) dead space and consequently the alveolar PCO_2 ($PACO_2$) (which is equivalent to and can be measured by the end-tidal PCO_2) is equal to the arterial PCO_2 ($PaCO_2$). Thus, the alveolar-arterial PCO_2 difference ($P(A-a)CO_2$] is normally zero.

Increasing alveolar dead space tends to cause a rise in the arterial PCO_2 and tends to lower the expired and alveolar $PACO_2$, thereby increasing the $P(A-a)CO_2$ or alveolar-arterial carbon dioxide difference.

The relationship between these gases and the dead space is relatively constant and can be used to calculate the amount of dead space present. This can be done relatively easily with the $PaCO_2$ in arterial blood if one has a capnograph to analyze the average expired $PECO_2$ and the $PACO_2$. If alveolar dead space increases, the end-tidal or alveolar PCO_2 ($PACO_2$) will be significantly lower than the arterial PCO_2 ($PaCO_2$), and the average expired PCO_2 ($PECO_2$) will also be lower than normal. For example, if a patient has a tidal volume (V_t) of 500 ml, $PaCO_2$ of 40 mm Hg, $PACO_2$ of 30 mm Hg, and $PECO_2$ of 21 mm Hg, the $P(A-a)CO_2$ is 10 mm Hg and:

$$V_d \text{ (anatomic)} = \frac{PACO_2 - PECO_2}{PACO_2} \times 500 = \frac{(30 - 20)\,(500)}{30} = 167 \text{ ml}$$

$$V_d \text{ (total)} = \frac{PaCO_2 - PECO_2}{PaCO_2} \times 500 = \frac{(40 - 20)\,(500)}{40} = 250 \text{ ml.}$$

Thus, the patient would have 83 ml of pathologic (alveolar) dead space. Note that the P_{ACO_2} is used to calculate anatomic dead space and the P_{aCO_2} is used to calculate total dead space.

e. Effects of Alveolar Ventilation on PaCO₂

If dead space and the rate of carbohydrate metabolism are kept constant, the P_{aCO_2} provides a relatively accurate indication of the quantity of alveolar ventilation. With a normal alveolar ventilation of about 4 liters/min, the P_{aCO_2} averages about 40 mm Hg. If the alveolar ventilation falls to 2 liters/min, the P_{aCO_2} tends to rise to about 80 mm Hg. On the other hand, if alveolar ventilation is increased to 8 liters/min, the P_{aCO_2} tends to fall to about 20 mm Hg.

5. Compliance

One of the main factors affecting ventilation is the compliance or distensibility of the lungs. In strict terms, pulmonary compliance refers to the volume of air or gas that can move into the lung for each unit of pressure change.

A significant proportion of total lung recoil is caused by surface tension in the air-fluid interface of alveoli and airways. Surface tension is the force generated in a fluid surface which tends to minimize the area of an air-fluid interface. If a surface is spherical, as in a bubble, surface tension generates pressures within the sphere, according to Laplace's law:

$$\Delta P = 2T/R \qquad or \qquad T = \frac{\Delta PR}{2},$$

where ΔP is pressure between the inside and outside of the sphere, T is surface tension, and R is radius of the sphere.

One can consider alveoli to be a large number of interconnected bubbles exhibiting a tendency to minimize surface area and to collapse. This tendency would seem to account for overall lung recoil. However, the Laplace equation dictates that surface tension should be reduced as alveoli become larger and that small alveoli (with high surface tension) empty into the larger alveoli (which have lower surface tension). However, surfactant, which lowers surface tension, keeps this from happening and helps to stabilize small alveoli and reduce their tendency to collapse.

AXIOM

Surfactant is essential for preventing atelectasis in smaller alveoli, especially in the dependent portions of the lung.

Ideally, compliance is determined while the lung is at its FRC. Reduction of FRC decreases lung recoil, promoting airway closure and atelectasis. Subsequently, a higher transmural pressure gradient is required to reopen the collapsed air spaces than would be necessary to expand normal nonatelectatic lung tissue.

Compliance is generally expressed in milliliters per centimeter H_2O pressure change. The normal value for lung compliance is about 200 ml/cm H_2O. For lung and chest wall together, the compliance is normally 100 ml/cm H_2O. Resistance is the reciprocal of compliance and is generally expressed in terms of centimeters H_2O pressure per liter of inflation. Thus, the normal resistance for the lung is 5 cm H_2O/liters, and the resistance for the lung plus the chest wall would be 10 cm H_2O/liters.

In general, the total resistance to ventilation (Rt) can be divided into three parts: airway resistance (Raw), lung resistance (RL), and chest-wall resistance (Rcw) (Fig. 8.9). For example, it normally takes about 15 cm H_2O pressure to passively ventilate a normal adult with a tidal volume of 1000 ml. Of this total pressure, approximately 5 cm H_2O pressure (with air flow at about 1.0 liter/sec) is needed to overcome airway resistance, 5 cm H_2O pressure to overcome the

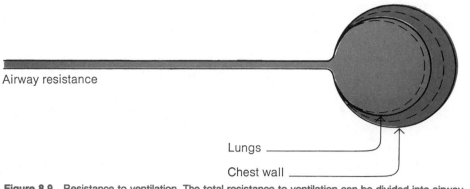

Airway resistance

Lungs ⎯⎯

Chest wall ⎯⎯

Figure 8.9 Resistance to ventilation. The total resistance to ventilation can be divided into airway resistance (represented here by a long, thin tube) and the lung and chest wall resistance (depicted by two semielastic containers, one within the other).

resistance of the lung, and 5 cm H_2O to overcome the resistance of the chest wall.

a. Airway Resistance (Conductance)

Resistance to gas flow is influenced by flow rate, flow character, and airway geometry. At low flow rates through smooth straight tubes, gas molecules move in a uniform, parallel streamlined manner characteristic of laminar flow. The relations between flow and pressure were first accurately described by the French physician, Poiseuille in 1846. Under the conditions of his experiments, the volume flow (Q) through a cylindrical tube was determined by:

$$Q = \frac{P\pi r^4}{8\, l\mu},$$

where P is the perfusion pressure, r is the internal radius of the cylinder, l is the length of the cylinder, and μ is the viscosity of the fluid.
Since

$$\frac{P}{Q} = \text{resistance} = R$$

$$R = \frac{8 \times \text{tube length} \times \text{gas viscosity}}{\text{radius}^4}.$$

Thus, according to Poiseuille's law, if the radius is reduced by half, resistance to flow is increased 16-fold.

The pressure required to maintain laminar flow is proportional to the velocity; however, when the flow becomes turbulent, the pressure required to maintain the same air flow is proportional to the square of the velocity.

AXIOM

In rapid turbulent breathing, airway resistance is inversely proportional to the fourth power of the radius of the air tubes and the square of the velocity of air flow.

Airway resistance (Raw) can also be calculated much more simply by dividing the pressure to overcome airway resistance (Paw) by the rate of air flow (F). If the rate of air flow is 1000 ml/sec or 1.0 liter/sec (which is double the flow rate normally seen with quiet, spontaneous breathing), the airway resistance (Raw) can be calculated as follows:

$$Raw = \frac{Paw}{F} = \frac{5 \text{ cm } H_2O}{1.0 \text{ L/sec}} = 5 \text{ cm } H_2O \cdot L^{-1} \cdot sec^{-1}.$$

The airway resistance tends to be lower in patients who are breathing spontaneously compared to patients who are being passively ventilated.

b. Lung Resistance

Lung resistance (R_L) can be calculated by dividing the pressure required to overcome the resistance of the lung (P_L) by the volume (V) to which the lung is inflated. Thus, normally

$$R_L = \frac{P_L}{V} = \frac{5 \text{ cm } H_2O}{1 \text{ L}} = 5 \text{ cm } H_2O/L.$$

c. Chest-Wall Resistance

Similarly, chest-wall resistance (R_{CW}) can be calculated by dividing the pressure required to overcome the resistance of the chest wall (P_{CW}) by the volume (V) of inflation. Thus, normally

$$R_{CW} = \frac{P_{CW}}{V} = \frac{5 \text{ cm } H_2O}{1 \text{ L}} = 5 \text{ cm } H_2O/L.$$

To differentiate between lung and chest-wall resistance or compliance, it is necessary to use an esophageal or intrapleural catheter to determine the intrapleural pressure changes with ventilation. The intrapleural pressure changes reflect lung resistance, which then can be subtracted from total static resistance to calculate chest-wall resistance.

d. Static Resistance

To determine how much of the tidal resistance to air flow is due to the airways, the term static resistance (R_s) is used to quantify the chest-wall and lung resistance together while there is no air flow. Thus, after the lungs are inflated and there is no air flow, the static resistance (R_s) of the lungs plus chest wall would be:

$$R_s = R_L + R_{CW}$$
$$= 5 \text{ cm } H_2O/L + 5 \text{ cm } H_2O/L$$
$$= 10 \text{ cm } H_2O/L.$$

Static compliance, which is the reciprocal of static resistance, would then be:

$$C_s = 1/R_s = 1/10 \text{ cm } H_2O/L$$
$$= 0.1 \text{ L/cm } H_2O$$
$$= 100 \text{ ml/cm } H_2O.$$

e. Effective Resistance and Effective Compliance

Although they are not strictly accurate, the terms total resistance (R_t), effective resistance, or dynamic resistance are sometimes used to include the sum of the resistances of the airways, lungs, and chest wall. For example:

$$R_t = R_{aw} + R_L = R_{CW}$$

$$R = \frac{5 \text{ cm } H_2O}{1 \text{ L}} + \frac{5 \text{ cm } H_2O}{1 \text{ L}} + \frac{5 \text{ cm } H_2O}{1 \text{ L}} = \frac{15 \text{ cm } H_2O}{1 \text{ L}}.$$

In this instance, R_{aw} is calculated as pressure change (rather than air flow) divided by the volume change.

Total compliance (C_t), also known as effective compliance or dynamic compliance, is the reciprocal of the total resistance:

$$C_t = 1 \text{ L}/R_t = 1 \text{ L}/15 \text{ cm } H_2O = 67 \text{ ml/cm } H_2O.$$

f. Causes of Increased Total Resistance

It is important to follow total resistance or compliance when the patient is on a ventilator.

AXIOM

Pneumothorax or airway obstruction should be suspected in any patient having difficulty breathing on a ventilator. Obviously, such problems must be corrected as soon as possible. If these mechanical problems can be ruled out, the rising inflation pressure is likely to be due to increased stiffness of the lung itself. For example, if a patient with a tidal volume of 1000 ml has a systems or peak inflation pressure (PIP) of 20 cm H_2O, and the PIP rises to 25 cm H_2O with no apparent mechanical cause, and if Raw and Rcw are constant, one can estimate that lung resistance R_L has probably increased about 50% by the following calculations:

$$Rt_1 = \frac{PIP}{Vt} = Raw + Rcw + R_L = 5 + 5 + R_{L_1} = 20 \text{ cm } H_2O/L$$

$$R_{L_1} = 10 \text{ cm } H_2O/L$$

$$Rt_2 = \frac{PIP_2}{Vt} = 25 = 5 + 5 + R_L$$

$$R_{L_2} = 15 \text{ cm } H_2O/L.$$

Since some ventilators are now capable of providing an inspiratory hold of 0.5 to 1.0 second, the static compliance or resistance of the lungs plus chest wall can be calculated directly from the ventilator pressure during the inspiratory hold.

Although some assumptions are made in deriving these figures, they can provide some guidelines for evaluating changes in airway and lung resistance. It must also be emphasized that changes or trends are far more important than absolute numbers.

g. Work of Breathing

During normal quiet ventilation, respiratory muscle contraction occurs only during inspiration. Expiration is usually a passive process caused by elastic recoil of the lung and chest wall. Thus, the respiratory muscles normally perform "work" only to cause inspiration and not at all to cause expiration.

The work of inspiration can be divided into three different fractions: (1) that required to expand the lungs against its elastic forces, called "compliance work" or "elastic work;" (2) that required to overcome the viscosity of the lung and chest-wall structures, called "tissue-resistance work;" and (3) that required to overcome airway resistance during the movement of air into lungs, called "airway-resistance work" (Fig. 8.10).

(1) Compliance Work

The compliance work is the work required to expand the lungs against the elastic forces in the surrounding tissues. This can be calculated by multiplying the volume of expansion times the average pressure required to cause the expansion. That is, compliance work $= (V \times P)/2$, where V is the increase in volume and P is the increase in intrapleural pressure.

(2) Tissue-Resistance Work

Tissue-resistance work is the work required to overcome the tissue resistance (tissue viscosity) of the lungs and chest cage.

(3) Airway-Resistance Work

This is the work required to overcome the resistance to airflow through the upper airway and bronchi.

(4) Types of Work

During normal quiet breathing most of the work performed by the respiratory muscles is used simply to expand the lungs. A small amount, normally only a

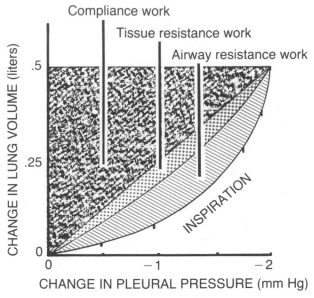

Figure 8.10 Graphical representation of the three different types of work accomplished during inspiration: (1) compliance work (2) tissue-resistance work, and (3) airway-resistance work.

few percent of the total work, is used to overcome tissue resistance (tissue viscosity), and somewhat more is used to overcome airway resistance. On the other hand, during very heavy breathing, when air must flow through the respiratory passageways at very high velocity, a much larger proportion of this work is used to overcome airway resistance. In pulmonary disease, all three types of work tend to be increased.

h. Energy Required for Ventilation

AXIOM

During normal quiet ventilation, only 2% to 3% of the total energy expended by the body is required for the pulmonary ventilatory process.

During heavy exercise, the absolute amount of energy required for pulmonary ventilation can increase as much as 25-fold. However, this still does not represent a significant increase in percentage of total energy expenditure because the total energy release by the body increases at the same time as much as 15- to 20-fold. Thus, even in heavy exercise, only 3% to 5% of the total energy expended is used for ventilation.

Pulmonary diseases can markedly increase the work of breathing by (1) decreasing pulmonary compliance, (2) increasing airway resistance, and (3) increasing tissue viscosity in the lung. This combination of factors can increase the work of breathing to more than one-third the total energy expended by the body. With some pulmonary conditions this excess work load alone may be the cause of death.

The relative increase in the work of breathing can be estimated to a certain extent clinically by observing the amount of patient effort required with each breath and the number of breaths per minute. As a rough, general rule, if it appears that patients are working at all to breath, their energy expenditure is doubled, and if they look like they are working hard, energy expenditure per breath is at least tripled. If the respiratory rate is 20 to 24 per minute, ventilatory work is doubled, and if the respiratory rate is 30 to 35 per minute, the work of breathing is tripled. Thus, if patients appear to be working hard and are breathing at 30 to 35 times per minute their work of breathing is probably at least nine times normal. As a general rule, a patient cannot sustain work of breathing of more than six times normal for more than a few hours without developing an acute ventilatory arrest.

AXIOM

A ventilatory rate of more than 30 to 35 per minute with increased effort with each breath is usually an indication to intubate the patient and begin ventilatory assistance.

B. DISTRIBUTION

The distribution of ventilated gas in the various lobe segments and alveoli is determined largely by local changes in the transpulmonary or distending pressures. Other factors that can alter gas distribution include airway closure, loss of surfactant, decreased elasticity of portions of the lung, partial or complete obstruction of bronchi, and increased lung water.

1. Transpulmonary Pressure

Transpulmonary or distending pressure is equal to the alveolar pressure minus pleural pressure. Alveolar pressure is the pressure that reaches the alveoli after the airway resistance is overcome; it is generally considered to be the same throughout the lung. Pleural pressure (which tends to resist alveolar inflation) is determined primarily by gravity; each centimeter change in position, up or down, results in a corresponding decrease or increase in the pleural pressure of 0.2 to 0.3 cm H_2O. Thus, the pleural pressure is usually 4 to 6 cm higher at the lung base than in the apex.

AXIOM

Because of higher pleural pressure and lower transpulmonary (distending) pressures at the base of the lung, lower-lobe alveoli are smaller. However, they distend better during inspiration because they are on a more favorable position on the pressure-volume curve for the lung.

Because pleural pressure is greater in the lower portions of the lung, there is a lower net distending or transpulmonary pressure in that area. As a consequence, the dependent alveoli are smaller than the alveoli at the apex. However, during inspiration the dependent alveoli expand relatively more than the alveoli at the apex. This occurs because the smaller alveoli are in a more favorable position on the pressure-volume curve, which describes the relationship between alveolar size and their distending pressure (Fig. 8.11). The small airways to the dependent alveoli also tend to close earlier during expiration and open later during inspiration than those associated with the larger apical alveoli. Because the small bronchi to the lower lobes close earlier, the associated alveoli do not contract to too small a volume during expiration. This also helps to prevent lower lobe atelectasis.

2. Airway Closure

Ordinarily, all airways are open at the end of a full inspiration. During expiration, however, some of the small airways (0.5 to 0.9 mm in diameter) close relatively early, especially in the lower lobes. This phenomenon has given rise to the concept of "closing volume," which is the lung volume present when a significant number of small airways have begun to close. The important corollary is that the airways that close earliest during expiration also open latest during inspiration. Since the pathologic processes that increase closing volumes tend to have their greatest effect on the more dependent portions of the lung, ventilation is distributed away from these areas in the most critically ill or injured patients, increasing the ventilation-perfusion ($\dot{V}/\dot{Q}$) mismatch.

AXIOM

If closing volume exceeds FRC, there is a progressive tendency to atelectasis.

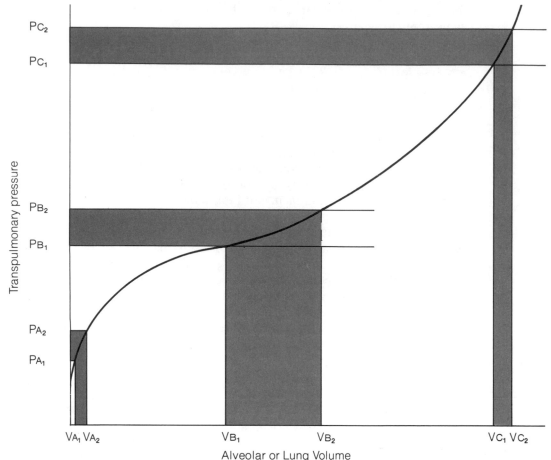

Figure 8.11 Effects of standard pressure changes on distention or volume. Depending upon the initial diameter or volume of an alveolus, a standard pressure change may produce widely different amounts of distention or volume change. When lung or aveolar volume is very low (VA_1), as in atelectasis, a certain pressure change ($PA_2 - PA_1$) will produce only minimal expansion of the alveoli or lung ($VA_2 - VA_1$). When the alveoli are open but small, as in the lung bases, the same pressure change ($PB_2 - PB_1$) will produce a rather significant volume increase ($VB_2 - VB_1$). In larger alveoli in the apex of the lung, the same pressure change ($PC_2 - PC_1$) will produce less expansion ($VC_2 - VC_1$) than in the basilar alveoli.

Closing volume increases with age, with the patient in the supine position, with obesity, and with abdominal distention, but it is decreased by spontaneous sighing. If functional residual capacity plus tidal volume are less than the closing volume, as often happens in ARDS, there is a progressive tendency to atelectasis as the gases in unventilated alveoli are absorbed. This is particularly apt to occur if the alveoli are filled with oxygen, which is absorbed much more readily than nitrogen.

AXIOM

The more severe the ARDS, the higher the tidal volumes and PEEP have to be in order to prevent a progressively severe atelectasis.

3. Surfactant

Surfactant is a surface-active material secreted by type II alveolar lining cells. It contains a number of phospholipids, including lecithin, sphingomyelin, phosphatidylglycerol, and phosphatidylinositol. A thin layer of surfactant floats on the alveolar lining fluid and reduces its surface tension. Without surfactant, small alveoli would tend to collapse completely and become atelectatic. Because of surfactant, small alveoli are stable, and total lung recoil increases with increased lung volume.

AXIOM

Surfactant is essential for preventing atelectasis in small alveoli.

Although surfactant production by type II (granular) pneumocytes appears to be decreased in experimental shock, surfactant metabolism can apparently be maintained without perfusion of the pulmonary capillaries as long as there is adequate alveolar ventilation. Interestingly, mild-to-moderate overdistention of alveoli, as may occur with sighing, tends to increase surfactant production; however, excessive distention of alveoli has the opposite effect.

Some of the clinical situations associated with decreased surfactant production include high concentrations of inhaled oxygen, cardiopulmonary bypass, and prolonged ventilator assistance. Although there have been some suggestions that decreased surfactant might be an etiologic factor in ARDS, decreased surfactant in such circumstances is apparently more a result than a cause of the altered pathophysiology.

C. DIFFUSION

The movement of gases back and forth between the alveoli and the plasma and red blood cells is accomplished largely by the process of diffusion. Since carbon dioxide diffuses so readily (about 20 times as fast as oxygen), hypercarbia due to impaired diffusion alone is extremely unlikely. Oxygen, on the other hand, is much less diffusible, and impaired diffusion may be a significant cause of hypoxemia, particularly at low oxygen concentrations.

AXIOM

Hypercarbia is virtually never due to a diffusion abnormality in the lung.

The most common cause of impaired or decreased diffusion in the lung is interstitial edema causing increased distance between the alveolar and capillary membranes. This is particularly apt to be seen in ARDS and congestive heart failure. Under ordinary circumstances, the thickness of the alveolar capillary membrane is about 0.2 μm and the distance between the alveolus and the interior of the red cell is less than 0.5 to 1.0 μm. However, even mild changes in capillary permeability may cause a severe increase in the amount of interstitial fluid and an abrupt drop in the Pao_2.

D. PERFUSION

1. Volume and Pressure

Three hypothetical "zones" can be delineated when considering the interaction between alveolar pressure and microvascular blood flow. In zone 1 which is at the apex of the lung if someone is standing, alveolar pressure (PA) during inspiration exceeds pulmonary artery (Pa) pressure and pulmonary venous (Pv) pressure, producing septal capillary collapse and cessation of blood flow. In zone 2, alveolar pressure (PA) is less than pulmonary artery (Pa) pressure, but greater than Pv. Consequently, blood flow in zone 2 should be intermittent and will cease during passive inspiration or diastole. In zone 3, both pulmonary artery and pulmonary venous pressures exceed alveolar pressure, and blood flow occurs throughout the cardiac cycle.

Most healthy lower-lobe lung tissue is of the zone 3 type, unless alveolar pressure is elevated significantly above atmospheric by a positive-pressure ventilator. In physiologic terms, zone 1 represents pulmonary dead space (ventilation without perfusion); zone 2 contains high V/Q units (ventilation in excess of perfusion); and zone 3 contains well-matched V/Q units.

AXIOM

Pulmonary artery wedge pressure catheters must be in lung zone 3, preferably below the mitral valve, to properly reflect left atrial filling pressure.

The total volume of blood in the pulmonary arteries, veins, and capillaries is about 500 to 750 ml, or about 10% to 15% of the total blood volume in an average adult male. In patients who are extremely vasoconstricted peripherally, the central blood volume (in the heart, lungs, and great vessels of the thorax) is increased, whereas the reverse is true in peripheral vasodilation.

Of the blood in the pulmonary circuit, approximately 60% to 65% is present in the pulmonary veins, with about 20% to 25% in the pulmonary arteries and 10% to 20% in the pulmonary capillaries. Pulmonary arteries are much more compliant than systemic arteries, and blood flow through the pulmonary vascular bed can often increase up to fourfold with no significant increase in pulmonary artery pressure.

Pressures in the right side of the heart, pulmonary vessels, and left atrium are usually much lower than those in the systemic circuit. The normal pressures in the various chambers and vessels are right atrium, 0 to 5 mm Hg; right ventricle, (RV) 15 to 25/0 to 5; and pulmonary artery, (PA) 15 to 25/5 to 10. The pressures in the pulmonary capillaries, pulmonary veins, and left atrium average about 5 to 10 mm Hg. Although the normal RV and PA systolic pressures are often said to be 25 mm Hg, in young adult males, they are usually much lower and in the range of 10 to 15 mm Hg.

2. Flow

Blood flow through the lung can be estimated using the Fick principle, which correlates oxygen consumption (V_{O_2}) by the tissues with cardiac output (Q) and arteriovenous oxygen difference [$C(a-v)O_2$].

$$Q = \frac{V_{O_2}}{C(a-v)O_2}.$$

Thus, if V_{O_2} is 250 ml/min and the a-v O_2 difference is 5 vol% (50 ml/L),

$$Q = \frac{250 \text{ ml/min}}{5 \text{ vol\%} \times 10}$$
$$= 250/50$$
$$= 5 \text{ L/min.}$$

At sea level, the average oxyhemoglobin saturation is approximately 70% to 75% in the pulmonary artery, 98% to 100% in pulmonary venules, and 95% to 98% in systemic arteries. Blood from the superior vena cava ordinarily has an oxygen saturation similar to that of the mixed venous blood in the pulmonary artery. Inferior vena cava blood generally has a higher oxygen saturation than superior vena cava blood. However, this is usually balanced fairly well by the very low (30% to 35%) oxygen saturation in coronary sinus blood so that the oxygenation of mixed venous and superior vena caval blood are quite similar if cardiac output is relatively normal (Table 8.4).

3. Vascular Resistance

Vascular resistance in the pulmonary circuit normally is only about one fifth to one tenth of that calculated for systemic arteries. Since the mean pressure is normally 10 to 15 mm Hg in the pulmonary artery and about 5 mm Hg in the pulmonary veins, the pressure drop across the pulmonary arterioles is approximately 5 to 10 mm Hg. If the pressure difference in millimeters of mercury across a vascular bed is divided by the blood flow in liters per minute, the result (if multiplied by 80 to convert the units into the metric system) is equal to the vascular resistance in the circuit in $dyne \cdot sec^{-1} \cdot cm^{-5}$. Using these calculations, the normal pulmonary arteriolar resistance (PaR) is about 80 to 160 $dyne \cdot sec^{-1} \cdot cm^{-5}$. This may be shown mathematically as:

Table 8.4

PRESSURE AND OXYGEN SATURATION IN VARIOUS CHAMBERS OF THE HEART	Pressure, mm Hg	O_2 Saturation, %
Superior vena cava	0–5	70–75
Inferior vena cava	0–5	75–80
Coronary sinus	—	30–40
Right atrium	0–5	70–75
Right ventricle	25/0–5*	70–75
Pulmonary artery	25/10(15)*†	70–75
Pulmonary capillaries	6–12	98–100
Left atrium	5–10	95–98
Left ventricle	120/0–5	95–98
Aorta	120/80(90)†	95–97

*These are the values of older adults. RV and Pa systolic pressure in young healthy individuals may be less than 12 to 15 mm Hg.
†Parentheses ( ) indicate the mean pressure.

$$\text{PaR dyne}\cdot\text{sec}^{-1}\cdot\text{cm}^{-5} = \frac{\text{pressure change (mm Hg)}}{\text{blood flow (L/min)}} \times 80$$

$$= \frac{[(10 \text{ to } 15) - 5]\,(80)}{5} = \frac{(5 \text{ to } 10)\,(80)}{5}$$

$$= 80 \text{ to } 160.$$

Normal systemic vascular resistance is $800-1600$ dyne$\cdot$sec$^{-1}\cdot$cm^{-5}.

4. Pulmonary Edema

Pulmonary edema refers to a situation in which there is a pathologically increased amount of water in the lungs. Such water usually accumulates initially in the peribronchial interstitial fluid spaces and later in the alveoli. Clinically, pulmonary edema is characterized by severe dyspnea and diffuse bubbly rales because of increased alveolar fluid. This may progress until frothy pink secretions begin to accumulate in the trachea and major bronchi.

The dynamics of fluid exchange between the capillaries and the interstitial fluid space of the lungs are similar to those involved in the systemic circulation, and can be described by the following (Starling's) equation:

$F = KA\,[(P_c - P_t) - \sigma\,(\pi_c - \pi_s)]$
F = rate of flow from the vascular space (capillary) to the interstitial space
K = a permeability factor (often increased in critically ill patients, particularly those with sepsis)
A = area of the capillaries involved
P_c = capillary hydrostatic pressure (normally averages about 9 to 10 mm Hg at the arteriolar end and 5 to 6 mm Hg at the venous end of pulmonary capillaries)
P_s = interstitial hydrostatic pressure (normally averages about −7 to −8 mm Hg)
σ = the reflective coefficient for protein
π_c = plasma oncotic pressure (about 22 to 28 mm Hg)
π_s = interstitial oncotic pressure (estimated to average about 3 to 6 mm Hg in the lungs).

Movement of fluid out of the capillaries into the pulmonary interstitial tissue is favored by factors that (1) increase capillary permeability (shock, sepsis), (2) increase the capillary hydrostatic pressure (congestive heart failure or administration of excess crystalloids), or (3) decrease the plasma oncotic pressure (cirrhosis or hypoalbuminemia).

AXIOM

The increased lung water in ARDS is largely due to increased pulmonary capillary permeability. However, any increase in capillary hydrostatic pressure will severely aggravate the situation.

E. VENTILATION-PERFUSION RATIOS

AXIOM

Reduced functional residual capacity (FRC) with (V/Q) imbalance is generally considered to be the main cause of abnormal blood gases in critically ill ICU patients.

Under normal circumstances, the average alveolar ventilation is about 4 liters/min and the perfusion is approximately 5 liters/min so that the average V/Q for the entire lung is about 0.8. Perfusion in the lungs is largely determined by gravity. Thus, a large fraction of the pulmonary circulation goes to dependent areas of the lung. Consequently, in the erect subject there is a very high V/Q ratio at the apices and a lower V/Q at the bases. However, as a general rule, the lung, through its own autoregulation (with bronchoconstriction in areas of poor blood flow and vasoconstriction where there is poor air flow) tends to maintain a relatively good match between perfusion and ventilation.

AXIOM

Mismatching of ventilation and perfusion or greatly increased areas of shunting or dead space are the main cause of hypoxemia in the ICU.

ABBREVIATIONS

P_{AO_2}	= alveolar oxygen tension
Pa_{O_2}	= arterial oxygen tension
$P\bar{v}_{O_2}$	= average oxygen tension in mixed venous blood
P_{ACO_2}	= alveolar oxygen tension
Pa_{CO_2}	= arterial carbon dioxide tension
P_{ECO_2}	= average carbon dioxide tension in expired gases
F_{IO_2}	= fraction of inspired oxygen (100% O_2 = F_{IO_2} of 1.0; room air = F_{IO_2} of 0.21)
$P_{(A-a)O_2}$	= alveolar-arterial oxygen difference or gradient
$P_{(A-a)CO_2}$	= alveolar-arterial carbon dioxide difference
V_d/V_t	= ratio of dead space (V_{DS}) to tidal volume (V_T)

SUMMARY POINTS

1. Since a tracheostomy can limit upward motion of the larynx during swallowing, it may increase the tendency to aspiration of swallowed liquid or food.
2. A coniotomy is the preferred method for rapidly establishing an emergency airway if an endotracheal tube cannot be inserted.
3. The most frequent cause of upper airway obstruction in comatose patients is prolapse of the tongue into the posterior pharynx. Pulling the mandible forward is the best way to relieve this type of airway obstruction.
4. The area between the vocal cords is the narrowest portion of the upper respiratory tract in an adult and is the most frequent site of upper airway obstruction.
5. Inspiratory stridor indicates a high-grade obstruction of the airway and is an indication for emergency endotracheal intubation or tracheotomy in the operating room.
6. Allowing a slight air leak during inspiration helps to ensure that a balloon in the trachea is not overinflated.
7. Excessive pulsation of a tracheostomy tube is often due to increased pressure of the cuff or tip of the tube against the innominate artery.
8. As respiratory muscle fatigue progresses, ventilation tends to cease abruptly rather than gradually decline.

9. If closing volume exceeds the functional residual capacity because of pulmonary disease, old age, pain, or the recumbent position, there is an increased tendency to atelectasis.

10. Early pulmonary edema will often produce a butterfly appearance on a chest x-ray because of the increased interstitial fluid around the segmental and subsegmental vessels extending out from the hilum.

11. The four main processes related to gas exchange in the lungs include ventilation (movement of air in and out of the lungs); distribution of ventilated gases into the various lobes, segments, and lobules; diffusion of gases back and forth between the alveoli and plasma; and perfusion of blood through the pulmonary capillaries.

12. The term *respiration* (often erroneously confused with the term *ventilation*) involves not only movement of gases in and out of the lung, but also all of the physiologic mechanisms involved in gas exchange, from inhalation of oxygen to its utilization at the cellular level.

13. Increased carbon dioxide in the blood (through its effect on brain pH) is normally the most powerful stimulus to which the respiratory center is exposed. Relatively small increases in arterial PCO_2 may cause dramatic increases in minute ventilation.

14. Persistently high arterial carbon dioxide concentrations, in the range of 60 to 70 mm Hg or higher, decreases the sensitivity of the respiratory center to carbon dioxide changes. Consequently, patients with chronic severe hypercarbia often must rely on hypoxemic stimulation of peripheral chemoreceptors to maintain adequate ventilation.

15. A severe respiratory alkalosis may cause the respiratory control center to increase ventilation even more.

16. Hypoxia indirectly stimulates the respiratory center through specific chemoreceptors in the carotid and aortic bodies.

17. If oxygen is administered to a patient with severe chronic hypercarbia, the patient's ventilation must be watched closely.

18. Any hospitalized patient who begins to hyperventilate without obvious cause should be considered to have hypoxemia, sepsis, or a pulmonary embolus until proven otherwise.

19. If the FVC is more than 25% lower than expected for the patient's age, height, weight, and sex, the patient is said to have a restrictive pulmonary defect.

20. In ARDS, the best correlation with increased shunting in the lung is the reduction in FRC.

21. At high tidal volumes, dead space increases relatively little; therefore, the V_d/V_t (dead space/tidal volume ratio) decreases and alveolar ventilation increases.

22. A rise in the $P(A-a)CO_2$ may indicate an increased dead space, usually due to alveoli that are not adequately perfused.

23. Surfactant is essential for preventing atelectasis in smaller alveoli. Especially in the dependent portions of the lung.

24. In rapid turbulent breathing, airway resistance is inversely proportional to the fourth power of the radius of the air tubes and the square of the velocity of air flow.

25. If the peak inflation pressure required to mechanically ventilate a patient rises rapidly, it should make one suspect (1) partial airway obstruction or (2) a pneumothorax, possibly under tension.

26. During normal quiet ventilation, only 2% to 3% of the total energy expended by the body is required for the pulmonary ventilatory process.

27. A ventilatory rate of more than 30 to 35 per minute with increased effort with each breath is usually an indication to intubate the patient and begin ventilatory assistance.

28. Because of higher pleural pressure and lower transpulmonary (distending) pressures at the base of the lung, lower-lobe alveoli are smaller. However, they distend better during inspiration because they are in a more favorable position on the pressure-volume curve for the lung.

29. If closing volume exceeds FRC, there is a progressive tendency to atelectasis.

30. The more severe the ARDS, the higher the tidal volumes and PEEP have to be in order to prevent progressively severe atelectasis.

31. Surfactant is essential for preventing atelectasis in small alveoli.

32. Hypercarbia is virtually never due to a diffusion abnormality in the lung.

33. Pulmonary artery wedge pressure catheters must be in lung zone 3, preferably below the mitral valve, to properly reflect left atrial filling pressure.

34. The increased lung water in ARDS is largely due to increased pulmonary capillary permeability. However, any increase in capillary hydrostatic pressure will severely aggravate the situation.

35. Reduced functional residual capacity (FRC) with ($\dot{V}/\dot{Q}$) imbalance is generally considered to be the main cause of abnormal blood gases in critically ill ICU patients.

36. Mismatching of ventilation and perfusion or greatly increased areas of shunting or dead space are the main causes of hypoxemia in the ICU.

BIBLIOGRAPHY

1. Angus, GE and Thurlebeck, WM: Number of alveoli in the human lung. J Appl Physiol 32:483, 1972.
2. Arbonelius, M, Lilja, B, and Senyk, J: Regional and total lung function in patients with hemidiaphragmatic paralysis. Respiration 32:253, 1975.
3. Bloom, SA, et al: Spurious assessment of acid-base status due to dilutional effect of heparin. Am J Med 70:528, 1985.
4. Clements, JA: Functions of the alveolar lining. Am Rev Respir Dis 115:67, 1977.
5. Clements, JA: Pulmonary surfactant. Am Rev Respir Dis 101:984, 1970.
6. Cohen, MI: Central determinants of respiratory rhythm. Annu Rev Physiol 43:91, 1981.
7. Comroe, JH, Jr, et al: The lung: Clinical Physiology and Pulmonary Function Test, ed 2. Year Book Medical Publishers, Chicago, 1962.
8. Dawson, CA: Role of pulmonary vasomotion in physiology of the lung. Physiol Rev 64:544, 1984.
9. Dempsey, JA and Forster, HV: Mediation of ventilatory adaptations. Physiol Rev 62:262, 1982.
10. Eisenkraft, JB: Pulse oximeter desaturation due to methemoglobinemia. Anesthesiology 68(2):234, 1984.
11. Ellis, JH, Perera, SP, and Levin, DC: A computer program for calculation and interpretation of pulmonary function studies. Chest 68:209, 1975.
12. Gil, J: Organization of microcirculation in the lung. Annu Rev Physiol 42:177, 1980.
13. Gleb, AF and Zamel, N: Effect of aging on lung mechanics in healthy nonsmokers. Chest 68:538, 1975.
14. Green, M and Moxham, J: The respiratory muscles. Clin Sci 68:1, 1985.
15. Guyton, AC: Textbook of Medical Physiology, ed 4. WB Saunders, Philadelphia, 1971.
16. Hildehan, JW, Goerle, J, and Clements, JA: Pulmonary surface film stability and composition. J Appl Physiol 47:604, 1979.
17. Hoppin, FG, Jr, Green, ID, and Mead, J: Distribution of pleural surface pressure in dogs. J Appl Physiol 28:863, 1969.
18. LeBlanc, P, Ruff, F, and Milic-Emili, J: Effects of age and body position on "airway closure" in man. J Appl Physiol 28:448, 1970.
19. Macklem, PT: Normal and abnormal functions of the diaphragm. Thorax 36:161, 1981.
20. Macklem, PT: Respiratory mechanics. Annu Rev Physiol 40:157, 1978.
21. Mecca, RS: Respiratory: Essential physiologic concerns. In Civetta, J, Taylor, R, and Kirby, R (eds): Critical Care. JB Lippincott, Philadelphia, 1988, p 1023.
22. Milic-Emili, J, et al: Regional distribution of inspired gas in the lungs. J Appl Physiol 21:749, 1966.
23. Mithoefer, JC and Karetsky, MS: The cardiopulmonary system in the aged. In Powers, JS (ed): Surgery of the Aged and Debilitated Patient. WB Saunders, Philadelphia, 1968.
24. Morgan, TE: Pulmonary surfactant. N Engl J Med 284:1185, 1971.
25. Nunn, JF: Applied Respiratory Physiology. Butterworth & Co, London, 1987, p 46.
26. Ordog, GJ, Wasserberger, J, and Balasubramaniam, S: Effect of heparin on arterial blood gases. Ann Emerg Med 14:233, 1985.

27. Raffin, TA: Indications for arterial blood gas analysis. Ann Intern Med 105:390, 1986.
28. Rose, CC and Wolfson, AB: Respiratory physiology. Emerg Med Clin North Am 7;2:187, 1989.
29. Roumos, C and Macklem, PT: Respiratory muscles. N Engl J Med 307:786, 1982.
30. Ruch, TC and Patton, HD: Physiology and Biophysics. WB Saunders, Philadelphia, 1974, p 304.
31. Sigrist, S, et al: The effect of amnophylline on inspiratory muscle contractility. Am Rev Respir Dis 126:46, 1982.
32. Thurlbeck, WM: The internal surface of nonemphysematous lungs. Am Rev Respir Dis 95:765, 1967.
33. Wagner, PD: Ventilation-perfusion relationships. Annu Rev Physiol 42:235, 1980.
34. West, JB: Pulmonary gas exchange. Int Rev Physiol 14:83, 1977.
35. West, JB, Dollery, CT, and Naimar, A: Distribution of blood flow in isolated lung: Relation to vascular and alveolar pressures. J Appl Physiol 19:713, 1964.
36. Whipp, BJ: Ventilatory control during exercise in humans. Annu Rev Physiol 45:393, 1983.

CHAPTER 9

Blood Gases: Pathophysiology and Interpretation

I. INTRODUCTION	Maintenance of an adequate gas exchange in the lungs and at the tissue level is vital in critically ill patients. Any factor that interferes with these processes must be diagnosed and corrected as soon as possible.

To understand these phenomena one must know (1) the major physical factors that determine alveolar concentration, (2) the factors that determine the rate at which gases diffuse through the respiratory membrane, (3) how gases are transported to and from the tissues, and (4) the factors involved in gas exchange at the tissue level. The changes that occur with various clinical pulmonary and cardiovascular problems should also be known.

II. THE PHYSICS OF GASES

A. GAS PRESSURES

Pressure is caused by repeated impact of kinetically moving molecules against a surface. Therefore, the pressure of a gas acting on the surfaces of the respiratory passages and alveoli is proportional to the summated force of impaction of all the molecules striking the surface at any given instant. In the lungs, one deals with mixtures of gases, particularly oxygen, nitrogen, and carbon dioxide. The rate of diffusion of each of these gases is directly proportional to their partial pressure.

B. RELATIONSHIP OF PRESSURE TO VOLUME (BOYLE'S LAW)

AXIOM

Boyle's law states that if the mass and temperature of a gas in a chamber remain constant but the pressure (P) increases or decreases, the volume (V) of the gas varies inversely with the pressure.

In other words,

$$V = \frac{K}{P},$$

where K is a constant.

Thus, 1.0 gmol of gas at 1 atm pressure will occupy 22.4 liters. However, if the pressure is increased to 2.0 atm, 1.0 gmol of gas will only occupy 11.2 liters of space. Atmospheric pressure drops about 3.12% per 1000 ft above sea level.

AXIOM

Air trapped in a pneumothorax or obstructed bowel will tend to expand 3.12% for each 1000 ft the patient is raised above sea level.

C. RELATIONSHIP OF TEMPERATURE TO VOLUME (CHARLES LAW)

AXIOM

Charles law (also known as Guy-Lassac's law) states that if the pressure of a given quantity of gas remains constant, the volume (V) of the gas increases in direct proportion to the rise in absolute temperature (T).

Absolute (kelvin) temperature is 273 K more than the temperature in degrees Centrigrade. In other words:

$$O°C = 273 \text{ K.}$$

Thus, room temperature (20°C) is 293 K and normal body temperature (37°C) is 310 K.

Using Charles law, a mole of gas occupying 22.4 liters at O°C would occupy $22.4 \times 310/273$ or 25.4 liters at a normal body temperature of 37°C.

D. THE GAS LAW

Combining Boyle's and Charles laws, the following relationship between volume (V) of a gas and its pressure (P) and absolute temperature (T) can be expressed by the following formula:

$$V = \frac{KT}{P}.$$

If the constant K is changed to nR (with n equal to the quantity of gas in gram-moles and R equal to a constant that depends on the units used), and if P is in millimeters of mercury, V is in liters, and T is in degrees kelvin, R is equal to 62.4. Therefore, at O°C at 1 atm pressure (760 mm Hg), the volume of 1.0 gmol of gas will be:

$$V = \frac{62.4 \, nT}{P}$$

$$= \frac{(62.4) \, (1.0) \, (273)}{760} = 22.4 \text{ L.}$$

III. THE VAPOR PRESSURE OF WATER

When air enters the respiratory passageways, water immediately evaporates from the surfaces of these passages and humidifies the inhaled air. This results from the fact that water molecules, like other dissolved gas molecules, are continually escaping from the surface of the lipid phase into the gas phase. The pressure that the water molecules exert to escape through the surface is called the vapor pressure of the water.

At O°C, water vapor pressure (P_{H_2O}) is 4.6 mm Hg, and at room temperature (20°C), the P_{H_2O} is 17.4°C. At 37°C, this vapor pressure is 47 mm Hg. Therefore, once air enters the upper respiratory tract and has become fully humidified, the partial pressure of the water vapor in the gas mixture is 47 mm Hg (Table 9.1).

Table 9.1

PARTIAL PRESSURES OF GASES (mm Hg) WHILE BREATHING ROOM AIR AT SEA LEVEL AND 20°C	Air	Inspired Air in Trachea	Average Alveolar Gas	Average Expired Gas
P_{O_2}	159.0	149.3	104.0	120.0
P_{CO_2}	0.3	0.3	40.0	28.0
P_{N_2}	583.3	563.4	569.0	565.0
P_{H_2O}	17.4	47.0	47.0	47.0
Total	760.0	760.0	760.0	760.0

AXIOM

Rapid inhalation of cold gases could quickly dry the passages of the upper airway.

IV. PRESSURES OF GASES IN WATER AND TISSUE

The concentration of a gas in a solution is determined not only by its pressure but also by its solubility coefficient. Some molecules, especially carbon dioxide, are physically or chemically attracted to water molecules while others are repelled. When molecules are attracted, far more of them can then become dissolved without building up excess pressure with the solution. On the other hand, those that are repelled will develop excessive pressures with little solubility.

AXIOM

Henry's law states that both the partial pressure and solubility coefficient determine the volume of gas that will be dissolved in a given volume of fluid.

The solubility coefficients from the important respiratory gases at body temperature are:

Oxygen	0.024
Carbon dioxide	0.57
Carbon monoxide	0.018
Nitrogen	0.012
Helium	0.008

Thus, carbon dioxide is more than 20 times as soluble as oxygen, and oxygen is more soluble than the other three major gases. These different solubilities are important because they help determine the quantity of the gas that becomes physically dissolved in the fluids of the body. This, in turn, is one of the major factors determining the rate at which the gas can be diffused through tissues.

V. DIFFUSION OF GASES THROUGH FLUIDS

The major factors that affect the rate of gas diffusion in a fluid include (1) the partial pressure of the gas, (2) the solubility of the gas in the fluid, (3) the cross-sectional area of the surface for diffusion, (4) the distance through which the gas must diffuse, (5) the molecular weight of the gas, and (6) the temperature of the fluid.

The greater the solubility of the gas and the greater the surface area for diffusion, the greater will be the number of molecules available to diffuse for any given pressure difference. On the other hand, the greater the distance that the molecules must diffuse, the longer it will take for the diffusion to occur. Finally, the greater the velocity of kinetic movement of the molecules, which at any given temperature is inversely proportional to the square root of the molecular weight, the greater the rate of diffusion of the gas. All of these factors can be expressed in a single formula:

$$D = \frac{(P)(A)(S)}{d \sqrt{MW}},$$

in which D is the diffusion rate, P is the pressure difference between the two ends of the diffusion pathway, A is the cross-sectional area of the pathway, S is the solubility of the gas, d is the distance of diffusion, and MW is the molecular weight of the gas.

Thus, the characteristics of the gas itself determine two factors of the formula, solubility and molecular weight, and these together are called the diffusion coefficient of the gas. Thus, the diffusion coefficient, which equals

$S/\sqrt{MW}$ determines the relative rates at which different gases at the same pressure levels will diffuse.

If the diffusion coefficient for oxygen is designated as 1.0, the relative diffusion coefficients for the gases of respiratory importance are:

Oxygen	1.0
Carbon dioxide	20.3
Carbon monoxide	0.81
Nitrogen	0.53
Helium	0.95

AXIOM

The diffusion coefficient for carbon dioxide is 20 times greater than for oxygen. Thus, diffusion seldom, if ever, interferes with carbon dioxide exchange in the lung.

VI. DIFFUSION OF GASES THROUGH TISSUE

The gases that are of respiratory importance are highly soluble in lipids and, consequently, are also highly soluble in cell membranes. Because of this, these gases diffuse through the cell membranes with very little impediment. The major limitation to the movement of gases in tissues is the rate at which the gases can diffuse through tissue water.

VII. DIFFUSION OF GASES THROUGH THE RESPIRATORY MEMBRANE

A. THE RESPIRATORY UNIT

The respiratory unit is composed of a respiratory bronchiole and its associated alveolar ducts, atria, and alveoli. There are about 300 million alveoli in the two lungs, each alveolus having an average diameter of about 0.2 mm (200 μm). The alveolar walls are extremely thin, and are closely approximated to an almost solid network of interconnecting capillaries. Because of the extensiveness of the capillary plexus, the movement of blood past the alveoli has been described as a "sheet" of flowing blood. The membrane through which gaseous exchange between the alveolar air and pulmonary capillary blood occurs is known as the respiratory membrane.

B. THE RESPIRATORY MEMBRANE

For oxygen to get from the alveolus into the pulmonary capillary bed, it must pass through four separate layers often referred to collectively as the alveolar-capillary or respiratory membrane. These four layers include:

1. A layer of fluid lining the alveolus. This fluid contains surfactant that reduces the surface tension of the alveolar fluid.

2. The alveolar epithelium comprised of very thin epithelial cells and a basement membrane.

3. A very thin interstitial space between the alveolar epithelium and capillary membrane.

4. The capillary endothelial membrane and its basement membrane, which fuses with the epithelial basement membrane in many places.

Despite all these layers, the overall thickness of the respiratory membrane averages about 0.6 μm, and in the thinnest areas, it is only 0.2 μm in thickness.

From histologic studies, it has been estimated that the total surface area of the respiratory membrane in the normal adult is approximately 160 m^2, or about the size of a tennis court. Although the lungs may contain about 700 ml of blood, the total quantity in the pulmonary capillaries at any given instant is only 60 to 140 ml.

The average diameter of the pulmonary capillaries is less than 8 μm, which means that red blood cells must actually squeeze through them. Therefore, the red blood cell membrane is often in intimate contact with the capillary wall. Consequently, oxygen and carbon dioxide may not have to pass through significant amounts of plasma as they diffuse between the alveolus and the red blood cells. This helps increase the rapidity of diffusion of gases between the alveolus and red blood cells.

VIII. FACTORS AFFECTING GAS DIFFUSION THROUGH THE RESPIRATORY MEMBRANE

The factors that determine how rapidly a gas will pass through the respiratory membrane are (1) the thickness of the membrane, (2) the surface area of the membrane, (3) the diffusion coefficient of the gas in the water of the membrane, and (4) the pressure difference between the two sides of the membrane.

The thickness of the respiratory membrane occasionally increases, usually as a result of edema fluid in the interstitial space. Also, some pulmonary diseases cause fibrosis of the lungs, which can further increase the thickness of some portions of the alveolar-capillary membrane. Because the rate of diffusion through the membrane is inversely proportional to its thickness, any factor that increases the thickness of the membrane to more than two to three times normal can interfere significantly with oxygenation of blood. Diffusion is virtually never a problem with carbon dioxide.

AXIOM
Interstitial pulmonary edema may cause hypoxemia, but it does not cause hypercarbia.

In pathologic states characterized by "thickening" of the alveolar-capillary membrane, oxygen diffusion may be severely impeded. Consequently, the red cell Po_2 may not reach equilibrium with the alveolar Po_2 during the time that it is in the pulmonary capillary. As a consequence, the arterial Po_2 falls.

Exhausting exercise at high altitude is one of the few situations in which impairment of oxygen diffusion can be readily demonstrated in apparently normal subjects. Similarly, patients with "thickening" of the alveolar-capillary membrane are most likely to show evidence of diffusion impairment when exercising, especially when exposed to low ambient oxygen concentrations, as at high altitudes.

The surface area of the respiratory membrane may be greatly decreased by many different conditions, such as atelectasis or resection of lung tissue. In emphysema, many of the alveoli coalesce with dissolution of alveolar walls. The new alveolar chambers are much larger than the original alveoli, but the total surface area of the respiratory membranes is considerably decreased. When the total surface area of the lung is decreased to approximately one third to one fourth of normal, exchange of gases through the membrane is impeded to a significant degree, even under resting conditions. During competitive sports and other strenuous exercise, modest decreases in the surface area of the alveoli can be a serious deterrent to oxygen uptake.

The pressure difference across the respiratory membrane is the difference between the pressure of the gas in the alveoli and the pressure of the gas in the blood. In room air, the normal alveolar-arterial oxygen difference ($P[A-a]o_2$) is 5 to 15 mm Hg. The normal alveolar-arterial carbon dioxide difference ($P[A-a]co_2$) is zero.

IX. DIFFUSING CAPACITY OF THE RESPIRATORY (ALVEOLAR-CAPILLARY) MEMBRANE

The ability of the respiratory membrane to exchange a gas between the alveoli and the pulmonary blood can be expressed in quantitative terms by its diffusing capacity. This is defined as the volume of a gas that diffuses through the membrane each minute for a pressure difference of 1 mm Hg. In normal young adults, the diffusing capacity for oxygen under resting conditions averages 21 $ml \cdot min^{-1} \cdot mm\ Hg^{-1}$. Investigators studying diffusion capacity found that the mean oxygen pressure difference across the respiratory membrane during normal, quiet breathing is approximately 12 mm Hg. Multiplication of this pressure by the diffusing capacity (21 × 12) gives a total of about 250 ml of oxygen diffusing through the respiratory membrane each minute. This is approximately equal to the rate at which an average adult uses oxygen under resting conditions.

During strenuous exercise or during other conditions that greatly increase pulmonary blood flow and alveolar ventilation, the diffusing capacity for oxygen in young male adults can increase to a maximum of about 65 ml·min^{-1}·mm Hg^{-1}, which is three times the diffusing capacity under resting conditions. This increase is due to (1) opening up of previously dormant pulmonary capillaries, thereby increasing the surface area of the blood into which the oxygen can diffuse, and (2) dilatation of pulmonary capillaries that were already open, thereby further increasing the surface area.

The diffusing capacity for carbon dioxide has not been measured because carbon dioxide diffuses through the respiratory membrane so rapidly that the average difference between the P_{CO_2} in the pulmonary capillary blood and in alveoli is less than 1 mm Hg. However, since the diffusion coefficient of carbon dioxide is 20 times that of oxygen, one would expect the diffusing capacity for carbon dioxide under resting conditions to be about 400 to 450 ml·min^{-1}·mm Hg^{-1}. During exercise the diffusing capacity for carbon dioxide should be about 1200 to 1300 ml·min^{-1}·mm Hg^{-1}.

The oxygen diffusing capacity can be calculated from measurements of (1) alveolar P_{O_2}, (2) P_{O_2} in the pulmonary capillary blood, and (3) the rate of oxygen uptake by the blood. Because of difficulties encountered in measuring oxygen diffusing capacity, physiologists prefer to measure carbon monoxide diffusing capacity, and then to use that to calculate the value for oxygen.

With the carbon monoxide method, a small amount of carbon monoxide is breathed into the alveoli, and the partial pressure of the carbon monoxide in the alveoli is measured from alveolar air samples. By measuring the volume of carbon monoxide absorbed over a period of time and dividing this by the partial pressure of carbon monoxide in end-tidal gas, one can determine carbon monoxide diffusing capacity.

X. FACTORS AFFECTING BLOOD GASES

Air at sea level has an average barometric pressure of 760 mm Hg and contains approximately 20.93% oxygen and 0.04% carbon dioxide, with nitrogen making up most of the remainder. Thus, the partial pressures of O_2 and CO_2 in the air at sea level are 159 and 0.3 mm Hg, respectively (Table 9.1).

A. ALVEOLAR GASES

1. Inspired Gases

Alveolar air does not have the same concentrations of gases as atmospheric air because (1) dry atmospheric air that enters the respiratory passages is humidified before it reaches the alveoli, (2) alveolar air is only partially replaced by atmospheric air with each breath, (3) oxygen is constantly being absorbed from the alveolar air, and (4) carbon dioxide is constantly diffusing from the pulmonary blood into the alveoli.

2. Humidification of Inspired Air

When air enters the upper airway, it is warmed and saturated with water, reducing the total pressure of the inhaled gases by 47 mm Hg to about 713 mm Hg. Thus, the inspired oxygen pressure (P_{IO_2}) in the trachea and bronchi falls to (713)(0.2093) or 149 mm Hg. If the patient is breathing 60% oxygen ($F_{IO_2} = 0.6$), the P_{IO_2} in the trachea or bronchi will be (713)(0.6) or 428 mm Hg:

$$P_{IO_2} = (P_B - P_{H_2O})(F_{IO_2})$$
$$= (760 - 47)(0.6)$$
$$= (713)(0.6)$$
$$= 427.8.$$

3. Rate at Which Alveolar Air Is Renewed by Atmospheric Air

The functional residual capacity (FRC) of the lungs, which is the amount of air remaining in the lungs at the end of normal expiration, in normal young 70-kg adults is about 2500 to 3000 ml. Approximately 350 ml of new air is brought into the alveoli with each new tidal volume, and the same amount of old alveolar air is expired. Therefore, the amount of alveolar air replaced by new atmospheric air with each breath is only about 12% to 16% of the total gas usually present in the lungs. With normal alveolar ventilation, approximately half the old alveolar gas is exchanged in 17 seconds. When a person's rate of alveolar ventilation is only half normal, half the gas is exchanged in 34 seconds. When the rate of ventilation is two times normal, half is exchanged in about 8 seconds.

AXIOM

If the PAO_2 is 480 mm Hg when one stops breathing, it should take approximately 2 minutes (about 136 seconds) for the PAO_2 to fall to about 60 mm Hg.

This relatively slow replacement of alveolar air is of particular importance in preventing sudden changes in gas concentrations in the blood. This makes blood gases much more stable than they would be otherwise and helps to prevent excessive decreases in tissue oxygenation and tissue pH when respiration is temporarily interrupted.

4. Oxygen Concentration and Partial Pressure in the Alveoli

Oxygen is continually being absorbed into the blood of the lungs, and new oxygen is continually entering the alveoli from the atmosphere. The more rapidly oxygen is absorbed, the lower its concentration becomes in the alveoli. On the other hand, the more rapidly new oxygen is brought into the alveoli from the atmosphere, the higher its concentrations becomes. Therefore, oxygen concentration in the alveoli is controlled by the rate of absorption of oxygen into the blood and the rate of entry of new oxygen into the lungs by ventilation.

5. Carbon Dioxide Concentration in the Alveoli

Carbon dioxide is continually being formed in the body, discharged into the alveoli, and removed from the alveoli by the process of ventilation. Therefore, the two factors that determine the partial pressure of carbon dioxide in the alveoli ($PACO_2$) are (1) the rate of excretion of carbon dioxide from the blood into the alveoli and (2) the rate at which carbon dioxide is removed from the alveoli by alveolar ventilation.

The relationship between carbon dioxide production by the body (VCO_2), the arterial PCO_2 ($PACO_2$), and alveolar ventilation (VA) can be expressed by the following equation:

$$PaCO_2 = \frac{VCO_2}{KVA}.$$

If VCO_2 is expressed as milliliters per minute, $K = 0.84$. Thus, if the VCO_2 is 200 ml/min and VA is 4.2 liters/min, then,

$$PaCO_2 = \frac{(0.84)(200)}{4.2} = \frac{168}{4.2} = 40 \text{ mm Hg.}$$

If alveolar ventilation is increased to 8.4 liters/min,

$$PaCO_2 = \frac{(0.84)(200)}{8.4} = \frac{168}{8.4} = 20 \text{ mm Hg.}$$

Since alveolar ventilation (VA) is equal to minute ventilation (VE) multiplied by $(1 - V_d/V_t)$, dead space (V_d/V_t) can be added into the equation. Thus,

$$PaCO_2 = K\frac{VCO_2}{VE(1 - V_d/V_t)}.$$

Thus, if $V_{CO_2} = 200$ ml/min, $V_E = 6$ liters/min, and $V_d/V_t = 0.3$,

$$P_{ACO_2} = \frac{(0.84)\,(200)}{(6)\,(1-0.3)} = \frac{168}{(6)\,(0.7)} = \frac{168}{4.2} = 40 \text{ mm Hg.}$$

It is not unusual for the V_d/V_t in ARDS to rise to 0.65. If the V_{CO_2} is still 200 ml/min, what minute ventilation is needed to maintain a P_{aCO_2} of 40 mm Hg?

$$P_{aCO_2} = \frac{(0.84)\,(200)}{V_E\,(1-0.65)} = 40 = V_E\frac{168}{(0.35)}$$

$$V_E = \frac{168}{(40)\,(0.35)} = \frac{168}{14} = 12 \text{ L/min.}$$

Thus, minute ventilation (V_E) would have to be doubled if the V_{DS}/V_T increased from 0.3 to 0.65.

6. Alveolar Gas Equation

Inspired gas in the trachea has a P_{O_2} of about 149 mm Hg and P_{CO_2} of about 0.3 mm Hg. As the water-saturated warmed air enters the alveoli, oxygen diffuses through the alveolar capillary membranes into the plasma and carbon dioxide diffuses from the blood into the alveoli. The mixed venous blood brought to the pulmonary capillaries normally has a P_{O_2} of about 40 mm Hg and a P_{CO_2} of 46 mm Hg. Under normal circumstances, 0.8 ml of carbon dioxide enters the alveoli from the capillaries for each 1.0 ml of oxygen that leaves the alveoli and enters the pulmonary capillaries. This relationship is expressed as the respiratory quotient (RQ).

AXIOM

The respiratory quotient is the ratio of the volume of carbon dioxide released by the lungs to the volume of oxygen taken up by the lungs.

This may be expressed by the formula:

$$RQ = \frac{V_{CO_2}}{V_{O_2}}$$

The RQ on a normal diet is about 0.8. To estimate alveolar oxygen (P_{AO_2}) from the fraction of inhaled oxygen (F_{IO_2}) and alveolar P_{CO_2} (P_{ACO_2}) (which is assumed to be equal to the arterial P_{CO_2} (P_{aCO_2}), one needs a correction factor (1/RQ) to determine how much oxygen is consumed for each millimeter of mercury of P_{CO_2} that enters the alveoli. If the RQ is 0.8, the correction factor is 1.25, and if the RQ is 1.0, the correction factor is 1.0.

For the usual circumstances where the RQ is 0.8, the alveolar gas equation is:

$$P_{AO_2} = (P_B - P_{H_2O})\,(F_{IO_2}) - (P_{aCO_2})\,(1/RQ).$$

Thus, in room air ($F_{IO_2} = 0.21$) at sea level with a P_{aCO_2} of 40 mm Hg, the P_{AO_2} is expected to be:

$$P_{AO_2} = (760 - 47)\,(0.21) - (40)\,(1/0.8)$$
$$= 150 - 50 = 100.$$

7. Estimating the Alveolar PO₂

When breathing room air, one can estimate the P_{AO_2} by subtracting the P_{aCO_2} from 145. Thus, if the arterial P_{CO_2} is 40 mm Hg, the P_{AO_2} should be about 105 mm Hg.

AXIOM

The alveolar P_{O_2} on supplemental oxygen is approximately equal to the percentage of inhaled oxygen multiplied by six.

Thus, a patient on 40% oxygen would be expected to have a P_{AO_2} of about 240, and a patient on 60% oxygen would be expected to have a P_{AO_2} of about 360 mm Hg. Using the alveolar gas equation with a Pa_{CO_2} of 40 and RQ of 0.8, the P_{AO_2} would actually be 235 and 378 mm Hg, respectively.

8. Expired Air

Expired air is a combination of dead space air and alveolar air, and its overall composition is determined by the proportion of each that is present. The very first portion exhaled is entirely dead space air. Then, progressively more and more alveolar air is exhaled with diminishing amounts of dead space air until nothing but alveolar air remains at the end of expiration. Therefore, if one wishes to collect alveolar air for study, one simply collects "end-tidal" gas.

AXIOM
End-tidal gas is generally a close approximation of alveolar gas.

B. Pa_{CO_2}

AXIOM
The Pa_{CO_2} can be increased by decreased minute ventilation, increased carbon dioxide production, or increased dead space.

1. Alveolar Ventilation (VA)

Carbon dioxide diffuses so rapidly that the Pa_{CO_2} usually provides an excellent index of the adequacy of overall ventilation of perfused alveoli. If the Pa_{CO_2} is greater than normal, one can usually assume that ventilation of perfused alveoli is reduced or carbon dioxide production is increased. If the Pa_{CO_2} is lower than normal, one can usually assume that alveolar ventilation is increased or carbon dioxide production is decreased. If the patient has increased dead space (due to emphysema, pulmonary emboli, or sepsis), then the patient will need an increased minute ventilation to maintain a normal Pa_{CO_2}.

AXIOM
One cannot usually correlate the Pa_{CO_2} with the adequacy of ventilation unless the patient is acidotic.

An elevated Pa_{CO_2} in the presence of metabolic alkalosis usually reflects a compensatory effort to restore arterial pH to normal. However, an elevated Pa_{CO_2} in a patient with metabolic acidosis generally indicates severe pulmonary insufficiency. As a rule, for each 1.0 mEq/liter that arterial bicarbonate (HCO_3) falls below 24.0 mEq/liter, the P_{CO_2} should eventually fall by about 1.4 mm Hg. Otherwise one can assume that the patient has impaired minute ventilation, increased dead space, or increased carbohydrate metabolism.

Another rule of thumb is that with proper ventilatory compensation for a metabolic acidosis, the Pa_{CO_2} should be equal to or less than the last two digits of the pH. Thus, with a pH of 7.35, the Pa_{CO_2} should be 35 mm Hg or less, and with a pH of 7.30, the Pa_{CO_2} should be 30 mm Hg or less.

Arterial pH is affected by both bicarbonate and Pa_{CO_2}, and the Pa_{CO_2} can change more than 200 times faster than bicarbonate can. Thus, one can often gain some impression of the acuteness of various respiratory changes by noting the effects of the Pa_{CO_2} on the pH. For each 1 mm Hg acute rise or fall in the Pa_{CO_2}, the pH decreases or increases by approximately 0.01. This assumes that the plasma bicarbonate levels remain relatively constant, as they often will for a few hours after an acute Pa_{CO_2} change.

If a patient with a pH of 7.40, Pa_{CO_2} of 40 mm Hg, and plasma bicarbonate of 24 mEq/liter were suddenly to stop ventilating and thereby rapidly increase the Pa_{CO_2} to 50 mm Hg, the plasma bicarbonate would change only minimally and the pH would fall to about 7.30. On the other hand, if the patient's Pa_{CO_2} change were present for more than a few hours, the plasma bicarbonate would have a chance to compensate, and the pH change would be less than expected.

For example, if the Pa_{CO_2} suddenly rose to 60 mm Hg, the pH would be about 7.22. However, if the P_{CO_2} is 60 mm Hg and the pH is 7.35, one can generally assume that the hypercarbia has been present for some time and that the plasma bicarbonate has risen to partially compensate for the respiratory acidosis.

2. Dead Space (V_d/V_t)

When the ventilation of an alveolar-capillary unit is normal but perfusion of the alveolar capillary is absent, the unperfused alveoli are referred to as dead space. The size of the dead space can be determined in the clinical pulmonary function laboratory by measuring the P_{CO_2} in arterial blood (Pa_{CO_2}) and the average expired gas ($P_E_{CO_2}$) and using the following (Bohr) equation:

$$\frac{V_d}{V_t} = \frac{Pa_{CO_2} - P_E_{CO_2}}{Pa_{CO_2}}.$$

The normal for $P_E_{CO_2}$ is 28 mm Hg when the Pa_{CO_2} is 40 mm Hg. Thus,

$$\frac{V_d}{V_t} = \frac{40 - 28}{40} = \frac{12}{40} = 0.3.$$

Under normal circumstances, with the $V_{DS}/V_T = 0.3$, the alveolar P_{CO_2} (PA_{CO_2}) and the arterial P_{CO_2} (Pa_{CO_2}) are equal so that the $P(A-a)_{CO_2} = 0$. If dead space increases, the Pa_{CO_2} will be higher than the end-tidal (alveolar) P_{CO_2}. By calculating the Bohr equation for V_{DS}/V_T with the Pa_{CO_2} and then the PA_{CO_2}, one can determine how much pathologic dead space (due to unperfused alveoli) is present. Thus, if the tidal volume is 600 ml, the Pa_{CO_2} is 40 mm Hg, the PA_{CO_2} is 30 mm Hg, and the average expired P_{CO_2} ($P_E_{CO_2}$) is 20 mm Hg:

$$\frac{V_d}{V_t}(total) = \frac{Pa_{CO_2} - P_E_{CO_2}}{Pa_{CO_2}} = \frac{40 - 20}{40} = 0.5$$

$$\frac{V_d}{V_t}(anatomic) = \frac{PA_{CO_2} - P_E_{CO_2}}{PA_{CO_2}} = \frac{30 - 20}{30} = 0.33.$$

The actual total dead space = (0.5)(600) = 300 ml and the "anatomic" dead space = (0.33)(600) = 200 ml. The difference between the total and anatomic dead space is the pathologic dead space: 300 − 200 = 100 mL.

3. Carbohydrate Metabolism

If the patient has to metabolize more than 450 g of carbohydrate per day, a greatly increased alveolar ventilation may be required to excrete the increased carbon dioxide produced by the carbohydrate metabolism.

The amount of extra ventilation required can be estimated by the following assumptions and calculations. The patient was probably metabolizing about 150 g of carbohydrate plus some protein and fat to have a previous carbon dioxide excretion (V_{CO_2}) of 200 ml/min. The extra 300 g of carbohydrate represent approximately 300/180 or 1.67 mol or 1667 mmol of glucose. The metabolism of each mmol of glucose will result in the production of 6 mmol of carbon dioxide by the following equation:

$$C_6H_{12}O_6 + 6O_2 \longrightarrow 6CO_2 + 6H_2O.$$

Therefore, 1667 × 6 or 10,000 mmol of carbon dioxide will be produced. Each mmol of carbon dioxide is equivalent to 22.4 ml so that 224,000 ml of carbon dioxide will be produced in 1 day or 156 ml of carbon dioxide each minute. This added to the baseline carbon dioxide production of 200 ml/min makes a total of 356 ml of carbon dioxide that would have to be excreted each minute. This may be a problem in some patients with chronic obstructive pulmonary disease (COPD) who have an increased dead space and limited minute ventilation.

For example, if the V_{CO_2} is 356 ml, the V_d/V_t is 0.5 and we would like the Pa_{CO_2} to stay at 40 mm Hg, the minute ventilation will have to be:

$$P_{CO_2} = \frac{(0.84)\,(V_{CO_2})}{V_E\,(1 - V_d/V_t)}$$

$$40 = \frac{(0.84)\,(356)}{V_E\,(0.5)}$$

$$20\,V_E = 299$$

$$V_E = 15 \text{ L/min.}$$

Since normal minute ventilation is considered to be about 6 liters/min, this is 2½ times normal. In a critically ill patient with COPD, this may be too great a ventilatory requirement without ventilator assistance.

AXIOM
Increased carbohydrate metabolism may be too great a ventilatory burden in a patients with COPD.

Obviously, when the physiologic dead space is very great, much of the work of ventilation is wasted effort because a large fraction of the ventilated air never reaches the blood.

4. Transport of Carbon Dioxide in the Blood

Transport of carbon dioxide by the blood is not nearly as great a problem as transport of oxygen because, even in the most abnormal conditions, carbon dioxide can usually be transported in far greater quantities than can oxygen. However, the amount of carbon dioxide in the blood does affect acid-base balance. Under normal resting conditions, each 100 ml of the blood carries an average of 4 ml of carbon dioxide from the tissues to the lungs to be released in the alveoli.

a. Chemical Forms in Which Carbon Dioxide Is Transported

Carbon dioxide diffuses out of the tissue cells in the form of carbon dioxide without bicarbonate because the cell membrane is almost totally impermeable to bicarbonate ions. As the carbon dioxide enters the capillary, it initiates a number of almost instantaneous physical and chemical reactions that are essential for carbon dioxide transport.

(1) Transport of Carbon Dioxide In the Dissolved State

A small portion of the carbon dioxide is transported to the lungs dissolved in plasma. The amount of carbon dioxide dissolved in plasma at 46 mm Hg is about 2.76 ml/dl (2.8 vol%). The amount dissolved at 40 mm Hg is about 2.40 ml. Therefore, only about 0.36 ml of new carbon dioxide is transported to the lungs in the form of dissolved carbon dioxide by each 100 ml of blood. This is only about 9% of all the carbon dioxide transported to the lungs and released there.

(2) Transport of Carbon Dioxide as Bicarbonate

Much of the dissolved carbon dioxide in the blood reacts with water to form carbonic acid. However, this reaction would occur much too slowly to be of importance were it not for the fact that the enzyme called carbonic anhydrase inside the red blood cells speeds up the reaction about 500-fold. The reaction occurs so rapidly in red blood cells that it reaches almost complete equilibrium within a fraction of a second. This allows tremendous amounts of carbon dioxide to react with red blood cell water even before the blood leaves the tissue capillaries.

In another fraction of a second, the carbonic acid formed in the red cells dissociates into hydrogen and bicarbonate ions. Most of the hydrogen ions then combine with the hemoglobin in the red blood cells because hemoglobin is a powerful buffer. At the same time, some of the bicarbonate ions diffuse into the plasma. To offset this ionic shift, chloride ions diffuse into the red blood cells.

This rapid shift is made possible by the presence of a special bicarbonate-chloride carrier protein in the red cell membrane. The phenomenon causing the chloride content of red blood cells in veins to be greater than that of red blood cells in arteries is called "the chloride shift."

The reversible combination of carbon dioxide with water in the red blood cells under the influence of carbonic anhydrase accounts for at least 70% of all the carbon dioxide transported from the tissues to the lungs.

AXIOM

When a carbonic anhydrase inhibitor (acetazolamide) is administered, carbon dioxide transport from the tissues becomes significantly impaired and the tissue PCO_2 can rise abruptly.

(3) Carbaminohemoglobin and Carbaminoproteins

In addition to reacting with water, carbon dioxide also reacts directly with hemoglobin to form the compound carbaminohemoglobin ($HbCO_2$). This combination of carbon dioxide with hemoglobin in readily reversible, and the carbon dioxide attached to hemoglobin in easily released into the alveoli. A small amount of carbon dioxide (usually equivalent to about 0.5 to 1.0 mEq/liter of bicarbonate) also combines with plasma proteins while en route to the lungs.

The theoretical quantity of carbon dioxide that can be carried from the tissues to the lungs in combination with hemoglobin and plasma proteins is approximately 30% of the total quantity transported, or about 1.5 ml of carbon dioxide in each 100 ml. However, this reaction is much slower than the reaction of carbon dioxide with water inside the red blood cells. Therefore, it is doubtful that the combinations of carbon dioxide with hemoglobin and proteins accounts for more than 15% to 25% of the total quantity of carbon dioxide transported from the tissues to the lungs.

b. The Carbon Dioxide Dissociation Curve

Carbon dioxide can exist in the blood as free carbon dioxide and in chemical combinations with water, hemoglobin, and plasma proteins. The total quantity of carbon dioxide combined with the blood in all these forms depends on the PCO_2.

The normal blood PCO_2 averages about 40 mm Hg in arterial blood and 46 mm Hg in mixed venous blood. Although the normal total concentration of carbon dioxide in the blood is about 5.0 vol% (5 ml/dl), only 0.4 vol% of this is actually exchanged as blood passes through the tissues or the lungs. That is, the concentration rises to about 5.2 vol% after the blood passes through the tissues, and falls to about 4.8 vol% after the blood passes through the lungs.

AXIOM

Although 25% or more of the oxygen carried by arterial blood is released to the tissues, only about 8% of the carbon dioxide carried by venous blood is released to the lungs.

5. Effect of the Oxygen-Hemoglobin Reaction on Carbon Dioxide Transport—the Haldane Effect

An increase in carbon dioxide in the blood will cause oxygen to be displaced from the hemoglobin. This is an important factor in promoting oxygen delivery to tissues at the capillary level. The reverse is also true; binding of oxygen with hemoglobin in the pulmonary capillaries tends to displace carbon dioxide from the blood. This effect, called "the Haldane effect," is quantitatively far more important in promoting carbon dioxide release in the lung than is the Bohr effect in promoting oxygen release in the tissues.

AXIOM

The addition of oxygen to hemoglobin in the lungs increases the release of carbon dioxide there (Haldane effect).

AXIOM

The addition of carbon dioxide to hemoglobin in the tissues increases the release of oxygen there (Bohr effect).

The Haldane effect occurs because the combination of oxygen with hemoglobin causes hemoglobin to become a stronger acid. This displaces carbon dioxide from the blood in two ways: (1) the highly acidic oxyhemoglobin has less tendency to combine with carbon dioxide to form carbaminohemoglobin, thus releasing much of the carbon dioxide that is present in the RBCs into the blood, and (2) the increased acidity of oxyhemoglobin causes it to release hydrogen ions, and these in turn bind with bicarbonate ions to form carbonic acid. The carbonic acid then dissociates into water and carbon dioxide, and the carbon dioxide is released from the blood into the alveoli. Thus, in the presence of oxygen, much less carbon dioxide can bind with the hemoglobin. In tissue capillaries, the Haldane effect allows increased pickup of carbon dioxide as oxygen is removed from the hemoglobin. In the lungs, carbon dioxide is released as oxygen is picked up by the hemoglobin.

a. Change in Blood Acidity during Carbon Dioxide Transport

The carbonic acid formed when carbon dioxide enters the blood in the tissues decreases the blood pH. However, the buffers present in the blood prevent the hydrogen ion concentration from rising greatly. Ordinarily, arterial blood has a pH of approximately 7.40, P_{CO_2} of 40 mm Hg, and bicarbonate of 24 mEq/liter, and as the blood acquires carbon dioxide in the tissue capillaries, the pH falls to approximately 7.35, P_{CO_2} rises to 46 mm Hg, and the HCO_3 rises to 25.1 mEq/liter. The reverse occurs when carbon dioxide is released from the blood in the lungs. In exercise or other conditions of high metabolic activity, or when blood flow through the tissues is very sluggish, the decrease in pH in the blood as it leaves the tissues can be 0.30 or more.

AXIOM

The arterial-central venous pH difference rises as cardiac output falls.

6. The Respiratory Exchange Ratio

Normally the tissues extract about 5 ml of oxygen from every 100 ml of blood brought to them, and release 4 ml of carbon dioxide back. The ratio of carbon dioxide output to oxygen uptake is called the respiratory exchange ratio or respiratory quotient (RQ). That is,

$$RQ = \frac{\text{Rate of carbon dioxide output}}{\text{Rate of oxygen uptake}} = \frac{V_{CO_2}}{V_{O_2}}.$$

In normal based conditions in an adult, the V_{CO_2} is 200 ml/min and the V_{O_2} is 250 ml/min. Therefore the RQ is 0.8; however, the value for RQ changes under different metabolic conditions.

When a person is utilizing only carbohydrates for body metabolism, the RQ rises to 1.00. On the other hand, when the person is utilizing only fats for metabolic energy, the level falls to as low as 0.7. The reason for this difference is that when oxygen is metabolized with carbohydrates, one molecule of carbon dioxide is formed for each molecule of oxygen consumed. However, when oxygen reacts with fat, a large share of the oxygen combines with hydrogen atoms from the fats to form water instead of carbon dioxide.

For a person on a normal diet consuming average amounts of carbohydrates, fats, and proteins, the value for RQ is considered to be about 0.83. If too much carbohydrate is being given and some is being converted to fat, the RQ is greater than 1.0. If ketones are being made in the liver but excreted in the urine before they can be metabolized, the RQ is less than 0.7.

C. MONITORING OXYGENATION AND VENTILATION

1. Clinical

a. CNS Function

The patient who is awake, alert, comfortable, and cooperative and has normal vital signs is generally oxygenating and ventilating adequately. However, if the patient is tachypneic and/or tachycardiac and appears to be anxious and/or confused, one should suspect a problem with the patient's ventilation or oxygenation and correct it as soon as possible. In comatose patients, it can sometimes be very difficult to judge how well the patient is oxygenating or ventilating without serial blood gas determinations.

AXIOM
Restlessness in a patient is due to hypoxemia until proven otherwise.

b. Cyanosis

Cyanosis, or a bluish discoloration of the skin and mucous membranes, requires at least 5.0 g of reduced (unoxygenated) hemoglobin or 3.5 g/dl of either sulfhemoglobin or methemoglobin, to be apparent under normal conditions. However, because the recognition of cyanosis depends on variables such as lighting conditions and skin pigmentation, it cannot be considered a reliable indicator of mild desaturation.

Cyanosis as a sign of inadequate oxygenation is almost worthless if the hemoglobin is less than 10 g/dl. Under such circumstances, the Sao_2 must usually be less than 65% (Pao_2 of 30 to 35 mm Hg) before the patient looks cyanotic.

AXIOM
Under most circumstances, patients will not look cyanotic unless they have at least 5 g of reduced (unoxygenated) hemoglobin at the capillary level.

It is generally true that the oxyhemoglobin saturation in venous blood seldom falls below 40% except in the coronary sinus and internal jugular bulb. Thus, in a patient with a Hb of 15.0 g/dl, good lungs and a normal cardiac output, the arterial Hbo_2 saturation would be about 100%, and the mixed venous oxygen saturation ($S\bar{v}o_2$) would be about 75%. The capillary Hbo_2 saturation would be halfway between or 87.5%. Thus, only 1.875 g of hemoglobin would be reduced or unsaturated at the capillary level.

If the cardiac output fell to 2.5 liters/min and everything else stayed constant, including the oxygen consumption (Vo_2) of 250 ml/min, the $S\bar{v}o_2$ would be about 50% and the capillary Hbo_2 saturation would be about 75%. Thus, 3.75 g of hemoglobin would be reduced or unsaturated at the capillary level and the patient would not look cyanotic. However, if the cardiac output is 3.0 liters/min, Hb = 15.0 g/dl, and Sao_2 is 80% (Pao_2 = 49 mm Hg), the $S\bar{v}o_2$ would be 40% and the capillary oxygen saturation would be 60%. As a consequence, 40% of the hemoglobin in the capillaries or 6.0 g of hemoglobin will be desaturated and the patient will appear to be cyanotic.

If a patient with a hemoglobin of only 10.0 g/dl had the same problems (i.e., an Sao_2 of 80% and $S\bar{v}o_2$ of 40%), the capillary Hbo_2 would be 60% and the amount of reduced hemoglobin would be 4.0 g/dl, which is less than the 5.0 g/dl of reduced hemoglobin needed to look cyanotic. Indeed, in a patient with hemoglobin of 10.0 g/dl, the arterial Hbo_2 saturation would have to fall below 60% (with a Pao_2 of about 30 to 32 mm Hg) before cyanosis would be evident.

AXIOM
Cyanosis as a sign of hypoxemia is helpful if the hemoglobin is ≥15 g/dl and almost worthless if the hemoglobin is <10 g/dl.

XI. BLOOD GASES

Our electrochemical methods for analyzing blood oxygen, carbon dioxide, and hydrogen ion concentrations can be traced to establishment of the work's first physical chemistry laboratory in 1887. However, the beginning of our ability to measure clinical use of blood gases can be specifically dated to April 18, 1956, when Leland Clark disclosed his polyethylene-covered oxygen electrode.

A. ARTERIAL PO_2

The arterial PO_2 (PaO_2) in normal, healthy young adults under ideal conditions is considered to be about 95 to 100 mm Hg. The PaO_2 is extremely important because it not only reflects the functional capabilities of the lungs, but also determines the rate at which oxygen can enter the tissues cells.

AXIOM
Although the PO_2 is usually only a small fraction of the oxygen content of arterial blood, it determines the rate and distance oxygen can diffuse into tissues from the capillary.

Multiple factors affect the level of the PaO_2. These include the amount of alveolar ventilation, the concentration of oxygen in the inhaled gases (FIO_2), the functional capabilities of the lungs, and the oxyhemoglobin dissociation curve.

B. ALVEOLAR VENTILATION

If the patient hyperventilates, the alveolar PCO_2 tends to fall and the alveolar PO_2 tends to rise. If the $PACO_2$ falls by 1 mm Hg, the PAO_2 rises by about 1.0 to 1.2 mm Hg. Thus, the lungs can make up for a certain degree of pulmonary dysfunction by hyperventilating. For example, if the patient hyperventilates on room air and decreases his $PACO_2$ to 20 mm Hg, his PAO_2 is raised by about 15 to 20 mm Hg to 115 to 125 mm Hg.

C. FRACTION OF INSPIRED OXYGEN

Unfortunately, the concentration, or fraction, of oxygen in the inspired gases (FIO_2) is often not considered adequate for evaluating the PaO_2. If a patient is receiving oxygen through a nasal cannula, the actual delivered FIO_2 is usually only 25% to 30%. If a properly fitting face mask is applied, the inhaled FIO_2 is still usually 10% to 15% less than that delivered to the mask. The approximate PaO_2 values that might be expected in normal persons who are inhaling various concentration of oxygen are listed in Table 9.2.

The expected alveolar or arterial PO_2 when the patient is being given oxygen can also be estimated by multiplying the actual delivered percentage of oxygen by six. Thus, a patient getting 60% oxygen would be expected to have a PaO_2 of about 60×6, or 360 mm Hg.

D. ALTITUDE

The PaO_2 that can be expected when a patient is breathing room air varies greatly with the height above sea level. The greater the altitude, the lower the PO_2 in the air and the greater the tendency for the patient to hyperventilate (Table 9.3). Atmospheric pressure and its PO_2 drops about 3.12%, or 7.5 mm Hg for each

---

Table 9.2

EXPECTED PaO_2 IN PATIENTS INHALING VARIOUS CONCENTRATIONS OF OXYGEN	FIO_2	0.21 (room air)	0.4	0.6	0.8	1.0
	Expected PaO_2*	100	227	370	512	655

*Assuming a $P(A-a)O_2$ of 10 mm Hg and PCO_2 of 40 mm Hg.

Table 9.3

CHANGES IN PO_2 AT VARIOUS ALTITUDES

Altitude (Feet above Sea Level)	Atmospheric Pressure (mm Hg)	PO_2 in Air (mm Hg)	PO_2 in Alveoli (mm Hg)	PO_2 in Arterial Blood* (mm Hg)
0	760	159	105	100
2,000	707	148	97	92
4,000	656	137	90	85
6,000	609	127	84	79
8,000	564	118	79	74
10,000	523	109	74	69
20,000	349	73	47	42
30,000	226	47	21	19

*Assuming ideal circumstances with a $P(A-a)O_2$ of 5 mm Hg or less.

1000-ft rise above sea level. On the top of Mt. Everest (29,028 ft), the atmospheric pressure is only 238 mm Hg and the PO_2 in the air is only about 50 mm Hg. In healthy young adults, this results in a PaO_2 of about 28 to 30 mm Hg. Because of the respiratory alkalosis, the SaO_2 at this PaO_2 is about 70%.

AXIOM

If patients are breathing room air, their PaO_2 will drop about 3 mm Hg for each 1000-ft rise above sea level.

Up to an altitude of approximately 10,000 ft, the arterial oxygen saturation (SaO_2) remains above 90%. However, above 10,000 ft, the SaO_2 progressively falls about 1% for each 1 mm Hg drop on PO_2, until at a 20,000-ft altitude, the PaO_2 is about 35 mm Hg and SaO_2 is only about 65%.

When a person breathes air at 30,000 ft, where the barometric pressure is about 226 mm Hg, PaO_2 will be only about 21 mm Hg. However, if the person breathes pure oxygen instead of air, most of the space in the alveoli formerly occupied by nitrogen now becomes occupied by oxygen. Even if the person is breathing 100% oxygen at 30,000 ft, the PaO_2 is only about 139 mm Hg.

E. AGE

Even in healthy individuals with no apparent problems, pulmonary changes occur with advancing age that cause a gradual fall in the PaO_2. On the average, the PaO_2 falls about 3 to 4 mm Hg per decade after the patient reaches 20 years of age. Thus, an otherwise normal 20-year-old patient with a PaO_2 of about 95 (on room air at sea level) might be expected to have a PaO_2 of about 74 mm Hg or less when he becomes 80 years of age.

F. ALVEOLAR-ARTERIAL OXYGEN DIFFERENCES

Another method for determining the degree to which lung function is impaired is to determine the alveolar-arterial oxygen gradient ($P[A-a]O_2$). Arterial blood samples can be obtained relatively easily. If there is a technique for trapping the end-expiratory gases (which generally represent average alveolar gases), the PAO_2 can be measured and $P(A-a)O_2$ calculated easily.

If alveolar gases cannot be measured, one can still estimate the PAO_2 by the alveolar gas equation. One can also estimate alveolar oxygen in patients with a normal cardiac output breathing room air by subtracting the $PaCO_2$ from 145. This is possible because the PAO_2 and $PACO_2$ add up to about 145 when a patient breathes room air at sea level. Since the $PACO_2$ is usually the same as the $PaCO_2$, the PAO_2 can be estimated from the arterial gas pressure by the following formula (assuming an RQ of 1.0).

$$PAO_2 = 145 - PaCO_2.$$

If the patient has a $Paco_2$ of 40 mm Hg,

$$Pao_2 = 145 - 40$$
$$= 105 \text{ mm Hg.}$$

If the Pao_2 were 90 mm Hg, the $P(A-a)o_2$ would be 15 mm Hg, which is relatively normal. A $P(A-a)o_2$ of 20 to 30 mm Hg on room air usually indicates mild pulmonary dysfunction, and a $P(A-a)o_2$ greater than 55 mm Hg on room air usually indicates severe pulmonary dysfunction.

AXIOM

On room air, a $P(A-a)o_2$ <20 mm Hg is normal, and a $P(A-a)o_2$ of 35 to 55 mm Hg indicates moderate pulmonary dysfunction.

G. OXYHEMOGLOBIN SATURATION

1. Normal Relationships

It can be seen from oxyhemoglobin dissociation curves that even when the Pao_2 is decreased to 59 mm Hg, the arterial hemoglobin is still about 90% saturated with oxygen. Furthermore, if the hemoglobin level is 15.0 g/dl and the tissue removes 5.0 ml of oxygen from each 100 ml of blood, the Po_2 of the venous blood falls to about 36 mm Hg, which is only 4 mm Hg below the normal value. Thus, if the Pao_2 is high to start with, the mixed venous Po_2 often changes minimally despite a substantial fall in Pao_2.

On the other hand, if the Pao_2 rises far above the upper limit of normal (90 to 100 mm Hg), the maximum oxygen saturation of hemoglobin cannot rise above 100%. Therefore, even if the Pao_2 should rise to 600 mm Hg or more, the saturation of hemoglobin would increase only 1% to 2% because at a Pao_2 of 100 mm Hg, the arterial oxygen saturation is about 98.4%.

Under circumstances of normal body temperature (37°C [98.6°F] and pH 7.40), certain standard relations exist between oxyhemoglobin saturation and the plasma Po_2 (Table 9.4).

Thus, the relation between arterial oxygen saturation (Sao_2) and plasma Po_2 is almost linear when the Sao_2 is 60% to 90%. However, as the Sao_2 rises above 90%, the Po_2 begins to rise much faster than the saturation, and below a saturation of 60%, saturation falls much more rapidly than the Po_2.

2. Factors Affecting Oxyhemoglobin Dissociation

AXIOM

The oxyhemoglobin dissociation curve is set up so that a "shift to the right" is associated with a higher Po_2 at a certain saturation and a "shift to the left" causes a lower Po_2 at that same saturation (Fig. 9.1).

The best known of the factors affecting the oxyhemoglobin dissociation curve are pH, temperature, and the amount of 2,3-diphosphoglycerate (2,3-DPG) in the red blood cells.

Table 9.4

RELATIONSHIP BETWEEN OXYHEMOGLOBIN SATURATION AND PLASMA Po_2	Oxygen Saturation, %	Po_2 (mm Hg)
	100.0	677
	98.4	100
	95	80
	90	59
	73	40
	50	26.2
	33	20
	30	18

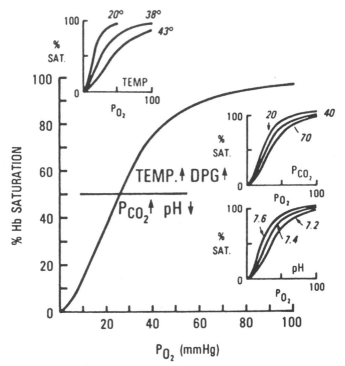

Figure 9.1 Shift of the oxygen dissociation curve by pH P_{CO_2}, temperature, and 2, 3-diphospho-glycerate (DPG). Note that shifts to the left tend to lower the P_{O_2} at a given oxyhemoglobin saturation. In contrast, a shift to the right tends to raise the P_{O_2}. (From West, JB: Respiratory Physiology, ed 3. Williams & Wilkins, Baltimore, 1985, with permission.)

a. pH

The more acidic the blood, the more readily hemoglobin gives up its oxygen and the higher the Pa_{O_2} will be for a particular oxyhemoglobin saturation. In contrast, alkalosis makes hemoglobin hold onto its oxygen more tightly, thereby lowering the Pa_{O_2} that would be present at a particular oxyhemoglobin saturation. In general, a rise or fall in pH of 0.10 causes a fall or rise (i.e., an opposite change) in the Pa_{O_2} of about 10% (Table 9.5).

AXIOM

Heat, acidosis, and increased 2,3-DPG shift the oxyhemoglobin dissociation curve to the right (i.e., raise the P_{O_2}).

AXIOM

Cold, alkalosis, and decreased 2,3-DPG shift the oxyhemoglobin dissociation curve to the left, lowering the P_{O_2} and reducing oxygen availability to tissue.

b. The P_{CO_2}

Shift of the oxyhemoglobin dissociation curve by changes in the blood levels of carbon dioxide and hydrogen ions is important to enhance release of oxygen from the blood in the tissues. This is called the Bohr effect.

As the blood passes through the lungs, carbon dioxide diffuses from the blood into the alveoli. This reduces the P_{CO_2} of the blood. This also decreases the hydrogen ion concentration and raises pH because of the resulting decreased amount of carbonic acid in the blood. Both of these changes shift the oxyhemoglobin dissociation curve to the left. With a shift to the left, the quantity of oxygen binding to hemoglobin at any given Pa_{O_2} is increased, thus allowing greater oxygen transport to the tissues. Then, when the blood reaches the tissue capillaries, exactly the opposite effect occurs. Carbon dioxide entering the blood from the tissues shifts the oxyhemoglobin dissociation curve to the right. The

Table 9.5

CHANGES IN PO₂ PRODUCED BY CHANGES IN pH	pH	7.60	7.50	7.40	7.30	7.20	7.10	7.00
	PaO₂ (mm Hg)*	80	90	100	111	122	134	148

*Assuming a temperature of 37°C and a hemoglobin saturation of 98.4%.

oxygen is displaced from the hemoglobin and delivered to the tissues at a higher P_{O_2} than would otherwise occur (Fig. 9.2).

c. Temperature

AXIOM

An increased temperature of 10°C raises the P_{O_2} about 5%.

As the temperature of blood increases, hemoglobin gives up oxygen more readily, raising the P_{O_2} in the plasma. The opposite occurs during cooling. For each 1°C rise in temperature, the P_{aO_2} rises about 5% (Table 9.6). With hypothermia, the P_{aCO_2} falls by about the same amount.

d. Exercise

During strenuous exercise, several factors can shift the oxyhemoglobin dissociation curve to the right so as to raise the P_{O_2}. Exercising muscles release large quantities of carbon dioxide and lactic acid. This increases the hydrogen ion concentration in muscle capillary blood. In addition, the temperature of the muscle often rises as much as 3° to 4°C, and phosphate compounds are also released. All these factors acting together shift the oxyhemoglobin dissociation curve of the blood in the muscle capillaries considerably to the right. Therefore, oxygen can sometime be released to the muscle at a P_{O_2} as high as 40 mm Hg

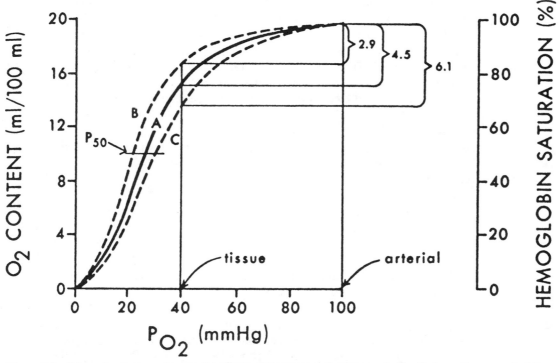

Figure 9.2 Schematic diagram showing the effects of increases and decreases in O₂ affinity on the amount of O₂ available at the PO₂ values prevailing in arterial blood and at the tissues. P₅₀ = PO₂ at which hemoglobin saturation is 50%. Hemoglobin concentration is assumed for convenience to be 14.9 g/100 ml; therefore, O₂ content at 100% saturation is 20 ml/100 ml. Curve A = normal blood; curve B = blood with increased affinity (decreased P₅₀); curve C = blood with decreased affinity (increased P₅₀). (From Murray, JR: The Normal Lung. WB Saunders, Philadelphia, 1986, p. 175, with permission.)

Table 9.6

PO$_2$ LEVELS AT VARIOUS TEMPERATURES*	Temperature °F	104.0	102.2	100.4	98.6	95.0	86.6
	Temperature °C	40	39	38	37	35	32
	PaO$_2$ (mm Hg)*	117	111	105	100	90	76

*Assuming a pH of 7.40 and a hemoglobin saturation of 98.4%.

even though as much as 75% of the oxygen has been removed from the hemoglobin. In the lungs the shift occurs in the opposite direction, thus allowing the hemoglobin in the red blood cells to pick up increased oxygen from the alveoli.

e. 2,3-DPG

Except for hemoglobin the compound present in greatest quantity in red blood cells is 2,3-DPG. A normal concentration of 2,3-DPG in the red blood cell keeps the oxyhemoglobin dissociation curve shifted slightly to the right. In addition, in hypoxic conditions that last longer than a few hours, the quantity of 2,3-DPG can increase considerably, thereby shifting the oxyhemoglobin dissociation curve even farther to the right. This can cause the PO$_2$ in the plasma to be as much as 10 mm Hg higher than it would have been otherwise.

AXIOM
Increased 2,3-DPG, as may occur with hypoxia or ischemia, tends to shift the oxyhemoglobin dissociation curve to the right and raise the PO$_2$.

For several years it was taught that the increase in red cell 2,3-DPG with hypoxia was an important adaptive mechanism for homeostasis. However, the presence of increased 2,3-DPG makes it more difficult for the hemoglobin to combine with oxygen in the lungs. Consequently, it is questionable whether the increased 2,3-DPG in hypoxia is as beneficial as had been believed.

If the concentration of 2,3-DPG falls, as it does in stored blood or during sepsis, the hemoglobin holds onto its oxygen more tightly and the PaO$_2$ tends to fall. In old bank blood, the 2,3-DPG may be very low, and it may take 6 to 24 hours after transfusion for the 2,3-DPG in the viable transfused red cells to return to normal. Thus, after massive transfusions, a patient may have a good hemoglobin level (>10 to 12 g/dl) and a good oxygen saturation (95% or more), and yet the PO$_2$ and oxygen delivery to the tissues may be reduced.

AXIOM
Some of the factors that reduce 2,3-DPG and shift the oxyhemoglobin curve to the left include sepsis, blood transfusions, severe malnutrition, severe phosphate deficiency, and carbon monoxide poisoning.

A shift to the left can significantly reduce the arteriovenous oxygen difference possible at certain fixed PO$_2$'s. For example, if the arterial PO$_2$ is 100 mm Hg and the venous PO$_2$ is 40 mm Hg, a shift to the left results in a C(a-v)O$_2$ of 2.9 ml/dl, whereas a shift to the right results in a C(a-v)O$_2$ of 6.1 ml/dl. If the cardiac output were 5 liters/min, the two oxygen consumptions would be 145 ml/min and 310 ml/min, respectively.

3. PaO$_2$/FIO$_2$ Ratio

A quick way to estimate the impairment of oxygenation, particularly if the patient is being given extra oxygen, is to calculate the PaO$_2$/FIO$_2$ ratio. That is, if a patient had a PaO$_2$ of 200 mm Hg on 40% oxygen, the PaO$_2$/FIO$_2$ ratio would be 200/0.40, or 500. Normally, the ratio is about 500 to 600, which usually correlates with a pulmonary shunt (Qs/Qt) of about 3% to 5%.

If a patient had a PaO$_2$ of 80 mm Hg on 40% oxygen, the PaO$_2$/FIO$_2$ ratio would be 80/0.4, or 200. A PaO$_2$/FIO$_2$ ratio of less than 200 corresponds with a

Table 9.7

RELATIONSHIP BETWEEN THE
PHYSIOLOGIC SHUNT (Qs/Qt)
AND PaO$_2$ WHILE BREATHING
100% OXYGEN

Arterial PO$_2$ (PaO$_2$)	Qs/Qt, %		
	If CO = 2.5 L/min; C(a-v)O$_2$ = 10	If CO = 5 L/min; C(a-v)O$_2$ = 5	If CO = 10 L/min; C(a-v)O$_2$ = 2.5
600	2	4	8
500	5	10	17
400	8	16	25
300	11	19	32
200	13	24	38
150	14	26	42
100	18	31	47
90	20	34	50
80	22	36	53
70	24	39	56
60	28	44	61
50	33	50	67

*Assuming an oxygen consumption of 250 ml/min and Hb of 10.0 g/dl.

Qs/Qt of about 20% and generally indicates a need for ventilatory support. The usual relationship between PaO$_2$/FIO$_2$ ratio and the Qs/Qt in patients with a normal cardiac output can be tabulated (Table 9.7).

4. Respiratory Index

Another method for evaluating the PaO$_2$ in relation to the FIO$_2$ is to calculate the respiratory index (RI) which is the alveolar-arterial oxygen difference [P(A-a)O$_2$] divided by the PaO$_2$. The alveolar PO$_2$ (PAO$_2$) can be calculated by the alveolar gas equation or estimated as six times the percentage of oxygen in the inhaled gas. The alveolar gas equation to determine PAO$_2$ is:

$$PAO_2 = (PB - PH_2O)(FIO_2) - PaCO_2(1/RQ).$$

One can assume PB = 760 and PH$_2$O = 47 at sea level. Thus, if the FIO$_2$ is 0.40, the PaCO$_2$ is 40, and RQ is 0.8,

$$PAO_2 = (760 - 47)(0.4) - (40)(1.25)$$
$$= (713)(0.4) - 50$$
$$= 285 - 50 = 235 \text{ mm Hg.}$$

Using the estimate that the PAO$_2$ is six times the percentage of oxygen in the inhaled gas, the PAO$_2$ on 40% oxygen is 40 × 6 or 240 mm Hg.

If the patient has a PaO$_2$ of 80 mm Hg on 40% oxygen, the P(A-a)O$_2$ could be estimated as 240 − 80 = 160 mm Hg and the respiratory index (RI) would be 160/80 = 2.0. If the PaO$_2$ is 60 on 40% oxygen, the RI is (240 − 60)/60 = 180/60 = 3.0.

Laghi and associates have determined that a patient with an RI of 1.0 and a cardiac index of 3.0 liters·min^{-1}·m^{-2} has a Qs/Qt of about 15%. That is, if the patient has a PaO$_2$ of 120 mm Hg on 40% oxygen, the RI would be (240 − 120)/120 = 120/120 = 1.0.

If the RI is 2.0 (PaO$_2$ of 80 on 40% oxygen) with a cardiac index of 2.0 liters·min^{-1}·m^{-2}, the Qs/Qt is about 22% to 25%.

5. Physiologic Shunting in the Lung (Venous-Arterial Admixture) (Qs/Qt)

Although problems with gas diffusion or distribution in the lungs can cause abnormal blood gases, the most important cause of hypoxia is usually ventilation-perfusion (V/Q) mismatching. When considering ventilation and perfusion, there can be four types of alveolar-capillary units. If ventilation and perfusion

409

are normal, the unit is normal. If there is ventilation without perfusion, the unit is considered to be dead space. If there is perfusion without ventilation, the unit is considered to be a (right-to-left) shunt. If there is neither ventilation nor perfusion, the unit is silent.

AXIOM

The amount of physiologic shunting in the lung (or venous-arterial admixture) (Qs/Qt) is the most sensitive and accurate guide to the onset and progression of acute respiratory failure.

If there is no ventilation in a portion of the lung that is perfused, a shunt is said to be present. If the ventilation is very low and perfusion is normal, a $\dot{V}/\dot{Q}$ mismatch is said to be present.

AXIOM

The physiologic shunt in the lungs is generally considered to be the most accurate index of the amount of pulmonary dysfunction in patients with acute respiratory failure.

Physiologic shunting in the lungs refers to that fraction of blood passing through the lungs without being oxygenated. Normally, the amount of venous-arterial admixture (shunt) in the lungs is about 3% to 5% of the cardiac output. This small amount of shunting is largely due to desaturated blood from bronchial veins draining into fully saturated pulmonary veins.

Physiologic shunting is somewhat harder to determine than alveolar-arterial oxygen differences because it requires drawing both arterial and mixed venous (pulmonary artery) blood samples and determining their oxygen contents. Mixed venous samples from the pulmonary artery are preferable to those obtained from central venous pressure catheters. However, central venous blood can be used to provide a reasonable estimate of the amount of shunting present if cardiac output is normal.

Although an F_{IO_2} of 1.0 was generally used in the past to determine the amount of physiologic shunting in the lung, the high F_{IO_2} in itself may cause increased shunting. Now the shunt present with an F_{IO_2} of 0.4 is considered to be a better indicator of lung function.

The Qs/Qt can be calculated from a modification of Berggren's formula:

$$Qs/Qt = \frac{Cc_{O_2} - Ca_{O_2}}{Cc_{O_2} - C\bar{v}_{O_2}},$$

where Cc_{O_2} is the pulmonary capillary oxygen content, Ca_{O_2} is the arterial content, and $C\bar{v}_{O_2}$ is the mixed venous oxygen content.

The Cc_{O_2} is calculated from the F_{IO_2} concentration of hemoglobin and the estimated alveolar Pa_{O_2} by the following formula:

$$Cc_{O_2} = [Hb](1.34) + (Pa_{O_2})(0.003).$$

The arterial oxygen content (Ca_{O_2}) and venous oxygen content ($C\bar{v}_{O_2}$) are calculated from the hemoglobin and their respective oxygen saturations and Po_2. If mixed venous blood is not available, the $C\bar{v}_{O_2}$ can be estimated from the Fick equation:

$$Ca_{O_2} = [Hb](1.34)(Sa_{O_2}/100) + (Pa_{O_2})(0.003)$$
$$C\bar{v}_{O_2} = [Hb](1.34)(S\bar{v}_{O_2}/100) + (P\bar{v}_{O_2})(0.003),$$

where [Hb] is the hemoglobin concentration, Sa_{O_2} and $S\bar{v}_{O_2}$ are the arterial and mixed venous oxygen saturation, and Pa_{O_2} and $P\bar{v}_{O_2}$ are the arterial and mixed venous oxygen tensions.

410

If the Cco_2 is 20 ml/dl, the Cao_2 is 19 ml/dl, and the $C\bar{v}o_2$ is 14 ml/dl, the shunt (Qs/Qt) is:

$$\frac{Qs}{Qt} = \frac{20 - 19}{20 - 14} = \frac{1}{6} = 17\%.$$

If it clinically appears that cardiac output and oxygen consumption are normal, the amount of shunting in the lung can also be estimated from arterial blood alone by assuming that the venous oxygen content (Cvo_2) is 5.0 ml/dl less than the arterial oxygen content (Cao_2). If the patient is septic, one should probably assume that the $C(a-v)O_2$ is only 3.0 ml/dl.

In general, if cardiac output doubles, the amount of shunt associated with a particular $P(A-a)o_2$ increases by about 50% (Table 9.7). This is related to the fact that if only a small amount of blood is going through the lung, the blood flow tends to go to well-ventilated alveoli. If cardiac output increases, more of the blood will go through less well-ventilated lung tissue.

Thus, if cardiac output is high, a relatively mild hypoxemia can result in a rather high shunt. For example, at a Po_2 of 300 mm Hg on 100% oxygen, if $\dot{V}o_2$ is 250 ml/min and the cardiac output is 2.5 liters/min, the shunt would be 11%, but at a cardiac output of 10.0 liters/min, the shunt would be 32% (Table 9.7).

AXIOM
A low arterial Po_2 in a patient with a low cardiac output often indicates more pulmonary dysfunction than the same Po_2 in a patient with a high cardiac output.

6. Shunt Index

To factor in the changes due to an increased or decreased cardiac output, we have sometimes utilized the concept of shunt index. The shunt index (SI) is the percentage of shunt divided by the cardiac index. For example, at a normal cardiac index of 3.5 $liters \cdot min^{-1} \cdot m^{-2}$ and a normal shunt of 5.0%, the SI is $5.0/3.5 = 1.4$. If a patient has a shunt of 20%, with a cardiac index of 2.5 $liters \cdot min^{-1} \cdot m^{-2}$, the SI is 8.0. If the cardiac index were 5.0 $liters \cdot min^{-1} \cdot m^{-2}$ at the same shunt, the SI would be 4.0. Patients with an SI above 5.0 usually require ventilatory support.

If the cardiac index is not known, the critical Qs/Qt is about 20% to 25%. Above these values, the patient usually has enough of a $\dot{V}/\dot{Q}$ abnormality to warrant aggressive ventilatory support and positive end-expiratory pressure (PEEP), particularly if the patient is septic or has had recent trauma or surgery.

7. Continuous Estimated Shunt Measurements

Calculation of the intrapulmonary shunt fraction (Qs/Qt) is generally recognized as the most reliable way to quantitate the extent to which pulmonary disease is contributing to arterial hypoxemia. This calculation requires analysis of mixed venous (PA) blood. The unavailability of PA blood samples in many critically ill patients has led to the description of a number of Pao_2 indices including $P(A-a)o_2$, Pao_2/PAo_2, Pao_2/Fio_2, and $P(A-a)o_2/Pao_2$. All of these indices may indirectly reflect Qs/Qt.

An oxygen content-based index, such as the estimated shunt, can be derived by mathematical manipulation of the classic shunt equation, and it allows estimation of the pulmonary shunt when PA blood samples are not available. This estimated shunt calculation is based on the use of an assumed $C(a-v)O_2$ of 3.5 ml/dl. The estimated shunt has been demonstrated by Cane and associates to be superior to the arterial Po_2-based indices for following the intrapulmonary shunt fraction.

Hess, Maxwell, and Shefet have shown that simultaneous monitoring of the cardiac index and $P(A-a)o_2$ not only allows for verification of the adequacy of cardiac output and peripheral perfusion, but also confirms the reliability of the estimated shunt.

8. Oxygen Content

The oxygen content of blood is determined primarily by the hemoglobin level and the oxyhemoglobin saturation. Each gram of hemoglobin measured clinically, when fully saturated, can carry 1.34 ml of oxygen. "Pure" hemoglobin can carry 1.39 ml of oxygen per gram, but clinically measured hemoglobin includes about 4% other compounds not carrying oxygen. Thus, a patient with a hemoglobin concentration of 15.0 g/dl can carry about 20.1 ml of oxygen per 100 ml in the red blood cells when the hemoglobin is fully saturated. Although the Pao_2 determines the rate at which oxygen enters the tissues, it contributes very little to the total oxygen content of blood. Each millimeter of mercury of Pao_2 represents only 0.0031 ml of oxygen in 100 ml of blood. Thus, a patient with a normal PAO_2 of 100 mm Hg has only 0.31 ml of oxygen dissolved in the plasma.

The oxygen content of arterial blood (Cao_2) can be calculated from the following formula:

$$Cao_2 = \frac{[Hb](1.34)(Sao_2)}{100} + (Pao_2)(0.003).$$

Thus, in a patient with a hemoglobin concentration of 15.0 g/dl, an Sao_2 of 98%, and a Pao_2 of 100 mm Hg,

$$Cao_2 = (15)(1.34)(98/100) + (100)(0.003)$$
$$= 20.0 \text{ ml of } O_2 \text{ per dl of blood.}$$

If the hemoglobin concentration falls to 10.0 g/dl, even if Sao_2 and Pao_2 remain the same, Cao_2 falls by about one third. For example:

$$Cao_2 = (10)(1.34)(98/100) + (100)(0.003) = 13.132 + 0.300$$
$$= 13.4 \text{ ml of } O_2 \text{ per dl of blood.}$$

AXIOM

Even with only 10 g/dl of full saturated hemoglobin, the red blood cells are carrying over 40 times as much oxygen as the plasma.

9. Oxygen Delivery (DO_2)

Oxygen content (in milliliters per liter of blood) multiplied by cardiac output (in liters per minute) is equal to oxygen delivery (Do_2), or the amount of oxygen brought to the tissues.

Thus, if the cardiac output (Q) is 5 liters/min and the arterial oxygen content (Cao_2) is 20 ml/dl or 200 ml/liter,

$$Do_2 = Q \cdot Cao_2$$
$$= (5)(200)$$
$$= 1000 \text{ ml/min.}$$

Note that the Cao_2 must be converted from ml/dl to ml/liter. This is done by multiplying the value in ml/dl by 10.

Increasingly, Do_2 is "indexed" or defined by square meters of body surface area (BSA). If the normal BSA is 1.73 m^2, then $Do_2I = (Q)(Cao_2)BSA$. In the patient above, the Do_2I is 1000 divided by 1.73 = 578 $ml \cdot min^{-1} \cdot m^{-2}$.

Whenever possible, one should try to keep the Do_2I in critically ill or injured patients above 500 $ml \cdot min^{-1} \cdot m^{-2}$, or preferably above 600 $ml \cdot min^{-1} \cdot m^{-2}$ particularly if the patient is septic. To a certain extent a good heart, which can increase cardiac output appropriately, can make up for bad lungs and a low hemoglobin level. The reverse is also true. However, a combination of poor oxygenation, low hemoglobin level, and low cardiac output may be rapidly fatal.

10. Oxygen Dissociation at the Tissue Level

The amount of delivered oxygen that can actually be released at the tissue level depends to a large extent upon the oxyhemoglobin saturation at a Po_2 of 20 mm Hg. This is often referred to as the S_{20}. In general, the Po_2 gradient between tissue capillaries and the mitochondria in the tissues is about 20 mm Hg. In other words, the capillary Po_2 usually does not fall below 20 mm Hg. A Po_2 of 20 mm Hg is found routinely only in the coronary sinus, and occasionally it is found in the jugular venous bulb at the base of the brain. If the Po_2 in the jugular venous bulb is less than 20 mm Hg, the patient is usually comatose.

The oxyhemoglobin saturation usually present at a Po_2 of 20 mm Hg is 33%. Thus, under normal circumstances, at least one third of the delivered oxygen is not available to the tissues and is returned to the lungs.

If the oxyhemoglobin curve is shifted to the right, as with fever or acidosis, the Po_2 tends to rise for a particular saturation, or conversely, the saturation for a particular Po_2 tends to fall. Thus, at a temperature of 39°C and pH of 7.00, the S_{20} is about 18%, and consequently much more of the delivered oxygen (up to 82%) is available to the tissues.

In actual practice, the Po_2 of mixed venous blood seldom falls below 23 mm Hg, and this is usually associated with an oxyhemoglobin saturation of 40%. Thus, generally, even in very low flow states, only 60% of the total oxygen delivery to the body is available for use. However, if the patient is febrile and acidotic, oxygen availability will tend to increase. The converse is also true; if the patient is cold and/or alkalotic, less oxygen is available to the tissues.

11. Oxygen Reserve

The ability of blood to give up more oxygen (increasing the arterio-venous oxygen difference) as cardiac output falls is an important homeostatic defense mechanism sometimes referred to as oxygen reserve. For example, if oxygen consumption (Vo_2) is 250 ml/min, arterial oxygen content (Cao_2) is 20 ml/dl or 200 ml/liter, and cardiac output (Q) is 5 liters/min, the venous oxygen content can be calculated by the Fick equation:

$$Q = \frac{Vo_2}{Cao_2 - C\bar{v}o_2}$$
$$5 = \frac{250}{200 - C\bar{v}o_2}$$
$$1000 - 5\, C\bar{v}O_2 = 250$$
$$5\, C\bar{v}o_2 = 750$$
$$C\bar{v}o_2 = 150 \text{ ml/L or } 15.0 \text{ ml/dl.}$$

If the Sao_2 were 100%, the mixed venous oxygen saturation ($S\bar{v}o_2$) would be about 75% (15/20).

If the cardiac output fell to 2.1 liters/min, the patient could still maintain an oxygen consumption of 250 ml/min by reducing the mixed venous oxygen content ($C\bar{v}o_2$) to 80 ml/liters or 8 ml/dl, which would result in an $S\bar{v}o_2$ of about 40%. This is about as low as mixed venous oxygen saturation ever gets even with a very low cardiac output.

12. Combination of Hemoglobin with Carbon Monoxide

Carbon monoxide accounts for more than 50% of the approximately 12,000 deaths from fire each year in the United States. This, plus the carbon monoxide poisonings due to faulty indoor heaters and exhausts from internal combustion engines, accounts for more than half of the deaths due to poisoning in the United States.

Carbon monoxide combines with hemoglobin at the same point on the hemoglobin molecule that oxygen does. Furthermore, it binds 230 times more strongly to hemoglobin than oxygen does. Therefore, an alveolar carbon monoxide level of only 0.4 mm Hg, which is only 1/230 that of the Pao_2, allows the carbon monoxide to compete equally with oxygen for combination with hemoglobin. This would cause one half the hemoglobin in the blood to bind with carbon monoxide instead of with oxygen. Under these circumstances, the Pao_2

413

could still be 90 to 100 mm Hg, but the Hbco would be 50% and the HbO_2 saturation would be 50%. If the Pao_2 is all that is measured, one might not even know that the arterial oxyhemoglobin saturation is only 50%. Interestingly, smoking one cigarette can raise carboxyhemoglobin (Hbco) levels to 10% to 12%, which is equivalent to an alveolar CO concentration of about 0.08 to 0.1 mm Hg. An alveolar carbon monoxide level of 0.7 mm Hg (about 0.1% in air) can be lethal.

AXIOM

A relatively normal arterial PO_2 but a very low oxyhemoglobin saturation should make one consider carbon monoxide poisoning.

A patient severely poisoned with carbon monoxide should be treated by administering 100% oxygen. The oxygen at alveolar pressures over 600 mm Hg displaces carbon monoxide from hemoglobin much more rapidly than atmospheric oxygen can. The half-life of Hbco in a patient breathing room air is 2 to 3 hours; if the patient is breathing 100% oxygen, the half-life is about 20 to 30 minutes.

The patient can also benefit by simultaneous administration of 4% to 5% carbon dioxide because this strongly stimulates the respiratory center. This increases alveolar ventilation, reduces the alveolar carbon monoxide concentration, and allows increased carbon monoxide to be released from the blood. With 96% oxygen and 4% carbon dioxide therapy, carbon monoxide can be removed from the blood 10 to 20 times more rapidly than by just breathing room air.

H. OTHER METHODS FOR EVALUATING BLOOD GASES

1. Pulmonary Artery Catheters

A number of pulmonary artery catheters have been developed to continuously monitor mixed venous oxygen saturation ($S\bar{v}o_2$). The normal $S\bar{v}o_2$ is about 70% to 75%. If cardiac output or arterial oxygen content falls or if oxygen consumption increases, the mixed venous oxygen saturation will tend to fall. Thus, changes in the $S\bar{v}o_2$ can provide early warning of problems with the lungs or cardiovascular system.

If the $S\bar{v}o_2$ rises to 80% or higher, the catheter tip may have wedged into a small pulmonary artery so that pulmonary capillary (oxygenated) blood is being analyzed. The other possibilities are a rise in cardiac output (as from sepsis or use of a vasodilator) or a drop in oxygen consumption (as with excess sedation or hypothermia).

A fall in $S\bar{v}o_2$ below 50% to 60% is usually due to a significant decrease in cardiac output or lung function so that oxygen delivery to the tissues is reduced. It could also be due to an increase in oxygen consumption, and all of these changes require urgent investigation. Although a sudden decrease in $S\bar{v}o_2$ often indicates important physiologic changes, the patient's condition can deteriorate seriously sometimes without any change in the $S\bar{v}o_2$.

PITFALL

Assuming that a patient's cardiovascular and pulmonary systems are stable because the $S\bar{v}o_2$ hasn't changed.

A rise in $S\bar{v}o_2$ above 80% may be due to an increased oxygen delivery (Do_2) or a fall in oxygen consumption (Vo_2) or both. It might also be due to the catheter tip wedging and thus elevating pulmonary capillary, rather than pulmonary arterial, blood. Development of a left-to-right shunt or severe hypoxia (Pao_2 >500 to 600 mm Hg) might also make the $S\bar{v}o_2$ rise. Causes of a decreased Vo_2 include paralysis, excess sedation, or hypothermia. In some instances sepsis will also cause a drop in Vo_2 in spite of a normal or increased Do_2.

AXIOM

There are many reasons that $S\bar{v}o_2$ will not fall as it should with impaired pulmonary or cardiac function.

2. Dual Oximetry

Another advance in continuous pulmonary monitoring is the combined use of arterial and PA oximetry (dual oximetry), which allows continuous calculation of the oxygen extraction index (EI) ($O_2EI = Sao_2 - S\bar{v}o_2/Sao_2$). Rasanen and associates demonstrated that a reasonable correlation exists between total body oxygen utilization and the oxygen extraction index (O_2EI) as long as the $S\bar{v}o_2$ remains >89%. Rasanen and associates have also suggested the use of dual oximetry to trend changes in Qs/Qt by calculation of a ventilation to perfusion index [$(\dot{V}/\dot{Q})I = (1 - Sao_2)/1 - S\bar{v}o_2$].

$$(\dot{V}/\dot{Q})I = \frac{1 - Sao_2}{1 - S\bar{v}o_2}.$$

Thus, a normal Sao_2 of 98% and $S\bar{v}o_2$ of 73% would produce

$$(\dot{V}/\dot{Q})I = \frac{1 - 0.98}{1 - 0.73} = \frac{0.02}{0.27} = 7.4\%.$$

3. Systemic Arterial Probes

A further development in the area of blood gas analysis is the intravascular probe. Although intravascular oxygen sensors have been available for some time, their usefulness has been limited by a progressive loss of sensitivity of the electrode as protein deposits accumulate on its membrane.

Recently, intravascular probes using fiberoptic light channels and special fluorescent compounds have been developed to continuously measure pH, Pao_2, and $Paco_2$. Some of the more recently developed probes are so small that they will pass through a 20-gauge catheter and still leave sufficient clearance for pressure measurements and blood sampling. Clinical experience with these fiberoptic "intravascular blood gas machines" is limited; however, these catheters should find wide acceptance as the technology is perfected.

4. Noninvasive Monitoring

a. Pulse Oximetry

The use of pulse oximetry for monitoring oxygen saturation and pulse amplitude in the fingers, nose, or toes can provide early warning of pulmonary or cardiovascular deterioration before it is clinically apparent. This technique employs a photosensor connected with a microprocessor that continuously determines pulse rate and oxyhemoglobin saturation. The photosensor is not heated and does not require calibration.

Oxyhemoglobin (Hbo_2) is red and reduced hemoglobin (Hb) is blue, each of which has a different absorption of light at a given wavelength. Because the ratio of transmittance at each of the two wavelengths (660 nm, red; 940 nm, infrared) varies according to the percentage of Hbo_2, pulse oximeters can be programmed to calculate and display the percentage of oxyhemoglobin saturation at each pulse.

Pulse oximetry has many advantages that make it ideal for use in the ICU. However, a number of factors can limit the effectiveness and accuracy of pulse oximetry. These include impaired local perfusion, abnormal hemoglobins, and very high Po_2's. For example a fall in Po_2 from 300 mm Hg to 90 mm Hg while inhaling 50% oxygen can be very important, but the pulse oximeter will still record a 100% saturation. Carboxyhemoglobin and fetal hemoglobin falsely raise oxyhemoglobin saturation readings while methemoglobin lowers them.

PITFALL

Assuming that blood gases are satisfactory if pulse oximeter readings don't change.

Pulse oximetry helps to reduce the number of arterial blood gas determinations and can provide rapid feedback on therapeutic interventions. In spite of its limitations, it is increasingly becoming the standard of care in emergency departments and neonatal, pediatric, and adult intensive care units.

b. Capnography

Capnography, by providing a real-time estimate of expired P_{CO_2}, is a useful and accurate means of assessing ventilatory adequacy, respiratory gas exchange, carbon dioxide production, and cardiovascular status (primarily cardiac output). Although the measurement of end-tidal carbon dioxide partial pressure ($ETCO_2$) usually underestimates Pa_{CO_2} by about 1 to 2 mm Hg, the difference is constant for a given patient provided the dead space/tidal volume (V_d/V_t) ratio, airway resistance, and rate of carbohydrate metabolism are not changing.

Mainstream and sidestream infrared capnometers are commercially available. A mainstream capnometer connects directly to the endotracheal tube, thus providing real-time, breath-by-breath analysis. The major disadvantage of this system is its size and bulk and the fact that it cannot be used in nonintubated patients. Sidestream capnometers aspirate gas from a port on the side of the ventilatory tubing. The principle advantages of this system are that it reduces mechanical dead space and can be used in nonintubated patients. However, there are many mechanical factors related to gas sampling which can affect the results and can require much expert attention and time.

Because carbon dioxide production is directly dependent on metabolic rate and the type of fuel burned, there are a large number of conditions that can lower $ETCO_2$. However, sudden decreases in $ETCO_2$ suggest mechanical problems in the airway, hypoventilation, increased dead space, or a sudden decrease in cardiac output. A gradual decrease in $ETCO_2$ is usually due to changes in the lung itself. Increases in the $ETCO_2$ are generally due to hypermetabolic states.

AXIOM

A sudden decrease in expired P_{CO_2} usually indicates that the patients are not eliminating of carbon dioxide as they should.

If a simultaneous arterial P_{CO_2} (Pa_{CO_2}) is available, one can use the end-tidal CO_2 to estimate the alveolar P_{CO_2} and then calculate the alveolar-arterial P_{CO_2} difference [$P_{(A-a)CO_2}$]. Normally this is zero, and if it suddenly increases, one should suspect either a pulmonary embolus or some other problem abruptly increasing dead space or causing a drastic reduction in cardiac output.

The most frequent use of $ETCO_2$ is to evaluate the adequacy of ventilation. Inadvertent esophageal intubation, tracheal extubation, and endotracheal tube obstruction can usually be readily detected. These monitors can reduce the number of arterial blood gas determinations obtained and be very useful in weaning patients from mechanical ventilatory support.

A capnograph can also be useful in determining the adequacy of circulation during CPR. The lower the blood flow, the lower the $ETCO_2$. If the mean $ETCO_2$ rises above 3.0% to 3.5%, cardiac output has probably become relatively normal. If the $ETCO_2$ suddenly falls below 1.0%, effective cardiac output has probably ceased.

In general, capnographs are accurate, easily handled, and relatively inexpensive. They are also reliable in a wide variety of clinical settings. We will probably see an increasing use wherever there are critically ill or injured patients.

c. Transcutaneous Monitoring of Oxygen and Carbon Dioxide

In 1951, Baumberger and Goodfriend discovered that a finger immersed in a 45°C electrolyte solution had a partial oxygen pressure (P_{O_2}) equal to the Pa_{O_2}. As a consequence, a great deal of effort has been spent to develop electrochemical sensors that can accurately detect the partial pressure of oxygen and carbon dioxide at the skin surface.

Transcutaneous oxygen and carbon dioxide tension ($Ptco_2$ and $Ptcco_2$) can be important variables for early warning of disturbed pulmonary or cardiovascular function, as well as for the evaluation of local tissue perfusion. Comparative studies indicate that $Ptco_2$ and $Ptcco_2$ are more sensitive indicators of circulatory changes than conventional monitoring variables such as arterial pressure, heart rate, CVP, ECG, and urine output. If tissue perfusion is severely reduced, $Ptco_2$ and $Ptco_2$ values deviate from their relationship with arterial partial pressures and become flow dependent, thereby providing only some qualitative information on local blood flow.

(1) Transcutaneous Oxygen

In adults, $Ptco_2$ is nearly always substantially lower than Pao_2, largely because the skin acts as a barrier to oxygen diffusion. Rithalia has noted that heating of the skin under the $Ptco_2$ monitor produces three major effects: (1) vasodilation of the cutaneous blood vessels; (2) right shift of the oxyhemoglobin dissociation curve increasing the Po_2; and (3) altered lipid structure of the stratum corneum, allowing more rapid diffusion of oxygen. Oxygen molecules that diffuse from the "arterialized" capillary bed to the skin surface are consumed at the electrode in an electrochemical reaction that alters current flow between a cathode and anode, proportional to the oxygen tension present. Unfortunately, heating the skin can be irritating or even damaging.

(2) Transcutaneous Carbon Dioxide

The transcutaneous carbon dioxide electrode is separated from skin by a thin hydrophobic membrane that is permeable to carbon dioxide. Carbon dioxide molecules diffuse through the membrane and form carbonic acid (H_2CO_3), which alters the pH of a conventional pH-sensitive glass electrode.

Carbon dioxide diffuses fairly rapidly through the skin. Heating the skin causes (1) faster diffusion of carbon dioxide to the skin surface, (2) decreased solubility of carbon dioxide, and (3) increased local metabolism and carbon dioxide production. These three heating effects cause transcutaneous CO_2 readings to be 1.2 to 2 times greater than arterial values.

(3) Advantages

In critically ill adults, $Ptco_2$ responds rapidly to changes in Pao_2 and cardiac output. Its 95% response time is less than 2 minutes, even in patients with low-flow circulatory shock. In a study of high-risk surgical patients monitored perioperatively with $Ptco_2$ sensor and pulmonary artery catheters, Nolan and Shoemaker found that decreases in cardiac output, oxygen delivery, oxygen consumption, and $Ptco_2$ were the earliest warning signs of impending circulatory deterioration.

(4) Disadvantages

Although transcutaneous monitoring is a noninvasive technique and can provide constant real-time monitoring, it has a number of disadvantages. If the electrode site is not changed every 2 to 6 hours, there is a risk of burns from the heated electrode. There may also be skin irritation from the adhesive ring.

d. Conjunctival Oxygen and Carbon Dioxide Measurements

In 1971, Kawan and Fatt attached a Clark Po_2 electrode to the anterior surface of a scleral contact lens as a means of continuously monitoring conjunctival oxygen tension ($Pcjo_2$). More recently, miniaturized fiberoptic electrodes have been developed for conjunctival CO_2 ($Pcjco_2$) and pH monitoring.

If cardiac output is adequate, $Pcjo_2$ tracks Pao_2 during variations in blood oxygenation. However, during hemorrhagic shock, $Pcjo_2$ tracks cardiac output. If Pao_2 is adequate, the $Pcjo_2$, like $Ptco_2$, follows local oxygen delivery. $Pcjo_2$ does not require a heated electrode because the conjunctiva does not have a stratum corneum that impedes oxygen diffusion. Since the conjunctiva is supplied by the ophthalmic branch of the internal carotid artery, $Pcjo_2$ may also reflect carotid arterial oxygen transport.

$Pcjo_2$ monitoring has been used to manage patients on mechanical ventilation, during extubation, and during therapeutic interventions. Kram and Shoemaker found that abrupt alterations in $Pcjo_2$ can rapidly reflect changes in ventilator mode, Fio_2, therapy with fluids, vasopressors and vasodilators, or endotracheal tube suctioning. A sudden drop in $Pcjo_2$ may be due to hypoxemia, pneumothorax, reduced cardiac output, or altered local perfusion.

e. Mass Spectrometry

Mass spectrometry allows measurement of all respiratory gases (carbon dioxide, oxygen, and nitrogen) and anesthetic gases on a breath-by-breath basis. Analysis of inspired and expired respiratory gases by mass spectrometry is rapid and accurate to 0.1% of the measurement value.

Mass spectrometry can be used to continuously monitor several patients at a time. However, as the number of monitored beds increases, so does the time between analysis and results. Data analyzed by the mass spectrometer are not real-time but are generally delayed by at least 9 to 22 seconds. This delay results from the aspirated sample having to traverse up to 150 ft of the catheter tubing before reaching the mass spectrometer. In a system with more than 10 monitoring stations, sample determinations may be delayed by more than 2 minutes.

A mass spectrometer can evaluate the carbon dioxide partial pressure curve in order to determine inspired and expired gas values. Sudden changes may indicate mechanical changes in the ventilatory system or airway. Slower changes may indicate important changes in cardiopulmonary function.

Some of the disadvantages of mass spectrophotometers are their high cost (at least $35,000) and their size. If used to monitor many patients, sample data may be provided too infrequently to prevent serious injury to the patient. Unless sampling from each patient can occur at least once a minute, alarms for low oxygen levels and low ventilator pressures and flow should be included.

ABBREVIATIONS USED IN RESPIRATORY STUDIES

PAO_2 = alveolar oxygen tension

PaO_2 = arterial oxygen tension

$P\bar{v}O_2$ = average oxygen tension in mixed venous blood

$PaCO_2$ = alveolar carbon dioxide tension

$PECO_2$ = average carbon dioxide tension in expired gases

FIO_2 = fraction of inspired oxygen (100% $O_2 \rightarrow FIO_2$ of 1.0 and room air $\rightarrow FIO_2$ of 0.21)

$P(A-a)O_2$ = alveolar-arterial oxygen difference or gradient

V_d/V_t = ratio of dead space (V_d) to tidal volume (V_t)

SUMMARY POINTS

1. Boyle's law states that if the mass and temperature of a gas in a chamber remain constant, but the pressure (P) increases or decreases, the volume (V) of the gas varies inversely with the pressure.
2. Air trapped in a pneumothorax or obstructed bowel will tend to expand 3% for each 1000 ft the patient is raised above sea level.
3. Charles law (also known as Guy-Lassac's law) states that if the pressure of a given quantity of gas remains constant, the volume (V) of the gas increases directly in proportion to the rise in absolute temperature (T).
4. Henry's law states that both the partial pressure and solubility coefficient determine the volume of gas that will be dissolved in a given volume of fluid.
5. The diffusion coefficient for carbon dioxide is 20 times greater than for oxygen. Thus, diffusion seldom, if ever, interferes with carbon dioxide exchange in the lung.
6. Interstitial pulmonary edema may cause hypoxemia, but it does not cause hypercarbia.

7. If the P_{AO_2} is 480 mm Hg when one stops breathing, it should take over 2 minutes (about 136 seconds) for the P_{AO_2} to fall to about 60 mm Hg.

8. The respiratory quotient is the ratio of the volume of carbon dioxide released by the lungs to the volume of oxygen taken up by the lungs.

9. The alveolar P_{O_2} on supplemental oxygen is approximately equal to the percentage of inhaled oxygen multiplied by six.

10. End-tidal gas is generally a close approximation of alveolar gas.

11. The P_{aCO_2} can be increased by decreased minute ventilation, increased carbon dioxide production, or increased dead space.

12. One cannot usually correlate the P_{aCO_2} with the adequacy of ventilation unless the patient is acidotic.

13. Increased carbohydrate metabolism may be too great a ventilatory burden in a patient with COPD.

14. When a carbonic anhydrase inhibitor (acetazolamide) is administered, carbon dioxide transport from the tissues becomes significantly impaired and the tissue P_{CO_2} can rise abruptly.

15. Although 25% or more of the oxygen carried by arterial blood is released to the tissues, only about 8% of the carbon dioxide carried by venous blood is released to the lungs.

16. The addition of oxygen to hemoglobin in the lungs increases the release of carbon dioxide there (Haldane effect).

17. The addition of carbon dioxide to hemoglobin in the tissues increases the release of oxygen there (Bohr effect).

18. Restlessness in a patient is due to hypoxemia until proven otherwise.

19. The arterial-central venous pH difference rises as cardiac output falls.

20. Under most circumstances, patients will not look cyanotic unless they have at least 5 g of reduced (unoxygenated) hemoglobin at the capillary level.

21. Cyanosis as a sign of hypoxemia is helpful if the Hb is $\geq$15 g/dl and almost worthless if the Hb is <10 g/dl.

22. Although the P_{O_2} is usually only a small fraction of the oxygen content of arterial blood, it determines the rate and distance that oxygen can diffuse into tissues from the capillaries.

23. If a patient is breathing room air, the P_{aO_2} will drop about 3 mm Hg for each 1000-ft rise above sea level.

24. On room air, a $P_{(A-a)O_2}$ <20 mm Hg is normal and a $P_{(A-a)O_2}$ of 35 to 55 mm Hg indicates moderate pulmonary dysfunction.

25. The oxyhemoglobin dissociation curve is set up so that a "shift to the right" is associated with a higher P_{O_2} at a given oxyhemoglobin saturation and a "shift to the left" indicates a lower P_{O_2} at that saturation.

26. Heat, acidosis, and increased 2,3-DPG shift the oxyhemoglobin dissociation curve to the right (i.e., raise the P_{O_2}).

27. An increased temperature of 1.0°C raises the P_{O_2} about 5%, and an increase of 0.10 in the pH lowers the P_{O_2} by about 10%.

28. Hypoxia and ischemia tend to increase 2,3-DPG, shift the oxyhemoglobin dissociation curve the right, and raise the P_{O_2}.

29. Cold, alkalosis, and decreased 2,3-DPG shift the oxyhemoglobin dissociation curve the left, lowering the P_{O_2} and reducing oxygen availability to tissue.

30. Some of the factors that reduce 2,3-DPG and thereby shift the oxyhemoglobin curve to the left include sepsis, blood transfusions, severe acute malnutrition, severe phosphate deficiency, and carbon monoxide poisoning.

31. The amount of physiologic shunting in the lung (or venous-arterial admixture) (Qs/Qt) is the most sensitive and accurate guide to the onset and progression of acute respiratory failure.

32. A P_{aO_2}/F_{IO_2} ratio >200 (i.e., a P_{aO_2} <80 on 40% oxygen) usually indicates a physiologic shunt in the lung of 20%.

33. A low arterial PO_2 in a patient with a low cardiac output usually indicates more pulmonary dysfunction (i.e., a higher shunt index) than the same PO_2 in a patient with a high cardiac output.

34. Even with only 10 g of full saturated hemoglobin, the red blood cells are carrying over 40 times as much oxygen as the plasma.

35. A relatively normal arterial PO_2 but a very low oxyhemoglobin saturation should make one consider carbon monoxide poisoning.

36. One should not assume that a patient's cardiovascular and pulmonary systems are stable because the $S\overline{v}O_2$ hasn't changed.

37. One should not always assume that the patient's blood gases are satisfactory if the pulse oximeter reading is high and doesn't change.

38. A sudden decrease in expired PCO_2 generally indicates that the patient is not eliminating carbon dioxide as well as he or she should, usually because of a sudden severe decrease in cardiac output.

BIBLIOGRAPHY

1. Andrews, JL: Physiology and treatment of hypoxia. Clin Notes Respir Dis 13:5, 1974.
2. Barker, SJ, Tremper, KK, and Heitzmann, HA: A clinical study of fiberoptic arterial oxygen tension. Crit Care Med 15:403, 1987.
3. Baumberger, JP and Goodfriend, RB: Determination of arterial oxygen tension through intact skin. Fed Proc Am Soc Exp Biol 10:10, 1951.
4. Bone, RC and Balk, RA: Non-invasive respiratory care unit. Chest 93:390, 1988.
5. Cane, RD, et al: Unreliability of oxygen tension-based indices in reflecting intrapulmonary shunting in critically ill patients. Crit Care Med 16:1243, 1988.
6. Clark, LC, Jr: Measurement of oxygen tension: A historical perspective. Crit Care Med 9:960, 1981.
7. Clements, JA: Pulmonary surfactant. Am Rev Respir Dis 101:984, 1970.
8. Comroe, JH, Jr, et al: The Lung: Clinical Physiology and Pulmonary Function Test, ed 2. Yearbook Medical Publishers, Chicago, 1962.
9. Foster, RE and Crandall, LED: Pulmonary gas exchange. Annu Rev Physiol 38:69, 1976.
10. Gil, J: Organization of microcirculation in the lung. Annu Rev Physiol 42:177, 1980.
11. Green, GE, Hassell, KT, and Mahutte, CK: Comparison of arterial blood gas with continuous intra-arterial and transcutaneous PO_2 sensors in adult critically ill patients. Crit Care Med 15:491, 1987.
12. Hess, D, Maxwell, C, and Shefet, D: Determination of intrapulmonary shunt: Comparison of an estimated shunt equation and a modified shunt equation with the classic equation. Respir Care 32:268, 1987.
13. Hock, RJ: The physiology of high altitude. Sci Am 222:52, 1979.
14. Katayama, M, et al: Intra-arterial continuous PO_2 monitoring by an ultra-fine microelectrode. Crit Care Med 15:357, 1987.
15. Killian, KJ and Campbell, EJM: Dyspnea and exercise. Annu Rev Physiol 45:465, 1983.
16. King, TKC, et al: Oxygen transfer in catastrophic respiratory failure. Chest 65:405, 1974.
17. Kram, HB and Shoemaker, WC: Transcutaneous, conjunctival, and organ PO_2 and PCO_2 monitoring in the adult. In Shoemaker, WC, et al (eds): Textbook in Critical Care. WB Saunders, Philadelphia, 1989, p 283.
18. Kram, HB, et al: Noninvasive conjunctival oxygen monitoring during carotid endarterectomy. Arch Surg 121:914, 1986.
19. Kram, HB, et al: Noninvasive measurement of tissue carbon dioxide tension using a fiberoptic conjunctional sensor: Effects of respiratory and metabolic alkalosis and acidosis. Crit Care Med 16:280, 1988.
20. Kwan, M and Fatt, I: A noninvasive method of continuous arterial oxygen tension estimation from measured palpebral conjunctival oxygen tension. Anesthesiology 35:309, 1971.
21. Laghi, F, et al: Respiratory index/pulmonary shunt relationship: Quantification of severity and prognosis in the post-traumatic adult respiratory syndrome. Crit Care Med 17:1121, 1989.
22. Lecky, JH and Ominsky, AJ: Postoperative respiratory management. Chest 62:505, 1972.
23. Lilienthal, JL, et al: An experimental analysis in man of the oxygen pressure gradient from alveolar air to arterial blood. Am J Physiol 147:199, 1946.
24. McConn, R and Del Guercio, LRM: Respiratory function of blood in the acutely ill patient and the effect of steroids. Ann Surg 174:436, 1971.
25. Mecca, RS: Respiratory: Essential physiologic concerns. In Civetta, J, Taylor, R, and Kirby, R (eds): Critical Care. JB Lippincott, Philadelphia, 1988, p 1023.
26. Milic-Emili, J, et al: Regional distribution of inspired gas in the lungs. J Appl Physiol 21:749, 1966.
27. Murray, JF: The normal lung. The Basis for Diagnosis and Treatment of Pulmonary Disease, ed 2. WB Saunders, Philadelphia, 1986, p 175.

28. Nolan, LS and Shoemaker, WC: Transcutaneous O_2 and CO_2 monitoring of high risk surgical patients during the perioperative period. Crit Care Med 10:762, 1982.
29. Nunn, JF: Applied Respiratory Physiology. Butterworth & Co, London, 1987, p 46.
30. Peris, LV, et al: Clinical use of the arterial/alveolar oxygen tension ratio. Crit Care Med 11:888, 1983.
31. Rasanen, J, Downs, JB, and Dehaven, B: Titration of continuous positive airway pressure by real time dual oximetry. Crit Care Med 15:395, 1987.
32. Rasanen, J, et al: Estimation of oxygen utilization by dual oximetry. Crit Care Med 15:404, 1987.
33. Rasanen, J, et al: Oxygen tensions and oxyhemoglobin saturations in the assessment of pulmonary gas exchange. Crit Care Med 15:1058, 1987.
34. Schena, J, Thompson, J, and Crone, RK: Mechanical influences on the capnogram. Crit Care Med 12:672, 1984.
35. Seigel, JH, et al: Cardiorespiratory interactions as determinants of survival and the need for respiratory support in human shock states. J Trauma 13:602, 1973.
36. Severinghaus, JW and Astrup, PB: History of blood gas analysis. Int Anesthesiol Clin 25:12, 1987.
37. Severinghaus, JW and Naireh, KH: Accuracy of response of several pulse oximeters to profound hypoxia. Anesthesiology 67:551, 1987.
38. Shapiro, BA and Cane, RD: Blood gas monitoring: Yesterday, today and tomorrow. Crit Care Med 17:966, 1989.
39. Shapiro, BA, et al: Preliminary evaluation of an intra-arterial blood gas system in dogs and humans. Crit Care Med 17:455, 1989.
40. Stasis, AF: Continuous evaluation of oxygenation and ventilation. In Civetta, JM, Taylor, RW, and Kirby, RR (eds): Critical Care. JB Lippincott, Philadelphia, 1988, p 317.
41. Sutton, JP, et al: Exercise at altitude. Ann Rev Physiol 45:427, 1983.
42. Sutton, RN, Wilson, RF, and Walt, AJ: Differences in acid-base levels and oxygen-saturation between central and arterial blood. Lancet 2:748, 1967.
43. Taylor, MB and Witman, JG: The current status of pulse oximetry. Anesthesia 41:943, 1986.
44. Temper, KK, Waxman, K, and Shoemaker, WC: Effects of hypoxia and shock on transcutaneous Po_2 values in dogs. Crit Care Med 7:526, 1979.
45. Triner, L and Sherman, J: Potential value of expiratory carbon dioxide measurement in patients considered to be susceptible to malignant hyperthermia. Anesthesiology 55:482, 1981.
46. Viale, JP, et al: Arterial-alveolar oxygen partial pressure ratio: A theoretical reappraisal. Crit Care Med 14:153, 1986.
47. Wagner, PD: Ventilation-perfusion relationships. Annu Rev Physiol 42:235, 1980.
48. West, JB: Pulmonary gas exchange. Int Rev Physiol 14:83, 1977.
49. Whipp, BJ: Ventilatory control during exercise in humans. Annu Rev Physiol 45:393, 1983.
50. Wilson, RF, et al: Arterial-central venous differences in critically ill and injured patients. Trauma 14:924, 1974.
51. Wilson, RF, et al: Oxygen consumption in critically ill surgical patients. Ann Surg 176:801, 1972.
52. Wilson, RF, et al: Severe alkalosis in critically ill patients. Arch Surg 105:197, 1972.

CHAPTER 10

Acute Respiratory Failure

I. DEFINITION

AXIOM
A PaO_2 <50 mm Hg and/or a $PaCO_2$ >50 mm Hg (with a pHa <7.35) developing within minutes or days can be called acute respiratory failure.

Defining acute respiratory failure can be extremely difficult. In general, acute respiratory failure or insufficiency refers to a rapidly developing impairment in the lungs' ability to maintain adequate oxygen and carbon dioxide homeostasis. It is also assumed that the impairment is so severe that it would not be compatible with life if it were maintained for more than a few hours or days. Respiratory failure has also been defined as a Pao_2 less than 50 mm Hg or a Pco_2 greater than 50 mm Hg (with a pHa $\leq$ 7.35) on room air at sea level. Even this, however, is a problem because the degree of respiratory failure will also depend on the patient's age and his prior blood gas status.

Acute respiratory failure may be classified by its pathophysiology, duration, and etiology.

II. PATHO-PHYSIOLOGY

Classification by pathophysiology divides respiratory failure into two main subsets: hypoxemic respiratory failure and hypoxemic-hypercapnic respiratory failure. Hypoxemic respiratory failure is characterized by a low Pao_2 associated with a normal or low $Paco_2$. It has also been labeled type I respiratory failure and type II or nonventilatory respiratory failure. Clinical causes of hypoxemia can be divided into three main groups: ventilation/perfusion ($\dot{V}/\dot{Q}$) mismatch, right-to-left intrapulmonary shunt (Qs/Qt), and diffusion abnormality (DL).

AXIOM
The most common abnormality in nonventilatory respiratory failure is $\dot{V}/\dot{Q}$ mismatch.

This $\dot{V}/\dot{Q}$ mismatch is generally associated with diseases directly affecting the lower airways and lung parenchyma. Increased shunting may be due to an anatomical shunt in the heart or lungs or a physiological shunt, especially in the adult respiratory distress syndrome (ARDS). However, using echocardiography, shunting through a probe patent foramen ovale may occur in more than 15% to 35% of patients who develop very high right atrial pressures. Diffusion impairment usually is a factor only in high cardiac output states in which there is insufficient time for hemoglobin to combine with oxygen through a thickened alveolar-capillary membrane. Hypoxemic respiratory failure is associated with a widened alveolar-arterial oxygen partial pressure gradient ($P[A-a]O_2$).

Hypoxemic-hypercapnic respiratory failure with a low Pao_2 and a high $Paco_2$ is also known as either type II respiratory failure or ventilatory failure.

This type of respiratory failure develops when carbon dioxide elimination is impaired due to alveolar hypoventilation or $\dot{V}/\dot{Q}$ mismatch. Alveolar hypoventilation usually results from impaired central ventilatory drive, peripheral neuromuscular control, or any condition producing complete or partial blockage to airflow.

Significant hypercapnia is always associated with hypoxemia unless the patient receives supplemental oxygen. Hypoxemic-hypercapnic respiratory failure produced by alveolar hypoventilation may be associated with a relatively normal $P(A-a)O_2$, while respiratory failure produced by $\dot{V}/\dot{Q}$ mismatching is usually associated with a greatly widened $P(A-a)O_2$, especially if the patient is on supplemental oxygen.

It should be noted that tissue hypoxia, may not only be due to a pulmonary problem causing a low arterial PO_2 (hypoxic hypoxia), but also to (1) a reduced ability of blood to carry oxygen, as in anemia or carbon monoxide poisoning (anemic hypoxia); (2) a reduction in tissue blood flow, either generalized, as in shock, or secondary to a local obstruction (circulatory hypoxia); or (3) interference by a toxin with the ability of tissues to utilize the oxygen brought to it (histotoxic hypoxia).

A. DURATION

Respiratory failure may be classified according to its duration into acute or chronic respiratory failure. Acute respiratory failure usually develops over minutes or days and indicates a degree of hypoxemia or hypercapnia that can be rapidly lethal. Chronic respiratory failure develops over a period of months or years and usually involves a certain degree of metabolic compensation with an elevated bicarbonate to keep the pHa between 7.30 and 7.35.

B. ETIOLOGY

Respiratory failure may be etiologically classified according to the anatomic or physiologic aspects of the respiratory system affected or the specific cause of the disorder (i.e., drugs, metabolic, neoplastic, infectious, or traumatic).

In general, diseases affecting the neuronal control of breathing or the chest bellows function produce ventilatory failure, whereas diseases interfering with gas exchange in the pulmonary parenchyma result in nonventilatory respiratory failure.

C. VENTILATORY FAILURE

Inadequate ventilation of the lungs may be due to (1) neurologic problems involving the brain, spinal cord, phrenic nerves, or intercostal nerves; (2) airway problems involving the nose, mouth, pharynx, trachea, or bronchi; (3) chest wall and diaphragmatic problems; and (4) pleural problems, including hydropneumothorax and/or fibrosis.

D. NEUROLOGIC PROBLEMS

1. Brain

AXIOM

If the patient is making no effort to breathe (in spite of a low PO_2 and/or high PCO_2), a neurologic problem or drug intoxication should be suspected and ventilatory assistance begun immediately.

Injury to the brain or intoxication by various drugs may severely reduce the respiratory center's drive to maintain adequate ventilation. If this problem is suspected and the respiratory efforts do not improve rapidly with oxygen, glucose, and naloxone, one should promptly intubate the patient and begin mechanical ventilation.

2. Spinal Cord

Injury to the spinal cord at C-4 or higher can effectively prevent any movement of the diaphragm or intercostal nerves. If the injury is below C-4 but above T-4 or T-5, the chest and abdominal wall will move paradoxically because of paralysis of the abdominal wall and lower intercostal muscles. The chest will retract inward and the abdomen will expand out during inspiration with the opposite occurring during expiration. This will produce a rocking horse appearance to the chest and abdomen during spontaneous ventilation.

AXIOM
A rocking horse motion of the chest and abdomen with spontaneous ventilation can be a sign of a high spinal cord injury.

3. Phrenic Nerves

The phrenic nerves are most likely to be injured by surgery or trauma in the neck and by cardiac surgery. Cooling the heart with ice can also cause phrenic nerve paralysis. Unilateral paralysis is often overlooked, but bilateral phrenic nerve paralysis can produce severe ventilatory insufficiency.

E. AIRWAY PROBLEMS

AXIOM
If the patient is making an effort to breathe, but there is inspiratory stridor or noisy air movement, an upper airway problem should be suspected.

1. Nose

Occlusion of the nose can cause severe upper airway problems in newborn infants. This is seldom a major problem in adults, but even in older individuals, occlusion of the nose tends to reduce the filtration, warming, and moistening of air reaching the trachea.

2. Pharynx

AXIOM
The most common cause of upper airway obstruction in unconscious patients is prolapse of the tongue into the pharynx.

Unconscious patients may relax all of their muscles and when a patient is lying on his or her back, the tongue tends to fall back into the pharynx. Any maneuver that pulls or pushes the jaw (mandible) forward will also move the tongue forward because of the attachment of the genioglossus muscle to the anterior mandible. The tongue can also be pulled forward with an oral airway, but if the patient wakes up, he or she may vomit.

3. Larynx

AXIOM
The narrowest part of the upper airway in adults is at the glottis (vocal cords).

Occlusion of the larynx can occur from a wide variety of problems. It is particularly important to examine the area of the glottis if there is any inspiratory stridor or other evidence of upper airway obstruction.

4. Trachea

The trachea is particularly apt to become occluded as a result of prolonged endotracheal or tracheostomy intubation. This may be due to excess granulation tissue or stenosis because of tracheomalacia from excessive pressure against the tracheal cartilages.

5. Bronchi

AXIOM
The most frequent cause of pulmonary problems in critically ill patients is atelectasis due to inadequate removal of bronchial secretions.

Inadequate coughing and deep breathing due to excess sedation or pain from recent trauma or surgery are the major causes of atelectasis. If the patient cannot be encouraged to cough or breathe deeply enough, nasotracheal suction may remove the secretions and help stimulate a cough. Relief of pain with intercostal blocks or epidural analgesia may be very helpful in patients. Occasionally bronchoscopy to remove excess secretions is required.

6. Chest Wall

Fractured ribs may severely limit ventilation because of the pain associated with movement of the bone ends and the associated muscle spasm. If there are segmental fractures of three or more ribs or the sternum, a flail chest with paradoxical movement of the injured portion of the chest may make ventilation extremely inefficient.

7. Pleural Cavity

AXIOM
Reduced breath sounds in one chest plus respiratory difficulty in a spontaneously breathing patient is indicative of a major airway obstruction or hydropneumothorax until proven otherwise.

Collections of air in the pleural cavity will reduce the capacity of the lung by an equivalent amount, and such collections should be drained with a chest tube as soon as possible. Collections of fluid due to heart failure should also be drained if they are large and/or the patient is moderately-severely symptomatic. A fibrothorax due to an adequately treated empyema or hemothorax may also restrict ventilation.

F. GAS-EXCHANGE PROBLEMS

The factors involved in gas exchange can be divided into three main groups: (1) perfusion, (2) diffusion, and (3) distribution.

1. Perfusion

Impairment of blood flow to alveoli results in increased "dead space" in the lungs. This problem is seen most frequently with pulmonary emboli chronic obstructive lung disease (COPD), or a low cardiac output. The excessive dilation of alveoli in COPD can cause loss of alveolar septae so that the amount of capillary surface area exposed to alveolar gas is reduced. The normal dead space/tidal volume ratio (V_d/V_t) is about 0.3. In ARDS, not only is the shunt (Qs/Qt) increased, but dead space is often more than doubled.

2. Distribution

If there are localized anatomic defects or partial obstructions in the large- or medium-sized airways, the inhaled gases may not be distributed throughout the lungs in an appropriate manner. Some portions of the lung will receive too much ventilation and others not enough. This can contribute to a ventilation/perfusion ($\dot{V}/\dot{Q}$) mismatch and significant hypoxemia.

3. Diffusion

Increases in the distance between alveoli and their associated capillaries, usually because of interstitial edema, can result in impaired transfer of oxygen to the capillaries. This may be aggravated by any problem, such as increased cardiac output, which limits the amount of time that red blood cells in the pulmonary capillaries are in contact with functional alveoli.

III. SPECIFIC CLINICAL PROBLEMS CAUSING RESPIRATORY FAILURE

Some of the specific clinical entities that can cause acute respiratory failure include atelectasis, aspiration, pneumonia, and pulmonary emboli. Other causes of acute respiratory failure that are seen primarily with trauma include pneumothorax, smoke inhalation, pulmonary contusion, and flail chest.

A. ATELECTASIS

Atelectasis is derived from a Greek term meaning "airless" and refers to collapse of a portion of lung. The main causes of atelectasis include (1) absorption atelectasis following obstruction of a bronchus, usually by a mucous plug, with subsequent resorption of the air in the distal lung; (2) passive or compression atelectasis due to a space-occupying lesion, such as a pneumothorax; (3) adhesive atelectasis (in spite of patent bronchi), which is presumably due to surfactant deficiencies in association with pneumonia and other inflammatory pulmonary problems; and (4) cicatrization atelectasis caused by pulmonary fibrosis.

The major clinical factors increasing the tendency to atelectasis include (1) reduced deep breathing or coughing, (2) increased quantities or thickness of sputum, and (3) reduced bronchial diameter due to edema or broncho-constriction.

Studies on the incidence of postoperative pulmonary complications indicate that they occur in at least 2.5% to 5.0% of all operations. Pulmonary complications occur in 5% to 10% of lower abdominal operations, 10% to 20% of upper abdominal procedures, and 15% to 40% of all thoracotomies. A patchy atelectasis involving smaller airways (microatelectasis) may not be diagnosed clinically or by chest radiography, but is probably present much more frequently than "macroatelectasis," which can be detected clinically or on chest x-rays.

The clinical hallmarks of atelectasis are moist rales or rhonchi at the lung bases with decreased breath sounds that tend to clear, at least partially, with a good cough. Atelectasis may be manifested by tachypnea, fever, and tachycardia, but these are often late signs secondary to bacterial proliferation in the atelectatic area of the lung. Shields, in 1949, demonstrated that intravenously administered bacteria tend to localize at sites of atelectasis.

PITFALL
Treating fever immediately after surgery with antibiotics rather than bronchial toilet.

Successful treatment of atelectasis depends on prompt mobilization of bronchial secretions by deep breathing, coughing, and nasotracheal suctioning if necessary. In patients with major areas of collapse or excessive secretions not removed by other means, therapeutic bronchoscopy is indicated. Pain medication should be judiciously used to help alleviate postoperative or post-traumatic pain without producing harmful respiratory depression. For patients with multiple injuries and a great deal of pain, epidural analgesia can be extremely helpful.

1. Aspiration

Aspiration of infected oropharyngeal contents or acidic gastric contents (with or without food particles) can create extremely severe pneumonia, which may be necrotizing and go on to form lung abscesses.

AXIOM
One should assume that all patients with seizures or a sudden loss of consciousness have aspirated.

Some of the conditions that predispose to aspiration include (1) alteration of consciousness, head injury, seizures, alcohol intoxication, drug overdose; (2) impaired swallowing, tracheostomy, esophageal obstruction, incompetent lower esophageal sphincter, tracheoesophageal fistula, nasogastric intubation; and (3) defective cough and gag reflexes.

PITFALL
Leaving a nasogastric tube in longer than is really necessary.

Efforts to minimize the likelihood of aspiration of oropharyngeal and gastric contents are important. As soon as possible, one should remove all tubes that pass through the upper airways, particularly nasogastric tubes. One should also discontinue drugs that depress the central nervous system.

Prevention of aspiration of gastric contents may be especially difficult in patients who require a nasogastric tube and are given antacids to prevent stress ulcer formation. The alkalinized stomach can quickly become a reservoir for the overgrowth of Gram-negative intestinal organisms. These organisms can move up along the nasogastric tube because it impairs function of the gastroesophageal sphincter. Aspiration of retained gastric contents can cause severe respiratory

427

tract infection. If the patient aspirates highly acid gastric contents, a severe chemical pneumonitis may evolve, and this is also likely to become infected.

If aspiration of gastric contents is thought to have occurred, the tracheobronchial tree should be suctioned out as soon as possible, preferably through an endotracheal tube with a flexible bronchoscope. If large particles of food are found, they are usually best removed with rigid bronchoscopy. Bronchoscopy, unless performed immediately, has little, if any, role in the removal of acid from the tracheobronchial tree since acid absorption through bronchial mucosa and the alveoli occurs very rapidly.

Corticosteroids for the treatment of aspiration are extremely controversial, and they are seldom used now. If they are used, they must be given very early.

Cultures should be obtained on any available sputum, but there is controversy as to whether antibiotics should be used prophylactically. Many clinicians now feel that antibiotics should not be used until clinical and/or radiologic evidence of pneumonitis exists.

PITFALL

Early use of antibiotics with aspiration may not reduce infection rates, but if infection does occur, resistant organisms are more likely to be involved.

Some clinicians feel that any episode of aspiration should be treated as though oropharyngeal contents have been aspirated and infection will ensue. Such antibiotics should be continued for approximately 3 days. If the clinical picture or chest x-ray does not indicate a developing pneumonia, the antibiotics can be discontinued. If an infiltrate is present on day 3, but the patient is afebrile, antibiotics are continued for a 7 to 10 day course. If the patient has an infiltrate and is febrile, culture and Gram stain of the sputum should be obtained to be certain that the correct antimicrobial agent is being administered.

The choice of antibiotics for the treatment of aspiration pneumonia is controversial. Penicillin G was once the mainstay of therapy, but up to 30% of these organisms are now penicillin resistant. Consequently, a beta-lactamase-stable antianaerobic antibiotic, such as clindamycin, is probably preferable.

B. PNEUMONIA

AXIOM

Fever developing soon after admission to an ICU is usually due to pneumonia or an IV catheter infection,

Pneumonia is one of the most common problems seen in ICU patients. In a patient hospitalized for community-acquired pneumonia, the typical signs of infection—productive cough, purulent sputum, fever, and rales—are usually present. Leukocytosis is the rule, and an infiltrate is generally present on the chest radiograph. However, pneumonias acquired in a hospital, especially in an ICU, may be more difficult to diagnose because the classic signs may be absent and because host defenses are altered by pre-existing conditions.

Some of the criteria used to make a diagnosis of pneumonia following trauma or surgery include (1) a new infiltrate seen on chest x-ray, (2) a temperature of at least 38°C for at least 24 hours, and (3) purulent sputum production plus cultured pathogens. An ideal sputum contains (1) few (<10) epithelial cells, (2) many (>25) polymorphonuclear leucocytes (PMNs) per high power field (HPF), and (3) has a preponderance of one type of organism.

Determining the source of pulmonary infiltrates in mechanically ventilated patients is a frequent and difficult clinical problem. Although bacterial pneumonia is often a primary consideration, ICU patients may develop pulmonary infiltrates, fever, leukocytosis, and purulent sputum because of a variety of noninfectious causes. There is also concern regarding the sensitivity and specificity of currently available diagnostic techniques used in identifying the responsible agent when pneumonia is suspected. Routine analysis of specimens gathered from an endotracheal tube is difficult to interpret because of tracheal colonization by potential pathogens, especially Gram-negative bacteria. Routine bronchoscopic specimens obtained from the lower airways are frequently inaccurate because of contamination by proximal tracheal and oral secretions.

Recent studies by Baughman and associates using semiquantitative culture techniques have shown that a protected brush specimen obtained through a flexible fiberoptic bronchoscope may be useful for the accurate assessment of bacterial pneumonia in intubated and ventilated patients.

AXIOM
Sputum cultures are best obtained with a protected brush or bronchoalveolar lavage.

Bronchoalveolar lavage (BAL) may also have a role in the assessment of opportunistic pulmonary infections. It has been found to have diagnostic value in evaluating acute bacterial pneumonia in nonintubated patients when semiquantitative culture techniques are used.

In a recent study, Guerra and Baughman evaluated the efficacy and safety of bronchoscopy with BAL in mechanically ventilated patients. Seventy-seven patients, 60 of whom underwent BAL, were analyzed according to the organisms found and the number of colony-forming units (cfu) growing on culture. Of 30 patients with clinical pneumonia having BAL, 18 (60%) had bacterial cultures felt to be diagnostic of bacterial pneumonia. These included two cases of *Legionella pneumophila*, and 16 cases with one or more organisms recovered at $>10^4$ cfu/ml of BAL fluid. No patient without the clinical diagnosis of pneumonia had a positive bacterial culture with $>10^4$ cfu/ml of BAL fluid. Although no patient died as a result of lavage, significant hypoxemia was encountered in several patients. In 35 patients with the same FIO_2 before and after bronchoscopy, the median change in PO_2 was -8.0 mm Hg (range -63.0 to $+29.0$).

Another method for determining if pneumonia is present is analysis of the pH of the respiratory mucus. Using a sterile 8-Fr suction catheter, Karnad, Mhaisekar, and Moralwar found that the average respiratory mucus pH was 7.3 to 7.4 on the day of intubation, 7.2 to 7.5 in 18 patients with colonization and 6.9 in 13 patients with later pneumonia. A decrease in the respiratory mucus pH ≥ 0.2 below the value on the day of intubation indicated the presence of pneumonia with a positive predictive value of 90%. This decrease in pH occurred before or on the same day as the development of radiologically detectable pneumonia in most cases. Thus, daily monitoring of the pH of tracheobronchial mucus may be of value in critically ill intubated patients.

The mortality rate for patients with postoperative pneumonia may exceed 50%, especially in ICU patients. Risk factors predicting a poor outcome include (1) Gram-negative pneumonitis, particularly with *Pseudomonas*; (2) signs of organ failure; (3) bilateral pneumonia; (4) positive blood cultures; (5) postoperative peritonitis; and (6) pneumonia acquired while receiving mechanical ventilation.

Another type of pneumonia that is being seen with increasing frequency in ICU patients are those due to opportunistic organisms in immunocompromised patients. Etiologic agents may be bacterial (especially *Pseudomonas* or *Mycobacterium*), fungal (including *Aspergillus, Cryptococcus, Candida,* or *Nocardia*), protozoan (*Pneumocystis*), or viral (e.g., cytomegalovirus or herpes). Patients with acquired immunodeficiency syndrome (AIDS) tend to have a high incidence of infection caused by *Pneumocystitis, Legionella,* and *Mycoplasma*. Neutropenic patients have a higher risk of *Pseudomonas* infection.

When a patient with an altered immune status develops pneumonia, vigorous diagnostic techniques should be used early in the process to obtain adequate specimens for special staining, cultures, light microscopy, and even electron microscopy to aid in establishing a specific diagnosis.

PITFALL
Any delay in efforts to diagnose the cause of a new pulmonary infiltrate in an immunosuppressed patient.

Acceptable diagnostic techniques include percutaneous needle biopsy, bronchoalveolar lavage, and transbronchial biopsy. In some cases a thoracotomy with open-lung biopsy may be needed. Empiric treatment often is necessary in these desperately ill patients and must be based on the likelihood of the patient's having a specific diagnosis.

C. PULMONARY EMBOLISM

The etiology, clinical findings, and treatment of pulmonary embolism are generally well recognized and will be dealt with in more detail in another chapter. The occlusion of pulmonary arteries by clots can cause (1) hyperventilation, (2) pulmonary restriction with a decreased vital capacity, (3) bronchoconstriction with a decrease in the FEV_1 and maximum midexpiratory flow rate, (4) hypoxemia secondary to ventilation-perfusion inequality, (5) variable degrees of pulmonary hypertension.

AXIOM
Since most pulmonary emboli occur in elderly patients with underlying cardiopulmonary disease, relatively small emboli can cause severe problems.

The redistribution of blood flow from unperfused areas may lead to a relative overperfusion of other alveoli, further increasing the ventilation-perfusion mismatch. Surfactant production may also be impaired after 24 hours, leading to local atelectasis and edema that may progress to a congestive atelectasis that grossly resembles pulmonary infarction.

AXIOM
Sudden development of tachypnea, tachycardia, and hypoxemia in a bedridden patient is due to a pulmonary embolism until proven otherwise.

D. PNEUMOTHORAX

Pneumothorax occurs when air escapes from the pulmonary parenchyma or through an opening in the chest wall and causes a portion of the lung to collapse. In simple pneumothorax, the mediastinal structures are not shifted, and the opposite lung is not compressed. In contrast, a tension pneumothorax, caused by the progressive accumulation of air within a pleural cavity, can lead to a shift in the mediastinal structures with possible compression of the contralateral lung and reduced venous return. Tension pneumothorax often results from a one-way valve phenomenon in which air enters the thoracic cavity from an opening in the pulmonary parenchyma or the chest wall. Air enters the pleural space during inspiration but cannot escape during expiration. Hypotension and circulatory collapse may occur within minutes if the condition is not promptly treated.

AXIOM
Most tension pneumothoraces should be diagnosed and treated on clinical criteria. Waiting for radiologic proof can be disastrous.

Blunt trauma may be associated with a pneumothorax caused by laceration of the lung from a rib fracture. However, a pneumothorax may also occur because of the sudden compression of the chest against a closed glottis, causing a rapid increase in the intrathoracic pressure leading to disruption of alveoli. A pneumothorax may also result from barotrauma, in which increased pressure in the airway (usually from positive-pressure mechanical ventilation) results in a "blow-out" type of alveolar injury.

Spontaneous pneumothorax often results from apical blebs that are apparently congenital in origin. Likewise, acquired conditions, such as bullous emphysema or pneumatocele following staphylococcal pneumonia, can result in a thinning of the pulmonary parenchyma that may leak air and cause a pneumothorax, particularly if high ventilatory pressures are used.

PITFALL
Assuming a small pneumothorax on a chest x-ray causes only a small decrease in lung capacity.

On plain chest x-rays showing <10% to 20% pneumothorax, the degree of physiologic insult may seem relatively mild. However, if the lung is regarded as a sphere with a volume of $\frac{4}{3}\pi r^3$, then the volume loss is determined by the third power of the radius. Thus, a diameter reduction from 20 to 16 cm causes a radius change from 10 to 8 cm and a theoretical volume loss from 3140 to 1608 ml (i.e., a net volume loss of 50% rather than just a 20% diameter loss). If the patient is symptomatic, has bilateral pneumothoraces, or will require positive-pressure ventilation (for surgery or mechanical ventilation), then a thoracostomy tube should be inserted and connected to an underwater seal to re-expand the lung.

E. SMOKE INHALATION

Direct heat injury below the vocal cords as a result of inhalation of hot gases is extremely rare except with superheated steam, which may have 4000 times the heat capacity of normal air.

The incomplete combustion of both natural and synthetic products can produce noxious gases that are inhaled and can cause local bronchial and alveolar, as well as systemic, effects. Corrosive acids and alkalis resulting from the reaction of sulfur and nitrogen oxides adherent to soot particles with lung surface water can also produce local and systemic injury. The magnitude of injury depends on the types of noxious gases inhaled, their concentration and solubility, and the duration of exposure.

Carbon monoxide inhalation is a special problem in fires involving wood, paper, and cloth from natural fibers. It has 230 times more affinity for hemoglobin than oxygen does. It binds with the hemoglobin molecule to form carboxyhemoglobin (Hbco), not only interfering with Hb carrying oxygen but also reducing the ability of hemoglobin to offload oxygen at the tissue level. The Pao_2 may be normal, but the Hbo_2 saturation, when directly measured, can be extremely low.

AXIOM
Patients with possible smoke inhalation must have both their arterial PO_2 and oxyhemoglobin saturation measured separately.

With levels of Hbco in the 20% to 40% range, the symptoms may be difficult to recognize but usually include headache, confusion, and other nonspecific central nervous system manifestations. Coma (from severe cerebral hypoxia) is likely to occur with Hbco levels in the range of 40% to 60%, and death tends to occur with levels greater than 60%.

PITFALL
Assuming that low carbon monoxide blood levels rule out smoke inhalation.

An increasing number of fires cause patients to inhale a variety of gases formed by burning of plastics and other synthetics. Water-soluble chemicals such as ammonia, sulfur dioxide, chlorine, and hydrogen chloride tend to dissolve in the upper respiratory tract, whereas lipid-soluble gases such as the aldehydes, phosgene, and nitric oxide tend to reach more distal lung radicals. Cyanide, a product of the combustion of synthetic materials such as polyurethane, produces its effect through systemic absorption and poisoning of the cytochrome electron transport systems.

The effect of inhaled toxic products includes direct epithelial destruction, mucosal edema, ciliary paralysis, and surfactant deficiency due to injury to type II alveolar epithelial cells. Injured and/or activated pulmonary alveolar macrophages secrete chemotoxins, producing local sequestration of PMNs. These PMNs in turn release proteolytic enzymes and oxygen-free radicals that potentiate the pulmonary injury.

Demling has noted a number of pulmonary effects that may result from peripheral burn wounds. Thromboxane A_2 released from burn tissue, in particular, has a number of potentially deleterious consequences, including bronchoconstriction, decreased lung compliance, and vasoconstriction with resultant pulmonary artery hypertension.

The diagnosis of smoke inhalation is based primarily on history and demonstration of soot in sputum or bronchoscopic specimens. Xenon clearance studies have also been used. The initial physical examination and chest x-rays may be deceptively normal.

With less severe inhalation injuries, treatment includes humidified air, vigorous pulmonary toilet, bronchodilators, and oxygen as needed. Direct upper airway injury with edema and the potential for airway obstruction may be of major concern after injuries due to fire in an enclosed space, especially if the face and mouth are burned and are apt to swell excessively.

Throughout the first 24 to 48 hours, the patient must be watched very closely for progressive swelling of mucosa that may cause airway obstruction. The need for high-volume fluid resuscitation to treat a major cutaneous burn increases the edema and the potential for obstruction. With severe inhalations, early intubation with a soft cuff nasotracheal tube and the use of a volume-cycled ventilator with carefully controlled positive end-expiratory pressure is probably indicated. Use of hypertonic saline may also reduce swelling of the mucosa of the airways.

The use of broad-spectrum antibiotics to try to prevent pulmonary infection is controversial.

F. PULMONARY CONTUSION

Any pulmonary infiltrate developing within 6 hours in an area of localized trauma to the lung is considered to represent pulmonary contusion. Pulmonary contusion histologically shows extravasation of protein-rich fluid and erythrocytes into alveoli and the interstitial spaces. In most instances, the extent of the pulmonary contusion as seen at surgery or on a CT scan, is at least two to three times greater than is apparent on the plain chest x-rays. In addition, the CT scan often shows pulmonary lacerations not apparent on plain chest films.

AXIOM
Pulmonary contusions are much more extensive than they appear on the initial x-rays.

Immediately after injury there is usually only interstitial and alveolar hemorrhage with relatively little edema in the contused area. However, within a few hours there is increasing edema with a marked thickening of alveolar walls. By 24 hours there may be loss of normal alveolar architecture, plus extensive PMN and round cell infiltration into the interstitial tissues and alveoli.

Nichols showed that surfactant was decreased in the area of lung contusion between 24 and 48 hours, causing a decreased compliance and worsening of lung mechanics. If saline is rapidly infused, there is increasing interstitial and alveolar edema with a rise in pulmonary artery pressure, causing the Po_2 to fall even further.

Recommendations on the management of pulmonary contusion and flail chest now include (1) cautious use of sodium-containing solutions and (2) use of blood to limit the amount of crystalloid resuscitation. Although corticosteroids may limit the size of pulmonary contusions experimentally, there is concern about their effect on lung defenses and they usually are not given.

G. FLAIL CHEST

A flail chest occurs when the sternum is fractured or at least three ribs are fractured in more than one area, resulting in paradoxical motion of the chest wall. The paradoxical motion involves the flail segment moving inward during inspiration and outward during expiration. The hypoxemia associated with flail chest has at least three causes: (1) underlying pulmonary contusion, (2) decreased efficiency and effectiveness of chest-wall motion, and (3) hypoventilation and atelectasis from chest-wall pain. In many cases, the most important cause of the hypoxemia is the underlying pulmonary contusion.

Treatment of flail chest has gone through several phases. Initially physicians relied on external mechanical stabilization with traction devices or belts. The introduction of the piston-driven ventilators in 1956 led to the development of the concept of internal pneumatic stabilization, in which the patient's respiratory drive was eliminated by rendering the patient alkalotic and allowing the ventilator to "stabilize" the flail segment.

More recently there has been a trend toward a more selective management of flail chest with ventilators. The mainstays of therapy now include (1) avoidance of overresuscitation with crystalloids, (2) appropriate pain relief so that vigorous pulmonary toilet can be used effectively to control secretions and prevent atelectasis, and (3) selective use of endotracheal intubation for multiple associated injuries or persistent hypoxemia (Po_2 <80 mm Hg on 40% oxygen). If the patient is given ventilatory assistance, there is also emphasis on early weaning from the ventilator based on physiologic parameters rather than chest-wall instability.

AXIOM
Patients with a flail chest plus severe head injuries, shock, or massive transfusions should probably be placed on a ventilator prophylactically. Any delay in beginning ventilatory assistance in such patients can greatly increase mortality rates.

IV. FAT EMBOLISM SYNDROME

A. THE CLASSIC SYNDROME

Fat embolism syndrome (FES) was first noted at autopsy in 1862 by Zenker. He described the presence of fat droplets in the lungs of a patient who died following a crush injury of the chest and abdomen. The first clinical case was diagnosed in 1874 by Von Bergman. Early descriptions focused on the triad of dyspnea, confusion, and petechiae. In more recent years, attention has been directed to the pulmonary dysfunction that develops.

AXIOM
CNS and pulmonary dysfunction occurring 12 to 72 hours after long-bone fractures is often due to fat emboli.

Classic FES is generally described as cerebral and respiratory dysfunction developing approximately 12 to 60 hours after severe injury, which usually includes long-bone and/or pelvic fractures. Most of the fat embolizing to the lung comes from the marrow of fractured bones. Some investigators, however, have found that some of the fat found in the lung is chemically different from marrow fat, especially in cholesterol content, and may come from excessive mobilization of fat by catecholamines. Furthermore, fat emboli can occur or develop after trauma or surgery involving only soft tissue.

Because the solubility of the fat is decreased following trauma, triglycerides tend to precipitate out as discrete fat particles or droplets in the blood. Peltier was one of the earliest investigators to demonstrate that it usually takes at least 12 to 48 hours for the lipoprotein lipase in the lungs to convert the relatively innocuous neutral triglycerides in fat emboli into fatty acids, and it is the free fatty acids that cause the inflammatory changes in the lung. In addition, activated platelets rapidly adhere to the fat emboli and are carried to the lungs. These provide a rich source of vasoactive materials, including serotonin, which can cause arterial vasoconstriction and further damage to the pulmonary capillaries.

AXIOM

The main laboratory changes in fat embolism syndrome include hypoxemia and thrombocytopenia.

There has been increasing attention to the association of intravascular coagulation with the fat emboli, as demonstrated by increased fibrin-split products together with reductions in the platelet count and the concentrations of various clotting factors in the blood. The thrombocytopenia may at least partially account for the petechiae that are occasionally found in the skin of the axilla or chest and in the conjunctivae of some patients with full-blown FES.

Fabian et al. recently reported on a 12-month prospective study of 92 patients with long-bone or pelvic fractures admitted to a level I trauma center. Arterial blood gases, Hct, platelet count, serum fibrinogen, serum lipase, and urinary fat bodies were determined serially from admission through the fifth hospital day. Patients were also evaluated daily by chest x-ray, vital signs, mental status, and presence of petechiae. Patients were felt to have an increased pulmonary shunt if the $P(A-a)O_2$ on 100% oxygen exceeded 100 mm Hg. Ten (11%) patients were felt to have the fat embolism syndrome because of an increased $P(A-a)O_2$. However, only four of these patients had petechiae.

B. SUBCLINICAL FAT EMBOLISM

The incidence of FES has been reported at 0.5% to 10% of fracture patients and seems to vary with the type and number of fractures. Prospective analyses by McCarthy and colleagues and then by Shier and associates have suggested that the syndrome often develops in mild or subclinical forms.

AXIOM

Many patients with fractured bones have no pulmonary symptoms but have an increased $P(A-a)O_2$ and thrombocytopenia.

Even patients with apparently uncomplicated extremity fractures may have significant pulmonary changes as reflected by an increased $P(A-a)O_2$ and decreased platelet counts. A study of patients admitted to an orthopedic service with uncomplicated extremity fractures showed that the great majority of patients had respiratory alkalosis (Fig. 10.1) and pulmonary changes, which were reflected by a slight-moderately decreased arterial PO_2 and PCO_2 and moderate-severely increased alveolar-arterial oxygen differences. Many of these patients also had decreased platelet counts and other coagulation changes characteristic of a consumptive coagulopathy. Even more important, there was relatively good correlation between the drop in the platelet count (presumably due to platelet trapping on fat emboli in the lung) and the increases in the alveolar-arterial oxygen differences (Fig. 10.2). These changes together with increased fat in the urine in over 80% of the patients tested suggested that, even with uncomplicated

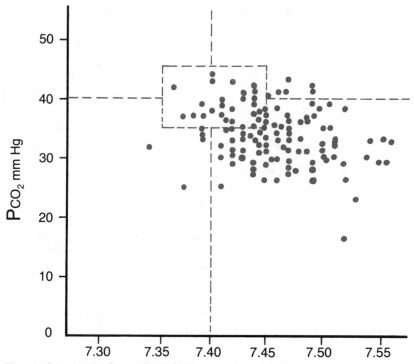

Figure 10.1 Arterial Pco₂ values of patients with uncomplicated extremity fractures.

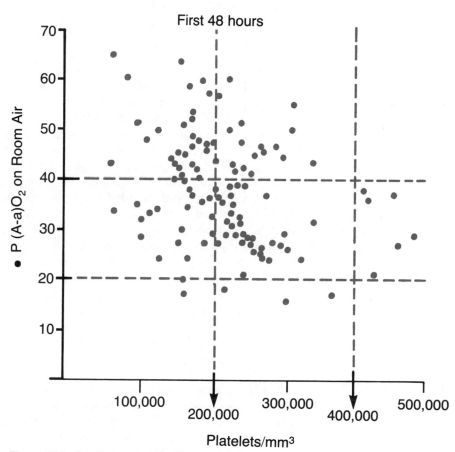

Figure 10.2 Correlations between blood gas determinations of coagulation changes in patients with uncomplicated extremity fractures.

extremity fractures, some of the changes characteristic of fat embolism may occur.

During the first few minutes following experimental fractures in dogs, fibrinogen and platelet concentrations in blood drop precipitously. However, within 24 hours fibrinogen levels usually return to normal. The fibrinogen levels continue to rise so that, by the sixth to eighth day following injury, fibrinogen levels are often two to three times normal. These increases in fibrinogen concentrations may contribute to the high incidence of venous thrombosis and pulmonary emboli in patients with fractures.

1. Hepatic Cirrhosis

It has been known for many years that severe hepatic cirrhosis is often associated with a reduced Po_2 and Pco_2. As a consequence, the $P(A-a)o_2$ is elevated and usually averages at least 40 to 50 mm Hg. The bulk of published data points to a ventilation-perfusion (V/Q) mismatch as the main cause for the "hypoxemia of liver cirrhosis." Cirrhotics, however, also commonly present with reduced hemoglobin levels, ascites, an increased P_{50}, abnormal cardiac output, and an increased minute ventilation.

The V/Q mismatch in hepatic cirrhosis is believed to be due to either an altered distribution of ventilation caused by an increase in closing volume or a blunted pulmonary vascular reactivity to hypoxia. Rodriguez-Roisin and co-workers have shown that patients with more advanced hepatic disease exhibit less pulmonary vascular reactivity to hypoxia, lower arterial Po_2, and more V/Q mismatching, as assessed by the multiple inert gas elimination technique.

In a more recent study, Melot and colleagues showed that there is no close correlation between the severity of the liver disease and the abnormal pulmonary vascular reactivity to hypoxia. They also determined that the "hypoxemia of liver cirrhosis" is explained by a V/Q mismatch, but this could not be explained by blunted hypoxic pulmonary vasoconstriction, except in an occasional patient.

V. ADULT RESPIRATORY DISTRESS SYNDROME

Probably the most frequent and serious type of acute respiratory failure seen in the ICU is the adult respiratory distress syndrome (ARDS). Raffin has estimated that up to 250,000 cases of ARDS may develop annually in the United States. The average mortality rate is about 50% to 65%, and if the ARDS is due to sepsis, the mortality rate is probably closer to 80% to 90%.

In 1967, Ashbaugh and Petty presented data on 12 patients with acute respiratory failure of diverse etiology. A similar pattern of respiratory failure was seen in all patients and included dyspnea, tachypnea, noncompliant lungs, and diffuse panacinar infiltrates on chest x-ray. All patients remained hypoxemic despite supplemental oxygen and other "usual" methods of respiratory support.

Ashbaugh and associates first used the term "acute respiratory distress in adults," because the clinical, physiologic, and pathologic course of events was remarkably similar to the infantile respiratory distress syndrome (hyaline-membrane disease). However, it is now clear that the reduction in surfactant seen in ARDS is a result of the process and not its cause. The reduction in surfactant in ARDS, nevertheless, does increase the tendency to diffuse microatelectasis.

The term ARDS was later coined by these investigators, and specific criteria for making the diagnosis were described.

A. DEFINITION

ARDS is difficult to define accurately because of the multiple circumstances in which it may develop and the variety of signs, symptoms, and laboratory values with which it may be associated. However, it is usually defined as a noncardiogenic permeability type of acute pulmonary edema. In articles dealing with ARDS, the usual definitions include (1) severe hypoxemia with a Po_2 of less than 50 to 60 mm Hg on 40% to 50% oxygen, (2) diffuse bilateral infiltrates that are not due to pneumonia; (3) typical initiating cause, such as sepsis; and (4) PAWP less than 12 to 15 mm Hg.

One of the newer definitions for ARDS was developed by Murray and coworkers in 1988. They defined ARDS as the presence of diffuse infiltrates involving all four quadrants of the anteroposterior chest roentgenogram, severe hypoxemia (Pao_2/PAo_2 <0.30), and a pulmonary arterial wedge $\leq$18 mm Hg. They also quantified severity of the parenchymal lung injury daily by the use of a lung injury score with three components: (1) a chest radiograph score, (2) a Pao_2/PAo_2 score, and (3) a positive end-expiratory pressure (PEEP) score (Table 10.1). The daily lung injury score was obtained by dividing the aggregate sum by the number of components available.

B. TERMS

Many terms have been used to describe the acute respiratory failure that develops in critically ill or injured patients. Terms such as shock lung, traumatic wet lung, and septic lung refer to respiratory distress in association with certain well-defined clinical situations. Other terms, such as congestive atelectasis and hemorrhagic atelectasis, refer to pathologic changes noted by various investigators.

The lung is very limited in the ways it can respond to various mechanical and chemical injuries. Virtually all types of ARDS have essentially the same pathophysiology, consisting of increased lung water and a decreased functional residual capacity (FRC) due to diffuse congestion and microatelectasis. The only major pathologic differences between the various entities may be the severity of the increased pulmonary capillary permeability, the pulmonary capillary pressures, and the severity of the congestive atelectasis.

C. ETIOLOGY OF ADULT RESPIRATORY DISTRESS SYNDROME

AXIOM

The most frequent cause of severe, progressive ARDS is sepsis.

Some of the more frequently mentioned causes of ARDS include sepsis, shock, fat embolism, massive transfusions, and aspiration. The pulmonary ef-

Table 10.1

COMPONENTS AND INDIVIDUAL VALUES OF THE LUNG INJURY SCORE

Score	Value*
Chest Roentgenogram	
No alveolar consolidation	0
Alveolar consolidation confined to 1 quadrant	1
Alveolar consolidation confined to 2 quadrants	2
Alveolar consolidation confined to 3 quadrants	3
Alveolar consolidation in all 4 quadrants	4
Hypoxemia Score (PaO_2/PAO_2)	
>0.40	0
0.30–0.30	1
0.20–0.29	2
0.10–0.10	3
<0.10	4
PEEP Score (When Ventilated), cm H_2O	
<5	0
6–8	1
9–11	2
12–14	3
>k5	4

*The final value is obtained by dividing the aggregate sum by the number of components that were used.
PEEP = positive end-expiratory pressure.

fects of cerebral hypoxia have also been suggested as an important etiologic factor.

1. Sepsis

The critical role of sepsis in the etiology of ARDS was defined by Fulton and Jones when they noted that of 44 trauma patients who developed ARDS, 40 (91%) had sepsis. The important role of sepsis has been confirmed by Walker and Eiseman and a large number of other investigators. It has been our feeling, ever since we first began to study this problem in 1965 and 1966, that sepsis was virtually always present with ARDS and that if sepsis wasn't seen, you weren't looking hard enough.

AXIOM

One should look for inadequately controlled sepsis in any patient developing ARDS.

Most pulmonary changes following severe sepsis, shock, or trauma are related to superoxide radicals, lysosomal enzymes, and various vasoactive substances released from activated macrophages and damaged, necrotic, or infected tissues. These substances can adversely affect the function of pulmonary capillaries and their associated alveoli. Some of the vasoactive substances that have been implicated in the development of the respiratory distress syndrome include catecholamines, serotonin, histamine, and vasoactive polypeptides, such as bradykinin.

2. Shock

ARDS was initially called shock lung by some investigators. However, only 2% to 7% of patients presenting with hemorrhagic shock will develop ARDS. Trauma has also been an important etiologic factor for ARDS in some series. Severe prolonged shock may damage the lungs by causing (1) ischemic damage to the pneumocytes and supporting structures of the lung and (2) damage to peripheral tissues, which in turn can liberate a wide variety of noxious substances that can interfere with pulmonary blood flow and function.

Pulmonary ischemia interferes with cellular metabolism by the pneumocytes and causes atelectasis by reducing mucociliary clearance in the tracheobronchial tree and by decreasing surfactant production by the type II granular pneumocytes. Since the half-life of surfactant is about 12 to 18 hours, it has been postulated that failure of continued surfactant production may account for some of the respiratory distress that appears 24 to 48 hours following shock or injury. However, we found that if the blood supply to one lung in an experimental animal is clamped off during a period of shock or infection, the lung deprived of circulation is relatively well preserved for at least 1 to 2 hours. However, the other lung, which is still perfused, deteriorates rapidly. Thus, it appears that blood-borne substances and emboli are far more damaging than 1 to 2 hours of pulmonary ischemia. Furthermore, in spite of ischemia, pneumocytes may get enough oxygen from aerated alveoli to maintain their metabolism.

3. Trauma

Trauma can cause ARDS or contribute to its development in a wide variety of ways, including pulmonary contusions, flail chest, shock, head injury, fat embolism syndrome, aspiration of gastric contents, and massive transfusions. Fulton and Jones found post-traumatic pulmonary insufficiency in 22% of patients with multiple trauma with chest involvement and in 14% without chest involvement.

If the patient had a pulmonary infiltrate immediately after or within 6 hours of blunt chest trauma, one can usually assume that an element of lung contusion is present. In a recent series at our institution, the presence of moderate-severe pulmonary contusion significantly increased the incidence of later pneumonia.

4. Fat Embolism Syndrome

In patients with severe trauma and multiple long-bone fractures, the major cause of ARDS may be fat embolism syndrome. Stabilization of lower extremity

438

fractures within the first 24 hours, so that the patient may be gotten out of bed, significantly reduces the incidence of ARDS and death in most series.

5. Fluid Overload and Congestive Heart Failure

AXIOM

Any tendency toward fluid overload greatly increases the tendency to the pulmonary edema and congestion that can develop in patients with shock, sepsis, or trauma.

Even without fluid overload, an increase in capillary permeability can cause a greatly increased water content in the lungs, thereby making them stiffer and less efficient in the oxygenation of blood. If the plasma oncotic pressure is reduced by administration of excessive quantities of crystalloids, the likelihood of extravasation of fluid into the lungs is increased even further.

6. Massive Transfusions

Stored blood contains increased quantities of aggregated platelets, white blood cells, red blood cells, fibrin, and other particulate matter. If more than four blood transfusions are required, some physicians feel that a microfilter should be used to remove the abnormal aggregates while the blood is being administered. Leukoagglutinins may be particularly important in causing lung damage. If the resulting aggregates are not filtered out properly as blood is administered, they can cause damage to the lung, both mechanically by obstructing small arterioles and capillaries and chemically by the effect of various vasoactive amines. However, pulmonary involvement is generally not a problem unless 20 or more units is given rapidly. It is likely that it is the combination of shock with the transfusions which is important, and that the appearance of disseminated intravenous coagulation (DIC) is especially significant. DIC in 7 (23%) of 30 patients with ARDS was noted by Bone.

7. Aspiration of Gastric Contents

Aspiration of gastric contents occurs far more frequently than is usually recognized clinically. Aspiration may occur during anesthetic induction or following trauma, particularly if the patient has been unconscious. This can also occur during or following the insertion of a nasogastric tube, especially if it does not function well. Nasogastric tubes render the lower esophageal sphincter incompetent and can act as a wick for gastric contents to move up the esophagus into the pharynx and larynx.

AXIOM

A poorly functioning nasogastric tube is usually far more of a risk to the lungs than no nasogastric tube.

8. Centroneurogenic Reflexes

Insults to the central nervous system (CNS) such as head trauma, subarachnoid or intracerebral hemorrhage, and grand mal seizures, can cause neurogenic pulmonary edema (NPE). Acute fulminant NPE is rare, but increased extravascular lung water (EVLW) occurs rather frequently after head injury or subarachnoid hemorrhage.

Originally NPE was considered to result from an acute increase of intracranial pressure (ICP) or a direct injury to the hypothalamus or medulla, causing a massive discharge of catecholamines. The ensuing "sympathetic storm" can cause marked elevation of pulmonary capillary pressure (P_{mv}). The sudden increase in P_{mv} was thought to cause a permeability increase by endothelial damage and pore stretching. This allowed large molecules, such as protein, to be present in the pulmonary edema fluid in NPE. Although the permeability defect may cause formation of large quantities of pulmonary edema with a high protein content fluid, NPE may resolve over 24 hours.

This classic theory has been challenged because of numerous experimental and clinical reports in which NPE developed without any increases in hydrostatic pressure. Consequently, an alternative mechanism of a neurally mediated independent increase in permeability has been postulated.

Pulmonary edema that appears in the immediate postoperative period in previously healthy patients may also be related to a sudden sympathetic discharge caused by severe pain. Such patients usually have no narcotics included in their anesthetic management. This postoperative stress may be especially harmful in patients with pre-existing heart disease. A similar form of pulmonary edema occasionally appears after the postoperative administration of naloxone and may be explained by the sudden experience of pain that causes a sympathetic storm. Pretreatment of brain-injured or scaled rats with neurodepressant drugs such as morphine, pentobarbital sodium, haloperidol, diazepam, chlorpromazine, or urethane can result in significant attenuation of the development of an ARDS-like syndrome.

Other forms of catecholamine-associated pulmonary edema occur in pheochromocytoma and toxemia of pregnancy. However, high PAWPs, indicating a cardiogenic origin, are often reported in toxemic patients.

9. Smoke Inhalation

AXIOM

The pulmonary injury caused by smoke inhalation is now the major killer of burn patients.

Injury from inhalation of smoke can be due to swelling of the airway mucosa, chemical changes in the lung, and systemic absorption of inhaled toxins, especially carbon monoxide, cyanide gases, and other products of the combustion of plastics.

Early increase in extravascular lung water (EVLW) after burns is primarily due to the chemical toxicity of the inhaled gases. The worst pulmonary changes, however, are often delayed for several days and are generally due to systemic or pulmonary sepsis.

10. Oxygen Toxicity

Excessive concentrations of inspired oxygen are both wasteful and dangerous. Concentrations of oxygen over 60% can damage the lung within 3 to 4 days, causing increasing alveolar collapse, type II granular pneumocyte dysfunction, and impaired mucociliary clearance. However, the lung appears to tolerate oxygen concentrations of less than 40% to 50% indefinitely.

11. Multiple Risk Factors

A number of risk factors for ARDS were noted by Norwood and Civetta in 1985. These included systemic sepsis, pulmonary contusion, aspiration, inhalation of toxic substances, near drowning, fractures of long bones, severe pancreatitis, diffuse pneumonia, and multiple emergency blood transfusions. Pepe noted that the risk factors involved appear to be additive. The incidence of ARDS was 25% with one risk factor, 42% with two risk factors, and 85% with three risk factors.

Henao, Daes, and Dennis found that shock, sepsis, and time from onset of trauma or disease to treatment were independent risk factors for the development of multiple organ failure, of which respiratory failure was the most frequent.

D. MECHANISMS OF ACUTE LUNG INJURY

1. Noncardiogenic Pulmonary Edema

The normal lung weight at autopsy is usually less than 550 g on the right and 500 g on the left. With ARDS, each lung often weighs more than 1000 to 1200 g and when cut looks more like liver than lung. Much of the increased lung weight appears to be extravascular lung water (EVLW).

The hypothesis of the famous English physiologist, Ernest Henry Starling (1866–1927), was that the direction and rate of fluid flow between capillaries and tissue spaces varied with the hydrostatic and osmotic pressures on each side of the capillary and the properties of the capillary. These principles have been incorporated into the Starling equation as:

$$Q_f = K_f A \ [(P_{mv} - P_{pmv}) - \sigma(\pi_{mv} - \pi_{pmv})],$$

where Q_f = the net transvascular fluid flow
K_f = the permeability of the capillary to water and solutes
A   = the area of the capillary
P_{mv} = the microvascular (capillary) hydrostatic pressure
P_{pmv} = the perimicrovascular (interstitial space) hydrostatic pressure
σ = reflection coefficient
π_{mv} = microvascular oncotic pressure
π_{pmv} = perimicrovascular oncotic pressure

2. Microvascular Hydrostatic Pressure

The main determinant of filtration across capillaries is the microvascular hydrostatic pressure (P_{mv}). In cardiogenic pulmonary edema, the end-diastolic volume of the left ventricle increases due to incomplete ejection. The resultant elevated pressure leads to increased left atrial, pulmonary venous, and pulmonary microvascular pressures.

Clinically, the P_{mv} usually is estimated by the PAWP, although it may be more accurately calculated as:

$$P_{mv} = LAP + 0.4\,(PAP - LAP),$$

where LAP and PAP are the mean left atrial and pulmonary artery pressures, respectively. The constant, 0.4, denotes the estimated fraction of pulmonary vascular resistance that is downstream from the exchange vessels. In young healthy individuals the pulmonary capillary pressure is probably only 1 to 2 mm Hg higher than the PAWP and averages about 5 to 7 mm Hg.

The P_{mv} is influenced by gravity. In the upright position, it may be as much as 30 cm H_2O higher at the bottom than at the apex of the lung.

Pulmonary arterial hypertension is a frequent finding in patients with severe ARDS, but it is not generally considered to be a major determinant of transcapillary fluid movement. However, an increased PAP or PAWP can probably greatly increase edema formation if permeability is increased. Moreover, an increase in pulmonary blood flow will increase EVLW formation when PAWP is high, even in the absence of an increased permeability.

Very high perfusion pressures increase the passage of tracer substances from the capillary lumen into the interstitium. This observation forms the basis for the "stretched pores" theory, which suggests that high pressure within capillaries and small veins may cause physical (shear) damage to the endothelium. Although such pores have not been demonstrated, this concept blurs the distinction between high pressure and increased permeability as the etiologies of the pulmonary edema. However, recent experiments in which the entire cardiac output was directed into only a portion of the pulmonary vasculature revealed that the ensuing pulmonary edema was due only to high pressure, with no evidence of increased permeability.

AXIOM

A high PAWP not only increases movement of fluid into the interstitium because of the increased filtration pressure, but also because a dilated capillary is more permeable.

3. Interstitial Hydrostatic Pressure

The hydrostatic interstitial pressure or perimicrovascular pressure (P_{pmv}) is a subject of much debate, since its direct measurement is extremely difficult. Most researchers claim that it is negative, with the P_{pmv} being more negative near the hilum of the lungs than in the periphery. The value generally used is about -7 to -9 mm Hg. This gradient within the interstitium is probably a major factor in the early perihilar formation of interstitial edema. It acts in concert with the P_{mv} in increasing filtration from the microvessels into the interstitium. Loss of surfactant will tend to make the interstitial pressure more negative and increase the severity of interstitial edema.

4. Plasma Colloid Oncotic Pressure

The oncotic pressure (π_{mv}) generated by plasma proteins against the semipermeable capillary membrane draws water into the capillaries. Its value can be calculated or it can be directly measured. In young healthy individuals with normal plasma protein levels, it probably averages about 22 to 28 mm Hg. Because π_{mv} tends to "offset" the P_{mv}, this gradient is frequently used in clinical studies of critically ill patients as an approximation of the net pulmonary fluid balance. With a normal COP of 22 to 28 mm Hg and a PAWP of 5 to 10 mm Hg, the osmotic wedge pressure gradient is about 15 to 20 mm Hg. If the COP falls and PAWP rises so that the osmotic wedge pressure gradient is less than 4 mm Hg, the incidence and severity of pulmonary edema in congestive heart failure is greatly increased. Although hypoproteinemia by itself does not affect steady-state filtration across the endothelial membranes, it makes the lungs more susceptible to pulmonary edema if P_{mv} is elevated.

5. Interstitial Colloid Oncotic Pressure

Data concerning interstitial or perimicrovascular colloid oncotic pressures (π_{pmv}) come mainly from the analysis of lung lymph. Since the endothelial membrane acts as a partial sieve for plasma proteins, the interstitial protein concentration is lower. The ratio of the total protein concentration of the lymph to that of the plasma (L/P ratio) is normally about 0.6. However, it varies with protein molecules of different sizes.

6. Reflection Coefficient σ

Properties of the endothelial membrane responsible for the selective transmission of protein molecules are expressed by the reflection coefficient of Staverman, which is represented by the Greek letter, sigma (σ). This coefficient is a measure of the membrane impediment to the passage of specific protein molecules. Its value is 1.0 when the membrane is totally impermeable, and zero when the membrane allows free passage of those protein molecules.

Dilution of interstitial protein and reduction of π_{pmv} are important mechanisms in the readjustment of the pulmonary fluid balance during hydrostatic pulmonary edema. When P_{mv} is high and water traverses the endothelial membrane, there is dilution of interstitial proteins and a consequent reduction in π_{pmv} by as much as 50%. Like P_{mv} and P_{pmv}, π_{pmv} is not the same everywhere in the pulmonary interstitium, because the interstitial proteins are not distributed homogeneously.

In sepsis, and especially in ARDS, this protein reflection coefficient may fall to close to zero so that the plasma proteins are not very helpful in preventing flow of fluid into the interstitium. Initially the pulmonary lymphatics can carry away this fluid quite well, but as the ARDS progresses, they may not be able to keep pace.

E. CAUSES OF CAPILLARY AND ALVEOLAR DAMAGE

1. Excess Complement Activation

The initial inciting event in the production of ARDS is believed to occur from a capillary leak, presumably resulting from damage to the pulmonary capillary endothelium. Much of this damage is thought to be caused by substances released by neutrophils which aggregate in the lungs under the influence of complement, especially C5a.

AXIOM

Excess complement activation acting on neutrophils is probably the cause of many, if not most, cases of ARDS.

In 1968 Kaplow and Goffinet reported that leukopenia developed rapidly during hemodialysis in four patients with chronic renal failure. The fall in the white blood cell (WBC) count began within minutes of the onset of dialysis and disappeared within an hour. It was initially supposed that the leukocytes were trapped on the cellophane membrane of the dialyzer; however, it was later observed that many of these patients had a marked decrease in Po_2 at the time the leukocyte count decreased. Craddock and associates in their landmark report in 1977 noted that the pulmonary vascular bed was the hiding place of the disappearing leukocytes.

A search for the mechanism of this sequence of events prompted a series of laboratory experiments reported by Jacob in 1983. In these studies, sheep plasma exposed to a hemodialyzer was reinfused into the animals. These animals developed sudden profound leukopenia and pulmonary dysfunction. Examination of fresh lung specimens from these sheep showed that the pulmonary capillaries were filled with leukocytes, particularly granulocytes and monocytes.

Staub, using the sheep lymph fistula model, observed that the infusion of activated complement components resulted in pulmonary artery hypertension, profound neutropenia, arterial hypoxemia, and increased pulmonary lymph flow, suggesting a capillary leak. Furthermore, if the sheep were rendered granulocytopenic before the infusion of activated complement, the effects of the complement could be prevented.

It is now felt that aggregation of leukocytes occurs in this setting because complement is activated by the cellophane coil, and C5a is generated. C5a and C3a, also known as anaphylatoxins, cause leukocyte aggregation and margination and promote their embolization to pulmonary capillaries. Neutropenic animals and animals that are deficient in C5a do not develop an alveolar-capillary leak. Thus, neutrophils are not absolutely necessary for the development of ARDS.

Becker and Ward have noted that other chemotaxins that may lure the neutrophil to the pulmonary microvasculature include a wide variety of bacterial factors, lymphokines, prostaglandins, leukotrienes, and immunoglobulin fragments.

The current hypothesis regarding the pathogenesis of ARDS is that some noxious process, such as sepsis, activates four proteolytic cascades including complement, coagulation, kallikrein, and fibrinolysis, resulting in leukoagglutination, capillary leak, and creation of a fibrin network.

a. Role of the Neutrophil in ARDS

Numerous studies have shown large numbers of neutrophils in the pulmonary microvasculature of patients with ARDS and in laboratory animals given pancreatitis, infusions of endotoxin or live bacteria, and particulate microembolization. The same experiments in animals that are rendered neutropenic produce none of the sequelae noted in intact animals. Furthermore, bronchoalveolar lavage (BAL) in patients with ARDS has retrieved fluid that is rich in elastase and oxidants (presumably released from neutrophils), which are known to be directly toxic to the lung.

Marginating neutrophils are normally innocuous. However, if they become activated by complement or other substances, they adhere to pulmonary capillary endothelium, migrate across the basement membrane, and degranulate, causing severe tissue injury. The adherence of activated neutrophils and endothelial cells has been shown to be mediated in part by cell surface receptors, including the Mac-1 glycoprotein family on human neutrophils and intercellular adhesion molecule-1 and endothelial leukocyte adhesion molecule-1 glycoprotein receptors on endothelium.

There are a number of mechanisms whereby neutrophils can damage the lungs. Under aerobic conditions, neutrophils can increase their oxygen uptake up to 100-fold. During this "metabolic burst," using neutrophil plasma membrane bound NADPH oxidase, neutrophils produce a group of destructive toxic oxygen metabolites including superoxide, hydrogen peroxide, and hydroxyl radical. All of these, particularly the hydroxyl radical, can damage lipid membranes, lung fibroblasts, parenchymal cells, endothelial cells, and a variety of enzymes. Normal lung defense mechanisms such as alpha$_1$-antitrypsin may also be inactivated by superoxide radicals.

All of these oxygen by-products are capable of being produced by neutrophils. Studies of cultured lung endothelial cells exposed to granulocytes and activated complement show direct cellular injury. Accumulating evidence also suggests that "free radical scavengers," such as superoxide dismutase and catalase, may ameliorate some of the effects.

Neutrophil granules contain protease, elastase, collagenase, cathepsins, cationic proteins, lysozymes, lactoferrin (to chelate microbial iron), and myeloperoxidase. Collagenase destroys basement membrane, and elastase destroys elastic tissue in arterial walls and lung tissue.

The intensity of complement activation and the blood levels of elastase tend to correlate with injury severity (especially the severity of limb injury), development of adult respiratory distress syndrome, development and severity of multiple organ failure, and probability of a fatal outcome. In at least one study, the plasma elastase level seemed to be the best predictor of the development of the adult respiratory distress syndrome. Of a number of substances studied, it correlated the best with the injury severity score and multiple organ failure severity. This supports the hypothesis that post-traumatic activation of the complement system leads to activation of granulocytes, followed by microvascular injury and eventual organ failure.

Additional evidence of endothelial damage in ARDS is increased levels of angiotensin-converting enzyme (ACE) in blood and alveolar fluid in ARDS. ACE is normally present in the endothelial calls of the lung where it converts angiotensin I to angiotensin II and also inactivates bradykinin. It has been suggested that with endothelial injury, increased amounts of ACE get into the blood, and if enough alveolar capillary membrane is injured, ACE will also appear in alveolar fluid.

Proteases digest enzymes and structural proteins, activate complement Hageman factor and plasminogen, and cleave fibrinogen. Thus, it appears that protease can produce direct pulmonary injury and can also activate other deleterious substances that can produce pulmonary endothelial damage.

Neutrophils also release various metabolites of arachidonic acid, including prostaglandins, thromboxanes, and leukotrienes. These substances may promote vasoconstriction, alter capillary permeability, and act as chemoattractants for other neutrophils. Neutrophils also release the platelet activating factor, which promotes platelet and neutrophil agglutination and increased vascular permeability.

AXIOM

Although the neutrophil is often the main cause of the acute lung injury in ARDS, it is becoming increasingly clear that it is not absolutely essential.

Some patients with ARDS fail to demonstrate neutrophil aggregation histologically. Furthermore, Maunder and associates report the occurrence of ARDS in neutropenic patients. Consequently, other processes, especially disseminated intravascular coagulation and platelet aggregation, which are often found in patients with ARDS and probably also have important roles in acute lung injury.

b. Role of Coagulation Injury in ARDS

The initial pathologic differences between sepsis-induced and trauma-induced ARDS seem to be that in sepsis, complement activation and aggregation of granulocytes in the lungs are particularly important. In trauma, activation of the clotting system often appears to be the major factor.

AXIOM

Excess activation of the coagulation system, especially in trauma patients, may be an important contributing factor to the development of ARDS.

The coagulation system is involved in ARDS, but it is not clear whether this involvement is a primary or secondary event. It has been known for a number of years that patients with ARDS have a high incidence of pulmonary vascular occlusion as measured angiographically. Furthermore, increased platelet consumption and sequestration in the lung are noted in ARDS.

A variety of experiments conducted by Malik and coworkers indicate that complement, neutrophil, fibrin, and fibrin degradation products are essential components for the development of ARDS following microembolization. Platelets do not appear pivotal in the genesis of ARDS but are believed to release serotonin and other arachidonic acid metabolites that can cause pulmonary vasoconstriction.

The observation that heparin and fibrinogen depletion do not block the development of ARDS in experimental animals shows that not every portion of the coagulation system is equally important in ARDS. Additionally, certain coagulation products may produce direct lung injury. Manwaring, Thorning, and Curreri show that the infusion of thrombin and "antigen D" (one of the fibrin degradation products) causes increased capillary permeability and hypoxemia.

In normal animals, the reticuloendothelial system (RES) plays a major role in the clearance of both aggregates and products of fibrin degradation (FDP). Saba and colleagues have shown that fibronectin is a particularly important component of this RES function. Fibronectin is a glycoprotein with a molecular weight of 450,000. This substance is present on platelet membranes and throughout the RES, where it appears to function as a nonspecific opsonin in the removal of FDP, platelets, and other aggregates. Patients with ARDS usually have low levels of fibronectin. Since cryoprecipitate has a large amount of fibronectin, it was hoped that this material might be beneficial in the treatment of ARDS. Although there was an initial wave of enthusiasm for the therapeutic effects of cryoprecipitate, clinical confirmation of its value has not been forthcoming.

c. Role of Arachidonic Acid Metabolites in ARDS

Arachidonic acid is found in endothelial cells, platelets, neutrophils and other types of macrophages and may be converted through the cyclo-oxygenase pathway to prostaglandins or thromboxanes or through the lipoxygenase pathway to the leukotrienes. These products of arachidonic acid metabolism, together with mechanical obstruction of pulmonary capillaries by leukocytes, platelets, and fibrin thrombi, probably account for much of the pulmonary artery hypertension that is often seen in patients with ARDS.

AXIOM

Excess production of thromboxane and leukotrienes can contribute to the development and progression of ARDS.

Thromboxanes can cause bronchoconstriction and severe pulmonary vasoconstriction, which can lead to increased pulmonary vascular permeability. Pulmonary vasoconstriction can also be produced by several other arachidonic acid metabolites, including prostaglandins E_2, F_2, and H_2.

There is a two-phased pulmonary vascular response to infused endotoxin in experimental animals. In the first phase, an acute rise in pulmonary vascular resistance begins approximately 1 hour following infusion, and this rise in pulmonary vascular resistance can be blocked by thromboxane synthetase inhibitors. The second phase of pulmonary vasoconstriction begins within 3 to 5 hours and does not respond to arachidonic acid inhibitors, suggesting that this phase is not related to thromboxane.

For each action mediated by a prostaglandin, there is an opposite or antagonistic function mediated by another prostaglandin. The lung is no exception, and prostaglandins E_1 and I_2 (prostacyclin) counteract the deleterious effects of thromboxane. Prostacyclin (PGI_2) is a powerful vasodilator and is an antagonist to platelet and neutrophil aggregation.

There has been increased interest recently in the role of leukotrienes in ARDS. Samuelsson's work with pure leukotrienes has shown a variety of biologic effects including (1) bronchoconstriction (leukotrienes C_4, D_4, E_4); (2) arteriolar vasoconstrictor and leakage of macromolecules (leukotrienes C_4, D_4); (3) increased leukocyte adhesion to small vessel endothelium, interstitial migration, and activation causing aggregation, degranulation, and superoxide production (leukotriene B_4).

Recently Fink and associates studied the roles of leukotriene C_4 and platelet activating factor (PAF) in nine patients with ARDS and 84 control subjects. An assay of leukocyte adherence inhibition (LAI) induced by each of these ligands was used to monitor the subjects. LAI for both ligands was negative in all healthy subjects. In the studies on the nine ARDS patients, the LTC_4-induced LAI was positive in all nine, and the PAF-induced LAI was positive in three of the nine patients. All three patients in whom the ARDS was caused by sepsis responded to both LTC_4 and PAF. The results of this study suggest that LTC_4 and PAF may be involved in the pathogenesis of ARDS, especially by sepsis, and suggest that the LAI assay may be useful for early diagnosis and monitoring of septic ARDS.

VI. PATHOLOGIC CHANGES IN ARDS

The basic pathophysiologic processes involved in ARDS are interstitial and alveolar pulmonary edema and a decreased FRC due to a diffuse congestive microatelectasis. The sequential changes in the lung in ARDS on electron microscopic examination can be divided into an exudative phase resulting in increased interstitial and alveolar edema and a proliferative phase with increasing numbers of macrophages and fibroblasts resulting in increasing interstitial fibrosis.

A. EXUDATIVE PHASE

The main pathological changes in the exudative phase of ARDS include (1) aggregation of PMNs in the lung and disruption of pulmonary capillary endothelium, (2) interstitial edema, (3) congestive atelectasis, and (4) alveolar edema and disruption.

1. PMN Aggregation and Pulmonary Capillary Changes

Very early in ARDS, increased numbers of PMNs can be found in the lung, adhering to pulmonary capillary endothelium. Almost simultaneously, there is swelling and disruption of mitochondria in the pulmonary capillary endothelial cells. This appears to be at least partially related to release of superoxide radicals and lysosomal enzymes from the PMNs that have aggregated in the pulmonary capillaries. The capillary endothelial cells then begin to swell and retract from adjoining cells, leaving progressively enlarging intercellular spaces.

2. Interstitial Edema

The second step in the exudative phase consists of fluid moving from the capillaries into the interstitial space through defects in and between the pulmonary capillary endothelial cells. This interstitial edema begins in peribronchial tissues and makes the lung stiffer and more difficult to ventilate. It also reduces oxygen diffusion from alveoli into the capillaries and causes bronchiolar mucosal swelling, which further increases the tendency to atelectasis.

3. Congestive Atelectasis

The third step in the exudative phase is increasing congestive atelectasis, and it is at this point that the respiratory problem is usually first clinically recognized. The pulmonary capillaries become progressively more dilated and filled with red blood cells, and there is an increasingly severe diffuse microatelectasis throughout the lungs. The disruption of the pulmonary capillary endothelium may become so great that even red blood cells may migrate into the interstitial space, producing an appearance of peribronchial hemorrhage.

4. Alveolar Disruption and Edema

In the fourth step in the exudative phase, increasing disruption of the alveolar lining is recognized and fluid begins to move from the interstitial space into the alveoli. Proteins, particularly fibrinogen, begin to accumulate in the alveolar fluid and may inactivate the surfactant present, further increasing the tendency to atelectasis. Type I (flat) alveolar cells are rapidly destroyed, leaving a denuded alveolar basement except where the cuboidal type II cells are present. Protein and other debris in the alveolae may begin to precipitate out as a hyalinelike membrane.

5. Pneumonitis

At the end of the exudative phase, increasing numbers of bacteria can often be found in the involved areas of lung. The atelectasis and alveolar fluid seem to offer an ideal milieu for bacteria to grow and multiply.

B. EARLY PROLIFERATIVE PHASE

The early proliferative phase is characterized by increased numbers of inflammatory cells and erythrocytes in the interstitial tissue and alveoli. Within about 48 to 72 hours of injury, the cuboidal type II alveolar cells begin to proliferate, covering the previously denuded basement membrane. Aggregates of plasma proteins, cellular debris, and fibrin increasingly condense and adhere to the denuded alveolar surface, forming hyalinelike membranes that progressively organize to line the alveoli and their associated ducts.

The alveolar septum thickens markedly over the next 3 to 10 days as it is infiltrated by increasing numbers of fibroblasts, plasma cells, leukocytes, and histiocytes. Capillary injury becomes increasingly apparent at this stage, and increasingly severe diffuse microatelectasis is seen.

C. LATE PROLIFERATIVE PHASE

The late proliferative phase usually begins after a week to 10 days and is characterized by increasing interstitial and alveolar fibrosis. This often occurs first in alveolar septa and in the hyalinelike membranes. The fibrosis then progressively becomes most apparent in the respiratory ducts and bronchioles. Eventually the alveolar structures may become virtually unrecognizable.

D. RESOLUTION AND OUTCOME

Not all patients with ARDS progress through this entire pathologic process. Some patients recover within days and never develop fibrosis, whereas others progress to end-stage fibrosing alveolitis. However, even the extensively involved lung may resolve a large portion of this pulmonary fibrosis over time.

VII. DIAGNOSIS OF ARDS

A. HISTORY

A history of sepsis, prolonged shock, or severe trauma preceding the onset of increasing respiratory difficulty should arouse suspicion of ARDS. Norwood and Civetta note six clinical conditions that they thought were definite risk factors for the development of ARDS. These include systemic sepsis, pulmonary contusion, aspiration of gastric contents, inhalation of toxic substances (especially NO_2, NH_3, chlorine, and SO_2), near drowning, and fractures of long bones. We would modify this list to be systemic sepsis, multiple trauma (especially with coma, flail chest, or multiple long-bone fractures), prolonged shock, prolonged ventilatory support, aspiration of gastric contents, toxic inhalations, and near drowning. Other risk factors may include multiple emergency blood transfusions, diffuse pneumonia, and acute severe pancreatitis. A delay of at least 24 to 48 hours from the onset of severe prolonged shock, trauma, or sepsis to the development of signs and symptoms of ARDS is quite characteristic.

B. PHYSICAL EXAMINATION

AXIOM

By the time the patient with ARDS shows signs of respiratory difficulty, the process is quite far advanced.

The physical examination of patients with early or impending acute respiratory failure may be remarkably unrevealing. In phase I (acute injury), the only abnormality noted may be slight tachypnea and tachycardia. This is a relatively nonspecific sign, but it may be very important evidence of developing shock, sepsis, or respiratory failure, and its cause must always be sought after diligently.

In phase II (latent period) which lasts about 6 to 48 hours, the patient is clinically stable, but hyperventilation increases slightly, and there is a slight increase in the work of breathing. Some basilar rales may be heard.

In phase III (acute respiratory failure) there is marked tachypnea and dyspnea and diffuse rales are heard.

In phase IV (severe acute respiratory failure), the patient must usually be on a ventilator to be alive, and there is clinical evidence of increasing pulmonary edema and consolidation (Table 10.2).

It is very difficult to judge a patient's blood gases merely by appearance. For example, a patient with a hemoglobin of less than 10 g/dl usually does not appear to be cyanotic unless skin perfusion is extremely poor. There must generally be at least 5.0 g/dl of reduced hemoglobin at the capillary level before a patient begins to look cyanotic. Since mixed venous oxygen saturation seldom falls below 40% to 50%, if the hemoglobin is less than 10 g/dl, the arterial oxygen saturation to cause cyanosis would have to be 50% to 60% or less.

PITFALL

Assuming that ARDS developed suddenly.

Patients frequently seem to develop clinical signs of ARDS rather suddenly; however, retrospective analysis of blood gases will often show that the process had been developing for at least 24 to 48 hours previously. Unless the patient is hyperventilating excessively or the arterial Po_2 is less than 55 to 60 mm Hg, many patients will not appear to have a serious pulmonary problem until rather late.

Table 10.2

ACUTE RESPIRATORY FAILURE

Blood Gas Changes during the Phases of Adult Respiratory Distress Syndrome
(Assuming Normal or Increased Cardiac Output)

Phases	Clinical Evidence of Respiratory Distress	Chest X-Ray	While Breathing Room Air (FIO_2 = 0.21)			
			PaO_2 (mm Hg)	$PaCO_2$ (mm Hg)	$P(A\text{-}a)O_2$ (mm Hg)	Qs/Qt, %
Normal	—	—	80–100	35–45	5–10	3–5
I: Injury and resuscitation	None	Normal	70–90	30–40	20–40	5–14
II: Subclinical respiratory distress	Mild-to-moderate tachypnea	Minimal or no infiltrate	68–80	25–35	30–50	10–15
III: Established respiratory distress	Increasing tachypnea	Increasing edema and confluence of infiltrates	50–60	20–35	40–60	20–30
IV: Severe respiratory failure three stages	Obvious respiratory failure	Increasing opacifications of the lungs	35–50	30–60	50–80	30–50

AXIOM

By the time it is evident that the patient has the classic signs of respiratory failure, such as the use of accessory muscles of respiration or flaring of the alae nasae, ARDS is usually far advanced and difficult to reverse.

C. X-RAY EXAMINATION

PITFALL

Using a normal chest x-ray to rule out early ARDS.

Roentgenographic features of adult respiratory distress syndrome are not present in phase I and most of phase II. The changes in phase II resemble those of early pulmonary edema. This is followed by increasing amounts of diffuse interstitial infiltrates which progress on to a diffuse, fluffy, panacinar pattern.

AXIOM

There is often a 12 to 36 hour delay in the appearance of the x-ray changes of ARDS. The x-ray changes are also slow to leave as the patient improves.

Computed tomographic (CT) scans may show patchy infiltrates interspersed with areas of normal-appearing lung. The fact that ARDS spares some regions of lung parenchyma can help one to understand the gas exchange abnormalities of ARDS, the variable responsiveness to positive end-expiratory pressure (PEEP), and the occurrence of oxygen toxicity. It also helps in interpreting lung biopsy specimens or bronchoalveolar lavage fluid in patients with ARDS.

At least one study has shown that, under controlled conditions, there is an excellent correlation between the amount of extravascular lung water (EVLW) and x-ray scoring of the amount of lung water in cardiac patients. In another study, however, the correlation was very poor.

VIII. BLOOD GAS STUDIES IN ARDS

A. pH

The typical patient with ARDS has a respiratory alkalosis initially. However, many have a metabolic alkalosis prior to the development of ARDS. If the patient has a metabolic alkalosis, the Pao_2 and $Paco_2$ may be low as a compensatory response rather than because of any pulmonary changes. In contrast, a normal Pco_2 in the presence of moderate-severe metabolic acidosis can be an important indication of severe ventilatory insufficiency, and this is not usually seen until the last phase of ARDS, unless the patient has an underlying COPD.

B. PaCO$_2$

In most patients with ARDS, the arterial Pco_2 is in the range of 25 to 35 mm Hg. When the $Paco_2$ rises above 45 mm Hg, in spite of a minute ventilation that is two to three times normal, the prognosis is extremely poor. Under such circumstances, the number of perfused functioning capillaries in the pulmonary parenchyma may be so critically reduced that it is impossible for the patient to eliminate carbon dioxide adequately through the lungs, no matter how great the ventilation (Table 10.3).

AXIOM

If the $PaCO_2$ is low but begins to rise in a patient in whom the Pao_2 and/or the pH is falling, the patient probably requires ventilatory support.

C. PaO$_2$

A falling Pao_2, which responds poorly to an increased Fio_2, is characteristic of the increased shunt in ARDS. Thus, a patient with a large physiologic shunt might have a Pao_2 of 50 mm Hg when breathing room air and a Pao_2 of only 80 to 100 mm Hg when breathing 100% oxygen. One should also be aware that the amount of psychological shunting in the lung may be quite varied at any particular Pao_2 (Fig. 10-3).

449

Table 10.3

INDICATIONS FOR VENTILATORY ASSISTANCE*			Ventilatory Assistance	
		Normal Values†	Is Suggested If*	Is Generally Mandatory If*
PCO_2 and dead space	$PaCO_2$ (mm Hg)	30–40*	45–55	>55
	VDS/VT	0.3–0.4	0.50–0.60	>0.60
Oxygenation	PaO_2 (mm Hg) $FIO_2 = 0.21$	80–90	50–60	<50
	PaO_2 (mm Hg) $FIO_2 = 1.0$	550–630	200–300	<200
	$P(A\text{-}a)O_2$ $FIO_2 = 0.21$	5–20	55–60	>60
$P(A\text{-}a)O_2$	$P(A\text{-}a)O_2$ $FIO_2 = 1.0$	20–60	350–450	>450
	Qs/Qt (%)	3–5	15–25	>25
Mechanics of ventilation	Respiratory rate	10–12	30–35	>35
	Tidal volume (ml/kg)	5–8	3.5–4.0	<3.5
	Vital capacity (ml/kg)	50–70	10.0–15.0	<10.0

*In previously healthy individuals with sepsis and/or trauma.
†In middle-aged or older hospitalized patients.

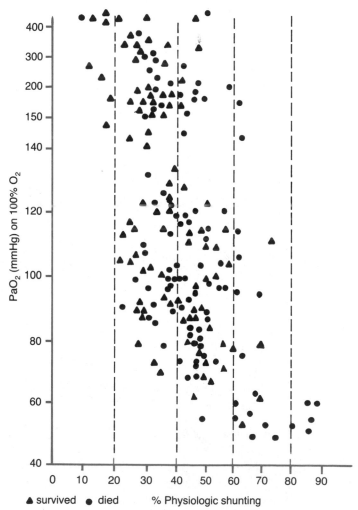

▲ survived ● died   % Physiologic shunting

Figure 10.3 Correlation between PaO_2 on 100% oxygen and physiologic shunting.

D. ALVEOLAR-ARTERIAL OXYGEN DIFFERENCE

The alveolar-arterial oxygen difference in a patient with previously normal lungs and a normal cardiac output at sea level while breathing room air, may be estimated by subtracting the sum of the arterial Po_2 and Pco_2 from 145 (i.e., $P[A\text{-}a]o_2 = 145 - [Pao_2 + Paco_2]$). Thus, a patient with a $Paco_2$ of 20 and Pao_2 of 60 mm Hg would have a $P(A\text{-}a)o_2$ of about 60 to 65 mm Hg.

AXIOM

A $P(A\text{-}a)o_2$ of 55 mm Hg or more in young healthy adults breathing room air at sea level is generally evidence of severe respiratory failure.

According to the alveolar gas equation, the alveolar Po_2 (Pao_2) expected at sea level while breathing 100% oxygen is equal to the barometric pressure (P_B) of 760 mm Hg minus the water vapor pressure (P_{H_2O}) of 47 mm Hg and the $Paco_2$ divided by the RQ. Thus, if the Pco_2 were 40 mm Hg and the RQ were 0.8 on 100% oxygen at sea level, the Pao_2 would be about 663 mm Hg. For example,

$$
\begin{aligned}
PAO_2 &= [(P_B - P_{H_2O})\,(FIO_2)] - Paco_2/RQ \\
&= [(760 - 47)\,(1.0)] - 40/0.8 \\
&= 713 - 50 \\
&= 663.
\end{aligned}
$$

If one obtains an arterial sample after the patient has been breathing 100% oxygen ($FIO_2 = 1.0$) for 20 to 30 minutes, one can simply apply the formula for calculating the PAO_2 and subtract the measured Pao_2. For example, if the Pao_2 is 300 mm Hg on an FIO_2 of 1.0, the $Paco_2$ is 40 and the RQ is 0.8,

$$
\begin{aligned}
P(A\text{-}a)o_2 &= PAO_2 - pao_2 \\
&= 663 - 300 \\
&= 363.
\end{aligned}
$$

A $P(A\text{-}a)o_2$ of more than 300 mm Hg usually indicates that ventilatory assistance with PEEP is required.

E. Pao_2/FIO_2 RATIO

A Pao_2/FIO_2 ratio that is less than 200 is equivalent to a physiologic shunt in the lung of about 20% and indicates a need for ventilatory assistance. The lower the Pao_2/FIO_2 ratio below 200, the greater the need for PEEP.

F. PHYSIOLOGIC SHUNT

If the physiologic shunt in the lung exceeds 20% to 25% in the presence of acute sepsis or trauma, the patient should receive ventilatory assistance. If the shunt exceeds 25% to 30% or if the patient is not responding to aggressive ventilatory assistance, one should probably use increasing amounts of positive end-expiratory pressure (PEEP) to get the FIO_2 to less than 0.4 to 0.5.

G. SHUNT INDEX

AXIOM

As cardiac output increases, the physiologic shunt in the lung will also increase.

If blood flow through the lung is very low, it will tend to go through the better ventilated portions of the lung. Consequently, for the same amount of pulmonary pathology, the shunt will tend to be lower with a lower cardiac output. With a higher cardiac output, increased amounts of the blood will go through poorly ventilated areas and increase the shunt. As a consequence, any factor increasing cardiac output tends to increase the amount of shunting in the lung.

To take the effect of blood flow on shunt into account, we occasionally calculate the shunt index. This is the percentage of shunt divided by the cardiac index. Thus, if the Qs/Qt is 24% and the cardiac index is 3.0 liters $\cdot$ min^{-1} $\cdot$ m^{-2}, the SI is 8.0. A patient with a shunt of 30% and a cardiac index of 5.0, has an SI of 6.0 and usually has less pulmonary dysfunction than the patient with an SI of

8.0. In most instances an SI of more than 5.0 probably requires PEEP and aggressive ventilatory support.

XI. CLINICAL PHASES OF ARDS

The development of respiratory insufficiency following injury may be divided into four phases (Table 10.2): injury and resuscitation, subclinical respiratory distress, established respiratory distress, and severe respiratory failure.

A. PHASE I (INJURY AND RESUSCITATION)

The injury and resuscitation phase of ARDS is characterized by altered tissue perfusion and metabolism. Unless there is a problem with CNS depression or damage to the airway, chest wall, or lungs, a mild-moderate respiratory alkalosis is generally present. The arterial Po_2 in previously healthy individuals will be about 70 to 80 mm Hg. The $Paco_2$ is usually in the range of 30 to 40 mm Hg. The Qs/Qt is only about 8% to 12%. The lungs are frequently clear on physical examination except for a few basilar rales or rhonchi. The chest x-ray generally appears to be normal.

B. PHASE II (SUBCLINICAL RESPIRATORY DISTRESS)

In this phase, the hyperventilation continues and the $Paco_2$ is often in the range of 25 to 35 mm Hg. The alveolar-arterial oxygen difference while a patient breathes room air may increase to 35 to 50 mm Hg, but there is still relatively little clinical evidence of a significant respiratory problem. X-rays at this time may again be normal or there may be mild diffuse infiltrates, compatible with multiple small areas of atelectasis and perihilar pulmonary congestion.

C. PHASE III (ESTABLISHED RESPIRATORY DISTRESS)

During this phase, it becomes clinically apparent that the patient is developing a significant respiratory problem. Although it often seems as if the problem had developed rather suddenly, serial blood gas determinations usually indicate that the problem had been developing progressively and the only thing that was sudden was the recognition of the problem. The patient tends to hyperventilate even more with a further drop in the $Paco_2$ to 20 to 35 mm Hg, and the Pao_2 may begin to fall to 50 to 60 mm Hg or lower. The $P(A-a)o_2$ on room air is often 50 to 70 mm Hg or more, and the pulmonary shunt is generally 20% to 30% or greater. Increasing pulmonary edema and progressive confluence of the previously scattered diffuse infiltrates is noted on the chest x-ray.

D. PHASE IV (SEVERE RESPIRATORY FAILURE)

This phase is characterized by increasingly severe hypoxia with a shunt of 30% to 40% or more. An Fio_2 of 0.8 to 1.0 is often required to maintain a $Pao_2 \geq 60$ mm Hg. The $Paco_2$ may gradually rise back toward normal or higher in spite of a minute ventilation that may exceed 15 to 20 liters. This is usually associated with a dead space/tidal volume ratio (V_d/V_t exceeding 0.60 to 0.65.

This combination of a greatly increased shunt and dead space is often associated with multiple organ failure and is usually lethal unless it can be reversed fairly rapidly. During this phase, increasing metabolic acidosis may also be noted, and the lungs may become almost completely opaque (whited-out) on chest x-ray.

X. TREATMENT OF ACUTE RESPIRATORY FAILURE

Therapy for acute respiratory failure is most effective when the problem is anticipated and vigorous prophylactic measures are instituted early. A patient with a high cardiac output and normal hemoglobin can generally tolerate a moderately low Pao_2 relatively well because oxygen delivery (Do_2) will be only mildly reduced. However, a patient with severe anemia and/or a low cardiac output tends to tolerate a low Pao_2 poorly.

A. NURSING CARE

Nursing care for patients who are apt to develop respiratory complications should include stimulation of the patient to cough and take deep breaths, position changes every 30 to 60 minutes, elevation of the head and chest as much as possible, and frequent chest physiotherapy. Early ambulation, coughing, and use of an incentive spirometer, such as the Tri-Flo, can be particularly helpful. Such preventive measures should be instituted early when they are most apt to be beneficial.

1. Encouraging Coughing and Deep Breathing

AXIOM

Proper coughing is the best method for preventing or treating atelectasis.

Whenever possible, proper coughing should be taught to patients preoperatively. According to Chevalier Jackson, the father of bronchoesophagology, the process of coughing can be divided into three phases: deep inhalation, bearing down with a closed glottis (ptussive squeeze), and the cough itself (blephic blast). If patients have such severe pain that they are unable to inhale deeply, they usually cannot produce an effective cough. Bearing down helps to "squeeze" secretions out of the alveoli and smaller bronchioles into the larger bronchi, where the subsequent blast of air may carry the material out of the lungs.

Judicious use of pain medication is required postoperatively and in the ICU. Enough analgesic should be given to facilitate coughing and proper breathing, but if too much is given, it may depress the cough reflex and ventilation.

AXIOM

If pain is quantified on a scale of 0 (no pain) to 10 (the worst pain imaginable), one should try to get the patient's pain down to a 3. One should not give enough analgesic for the patient to have no pain, but only enough so that the pain does not bother the patient.

Epidural analgesia is particularly helpful for relieving pain from surgical incisions or fractured ribs. However, with epidural analgesia, apnea monitoring in an ICU or step-down ICU environment is required. Apnea may occur up to 16 to 24 hours after a dose of epidural analgesia. For incisions in the chest or upper abdomen, properly performed intercostal nerve block with 0.5% bupivacaine (Marcaine) may provide pain relief for 6 to 12 hours.

Bragg, in a recent review of interpleural analgesia with injection of 20 to 30 ml of 0.25% to 0.5% bupivacaine with 1 : 200,000 epinephrine, found that this technique could produce analgesia of rapid onset and long duration in the great majority of postoperative and post-trauma patients with much less problem than IV or epidural analgesia. Baker and Tribble have also reported success with this procedure, using a pleural catheter inserted through a chest tube. Pleural effusions, pneumonia, bullous emphysema, and PEEP are the only major contraindications.

It is not unusual for intubated patients to have many rales or rhonchi, but little or no secretions recovered on aspiration of the trachea and major bronchi. In such patients, an effective cough may sometimes be obtained by temporarily occluding the tube after a deep inspiration. An effect similar to the normal process of bearing down may then be achieved so that a better blast phase can be obtained.

AXIOM

Operative stabilization of lower extremity fractures within 24 hours of injury can decrease the incidence of pulmonary infections, fat embolism syndrome, and ARDS.

In one study of 132 consecutive patients with multiple musculoskeletal injuries, the length of time from injury to the operative stabilization of the lower extremity fractures correlated with the incidence of ARDS. A delay in fracture-stabilization surgery greater than 24 hours was associated with a fivefold increase in the incidence of ARDS ($P < 0.001$). For the more severely injured patients (Injury Severity Score greater than 40), the ARDS rates were 17% with early fracture stabilization and 75% with delayed surgery ($P < 0.001$).

AXIOM
Severe hypophosphatemia can impair ventilatory effort.

Since hypophosphatemia can impair muscle function, its effects on diaphragmatic function were studied in eight patients who had acute respiratory failure and required ventilatory assistance. The mean serum phosphorus level was 0.55 ± 0.18 mmol/liter (normal 1.20 ± 0.10). After phosphate infusion, the mean serum phosphorus level increased significantly to 1.33 ± 0.21 mmol/liter. The increase in serum phosphorus was accompanied by a marked increase in the transdiaphragmatic pressure after phrenic nerve stimulation (17.3 ± 6.5 versus 9.8 ± 3.8 cm H_2O) ($P < 0.001$). The increase in the serum phosphorus levels correlated fairly well with the increases in transdiaphragmatic pressure ($r = 0.73$).

2. Frequent Position Changes

AXIOM
Whenever possible, bedridden critically ill patients should be turned as far prone as possible at least once every 2 hours.

Frequent position changes of all types to change the ventilation and perfusion patterns within the lung can significantly reduce the tendency to atelectasis. At any one time, at least a third of the patients in the intensive care unit should be on one side or the other or sitting relatively upright.

3. Elevation of the Head and Chest

Elevation of the head and chest decreases the pressure put on the diaphragm by the abdominal viscera. The upright position for the chest produces the best overall ventilation/perfusion ratios for the lung. All too often these maneuvers are given too low a priority in the patient care plan. Monitoring lines, intravenous lines, drains, and ventilation tubing should be placed so that they will not interfere with turning patients or sitting them up.

Proper positioning of obese patients is particularly important. When an obese patient is lying flat, the weight of the anterior chest and abdominal viscera press against the diaphragm and can greatly increase the work of breathing. Such an individual should, therefore, either be kept sitting up or lying on the side as much as possible.

4. Chest Physiotherapy

Chest percussion and dependent drainage (CPDD) is becoming increasingly popular in the United States as a method to prevent or treat atelectasis. Vibration therapy with the patient in various positions may also be helpful in removing mucous plugs.

B. GENERAL MEASURES

Some general measures that should be performed to help reduce the tendency toward pulmonary complications in critically ill or injured patients include early recognition and control of infection, reduction of abdominal distention, reduction of oxygen demand, and, in selected instances, chest tube drainage of the pleural cavities.

1. Prevention and Control of Infection

Prevention or control of infection is extremely important in any patient with a tendency to ARDS. In patients with increasing pulmonary insufficiency of unknown etiology, special efforts must be made to diagnose occult infection.

AXIOM

The most common reason for increasing respiratory failure in spite of optimal therapy is uncontrolled infection.

Cultures of the blood and all possible infected or contaminated sites must be taken, and all intravenous catheters should be changed if the patient is running a temperature >101.4°F without obvious cause. If the patient has had abdominal surgery, a CT scan of the abdomen and pelvis may be particularly helpful.

2. Reduction of Abdominal Distention

Abdominal distention should be prevented and vigorously treated by nasogastric suction. Once swallowed air reaches the small bowel and ileus develops, it is very difficult to relieve abdominal distension. The patency of the nasogastric tube must be checked frequently.

AXIOM

If a nasogastric tube is not functioning, its presence does more harm than good.

Not only do nasogastric tubes irritate the pharynx and create increased upper respiratory tract secretions, but if it is not working properly, it increases the incidence of aspiration of gastric contents. When the patient is lying flat, retained gastric contents can move up alongside the nasogastric tube to the pharynx and larynx, where they subsequently can be aspirated into the lungs. In patients who will require prolonged gastrointestinal intubation and who have pre-existing severe pulmonary disease, it may be wise to insert a jejunostomy tube and/or gastrostomy tube rather than rely on prolonged nasogastric intubation.

If ascites is present, careful removal of excessive intraperitoneal fluid may help reduce the pressure against the diaphragm. However, proper attention must be given to blood pressure and pulse rate during paracentesis to ensure that hypovolemia or hypotension does not develop. If repeated taps are required, one must also be concerned about the effects of the protein loss.

3. Reduction of Fever, Pain, and Restlessness

If the patient has a fever or is restless, antipyretics and careful use of analgesics and/or sedatives in small IV doses may help to reduce excessive oxygen demands. However, excess sedatives or analgesics in critically ill or injured patients may drastically reduce their efforts to breathe, and ventilation must be either controlled or watched very carefully if such agents are used.

AXIOM

One should always look for hypoxia or hypotension after an analgesic or sedative is given.

The nurse must be aware of the effects of analgesics or sedatives administered to any sick, injured, or postoperative patient and must observe such individuals extremely carefully. Frequently, patients who have suffered severe trauma or have just had an operation will appear to be restless because of severe pain. However, the restlessness or confusion may be due to hypoxia. If an analgesic, particularly a large dose of morphine or meperidine, is given when hypoxia is present, the resultant decrease in ventilation and additional hypoxia could be fatal.

AXIOM

Restlessness should be considered due to hypoxia until proven otherwise.

Narcotics and sedatives are contraindicated in restless patients until it has been shown that the patient's ventilation and oxygenation are adequate.

4. Thoracentesis for Excessive Pleural Fluid

Increased pleural fluid is frequent in patients with ARDS, especially those who have abdominal sepsis. This fluid should be drained; however, insertion of subclavian vein catheters or thoracentesis in intubated patients must be done very cautiously. Even a minimal lung puncture in a patient requiring ventilatory assistance greatly increases the tendency to develop a tension pneumothorax, particularly if high ventilatory pressures and PEEP are being used.

5. Thoracotomy Tubes for Pleural Fluid or High Ventilatory Pressures

AXIOM

Greatly increased inflation pressures often indicate that increased tracheobronchial secretions or significant amounts of pleural fluid are present.

Many patients with ARDS, particularly those with peritonitis, have increased pleural fluid, which is often missed on plain chest x-rays if the patient is supine. If high ventilatory pressures are required, one should suspect that a pleural effusion is present. Bilateral chest tubes in patients with high ventilatory pressures (>50 to 60 cm H_2O) also help to prevent sudden death if a pneumothorax develops.

C. FLUID THERAPY

AXIOM

Any rise in pulmonary capillary pressure will tend to make ARDS worse.

Because most patients with ARDS have excessive lung water, particularly in the pulmonary interstitial space, careful dehydration can be extremely helpful. Therefore, once the patient has been properly resuscitated and oxygen delivery (Do_2) is known to be adequate, gradual dehydration should be initiated. This, however, must be done very cautiously so that the patient's vital signs, urine output, and Do_2 are well maintained. Sudden or severe dehydration may impair tissue perfusion and cause even more cardiopulmonary deterioration. Careful, gradual dehydration can often pull relatively large quantities of fluid from the interstitial space with relatively little decrease in preload to the heart.

Even if a patient is on TPN or requires fairly large amounts of fluid to maintain an adequate urine output, it is still possible to dehydrate her or him. To accomplish this, one must strive, using diuretics as needed, to make the measured hourly fluid output equal to or slightly greater than the hourly fluid intake. This allows the patient to be dehydrated by at least the insensible water loss. In most normal adults on a ventilator with maximal humidification, this averages to 20 to 30 ml/h. Thus, if an adequate urine output is maintained with diuretics and the fluid intake is equal to or slightly less than the measured fluid output (including urine), the patient will be gradually dehydrated by approximately 500 to 1500 ml a day. One method for determining the effectiveness of dehydration efforts is to follow the serum osmolarity. If the serum osmolarity rises progressively until it approaches or exceeds 300 mOsm/liter, this is evidence that the efforts at dehydration are successful.

AXIOM

Although dehydration will tend to improve most patients with ARDS, it must be done carefully so as to not interfere with oxygen delivery.

If the patient is septic, it may be extremely difficult to remove fluid without interfering with tissue perfusion. Septic patients often have greatly increased capillary permeability and require over 200 to 300 ml of IV fluid each hour over and above measured output to maintain an adequate intravascular volume. A restricted fluid intake in such patients can quickly cause hypotension and oliguria, resulting in further pulmonary and renal deterioration.

There is much controversy about the use of colloids in patients with ARDS. If the pulmonary capillary permeability is normal, an increased colloid osmotic pressure may help to draw fluid from the interstitial space into the vascular space. However, because the capillary permeability is generally increased in ARDS, infused colloids (particularly albumin) may quickly leave the capillary space and enter the interstitial fluid space, where they can then draw in even more interstitial fluid. As a consequence, colloids (particularly albumin) are given cautiously, if at all, in ARDS, even if there is moderate-to-severe hypoproteinemia.

1. Continuous Arteriovenous Hemofiltration

One method for removing excess water, particularly in patients with acute renal failure, is continuous arteriovenous hemofiltration (CAVH). In one study, continued deterioration due to fluid overload was treated very successfully by CAVH, which produced a dramatic improvement in 22 of 24 patients.

The characteristics of the peptides that cause permeability pulmonary edema are such that many of these substances are cleared during one pass through the hemofiltration device. Thus, hemofiltration may be very helpful in the treatment of ARDS, especially if there is concurrent renal failure.

2. Hemoglobin Levels

AXIOM
Critically ill patients with severe sepsis and/or ARDS tend to do better with higher hemoglobin levels (11.0 to 12.5 g/dl).

In most centers, the hematocrit in critically ill patients is kept around 30% to 35%, and this level generally provides adequate oxygen transport. However, a hemoglobin level of 12.0 to 14.0 g may be preferable in septic patients, especially those with ARDS. The mortality rates and the amount of physiologic shunting in the lung in our patients appear to be decreased by the higher hemoglobins. We also found that the Do_2 and Vo_2 were increased significantly as hemoglobin levels were raised from below 10.0 g/dl to above 12.5 g/dl.

D. DRUGS

1. Bronchodilators

AXIOM
Any past or present evidence of bronchospasm should be an indication for carefully trying bronchodilators in patients developing any symptoms or signs of respiratory distress.

Bronchodilators should be given if there is any evidence of bronchospasm or increased airway resistance. Since airway resistance often has to be increased to more than four times normal before it becomes clinically evident, it may be wise to give a bronchodilator on a trial basis to patients with high ventilatory pressures and note the response. If the patient is on a ventilator, one can estimate changes in airway resistance by computing the dynamic compliance (tidal volume divided by the peak inflation pressure, or PIP) before and after the bronchodilators. One can also determine how much of the PIP is due to airway resistance by noting the difference between the PIP and plateau pressure if a 0.5-second inspiratory hold is applied (Fig. 10.4).

Recently it has been found that some bronchodilators may have benefits other than just bronchodilation. Increased pulmonary vascular permeability leading to increased plasma protein extravasation and accumulation (PPA) in the interstitial fluid is a characteristic feature of acute lung injury. Interestingly, beta$_2$-agonists, such as terbutaline, in therapeutic doses can reduce the increased lung vascular permeability and reduce PPA in some patients.

457

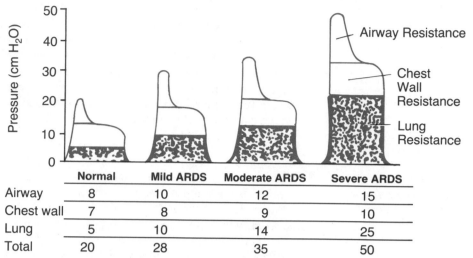

Figure 10.4 Ventilatory pressures required to overcome airway resistance, chest wall resistance, and lung resistance in normal individuals and in patients with ARDS.

	Normal	Mild ARDS	Moderate ARDS	Severe ARDS
Airway	8	10	12	15
Chest wall	7	8	9	10
Lung	5	10	14	25
Total	20	28	35	50

2. Digitalis and Diuretics

Diuretics should be used, as needed, if there is evidence of overt heart failure, and digoxin may also be helpful, especially with atrial fibrillation. Diuretics in multiple small doses may also be required to help dehydrate patients with ARDS, even if there is no evidence of congestive heart failure (CHF).

3. Steroids

Since aspiration of gastric contents may produce a severe chemical pneumonitis, some physicians believe that hydrocortisone should be started as soon as there is evidence that aspiration has occurred. The data, however, are conflicting, and most investigators believe that there is no good evidence for the use of hydrocortisone under such circumstances. If steroids are given, a suggested dose is 50 to 100 mg of hydrocortisone or 4 to 6 mg of dexamethasone every 4 to 6 hours.

In the fat embolism syndrome, multiple studies have shown benefit from early administration of steroids. Given prophylactically, they have been found to reduce the amount of hypoxemia that develops. Steroids have also shown some benefit when administered after clinical signs of FES have developed.

AXIOM

Steroids in ARDS are very controversial, but they may be helpful in selected patients in the late proliferative (increasing fibrosis) stage if no bacterial infection is present.

In established ARDS, high-dose corticosteroids often increase mortality and morbidity. However, Ashbaugh and Maier successfully used corticosteroids in patients who had established ARDS as their primary clinical problem. Hooper and Kearl have noted that, in the studies that did not demonstrate benefit from high-dose corticosteroid therapy, the duration of ARDS before treatment was brief and the state of the process that initiated the ARDS was not mentioned. These authors report 10 patients with established ARDS and no infection who were treated with prolonged courses of adrenocortical steroids. Eight of the 10 patients had uninterrupted courses of the steroids for greater than 21 days, and for 12 days, the dose of methylprednisolone was greater than 40 mg/d. Eight (80%) of these 10 patients survived. Thus, corticosteroids may be of benefit in selected ARDS patients in the late proliferative phase, if there is no bacterial infection present.

4. Prostaglandin E₁

PGE₁ markedly decreases pulmonary artery pressure, pulmonary and systemic vascular resistance, and venous pressures, while increasing cardiac output, Pa_{O_2}, oxygen delivery, and oxygen consumption in experimental animals. The data are consistent with the concept that this drug reduces vasoconstriction in the pulmonary and systemic circulations. One study in septic patients shows some improvement with PGE₁, but a more recent large multicenter study by Bone, Francis, and Pierce shows no significant benefit.

5. Ketanserin

Ketanserin is a new experimental drug that is an antagonist of serotonin receptors in blood vessels, platelets, and bronchial tissue. This agent can reduce the increase in pulmonary and systemic vascular resistance that occurs experimentally after infusion of endotoxin. However, no good clinical data is available on this agent at this time.

E. INHALATION THERAPY

Proper aerosolization and nebulization may help reduce the viscosity of mucoid material in the bronchi, making it easier for the patient to cough up secretions. Intermittent positive-pressure breathing (IPPB) may also be very helpful if it stimulates the patient to breathe and cough properly or if it carries needed moisture or medication into the tracheobronchial tree. However, if it accomplishes none of these, it will actually tend to cause bronchoconstriction and impair pulmonary function, unless given with a bronchodilator.

It is now well recognized that the routine use of IPPB postoperatively probably does not reduce the incidence of pulmonary complications. However, any technique (whether it is "blow bottles" or blowing up gloves) that causes the patient to breathe and cough deeper is of value. An incentive spirometer, such as the Tri-Flo, if used properly, may be particularly beneficial.

F. VENTILATORY ASSISTANCE

AXIOM

If ventilatory assistance in critically ill or injured patients is delayed until there is clinical evidence of severe respiratory failure, correction of the pulmonary insufficiency can be extremely difficult and the prognosis is much poorer.

1. Clinical Indications for Ventilatory Support

Clinical situations in which early ventilatory assistance may benefit critically ill or injured patients (even those with relatively normal ventilation and blood gases) include severe flail chest (particularly if there are two or more associated injuries), coma, generalized peritonitis, and previous severe pulmonary disease. Severe smoke inhalation or aspiration of large amounts of gastric acid may also be indications for early ventilatory assistance, even if no other problems are present.

A ventilatory rate >30 to 35 per minute with obvious increased efforts to breathe indicates a ventilatory work load more than six times normal. Delay in ventilating such a patient may result in a sudden respiratory arrest.

2. Laboratory Indications

Some of the laboratory indications for ventilatory assistance (Table 10.3) include (1) an arterial P_{O_2} less than 55 or 60 mm Hg on room air, (2) a Pa_{O_2} <80 mm Hg on 40% oxygen, (3) an arterial P_{CO_2} >45 mm Hg and pH <7.35, (4) an alveolar-arterial oxygen difference on room air greater than 55 to 60 mm Hg, (5) a physiologic shunt in the lung exceeding 20% to 25%, (6) greatly increased respiratory effort, (7) V_{DS}/V_T >0.60, (8) persistent rapid respiratory rates (>35 to 40 per minute), and (9) extensive chest x-ray changes.

Trends in the patient's blood gases or clinical condition are much more important than isolated or single laboratory values or examinations. A patient should be given ventilatory support if his or her general condition, blood gases, or ventilation are progressively deteriorating, or if the work of breathing is increasing, particularly if underlying sepsis has not been adequately controlled.

459

G. MECHANICAL VENTILATION

1. Monitoring Ventilatory Assistance

2. Clinical

The most frequent reason for admission to an ICU after trauma is ventilatory support. Development of ARDS can be highly lethal. In one report, 50% of all trauma victims who developed ARDS died, and of those with clinical evidence of aspiration of gastrointestinal contents, 60% died. Consequently, trauma patients requiring ventilatory support must be monitored carefully to prevent these complications.

AXIOM

If the patient is awake, alert, comfortable, and cooperative, and has normal vital signs, the ventilator is usually functioning properly.

If the patient is tachypneic and/or tachycardic and appears to be anxious or fighting the ventilator, something is usually wrong with the airway, the ventilator, or its settings, and should be corrected as soon as possible. However, in comatose patients, it can be very difficult to judge how well the patient is tolerating ventilatory support.

The patient and the ventilatory equipment should be monitored at least every 2 hours. This includes auscultation of the chest for bilateral air entry and the location of rales and rhonchi. The balloon cuff on the endotracheal or tracheostomy tube is inflated until there is just a small air leak during peak inspiration.

Cyanosis as a sign of inadequate oxygenation is almost worthless if the hemoglobin is less than 10 g/dl. Under such circumstances, the Sao_2 must usually be less than 60% to 65%, corresponding to a Pao_2 of about 30 to 35 mm Hg, before the patient looks cyanotic.

3. Monitoring the Ventilator

A number of factors can reduce the delivered gas volume to inadequate levels. These are high-flow rates, undetected circuit leaks, and high temperature of the water in the humidifier. Consequently, it is important to monitor delivered V_T by inserting a respirometer in the circuit.

Other parameters requiring frequent monitoring are ventilatory rate, ventilatory pressures (both peak airway and PEEP), Fio_2, minute ventilation, and heat level of the humidifier.

AXIOM

Any sudden rise in peak inflation pressures must be corrected promptly, usually by improving the airway or relieving a pneumothorax.

Peak inflation pressures (PIP) should be monitored especially closely. Use of an inspiratory hold of 0.5 second will permit calculation of dynamic and static pulmonary compliance. A rapid increase in PIP may be the result of (1) a mucus plug, (2) endotracheal tube (ETT) kinking, (3) the ETT slipping into the right mainstem bronchus, or (4) a pneumothorax. A slight and/or slow increase in airway pressure may be an indication of increased lung water with decreased compliance. A rapid decrease in pressure usually indicates a ventilator or circuit disconnection or an endotracheal cuff leak. A very slow decrease in airway pressure may indicate improvement in lung compliance, a decrease in airway resistance, or a slow air leak.

AXIOM

If an increase in minute ventilation (VE) increases the Pco_2, one should suspect the presence of auto-PEEP.

In patients with a high minute ventilation and rapid respiratory rates, a phenomenon known as auto-PEEP may develop because the gas in the lungs does not have enough time to escape during expiration. This will tend to progressively increase inflation pressures, dead space, and the P_{CO_2}. A quick way to determine if auto-PEEP is present is to stop the ventilator at the end of expiration and note the pressure in the system. If no auto-PEEP is present, the pressure in the tracheobronchial tree will fall to whatever level of PEEP is being used.

4. Blood Gases

With adequate alveolar ventilation, the Pa_{CO_2} will be closely related to the pHa. As a rough rule, the Pa_{CO_2} should be equal to or less than the last two digits of the pHa. Thus, if the pHa is 7.40, the Pa_{CO_2} should be 40 mm Hg or less. If the pHa is 7.30, the Pa_{CO_2} should be 30 mm Hg or less.

When evaluating the Pa_{O_2}, it is essential to know the actual inspired FI_{O_2}. Using the ratio of the Pa_{O_2} to the FI_{O_2} can provide much useful information (Table 10.4). However, calculation of the physiologic shunt (Qs/Qt) on 40% to 50% oxygen from arterial and mixed venous blood generally provides the most accurate indication of how the patient's lungs are progressing. If cardiac index is changing, calculation of the shunt index may be more accurate.

5. Mixed Venous Oxygen Saturation

AXIOM

The arterial P_{CO_2} and P_{O_2} reflect pulmonary function, but venous gases tend to reflect tissue perfusion and metabolism.

Pulmonary artery catheters equipped to continuously monitor mixed venous oxygen saturation ($S\bar{v}_{O_2}$) can be very helpful in monitoring cardiopulmonary performance on a ventilator. The normal $S\bar{v}_{O_2}$ is 70% to 75%. In patients with sepsis or cirrhosis with a high cardiac output, the $S\bar{v}_{O_2}$ may be 80% to 85% or even higher. Nevertheless, a sudden or rapid change in $S\bar{v}_{O_2}$, especially a decrease of more than 5% to 10%, indicates that something is wrong and should initiate a rapid search for a problem with ventilation, oxygenation, or cardiac output.

6. Noninvasive Monitoring

a. Pulse Oximetry

The use of pulse oximetry for monitoring oxygen saturation and pulse rate can provide early warning of pulmonary or cardiovascular deterioration before it is clinically apparent. It is of most value if the Sa_{O_2} is between 90% and 95%. Any sudden change in the oxygen saturation, particularly a drop of >5% indicates a need for an emergency assessment of the ventilator and the patient's cardiopulmonary function.

b. Capnography

Sudden decreases in end-tidal carbon dioxide (ET_{CO_2}) suggest a mechanical problem in the airway, hypoventilation, or increased dead space. A gradual decrease in ET_{CO_2} is usually due to changes in the lung itself. Increases in the ET_{CO_2} are generally due to hypermetabolic states.

If a simultaneous Pa_{CO_2} is available, one can estimate the alveolar-arterial

Table 10.4

INTERPRETATION OF $Pa_{O_2}:FI_{O_2}$ RATIO

Pa_{O_2}	FI_{O_2}	Ratio	Qsp/Qt, %	Abnormality
240	0.4	600	5	None
120	0.4	300	10	Minimal
100	0.4	250	15	Mild
80	0.4	200	20	Moderate
60	0.4	150	30	Severe*
40	0.4	100	40	Very severe*

*In trauma or septic patients, ventilatory assistance and positive end-expiratory pressure (PEEP) to reduce the Qs/Qt to 1% should be considered. The higher the Qsp/Qt, the greater the need for ventilatory assistance and PEEP.

P_{CO_2} difference ($P[A-a]_{CO_2}$). Normally this is zero, and if it suddenly increases, one should suspect a pulmonary embolus or drastic reduction in cardiac output.

H. TYPES OF VENTILATORY ASSISTANCE

1. Pressure-Cycled Ventilators

The Bird MK VIII is an example of a pressure-cycled ventilator that will deliver gas until the pressure limit selected is reached, at which point the exhalation valve opens, unless inflation hold is employed. The delivered volume varies with changes in airway resistance, lung compliance, and the ventilator circuit. Consequently, delivery of a specific volume of gas with each breath is difficult. However, by assessing the airway resistance encountered and the dynamic compliance of the patient's lungs, the flow rates and pressure limits can usually be adjusted to provide adequate tidal volumes and minute ventilation.

AXIOM
Pressure-cycled ventilators may not adequately inflate the lungs which have become very noncompliant.

Pressure-cycled ventilators are suitable for use in patients who do not have severe pulmonary pathology or high airway resistance. Pressure-cycled machines can be helpful in emergency situations because they are relatively simple to operate, quick to set up, and easy to move with a patient. They can also operate from a pressurized gas source and can be used for transport or if electrical power becomes shut down.

2. Time-Cycled Ventilators

The Siemens Servo 900, the Monaghan 225 Fluidic Ventilator, and the Bourns BP-200 are time-cycled ventilators that allow gas flow to the patient until a preset inspiratory time is achieved. The desired tidal volume can be attained by adjusting inspiratory time and flow rate or by settling the minute ventilation and the respiratory rate. The BP-200 can be used to provide intermittent mandatory ventilation. With intermittent mandatory ventilation (IMV), gas flow is continuous across the patient's airway, and as the number of mandatory ventilations from the ventilator are reduced during weaning, the patient supplements the $\dot{V}_E$ by breathing spontaneously from the passing flow of fresh gas.

3. Volume-Cycled Ventilators

AXIOM
Volume-cycled ventilators are usually needed to adequately ventilate patients with ARDS.

The Bennett MA1 is an example of a volume-cycled ventilator in which inspiration is terminated by delivery of a preset tidal volume. Volume ventilators are far more suitable than pressure-cycled machines for patients with "stiff lungs," since they will deliver a preset tidal volume regardless of the pressure required. However, they have a pressure limit control or "pop-off" that can be adjusted as needed to a level slightly higher than the peak airway pressure generated by delivery of the preset volume.

The presence of a leak in the ventilatory circuit is detected by monitoring exhaled volume. The exhaled volume will include some gas compressed in the ventilating cycle during inspiration and, therefore, will be less than the volume delivered by the ventilator. A reduction in lung compliance will decrease the volume delivered to the patient and increase the volume of gas compressed within the circuit. This will often go undetected because the total volume of gas measured by the spirometer on the expiratory limb of the circuit may show no change.

4. High-Frequency Ventilators

In 1967, Borg and colleagues developed high-frequency ventilation (HFV) in an effort to reduce the barotrauma and cardiac compressive effects of high tidal volumes. HFV involves several different methods by which the lung is ventilated at a frequency exceeding 60 cycles per minute (cpm). These include high-frequency positive-pressure ventilation (HFPPV) (60 to 100 cpm), high-frequency jet ventilation (HFJV) (60 to 200 cpm), and high-frequency oscillation (HFO) (600 to 3000 cpm).

Compared to conventional ventilatory modes, HFV offers several theoretical advantages. Using a very low tidal volume, it reduces both mean and peak airway pressures. This results in less impairment of venous return and a reduced right ventricular afterload. The likelihood of pulmonary barotrauma is also reduced. The techniques of HFV have proven suitable for bronchoscopy, laryngoscopy, and laryngeal or tracheal surgery. It also appears to be helpful in treating bronchopleural fistulas and controlling increased intracranial pressure (Table 10.5).

AXIOM

High-frequency ventilators have no advantage in ARDS, but may be useful in upper airway surgery or patients with bronchopleural fistulas.

A modification of HFV is high-frequency positive-pressure ventilation (HFPPV). HFPPV uses a relatively standard setup with low compliance, nondistensible circuitry, usually directly attached to a bronchoscope or endotracheal tube. The usual ventilatory rate is 60 to 100 cpm with correspondingly low tidal volumes. Gas is insufflated using a pneumatic valve principle without external air entrapment. Exhalation occurs around the tube if it is uncuffed or through sensitive exhalation valves. The advantages of HFPPV include easy adaptability to conventional machines and simple circuitry. However, as tidal volume and frequency increase, so do mean and peak airway pressures. Also, humidification during long-term use remains a problem.

HFJV delivers gas through a small catheter, either a 14 or 16 gauge intracath within the trachea, or a similar size channel incorporated into the wall of the endotracheal tube opening at its tip. The gas is delivered under high pressure (10 to 60 psi) at frequencies of 60 to 200 cpm. Unlike HFPPV, HFJV entrains gas through the Bernoulli principal, thus enhancing alveolar ventilation. Both HFPPV and HFJV use a compressed gas source and an on-off valve with variable frequency and insufflation time. They also require a circuit in which compressible volume is virtually eliminated. The systems generally remain open to allow continuous egress of gas at high volumes from the lungs.

HFO differs from the other HFV techniques in that it moves a volume of gas to and from the airway without bulk flow at rates of 10 to 50 Hz (600 to 3000 cpm). Oxygen is added through a bias flow system as required by metabolic rate, and carbon dioxide is removed by an absorber or bypass circuit.

The presumed decrease in peak airway pressure with HFV has provided

---

Table 10.5

GUIDELINES FOR VENTILATORY THERAPY FOR PATIENTS WITH ARDS

1. Volume-cycled ventilators are preferred.
2. Maintain high tidal volumes, usually at least 12 ml/kg.
3. Keep peak inflation pressure less than 50 cm H_2O.
4. Start with assist control and switch to IMV when feasible.
5. Reduce IMV rate gradually as long as pHa $\geq$7.35 and $PaCO_2$ $\leq$45 mm Hg.
6. Keep FIO_2 as low as possible, preferably less than 0.40 to 0.50, but keep PaO_2 >60 mm Hg.
7. Sigh 6 to 12 times per hour with a sighing volume 1.5 to 2.0 times the patient's tidal volume.
8. Use maximum nebulization and humidification.
9. Provide PEEP, usually at least 5 to 10 cm H_2O preferably with IMV, if ARDS is severe or increasing.

ARDS = adult respiratory distress syndrome; IMV = intermittent mechanical ventilation; PEEP = positive end-expiratory pressure.

some increased success in managing bronchopleural and tracheoesophageal fistulas. Reducing mean airway pressure also decreases the unfavorable effects that mechanical ventilation can have on cardiac output. However, a PEEP of 5 to 8 cm H_2O is generated by HFJV, so that mean airway pressure may be higher with HFJV than with conventional ventilators. In the only published controlled comparison of HFJV and conventional ventilation in humans, peak airway pressure was lower with HFJV, but mean airway pressure and arterial oxygen and carbon dioxide tensions were similar.

HFV has been extensively employed for ventilatory support during laryngoscopy, bronchoscopy, and microlaryngeal and tracheal surgery. Because HFV may be applied through an uncuffed endotracheal tube or without a tube, cuff trauma to the trachea might be reduced and aspiration may be minimized or prevented by the high-velocity egress of expiratory gas.

Cessation of spontaneous respiration with HFV, possibly caused by the stimulation of muscle spindle or stretch receptors, has been described by Borg and associates as an advantage during thoracoabdominal surgery and as a facilitator in weaning patients who breathe out of phase with the ventilator. However, other investigators have noted that spontaneous respiration continues during HFV.

Perhaps one of the more attractive features of HFJV is its application in patients with a predictable difficult intubation. A catheter can be inserted percutaneously through the cricothyroid membrane allowing oxygen administration and ventilation by jet insufflation. A similar system can be adapted when endotracheal tubes are changed in unstable patients by the use of a shortened nasogastric tube as a guiding stylet through which jet ventilation is delivered.

Several problems exist with HFV. It is more difficult to predict the effect of selected ventilator settings on gas exchange with HFV than with conventional ventilation. Catheter kinking and obstruction may also occur rather easily with HFJV. A satisfactory system to humidify rapidly flowing gases remains to be developed. The small VT cannot be measured by conventional equipment, and system pressures may be inaccurate because technology for measuring such pressures is inadequate. Restriction of exhalation during HFJV dramatically increases airway pressure because of the high minute volumes delivered. A similar problem may occur during application of HFJV to patients who do not have an endotracheal tube and who intentionally or reflexly close their larynx.

Displacement of the insufflating jet catheter may produce rapid insufflation of the gastrointestinal tract with resulting tension pneumoperitoneum.

Combined HFV (CHFV) was introduced in 1983, utilizing a base rate of 60 breaths per minute and a HFO rate of 50 Hz (3000 cpm) superimposed during each base cycle. The superimposed 50-Hz pulses are thought to improve gas distribution through enhanced convection, while the basal breath rate provides sufficient pressure to open and stabilize the airways. In a prospective clinical trial of 35 patients suffering from severe post-traumatic and/or septic ARDS who were refractory to conventional controlled mechanical ventilatory (CMV) support, Borg and associates found that combined high-frequency ventilation (CHFV) resulted in improved survival of patients who were clinically and physiologically indistinguishable from the ARDS nonsurvivors treated with CMV. In surviving CHFV patients, the decrease in airway pressures permitted an increased cardiac output with a rise in the oxygen delivery. Unfortunately, the base rate of 60 breaths per minute combined with an HFV rate at a higher level tended to increase end-expiratory and airway pressures to unacceptable levels in patients with noncompliant lungs.

I. VENTILATOR MODES

1. Controlled Mechanical Ventilation

During controlled mechanical ventilation (CMV), the ventilator delivers a preset tidal volume a preset number of times per minute. The patient cannot trigger additional breaths, as in the case of assist-control (AC) mode, or achieve successful spontaneous respiration, as in the case of intermittent mandatory ventilation.

If the patient attempts to breathe spontaneously, an asynchronous ventilatory pattern results because the ventilator will not respond to the patient's efforts, and this can cause the patient to develop apprehension and air hunger. Because of these disadvantages, CMV is restricted to patients who are apneic as a result of brain damage, sedation, or muscle paralysis. Properly functioning ventilator alarms are crucial to the safe employment of CMV.

2. Assist-Control Ventilation

In the assist-control (AC) mode, the ventilator delivers a breath either when triggered by the patient's inspiratory effort or independently if such an effort does not occur within a preselected time period. All breaths are delivered under positive pressure by the machine, but unlike CMV, the preset rate can be exceeded by the patient's triggering efforts. If the patient's spontaneous rate falls below the preset "backup" rate, controlled ventilation is provided until the patient's spontaneous rate exceeds the "backup" rate again.

Clinical experience with AC indicates that it is a considerable improvement over CMV. However, particular attention must be paid to proper adjustment of the sensitivity of the triggering mechanism. If the ventilator is too sensitive, it may autocycle. If the ventilator is too insensitive, a very large negative pressure may be required to trigger the ventilator.

3. Intermittent Mandatory Ventilation

IMV was proposed by Downs and colleagues to help wean adults from mechanical ventilators. It allows the patient to breathe spontaneously, with mechanical inflations supplied at regular preset intervals. The mechanical ventilatory rate is set by the operator and cannot be influenced by the patient. Between sequential mechanical breaths, an unrestricted flow of gas, which is equal to or greater than the patient's peak inspiratory demand, must be provided to minimize the work of any spontaneous breathing done between the mechanical breaths.

AXIOM

IMV may have three advantages over standard assist-controlled ventilation: (1) earlier weaning, (2) improved cardiac output, and (3) better $\dot{V}/\dot{Q}$ matching.

The earlier weaning with IMV results from the patient progressively taking over the work of breathing. This spontaneous breathing while on the ventilator acts as a means of exercising and preserving muscle tone and function. Other advantages noted by Weisman and associates include avoidance of respiratory alkalosis, decreased need for sedation, lower mean airway pressure, and prevention of respiratory muscle atrophy. They also note some potential disadvantages which include increased risk of carbon dioxide retention, increased work of breathing, respiratory muscle fatigue, prolonged weaning if the IMV rate is decreased too slowly, and increased likelihood of cardiovascular decompensation during weaning. As a general rule, the mandatory rate for the ventilator can be dropped about 2 per minute every 1 to 2 hours as long as (1) the Pa_{CO_2} is less than 45 mm Hg, (2) the pHa is 7.35 or higher, and (3) the combined rate for the ventilator plus the patient is less than 30 per minute. The lower inspiratory intrapleural pressure (PPL) that occurs during spontaneous ventilatory efforts results in better right ventricular filling and cardiovascular function. The spontaneous breathing with IMV also promotes more normal matching of ventilation to perfusion ($\dot{V}/\dot{Q}$) than continuous mandatory ventilation (CMV). With CMV, only the nondependent lung is ventilated, but with spontaneous breaths, the movement of the diaphragm ensures a more uniform ventilation.

4. Synchronized Intermittent Mandatory Ventilation

This technique allows spontaneous breathing between mechanically delivered ventilator breaths. At regular intervals, the mandatory breath is synchronized to begin with the patient's next spontaneous inspiratory effort in the same fashion as the pressure-cycled (assisted) termination of exhalation. This technique was introduced because of concern that a mechanical breath might be superimposed on a spontaneous breath, causing "stacking" with increases in peak inspiratory pressure, mean airway pressure, and mean intrapleural pressure. Similar concerns existed if the mechanically delivered volume was added at the peak of spontaneous exhalation.

Indeed, Shapiro, Harrison, and Walton note that mean P_{PL}, assessed with an esophageal balloon, was substantially lower with SIMV than with IMV in normal volunteers. Hasten, Downs, and Heenen found that although peak inspiratory pressure was greater with IMV than with SIMV, it had no significant effect on cardiovascular function. In another study, Heenen, Downs, and Douglas found no cardiac or pulmonary differences at all between IMV and SIMV. Thus, SIMV does not seem to offer any consistent physiologic advantages over IMV.

In a recent study, Groeger, Levinson, and Carlson compared SIMV and AC, using a crossover protocol in 40 patients requiring mechanical ventilation and PEEP for acute respiratory failure. They found that SIMV was associated with significant increases in systemic BP, pulmonary artery wedge pressure, cardiac output, and left ventricular stroke work. Mean airway pressure, peak airway pressure, ventilator rate, and pHa were lower with SIMV, and $Paco_2$ was higher. Minute ventilation, resting energy expenditure, oxygen consumption (Vo_2), carbon dioxide production (Vco_2), Pao_2, pulmonary artery pressure, CVP, and peripheral vascular resistance were unchanged.

Kirby in an accompanying editorial was apparently surprised by the authors' conclusions that they "found no evidence to support any clear-cut advantage of SIMV or AC in the acute management of respiratory failure." Kirby felt that this suggested a bias for AC, notwithstanding the fact that SIMV is the preferred mode of ventilation at their center.

5. Positive End-Expiratory Pressure

AXIOM

Ventilatory assistance with positive end-expiratory pressure (PEEP) is felt by many to be the most effective supportive therapy for ARDS.

A small amount of PEEP (3 to 5 cm H_2O) is added routinely in some centers whenever a patient is put on a ventilator to provide the "physiologic PEEP" that is thought to be present in the normal upper airway. If the pulmonary problem is not rapidly improving with other vigorous therapy, larger amounts of PEEP may be used. PEEP helps prevent collapse of the alveoli during the expiratory phase of ventilation and also increases the lung's functional residual capacity (FRC) (Fig. 10.1). As increasing PEEP is added, the FRC and Pao_2 tend to rise and the Qs/Qt usually falls.

AXIOM

If the patient requires an $FIO_2 > 50\%$ to maintain a $PaO_2 \geq 60$ mm Hg, PEEP should probably be added as needed, while maintaining an adequate oxygen delivery.

Although PEEP has been used for almost 20 years since it was first described as such by Ashbaugh and associates, the "optimal" level of PEEP is still controversial. Initially "optimal PEEP" was felt by Suter, Fairley, and Isenberg to be that level of PEEP that provides the best overall lung compliance. The term "best PEEP" was felt to be that PEEP level achieving the lowest Qs/Qt without a physiologically significant reduction in cardiac output. The term "rational PEEP" has been used by some to indicate the level of PEEP that maintains an adequate oxygen delivery but allows the FIO_2 to be reduced to 0.5 or less.

A reasonable approach to the hypoxic patient with ARDS is to gradually increase the PEEP while maintaining adequate vital organ perfusion with oxygenated blood (i.e., normal or increased oxygen delivery) while reducing the FIO_2 to less than 0.4 to 0.5.

AXIOM

Although PEEP tends to be beneficial by increasing FRC and PaO_2, one must often add fluid and/or inotropes to maintain an adequate oxygen delivery and urine output.

Although there has been much enthusiasm for using PEEP in patients with ARDS, it should be emphasized that high levels of PEEP are not always beneficial. If FRC is low and blood volume is adequate, PEEP may greatly improve FRC and pulmonary function. However, PEEP does retard venous return somewhat and may cause an abrupt fall in cardiac output if the patient is hypovolemic. In some instances, the cardiac output reduction will be large enough to also cause a fall in the systolic blood pressure. Consequently, vital signs, skin perfusion, and urine output must be monitored closely in any patient on increasing amounts of PEEP. If tissue perfusion is impaired after PEEP has been applied and does not improve after appropriate administration of additional fluids or inotropic agents, PEEP should be reduced progressively until the patient's hemodynamic status improves. If inotropic agents are needed to offset the deleterious effects of PEEP, dobutamine is often superior to dopamine because of its greater reduction of afterload.

In a short-term study of the hemodynamic effects of dopamine and dobutamine in eight patients with acute hypoxemic respiratory failure, dopamine increased cardiac output almost 20%, but PAWP increased about 50%. In contrast, dobutamine increased cardiac output about 30% and the PAWP fell. Dopamine also increased left ventricular end-diastolic and end-systolic volumes while dobutamine decreased them. As expected, the intrapulmonary shunt tended to increase with the cardiac outputs.

If the systemic pulse pressure falls as PEEP is increased or if more than 10 cm H_2O PEEP is used, cardiac output and PAWP should be monitored. If cardiac output falls with PEEP, one should use fluid and/or inotropes to restore Do_2 back to at least 600 ml $\cdot$ min^{-1} $\cdot$ m^{-2}. Although we depend on the PAWP to a great extent to make decisions concerning therapy, the PAWP may be inaccurate when the patient is on high levels of PEEP.

AXIOM

As a general rule, for every 3.0 cm H_2O PEEP used above 10 cm H_2O, one can subtract 1.0 mm Hg from the PAWP to obtain a "corrected PAWP."

In some instances, PEEP, rather than expanding atelectatic or small alveoli, may overexpand relatively normal alveoli. This is particularly apt to occur in patients with pre-existing obstructive lung disease or unilateral lung problems. In advanced COPD, PEEP will tend to increase the dead space in the lungs even more. This can cause the Pao_2 to fall and the $Paco_2$ to rise. Thus, continuous end-tidal carbon dioxide monitoring with a capnograph, if available, can be used to measure expired concentrations in order to promptly detect any increases in dead space.

We tend to use at least 5.0 cm H_2O PEEP on anyone requiring ventilator assistance, unless the patient is severely hypovolemic, is hypercarbic, or has an elevated ICP. In patients with ARDS, the PEEP is increased by 2 to 3 cm H_2O approximately every 15 minutes, watching the pulse oximeter and with frequent reassessments of Pao_2 and $Paco_2$. If more than 10 cm H_2O PEEP is required, a PAWP catheter should be inserted so that Do_2, Vo_2, and Qs/Qt can be determined with each change in ventilatory settings or PEEP.

Fluid therapy is critical when PEEP is used to treat ARDS. As the PEEP is increased, venous return and cardiac output and oxygen transport tend to fall. One can reverse this by giving fluid or inotropic agents. We generally prefer to use mild doses of both dopamine and dobutamine to maintain an oxygen transport of at least 600 and preferably 700 ml $\cdot$ min^{-1} $\cdot$ m^{-2}. If at all possible, we would like to keep the patient "dry," with an adequate urine output (at least 0.5 ml·kg^{-1}·h^{-1}) but a PAWP <12 mm Hg. However, if more than 10 μg·kg^{-1}·min^{-1} of dopamine and dobutamine is needed, we give more fluid or blood, preferring to keep the hemoglobin ≥12.0 g/dl. Although giving blood to patients with a hemoglobin ≥10 g/dl is controversial, we have found that each unit of packed red cells in such individuals raises oxygen content by about 7% to 10% and increases oxygen transport by about 6% to 8%.

6. Auto-PEEP

Although PEEP may be very helpful in managing patients with severe pulmonary dysfunction, especially ARDS, auto-PEEP is a complication that should be avoided. Lung volume at end expiration approximates the relaxation volume of the respiratory system, that is, the lung volume determined by the static balance between the opposing elastic recoils of the lung and chest wall. However, in patients with airflow limitation, end-expiratory lung volume may exceed predicted functional residual capacity (FRC). This occurs when the rate of lung emptying is slowed and expiration is interrupted by the next inspiratory effort. This progressive increase in end-expiratory lung volume is called dynamic hyperinflation, auto-PEEP, or intrinsic PEEP.

The factors that determine the development of auto-PEEP include increased tidal volume, prolonged emptying of the lung, and a shortened expiratory time. Such hyperinflation has a number of adverse effects: (1) the respiratory muscles operate at an unfavorable position on their length-tension curve; (2) elastic recoil of the chest wall is directed inward, thereby causing an extra elastic load; and (3) breathing takes place at the upper, less compliant portion of the pressure-volume curve of the lung.

AXIOM

If the PCO$_2$ is rising in spite of an increasing minute ventilation, one should suspect the presence of auto-PEEP.

In patients receiving mechanical ventilation, dynamic hyperinflation has sometimes been termed occult-PEEP because, unlike externally applied PEEP, it is not registered on the ventilatory pressure manometer. If, however, the expiratory port of the ventilator circuit is occluded immediately before the onset of the next breath, the pressure in the lungs and ventilator circuit will equilibrate and the level of auto-PEEP will be displayed on the ventilator manometer. Alternatively, the level of auto-PEEP can be estimated from continuous recordings of airway pressure and flow during mechanical ventilation. Recently auto-PEEP has been detected by monitoring changes in end-expiratory volume using inductive plethysmography.

The increased work of breathing resulting from auto-PEEP can be decreased by several therapeutic measures including (1) bronchodilators, (2) a larger diameter endotracheal tube, (3) decreasing the minute ventilation by controlling fever or pain, and (4) minimizing the ratio of inspiratory time to expiratory time by increasing the inspiratory flow rate or using nondistensible tubing in the ventilator circuit. However, recently Walley and Schmidt reported a patient in whom an increase in the inspiratory/expiratory time ratio resulted in the development of intrinsic PEEP which beneficially reduced airway pressure.

7. Continuous Positive Airway Pressure

Continuous positive airway pressure (CPAP) was first used as positive-pressure oxygen breathing to help keep the lungs expanded in patients with crushed chest injuries and to treat infants with the neonatal distress syndrome. However, CPAP is now also widely used in adults with a wide variety of severe pulmonary problems.

AXIOM

Properly applied CPAP can greatly improve pulmonary function and reduce the need for ventilatory assistance.

CPAP provides continuous airway pressure to a patient breathing spontaneously. It is possible, with some difficulty, to provide CPAP through a mask to cooperative patients who do not have an endotracheal or tracheostomy tube. However, the mask must fit very exactly so as to prevent air leaks and patient discomfort.

With this technique, the patient breathes out against an increased pressure of up to 10 to 20 cm H_2O, but the mechanics of ventilation do not change. The lung, however, performs at a more favorable location on the pressure-volume curve, thereby increasing lung compliance and reducing the tendency to atelectasis. As a general rule, lung compliance is best at a volume equal to the lung's normal FRC. When CPAP is less than 10 cm H_2O, expiration is usually passive. At higher pressures, abdominal muscles must be used to increase intra-abdominal pressure to aid expiration.

A variety of mechanical devices can be used to deliver CPAP. A common and convenient method, with or without a ventilator, uses continuous gas flow (usually 10 to 20 liters/min at a specified FIO_2), a reservoir bag, a one-way valve, a humidifier, and an expiratory pressure valve. Both FIO_2 and gas flow rate are precisely regulated by an air-oxygen blender. The gas is directed into a 3-liter bag that acts as a reservoir for the patient's breathing. It then passes through a one-way valve, which opens during spontaneous inspiration and closes during expiration.

Studies in healthy volunteers and a large number of patients have demonstrated quite a bit of variability in the operational characteristics of commercially available demand-flow CPAP systems. In some of these reports, a continuous flow (60 liters/min) reservoir bag system with a low-resistance valve (Emerson) required less inspiratory effort, maintained higher inspiratory airway pressure, and was associated with less work of breathing than several other demand-flow systems.

8. Spontaneous Positive End-Expiratory Pressure

Spontaneous positive end-expiratory pressure (sPEEP), like CPAP, is a positive-pressure mode that can be used with spontaneous breathing. It can be used by itself or in conjunction with mechanical ventilation in the form of intermittent mandatory ventilation (IMV). With CPAP, both inspiratory and expiratory pressures are positive, although the inspiratory level is less. With sPEEP, airway pressure is zero or negative (subambient) during inspiration but increases at the end of expiration to a predetermined positive pressure. The level of CPAP or sPEEP used is designed to increase expiratory transpulmonary pressure and lung volume (functional residual capacity).

CPAP and sPEEP may be particularly useful in increasing the Pao_2 in patients with $\dot{V}/\dot{Q}$ abnormalities. The only difference between sPEEP and CPAP is that sPEEP may be interrupted periodically by a controlled ventilation from a ventilator.

9. Pressure Support Ventilation

Pressure support ventilation (PSV) is a form of mechanical ventilation in which the patient's spontaneous inspiratory effort is augmented with a clinician-selected level of positive airway pressure. PSV is, in fact, similar to intermittent positive-pressure breathing (IPPB), but PSV differs from IPPB in that airway pressure is held constant throughout the inspiratory period. The inspiratory pressure in PSV can range from 1 to 100 cm H_2O, is held constant through servocontrol of delivered flow, and is terminated when a certain minimum inspiratory flow is reached. PSV is clearly different from conventional volume-

469

cycled ventilation in that with PSV the clinician selects only the inspiratory pressure; the patient controls ventilatory timing and interacts with the delivered pressure to determine the inspiratory flow and tidal volume.

AXIOM

Pressure-support ventilation can improve blood gases at lower FIO_2 levels, increase patient comfort on the ventilator, and accelerate the weaning process.

Newer microprocessor-driven mechanical ventilators (e.g., Hamilton Veolar, Puritan-Bennett 7200, Bear-5, and Siemens 900C) include pressure support (PS) modes that operate in conjunction with their demand-flow valve systems. Two approaches have been described. The first employs a low level (5 to 10 cm H_2O) of PS as "assisted mechanical ventilation" between IMV breaths, to decrease spontaneous ventilatory work. Poorly designed demand-flow valve systems (low-flow on demand, long response time, low triggering pressure, highly resistant breathing circuit, and a flow-resistor expiratory pressure valve) and endotracheal tube resistance are two reasons often cited as the rationale for using PS. However, unless the PS level is set precisely to match the pressure drop necessitated by the circuit resistance and demand valve, positive-pressure ventilation results.

The second approach employs PS as a stand-alone mechanical ventilatory mode. Here, the PS level is adjusted to provide the desired tidal and minute volume. Since large variations in tidal and minute volume can occur at a set level of PS, determining the proper settings based on volume exchange is sometimes difficult. Capnography is useful in titrating the level of PS to an appropriate end-tidal Pco_2. When PS serves as a stand-alone technique, there is no safety or backup mechanism to ventilate the patient in the event of apnea (except with the Hamilton Veolar ventilator).

The patient's spontaneous work of breathing with PS is less than breathing with CPAP at the same pressure, but the technique is based on an entirely different concept than CPAP. In the PS mode, the ventilator is patient triggered on and it continues in the inspiratory phase to a preselected positive-pressure limit. As long as the patient's inspiratory effort is maintained, the preselected airway pressure is kept constant by a variable flow of gas from the ventilator. Inspiration then cycles "off" when the patient's inspiratory flow demand decreases to a preselected percentage of the initial peak mechanical inspiratory flow. The ventilator flow then cycles out of the PS mode, following which passive exhalation occurs. The airway pressure, flow, and lung volume changes during PS are more akin to assisted mechanical ventilation than to spontaneous breathing with CPAP. At constant levels of combined PS and CPAP, peak inspiratory flow rate, flow waveform, inspiratory time, tidal volume, mean airway pressure, and the airway pressure contour depend on the patient's breathing pattern.

AXIOM

The principle advantages of PSV are decreased patient work of breathing and improved subjective comfort.

Wong, Stemmer, and Gordon have noted that PSV can lower airway pressures compared with conventional positive-pressure volume ventilation. PSV can also enhance spontaneous tidal volume, thereby lessening the need for mechanical breaths. Reducing the required number of mechanical breaths will also decrease Paw. Therefore, PSV should be useful in ventilating patients with bronchopleural fistula.

Since PS is a form of mechanical ventilation, patients treated with it should not be considered to be breathing spontaneously. Fassoulaki and Eforakopoulou recently showed that energy expenditure with PSV is 10% to 18% less than with spontaneous ventilation. Patients receiving PS with CPAP may appear to be assuming the full workload of spontaneous ventilation. This plus good arterial blood gas tensions and pH values can lead the clinician to conclude erroneously that the patient has relatively little pulmonary dysfunction. Thus, a patient who still has decreased FRC and lung compliance may be treated with PS of 5 cm H_2O, CPAP of 5 or 10 cm H_2O, and a low inspired oxygen concentration and have "normal" blood gas values. However, if the patient is extubated, he may become dyspneic and hypercapnic while breathing without this support.

When conventional PPV fails to ventilate patients with barotrauma, high-frequency jet ventilation (HFJV) is often considered. However, pressure support ventilation (PSV) can also lower Paw compared with conventional positive-pressure volume ventilation. PSV can enhance spontaneous tidal volume (VT), thereby lessening the need for mechanical breaths. Reducing the required number of mechanical breaths will also decrease Paw. Like HFJV, PSV should be useful in ventilating patients with acute airleak. Wong, Stemmer, and Gordon recently described a patient who could not be ventilated with conventional positive-pressure volume ventilation but was ventilated successfully with PSV.

10. Mandatory Minute Volume

Hewlett, Platt, and Terry describe a technique called mandatory minute volume (MMV) in which the patient is guaranteed a preselected minute ventilation. If the entire amount is breathed spontaneously, there is no augmentation by the ventilator. If the spontaneous minute ventilation does not reach the preselected level, the portion that has not been breathed spontaneously is collected by the ventilator and delivered automatically. Ventilators incorporating MMV are the Hamilton Veolar, Bear-5, and Ohmeda CPU 1. If the patient's expected minute ventilation is still less than the preselected value, the ventilator automatically adds PS in 1 to 2 cm H_2O increments until the desired minute ventilation is reached. The Bear-5 and Ohmeda CPU 1 ventilators provide mandatory breaths if the patient fails to achieve the preselected minute ventilation during spontaneous breathing.

11. Reverse Inspiratory-Expiratory Ratios

If peak inspiratory pressures are very high, one way to reduce them is to reduce the inspiratory flow rate and prolong the inspiratory time. Intermittent positive-pressure ventilation (IPPV) with inspiratory time (I) longer than expiratory time (E) has been termed inversed ratio ventilation (IRV). This has been used successfully to treat a number of infants and adults with severe respiratory problems. IRV improves gas exchange by progressive alveolar recruitment. If very high (4/1) I:E ratios are used, gas exchange may be improved by air trapping without affecting peak airway pressures.

In a study of 18 adults with acute respiratory failure, Ravizza and colleagues found that 6 hours of IRV significantly improved Pao_2/Fio_2 ratios and static compliance more than CPPV. The only significant difference encountered between CPPV and IRV was a decrease in peak airway pressure, which should reduce the risk of barotrauma.

AXIOM

Reverse I:E ratios for 6 hours or more may improve pulmonary performance in selected patients, but one must watch carefully for the deleterious effects of auto-PEEP.

In the past, studies with only 30 minutes of IRV showed no improvements. The different effects of 30 minutes versus 6 hours of IRV can be explained by the fact that IRV improves gas exchange by progressive alveolar recruitment. Previous reports did not encounter any improvement of Pao_2 after IRV because the results were measured too soon (15 minutes). However, if there is any retardation of expiration, such as with COPD, if the minute ventilation is very high (>25 to 30 liters), or if ventilator rates exceed 30 to 40 minutes, the gas in the lung may not have time to be exhaled, and increasing dynamic hyperinflation (auto-PEEP) may occur.

12. Simultaneous Independent Lung Ventilation

AXIOM

Independent lung ventilation may be helpful with unilateral injuries, but it requires a great deal of ventilator expertise for the technique to work properly.

Significant unilateral lung disease or trauma is not infrequently encountered during the management of patients with severe respiratory dysfunction. In many of these patients, the standard forms of mechanical ventilation will make the ventilation-perfusion abnormality worse by overexpanding the more normal lung. In such instances, use of an appropriately sized, double-lumen endobronchial catheter and synchronous independent lung ventilation (SILV) can be much more effective. This technique has also been referred to as differential lung ventilation (DLV). SILV or synchronized DLV has been accomplished either by the use of a single ventilator and two breathing circuits or by the use of two synchronized ventilators. However, patients with unilateral lung injuries have also been managed successfully with two unsynchronized ventilators. In a recent study on dogs with unilateral acid lung injury, there was essentially no difference between synchronous and asynchronous DLV with 10 cm H_2O PEEP.

J. REGULATING THE VENTILATOR

When beginning ventilator assistance for ARDS, we generally use a volume-cycled ventilator with assist control and 50% to 100% oxygen. Additional changes are made according to certain guidelines and the patient's progress (Table 10.5).

1. Fraction of Inspired Oxygen

Whenever a patient is being started on a ventilator, an FIO_2 of 1.0 is generally used. However, after the patient's condition has stabilized, the lowest FIO_2 possible, preferably 0.4 or less, should be used to maintain an arterial oxygen saturation (Sao_2) of 90% or more or a Pao_2 of at least 60 to 70 mm Hg. Although there are minimal clinical data on the incidence of toxicity with prolonged oxygen administration, an FIO_2 of 0.4 or less does not seem to damage the lungs, whereas an FIO_2 of 0.6 administered for prolonged periods may be harmful. Nebulization and humidification are usually kept at the maximum possible with the selected FIO_2.

2. Tidal Volume

When mechanical ventilatory assistance is begun for patients with ARDS, the initial tidal volume is usually set at 12 ml/kg. This may gradually be increased to 15 ml/kg, depending upon the peak airway pressure and the patient's response. If the patient is hypovolemic, the higher tidal volumes may reduce venous return and cause a significant drop in cardiac output and blood pressure. If 5 to 10 cm H_2O PEEP are used, the tidal volume can usually be kept at 10 to 12 ml/kg.

All too often a low tidal volume, particularly if large amounts of oxygen are given, will provide relatively normal blood gases. With relatively normal blood gases, there may be some reluctance to use high tidal volumes and/or PEEP, even if increased physiologic shunting in the lung can be demonstrated.

AXIOM

Patients with acute respiratory failure are put on a ventilator primarily to obtain optimal alveolar distention. Achieving normal blood gases is a very secondary consideration.

Patients with severe sepsis have a strong tendency to develop a progressively severe congestive atelectasis. Ideally, the lungs should be inflated to have an FRC close to normal and higher than the closing volume. Tidal volumes that may be more than adequate in other patients may be too small to maintain proper alveolar inflation in ARDS.

AXIOM

A patient with increasing or severe ARDS is best followed with serial DO_2, VO_2, and Qs/Qt.

The only way to be sure that a particular ventilator setting is appropriate is by analysis of the patient's response. Simultaneous arterial and mixed venous gas analyses plus cardiac output determinations so as to calculate DO_2, VO_2, and Qs/Qt provide the best guides to optimal ventilator settings. Although clinical evaluation is important, small blood gas changes, which may provide important data on trends in the patient's condition, may not be apparent on physical examination or isolated blood gas analyses.

3. Respiratory Rate and Ventilator Mode

The respiratory rate should initially be at about 12 to 14 per minute with assist control as the ventilator mode to be sure that the patient is not air hungry or restless and is not fighting the ventilator. However, the combination of a fast respiratory rate and high tidal volume may cause a severe respiratory alkalosis, which can cause cerebral and cardiovascular deterioration, particularly if a metabolic alkalosis is already present.

As soon as the patient is stable and seems to be working the ventilator relatively well, we switch to IMV at a backup rate of 12 to 16 per minute. The IMV rate is then progressively dropped as long as the pHa is >7.45, the $Paco_2$ is <45 mm Hg, and the patient's spontaneous breath rate plus the IMV rate is >30 per minute. As the patient progressively takes over the task of breathing, the IMV rate can be progressively reduced to 2 to 4 breaths per minute.

4. PEEP

There is some controversy about whether 3 to 5 cm H_2O PEEP (so-called physiological PEEP) should be used on all patients on a ventilator, except perhaps those with a high ICP or COPD. However, we routinely will use at least 5 cm H_2O PEEP unless the patient is hypovolemic, or has a high Pco_2 or increased intracranial pressure.

We recommend that PEEP be increased to 2 to 3 cm H_2O approximately every 15 to 30 minutes, with frequent reassessment of arterial oxygen tension, intrapulmonary shunt fraction, and oxygen transport, until the Qs/Qt is <20%. If more than 10 cm H_2O PEEP is required, a PA catheter should probably be inserted so that oxygen transport can be determined with each change in ventilator settings.

5. Sighing

AXIOM

Appropriate sighing can help prevent atelectasis especially in patients receiving low tidal volumes, little or no PEEP, and low rates of ventilatory assistance.

Patients should generally sigh 6 to 12 times per hour. A sighing volume approximately 1.5 to 2 times the tidal volume should be used, but the inflation pressure usually should not exceed 50 to 60 cm H_2O. Although sighs can be of value in patients with low tidal volumes, especially less than 8 to 10 ml/kg, they are not as important with tidal volumes greater than 12 ml/kg, particularly if more than 5 to 10 cm H_2O PEEP is being used.

6. Inflation or System's Pressure

Although a high tidal volume in the range of 12 to 15 ml/kg is frequently used in the treatment of patients with ARDS, ventilation pressures greater than 50 to 60 cm H_2O should be avoided where possible because of the increased risk of

473

pneumothorax and hypoperfusion. While the patient is on the ventilator, it is very important to watch these pressures. A rapidly rising pressure may indicate obstruction to the free inflow of gases from the ventilator to the patient because of kinking or malpositioning of the endotracheal or tracheostomy tubes, excessive secretions, or a pneumothorax. If the rise in inflation pressure is relatively gradual and the above problems can be ruled out, the lung is probably becoming stiffer because of increasing congestive atelectasis and interstitial edema.

One can use the system or peak inflation pressures to calculate or estimate the so-called dynamic pulmonary compliance, which is equal to the tidal volume divided by the peak inspiratory pressure. This provides some indication of the total resistance of the airways, lungs, and chest wall. When possible, it is preferable to measure the end-inspiratory (plateau) pressure with an inspiratory hold for 0.5 to 1.0 seconds so as to calculate "static pulmonary compliance." Differences between dynamic and static resistances are primarily due to airway resistance (Fig. 10.4).

K. EXTRACORPOREAL MEMBRANE OXYGENATION

1. Definition

Extracorporeal membrane oxygenation (ECMO) is the term used to describe prolonged cardiopulmonary bypass achieved with a membrane oxygenator and extrathoracic vascular cannulation. A modified heart-lung machine is used, consisting of a venous blood drainage reservoir, a servoregulated roller pump, a membrane lung to exchange oxygen and carbon dioxide, and a heat exchanger to maintain temperature. The patient must be maintained with continuous heparin anticoagulation to prevent thrombosis within the circuit.

AXIOM

ECMO can be very helpful in selected patients, especially neonates, who have reversible pulmonary problems that respond poorly to standard ventilatory support.

Use of ECMO reduces the need for (1) high FIO_2 and positive end-expiratory pressure (PEEP) for oxygenation and (2) high tidal volumes with their resultant increased peak-inspiratory pressures and minute ventilation for carbon dioxide removal. Thus, ECMO may allow reversal of the underlying pulmonary problem and may promote recovery by minimizing the harmful effects of continuing high-pressure mechanical ventilation.

2. History

a. Neonatal Application

Extracorporeal circulation for respiratory failure was first attempted in newborns by Rashkind. Bartlett and his colleagues began clinical trials of ECMO in 1972 and reported the first successful use of ECMO in newborn respiratory failure in 1976. The technique has been used in the management of over 600 neonates in more than 20 centers in the United States, with an overall survival rate of 75% to 95%. The infants in these centers are treated only after they meet criteria predicting an 80% to 100% mortality without ECMO.

b. Pediatric Application

In the 1970s, concurrent with an adult collaborative study, ECMO was evaluated in children beyond the neonatal period. Bartlett and others reported an ECMO survival rate of 30% in selected children with acute respiratory failure (ARF) whose predicted survival rate with conventional therapy was thought to be less than 10%.

c. Adult Application

A multicenter prospective randomized study of ECMO in adults with ARF was reported in 1979 by Zapol, Snider, and Hill. Ninety adults with severe ARF were admitted into the study according to a strict protocol that specified continuing conventional mechanical ventilation for the control group and ECMO for the study group. The survival rate with ECMO was 9.5% compared to 8.3% in those receiving conventional treatment. Overall national experience with ECMO at that time was only marginally better, with a reported pooled survival rate of

15%. Thus, extracorporeal membrane oxygenation did not change the outcome in a group of patients with ARF for whom therapy was begun after several days of high-pressure mechanical ventilation and high oxygen concentration. The cause of death in patients in both the ECMO and control groups was pulmonary fibrosis or necrotizing pneumonitis. The study demonstrated that ECMO provided safe and stable life support, and suggested that it would be effective for high-risk patients if begun early before pulmonary fibrosis or necrosis occurred.

d. Patient Selection

The indications for ECMO support are acute reversible respiratory or cardiac failure unresponsive to optimal ventilator and pharmacologic management, but from which recovery can be expected within a reasonable period (<7 to 10 days) of extracorporeal support. However, if the patient has (1) extensive pulmonary fibrosis, (2) necrotizing pneumonitis, (3) an incurable disease, and (4) prolonged ventilator therapy with high inflation pressures and high oxygen concentrations for a week or more, it should not be used. The requirement for systemic heparinization also limits the population for whom ECMO is appropriate.

e. Neonates

ECMO should be considered for newborn infants over 34 weeks gestational age with severe respiratory failure unresponsive to conventional optimal management and with an expected mortality rate of 80% without ECMO. Persistent fetal circulation (PFC) or persistent pulmonary hypertension of the newborn (PPHN) is a major cause of hypoxemia in full-term infants, regardless of whether the primary condition is diaphragmatic hernia, meconium aspiration, respiratory distress syndrome, sepsis, or primary PFC. In this condition, pulmonary arteriolar spasm results in high pulmonary vascular resistance and right-to-left shunting through the ductus arteriosus and foramen ovale. Contraindications to ECMO include evidence of significant intracerebral hemorrhage, multiple congenital anomalies, and irreversible lung damage.

f. Adults

In adults, the challenge is to identify causes of ARF that may be reversible within the safe time limits of ECMO support. Conditions treated successfully by ECMO techniques have included selected cases of bacterial and viral pneumonia, fat and thrombotic pulmonary embolism, thoracic or extrathoracic trauma, shock, sepsis, and near drowning.

AXIOM

ECMO support in adults requires extensive resources, but it may be very helpful in carefully selected patients in special centers.

Many investigators now believe that because of several key factors including new equipment, better definition of patients for the study, earlier intervention, a lower fraction of inspired oxygen (FIO_2), and ventilator settings that are less traumatic to the lung, survival rates with ECMO can be improved. Gattinoni and associates, using a modified ECMO technique (low-frequency positive-pressure ventilation with extracorporeal carbon dioxide removal), achieved 49% survival in a group of adults with ARF.

3. Criteria for Ventilatory Weaning

a. Extubation versus Weaning

Indications to discontinue mechanical ventilation must not be confused with indications to remove an endotracheal tube. Patients with altered states of consciousness, recurrent aspiration, or copious secretions may achieve ventilator independence, yet still require continued airway protection.

b. General Condition of the Patient

There is little justification for performing tests to determine if weaning is possible if the patient is hemodynamically unstable. Furthermore, withdrawal of mechanical ventilation should not be considered until there is improvement in the problem that necessitated mechanical support. The patient should not have dysrrhythmias or a high fever. The chest x-ray should be improving or at least "stable." A hematocrit of at least 30% is helpful but not really necessary if cardiovascular function is normal.

PITFALL
Attempting weaning in poorly responsive, unstable patients.

Young, cooperative, otherwise healthy patients can often be successfully weaned even when their weaning parameters are only marginal. In elderly, less cooperative individuals with other organ system dysfunction, even the presence of the optimal criteria does not guarantee successful weaning.

Three physical findings seen during spontaneous ventilation tests that may predict weaning failure include rapid shallow breathing, respiratory alternans (alternating between abdominal and chest-wall breathing), and abdominal paradox (inward movement of the abdomen during inspiration in the supine position). All of these tend to indicate that the patient's ventilatory muscles are weak and/or fatigue easily.

c. Weaning Parameters

A number of tests have been proposed to determine whether a patient is ready for a gradual withdrawal of ventilatory support. Such criteria seek to minimize premature weaning attempts, while at the same time keeping the time on the ventilator to a minimum. Generally, these tests can be separated into three areas of assessment: ability to oxygenate, resting ventilatory needs, and ventilatory mechanical capability (Table 10.6).

(1) Oxygenation

AXIOM
Oxygenation should be reasonable before beginning weaning, but ventilatory support is needed more for poor mechanical function than for mild-moderate gas exchange problems.

In general, the lower the FIO_2 needed to maintain a Pao_2 of at least 60, and preferably 70 to 80 mm Hg, the more likely the weaning process is to be successful. A Pao_2 of 90 or higher on 30% oxygen is usually quite adequate. This is equivalent to a Pao_2/FIO_2 ratio of 300 and a Qs/Qt of less than 15%.

The venous admixture or shunting in the lungs (Qs/Qt) which is normally 3% to 5% should be less than 15% before ventilatory support is discontinued. Since patients with a low cardiac output have a lower shunt than patients with similar pulmonary dysfunction but a high cardiac output, patients with low

Table 10.6

TESTS FOR WITHDRAWAL OF VENTILATORY SUPPORT

Test	Weaning Criteria Minimal	Optimal
Qs/Qt	<20%	<10–15%
Pao_2/FIO_2	>200	>300–400
$P(A-a)O_2$ on FIO_2 1.0	<350	<250–300
PCO_2 with pH ≤7.40	7.45	7.35–7.40
V_d/V_t	<0.6	<0.45
Vital capacity	>10 ml/kg	≥15 ml/kg
Maximum inspiratory force	−20 cm H_2O	−30 cm H_2O
VT	≥5 ml/kg	≥6 ml/kg
Minimum ventilation (VT)	<12 liters	<10 liters
Respiratory rate	<30 per min	<20 per min

cardiac outputs (less than 2.5 liters$\cdot$min$^{-1}\cdot$m^{-2}) may not successfully wean even with a Qs/Qt of less than 10%.

While a marginal patient is being weaned, frequent blood gas analyses may be needed. However, ear or finger oximetry measurements may be substituted for Pao$_2$ values if the patient is on 30% oxygen or less and has a Po$_2$ of 60 to 80 mm Hg (i.e., 90% to 95% saturation).

AXIOM
In patients with severe chronic pulmonary disease, one should try to wean toward the PO$_2$ and PCO$_2$ that the patient is normally able to maintain.

(2) Resting Ventilatory Needs

(a) pH-PCO$_2$ relationship

Carbon dioxide tension and blood pH are dependent on alveolar ventilation. Increased carbon dioxide production must be matched with increased alveolar ventilation to maintain a steady-state Paco$_2$ and pH. Fever, sepsis, shivering, and high glucose loads during total parenteral nutrition may increase carbon dioxide production and ventilatory demands. A Pco$_2$ higher than expected from the pH generally indicates that weaning should not be attempted unless the patient has COPD and chronic hypercarbia.

(b) V$_{ds}$/V$_t$ ratio

Patients whose dead space/tidal volume ratio (V$_d$/V$_t$) exceeds 0.6 can be very difficult to wean from ventilatory support. Small increases in V$_d$/V$_t$ above 0.6 require large increases in minute ventilation (VE) in order to maintain a given Paco$_2$.

(c) Minute ventilation

AXIOM
Need for a high minute ventilation to maintain the patient's normal PCO$_2$ is a contraindication to aggressive weaning.

VE is determined by carbon dioxide production and the V$_d$/V$_t$. A patient whose V$_{ds}$/V$_t$ ratio is 0.3 to 0.4 will maintain a near normal Paco$_2$ with a VE of less than 10 liters/min. The maximal voluntary ventilation that a patient can achieve must be at least 2 to 2½ times his resting minute ventilation.

(3) Mechanical Capability

The two measurable parameters that we have used the most to evaluate a patient's ability to wean are the forced vital capacity and the (maximum) negative inspiratory pressure (NIP). Forced vital capacity (FVC) is dependent on neuromuscular strength, motivation, and respiratory system compliance. A FVC exceeding at least 10, and preferably >15 ml/kg, usually indicates that weaning may take place. The patient should also be able to develop at least 20, and preferably 30, cm H$_2$O negative pressure to be successfully weaned from a ventilator. In general, the FVC seems to be a more reliable test.

(4) Weaning Parameters in the Elderly

AXIOM
One must watch elderly patients after extubation with special care, even if they have had excellent weaning parameters.

Krieger and colleagues have noted that the usual weaning parameters (derived from middle-aged patients) are not entirely helpful in determining when to discontinue mechanical ventilatory support in elderly patients. Parameters studied included spontaneous respiratory rate, tidal volume, minute ventilation, maximal negative inspiratory pressure (NIP), pH, Paco$_2$, Pao$_2$, and Pao$_2$/Fio$_2$. Approximately 10% of patients averaging 80 years of age required reinstitution of mechanical support within 48 hours in spite of meeting all criteria prior to extubation.

d. Work of Breathing

Work of breathing (WOB) is estimated clinically by observing the spontaneous efforts of the patient without ventilatory assistance for a period of time. Clinical WOB can be calculated as respiratory rate divided by 10 multiplied by evidence of respiratory effort (ERE). ERE is 1.0 with normal quiet breathing, 2.0 with noticeable effort on the part of the patient, and 3.0 to 4.0 with increased effort. A WOB that is 6.0 or more indicates a need for continued ventilatory assistance.

Shikora and associates have determined WOB as the difference in oxygen consumption (Vo_2) between spontaneous and mechanical ventilation. Their studies were on 20 patients who were difficult to wean after 2 weeks of ventilatory support. If the Vo_2 while breathing spontaneously was more than 15% higher than the Vo_2 with the mechanical ventilation, none of 12 patients were able to be extubated. With a WOB <15% of the Vo_2 with mechanical ventilation, five of the eight patients were extubated within 2 weeks.

e. Techniques of Weaning

The two most frequent methods for weaning patients from mechanical ventilatory support are the traditional (trial-and-error) T-bar technique and the IMV technique. With the T-bar technique, the patient is forced to assume the work of breathing all at once during gradually increasing trial periods of spontaneous ventilation. During these periods, the patient breathes a humidified gas mixture, usually containing at least 25% or 30% oxygen, delivered by a T-tube attached to the endotracheal or tracheostomy tube.

With the IMV technique, the patient is allowed to assume the work of breathing gradually by regularly interspersing ventilator (mandatory) breaths between spontaneous respirations. Patients are closely observed for fatigue, increasing tachypnea or tachycardia, hypoxemia, and/or hypercarbia. At least once an hour, the patients lungs should be inflated to a volume at least 1.5 to 2.0 times the tidal volume to reduce the tendency to atelectasis that is inherent in this technique.

During weaning with IMV, the IMV rate is decreased by one or two breaths per minute, every 1 to 2 hours as long as (1) the pH_a remains above 7.35, (2) the $Paco_2$ is less than 45 mm Hg, and (3) the respiratory rate is less than 30 per minute. Arterial blood gas measurements should be obtained after each ventilator adjustment or if there is any question about the patient's status. A pulse oximeter can greatly reduce the number of arterial blood gas (ABG) determinations. If the patient remains clinically stable at an IMV rate of two to four breaths per minute, discontinuation of mechanical support and tracheal extubation can usually follow. Oxygen at a slightly higher concentration than was used with mechanical ventilation should be delivered by face mask as soon as the patient is extubated. If the patient is unable to progress beyond an IMV of two to four per minute, we will try further weaning on 5 to 10 cm H_2O with CPAP or with pressure support ventilation (PSV).

Both the T-bar and IMV techniques of weaning are used widely. No well-controlled objective prospective study has shown a superiority of one technique over the other. Although this author prefers the IMV technique, in some individuals, the T-bar technique seems to work better. Interestingly, progressively increased time on the T-bar seems to be the best way to wean patients with high spinal cord injuries.

(1) Failure to Wean

AXIOM

Failure to wean often implies inadequate control of the primary process (especially infections), inadequate dehydration, and/or inadequate restoration of the FRC with PEEP or PSV.

If there is a failure to wean, in spite of all other efforts to improve ventilation, one should also:

1. Improve nutrition, especially protein intake, using the enteral route if possible.

2. Reverse any potassium, calcium, phosphorous, or thyroid deficiencies.

3. Discontinue all sedatives.

4. Try theophylline in therapeutic doses.

5. Consider the use of progesterone as a respiratory center stimulant (20 mg Provera t.i.d. for 7 to 10 days).

6. Search for organic neuromuscular disease.

7. Consider reversing drug-induced neuromuscular dysfunction with Tensilon.

8. Consider methylprednisolone in COPD patients or those with evidence of pulmonary fibrosis (0.5 mg/kg daily for 1 to 3 days and then tapered over 1 to 2 weeks.

9. Reduce the carbohydrate intake.

AXIOM

Prolonged ventilation of a patient who cannot be weaned may require gradually retraining a patient's ventilatory muscles and allowing increasing periods of cardiovascular stress, much as one would do in training to run a marathon.

SUMMARY POINTS

1. A PaO_2 <50 mm Hg and/or a $PaCO_2$ >50 mm Hg (with a pHa <7.35) developing within minutes or days can be called acute respiratory failure.
2. The most common abnormality in nonventilatory respiratory failure is $\dot{V}/\dot{Q}$ mismatch.
3. If the patient is making no effort to breathe (in spite of a low PO_2 and/or high PCO_2), a neurologic problem or drug intoxication should be suspected and ventilatory assistance begun immediately.
4. A rocking horse motion of the chest and abdomen with spontaneous ventilation can be a sign of a high spinal cord injury.
5. If the patient is making an effort to breathe, but there is inspiratory stridor or noisy air movement, an upper airway problem should be suspected.
6. The most common cause of upper airway obstruction in unconscious patients is prolapse of the tongue into the pharynx.
7. The narrowest part of the upper airway in adults is at the glottis (vocal cords).
8. The most frequent cause of pulmonary problems in critically ill patients is atelectasis due to inadequate removal of bronchial secretions.
9. Reduced breath sounds in one chest plus respiratory difficulty in a spontaneously breathing patient is indicative of a major airway obstruction or hydropneumothorax until proven otherwise.
10. One should not treat fevers immediately after surgery with antibiotics rather than bronchial toilet.
11. One should assume that all patients with seizures or a sudden loss of consciousness have aspirated.
12. One should not leave a nasogastric tube in longer than is really necessary.
13. Early use of antibiotics with aspiration may not reduce infection rates, but if infection does occur, resistant organisms are more likely to be involved.
14. Fever developing soon after admission to an ICU is usually due to pneumonia or an IV catheter infection.
15. Sputum cultures are best obtained with a protected brush or bronchoalveolar lavage.
16. One should not delay in efforts to diagnose the cause of a new pulmonary infiltrate in an immunosuppressed patient.
17. Since most pulmonary emboli occur in elderly patients with underlying

cardiopulmonary disease, relatively small emboli can cause severe problems.

18. Sudden development of tachypnea, tachycardia, and hypoxemia in a bedridden patient is due to a pulmonary embolism until proven otherwise.

19. Most tension pneumothoraces should be diagnosed and treated on clinical criteria. Waiting for radiologic proof can be disastrous.

20. One should assume that a small pneumothorax on a chest x-ray causes only a small decrease in lung capacity.

21. Patients with possible smoke inhalation must have both their arterial PO_2 and oxyhemoglobin saturation measured separately.

22. One should not assume that low carbon monoxide blood levels rule out smoke inhalation.

23. One should assume that pulmonary contusions are much more extensive than they appear on the initial x-rays.

24. Patients with a flail chest plus severe head injuries, shock, or massive transfusions should probably be placed on a ventilator prophylactically. Any delay in beginning ventilatory assistance in such patients greatly increases mortality rates.

25. The main laboratory changes in fat embolism syndrome include hypoxemia and thrombocytopenia.

26. The most frequent cause of severe, progressive ARDS is sepsis.

27. One should look for inadequately controlled sepsis in any patient developing ARDS.

28. Any tendency toward fluid overload greatly increases the tendency to the pulmonary edema and congestion that can develop in patients with shock, sepsis, or trauma.

29. A poorly functioning nasogastric tube is usually far more of a risk to the lungs than no nasogastric tube.

30. The pulmonary injury caused by smoke inhalation is now the major killer of burn patients.

31. A high PAWP increases movement of fluid into the interstitium not only because of the increased filtration pressure but also because a dilated capillary is more permeable.

32. Excess complement activation acting on neutrophils is probably the cause of many, if not most, cases of ARDS.

33. Although the neutrophil is often the main cause of the acute lung injury in ARDS, it is becoming increasingly clear that it is not absolutely essential.

34. Excess activation of the coagulation system, especially in trauma patients, may be an important contributing factor to the development of ARDS.

35. Excess production of thromboxane and leukotrienes can contribute to the development and progression of ARDS.

36. By the time the patient with ARDS shows signs of respiratory difficulty, the process is quite far advanced.

37. One should not assume that ARDS developed suddenly.

38. By the time it is evident that the patient has the classic signs of respiratory failure, such as the use of accessory muscles of respiration or flaring of the alae nasae, ARDS is usually far advanced and difficult to reverse.

39. One should not use a normal chest x-ray to rule out early ARDS.

40. There is often a 12 to 36 hour delay in the appearance of the x-ray changes of ARDS. The x-ray changes are also slow to leave as the patient improves.

41. If the $PaCO_2$ is low but begins to rise in a patient in whom the PaO_2 and/or the pH is falling, the patient probably requires ventilatory support.

42. A $P(A-a)O_2$ of 55 mm Hg or more in young, healthy adults breathing room air at sea level is generally evidence of severe respiratory failure.

43. As cardiac output increases, the physiologic shunt in the lung will also increase.

44. Proper coughing is the best method for preventing or treating atelectasis.
45. If the pain is quantified on a scale of 0 (no pain) to 10 (the worst pain imaginable), one should try to get the patient's pain down to a 3. One should not give enough analgesic for the patient to have no pain, but only enough so that the pain does not bother him.
46. Operative stabilization of lower extremity fractures within 24 hours of injury can decrease the incidence of pulmonary infections, fat embolism syndrome, and ARDS.
47. Severe hypophosphatemia can impair ventilatory effort.
48. Whenever possible, bedridden critically ill patients should be turned as far prone as possible at least once every 2 hours.
49. The most common reason for increasing respiratory failure in spite of optimal therapy is uncontrolled infection.
50. If a nasogastric tube is not functioning, its presence does more harm than good.
51. One should always look for hypoxia or hypotension after an analgesic or sedative is given.
52. Restlessness should be considered due to hypoxia until proven otherwise.
53. Greatly increased inflation pressures often indicate that increased tracheobronchial secretions or significant amounts of pleural fluid are present.
54. Any rise in pulmonary capillary pressure will tend to make ARDS worse.
55. Although dehydration will tend to improve most patients with ARDS, it must be done carefully so as to not interfere with oxygen delivery.
56. Critically ill patients with severe sepsis and/or ARDS tend to do better with higher hemoglobin levels (11.0 to 12.5 g/dl).
57. Any past or present evidence of bronchospasm should be an indication for carefully trying bronchodilators in patients developing any symptoms or signs of respiratory distress.
58. Steroids in ARDS are very controversial, but they may be helpful in selected patients in the late proliferative (increasing fibrosis) stage if no bacterial infection is present.
59. If ventilatory assistance in critically ill or injured patients is delayed until there is clinical evidence of severe respiratory failure, correction of the pulmonary insufficiency can be extremely difficult and the prognosis is much poorer.
60. If the patient is awake, alert, comfortable, and cooperative, and has normal vital signs, the ventilator is usually functioning properly.
61. Any sudden rise in peak inflation pressures must be corrected promptly, usually by improving the airway or relieving a pneumothorax.
62. If an increase in minute ventilation (VE) increases the PCO_2, one should suspect the presence of auto-peep.
63. The arterial PCO_2 and PO_2 reflect pulmonary function, but venous gases tend to reflect tissue perfusion and metabolism.
64. Pressure-cycled ventilators may not adequately inflate lungs that have become very noncompliant.
65. Volume-cycled ventilators are usually needed to adequately ventilate patients with ARDS.
66. High-frequency ventilators have no advantage in ARDS, but may be useful in upper airway surgery or in patients with bronchopleural fistulas.
67. IMV may have three advantages over standard assist-control ventilation: (1) earlier weaning, (2) improved cardiac output, and (3) better V/Q matching.
68. Ventilatory assistance with positive end-expiratory pressure (PEEP) is felt by many to be the most effective supportive therapy for ARDS.
69. If the patient requires an $FIO_2 > 50\%$ to maintain a $PaO_2 \geq 60$ mm Hg, PEEP should probably be added as needed, while maintaining an adequate oxygen delivery.

70. Although PEEP tends to be beneficial by increasing FRC and PaO_2, one must often add fluid and/or inotropes to maintain an adequate oxygen delivery and urine output.

71. As a general rule, for every 3.0 cm H_2O PEEP used above 10 cm H_2O, one can subtract 1.0 mm Hg from the PAWP to obtain a "corrected PAWP."

72. If the PCO_2 is rising in spite of an increasing minute ventilation, one should suspect the presence of auto-PEEP.

73. Properly applied CPAP can greatly improve pulmonary function and reduce the need for ventilatory assistance.

74. Pressure support ventilation can improve blood gases at lower FIO_2 levels, increase patient comfort on the ventilator, and accelerate the weaning process.

75. The principle advantages of PSV are decreased patient work of breathing and improved subjective comfort.

76. Reverse I:E ratios for 6 hours or more may improve pulmonary performance in selected patients, but one must watch carefully for the deleterious effects of auto-PEEP.

77. Independent lung ventilation may be helpful with unilateral injuries, but it requires a great deal of ventilator expertise for the technique to work properly.

78. Patients with acute respiratory failure are put on a ventilator primarily to obtain optimal alveolar distention. Achieving normal blood gases is a very secondary consideration.

79. A patient with increasing or severe ARDS is best followed with serial DO_2, VO_2, and Qs/Qt.

80. Appropriate sighing can help prevent atelectasis, especially in patients receiving low tidal volumes, little or no PEEP, and low rates of ventilatory assistance.

81. ECMO can be very helpful in selected patients, especially neonates, who have reversible pulmonary problems that respond poorly to standard ventilatory support.

82. ECMO support in adults requires extensive resources, but it may be very helpful in carefully selected patients in special centers.

83. One should not attempt to wean poorly responsive, unstable patients.

84. Oxygenation should be reasonable before beginning weaning, but ventilatory support is needed more for poor mechanical function than for mild-moderate gas-exchange problems.

85. In patients with severe chronic pulmonary disease, one should try to wean toward the PO_2 and PCO_2 that the patient is normally able to maintain.

86. Need for a high minute ventilation to maintain the patient's normal PCO_2 is a contraindication to aggressive weaning.

87. One must watch elderly patients after extubation with special care, even if they have had excellent weaning parameters.

88. Failure to wean often implies inadequate control of the primary process (especially infections), inadequate dehydration, and/or inadequate restoration of the FRC with PEEP or PSV.

89. Prolonged ventilation of a patient who cannot be weaned may require gradually retraining a patient's ventilatory muscles and allowing increasing periods cardiovascular stress, much as one would do in training to run a marathon.

BIBLIOGRAPHY

1. Anderson, BO, et al: Marginating neutrophils are reversibly adherent to normal lung endothelium. Surgery 190:51, 1991.
2. Anderson, RR, et al: Documentation of pulmonary capillary permeability in the adult respiratory distress syndrome accompanying human sepsis. Am Rev Respir Dis 119:869, 1979.

3. Andreadis, N and Petty, TL: Adult respiratory distress syndrome: Problems and progress. Am Rev Respir Dis 132:1344, 1985.
4. Argov, Z and Mastaglia, FL: Disorders of neuromuscular transmission caused by drugs. N Engl J Med 301:409, 1979.
5. Ashbaugh, DG and Petty, TL: PEEP, physiology indications and contraindications. J Thorac Cardiovasc Surg 65:195, 1973.
6. Ashbaugh, DG and Maier, RV: Idiopathic pulmonary fibrosis in adult respiratory syndrome. Arch Surg 120:530, 1985.
7. Ashbaugh, DG, et al: Acute respiratory distress in adults. Lancet 2:319, 1967.
8. Aubier, M, et al: Effect of hypophosphatemia on diaphragmatic contractility in patients with acute respiratory failure. N Engl J Med 313:420, 1985.
9. Aubier, M, et al: Aminophylline improves diaphragmatic contraction. N Engl J Med 305:249, 1981.
10. Baker, JW and Tribble, CG: Pleural anesthetics given through an epidural catheter secured inside a chest tube. Ann Thorac Surg 51:138, 1991.
11. Baldwin, SR, et al: Oxident activity in expired breath of patients with adult respiratory distress syndrome. Lancet i:11, 1986.
12. Balk, R and Bone, RC: Classification of acute respiratory failure. Med Clin North Am 67:551, 1983.
13. Banner, MJ and Gallagher, TJ: Respiratory failure in the adult: Ventilatory support. In Kirby, RR, Smith, RA, and Desautels, DA (eds): Mechanical Ventilation. Churchill Livingstone, New York, 1985, p 209.
14. Banner, MJ and Smith, RA: Mechanical Ventilation. In Civetta, JM, Taylor, RW, and Kirby, RR (eds): Critical Care. JB Lippincott, Philadelphia, 1988, p 1168.
15. Bartlett, RH, et al: Extracorporeal membrane oxygenation for newborn respiratory failure: Forty-five cases. Surgery 92:872, 1983.
16. Bartlett, RH, et al: Extracorporeal membrane oxygenation (ECMO) cardiopulmonary support in infancy. Trans Am Soc Artif Intern Organs 22:80, 1976.
17. Basran, GS, et al: Beta-2-adrenoceptor agonists as inhibitors of lung vascular permeability to radiolabelled transferrin in the adult respiratory distress syndrome in man. Eur J Nucl Med 12:381, 1986.
18. Baughman, RP, et al: Use of the protected specimen brush in patients with endotracheal or tracheostomy tubes. Chest 91:233, 1987.
19. Baumann, WR, et al: Incidence and mortality of adult respiratory distress syndrome: A prospective analysis from a large metropolitan hospital. Crit Care Med 14:1, 1986.
20. Baumberger, JP and Goodfriend, RB: Determination of arterial oxygen tension in equilibrium through intact skin. Fed Proc Am Soc Exp Biol 10:10, 1951.
21. Becker, EL and Ward, PA: Chemotaxis. In Parker, CW (ed): Clinical Immunology. WB Saunders, Philadelphia, 1980, p 272.
22. Bevilacqua, MP, Stergelin, S, and Grimbrone, MA: Endothelial leukocyte adhesion molecule 1: An inducible receptor for neutrophils related to complement regulatory proteins and lectins. Science 243:1160, 1989.
23. Bohn, DJ, et al: Ventilation by high frequency oscillation. J Appl Physiol 48:710, 1981.
24. Bone, RC: Extracorporeal membrane oxygenation for acute respiratory failure (editorial). JAMA 256:910, 1986.
25. Bone, RC and Balk, RA: Non-invasive respiratory care unit. Chest 93:390, 1988.
26. Bone, RC, Francis, PB, and Pierce, AK: Intravascular coagulation associated with the adult respiratory distress syndrome. Am J Med 61:585, 1976.
27. Borg, UR, et al: Prospective evaluation combined high frequency ventilation in post-traumatic patients with adult respiratory distress syndrome refractory to optimized conventional ventilatory management. Crit Care Med 17:1129, 1989.
28. Bragg, CL: Intrapleural analgesia. Heart Lung 20:30, 1991.
29. Bragg, CL: Practical aspects of epidural and intrathecal narcotic analgesia in the intensive care setting. Heart Lung 18:599, 1989.
30. Bresler, MJ and Sternbach, GL: The adult respiratory distress syndrome. Emerg Med Clin North Am 7:419, 1989.
31. Bromage, PR, Caporesi, E, and Chestnut, D: Epidural narcotics for postoperative analgesia. Anesth Analg 59:473, 1980.
32. Bryan-Brown, CW: Tissue blood flow and oxygen transport in critically ill patients. Crit Care Med 3:103, 1975.
33. Burford, TH and Sampson, PC: Traumatic wet lung: Observations on certain physiologic fundamentals of thoracic trauma. J Thorac Cardiovasc Surg 14:415, 1945.
34. Burke, JF, Pontoppidan, H, and Welch, CE: High output respiratory failure: An important cause of death ascribed to peritonitis orileus. Ann Surg 158:581, 1963.
35. Butler, WJ, et al: Ventilation by high-frequency oscillation in humans. Anesth Analg 59:577, 1980.
36. Bynum, LJ and Pierce, AK: Pulmonary aspiration of gastric contents. Am Rev Respir Dis 114:1129, 1976.

37. Cameron, JL, Mitchess, WH, and Zuidema, GD: Aspiration pneumonia: Clinical outcome following documented aspiration. Arch Surg 106:49, 1973.
38. Chapman, RL, et al: Effect of continuous positive-pressure ventilation and steroids on aspiration of hydrochloric acid (pH 1.8) in dogs. Anesth Analg 53:556, 1974.
39. Clowes, GHA, et al: Septic lung and shock lung in man. Ann Surg 181:681, 1975.
40. Comroe, JH and Botelho, S: The unreliability of cyanosis in the recognition of arterial anoxemia. Am J Med Sci 215:1, 1947.
41. Connors, AF, McCaffree, DR, and Rogers, RM: The adult respiratory distress syndrome. DM 27:1, 1981.
42. Covelli, HD, Nessan, VJ, and Tuttle, WK, III: Oxygen derived variables in acute respiratory failure. Crit Care Med 11:646, 1983.
43. Covelli, HD, Weled, BD, and Beckman, JF: Efficiency of continuous positive airway pressure administered by face mask. Chest 81:147, 1982.
44. Covino, BG: Interpleural regional analgesia (editorial). Anesth Analg 67:472, 1988.
45. Craddock, PR, et al: Hemodialysis leukopenia: Pulmonary vascular leukostasis resulting from complement activation by dialyzer cellophane membrane. J Clin Invest 59:879, 1977.
45a. Demling, RH: Role of prostaglandins in acute pulmonary microvascular injury. Ann NY Acad Sci 384:517, 1982.
46. de Oliveira, GG, Shimano, LT, and de Oliveira, AMP: Acute respiratory distress syndrome (ARDS): The prophylactic effect of neurodepressant agents. J Trauma 26:451, 1986.
47. Dhainaut, JF, et al: Mechanisms of decreased left ventricular preload during continuous positive pressure ventilation in ARDS. Chest 90:74, 1986.
48. Downs, JB: New modes of ventilatory assistance. Chest 90:626, 1986.
49. Downs, JB, Klein, EF, and Modell, JH: The effect of incremental PEEP on Pao_2 in patients with respiratory failure. Anesth Analg 52:210, 1973.
50. Downs, JB, Klein, EF, and Desautels, D: Intermittent mandatory ventilation: A new approach to weaning patients from mechanical ventilators. Chest 64:331, 1973.
51. Downs, JB, et al: Intermittent mandatory ventilation: A new approach to weaning patients from mechanical ventilators. Chest 64:331, 1973.
52. Dreyfuss, D, et al: High frequency ventilation in the management of tracheal trauma. J Trauma 26:287, 1986.
53. East, TD, IV, Pace, NL, and Westenskow, DR: Synchronous versus asynchronous differential lung ventilation with PEEP after unilateral acid aspiration in the dog. Crit Care Med 11:441, 1983.
54. Eiseman, LWB: The changing pattern of post-traumatic respiratory distress syndrome. Ann Surg 181:693, 1975.
55. El-Baz, H, Faber, LP, and Doolas, A: Combined high-frequency ventilation for management of terminal respiratory failure: A new technique. Anesth Analg 62:39, 1983.
56. El-Naggar, M, et al: Factors influencing choice between tracheostomy and prolonged translaryngeal intubation in acute respiratory failure: A prospective study. Anesth Analg (Cleve) 55:195, 1976.
57. Eriksson, I, et al: The influence of the ventilatory pattern on ventilation, circulation and oxygen transport during continuous positive-pressure ventilation. Acta Anaesthesiol Scand (Suppl)64:149, 1981.
58. Fabian, TC, et al: Fat embolism syndrome: Prospective evaluation in 92 fracture patients. Crit Care Med 18:42, 1990.
59. Fantone, JC, Kunkel, SL, and Ward, PA: Chemotactic mediators in neutrophil-dependent lung injury. Annu Rev Physiol 44:283, 1983.
60. Fassoulaki, A and Eforakopoulou, M: Cardiovascular, respiratory, and metabolic changes produced by pressure-supported ventilation in intensive care unit patients. Crit Care Med 17:527, 1989.
61. Feeley, TW and Hedley-White, J: Weaning from controlled ventilation and supplemental oxygen. N Engl J Med 292:903, 1975.
62. Fink, A, et al: Adult respiratory distress syndrome: Roles of leukotriene C_4 and platelet activating factor. Crit Care Med 18:905, 1990.
63. Fisher, J, Nobel, WH, and Kay, CJ: Hypoxemia following pulmonary embolism. Anesthesiology 54:204, 1981.
64. Fisher, JE, et al: Massive steroid therapy in severe fat embolism. Surg Gynecol Obstet 667:132, 1971.
65. Fowler, AA, et al: Adult respiratory distress syndrome: Risk with common predispositions. Ann Intern Med 98:593, 1983.
66. Frank, E, et al: Comparison of intrapleural bupivacaine versus intramuscular narcotic for treatment of subcostal incision pain. Anesth Analg 67:266, 1988.
67. Fulton, RL and Jones, CE: The cause of post-traumatic pulmonary insufficiency in man. Surg Gynecol Obstet 140:179, 1975.
68. Gattinoni, L, et al: Low-frequency positive-pressure ventilation with extracorporeal CO_2 removal in severe acute respiratory failure. JAMA 256:881, 1986.

69. Gibney, RTN, Wilson, RS, and Pontoppidan, H: Comparison of work of breathing on high gas flow and demand valve continuous positive airway pressure systems. Chest 82:692, 1982.

70. Goldman, AL, Morrison, D, and Foster, LJ: Oral progesterone therapy: Oxygen in a pill. Arch Intern Med 141:574, 1981.

71. Goris, RJA, Nuytinck, HKS, and Redl, H: Scoring systems and predictors of ARDS and MOF. Prog Clin Biol Res 236B:3, 1987.

72. Goris, RJA, et al: Multiple-organ failure: Generalized autodestructive inflammation? Arch Surg 120:1109, 1985.

73. Gosling, HR and Pellegrini, VD: Fat embolism syndrome: A review of the pathophysiology and physiological basis of treatment. Clin Orthop 165:68, 1982.

74. Gotloib, L, et al: Hemofiltration in septic ARDS: The artificial kidney as an artificial endocrine lung. Resus 13:123, 1986.

75. Greaves, TH, et al: Inverse ratio ventilation in a 6-year-old with severe post-traumatic adult respiratory distress syndrome. Crit Care Med 17:588, 1989.

76. Groeger, JS, Levinson, MR, and Carlon, GC: Assist control versus synchronized intermittent mandatory ventilation during acute respiratory failure. Crit Care Med 17:607, 1989.

77. Guerra, LF and Baughman, RP: Use of bronchoalveolar lavage to diagnose bacterial pneumonia in mechanically ventilated patients. Crit Care Med 18:170, 1990.

78. Gurd, AR and Wilson, RI: The fat embolism syndrome. J Bone Joint Surg 56B:408, 1974.

79. Gurevitch, MJ, et al: Improved oxygenation and lower peak airway pressure in severe adult respiratory distress syndrome: Treatment with inverse ratio ventilation. Chest 89:211, 1986.

80. Hasten, RW, Downs, JB, and Heenen, TJ: A comparison of synchronized and nonsynchronized intermittent mandatory ventilation. Respir Care 25:554, 1980.

81. Heenan, TJ, Downs, JB, and Douglas, ME: Intermittent mandatory ventilation: Is synchronization important? Chest 77:598, 1980.

82. Henao, FJ, Daes, JE, and Dennis, RJ: Risk factors for multiorgan failure: A case-control study. J Trauma 31:74, 1991.

83. Henry, WC, West, GA, and Wilson, RS: A comparison of the oxygen cost of breathing between a continuous flow CPAP system and a demand-flow CPAP system. Respir Care 28:1273, 1983.

84. Hewlett, AM, Platt, AS, and Terry, VG: Mandatory minute volume: A new concept in weaning from mechanical ventilators. Anaesthesia 32:163, 1977.

85. Hickling, KG: Extracorporeal CO_2 removal in severe adult respiratory distress syndrome. Anaesth Intensive Care 14:46, 1986.

86. Hill, JD, et al: Prolonged extracorporeal oxygenation for acute post-traumatic respiratory failure (shock-lung syndrome). N Engl J Med 286:629, 1972.

87. Hoff, BH, et al: Intermittent positive pressure ventilation and high frequency ventilation in dogs with experimental bronchopleural fistula. Crit Care Med 11:598, 1983.

88. Hoffman, RA, Ershowsky, P, and Krieger, BP: Determination of auto-PEEP during spontaneous and controlled ventilation by monitoring changes in end-expiratory thoracic gas volume. Chest 96:613, 1989.

89. Holcroft, JW, Vassar, MJ, and Weber, CJ: Prostaglandin E_1 and survival in patients with the adult respiratory distress syndrome: A prospective trial. Ann Surg 203:371, 1986.

90. Holzapfel, G, et al: Static pressure-volume curves and effect of positive end-expiration pressure on gas exchange in adult respiratory distress syndrome. Crit Care Med 11:591, 1983.

91. Hooper, RG and Kearl, RA: Established ARDS treated with a sustained course of adrenocortical steroids. Chest 97:138, 1990.

92. Horowitz, HH, et al: Pulmonary response to major injury. Arch Surg 108:349, 1974.

93. Hudson, LD, et al: Does intermittent mandatory ventilation correct respiratory alkalosis in patients receiving assisted mechanical ventilation? Am Rev Respir Dis 132:1075, 1985.

94. Hurst, JM, DeHaven, CB, and Branson, RD: Comparison of conventional mechanical ventilation and synchronous independent lung ventilation (SILV) in the treatment of unilateral lung injury. J Trauma 25:766, 1985.

95. Idell, S, et al: Angiotensin converting enzyme in bronchoalveolar lavage in ARDS. Chest 91(1):52, 1987.

96. Irwin, RS and Demers, RR: Mechanical ventilation. In Rippe, JM, et al (eds): Intensive Care Medicine. Little, Brown & Co, Boston, 1985, p 462.

97. Jacob, HS: Complement-mediated leucoagglutination: A mechanism of tissue damage during extracorporeal perfusion, myocardial infarction, and in shock. Q J Med 207:289, 1983.

98. Jacobs, ER and Bone, RC: Clinical indicators in sepsis and septic adult respiratory distress syndrome. Med Clin North Am 70:921, 1986.

99. Janoff, A, et al: Pathogenesis of experimental shock: IV. Studies of lysosomes in normal and tolerant animals subjected to lethal trauma and endotoxemia. J Exp Med 116:541, 1962.

100. Johnson, AR, et al: Neutral endopeptidase in serum samples from patients with adult respiratory distress syndrome: Comparison with angiotensin-converting enzyme. Am Rev Respir Dis 132:1262, 1985.

101. Johnson, KD, Cadambi, A, and Seibert, GB: Incidence of adult respiratory distress syndrome

485

in patients with multiple musculoskeletal injuries: Effect of early operative stabilization of fractures. J Trauma 25:375, 1985.

102. Jonzon, A, et al: High frequency positive pressure ventilation by endotracheal insufflation. Acta Anesthesiol Scand (Suppl)43:1, 1971.

103. Kaplan, LS and Goffinet, JA: Profound neutropenia during the early phase of hemodialysis. JAMA 203:1135, 1968.

104. Karnad, DR, Mhaisekar, DG, and Moralwar, KV: Respiratory mucus pH in tracheostomized intensive care unit patients: Effects of colonization and pneumonia. Crit Care Med 18:600, 1990.

105. Kirby, PR: Limits and cautions with the use of high frequency ventilation. Crit Care Med 12:827, 1984.

106. Kirby, RR: Synchronized intermittent mandatory ventilation versus assist control: Just the facts, ma'am. Crit Care Med 17:706, 1989.

107. Kolton, M, et al: Oxygenation during high-frequency ventilation compared with conventional mechanical ventilation in two models of lung injury. Anesth Analg 61:323, 1982.

108. Kram, HB and Shoemaker, WC: Transcutaneous, conjunctival, and organ Po_2 and Pco_2 monitoring in the adult. In Shoemaker, WC, et al (eds): Textbook in Critical Care. WB Saunders, Philadelphia, 1989, p 283.

109. Kram, HB, et al: Noninvasive measurement of tissue carbon dioxide tension using a fiberoptic conjunctival sensor: Effects of respiratory and metabolic alkalosis and acidosis. Crit Care Med 16:280, 1988.

110. Kram, HB, et al: Noninvasive conjunctival oxygen monitoring during carotid endarterectomy. Arch Surg 121:914, 1986.

111. Krieger, BP, et al: Evaluation of conventional criteria for predicting successful weaning from mechanical ventilatory support in elderly patients. Crit Care Med 17:858, 1989.

112. Kwan, M and Fatt, I: A noninvasive method of continuous arterial oxygen tension estimation from measured palpebral conjunctival oxygen tension. Anesthesiology 35:309, 1971.

113. Laghi, F, et al: Respiratory index/pulmonary shunt relationship: Quantification of severity and prognosis in the post-traumatic adult respiratory syndrome. Crit Care Med 17:1121, 1989.

114. Laufe, MD, et al: Adult respiratory distress syndrome in neutropenic patients. Am J Med 80:1022, 1986.

115. LeQuire, VS, et al: A study of the pathogenesis of fat embolism based on human necropsy material and animal experiments. Am J Pathol 35:999, 1959.

116. Lewis, BM: Two simple tables for interpreting blood gas measurements. Postgrad Med 53:195, 1973.

117. Lindeque, BG, et al: Fat embolism and the fat embolism syndrome: A double blind therapeutic study. J Bone Joint Surg 69B:128, 1987.

118. Luce, JM, Pierson, DJ, and Hudson, LD: Intermittent mandatory ventilation. Chest 79:678, 1981.

119. Lukenheimer, PP, et al: Application of transtracheal pressure oscillations as a modification of "diffusion reaspiration." Br J Anaesth 44:627, 1972.

120. MacIntyre, NR: Pressure support ventilation: Effects on ventilatory reflexes and ventilatory muscle work loads. Respir Care 32:447, 1987.

121. MacIntyre, NR: Respiratory function during pressure support ventilation. Chest 89:677, 1986.

122. Mackenzie, CF: Compromises in the choice of orotracheal and nasotracheal intubation and tracheostomy. Heart Lung 12:485, 1983.

123. Malik, AB, et al: Role of blood components in mediating lung vascular injury after pulmonary vascular thrombosis. Chest 83:215, 1983.

124. Manwaring, O, Thorning, D, and Curreri, PW: Mechanism of acute pulmonary dysfunction produced by fibrinogen degradation products. Surgery 84:85, 1978.

125. Maunder, RJ, et al: Occurrence of the adult respiratory distress syndrome in neutropenic patients. Am Rev Respir Dis 133:313, 1986.

126. Maunder, RJ, et al: Preservation of normal lung regions in the adult respiratory distress syndrome: Analysis by computed tomography. JAMA 255:2463, 1986.

127. McBay, AJ: Carbon monoxide poisoning. N Engl J Med 272:252, 1965.

128. McCarthy, B, et al: Subclinical fat embolism: A prospective study of fifty patients with extremity fractures. J Trauma 13:9, 1973.

129. McEvoy, RD, et al: Lung mucus ciliary transport during HFV. Am Rev Respir Dis 126:452, 1982.

130. McMenamy, RH, Birkhahn, R, and Oswald, G: Multiple systems organ failure: I. The basal state. J Trauma 21:99, 1981.

131. Melot, C, et al: Pulmonary and extrapulmonary contributors to hypoxemia in liver cirrhosis. Am Rev Respir Dis 139:632, 1989.

132. Miller, TA: Protective effects of prostaglandins against gastric mucosal damage: Current knowledge and proposed mechanisms. Am J Physiol 245:G601, 1983.

133. Modig, J: Effectiveness of dextran 70 versus Ringer's acetate in traumatic shock and adult respiratory distress syndrome. Crit Care Med 14:454, 1986.
134. Modig, J: Adult respiratory distress syndrome: Pathogenesis and treatment. Trans Am Soc Artif Intern Organs 31:604, 1985.
135. Modig, J and Bagge, L: Specific coagulation and fibrinolysis tests as biochemical markers in traumatic-induced adult respiratory distress syndrome. Resus 13:87, 1986.
136. Molly, DW, et al: Hemodynamic management in clinical acute hypoxemic respiratory failure: Dopamine vs dobutamine. Chest 89:636, 1986.
137. Monaco, V, et al: Pulmonary venous admixture in injured patients. J Trauma 12:15, 1972.
138. Moore, FD, Lyon, JH, and Pierce, EC: Pathophysiology of respiratory failure and principles of respiratory care after surgical operations, trauma, hemorrhage, burns and shock. In Post-Traumatic Pulmonary Insufficiency. WB Saunders, Philadelphia, 1969.
139. Moss, G: Cerebral etiology of the acute respiratory distress syndrome: Diphenlhydantoin prophylaxis. J Trauma 15:39, 1975.
140. Mueleman, TR, et al: Ketanserin prevents platelet aggregation and endotoxin induced pulmonary vasoconstriction. Crit Care Med 11:606, 1983.
140a. Murray, JF: An expanded definition of the adult respiratory distress syndrome. Am Rev Resp Dis 138:720, 1988.
141. Neuhof, H, Seeger, W, and Wolf, HR: Generation of mediators by limited proteolysis during blood coagulation and fibrinolysis: its pathogenetic role in the adult respiratory distress syndrome (ARDS). Resus 14:23, 1986.
141a. Nichols, RT, Pearce, HJ, and Greenfield, LJ: Effects of experimental pulmonary contusion on respiratory exchange and lung mechanics. Arch Surg 96:723, 1968.
142. Nolan, LS and Shoemaker, WC: Transcutaneous O_2 and CO_2 monitoring of high risk surgical patients during the perioperative period. Crit Care Med 10:762, 1982.
143. Norwood, SH and Civetta, JM: Ventilatory support in patients with ARDS. Surg Clin North Am 65:895, 1985.
144. Nuytinck, JK, et al: Posttraumatic complications and inflammatory mediators. Arch Surg 121:886, 1986.
145. Ognibene, FP, et al: Adult respiratory distress syndrome in patients with severe neutropenia. N Engl J Med 315:547, 1986.
146. Pace, MI, et al: Differential lung ventilation following unilateral hydrochloric acid aspiration in the dog. Crit Care Med 11:17, 1983.
147. Peer, EM and Schwartz, SI: Development and treatment of post-traumatic pulmonary platelet trapping. Ann Surg 181:447, 1975.
147a. Peltier, LF: Fat embolism. Clin Orthop 187:3, 1984.
148. Pepe, PE, et al: Clinical predictors of the adult respiratory distress syndrome. Am J Surg 144:124, 1982.
149. Peris, LV, et al: Clinical use of the arterial/alveolar oxygen tension ratio. Crit Care Med 11:888, 1983.
150. Petty, TL: Adult respiratory distress syndrome: Definition and historical perspective. Clin Chest Med 3:3, 1982.
151. Pierce, EC: Is extracorporeal membrane oxygenation a viable technique? Ann Thorac Surg 31:102, 1981.
152. Pistolesi, N and Ginntini, C: Assessment of extravascular lung water. Radiol Clin North Am 16:551, 1978.
153. Raffin, TA: ARDS: Mechanisms and management. Hosp Pract [Off] 22:65, 1987.
154. Rashkind, WJK, et al: Evaluation of disposable plastic, low-volume, pumpless oxygenator as a lung substitute. J Pediatr 66:94, 1965.
155. Ravizza, AG, et al: Inversed ratio and conventional ventilators: Comparison of the respiratory effects. Anesthesiology 59:A523, 1989.
156. Rinaldo, JE: Mediation of ARDS by leukocytes: Clinical evidence and implications for therapy. Chest 89:590, 1986.
157. Riska, E, Von Bonsdorff, H, and Hakkinen, S: Primary operative fixation of long bone fractures in patients with multiple injuries. J Trauma 17:111, 1977.
158. Rithalia, SVS and Booth, S: Factors influencing transcutaneous oxygen tension. Intens Care World 126, 1985.
159. Robin, ED, et al: Capillary leak syndrome with pulmonary edema. Arch Intern Med 130:66, 1972.
160. Rodriguez-Roison, R, et al: Gas exchange and pulmonary vascular reactivity in patients with liver cirrhosis. Am Rev Respir Dis 135:1085, 1987.
161. Rosenblum, R: Physiologic basis for the therapeutic use of catecholamines. Am Heart J 87:527, 1974.
162. Rossing, TE, et al: Tidal volume and frequency dependence of carbon dioxide elimination by high frequency ventilation. N Engl J Med 305:1375, 1981.
163. Saba, TM, et al: Cryoprecipitate reversal of opsonic surface binding glycoprotein deficiency in septic surgical and trauma patients. Science 201:622, 1978.

164. Sacks, T, et al: Oxygen radicals mediate endothelial cell damage by complement-stimulated granulocytes. J Clin Invest 61:1161, 1978.
165. Safar, P, Grenvik, A, and Smith, J: Progressive pulmonary consolidation: Review of cases and pathogenesis. J Trauma 12:955, 1972.
166. Sahn, SA, Laushminarayan, S, and Petty, TL: Weaning from mechanical ventilation. JAMA 1976; 235:2208.
167. Sankaran, S and Wilson, RF: Factors affecting prognosis in patients with flail chest. J Thorac Cardiovasc Surg 60:402, 1970.
168. Schachter, EN, Tucker, D, and Beck, GJ: Does intermittent mandatory ventilation accelerate weaning? JAMA 246:1210, 1981.
169. Schena, J, Thompson, J, and Crone, RK: Mechanical influences on the capnogram. Crit Care Med 12:672, 1984.
170. Schonfeld, SA, et al: Fat embolism prophylaxis with corticosteroids. Ann Intern Med 99:438, 1983.
171. Seeger, W and Lasch, HG: Septic lung. Rev Infect Dis 9:S570, 1987.
172. Severinghaus, JW and Naireh, KH: Accuracy of response of several pulse oximeters to profound hypoxia. Anesthesiology 67:551, 1987.
173. Shapiro, BA: General principles of airway pressure therapy. In Shoemaker, WC, et al (eds): Textbook of Critical Care. WB Saunders, Philadelphia, 1989, p 505.
174. Shapiro, BA and Cane, RD: Blood gas monitoring: Yesterday, today and tomorrow. Crit Care Med 17:966, 1989.
175. Shapiro, BA, Cane, RD, and Harrison, RA: Positive end-expiratory pressure in adults with special reference to acute lung injury: A review of the literature and suggested clinical corrections. Crit Care Med 12:127, 1984.
176. Shapiro, BA, Harrison, RA, and Walton, JR: Intermittent demand ventilation (IDV): A new technique for supporting ventilation in critically ill patients. Respir Care 21:521, 1976.
177. Shapiro, BA, et al: Preliminary evaluation of an intra-arterial blood gas system in dogs and humans. Crit Care Med 17:455, 1989.
177a. Shields, RT: Pathogenesis of postoperative pulmonary atelectasis. Arch Surg 58:489, 1949.
178. Shier, MR, et al: Fat embolism prophylaxis: A study of four treatment modalities. J Trauma 17:621, 1977.
179. Shikora, SA, et al: Work of breathing: Reliable predictor of weaning and extubation. Crit Care Med 18:157, 1990.
180. Shoemaker, WC and Appel, PL: Effects of prostaglandin E_1 in adult respiratory distress syndrome. Surgery 99(3):275, 1986.
181. Shoemaker, WC and Hanser, CJ: Critique of crystalloid versus colloid therapy in shock and shock lung. Crit Care Med 7:117, 1979.
182. Singer, MM, Wright, F, and Stanley, LK: Oxygen toxicity in man: A prospective study in patients after open heart surgery. N Engl J Med 283:1473, 1970.
183. Sivak, ED, et al: Long term management of diaphragmatic paralysis complicating prosthetic valve replacement. Crit Care Med 11:438, 1983.
184. Sivak, ED, et al: Value of extravascular lung water measurement vs portable chest x-ray in the management of pulmonary edema. Crit Care Med 11:498, 1983.
185. Sjostrand, U: High frequency positive-pressure ventilation (HFPPV): A review. Crit Care Med 8:345, 1980.
186. Smith, CW, et al: Cooperative interactions of LFA-1 and Mac-1 with intercellular adhesion molecule-1 in facilitating adherence and transendothelial migration of human neutrophils in vitro. J Clin Invest 83:2008, 1989.
187. Smith, G, Cheney, FV, Jr, and Winter, PM: The effect of change in cardiac output on intrapulmonary shunting. Br J Anaesth 46:337, 1974.
188. Stasic, AF: Continuous evaluation of oxygenation and ventilation. In Civetta, JM, Taylor, RW, and Kirby RR (eds): Critical Care. JB Lippincott, Philadelphia, 1988, p 321.
189. Staub, NC: Pulmonary edema due to increased microvascular permeability to fluid and protein. Circ Res 43:145, 1978.
190. Steier, M, et al: Pneumothorax complicating continuous ventilatory support. J Thorac Cardiovasc Surg 67:17, 1974.
191. Stevens, JH and Rabbin, TA: Adult respiratory distress syndrome: etiology and mechanisms. Postgrad Med J 60:505, 1984.
192. Stoltenberg, JJ and Gustilo, RB: The use of methylprednisolone and hypertonic glucose in the prophylaxis of fat embolism syndrome. Clin Orthop 143:211, 1979.
193. Sugerman, HJ, Rogers, RM, and Miller, LD: Positive end-expiratory pressure indications and physiologic considerations. Chest 62:865, 1972.
194. Suter, PM, Fairley, HG, and Isenberg, MD: Optimum end-expiratory pressure in patients with acute pulmonary failure. N Engl J Med 292:284, 1975.
195. Tabeling, BB and Modell, JH: Fluid administration and increased oxygen delivery during continuous positive pressure ventilation after freshwater neardrowning. Crit Care Med 11:693, 1983.

196. Tahranainen, J, Salmenpera, M, and Nikki, P: Extubation criteria after weaning from intermittent mandatory ventilation and continuous positive airway pressure. Crit Care Med 11:702, 1983.
197. Taylor, MB and Whitman, JG: The current status of pulse oximetry. Anesthesia 41:943, 1986.
198. Temper, KK, Waxman, K, and Shoemaker, WC: Effects of hypoxia and shock on transcutaneous Po_2 values in dogs. Crit Care Med 7:526, 1979.
199. Thom, SR: Smoke inhalation. Emerg Clin North Am 7:371, 1989.
200. Thompson, PB, et al: Effect on mortality of inhalation injury. J Trauma 26:163, 1986.
201. Tobin, MJ and Lodato, RF: PEEP, auto-PEEP and water falls (editorial). Chest 96:449, 1989.
202. Tranbaugh, RF, et al: Effect of inhalation injury on lung water accumulation. J Trauma 23:597, 1983.
203. Triner, L and Sherman J: Potential value of expiratory carbon dioxide measurement in patients considered to be susceptible to malignant hyperthermia. Anesthesiology 55:482, 1981.
204. Trunkey, DD: Inhalation injury. Surg Clin North Am 56:1133, 1978.
205. Turnbull, AD, et al: High-frequency jet ventilation in major airway or pulmonary disruption. Ann Thorac Surg 32:468, 1981.
206. Van Besouw, JP and Hinds, CJ: Fat embolism syndrome. Br J Hosp Med 42:304, 1989.
207. Van Slyke, DD and Neill, JM: The determination of gases in blood and other solutions by vacuum extraction and manometric measurement. J Biol Chem 61:523, 1924.
208. Vedder, NB, et al: Role of neutrophils in generalized reperfusion injury associated with resuscitation from shock. Surgery 106:509, 1989.
209. Venus, B, et al: Prophylactic intubation and continuous management of inhalation injury in burn patients. Crit Care Med 9:519, 1981.
210. Viale, JP, et al: Arterial-alveolar oxygen partial pressure ratio: A theoretical reappraisal. Crit Care Med 14:153, 1986.
211. Walker, L and Eiseman, B: The changing patterns of posttraumatic respiratory distress syndrome. Ann Surg 181:693, 1975.
212. Walley, KR and Schmidt, GA: Therapeutic use of intrinsic positive end-expiratory pressure. Crit Care Med 18:336, 1990.
213. Walt, AJ and Wilson, RF: Clinical, hemodynamic and respiratory changes in sepsis due to peritonitis and methods of management. Proc R Soc Med (Suppl)63:31, 1970.
214. Ward, HN: Pulmonary infiltrates associated with leukoagglutinin transfusion reactions. Ann Intern Med 73:689, 1970.
215. Ward, PA, Johnson, KJ, and Til, GO: Current concepts regarding adult respiratory distress syndrome. Ann Emerg Med 14:724, 1985.
216. Weigelt, JA: Current concepts in the management of the adult respiratory distress syndrome. World J Surg 11:161, 1987.
216a. Weisman, IM, Rinaldo, JE, and Rogers, RM: Positive end-expiratory pressure in adult respiratory failure. N Engl J Med 307:1381, 1982.
217. Weiss, SJ: Tissue destruction of neutrophils. N Engl J Med 320:365, 1989.
218. Wilson, J: Pulmonary factors produced by septic shock: Cause or consequence of shock lung. J Reprod Med 8:307, 1972.
219. Wilson, RF, et al: Respiratory and coagulation changes after uncomplicated fractures. Arch Surg 106:395, 1973.
220. Wilson, RF, et al: Physiologic shunting in the lung in critically ill or injured patients. J Surg Res 10:571, 1970.
221. Wong, C, Flynn, J, and Demling, RH: Role of oxygen radicals in endotoxin-induced lung injury. Arch Surg 119:77, 1984.
222. Wong, DH, Stemmer, EA, and Gordon, I: Acute massive air leak and pressure support ventilation. Crit Care Med 18:114, 1990.
223. Worthen, GS, et al: Neutrophil-mediated pulmonary vascular injury: Synergistic effect of trace amounts of lipopolysaccharide and neutrophil stimuli on vascular permeability and neutrophil sequestration in the lung. Am Rev Respir Dis 136:19, 1987.
224. Yeston, NS and Niehoff, JM: Trauma and pulmonary insufficiency: Mediators and modulators of adult respiratory distress syndrome. Int Anesthesiol Clin 25:91, 1987.
225. Zapol, WM, Snider, MT, and Hill, JD: Extracorporeal membrane oxygenation in severe acute respiratory failure: A randomized prospective study. JAMA 242:2193, 1979.
226. Zwillich, CB, et al: Complications of assisted ventilation: A prospective study of 354 consecutive episodes. Am J Med 57:161, 1974.
227. Zwischenberger, JB and Bartlett, R: Extracorporeal circulation for respiratory or cardiac failure. In Civetta, JM, Taylor, RW, and Kirby RR (eds): Critical Care. JB Lippincott, Philadelphia, 1988, p 1629.

CHAPTER 11

Deep Vein Thrombosis and Pulmonary Embolism

I. INCIDENCE

A. PULMONARY EMBOLI

It has been estimated that each year, five to six million patients in the United States develop deep venous thrombosis. About 10% of these patients, (500,000 to 600,000) have a pulmonary embolus, and of those with an embolus, 10% to 20% (50,000 to 120,000) die. In some hospitals, it is the major cause of death after herniorrhaphy, cholecystectomy, and hysterectomy. With major abdominal or orthopedic surgery, the incidence of fatal pulmonary emboli may exceed 1% to 2%.

If one looks carefully for pulmonary emboli, even the smallest visible macroscopically, they can be found in almost two thirds of autopsies on patients over 40 years of age. Although only about 15% of the pulmonary emboli found at autopsy are diagnosed prior to death, many of them are too small to be clinically significant, except in patients with advanced cardiopulmonary disease.

AXIOM

Far more pulmonary emboli occur than are suspected clinically.

It has been estimated that 1 out of every 40 to 80 patients admitted to a hospital will have a pulmonary embolus during that hospitalization. Of these, up to 10% to 20% (i.e., 1 out of every 200 to 800 patients admitted) will die of a pulmonary embolus. Of those who survive, 30% or more of the untreated patients will have recurrent pulmonary emboli, and of these episodes of recurrent emboli, up to 20% will be fatal.

B. VENOUS THROMBOSIS

At least 90% to 95% of clinically significant pulmonary emboli originate in veins of the lower extremities or pelvis. However, less than one fourth of the venous thrombi causing pulmonary embolism produce clinical signs or symptoms in the legs, allowing diagnosis prior to autopsy. About 25% of patients without previous venous problems develop deep vein thrombosis (DVT) in the calf following abdominal surgery. If the patient had a previous episode of DVT, the incidence may rise to 68%. After myocardial infarction, the incidence of venous thrombi in the deep veins of the calf may be as high as 40%.

II. DEEP VEIN THROMBOSIS

A. PREDISPOSING FACTORS

AXIOM

Factors that appear to predispose patients to the formation of venous thrombi are often referred to as Virchow's triad and include stasis of blood, venous-wall injury or disease, and hypercoagulability.

1. Venous Stasis

Factors that tend to cause venous stasis include congestive heart failure, prolonged bed rest or sitting, varicosities, lower extremity and pelvic fractures, operations, pregnancy, obesity, and arteriosclerosis. Emptying of the legs' deep veins when an individual is upright takes 5 to 30 seconds depending on activity. When lying down, it may take 1 to 2 minutes for contrast material to be cleared from these veins. Following surgery, up to 25 minutes may be required. When sitting, there may be little or no clearing of the contrast material from deep leg veins, especially in the soleus muscle, for much longer periods or until the calf muscles are used. The culs-de-sac just proximal to the venous valves are the last areas to clear.

2. Abnormal Venous Wall

Abnormalities of veins may occur with trauma (particularly fractures), thrombophlebitis, arteriosclerosis, or diabetes mellitus. Vein damage from indwelling catheters and various intravenous solutions is potentially so hazardous in the lower extremities that leg veins, especially at the groin, are seldom used to establish IVs in adults.

3. Hypercoagulability

Trauma and surgery tend to increase the activation of factor X in the clotting cascade. In addition, the concentrations of fibrinogen, which is an acute-phase protein, tend to rise progressively after trauma. By the sixth to eighth day following uncomplicated extremity fractures, fibrinogen levels often average two to three times normal.

Because of the increase in blood coagulability after surgery, some surgeons administer minidose heparin (5000 units deep subcutaneously) just before surgery and every 12 hours for several days postoperatively or until the patient is ambulating well. This may be particularly important in patients who are elderly or have other factors that predispose them to deep vein thrombosis and pulmonary embolism.

Elevated levels of female hormones increase the risk of venous thromboembolism, particularly in women with type A blood. Risk of venous thrombosis or pulmonary embolism may be increased up to threefold by oral contraceptives and sixfold by pregnancy.

Visceral carcinomas, especially of the pancreas or prostate, are associated with an increased incidence of thrombophlebitis, venous thrombosis, and pulmonary embolism. Causative factors may include confinement to bed, pressure on the inferior vena cava by intra-abdominal masses, and increased platelet aggregation. One of Trousseau's signs refers to the migratory thrombophlebitis that may be seen with carcinomas of the abdominal viscera.

Thromboplastin generation is accelerated in cigarette smokers, resulting in an increased incidence of spontaneous arterial and venous thrombosis. Patients with diabetes mellitus have increased platelet aggregation, in addition to a high incidence of peripheral arterial disease.

A large number of other less frequent medical disorders can also cause a hypercoagulable state (Table 11.1).

B. SITES OF VENOUS THROMBOSIS

The most likely site for venous thrombosis to begin is in the deep veins of the calf, particularly within the soleus muscle. Veins in the soleus muscle are quite large and have an acute angle of entry into the peroneal and posterior tibial veins. Consequently, if the soleus muscle does not contract frequently, the blood in its veins tends to pool and is more apt to form thrombi.

In most patients, thrombi in the calf veins tend to remain localized there. However, if a thrombus extends up into the femoral and iliac veins, it is usually much larger and much more apt to break off and embolize to the lung.

AXIOM
Thrombi in calf veins rarely embolize. Iliac or femoral vein thrombi are much more apt to become pulmonary emboli.

Table 11.1

MEDICAL CAUSES OF HYPERCOAGULABLE STATES	*Primary* 1. Antithrombin III deficiencies 2. Protein C or S deficiencies 3. Abnormal fibrinogen 4. Decreased or abnormal plasminogen 5. Vascular plasminogen activator deficiency 6. Plasminogen activator inhibitor 7. Factor XII deficiency 8. Homocystinuria
	Secondary 1. Immobilization 2. Postoperative 3. Malignancy 4. Pregnancy 5. Oral contraceptives and estrogen therapy 6. Nephrotic syndrome 7. Heparin, epsilon aminocaproic acid, Konyne 8. "Lupuslike anticoagulant" 9. Platelet disorders 10. "Hyperviscosity" 11. Prosthetic surfaces

C. PATHOLOGY

1. Thrombophlebitis

Phlebitis refers to any inflammatory process involving a vein. If there is any associated thrombosis, the process is referred to as thrombophlebitis. Clinically this process is characterized by pain and swelling over the involved vein. Because the inflammatory process attaches the thrombus more firmly to the vein, it is less apt to embolize than a bland (noninflammatory) thrombosis.

2. Phlebothrombosis

Phlebothrombosis refers to thrombosis in a vein that has little or no inflammatory changes. Clinically there are few symptoms except possibly for some peripheral edema. The thrombus is more loosely attached than in thrombophlebitis and is more apt to result in a pulmonary embolus.

3. Phlegmasia Alba Dolens

Phlegmasia alba dolens, which means painful, swollen white leg, refers to an extremely edematous leg with pale skin due to thrombosis of iliofemoral veins. This problem is characteristically seen in late pregnancy. Blood flow is apparently adequate to prevent severe stasis, but the pressure in the veins is often high enough to cause moderate-to-severe edema.

4. Phlegmasia Cerulea Dolens

Phlegmasia cerulea dolens refers to a painful, swollen blue leg due to iliofemoral venous thrombosis. The tissue pressure due to occluded veins may become so high that the arterial blood flow may be inadequate to maintain the viability of the leg. Particularly at risk are muscles within the various fascial compartments in the lower legs. If the process does not improve rapidly with heparin and other supportive measures (such as leg elevation, etc.), surgical removal of the thrombi may be required to prevent gangrene. Early thrombolytic therapy may be of great benefit with this problem.

PITFALL
Failure to recognize and treat phlegmasia cerulea doleans early may result in compartment syndrome or leg loss.

5. Chronic Venous Insufficiency

Following episodes of thrombophlebitis, the valves in the deep veins and in the communicating veins (which join the superficial and deep venous system) may become fibrosed or contracted so that their function is impaired. The phlebitis may also occlude adjacent lymphatics. As a consequence, chronic venous stasis can result in a postphlebitic syndrome with an almost "woody" swelling of the lower leg and ankle plus hyperpigmentation and ulceration, particularly just above the medial malleolus. The woody feeling of the edematous tissue is due to protein and fibrin deposition.

D. DIAGNOSIS

1. History

AXIOM

Over 70% of patients with deep vein thrombosis in their legs have no symptoms, and when symptoms are present, they are usually nonspecific.

a. Symptoms

If the patient has calf pain during walking or develops swelling of the foot and leg on one side postoperatively, one should become very suspicious of DVT. Occasionally a superficial thrombophlebitis of the greater or lesser saphenous veins will present with localized pain and tenderness.

b. Predisposing Factors

A careful search in the patient's history must be made for any factors that increase the likelihood of deep vein thrombosis (Table 11.2).

AXIOM

Predisposing factors for DVT include age greater than 60 years, cardiovascular disease, prolonged bed rest, recent surgery, malignancies, and cerebrovascular accidents.

Trauma or disease involving the pelvis or lower extremities, particularly in association with hip fractures or amputations, should always be considered as having a high risk. There should be particular concern about deep vein thrombosis if the patient had been sitting for prolonged periods on a boat, bus, or plane, or if the patient is a young woman who is pregnant or taking oral contraceptives. Interestingly, there is some controversy on whether or not there is an increased tendency for morbidly obese patients to develop DVT and pulmonary embolism (PE).

2. Physical Examination

AXIOM

Most pulmonary emboli come from leg veins, but the DVT can be detected clinically only in a minority of patients.

Careful physical examination of the legs is important in anyone suspected of having DVT or pulmonary emboli, but it is not very helpful in most patients. Less than a third of patients with proven pulmonary emboli have any clinical evidence of deep vein thrombosis in their legs. On the other hand, of those who

---

Table 11.2

CLINICAL RISK FACTORS FOR VENOUS THROMBOEMBOLISM	Congestive heart failure
	Myocardial infarction
	Shock
	Obesity
	Estrogens; pregnancy
	Malignancy
	Surgery
	Immobility
	Trauma
	Previous pulmonary embolism or deep vein thrombosis
	Increasing age

have clinical evidence of deep venous disease, up to 50% have no abnormalities that can be demonstrated on venography.

The most frequent signs and symptoms of deep vein thrombosis include increased unilateral calf size (which is best checked with a tape measure and which is present in about 30% of patients); lower leg pain (usually greatest in the calf) in 25%; calf tenderness in 20%; and a positive Homans' sign (pain in the calf with dorsiflexion of the foot) in 10%.

3. Tests for Peripheral Venous Thrombosis

a. Venous Angiography (Phlebography)

AXIOM

Venous angiography is generally considered to be the most accurate diagnostic test of venous thrombosis and is the "gold standard" against which other tests are measured.

The usual technique for deep venous angiography involves injection of contrast material into a dorsal vein of the foot. A tourniquet is placed above the ankle to occlude superficial venous drainage. This forces the contrast material to drain into the deep venous system.

The most frequent findings with venous thrombi include filling defects in or occlusion of portions of the deep veins. Pelvic thrombi, particularly in the internal iliac vein, which may be the source of up to 5% to 10% of fatal pulmonary emboli, are not detected by this technique.

b. Labeled Fibrinogen

Fibrinogen labeled with radioactive iodine (fibrinogen ^{125}I) has been used extensively to document the development of venous thrombi in the legs. After this material is injected, scintigraphic scanning is performed over the legs at selected levels for several days. The tagged fibrinogen becomes incorporated into any clots that form, and if there is increasing radioactivity in an area, the diagnosis of thrombi in the underlying veins is almost certain and correlates with the phlebogram in up to 93% of cases.

Using this very sensitive technique, which can detect rather small thrombi, it has been shown that at least 25% to 30% of patients over 40 years of age having an abdominal operation under general anesthesia develop deep venous thrombi in their calves. Over 90% of these thrombi occur less than 48 hours after surgery. Fortunately, less than 10% of these thrombi propagate into the iliofemoral veins, where they are much more likely to detach and form pulmonary emboli.

AXIOM

Labeled fibrinogen is most useful for detecting DVT in calf veins.

Unfortunately, labeled fibrinogen is less sensitive for clots in the femoral veins and is almost totally insensitive for iliac vein thrombosis. In addition, it may take up to 72 hours after injection of the labeled fibrinogen before a result can be obtained. Furthermore, if there has been surgery on the lower extremity, a false-positive result is apt to be obtained because of the fibrinogen moving into the operative site. It must also be remembered that whenever fibrinogen is administered to a patient, there is risk of hepatitis unless the blood for obtaining the fibrinogen is taken from the patient or from specially selected donors.

c. Doppler Ultrasonography

Doppler ultrasonography has become an increasingly popular and accurate technique for evaluating the patency of leg veins. It is noninvasive and can be performed rapidly and easily. The Doppler depends upon the fact that a moving column of blood reflects an ultrasonic signal at frequencies that vary directly with the blood velocity. Compression of the leg increases blood flow toward the heart. If there are clots in these veins, frequencies that are different from normal are obtained. It is quite accurate if a common iliac or an external iliac vein is completely occluded, but it is much less reliable in identifying (1) incomplete

495

occlusions of iliac veins or (2) femoral or popliteal vein occlusion. False negatives, because of collateral venous drainage, can occur in up to 65% of tests.

AXIOM
Doppler studies for DVT are apt to be falsely negative if the proximal veins are not completely occluded or if the process involves distal veins.

d. Impedance Plethysmography

Impedance plethysmography can be useful as a bedside screening technique for venous thrombi, particularly if proximal veins are completely occluded. It is noninvasive and can be repeated as often as desired without danger to the patient. During inspiration, the impedance (electrical resistance) of the leg normally increases by at least 0.2% because the increased venous return causes decreased blood volume in the legs. If the veins are occluded, the volume of the legs does not decrease during inspiration. Although there are many false positives, few patients with deep venous thrombosis, except those with involvement only of minor veins of the calves, have a normal impedance tracing.

e. Indium-Labeled Platelet Imaging

A new technique of infusing platelets labeled with indium and imaging their uptake on clots in leg veins or in lung vessels has been found to be highly sensitive and specific when compared with other diagnostic tests. In one study of 23 patients, indium platelet imaging was found to have a sensitivity of 100% and specificity of 90%. However, this test is inconvenient and is not widely used.

E. PREVENTION

AXIOM
Prevention of DVT involves improved mechanical emptying of leg veins and use of anticoagulants.

Prevention of deep venous thrombosis and pulmonary embolism should be an integral part of the care of all critically ill, postoperative, and injured patients. These preventative measures are most effective if begun preoperatively in patients undergoing elective surgical procedures, particularly those involving the abdomen or lower extremities.

The methods used most frequently to prevent venous thrombosis and pulmonary embolism include various types of exercise, positioning of the legs, stockings or leg wraps, external compression devices, and various types of anticoagulation, particularly low-dose heparin. The type of prophylaxis used depends on the type of surgery being performed and the number of risk factors the patient has for developing DVT (Table 11.3).

1. Exercise

Most venous thrombi that produce pulmonary emboli begin in the lower leg, especially in veins within the soleus muscle. When the calf muscles contract actively or passively, blood is pushed out of these veins rather vigorously toward the heart (hence the name, soleus pump).

a. Active Exercise

There is no question that individuals who are actively walking immediately prior to and just after surgery are less apt to develop venous thrombosis. For this reason, great efforts are made to have hemodynamically stable individuals walking as soon as possible postoperatively, usually on the afternoon or night of surgery.

PITFALL
Feeling that just getting a patient "out of bed" is adequate DVT prophylaxis.

Just getting the patient out of bed is not DVT prophylaxis, particularly if the patient is "dragged" along between two nurses or physical therapists and does not actively use his or her calf muscles. It is also important that the patient's time

Table 11.3

AN APPROACH TO PROPHYLAXIS OF DEEP VEIN THROMBOSIS (DVT)	Type of Operation or Condition	Usual-Risk Patient	High-Risk Patient (e.g., Prior DVT or PE)
	General abdominothoracic surgery	Low-dose heparin, 5000 units SC q. 12 h, starting 2 h preop *plus* graded compression stockings	5000 units heparin SC q. 8 h *plus* intermittent calf muscle compression
	Eye or brain surgery or open prostatectomy	Intermittent calf muscle compression	(?) Add dextran
	Hip surgery	(?) 5000 units of SC heparin (q. 8 h), *or* (?) aspirin, *or* (?) dextran	(?) Warfarin *or* (?) caval interruption
	General medical patients, including nonhemorrhagic stroke	Low-dose heparin, 5000 units SC q. 12 h, *plus* graded compression stockings	Heparin 5000 units SC q. 8 h, *or* "full" heparin anticoagulation overlapping with therapeutic doses of warfarin
	Hemorrhagic stroke	Intermittent calf muscle compression	(?) Add dextran

PE = pulmonary embolism; SC = subcutaneous.

out of bed is not spent sitting in a chair for prolonged periods, particularly if the legs are bent at right angles to the thighs. However, efforts to have the patient exercise his or her legs in bed can be very helpful, particularly if the patient cannot or will not ambulate properly.

b. Passive Exercises

If the patient cannot exercise actively, there is some value in passively exercising the calf muscles by alternately flexing and extending the feet at the ankles. Various machines have been used to intermittently press against the soles of the feet, causing motion at the ankle. Other devices utilize intermittent squeezing of the calf muscles to encourage blood flow.

2. Position

Elevation of the lower extremities, particularly to 30° or more above the horizontal, may significantly improve the blood flow from the legs to the heart. Doing this every hour or so during surgery greatly reduces the incidence of postoperative DVT. One must be careful, however, not to lower the chest or head below the abdomen because this may interfere with ventilation and venous return from the head. In addition, there is often a tendency to bend the extremities at the knees when the legs are elevated. This may increase the pressure of pillows or sheets against the popliteal space in back of the knees, thereby retarding blood flow through the popliteal veins.

PITFALL

Allowing persistent pressure against the popliteal vein, especially in patients with a tendency to DVT.

3. Stockings

Properly fitting stockings or ace wraps over the entire lower extremity, from the toes to the groin, can greatly improve the rate of blood flow through the deep leg veins and thereby reduce the likelihood of deep vein thrombosis. In evaluating venous stasis and its relationship to intravascular thrombosis, velocity of blood flow (cm/sec) is more important than flow rate (ml/min). The cross-sectional area of the veins in the lower leg of an adult is normally about 2.5 to 3.0 cm², and the mean velocity of blood flow in the area is about 0.5 cm/sec. Well-fitted elastic stockings producing a uniform compression of about 10 to 15 mm Hg on the lower legs decrease the cross-sectional area of the veins to about one fifth of normal, thereby increasing the velocity of blood flow to about 2.5 cm/sec.

AXIOM

For elastic stockings or (ace) wraps to be effective, they must apply a uniform compression and facilitate venous return.

It must be emphasized that elastic stockings must fit properly to be effective. Ideally, the compression is greatest over the feet and is gradually reduced more proximally. Improperly fitting stockings, which are frequently seen when only one size of elastic stocking is used for all patients, can act as a tourniquet and make any tendency to stasis worse. Improperly applied ace wraps may also act as tourniquets and increase the tendency to DVT.

4. External Pneumatic Compression

External pneumatic compression devices have been shown to decrease the incidence of DVT in high-risk patients. Black, Baker, and Snook reported their experience with external pneumatic compression (EPC) therapy in preventing clinically evident deep venous thrombosis (DVT) and pulmonary emboli (PE) in 523 neurologic and neurosurgical patients. The authors felt that the low incidence of DVT (2.3%) and PE (1.8%) in these patients was good evidence that EPC can be extremely efficacious.

5. Prophylactic Anticoagulation

The use of anticoagulants to prevent deep vein thrombosis and pulmonary embolism has received a great deal of attention. Particular emphasis has been placed on low-dose heparin; however, warfarin, aspirin, dextran, and several other agents have also been used by some investigators.

a. Heparin

Deep subcutaneous administration of heparin in "low" doses of 5000 units preoperatively and every 12 hours postoperatively for 5 to 10 days does not usually cause any significant change in the standard coagulation studies. However, it does reduce the incidence and severity of deep vein thrombosis and pulmonary embolism following many types of general surgery. This is accomplished primarily by decreasing the activation of factor X, which is probably the most important cause of the hypercoagulability following surgery or trauma.

It has been thought for some time that minidose heparin does not protect patients who have a very high risk of thromboembolism or who have extensive surgery. In patients with major trauma, orthopedic surgery on the lower extremities, or extensive pelvic surgery for malignant disease, the rate of venous thrombosis in both protected and unprotected patients is 40% to 70%, and the rate of fatal pulmonary embolism is 1% to 5%.

In some studies, low-dose heparin appears to be less effective than warfarin, dextran, or aspirin. This is particularly true if there is a history of prior thromboembolism or prolonged best rest. In addition, many surgeons feel that low-dose heparin causes more blood loss during surgery and increases the incidence and severity of postoperative hematomas. Consequently, many surgeons reserve these agents for elective general surgical procedures on individuals who have a very strong predilection to venous thrombosis and are not apt to have much blood loss.

It has been shown in some randomized controlled prospective trials that the thrombotic tendency in high-risk patients can be overcome by increasing the dose of prophylactic heparin. The dose must be high enough to restore to normal the hemostatic equilibrium disturbed by the pathophysiologic response to surgery. Using the activated partial thromboplastin time (aPTT) as an index of activation of the coagulation cascade, Leyvraz and colleagues confirmed that the aPTT is decreased in the first postoperative week, signifying hypercoagulability. Increased subcutaneous heparin (an average of 18,000 units per day) was required to restore the activated partial thromboplastin time to normal. Patients in whom the heparin dose was adjusted to the response of the activated partial thromboplastin time had fewer thromboembolic complications and had no

Table 11.4

RECOMMENDATIONS OF THE AMERICAN HOSPITAL ASSOCIATION COUNCIL ON THROMBOSIS	*Preoperative Screening* No aspirin or other platelet antiaggregating drugs for 5 days preop No warfarin therapy at the time of surgery Hematocrit, PT, PTT, and platelets should be normal *Dose and Duration of Prophylaxis* 5000 units of heparin SC 2 hours preop and repeat every 12 h until hospital discharge *Limitations* The low-dose heparin regimen is of limited value in repair of femoral fractures, hip and knee joint reconstruction, and open prostatectomy The regimen is not currently recommended for operations on the eye, on the brain, or requiring spinal anesthesia The regimen is ineffective in patients with an active thrombotic process *Monitoring of Heparin Therapy* No laboratory tests (whole blood clotting time, PTT, thrombin time, antithrombin III assay) are necessary *Hemorrhage* Low-dose heparin may minimally increase operative hemorrhage *Role of Physician* There will be instances in which the physician will correctly decide not to employ low-dose heparin prophylaxis in special situations

PT = prothrombin time; PTT = partial thromboplastin time; SC = subcutaneous.

more hemorrhagic side effects than patients who received a constant arbitrarily fixed dose. Physicians following the recommendations of the American Hospital Association Council on Thrombosis may also have relatively few complications (Table 11.4).

In a special report published in 1988, Collins and associates reviewed more than 70 randomized trials in general, urologic, elective orthopedic, or traumatic orthopedic surgery. The outcome among patients assigned to receive standard therapy was compared with that among those assigned to receive the same standard therapy plus perioperative treatment with heparin (started a few hours before surgery or on admission, and injected subcutaneously every 8 to 12 hours for about a week, or until the patient was ambulant). In summary this review of more than 70 randomized trials in 16,000 patients demonstrated that the perioperative use of subcutaneous heparin can prevent about half of all pulmonary emboli and about two thirds of all deep vein thromboses. The reduction in deaths attributed to pulmonary embolism was particularly striking (19 occurred in the patients assigned to receive heparin as compared with 55 in the controls, $P < 0.0001$) and was not offset by any increase in deaths attributed to other causes; therefore, total mortality was also reduced significantly. Heparin appeared to reduce the risk of deep vein thromboses and deaths from pulmonary embolism for all types of surgery. These findings provide strong evidence that perioperative subcutaneous heparin can reduce mortality form pulmonary embolism in all these types of surgery. At present, however, many orthopedic and general surgeons do not routinely use any form of prophylactic anticoagulation. These findings suggest that policy should be reconsidered, at least in patients at high risk for thromboembolic events.

Low-dose heparin in combination with dihydroergotamine has been enthusiastically touted in Europe. Dihydroergotamine is able to constrict peripheral veins and should thereby enhance venous return. However, gangrene of digits due to ergotamine-induced spasm of digital vessels has been reported.

Several trials have shown that low molecular weight (LMW) heparin can be an effective antithrombotic agent with few side effects. In particular, LMW heparin is less likely to cause heparin-induced thrombocytopenia or thrombosis. Nevertheless, anyone receiving heparin, even in low doses, should have platelet counts done at least every other day.

AXIOM

Patients should have aPTT and platelet counts before starting heparin and at least every other day while receiving heparin.

b. Coumadin (Warfarin)

Although long-term, adequately controlled anticoagulation with Coumadin (warfarin) reduces both the incidence of deep vein thrombosis following hip surgery and the incidence of lethal pulmonary embolism following both hip and general surgery, it also increases the risk of bleeding. Consequently, it is used relatively infrequently. Nevertheless, Francis and colleagues reported a two-stage regimen for warfarin in which a dose large enough to prolong the prothrombin time by 1.5 to 3.0 seconds was given before surgery and enough postoperatively, when there was less likelihood of bleeding, to raise the prothrombin time to about 1.5 times control. This reduced the incidence of both DVT and bleeding complications.

c. Aspirin

Aspirin reduces platelet aggregation and the tendency to venous thrombosis. Aspirin alters the activity of all of the platelets it contacts for the life of those platelets, which is usually about 10 days. Nonsteroidal anti-inflammatory drugs (NSAIDs), such as ibuprofen, in contrast, alter the activity of platelets only for about 6 to 24 hours.

Although aspirin has decreased the incidence of DVT and PE in several experimental and clinical studies, it is not widely used clinically. It appears to be more effective if used with dipyridamole (Persantine); however, the combination can cause excessive bleeding. Although aspirin by itself usually increases the bleeding time by only 2 to 3 minutes, if the patient has any other disease or drugs that also interfere with platelet function, the bleeding time can rise to clinically significant levels.

AXIOM

Administration of aspirin to patients who have any other cause for platelet dysfunction can cause a significantly increased bleeding time for up to 10 days.

d. Dextran

Dextran is a name given to a wide group of polysaccharides formed by the action on sucrose of an enzyme produced by the bacterium *Leuconostoc mesenteroides*. Dextran 40 consists of a group of these polysaccharides with an average molecular weight of 40,000. It appears to reduce the incidence of deep venous thrombosis as demonstrated by phlebography but not by fibrinogen I 125 studies, which detect much smaller thrombi. In some studies the incidence of fatal pulmonary emboli fell from 2.1% in controls to 0.3% with dextran 40.

The antithrombotic effects of low molecular weight dextran appear to be due to (1) reduced platelet activation and aggregation, (2) changes in the structure of fibrin (because dextrans interfere with the activity of factor XIII, which is important for thrombus stability), and (3) improved blood flow, especially through capillaries. Some physicians feel strongly that the efficacy of dextran in orthopedic and gynecologic surgery is well established. However, its value in general surgery is less clear.

To be effective, dextran must be given on the same day as the surgery or trauma. During the first 24 hours, 500 to 1000 ml is given by continuous IV infusion followed by 500 ml daily until the patient is actively walking.

When the dextran is first started, one should look carefully for anaphylactoid reactions, which have been reported to occur in 0.008% to 0.08% of patients. If such a reaction is encountered, treatment usually includes epinephrine

(0.5 to 1.0 ml of 1:1000 solution IV or IM, depending on the severity of the reaction) and steroids (at least 250 mg of hydrocortisone). Antihistamines may also be of value.

AXIOM

If dextrans are used, the blood bank must be warned so that they can wash the dextran off of the red blood cells prior to typing and cross-matching the blood.

Dextrans, particularly dextran 70, may coat red blood cells and interfere with their aggregation by antigen-antibody reactions. Dextrans may also increase oozing from raw surfaces. Therefore, they should not be given to patients with large open wounds, marked thrombocytopenia or clotting defects. Renal damage may also occur if large amounts of dextran are given to dehydrated patients.

F. TREATMENT

1. Anticoagulation

The most important part of the treatment of deep venous thrombosis is adequate anticoagulation, so as to prevent formation of new thrombi while there is spontaneous or medical thrombolysis. This anticoagulation is usually begun with heparin and then continued with Coumadin for at least 3 to 6 months, depending upon the cause of DVT.

a. Heparin

Prior to considering initiating heparin therapy, a careful history and physical should be obtained, as well as appropriate laboratory studies (Table 11.5). There are few absolute contraindications to anticoagulation, particularly if dosage is controlled properly with coagulation studies. Bleeding from mucosal lesions, such as an active duodenal ulcer, is a clear contraindication to heparin therapy. Although the presence of a nonbleeding ulcer may not be a contraindication, heparin in such circumstances must be given with great care. Other individuals in whom heparin therapy is a special risk are those with surgery or trauma to the brain, eye, spinal cord, urinary tract, joints, or retroperitoneum within the past 4 to 7 days.

Other categories of patients who have an increased risk of bleeding with heparinization include the elderly (particularly obese females), those with blood dyscrasias, those with multiple indwelling catheters (nasogastric tube, urinary catheter, etc.), and those on immunosuppressive drugs.

Depending on the risk profile of the patient, one may or may not require a confirmation of the diagnosis of DVT before beginning therapy.

(1) Actions of Heparin

Heparin inhibits the coagulation mechanism in at least three sites: (1) activation of factor X, (2) formation of thrombin from prothrombin, and (3) conversion of

---

Table 11.5

PROCEDURE PRIOR TO INITIATING HEPARIN THERAPY	1. Obtain a careful history
	   a. History of prior thromboembolic or bleeding problems
	   b. Prior response to anticoagulation
	   c. Underlying diseases that might affect heparinization (e.g., recent surgery or trauma)
	   d. Concomitant drug therapy
	   e. Symptoms suggestive of an active bleeding disorder
	2. Physical examination to detect potential risk of bleeding
	   a. Blood pressure
	   b. Skin examination to exclude petechia and ecchymosis
	   c. Rectal examination with stool sample for occult blood
	3. Baseline laboratory evaluation
	   a. Complete blood count
	   b. Platelet count (qualitative assessment on blood smear will suffice)
	   c. Partial thromboplastin time and prothrombin time
	   d. Urine analysis (to detect hematuria)

fibrinogen to fibrin. These effects are produced by enhancing the effect of an alpha$_2$ globulin known as heparin cofactor or antithrombin III (AT-III). This heparinantithrombin complex appears to act most effectively by inhibiting activated factor X, thereby decreasing the formation of thrombin. It is now known that the heparin-antithrombin complex also inhibits activated factors IX, XI, XII, and kallikrein. In addition, heparin has been reported to have high affinity for platelet factor 4 (PF4), to the extent that PF4 can effectively compete with AT-III for heparin binding. Only a portion the unfractionated heparin (UH) used clinically has high AT-III affinity, and displays very high anticoagulant activity. The smallest polymers having this property are characterized by a MW = 1800 to 5500 d. These low molecular weight fractions may be separated from the larger molecules by gel filtration or AT-III affinity column chromatography. Partially modified low molecular weight fractions may also be obtained by cleavage of the larger molecules by chemical or enzymatic depolymerization. Low molecular weight fractions thus obtained have mean MW = 3000 to 6000 d; however, they retain a degree of heterogeneity present in the parent molecules.

The smaller fragments or low molecular weight heparin (LMWH) fractions appear to be different both from one another and from the parent molecule. Notable differences include greater subcutaneous bioavailability, greater in vitro inhibition of factor Xa than factor IIa.

Clinical studies of low molecular weight heparins have shown that they are generally less hemorrhagic for equivalent antithrombotic effect(s) than unfractionated heparins. In addition, several clinical studies have demonstrated their superiority in the prophylaxis of deep venous thrombosis formation following major surgery.

Since the possible adverse reactions of heparins may be related to the disease that they are used to treat, the effects of low molecular weight dextran (LMWD) were studied in normal subjects by Freedman and associates. They found that the agent worked well and was well tolerated. There was no evidence of thrombocytopenia.

AXIOM

In some instances, the improvement in pulmonary or leg symptoms following the administration of heparin may be so dramatic that it can be considered almost diagnostic.

Abrupt improvement in leg or pulmonary symptoms following a large dose of IV heparin is probably due to an inhibition of serotonin. It is most apt to occur if at least 5000 to 10,000 units of heparin is given rapidly IV. Although heparin does not in itself cause clot lysis, it facilitates the disappearance of clots by preventing additional thrombus formation while the patient's own lytic processes are active.

(2) Methods of Administration

(a) Continuous intravenous infusion

The safest and most effective method for administering heparin is by continuous IV infusion. An initial injection of heparin (100 U/kg) should be given IV as a bolus, immediately followed by a continuous IV infusion of whatever amount is needed, usually 750 to 1250 units per hour, to maintain the thrombin time or PTT at 1.5 to 2.0 times the upper limits of normal for that laboratory.

AXIOM

If antithrombin levels are low, much larger doses of heparin are needed to anticoagulate the patient.

Normal levels of antithrombin are needed for heparin to work properly. Although 20,000 to 30,000 units of heparin daily, given by continuous IV infusion, will adequately anticoagulate most patients, 5% to 10% of patients may require much larger doses. Sometimes as much as 60,000 to 80,000 units per day is needed for the first 2 to 3 days after a large embolus or thrombus has reduced the patient's antithrombin levels to less than 50% to 60% of normal. If such doses of heparin are required, coagulation tests should be performed every 6 to 8 hours to prevent overcoagulation as the antithrombin levels begin to spontaneously rise back to normal.

AXIOM
The first clinical evidence of excessive anticoagulation is often the presence of microscopic hematuria.

Patients often become much more responsive to heparin after the initial 2 or 3 days, as antithrombin levels begin to rise back toward normal. Giving fresh frozen plasma or cryoprecipitate can restore antithrombin levels to normal much faster, thereby reducing the amount of heparin needed for adequate anticoagulation.

(b) Intermittent intravenous injection	Although continuous IV infusion is usually the most effective and safest way to give heparin, in some patients the amount of fluid given simultaneously may be excessive and in some patients no veins are available for the infusion. Under such circumstances, heparin can be given by intermittent IV injection through what is called a "heparin lock" in a peripheral vein. This usually consists of a scalp vein needle attached to IV tubing which has its other end closed with a resealable diaphragm through which injections can be made. The doses are usually 5000 to 8000 units every 4 hours or 6000 to 10,000 units every 6 hours. This is a convenient technique, but the clotting time is often increased to infinity for at least an hour following each injection, thereby increasing the risk of bleeding complications.
(c) Intermittent subcutaneous injection	This technique consists of injecting very concentrated heparin (20,000 to 40,000 units per milliliter) deep into the subcutaneous fat through a long 25- to 26-gauge needle. The injection must be given atraumatically. The needle is wiped clean of heparin before injecting, and ice is applied over the site of injection for several minutes before and after each injection to reduce the incidence and severity of pain and hematoma at the injection site. The dose is usually 10,000 to 15,000 units every 8 hours or 15,000 to 20,000 units every 12 hours. This technique usually produces adequate heparin levels within 1 hour, followed by a high peak for 1 to 2 hours and then a gradual decline over the next 6 to 10 hours.
(3) Duration of Therapy	Once a patient is started on heparin, it should be given for at least 5 to 7 days or until all symptoms of the embolus or deep venous thrombosis have disappeared and full, stable oral anticoagulation has been achieved.
(4) Complications	The major complication of heparin therapy is bleeding either externally or internally into a hollow viscus or into closed spaces, such as the retroperitoneum. Such complications have been reported in 10% to 27% of patients receiving heparin. In about 5% of the patients receiving heparin, the bleeding is severe enough to require one or more blood transfusions. Older women are particularly prone to develop bleeding complications. In some hospitals heparin is the most frequent cause of drug-related death.

Approximately 5% of patients show an increased sensitivity to heparin and about 10% have an extremely increased resistance to heparin. Regulating dosage in these individuals may be very difficult. Even with frequent (every 6 to 8 hours) clotting tests and close regulation of dosage, preferably by constant IV infusion, the amount of anticoagulation may be extremely variable from day to day. In general, it is safer to be very cautious about increasing heparin dosage beyond 1000 to 1250 units per hour.

Up to 10% to 15% of patients receiving heparin may have an acute nonidiosyncratic reaction with a mild temporary thrombocytopenia that does not require stopping the heparin therapy. However, 3% to 9% of patients receiving heparin will have an idiosyncratic heparin-induced thrombocytopenia (HIT) due to an antigen-antibody reaction causing deposition of platelet aggregates in the microcirculation. This is mediated by a specific platelet-associated IgG antibody. Thrombosis has been reported in 1% to 20% of patients with HIT. This may result in acute myocardial infarction, CVA, pulmonary embolus, or peripheral artery thrombosis. Once idiosyncratic HIT is recognized, heparin should be discontinued and another anticoagulant should be used. Even the small amounts of heparin used in catheter flushes can cause the HIT syndrome in a sensitized patient.

AXIOM
Platelet counts should be performed daily or at least every other day on patients who are receiving heparin.

Heparin-induced thrombocytopenia is apparently nonexistent or very rare in patients on low molecular weight heparin.

b. Coumadin

Oral anticoagulant therapy with Coumadin may be started as soon as the signs and symptoms of DVT or pulmonary embolus have subsided with heparin. Beginning Coumadin early (within 3 days of starting the heparin) has significantly reduced the duration of hospitalization in some series.

Coumadin has no benefit in the acute phase of DVT. Its main role is prevention of further thrombus formation. This agent acts on the liver to inhibit hepatic production of prothrombin (factor II) and factors VII, IX, and X, all of which are involved in thrombin formation. Since factor VII has the shortest half-life (about 6 hours) of these factors, the prothrombin time (PT) usually becomes prolonged before the partial thromboplastin time becomes abnormal.

A dosage of 10 to 15 mg of Coumadin daily will usually cause the prothrombin time to rise to about 1.5 times normal in 3 to 5 days. After this effect has been achieved, a daily dose of 5.0 to 7.5 mg will usually be adequate to maintain this level of anticoagulation. Since most pulmonary emboli that recur do so within 3 months of hospitalization, Coumadin should be continued for at least that length of time. If the patient has a strong predisposition to venous thrombi and pulmonary embolus, it may be wise to continue oral anticoagulants indefinitely or to interrupt the inferior vena cava below the renal veins.

The hemorrhagic complications of long-term warfarin therapy increase linearly with the duration of treatment and the prothrombin time. Petitti, Strom, and Melmon confirmed this with their studies and suggested that intensive, long-term warfarin anticoagulation should not be used if it is the patient's first episode of venous thromboembolism and the patient has no predisposing conditions.

AXIOM
With long-term anticoagulation, the prothrombin time should not exceed 1.5 times control.

One must also be aware that a wide variety of conditions can alter the prothrombin time in spite of a constant dose of Coumadin (Table 11.6). Consequently, with any change in the patient's condition or medications, the PT should be watched much more closely.

Table 11.6

FACTORS ALTERING PROTHROMBIN TIME (PT)	
	Factors That Increase (Prolong) the PT Endogenous: hepatic failure, congestive heart failure, hyperthyroidism, fever, malignancies Exogenous: alcohol, antibiotics, cimetidine, ibuprofen, narcotics, pentoxifylline, phenytoin, salicylates
	Factors That Decrease (Shorten) the PT Endogenous: edema, hyperlipemia, hypothyroidism Exogenous: corticosteroids, antacids, antihistamines, barbiturates, oral contraceptives, vitamin C
	Factors That May Increase or Decrease the PT Exogenous: ranitidine, chloral hydrate, diuretics

c. Aspirin

If Coumadin cannot be used safely to treat DVT, aspirin in doses of 80 to 325 mg every 8 to 24 hours may be of some benefit. It is felt by some investigators that the smaller doses of aspirin may inhibit thromboxane without also inhibiting prostacyclin (PGI_2), thereby maximizing its effort.

Aspirin reduces platelet aggregation by inhibiting thromboxane release by the platelets. This is at least partly due to acetylation of the platelet membrane and inhibition of platelet factor 3 activation. Aspirin must be used cautiously in patients with peptic ulcer disease or any bleeding tendency. The patient must also be cautioned not to take aspirin if he or she is receiving Coumadin or heparin because of the increased risk of bleeding complications.

d. Persantine (Dipyridamole)

This drug, which is also an inhibitor of platelet aggregation, has been used, often with aspirin, to help prevent thrombus formation on prosthetic cardiac valves when the patient cannot take Coumadin safely. However, much data suggests that giving both Persantine and aspirin is no more beneficial than giving aspirin by itself, and the combination increases the risks of excessive bleeding.

2. Surgery

There are relatively few indications for surgery on acute deep venous thrombosis unless the viability of the leg is threatened, such as in phlegmasia cerulea dolens or compartment syndrome. If the leg is severely ischemic and surgery is not feasible, there may be some advantage to using thrombolytic agents, preferably as a low-dose local infusion.

a. Thrombectomy

If local anesthesia is used while the common femoral vein is being explored, the patient can be asked to perform a Valsalva maneuver when the vein is opened to help remove the proximal venous thrombi. One should also do this while the balloon catheter is being advanced up the iliac vein into the inferior vena cava. If the patient has a general anesthetic, one can accomplish a similar result by inflating the lungs to a pressure of 30 to 40 cm H_2O. This helps prevent embolization to the lungs. If there are bilateral iliac vein thromboses, a simultaneous exploration of both femoral veins is appropriate. Probably the best way to prevent pulmonary emboli during these procedures is to insert a vena cava filter prior to the thrombectomy.

Distal clots may have to be squeezed out of the thigh and legs by compression of the lower extremity. One may also try to flush the clots out by infusing a heparin solution through a foot vein with a tourniquet above the ankle to make the heparin flush go through the deep veins. After all possible clots have been removed, an IV with dilute heparin should be infused distally to keep the deep veins open.

b. Fasciotomy

If signs or symptoms of compartment syndrome develop, a fasciotomy should be performed. If one can accurately measure intracompartmental pressure, a pressure exceeding 30 mm Hg is also an indication for fasciotomy. If one cannot measure the compartment pressures, and there is clinical evidence of a compartment syndrome, one should probably open the anterior compartment slightly. If the muscle is under pressure and bulges out through the wound, a complete four-compartment fasciotomy should be performed.

III. PULMONARY EMBOLI

A. PATHOLOGY

1. Location and Size

In our autopsy series, the pulmonary emboli were lodged in the main pulmonary artery trunk in 20% of cases, the right or left main pulmonary arteries in 25%, lobar arteries in 33%, and segmental or smaller vessels in 20% to 25%. The right side is usually involved more than the left, and the lower lobes are usually involved more than the upper lobes. Most rapidly fatal emboli are 7 to 8 mm in diameter and occlude blood flow to at least one entire lung. Emboli less than 4.0 mm in diameter seldom cause a clinical problem unless they are multiple or the patient has pre-existing borderline cardiopulmonary function.

2. Parenchymal Changes

The usual pulmonary embolus without infarction causes only minimal pulmonary parenchymal changes. The alveoli in the distribution of the involved pulmonary arteries may be somewhat atelectatic, and the vessels distal to the emboli may be somewhat collapsed. The pleura is not involved, and there is usually only minimal pleural effusion unless heart failure has developed.

3. Pulmonary Infarction

The lung parenchyma has a double blood supply. The pulmonary arterial system brings in venous blood to be oxygenated, and the bronchial arterial system supplies oxygenated blood to the supporting structures of the lung. Pulmonary infarction is infrequent unless both the pulmonary artery and bronchial artery circulation are impaired. This is more apt to occur with pulmonary embolism in patients with pneumonia, systemic hypotension, pulmonary hypertension, or malignancies.

AXIOM

The presence of pleuritic chest pain and hemoptysis usually indicates the presence of a pulmonary infarction rather than a simple pulmonary embolus.

On autopsy, pulmonary infarcts are characteristically dark red, firm, hemorrhagic, and less than 5.0 cm in diameter. The parenchymal involvement extends out to include the visceral pleura, and apparently this is what causes the pleuritic pain. Frequently, hemorrhagic pleural fluid with a high protein content characteristic of an exudate is present. Four states in the evolution of a "complete" pulmonary infarction can often be recognized microscopically: congestion, extravasation (of red blood cells into the interstitial and alveolar spaces), necrosis, and cicatrization. The extravasation of red cells into the alveoli is apparently the source of hemoptysis in pulmonary infarcts. Infarcts that do not progress to the stage of necrosis are sometimes called "incomplete" and cause little or no scarring.

Although pulmonary infarcts can cause hemoptysis and severe chest pain, they usually involve only segmental or subsegmental pulmonary arteries and are generally associated with only mild overall impairment of pulmonary artery blood flow.

AXIOM

The main concerns with pulmonary infarction are relief of symptoms and prevention of additional emboli.

B. CARDIAC FINDINGS

Patients with pre-existing cardiac disease have a greatly increased incidence of PE, and large pulmonary emboli can cause cardiac changes. Some cardiac abnormality is found in most patients dying with pulmonary emboli. In one series, cardiac abnormalities were found in almost half of the patients and included right ventricular hypertrophy (45%) and myocardial infarction (13%).

Right ventricular dilatation due to acute right heart failure can be caused by sudden occlusion of a large portion of the pulmonary arterial tree. Right ventricular hypertrophy, on the other hand, is usually due to chronic obstructive pulmonary disease or recurrent pulmonary emboli.

C. PATHOPHYSIOLOGY

1. Pulmonary Changes

a. Gas Exchange

(1) PaCO₂

AXIOM

The typical blood gas changes with pulmonary emboli include a reduced PCO_2 and PO_2 and an increased $P(A-a)CO_2$.

Pulmonary emboli, by reducing perfusion to alveoli, increase pulmonary dead space. If minute ventilation were maintained at a constant level, the arterial PCO_2 ($PaCO_2$) would tend to rise. However, acute pulmonary emboli invariably also cause tachypnea and hyperventilation, which usually more than compensates for the increased dead space. Consequently, the $PaCO_2$ is usually decreased. However, because of the increased dead space, increased alveolar-arterial PCO_2 differences develop. This is most easy to determine if one is monitoring PCO_2 in arterial blood and end-tidal PCO_2 on a capnograph.

AXIOM

Any sudden increase in the $P(A-a)CO_2$ should make one suspect a pulmonary embolus.

(2) PaO₂

Arterial hypoxemia is characteristic of pulmonary embolism. This hypoxemia is so constant that a large pulmonary embolus can usually be ruled out if the arterial PO_2 (PaO_2) is 80 mm Hg or higher while the patient breathes room air. However, with a small pulmonary embolus, the PaO_2 may be normal or only minimally reduced. Indeed, up to 12% of the patients with proven pulmonary emboli may have a PO_2 of 80 mm Hg or more on room air.

Pulmonary function studies during an acute pulmonary embolus usually reveal decreased vital capacity, decreased ratio of the 1-second forced expiratory volume (FEV_1) to forced vital capacity (FVC), and decreased diffusing capacity. Bronchoconstriction has also been demonstrated by radiologic techniques.

Although there are many possible mechanisms for the hypoxemia of pulmonary embolism, the most likely cause is a ventilation-perfusion imbalance. In addition to the increased dead space resulting from the reduced pulmonary artery blood flow to the involved lung tissue, local neurologic reflexes and release of vasoactive substances, such as serotonin and histamine, from the embolic material may decrease ventilation in the adjacent normal well-perfused areas of the lung. Nevertheless, the main cause of the hypoxemia seen with pulmonary emboli is the mechanical reduction of blood flow to otherwise functioning lung tissue by the emboli themselves.

With pulmonary infarction, the involved pulmonary tissue has relatively little gas exchange or blood flow. Consequently, the areas tend to act as "silent units" with relatively little increase in dead space or physiologic shunting. Although the amount of pulmonary tissue involved in pulmonary infarction is usually rather small, aspiration of blood into otherwise normal alveoli in adjacent lung tissue together with splinting of the diaphragm and chest wall due to pain may cause enough hypoventilation or atelectasis to precipitate a significant drop in the arterial PO_2.

(3) P(A-a)O₂ and Qs/Qt

AXIOM

The major functional change in the lungs with pulmonary emboli appears to be an increased ventilation-perfusion imbalance.

Patients with pulmonary emboli almost invariably have an increased alveolar-arterial oxygen gradients [P(A-a)O$_2$] and increased physiologic shunting in the lung (Qs/Qt). The oxygen gradient between the alveoli and the pulmonary capillaries, which is usually only about 10 to 20 mm Hg while breathing room air, can rapidly rise to 40 mm Hg or higher. Normally the physiologic shunt in the lungs (i.e., the percentage of blood going through the lungs without being oxygenated properly) is about 3% to 5% of the cardiac output. With symptomatic pulmonary embolism, this figure is usually increased to at least 10% to 15%.

2. Cardiovascular Changes

The main cardiovascular changes that may occur after pulmonary embolism include increased pulmonary artery pressure and various degrees of acute right heart failure (acute cor pulmonale). If the pulmonary embolus is large, cardiac output may be significantly reduced, resulting in impaired coronary circulation and reduced left ventricular function.

a. Pulmonary Artery

AXIOM
The cardiovascular changes following pulmonary embolism are primarily due to mechanical occlusion of the involved portions of the pulmonary arterial tree.

In previously normal patients, obstruction of at least 25% of the pulmonary vascular bed is needed to raise the systolic pulmonary artery pressure (PAP) above 25 mm Hg. Right atrial pressure generally does not rise until there is angiographic obstruction of 35% of the pulmonary vascular bed and the PAP exceeds 30 mm Hg. Pulmonary blood flow and cardiac output in previously normal individuals generally do not fall until there is 50% to 75% occlusion of the pulmonary arterial tree and/or the PAP exceeds 40 mm Hg.

In general, healthy patients with pulmonary embolism have less severe physiologic changes than might be expected from the size of the emboli. In contrast, chronically ill patients tend to have relatively greater pathophysiologic changes with small emboli, because of significant pre-existing cardiac or pulmonary disease.

b. Right Heart Failure

AXIOM
A pulmonary artery systolic pressure >40 mm Hg is possible only if the right ventricle has become hypertrophied by pre-existing cardiac or pulmonary disease.

The right heart is normally not able to maintain a systolic pulmonary artery pressure above 40 mm Hg. If the PAP is greater than 40 mm Hg, right ventricular hypertrophy due to pre-existing cardiac or pulmonary disease is present. With a PAP greater than 40 mm Hg due to sudden occlusion of more than 60% to 70% of the pulmonary vasculature, the normal right ventricle will fail and become increasingly distended. As the right ventricle fails, its end-diastolic pressure will rise above 6 mm Hg, and the central venous pressure will often exceed 12 to 16 cm H$_2$O. The distention of the right heart may also cause dilation of the pulmonary and tricuspid valve rings, resulting in pulmonary and tricuspid insufficiency. All of these changes are most representative of what happens in patients with no prior cardiac or pulmonary disease. In patients with severe underlying cardiopulmonary problems, relatively small emboli can cause severe symptoms, hypotension, or death.

(1) Reduced Coronary Blood Flow

Large pulmonary emboli can greatly increase the work load of the right heart. In addition, since large pulmonary emboli can cause a severe decrease in cardiac output and aortic pressure, coronary artery blood flow can also fall, producing an increasing discrepancy between coronary blood flow and myocardial oxygen demands.

Table 11.7

INCIDENCE OF TYPES OF CLINICAL PRESENTATION OF PULMONARY EMBOLI	30%–60%	tachypnea-tachycardia
	30%–40%	asymptomatic
	10%–20%	acute cor pulmonale (right heart failure with or without systemic hypotension)
	5%–15%	pulmonary infarction (chest pain, hemoptysis)
	1%– 2%	acute left heart failure

c. Left Heart Failure

Left heart failure following pulmonary embolism is unusual in patients with a previously normal heart. However, the increased work load due to the pulmonary embolus can put an excessive strain on an already diseased heart, and if the hypoxemia is severe and/or coronary blood flow cannot keep pace, the left heart may rapidly become ischemic and fail. When this occurs, it may be very difficult at times to differentiate between an acute pulmonary embolus and an acute myocardial infarction.

D. DIAGNOSIS

Pulmonary emboli can be extremely difficult to diagnose because the clinical presentation is usually either silent or very nonspecific (Table 11.7). In fact, it is apparent from autopsy studies that most pulmonary emboli are clinically silent.

AXIOM
Any acute respiratory or cardiac signs or symptoms not readily explained, particularly in chronically ill or postsurgical patients, should be considered due to pulmonary emboli until proven otherwise.

The diagnostic approach to a patient with a possible pulmonary embolus involves a careful history, physical examination (looking for evidence of cardiac, pulmonary, peripheral venous changes, and various predisposing factors), and scan or angiographic evidence of occlusion of one or more portions of the pulmonary artery tree. Laboratory studies may be confirmatory, but they are nonspecific. Indeed, the list of differential diagnoses is quite long (Table 11.8).

1. History

Dyspnea is present to some degree in almost all patients with clinical evidence of pulmonary emboli (Table 11.9). However, dyspnea and tachypnea may be

Table 11.8

DIFFERENTIAL DIAGNOSIS OF CLINICAL FEATURES OF PULMONARY EMBOLISM	*Dyspnea* Atelectasis Pneumonia Pneumothorax Pulmonary edema Acute bronchitis Asthma Sepsis Metabolic acidosis *Pleuritic Chest Pain* Pneumonia Pneumothorax Pericarditis Pulmonary neoplasm Subdiaphragmatic irritation Muscle strain Rib fracture	*Hemoptysis* Pneumonia Bronchial neoplasm Acute bronchitis Tuberculosis *Right Heart Failure* Myocardial infarction Cardiac tamponade Myocarditis *Cardiovascular Collapse* Myocardial infarction Hemorrhage Sepsis Cardiac tamponade Tension pneumothorax

Adapted from Hirsh, J, Hull, RD, and Raskob, GE: Diagnosis of pulmonary embolism. J Am Coll Cardiol 8:128B, 1986.

509

Table 11.9

SYMPTOMS IN SYMPTOMATIC
PULMONARY EMBOLISM

Symptoms	Incidence, %
Dyspnea	90–95
Cough	50–70
Chest pain	20–50
Hemoptysis	10–25

a. Dyspnea

caused by a wide variety of disorders including congestive heart failure, atelectasis, or pneumonitis. It is also a very common nonspecific reaction to mental or physical stress of any type.

b. Cough

Cough is present in up to two thirds of patients with pulmonary emboli. It is particularly apt to occur in patients with a pulmonary infarction or underlying cardiac failure. In the presence of a pulmonary infiltrate, cough, and fever, differentiating between pneumonia and pulmonary embolism may be extremely difficult at times.

c. Chest Pain

Pleuritic chest pain is present in most patients with pulmonary infarction, particularly if the individual is young and otherwise healthy. However, chest pain is often either absent or rather vague in individuals who have pulmonary emboli without infarction, particularly if the patient is elderly and has underlying cardiac or pulmonary disease. In older individuals, pain due to a pulmonary embolus may be difficult to differentiate from pain caused by ischemic myocardium.

d. Hemoptysis

Hemoptysis, more than any other single symptom, is apt to stimulate the clinician to consider a diagnosis of pulmonary embolism. Although hemoptysis is characteristic of pulmonary infarction, it can also occur with severe heart failure of any cause.

e. Predisposing Factors

The presence of factors that predispose patients to the development of DVT are extremely significant. The more of these factors that are present, the more likely it is that DVT and PE have occurred. An acute, severe PE is unlikely if the patient is not postoperative or has not had an acute myocardial infarction (Table 11.10).

2. Physical Examination

AXIOM

The most frequent signs of pulmonary emboli are tachypnea and tachycardia.

Abnormal physical findings are often absent in patients with pulmonary emboli. The most frequent pulmonary signs found are tachypnea and some basilar rales. An accentuated pulmonic second sound (P_2) is less common but more suggestive of the diagnosis.

Table 11.10

CLINICAL CONDITIONS
ASSOCIATED WITH
DVT AND PE

Clinical Condition	Incidence of DVT, %	Incidence of Fatal PE, %
Orthopedic surgery	40–70	2–5
Myocardial infarction	30–40	1–2
Paralysis	15–60	<1
Major abdominal surgery	10–30	1–5
Medical aspects	5–15	<1

AXIOM

Wide expiratory splitting of the second heart sound, due to delayed emptying of the right ventricle, may be a particularly important clue to the diagnosis of pulmonary embolus.

With severe pulmonary emboli the major clinical signs are hypotension, excessive sweating, cyanosis, and pedal edema, usually due to concomitant heart failure. Except for the accentuated P_2, which usually indicates some degree of pulmonary hypertension, these are all nonspecific signs.

A pulmonary embolus large enough to produce severe right heart failure may cause jugular venous distension. Pulmonary or tricuspid insufficiency may also develop if the embolus causes severe dilatation of the right ventricle and its valves. Acute enlargement of the liver is unusual, but if a pulsating tender liver is found, the patient probably has acute severe right heart dilatation with tricuspid insufficiency and an extremely poor prognosis.

3. Laboratory Studies

Laboratory abnormalities found with pulmonary emboli are relatively nonspecific, but they may help to confirm a clinical suspicion.

a. Blood Count

The white blood cell count (WBC) is generally normal or only slightly elevated with pulmonary emboli. Since a leukocytosis exceeding $15,000/mm^3$ is found in only about 10% of patients with pulmonary emboli, a WBC above this value tends to favor a diagnosis of bacterial pneumonia.

b. Arterial Blood Gas Analysis

Hypoxia (Po_2 <80) following an acute pulmonary embolism will occur in 85% to 95% of patients. However, the diagnosis of pulmonary embolism cannot be excluded by a normal Po_2. Mechanisms accounting for this hypoxia include ventilation perfusion mismatch, decrease in lung volume secondary to bronchoconstriction, and inadequate respirations as a result of pleuritic chest pain.

Because the Pco_2 is almost always significantly decreased, thereby elevating the alveolar Po_2 (PAo_2), the alveolar (A)-arterial(a) oxygen gradient is a more sensitive reflection of the right-to-left cardiopulmonary shunt than the PAo_2 alone. An arterial blood gas is all that is needed for the calculation of the gradient.

$$PAo_2 = 145 - Pco_2$$
$$P(A\text{-}a)o_2 = PAo_2 - Pao_2.$$

An A-a gradient greater than 20 mm Hg on room air reflects a mild ventilation-perfusion mismatch and $P(A\text{-}a)o_2$ >55 on room indicates a severe $\dot{V}/\dot{Q}$ mismatch and is present in 80% to 90% of patients with a pulmonary embolism.

If the patient is receiving oxygen, one can calculate the Pao_2/Fio_2 ratio. A ratio of >200 (e.g., a Pao_2 <80 mm Hg on 40% oxygen) usually indicates a pulmonary shunt exceeding 20% and a need for ventilator assistance.

c. Capnography

Normally, there is no gradient for carbon dioxide across the alveolar membranes, so that the normal $P(A\text{-}a)co_2$ is almost zero. However, any increase in dead space (such as with pulmonary emboli, decreased cardiac output, or COPD), will raise the $P(A\text{-}a)co_2$. If capnography is available, one can quickly determine the $P(A\text{-}a)co_2$ from the blood gases and the end-tidal carbon dioxide concentration. Any sudden rise in the $P(A\text{-}a)co_2$, not clearly due to a sudden fall in cardiac output, may be almost diagnostic of a pulmonary embolus. Indeed, a recent successful pulmonary embolectomy at our hospital was diagnosed intraoperatively in this manner.

In patients with COPD, the $P(A\text{-}a)co_2$ is already increased. However, Chopin and colleagues recently noted that the alveolar–end-tidal carbon dioxide difference or $P(A\text{-}ET)CO_2$ is abolished by forced and prolonged expiration in COPD, but not in patients with pulmonary emboli. Of 34 adult COPD patients with suspected pulmonary emboli (PE), the 17 with PE had a $PaCO_2$ maximal expiration end-tidal PCO_2 gradient [$P(a\text{-}et)CO_2$] of 12 ± 7 mm Hg and the 17 without PE had a $P(a\text{-}et)CO_2$ of 1 ± 2 mm Hg. If a gradient difference of 5% or more was considered diagnostic, the positive predictive value of the test was 74% and the negative predictive value was 100%.

d. Chemistry Tests

It used to be said that pulmonary emboli characteristically produced an elevated lactic dehydrogenase (LDH) and bilirubin with an almost normal serum glutamic oxaloacetic transaminase (SGOT). While it is true that over 75% of patients with proven pulmonary emboli, have an elevated LDH, about 30% have a slight-to-moderately elevated bilirubin, and 10% to 15% have a slight-to-moderately-elevated SGOT. Thus, the most frequent combination of results seen with these tests in pulmonary embolism is actually an increased LDH with a normal bilirubin and SGOT (present in about 40% to 50% of patients).

e. Coagulation Studies

Increased levels of fibrin split products (FSP) in the serum have been reported to be present in the majority of angiographically proven emboli. In contrast, patients with thrombophlebitis or venous thrombosis and no pulmonary embolism have either low or no detectable FSP levels.

f. Pulmonary Artery Pressures

A flow-directed pulmonary artery catheter should probably be inserted in any patient who may have a hemodynamically significant pulmonary embolus. With such catheters, direct measurements of right ventricular, pulmonary artery, and pulmonary artery wedge pressures can be obtained.

AXIOM

Sudden development of high pulmonary artery pressures with a concomitant low pulmonary artery wedge pressure in a previously normal patient is almost diagnostic of an acute pulmonary embolus.

4. Electrocardiogram

AXIOM

Electrocardiographic (ECG) and x-ray changes with pulmonary emboli are usually nonspecific.

ECG changes may be suggestive and supportive of a clinical diagnosis of pulmonary embolism, but they are not diagnostic. In the urokinase trials, approximately 85% of the patients had ECG changes. The most common abnormality is nonspecific ST-T-wave changes. New-onset atrial fibrillation is present in 5% of patients. The most suggestive ECG changes (due to a sudden increase in right heart strain) are a deep S wave in lead I; a deep Q wave in leads III and aVF; T-wave inversion in leads III, aVF, and the right precordial leads; tall P waves; and a delay in right ventricular conduction (complete or incomplete right bundle branch block) (Fig. 11.1). The S_1Q_3 sign is most specific for pulmonary emboli but is present in only 3% to 4% of such patients. If large pulmonary emboli persist or recur, there may be evidence of right atrial and right ventricular hypertrophy (Fig. 11.2).

5. Radiologic Studies

a. Chest X-Rays

The chest x-ray is of relatively little help in the diagnosis of pulmonary emboli. Its main value is to help exclude other intrathoracic diseases. The chest x-ray remains normal in at least 25% to 30% of cases, and most of the abnormalities seen (pulmonary congestion, pneumonitis, atelectasis, or effusion) are nonspecific. The hemidiaphragm on the involved side is often slightly elevated, suggesting the presence of some atelectasis. With a large pulmonary embolus one might rarely see a bulging pulmonary artery with diminished peripheral pulmonary vascular markings distal to the embolus (Westermark's sign).

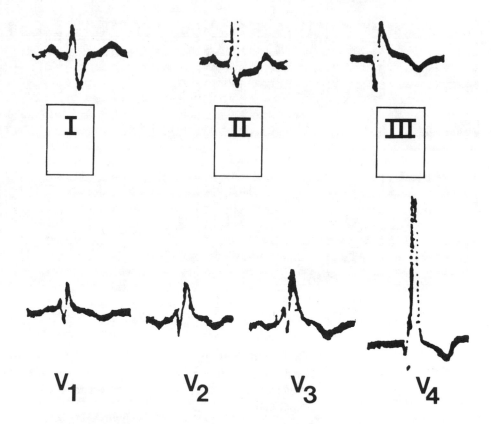

- **Transient Right B.B.B.**
- **T wave inversion V₁-V₄**

Figure 11.1 With pulmonary embolus infarction we may see a large S wave in lead I and Q wave in III. ST depression is usually present in lead II. There is also commonly a right bundle branch block and T wave inversion in V_1 through V_4.

Pulmonary infarction is more apt to cause x-ray changes than is a pulmonary embolus. These findings include an area of consolidation or infiltration, which occasionally has the shape of a truncated cone or wedge extending out to the pleura. The (hilar) side of the density is pointed. The lateral end of the cone or wedge is rounded (Hampton hump).

b. Perfusion Lung Scans Lung scanning after injection of macroaggregated radioiodinated serum particles (10 to 50 μm in diameter) is safe and can be extremely helpful, particularly as a screening test to exclude the diagnosis. There are few false-negative results.

AXIOM

If a perfusion lung scan is normal, it is fairly good evidence that a pulmonary embolus is not present.

Perfusion defects larger than a segment that are unmatched (i.e., the ventilation scan of that area is normal) and occur in two or more areas of the lung that are normal on the chest x-ray are strongly suggestive of the diagnosis of pulmonary embolus (Table 11.11). Unfortunately, there are many causes of impaired perfusion in the lung which can result in false-positive "cold" or "empty" areas on the lung scan. Pneumonitis, atelectasis, blebs, and tumors are just a few. In one study it was found that 60% of patients with positive-perfusion lung scans had a normal pulmonary arteriogram, and 10% of normal subjects

513

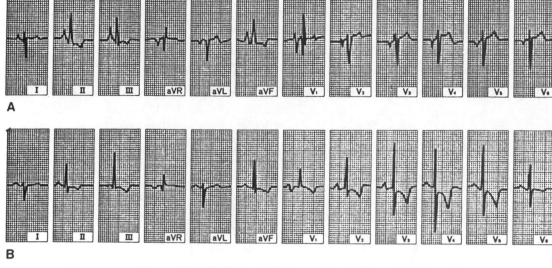

Figure 11.2 (*A*) Right atrial hypertrophy; (*B*) right ventricular hypertrophy.

showed defects on the perfusion scan. In addition, a significant number of perfusion scans are in the gray zone (i.e., not clearly positive or negative). Nevertheless, under certain circumstances, a lung scan can be virtually diagnostic.

AXIOM
Demonstration of large areas of decreased perfusion on a lung scan in a portion of the lung that has normal ventilation and is normal on chest x-ray can be considered almost diagnostic of pulmonary emboli.

If a pulmonary embolus produces changes that can be seen on the plain chest x-ray film, the lung scan is of no help in differentiating an embolus from other lesions in that area. In addition, small areas of decreased perfusion due to small emboli may not be appreciated on the lung scan. Furthermore, other lesions such as congestive heart failure or chronic lung disease not always readily apparent on the plain chest film, can also cause small defects on the lung scan. In addition, since the patient has to remain relatively still for 20 to 25 minutes while the scan is being performed, it may be difficult to get an adequate scan in restless patients.

c. Ventilation Lung Scans   Ventilation lung scans can help confirm the diagnosis of pulmonary embolism, particularly if the perfusion scan is abnormal. Inhaled radioactive xenon 133 rapidly distributes itself throughout all ventilated portions of the lung. Poorly

Table 11.11

PROBABILITY OF PULMONARY EMBOLISM ON VENTILATION-PERFUSION SCANS (ASSUMING NORMAL CHEST X-RAY)		
	High	≥2 large unmatched perfusion deficits (UPDs)*
		≥1 large and 1 moderate-sized UPD*
	Intermediate	≥4 moderate-sized UPDs†
	Low	1 large matched perfusion defect (MPD)
		<4 moderate-to-large MDPs
		>3 small MDPs‡

*Large defects = >75% of a segment
† = 25%–75% of a segment
‡Small defect = <25% of a segment

ventilated areas are manifested as "cold" spots, which do not emit radioactivity. A significant decrease in perfusion of an area of the lung usually produces some reduction in ventilation of that area. However, it is generally assumed that the perfusion defect will be much greater than the ventilation defect in an individual with a pulmonary embolus.

AXIOM
An area larger than a segment with poor perfusion and little or no impairment of ventilation is considered a high-probability scan, particularly if the chest x-ray is normal in that area.

Unfortunately, ventilation scans have poor spatial resolution and they are not particularly helpful in patients with small-to-medium-sized perfusion defects.

In a recent report on the prospective investigation of pulmonary embolism diagnosis (PIOPED), a random sample of 933 patients was studied: 931 underwent scintigraphy, and 755 of these had pulmonary angiography. Of 116 patients with high-probability scans and definitive angiograms, 102 (88%) had pulmonary embolism. However, only a minority of the patients with pulmonary emboli had high-probability scans (sensitivity 41%; specificity 97%).

Of 322 patients with intermediate probability scans, 105 (33%) had pulmonary embolism. Pulmonary embolism occurred in only 12% of patients with low probability scans. Thus, clinical assessment combined with the ventilation/perfusion scan established or excluded the diagnosis of pulmonary embolism in only a minority of patients.

d. Dynamic Radionuclide Studies

Hackbarth, Kuhns, and Sarniak recommend that if clinical suspicion of a pulmonary embolus is high, but the traditional V/Q scan is negative because the large embolus is nonocclusive and in central veins, a dynamic pulmonary flow study using ^{99m}Tc diethylenetriamine penta-acetic acid (DTPA) be performed in hemodynamically stable individuals. Pulmonary angiography is still necessary for hemodynamically stable patients considered for surgical embolectomy or for thrombolysis.

e. Pulmonary Arteriogram

AXIOM
The pulmonary arteriogram is the "gold standard" by which all other techniques for diagnosing pulmonary emboli are judged.

However, although it is the most accurate technique for determining the presence or absence of pulmonary emboli, it is frequently falsely negative for small emboli. When the pulmonary arteriogram is positive, it is very specific. Filling defects due to large- or medium-sized emboli are readily seen (Fig. 11.2). Unfortunately, small emboli may be difficult to discern, particularly if the arteriogram is delayed for several days and the emboli have lysed.

If there is any doubt concerning the presence of a hemodynamically significant pulmonary embolus and there is a reluctance to initiate therapy, a pulmonary arteriogram should be performed. This is particularly important in young, otherwise healthy individuals. Unnecessary therapy with heparin and Coumadin, which are potentially dangerous anticoagulants, may cause more harm than good when given to young individuals with few risk factors for DVT or PE.

If the patient is in moderate-to-severe shock, a pulmonary arteriogram can be obtained while the patient's circulation is being supported with partial (femoral vein-femoral artery) cardiopulmonary bypass using a portable machine.

Increasing experience is accumulating in the use of intravenous digital subtraction angiography for the diagnosis of pulmonary embolism. In one series, 33 patients suspected of pulmonary embolism received both a digital subtraction study after a right atrial injection and a standard pulmonary angiogram. In 31 of the 33 patients, an acceptable digital study was obtained, and these correctly identified pulmonary emboli in 12 cases. Emboli as peripheral as third-order pulmonary arteries were detected, and there was only one false-positive result.

AXIOM

If a pulmonary arteriogram is difficult to obtain, one should try to get IV digital subtraction pulmonary angiography.

f. Echocardiogram

An echocardiogram, especially a two-dimensional study, may occasionally be useful. Demonstration of an enlarged, volume-overloaded right ventricle in a hypoxic, and/or shock patient without right ventricular infarction is highly suggestive of a massive pulmonary embolus. In rare cases, thrombus may be visualized inside the heart and/or a pulmonary artery. Systolic fluttering from regurgitation as well as other abnormalities of tricuspid valve motion have been noted on M-mode studies.

g. Computed Tomographic Scan

Computed tomographic (CT) scans are not generally recommended for diagnosing pulmonary emboli, but there are a few reports of major emboli diagnosed when computed axial tomography was done with IV contrast.

E. THERAPY

The therapy available for pulmonary embolism or its complications includes general supportive measures, anticoagulation with or without thrombolysis, mechanical cardiovascular support, interruption of the inferior vena cava, and pulmonary embolectomy.

1. General Supportive Measures

a. Respiratory Support

(1) Oxygen

Because severe hypoxemia can rapidly develop in patients with pulmonary embolism, oxygen should be administered in a concentration to maintain an Pao_2 of at least 60 mm Hg and/or an oxyhemoglobin saturation ≥90%. If hypotension or impaired tissue perfusion develops, there is an even greater need for oxygen, and the Pao_2 should probably be kept at 80 mm Hg or higher.

(2) Bronchodilators

If there is clinical evidence of bronchospasm, aminophylline can be given slowly IV in a loading dose of 7 mg/kg followed by 0.5 to 1.0 $mg \cdot kg^{-1} \cdot h^{-1}$ by continuous IV infusion. This agent must be given with great care if there is any tendency to hypotension or arrhythmias. Steroids or nebulized bronchodilators may also be tried.

(3) Ventilator Assistance

If there is evidence of impaired ventilation or an inadequate response to oxygen, ventilatory assistance should be initiated without delay. This is particularly important if hypotension or a decrease in cardiac output develops.

b. Cardiovascular Support

(1) Fluids

Any concomitant hypovolemia should be rapidly corrected, particularly if hypotension develops. Pulmonary hypertension resulting from the pulmonary embolus may cause the central venous pressure (CVP) to be deceptively high in spite of a relative hypovolemia. Insertion of a Swan-Ganz catheter to measure the pulmonary artery wedge pressure (PAWP) may help to determine the patient's volume status, especially if there have been any significant hemodynamic changes. The PAWP also provides important information about filling pressures of the left heart and is a better guide to fluid administration than the CVP. However, if the PAWP catheter tip is in a pulmonary artery branch that is occluded with an embolus, the pulmonary artery wedge pressures will not accurately reflect left atrial pressures.

AXIOM

The hemodynamic response to a fluid challenge (a balanced electrolyte solution given at a rate of 3 ml/kg over 10 minutes) is often the best way to evaluate the patient's fluid status.

(2) Inotropic Agents

If there is acute right or left heart failure, intravenous digoxin may be given; however, it provides relatively little inotropic support. The inotropic effects of dopamine and dobutamine are much more rapid and stronger, and the dosage can be regulated more precisely and rapidly. Dopamine is usually preferable to dobutamine if the patient is hypotensive, because the vasodilating effects of dobutamine can further depress blood pressure. However, if the systemic BP is adequate and cardiac output is low, dobutamine is preferred.

Isoproterenol is of little value in the treatment of pulmonary embolism and is usually contraindicated because of its tendency to increase myocardial oxygen consumption and decrease coronary artery blood flow. However, in an occasional individual with a slow pulse rate and a low cardiac output, isoproterenol in a dose of 1 to 2 μg/min may be of benefit.

c. Acid-Base Balance

A moderate respiratory alkalosis ($Paco_2$ less than 30 mm Hg) may be due to hypoxemia, impaired tissue perfusion, excessive pulmonary congestion, or pain. Therapy, therefore, is directed toward improving oxygenation and tissue perfusion. Sedation to reduce tachypnea should be avoided until the patient is hemodynamically stable and should only be given if the patient's BP and cardiac output are stable and ventilation and oxygenation have been optimized.

Metabolic acidosis may occur if shock or severe hypoxemia develops. If the pH remains below 7.10 in spite of efforts to improve tissue perfusion, the acidosis should probably be partially corrected to a pHa of 7.25 with sodium bicarbonate. The bicarbonate deficit can be calculated using 30% of the body weight in kilograms as the bicarbonate space. The bicarbonate can generally be infused safely at 2.5 mEq/min, correcting only half the total deficit at any one time.

Respiratory acidosis, if acutely developed, should be aggressively managed with endotracheal intubation and ventilatory assistance. Pre-existing respiratory acidosis due to chronic lung disease must be corrected cautiously. One should not reduce a chronically elevated $Paco_2$ by more than 5 mEq/h.

d. Vasopressors

If hypotension (systolic BP less than 80 to 90 mm Hg) persists in spite of adequate fluids, inotropic agents, and correction of acid-base abnormalities, vasopressors may be required to maintain adequate coronary and cerebral blood flow, particularly in elderly patients. The dopamine infusion can be increased to 30 to 60 μg$\cdot$kg$^{-1}\cdot$min^{-1} for its vasoconstrictor action. If this is not adequate, norepinephrine (Levophed) may be used.

If norepinephrine must be used to maintain blood pressure, the addition of phentolamine (Regitine) or a similar alpha$_1$ antagonist can help reduce some of the excessive vasoconstriction in the pulmonary and systemic vasculature that would occur with norepinephrine alone. Two ampules (a total of 10 mg) of phentolamine added to each 4 to 8 mg of norepinephrine in 250 ml to 500 ml of solution is usually adequate to reduce the excessive vasoconstriction that can occur with norepinephrine alone.

e. Diuretics

If the urine output is low in spite of appropriate therapy (adequate fluids, blood pressure, and tissue perfusion), diuretics should be given as needed to maintain a urine output of at least 0.5 ml$\cdot$kg$^{-1}\cdot$h^{-1}. We prefer osmotic diuretics, such as mannitol, over the loop diuretics and will give up to 12.5 to 25 g of mannitol per hour (not to exceed 100 to 150 g in 24 hours) as needed. Mannitol also has some superoxide radical scavenging properties.

f. Pain Relief

If severe chest pain is present, frequent small IV doses (1 to 2 mg) of morphine may be required. However, analgesics must be used very cautiously because they can cause sudden severe hypoventilation or hypotension, particularly if the patient is not on a ventilator or is hypovolemic.

2. Anticoagulation

More than two thirds of patients with fatal pulmonary emboli have evidence at autopsy of emboli incurred during the previous several days or weeks. In addition, at least one third of patients with pulmonary emboli will have recurrences unless adequate anticoagulation is provided. Consequently, anticoagulation with heparin, followed in most instances by prophylactic oral anticoagulants such as Coumadin, should be provided to virtually all patients without contraindications to such agents. There are increasing data suggesting that if there is a reasonable likelihood that an acute pulmonary embolus has occurred, particularly in post-traumatic or postsurgical patients, heparin therapy should be begun immediately, without waiting for a definitive diagnosis.

AXIOM

The most important and effective treatment for PE is the early administration of heparin in full therapeutic dosage to prevent additional emboli while lysis of the emboli progresses.

With early adequate heparin therapy, the mortality rate of established pulmonary embolism has fallen in some hospitals from as high as 25% to 30% to less than 8%.

AXIOM

In young individuals, with no risk factors for pulmonary emboli, it is best to confirm the diagnosis of pulmonary embolism before beginning full heparin therapy.

If embolization of a DVT is prevented for 10 to 14 days, the remaining thrombus, particularly in the iliac or femoral veins, will often organize and attach firmly to the adjacent venous wall. After the clot is well attached, and particularly if it becomes covered with endothelium, the risk of that thrombus becoming an embolus is quite small. Long-term anticoagulation with agents such as Coumadin is not without risks. The incidence of morbidity and mortality due to hemorrhage in the brain after even minor trauma increases dramatically with the number of months of anticoagulant therapy. The risk-to-benefit ratio of chronic anticoagulation must be weighed carefully in each patient.

3. Thrombolytic Therapy

a. Indications

AXIOM

Thrombolytic therapy should be considered in individuals with large pulmonary emboli causing acute, severe cardiopulmonary dysfunction.

There has been increasing interest in using thrombolytic agents to accelerate lysis of large or severely symptomatic pulmonary emboli. Normally the lung has high concentrations of fibrinolysins that cause progressive lysis of any pulmonary thrombi or emboli. It has been found that at least 25% of pulmonary emboli disappear by 10 days, 67% by 28 days, and 95% by 60 days. In some patients an even faster rate of lysis may be highly desirable. Therapy with thrombolytic agents may be particularly important in patients with large or multiple emboli or severe underlying cardiopulmonary disease.

b. Agents Available

The three thrombolytic agents used most frequently are streptokinase (a soluble product of *Streptococcus pyogenes*), urokinase (a thrombolytic agent found in human urine), and recombinant human tissue-type plasminogen activator (TPA).

(1) Streptokinase

Streptokinase acts by first combining with plasminogen. This streptokinase-plasminogen complex then converts more plasminogen to plasmin, which is the naturally occurring fibrinolysin. Streptokinase is quite effective and is much less expensive than urokinase. However, if too much streptokinase is given, it may combine with most of the plasminogen, thereby leaving little free plasminogen to be converted to plasmin. Consequently, the dosage of streptokinase must be regulated carefully. Another disadvantage of streptokinase is that it frequently causes allergic reactions in patients with previous streptococcal infections. Consequently, hydrocortisone and/or prednisolone are usually given with and after the streptokinase. Streptokinase is known to have a 20% frequency of serious complications, most notably cerebral hemorrhage, which occurs in about 1% to 2% of patients. If streptokinase is given once, it usually cannot be given again.

(2) Urokinase

Urokinase acts by directly converting plasminogen in the blood to plasmin, and the dosage is easily regulated. Since urokinase is a naturally occurring enzyme, there are no antigenicity problems. However, it is extremely expensive.

(3) Tissue-Type Plasminogen Activator

Recombinant human tissue-type plasminogen activator works by lysing fibrin directly. A theoretical advantage of tPA over other thrombolytic agents is that it acts by first adhering to the clot and then lysing only the fibrin deposited within the clot. With proper dosing this can avoid the generalized fibrinolysis that occurs with other agents. However, this selective fibrinolysis is thought to occur only with the lower dosage protocols.

Two multicenter studies to evaluate the efficacy of treating angiographically proven pulmonary embolism with tPA have been performed. Patients were excluded from the study if they had intracranial disease, major bleeding problems, recent operation or organ biopsy, severe impairment of hepatic or renal function, pregnancy or lactation, or an inability to tolerate the initial diagnostic pulmonary angiographic investigation. The treatment was 100 mg of tPA administered through a peripheral vein over a period of 2 hours. No adjunctive therapy was used. Standard heparin therapy followed the tPA administration.

Goldhaber has reported that more than 80% of tPA-treated patients have clot lysis within 2 hours, compared with 48% of urokinase-treated patients. However, improvement in lung scan reperfusion at 24 hours was identical in the two treatment groups. The results indicate that, in the dose regimens employed, tPA acts more rapidly than urokinase in the treatment of PE. No instances of intracranial bleeding were observed.

(4) Results

Thrombolytic agents work best on thrombi that are less than 3 days old. Patients treated with urokinase for 12 hours and then heparin for 5 days have had a more rapid improvement in their hemodynamics and a more rapid disappearance of pulmonary emboli than those treated with only heparin. However, it is not clear if such changes reduce mortality and the incidence of bleeding problems. Results with streptokinase have been similar except for an increased incidence of fever and a 6% incidence of allergic reactions.

Increased bleeding to some degree is frequent with thrombolytic therapy and is due to the breakdown of fibrin and fibrinogen into "split products," which act as anticoagulants by (1) inhibiting fibrin polymerization, (2) competitively inhibiting thrombin, and (3) coating the surface of platelets, thereby rendering them less agreeable.

4. Venous Interruption

The great majority (90% to 95%) of pulmonary emboli arise from tributaries of the inferior vena cava below the renal veins, particularly the iliac and femoral veins. Although proper anticoagulation can prevent 80% to 90% of recurrent pulmonary emboli, about 10% to 20% of patients are better treated with some type of mechanical interruption of the infrarenal vena cava.

Table 11.12

INDICATIONS FOR INTERRUPTION OF THE INFERIOR VENA CAVA	Pulmonary embolism or extensive deep venous thrombosis and absolute contraindication for anticoagulation
	Major bleeding on anticoagulation for embolism or venous thrombosis
	Recurrent pulmonary emboli causing hemodynamic compromise
	Failure of adequate anticoagulation to prevent recurrent thromboembolic disease
	Chronic cor pulmonale due to multiple pulmonary emboli
	Recurrent or severe septic embolization (requires ligation of the inferior vena cava)
	Following pulmonary embolectomy
	Any pulmonary embolism causing severe hemodynamic compromise
	Massive pulmonary embolism in the absence of a reversible predisposing condition

a. Indications

The main indication for venous interruption in patients with significant pulmonary emboli are (1) situations in which the patient should not be or cannot be anticoagulated properly, (2) recurrent emboli in spite of adequate anticoagulation, (3) massive life-threatening emboli, (4) recurrent late emboli, and (5) continuing long-term presence of important predisposing factors (Table 11.12).

Most patients who have pulmonary emboli while on anticoagulants are not adequately anticoagulated. Furthermore, although there is a tendency to diagnose any recurrent chest pain in a patient with a proven pulmonary embolus as a recurrent pulmonary embolism, such pain may be due to other causes, including bleeding into a previous pulmonary infarct.

PITFALL

A tendency to automatically assume that all dyspnea and chest pain are due to a recurrence if a diagnosis of pulmonary embolus has ever been made in the past.

Patients who have had a pulmonary embolus large enough to cause hypotension or cor pulmonale with right heart failure should be strongly considered for inferior vena caval (IVC) interruption. These patients are particularly prone to develop recurrent pulmonary emboli, and even small additional emboli may be fatal.

Some patients have a continued strong predisposition to deep vein thrombosis and pulmonary embolism. Patients with chronic congestive heart failure, for example, are particularly prone to have pulmonary emboli and are also difficult to maintain on adequate anticoagulation. Patients who have recurrent pulmonary emboli in spite of anticoagulation therapy should also have IVC interruption. In such individuals, lifelong anticoagulation is usually the only other alternative.

Because of the high complication rate associated with anticoagulants in patients who have DVT or pulmonary emboli, Cohen and associates tried using Greenfield filters in these patients and found that they were a much safer primary treatment than anticoagulation.

b. Techniques

Multiple types of IVC interruption have been proposed, including ligation (Ochsner), plication (Spencer), one-lumen clips (Moretz), multiple-lumen clips (Miles), umbrellas (Mobin-Uddin), and filters (Greenfield). Complete ligation is more apt to cause complications related to venous stasis in the lower extremities than other types of IVC interruption, but it is necessary for recurrent or severe septic emboli, which are usually multiple and small.

Efforts to plicate the inferior vena cava with sutures can cause intimal damage which may result in bleeding or local thrombus formation, and the sutures or staples used to perform the plication may pull through the vessel wall. The one-lumen clips obviate these problems, but the 4-mm wide lumen that it leaves in the IVC may allow clots to slide through or propagate proximal to the clip. The multiple-lumen clips, which convert the IVC into four 4-mm channels separated by 4-mm bridges, appear to be the most successful of the various external clips.

Although the multiple-lumen clip appears to be as effective as ligation and less likely to cause venous stasis, ligation is probably necessary if the patient has multiple small pulmonary emboli, septic emboli, an actual or potential intracardiac right-to-left shunt, of if the caval clip has failed. Patients with a patent foramen ovale, the most common type of atrial septal defect, may develop a paradoxical embolus (a venous embolus that gets into the systemic arterial circuit) which, even if small, can cause death or severe disability if it occludes a major coronary or cerebral vessel.

Greenfield and associates have designed a cone-shaped stainless steel filter device designed to trap emboli without significant reduction in venous flow. Fixation is achieved by hooks that grasp the wall of the IVC, usually without penetrating the full thickness of the caval wall. This "fishhook" principle is designed to prevent proximal migration, and the filter becomes even more securely fixed when emboli become trapped. The filter may be inserted under local anesthesia through either the jugular or the femoral vein, and it appears that the Greenfield filter is less likely to promote thrombosis than other filters. Currently the Greenfield filter is the device most frequently used to provide IVC interruption to prevent pulmonary emboli.

c. Complications

There are certain risks and complications to IVC interruption that should always be considered. Because anticoagulation is often interrupted during any retroperitoneal dissection, pulmonary emboli may occur in the perioperative period. In addition, if blood volume or cardiovascular function is marginal, sudden interruption of the IVC can result in severe hypotension and may occasionally cause cardiac arrest.

Most of the severe leg swelling following IVC interruption is due to underlying venous disease. IVC interruption in patients with normal leg veins seldom causes severe prolonged swelling or other complications. Leg swelling following IVC interruption can be partially prevented by postoperative elevation of the legs and properly fitted elastic stockings. Anticoagulation may also be of some value, but should be reduced or discontinued for at least 6 to 12 hours if an intra-abdominal procedure was performed.

The Greenfield filter can usually be inserted under local anesthesia without interrupting anticoagulant therapy and has relatively few side effects.

d. Results

The incidence of recurrent emboli after IVC interruption varies from 12% to 35%. These recurrent emboli are frequently due to large collateral or aberrant venous pathways. Such pathways have been demonstrated in up to 20% of patients who have complete IVC interruption. However, the dilated collaterals for the IVC or its branches are usually less than 3.0 to 4.0 mm in diameter, so these emboli tend to be small.

5. Mechanical Support

AXIOM

If moderate-to-severe hypotension due to a pulmonary embolus persists in spite of all other measures, mechanical support with partial cardiopulmonary bypass should be instituted as rapidly as possible.

A portable cardiopulmonary bypass machine primed with a balanced electrolyte solution can be brought to the patient's bedside or inserted in the operating room. If the diagnosis of pulmonary embolus has been proven and there is continued deterioration, a pulmonary embolectomy should be performed. If a pulmonary arteriogram has not already been performed, one can be performed in the cardiac catheterization laboratory or radiology suite while the patient's circulation is supported by the cardiopulmonary bypass machine.

a. Pulmonary Embolectomy

AXIOM

Pulmonary embolectomy is the preferred treatment in patients with proven pulmonary emboli that cause persistent, severe shock in spite of all other therapeutic modalities.

Some studies have shown that with emboli in the main branches of the pulmonary artery, emergency surgical embolectomy provides a higher relative survival rate and a lower complication rate than full heparinization or thrombolytic therapy. However, pulmonary embolectomy is rarely performed. The patients with the largest emboli often die too quickly for bypass to be available, while those with smaller emboli will usually respond adequately to other supportive therapy. This procedure, done as an emergency, has an operative mortality rate ranging from 23% to 60%, primarily because of the advanced age and coincident medical problems present in most of these patients.

Some of the problems that delay or reduce the number of emergency pulmonary embolectomies performed include uncertainty of diagnosis (particularly when an acute myocardial infarction may also be present) and lack of facilities in many hospitals for rapid, accurate diagnosis and treatment. It takes most centers at least 2 to 3 hours to obtain a definite diagnosis of pulmonary embolus and to mobilize the people and facilities needed for a pulmonary embolectomy.

Although only a few transvenous catheter embolectomies have been performed, they have reported survival rates as good as open embolectomy. IVC interruption of some type should be performed with or soon after pulmonary embolectomy.

Occasionally, an elective pulmonary embolectomy may be of value in patients with chronic extensive emboli. Chronic large-vessel thromboembolic pulmonary hypertension is characterized by widespread obstruction of the main, lobar, and segmental pulmonary arteries that develops when thromboemboli fail to resolve and are incorporated into the arterial wall. Moser and associates feel that pulmonary thromboendarterectomy is the treatment of choice for this disorder because it greatly reduces pulmonary vascular resistance, improves cardiac output, and restores exercise tolerance. It also relieves hypoxemia, which is uniformly present by the time functional impairment is significant.

Kapitan, Clausen, and Moser recently reviewed gas exchange in nine such patients before and 8 to 18 months after pulmonary thromboendarterectomy. Preoperatively, all of the patients had pulmonary hypertension and were hypoxemic or had an exevated $P(A-a)O_2$. The V/Q distribution was widened with an elevated V_d/V_t and a low cardiac index. After thromboendarterectomy, significant improvement occurred. The V/Q distribution because almost normal, and the cardiac index increased. Kapitan, Clausen, and Moser concluded that thromboendarterectomy improved gas exchange both by improving V_A/Q relationships and by increasing cardiac output.

IV. SUMMARY

Deep vein thrombosis and pulmonary emboli occur frequently in critically ill patients. Unfortunately, these entities are easily missed clinically, and most of the diagnostic tests for them are nonspecific. A high index of suspicion, together with early and frequent blood gas analyses in patients with factors predisposing to deep vein thrombosis, is essential for early diagnosis. Early, well-controlled anticoagulation with heparin is the cornerstone of therapy. Most of these patients already have some impairment of pulmonary and cardiovascular function;

therefore, ventilatory and cardiovascular support must be instituted early and aggressively if shock or severe hypoxemia develops.

SUMMARY POINTS

1. At least 50,000 patients die of pulmonary emboli each year in the United States.
2. Only about 15% to 25% of pulmonary emboli found at autopsy are diagnosed prior to death.
3. Following abdominal surgery, 25% to 68% of adults will develop thrombi in the deep veins of the calf.
4. The three main factors that increase the tendency to deep vein thrombosis (DVT) are known as Virchow's triad and include stasis of blood, venous-wall injury, and hypercoagulability.
5. Thrombi in calf veins rarely embolize. Iliac or femoral vein thrombi are much more likely to become pulmonary emboli.
6. Failure to recognize and treat phlegmasia cerulea dolens early may result in compartment syndrome or leg loss.
7. Over 70% of patients with deep vein thrombosis in their legs have no symptoms, and when symptoms are present, they are usually nonspecific.
8. Predisposing factors for DVT include age greater than 60 years, cardiovascular disease, prolonged bed rest, recent surgery or trauma, malignancies, and cerebrovascular accidents.
9. Most pulmonary emboli come from leg veins, but the DVT can be detected clinically only in 10% to 25% of these patients.
10. Venous angiography is generally considered to be the most accurate diagnostic test for deep venous thrombosis and is the "gold standard" against which other tests are measured.
11. Labeled fibrinogen is most useful for detecting DVT in calf veins.
12. Doppler studies for DVT are apt to be falsely negative if the veins are not completely occluded.
13. Prevention of DVT involves improved mechanical emptying of leg veins and use of anticoagulants.
14. Getting a patient out of bed is not prophylactic for DVT unless the patient is actively using his or her leg muscles.
15. One should not allow pillows or anything else to persistently press against the back of the knees, especially in patients with a tendency to DVT.
16. For elastic stockings or (ace) wraps to be effective, they must apply a uniform compression to the extremity and facilitate venous return.
17. Patients should have PTT and platelet counts before starting heparin and at least every other day while heparin is being given.
18. Administration of aspirin to patients who have any other cause for platelet dysfunction can cause a significantly increased bleeding time for up to 10 days.
19. If dextrans are used, the blood bank must be warned so that they can wash the dextran off of the red blood cells prior to typing and cross-matching the blood.
20. In some instances, the improvement in pulmonary or leg symptoms following the administration of heparin may be so dramatic that it can be considered almost diagnostic.
21. If antithrombin levels are low, much larger doses of heparin are needed to anticoagulate the patient.
22. Slight underheparinization is generally easier to correct and safer than excessive bleeding.
23. Early oral anticoagulation, within 3 days of starting heparin, shortens hospitalization time for patients with DVT and/or pulmonary emboli.

24. With long-term oral anticoagulation, the prothrombin time should not exceed 1.5 times control.
25. A wide variety of factors and drugs may alter the PT. Consequently, the PT should be monitored very closely with any change in condition or medications.
26. Surgery is seldom required for DVT unless the limb is in jeopardy or a compartment syndrome is suspected.
27. The presence of pleuritic chest pain and hemoptysis usually indicates the presence of a pulmonary infarction rather than a simple pulmonary embolus.
28. The main concerns with pulmonary infarction are relief of symptoms and prevention of additional emboli.
29. The typical blood gas changes with pulmonary emboli include a reduced PCO_2 and PO_2 and an increased $P(A-a)CO_2$.
30. Any sudden increase in the $P(A-a)CO_2$ should make one suspect a pulmonary embolus or fall in cardiac output.
31. The main cause of the hypoxemia seen with pulmonary emboli is the mechanical reduction of blood flow to otherwise functioning lung tissue.
32. The major functional change in the lungs with pulmonary emboli appears to be an increased ventilation-perfusion imbalance.
33. Most pulmonary emboli are clinically silent.
34. Any acute respiratory or cardiac signs or symptoms that are not readily explained, particularly in chronically ill or postsurgical patients, should be considered due to pulmonary emboli until proven otherwise.
35. The most frequent signs of pulmonary emboli are tachypnea and tachycardia.
36. Wide expiratory splitting of the second heart sound, due to delayed emptying of the right ventricle, may be an important clue to the diagnosis of pulmonary embolus.
37. The typical results of laboratory tests in pulmonary emboli include a normal or slightly increased WBC, bilirubin, and SGOT, and a moderately elevated LDH.
38. Ventilatory assistance should be strongly considered with pulmonary emboli if the $P(A-a)O_2$ on room air is ≥ 55 mm Hg or the Qs/Qt on 40% to 50% oxygen is $\geq 20\%$ to 25%.
39. Sudden development of a high pulmonary artery pressure with a concomitant low pulmonary artery wedge pressure in a previously normal patient is almost diagnostic of an acute pulmonary embolus.
40. ECG and x-ray changes with pulmonary emboli are usually nonspecific.
41. If a perfusion lung scan is normal, it is fairly good evidence that a pulmonary embolus is not present.
42. Demonstration of large segments of decreased perfusion on a lung scan in areas of the lung that have normal ventilation and are normal on chest x-ray can be considered almost diagnostic of a pulmonary embolus.
43. The pulmonary arteriogram is the "gold standard" by which all other techniques for diagnosing pulmonary emboli are judged, but it tends to miss multiple small emboli.
44. If a pulmonary arteriogram is difficult to obtain, one should try to get IV digital subtraction pulmonary angiography.
45. The hemodynamic response to a fluid challenge (a balanced electrolyte solution given at a rate of 3 ml/kg over 10 minutes) is the best way to evaluate the patient's fluid status.
46. The most important and effective treatment for most pulmonary emboli is the early administration of heparin in full therapeutic dosage.
47. In young individuals with no risk factors for pulmonary emboli, one should confirm the diagnosis of pulmonary embolism before beginning full heparin therapy.

48. Thrombolytic therapy should be considered in individuals with large pulmonary emboli causing acute severe cardiopulmonary dysfunction.

49. It is an error to assume that all dyspnea and chest pain are due to a recurrence if a diagnosis of pulmonary embolus has been made in the past.

50. The main indication for IVC interruption in patients with significant pulmonary emboli are (a) situations in which the patient should not or cannot be anticoagulated properly, (b) recurrent emboli in spite of adequate anticoagulation, (c) massive life-threatening emboli, (d) recurrent late emboli, and (e) continuing long-term presence of important predisposing factors.

51. If moderate-to-severe hypotension due to a pulmonary embolus persists in spite of all other measures, mechanical support with partial cardiopulmonary bypass should be instituted as rapidly as possible.

52. Pulmonary embolectomy is the preferred treatment in patients with proven pulmonary emboli that cause persistent severe shock in spite of all other therapeutic modalities.

BIBLIOGRAPHY

1. Barrowcliffe, TW and Thomas, DP: Low molecular weight heparins: Antithrombotic and haemorrhagic effects and standardization. Acta Chir Scand [Suppl] 543:57, 1988.
2. Black, PM, Baker, MP, and Snook, CP: Experience with external pneumatic calf compression (EPC) therapy in preventing clinically evident deep venous thrombosis (DVT) and pulmonary emboli (PE) in neurological and neurosurgical patients. Neurosurgery 18:440, 1986.
3. Bruhn, HD. Biochemistry of tumor cell thrombosis: Thrombin as growth hormone. Behring Inst Mitt 79:31, 1986.
4. Chong, BH, et al: Heparin-induced thrombocytopenia: Studies with a new low molecular weight heparinoid, Org 10172. Blood 73:1592, 1989.
5. Chopin, C, et al: Use of capnography in diagnosis of pulmonary embolism during acute respiratory failure of chronic obstructive pulmonary disease. Crit Care Med 18:353, 1990.
6. Clark-Pearson, DL, et al: Indium III platelet imaging for the detection of deep venous thrombosis and pulmonary embolism in patients without symptoms after surgery. Surgery 98:98, 1985.
7. Cohen, JR, Tenenbaum, N, and Citron, M: Greenfield filter as primary therapy for deep venous thrombosis and/or pulmonary embolism in patients with cancer. Surgery 190:12, 1991.
8. Cohen, JR, et al: Regional anatomical differences in the venographic occurrence of deep venous thrombosis and long-term follow-up. J Cardiovasc Surg 29:547, 1988.
9. Collins, R, et al: Reduction in fatal pulmonary embolism and venous thrombosis by perioperative administration of subcutaneous heparin. N Engl J Med 318;18:1162, 1988
10. Ducas, J and Prewitt, RM: Pathophysiology and therapy of right ventricular dysfunction due to pulmonary embolism. Cardiovasc Clin 17:191, 1987.
11. Dunmire, SM: Pulmonary embolism. Emerg Med Clin North Am 7:339, 1989.
12. Fisher, MR and Higgins, CB: Central thrombi in pulmonary arterial hypertension detected by MR imaging. Radiology 158:223, 1986.
13. Francis, CW, et al: Two-step warfarin therapy: Prevention of postoperative venous thrombosis without excessive bleeding. JAMA 249:374, 1983.
14. Freedman, MD, et al: An evaluation of the biological response to Fraxiparine (a low molecular weight heparin) in the healthy individual. J Clin Pharmacol 30:720, 1990.
15. Friedell, ML, et al: Migration of a Greenfield filter to the pulmonary artery: A case report. J Vasc Surg 3:929, 1986.
16. Gallus, A, et al: Safety and efficacy of warfarin started early after submassive venous thrombosis or pulmonary embolism. Lancet 2:1293, 1986.
17. Goldhaber, SZ: Pulmonary embolism and deep venous thrombosis. WB Saunders, Philadelphia, 1985.
18. Goldhaber, SZ, et al: Randomized controlled trial of recombinant tissue plasminogen activator versus urokinase in the treatment of acute pulmonary embolism. Lancet II:293, 1988.
19. Goldhaber, SZ, et al: Acute pulmonary embolism treated with tissue plasminogen activator. Lancet 2:886, 1986.
20. Greenfield, LZ and Michna, BA. Twelve-year clinical experience with the Greenfield vena caval filter. Surgery 104:706, 1988.
21. Greenspan, RH, et al: Accuracy of the chest radiograph in the diagnosis of pulmonary embolism. Invest Radiol 17:539, 1982.
22. Hackbarth, R, Kuhns, L, and Sarniak, A: Central pulmonary embolism with normal ventilation/perfusion scan: Diagnosis by nuclear pulmonary artery flow studies. Ann Emerg Med 20:95, 1991.

23. Holmer, E, Kurachi, K, and Soderstrom, G: The molecular-weight dependence of the rate-enhancing effect of heparin on the inhibition of thrombin: Factor Xa, Factor IXa, Factor XIIa and kallikrein by antithrombin. Biochem J 193:393, 1981.

24. Huet, Y and Gouault-Heilmann, M: Low molecular weight heparin fraction PK 10169: A new therapeutic means for anticoagulant therapy? Haemostasis 16:165, 1986.

25. Kakkar, VV: The current status of low-dose heparin in the prophylaxis of thrombophlebitis and pulmonary embolism. World J Surg 2:3, 1978.

26. Kakkar, VV, et al: Prophylaxis for postoperative deep-vein thrombosis: Synergistic effect of heparin and dihydroergotamine. JAMA 241:39, 1979.

27. Kapitan, KS, Clausen, JL, and Moser, KM: Gas exchange in chronic thromboembolism after pulmonary thromboendarterectomy. Chest 98:14, 1990.

28. Kramer, FL, Teitelbaum, G, and Merli, GJ: Panvenography and pulmonary angiography in the diagnosis of deep venous thrombosis and pulmonary thromboembolism. Radiol Clin North Am 24:397, 1986.

29. Layvraz, PF, et al: Adjusted versus fixed-dose subcutaneous heparin in the prevention of deep-vein thrombosis after total hip replacement. N Engl J Med 309:954, 1983.

30. Leroy, J, et al: Treatment of heparin-associated thrombocytopenia and thrombosis with low-molecular-weight heparin (CY216). Semin Thromb Hemost 2:326, 1985.

31. Lund, O, et al: Treatment of pulmonary embolism with full-dose heparin, streptokinase or embolectomy: Results and indications. Thorac Cardiovasc Surg 34:240, 1986.

32. Mills, SR, et al: The incidence, etiologies, and avoidance of complications of pulmonary angiography in a large series. Diagn Radiol 136:295, 1980.

33. Moser, KM: State of the art: Venous thromboembolism. Am Rev Respir Dis 141:235, 1990.

34. Moser, KM, et al: Thromboendarterectomy for chronic, major vessel thromboembolic pulmonary hypertension. Ann Intern Med 107:560, 1987.

35. Petitti, DB, Strom, BL, and Melmon, KL: Duration of warfarin anticoagulant therapy and the probabilities of recurrent thromboembolism and hemorrhage. Am J Med 81:255, 1986.

36. Roussi, JH, Houbouyan, LL, and Goguel, AF: Use of low-molecular-weight heparin in heparin-induced thrombocytopenia with thrombotic complications. Lancet 1:1183, 1984.

37. Salzman, EW and Davies, GC: Prophylaxis of venous thromboembolism: Analysis of cost effectiveness. Ann Surg 191:207, 1989.

38. Salzman, EW, et al: Management of heparin therapy: Controlled prospective trial. N Engl J Med 292:1046, 1975.

39. Todd, GJ, et al: Recent clinical experience with the vena cava filter. Am J Surg 156:353, 1988.

40. The Urokinase Pulmonary Embolism Trial: A National Cooperative Study. (American Heart Assoc Monogr No 39). Circulation 47:1, 1973.

CHAPTER 12

Chronic Respiratory Failure

Chronic obstructive pulmonary disease (COPD) affects over 25% of the adult population and is responsible for an enormous cost in health care dollars, lost work, and frequent ventilator use. The course of the disease may extend over 20 to 30 years with a progressive downhill course. The estimated economic impact of this disorder in 1979 was $5.7 billion.

Some physicians feel that COPD is the most rapidly growing health problem in adult medicine today. Unfortunately, many of these patients do not seek medical advice until the disease is quite advanced and they have marked ventilatory disability. Another problem is that, in many of these patients, the disease appears to progress relentlessly regardless of the therapy.

I ETIOLOGY

Chronic respiratory insufficiency is a long-standing pathophysiologic abnormality resulting in an inability of the lungs to maintain an adequate Pao_2 and $Paco_2$ with a reasonable amount of work of breathing at rest and with ordinary activity. The etiology of chronic respiratory failure may be divided into nonpulmonary and pulmonary causes. The nonpulmonary causes include (1) central nervous system (CNS) disorders due to drugs, CNS infections, vascular problems, trauma; (2) peripheral nervous system diseases, such as amyotrophic lateral sclerosis, polio, and Guillian-Barré syndrome; (3) myopathies such as myasthenia gravis, muscular dystrophy, and amyotonia; (4) endocrine problems, such as myxedema; and (5) chest-wall abnormalities due to kyphoscoliosis, obesity, or surgery.

Pulmonary causes of chronic respiratory failure include (1) chronic lower airway obstruction due to foreign bodies, trauma, and neoplasms; (2) chronic obstructive pulmonary disease, such as emphysema and chronic bronchitis; (3) parenchymal diseases, such as emphysema, interstitial fibrosis, alveolar proteinosis, and tumors; (4) vascular problems, such as congestive heart failure and previous or recurrent pulmonary emboli; and (5) chronic pleural inflammation, fibrosis, or effusions. Some of the other more frequent chronic pulmonary problems that may progress to chronic respiratory failure include the various pneumoconioses, the nonspecific fibroses, and bronchiectasis. Healed bilateral extensive tuberculosis and surgical resections of lung tissue may also chronically impair pulmonary function.

The most common cause of chronic respiratory failure is chronic obstructive pulmonary disease (COPD), which is also called chronic airway obstruction (CAO), and includes emphysema and chronic bronchitis. COPD implies that an irreversible degree of small airway disease or obstruction is present. In contrast, true asthma is characterized by abnormal airway responsiveness or reactivity which results in reversible bronchospasm. Asthmatic bronchitis is a term sometimes used to describe increased airway reactivity in a patient who already has some degree of fixed airway obstruction.

AXIOM

Cigarette smoking is probably the single most frequent cause of COPD.

The current theory for the development COPD has been described by Flenley and is called the protease/antiprotease theory. According to this theory, cigarette smoke attracts alveolar macrophages to terminal bronchioles and alveoli. These alveolar macrophages release leukotrienes, complement, and other chemotactic factors, which then attract neutrophils. The macrophages and neutrophils release elastase, which attacks collagen, elastin, and other components of the alveolar and bronchial walls. Alpha$_1$ protease (a natural local defense measure) is inhibited by free radicals generated by the cigarette smoke.

II. PATHOLOGIC CHANGES

A. EMPHYSEMA

AXIOM

Pulmonary emphysema may be defined as a chronic respiratory disease characterized physiologically by partial obstruction to airflow in smaller bronchioles during expiration.

Pathologically, emphysema demonstrates abnormal enlargement of the distal air spaces and destructive changes of the alveolar walls interspersed with zones of interstitial and alveolar fibrosis. If dense fibrosis predominates, the lesion is often considered to be a chronic organizing pneumonia. If the alveolar dilatation is more prominent, the problem is considered to be emphysema. The alveolar dilatation appears to be primarily due to the partial airflow obstruction.

1. Types of Emphysema

Several types of emphysema have been described in relation to the portion of the acinus predominately involved.

a. Centrilobular or Centriacinar Emphysema

Centrilobular or centriacinar emphysema predominately involves the respiratory bronchioles in the proximal portions of the acinus. Proximal acinar or centrilobular emphysematous spaces are usually larger and are frequently found in the upper lobes and superior segments of the lower lobes. This type of emphysema, usually found only in smokers, is often associated with clinical evidence of chronic bronchitis.

b. Paraseptal or Periacinar Emphysema

Distal acinar (paraseptal or periacinar) emphysema is associated with congenital bullous disease of the lungs and spontaneous pneumothorax in young adults.

c. Panacinar (Panlobular) Emphysema

Panacinar emphysema involves the entire acinus uniformly. It tends to occur along the inferior and anterior portions of the lung. This change is found in familial emphysema associated with homozygous (ZZ) alpha$_1$-antitrypsin deficiency. Lower zonal panacinar emphysema also frequently occurs with upper zonal (proximal) acinar emphysema in smokers. Panacinar emphysema is also found in a variety of congenital and pediatric problems associated with bronchial or bronchiolar obliteration.

d. Irregular Emphysema

Irregular emphysema, in which there is random involvement of the acinus is most apt to be seen in association with scarring from trauma or previous inflammation.

2. BRONCHIAL CHANGES

Narrowing of bronchi and bronchioles in emphysema and chronic bronchitis may be due to intraluminal and extraluminal factors. Intraluminal narrowing can be caused by mucosal edema, inflammatory infiltration of the mucosa, hyperplasia of bronchial mucous glands and goblet cells, or excessive secretions. Persistent or excessive contraction of the smooth muscle in the bronchial wall due to various neurogenic and hormonal influences, particularly hypoxia, may further reduce lumen size. Outside the bronchi, the increased fibrous tissue that accumulates may contract with time and cause an irreversible reduction in the bronchial lumen.

a. Small Bronchioles

The major site of airway obstruction in patients with chronic bronchitis or emphysema is in the small bronchioles (2.0 mm or less in diameter). Since bronchi and bronchioles tend to dilate during inspiration, impairment of airflow during inspiration through the narrowed bronchioles is relatively mild. However, during expiration when pleural pressure exceeds airway pressure, the diameter of the bronchioles is reduced even further. Thus, there may be a greatly increased obstruction to airflow, particularly in the smallest bronchioles.

b. Large Bronchi

Although the emphasis in the past has been on the obstruction in the smallest bronchioles, it is now clear that airway obstruction may also occur in larger, more central bronchi. During expiration, a pressure differential from the alveoli to the mouth is needed for air to move out of the lung. As the expiratory effort is increased, an increased pressure is exerted on the lung tissue. This increased transmural pressure can narrow the airway enough to restrict airflow, especially in patients with weak, easily collapsible bronchi. In severe cases, the expiratory efforts can, in fact, close the airway before the alveolus can empty, thereby trapping air in the alveolus.

Thus, the transmural pressure required to collapse or compress the airways depends on the pressure outside the walls, the pressure within the airway, and the strength of the bronchial walls. Anything that lowers the intraluminal pressure tends to promote airway collapse at lower flow rates. For example, mucus in the smaller airways lowers airflow and decreases the intraluminal pressure in the larger central airways.

The term equal pressure point (EPP) denotes the point in the airways during expiration at which the intraluminal pressure equals the pleural pressure. This point must exist because, as air flows from the alveoli to the mouth during expiration, the pressure that causes the flow is above pleural pressure in the alveoli and below that at the mouth. As pleural pressure rises the EPP moves from central bronchi toward the alveoli. Thus, the airways have a tendency to collapse proximal to the EPP. One consequence of central airway collapse is impairment of secretion clearance, because coughing may cause more central bronchial collapse than less forceful expiratory efforts. In addition, bronchial collapse can impair ventilatory mixing and cause increasing hypoxia.

B. ASTHMA

Asthma by definition is an acute episodic respiratory problem due to reversible diffuse airway obstruction resulting from bronchial smooth-muscle constriction, mucosal edema, and inflammation and accumulation of bronchial secretions. Ordinarily, the changes it produces are reversible. However, if asthma continues for long periods, it may produce lung changes similar to those seen in emphysema.

The basic abnormality in many asthmatics is a lack of, or defect in, adenylate cyclase on the cell membrane, leading to a reduction in the formation of 3',5'-cyclic AMP from ATP. This results in partial beta-receptor blockade which is manifested as hyperresponsiveness of the bronchial tree to immunologic, physical, chemical, or psychic stimuli. These patients also often have a genetic predisposition to become sensitized to environmental antigens with the production of increased amounts of the immunoglobulin IgE (also known as skin-sensitizing antigen or reagin). When IgE, which is bound to mast cells and basophils, combines with its specific antigen, a number of pharmacologically active mediators, especially histamine and slow-reacting substance (SRS), which can induce asthma, are released.

C. CHRONIC BRONCHITIS

Chronic bronchitis is defined clinically as a chronic inflammatory process in the major bronchi characterized by productive cough, present on most days, for at least 3 months of the year, for at least 2 consecutive years. Pathophysiologically, it is characterized by excessive mucous secretion and mucous gland hypertrophy within the tracheobronchial tree. Mild forms usually show no abnormalities on x-ray or pulmonary function tests. The more advanced forms of chronic bronchitis, however, can have changes in pulmonary function and clinical findings similar to those seen with chronic obstructive pulmonary disease (COPD).

D. PNEUMOCONIOSES

Inhalation of noxious agents can result in either an acute pneumonitis or chronic granulomas with fibrosis. Particles larger than 10 microns do not get to the deeper portions of the lungs, but smaller particles, particularly those less than 5 microns in diameter, may reach the alveoli where they are engulfed by phagocytes. Some of these particles, such as marble or gypsum, are soluble and eventually disappear. Others remain in the lymphoid tissue. All cause some fibrosis. The most common pneumonoconioses include silicosis, anthracosis, berylliosis, and asbestosis.

1. Silicosis

Silicosis is a disease of the lungs caused by prolonged inhalation of free crystalline silica in quantities sufficient to produce clinically apparent pulmonary fibrosis. The silica particles stimulate a powerful local fibroblastic response in the lymphatics of the lung, resulting in nodules of fibrous tissue with a characteristic whorled appearance on cross section. This fibrosis can engulf and eventually occlude branches of the bronchial tree, producing a diffuse obstructive emphysema. Tuberculosis is a frequent complication in patients with silicosis and causes further pulmonary damage. Cor pulmonale is a frequent late complication and is the cause of death in many instances.

2. Anthracosis

Inhalation of coal dust without silica is seldom harmful, but quite rare. Pure anthracosis causes much less fibrosis than is usually seen with silicosis, but it may cause more severe focal emphysema.

3. Asbestosis

AXIOM
Exposure to asbestos greatly increases the risk of pulmonary fibrosis, cancer of the lung, and mesothelioma.

Asbestosis is quite different from silicosis. The lymphatic system is only involved slightly and usually rather late in the disease process. The early fibrosis, which is primarily peribronchial, is diffuse rather than nodular. Severe pleural involvement is very common, and inhalation of asbestos fibers is probably the most important etiologic factor in the development of pleural mesotheliomas. The characteristic physiologic disturbance is hypoxia due to impaired diffusion of oxygen across the thickened alveolar capillary membranes. Diffuse obstructive emphysema is not seen, but cor pulmonale or pleural or pulmonary malignancies frequently cause death.

4. Berylliosis

Inhalation of beryllium compounds may cause an unusual chronic granuloma of the lung, which may be manifested on x-ray as a diffuse ground-glass appearance of the lungs with enlargement of the hilar lymph nodes. Interference with oxygen diffusion is the characteristic physiologic defect, and cor pulmonale is the usual cause of death.

E. BRONCHIECTASIS

Bronchiectasis is a pathologic dilatation of bronchi and bronchioles due to necrotizing bronchitis, usually following one or more severe chronic childhood pulmonary infections. Pathologically, the diseased lung, usually the basilar segments of the lower lobes plus the middle lobe or lingula, has markedly dilated small- and medium-sized bronchi associated with chronic inflammation, fibrosis, and destruction of much of the bronchial wall. Large shunts may also develop between the pulmonary and bronchial vessels. These patients tend to have excessive quantities of bronchial secretions and are particularly prone to recurrent infection. Bronchiectasis sica is a form of bronchiectasis with dilated distal bronchi but no excess secretions or sputum. However, this type of bronchiectasis may be more apt to cause hemoptysis.

1. Chronic Granulomatous Infections

A variety of chronic granulomatous infections, due to mycobacteria and various fungi, may cause chronic fibrotic changes in the lung. Tuberculosis and the atypical mycobacterial infections in particular may form cavities that can act as sites of secondary infection. Tuberculosis is the most common cause of bronchiectasis in the upper lobes.

III. CHRONIC OBSTRUCTIVE LUNG DISEASE

AXIOM

The most characteristic lung volume change in COPD is an increased residual volume.

A. PHYSIOLOGIC EFFECTS

1. Ventilation and Gas Exchange

a. Changes in Lung Volume

The expiratory obstruction of emphysema results in gas retention in the lungs and a great increase in the residual volume. As a consequence, the functional residual capacity (FRC) is also increased, but the expiratory reserve volume (ERV) is usually decreased. Because of this, the patient has to breathe nearer and nearer to the limit of her or his lung capacity. Once the tidal volume exceeds 40% of the vital capacity, the patient tends to fatigue and may go into progressive ventilatory failure. The tidal volume is often increased initially but later tends to fall. The inspiratory reserve volume may be severely decreased early in the disease process. Total lung capacity tends to increase, but vital capacity is almost invariably decreased.

(1) Alveolar Dead Space

The increased size of the alveoli and loss of alveolar septa in emphysema result in increased alveolar dead space. An increase in dead space tends to cause carbon dioxide retention if minute ventilation remains constant. The increased Pa_{CO_2} initially stimulates a deeper tidal volume and increased respiratory rate, but later it may be difficult for the patient to maintain an increased tidal volume. In addition, the poor mixing of air in the lung and inefficient diffusion result in a reduction of the Pa_{CO_2}. In general, a rising Pa_{CO_2} is a powerful stimulus to the respiratory center. However, when the Pa_{CO_2} rises to levels exceeding 60 to 70 mm Hg, the respiratory center becomes relatively unresponsive to changes in the Pa_{CO_2} and, therefore, must depend largely on hypoxia for the respiratory drive.

AXIOM

COPD patients with chronic hypercarbia depend on hypoxemia to maintain an adequate ventilation.

(2) Responses to Carbon Dioxide and Oxygen

Administration of oxygen and correction of hypoxia in patients with severe emphysema may occasionally remove the hypoxic drive to the respiratory center, which has already become unresponsive to carbon dioxide. Thus, the patient may stop breathing for prolonged periods, and death from hypercarbia due to further retention of carbon dioxide may rapidly ensue. When oxygen is given to patients with severe hypercarbia, care must be taken to give it in small amounts (only 1 to 2 liters of oxygen per minute or in concentrations of only 24% to 28%) and to watch their ventilation carefully.

531

AXIOM

COPD patients receiving oxygen must be observed carefully for evidence of reduced ventilation or increasing respiratory acidosis.

(3) Respiratory Effort

In severe airway obstruction, the respiratory efforts (voluntary or involuntary) become progressively less efficient. Furthermore, in advanced COPD, the increased respiratory efforts against a high airway resistance may burn up more oxygen than is delivered by the small increase in minute ventilation that may result. On the other hand, when oxygen is given, the resultant high Po_2 in the alveoli plus the elevated Pco_2 which develops because of the impaired alveolar ventilation, provide larger alveolar-inspired gradients for both oxygen and carbon dioxide. These increased alveolar-inspired gradients allow larger volumes of oxygen and carbon dioxide exchange per liter of minute ventilation.

The idea that respiratory failure is often diaphragmatic failure or a disparity between energy input and work output by the diaphragm has received a lot of attention. The supply of oxygen to the diaphragm decreases with anemia or decreased cardiac output. Hypercapnia in congestive heart failure may be construed as a compensatory mechanism when stiff lungs, airways obstruction, and a limited cardiac output combine to make it impossible, in terms of energy intake and output, to maintain eucapnia. However, lower, flatter diaphragms make diaphragmatic work inefficient, and the work required for a given amount of ventilation is also increased by obstruction to airflow and by extreme obesity. Thus, it may be necessary for the cardiorespiratory systems to reach a new steady state at a higher $Paco_2$.

b. Sleep

AXIOM

Any tendency to hypoxemia or hypercarbia tends to become worse during sleep, especially in COPD patients.

Breathing is controlled by a brainstem center which in turn is acted on by higher neural influences. This center helps to stabilize breathing and compensates for various neuromechanical abnormalities. Loss of wakefulness-dependent descending influences during nonrapid eye movement (NREM) sleep can result in alternating hyperventilation and apnea, also known as periodic breathing. In addition, loss of the descending wakefulness influence can lead to loss of motor compensation, which in turn can cause a rise in upper airway resistance and obstructive sleep apnea or hypoventilation in patients with thoracic neuromuscular disorders.

REM sleep poses different problems for the respiratory control system owing to muscular atonia and suppression of chemical feedback. These changes are associated with respiratory deterioration in patients with compromised diaphragmatic function, such as with chronic obstructive pulmonary disease.

2. Circulatory Effects

AXIOM

Patients with COPD may develop a vicious cycle of increasing hypoxemia and pulmonary vasoconstriction.

Patients with increasingly severe emphysema eventually develop pulmonary hypertension and right heart failure, a combination often referred to as cor pulmonale. The pulmonary hypertension tends to develop because of increasing constriction or narrowing of the pulmonary arterioles and reduction in the size of the pulmonary capillary bed. The pulmonary arteriolar constriction is caused by reversible local hypoxia and an irreversible contraction of the fibrotic process around the arterioles. The reduction in the size of the capillary bed and the fibrosis in the periarteriolar tissue in patients with COPD are irreversible, but the pulmonary vasoconstriction due to hypoxia can often be reversed to some degree by careful administration of oxygen.

Another factor affecting circulation in emphysematous patients is the character of their respiration. As the disease progresses, expiration becomes more prolonged and forced. During this prolonged forced expiration, venous return to the chest may be greatly reduced. Then, during inspiration, the venous return may be large and abrupt, resulting in wide swings of the stroke volume and blood pressure during the respiratory cycle. When the systolic BP falls by more than 15 mm Hg during inspiration, the process is referred to as pulsus paradoxus. As cor pulmonale begins to develop, the right heart may be unable to handle the increased venous return during inspiration, causing even greater swings in pressure and flow. Since right ventricular muscle fiber bundles cross the interventricular septum and interdigitate with those from the left ventricle, severe right ventricular dysfunction in patients with COPD is often also associated with some left ventricular dysfunction.

Increasing hypoxemia, regardless of its etiology, also tends to cause a progressive rise in hematocrit. The resulting polycythemia, particularly if the hematocrit rises above 55%, not only increases the resistance to blood flow but also increases the tendency to thrombosis in deep leg veins and within the pulmonary arterial tree.

3. Metabolic Effects

The main metabolic effects of chronic airway obstruction are due to hypercarbia and hypoxia. Initially, COPD patients tend to hyperventilate and have a low $Paco_2$. However, as the disease progresses, alveolar dead space rises and effective alveolar ventilation decreases, both of which tend to increase carbon dioxide retention. Metabolically, the carbon dioxide retention causes an increased excretion of chloride by the kidneys and increased reabsorption of bicarbonate to produce a metabolic alkalosis. This metabolic alkalosis must be remembered if the patient with emphysema is placed on a ventilator. If chronic respiratory acidosis is corrected too rapidly, the low Pco_2 plus the pre-existing high bicarbonate levels can cause a severe combined alkalosis that may cause convulsions and/or dangerous arrhythmias. Some of these effects may be due to abrupt decreases in plasma-ionized calcium levels.

AXIOM

A rise in pH of 0.10 tends to cause a 4% to 8% decrease in ionized calcium and magnesium levels, a 0.5 mEq/liter decrease in potassium, and a 10% drop in the $Paco_2$.

In patients with very severe chronic hypercarbia, the $Paco_2$ may rise to over 90 mm Hg with a compensatory increase in bicarbonate levels to over 45 mEq/liter. It is important to emphasize, however, that ventilation is usually so impaired in patients with this much hypercarbia that they would generally not survive unless oxygen were given.

IV. DIAGNOSIS

For epidemiologic studies, chronic obstructive lung disease (which includes emphysema and severe chronic bronchitis) is usually characterized by one or more of the following criteria: (1) persistent expiratory wheezing, (2) shortness of breath causing patients to stop for breath when walking at their own pace on level ground, and (3) a forced expiratory volume in the first second (FEV_1) less than 60% of the total forced vital capacity (FVC). These findings, however, are nonspecific and may also be found in patients with heart disease or asthma.

A. CLINICAL

Most patients with chronic pulmonary disease show minimal clinical changes initially except for some dyspnea on exertion. However, coughing may be quite prominent and productive in patients with chronic bronchitis or bronchiectasis. In addition, patients with acute respiratory failure superimposed on COPD generally have had dyspnea and worsening of their chronic cough for several days. The sputum is usually thick and mucoid or purulent.

In advanced cases, severe hypoxia may cause confusion, disorientation, agitation, and restlessness alternating with somnolence and other mental changes. Acute hypercarbia may cause sweating and nonspecific cardiovascular stimulation, resulting in tachycardia and increased blood pressure.

In some instances, it has been noted that patients with chronic bronchitis tend to be edematous and cyanotic and have been referred to as "blue bloaters" as opposed to pure emphysema patients who tend to be asthenic and have sometimes been referred to as "pink puffers."

As inflammation and mucous secretion increase in patients with chronic bronchitis, there is an increasing tendency to hypoxemia and hypoventilation. Compensatory changes include increased pulmonary perfusion and polycythemia. Continued chronic hypoxemia leads to pulmonary artery hypertension and eventual cor pulmonale. Terminally, these patients become edematous (bloated) because of their heart failure and are cyanotic because of the polycythemia and hypoxemia.

Patients with pure emphysema have progressive lung destruction. Compensatory changes for the decrease in ventilatory capacity include further expansion of the chest cavity and an increased respiratory rate. Tachypnea and increased work of breathing develop. Because there is no polycythemia, the patients do not tend to become cyanotic.

Patients with moderate-to-severe chronic emphysema tend to have an increased anteroposterior diameter of the chest, elevated clavicles, and a high dorsal kyphosis. The chest wall and diaphragm tend to be fixed in an inspiratory position. The expiratory phase of ventilation tends to be prolonged and forced, often with wheezing. Manifestations of cor pulmonale include a loud pulmonary component to the second heart sound, a right ventricular heave, jugular venous distention, and lower extremity edema.

The absence of wheezing is an ominous finding in severe bronchospasm because it implies minimal air movement and is a harbinger of respiratory arrest. The presence of inspiratory wheezing implies that mucosal edema or bronchospasm is probably present in the proximal airways, causing impairment of both inspiratory and expiratory flow. Contraction of the sternocleidomastoid muscles and other accessory muscles is indicative of severe obstruction ($FEV_1 < 1.0$). With very severe bronchospasm, the patient may be unable to speak or may have an altered level of consciousness or central cyanosis.

Hyperinflation of the lungs and large swings in intrathoracic pressure can lead to pulsus paradoxus. The systolic blood pressure fall during inspiration normally is not greater than 10 mm Hg. A value greater than 15 mm Hg in acute bronchospasm is usually associated with an FEV_1 of <0.9 liter. However, pulsus parodoxus is nonspecific and occurs in other disease states, such as pericardial tamponade, cardiomyopathy, severe asthma, and acute hypovolemia.

B. Electrocardiography

Patients with cor pulmonale will often have evidence of right ventricular hypertrophy and a tall P-wave sometimes referred to as P-pulmonale.

C. X-RAY

On x-ray examination, COPD is recognized primarily by radiolucent lung fields, increased AP diameter of the chest, and depressed diaphragms. However, the chest x-ray may be relatively normal in many patients with moderate-to-advanced blood gas changes.

In patients with chronic bronchitis, increased peribronchial and bronchial marking may be noticed. Patchy areas of hyperluncency and fibrosis, a flat diaphragm, and attenuated pulmonary vasculature are also frequently seen in emphysematous patients.

The pneumoconioses and other fibrotic lung diseases may show evidence of increased bronchovascular marking with or without nodules along the bronchi and in the hila of the lungs.

D. BLOOD GAS STUDIES

In the initial phases, the blood gas studies may be relatively normal except for a mild-to-moderate decrease in the Pao_2 and $Paco_2$. In its most advanced stages, COPD is characterized by a partially compensated respiratory acidosis with a pH of 7.33 to 7.37, an elevated $Paco_2$ (45 to 65 mm Hg or higher), and a decreased Pao_2 (40 to 60 mm Hg). In patients with chronic respiratory failure and an elevated $Paco_2$, the kidneys retain bicarbonate to compensate. This results in a low-normal arterial pH, an increased serum bicarbonate concentration, and a proportionately decreased serum chloride level. Therefore, patients with acute respiratory failure will tend to have an elevated $Paco_2$ with a normal bicarbonate and a low pH. Patients with chronic respiratory failure will tend to have an elevated Pco_2 and bicarbonate and a low-normal pH. Patients with COPD and a superimposed acute respiratory failure will tend to have an elevated Pco_2 and bicarbonate and a low pH (Table 12.1).

AXIOM

If the pH is less than 7.30 in a patient with COPD, the patient has either a superimposed acute respiratory problem or a metabolic acidosis due to sepsis or impaired tissue perfusion.

Arterial blood gases may also be used to stage acute asthma (Table 12.2). Stage I is characterized by normal blood gases. Patients in stage II have a decreased $Paco_2$ and a normal Pao_2 (hyperventilation has led to normalization of Pao_2). Stage III is associated with a decrease in both $Paco_2$ and Pao_2 (hyperventilation is now unable to totally compensate for a widened $P[A-a]o_2$). Stage IV is characterized by a normal $Paco_2$ and a further decrease in Pao_2 (inspiratory fatigue is now prominent). Patients in stage V have respiratory failure with an increased $Paco_2$ and marked decrease in Pao_2. These findings indicate an impending respiratory arrest. This classification system is best applied after initial aggressive treatment of asthmatic patients and may be inappropriate if applied before the initial therapy.

AXIOM

A normal $PaCO_2$ in the presence of a very low PaO_2 should alert the physician to respiratory fatigue and the danger of an impending respiratory arrest.

E. PULMONARY FUNCTION STUDIES

The most characteristic pulmonary function change in emphysema is a greatly reduced ratio of FEV_1 to the total FVC. Normally this ratio is 75% to 85%, but in advanced CAO, it may be less than 50%.

Of the various lung changes, the most characteristic and earliest finding is an increase in residual volume. Associated changes include a decreased ERV and inspiratory capacity. The total FVC is decreased, particularly in advanced disease, even though total lung capacity is often significantly increased.

Table 12.1

EXAMPLES OF ARTERIAL BLOOD GAS CHANGES IN PATIENTS WITH CHRONIC OBSTRUCTIVE PULMONARY DISEASE AND HYPERCARBIA

Clinical Situation	pH	Pco_2 (mm Hg)	Hco_3 (mEq/L)
Normal	7.40	40	24
Acute respiratory acidosis	7.25	55	24
Chronic respiratory acidosis	7.35	55	29
Chronic respiratory acidosis with acute relapse	7.25	65	29
Chronic respiratory acidosis with acute metabolic acidosis	7.25	55	23

Table 12.2

STAGING OF ASTHMA BY BLOOD GASES	Stage	PO_2	PCO_2	$P(A-a)O_2$
	I	N	N	N
	II	N	---	+
	III	+	---	++
	IV	+++	N	+++
	V	+++	+	++++

AXIOM

Closing volume and the tendency to develop atelectasis increases early in COPD.

Although it is known that decreases in the FEV_1 are often used to identify CAO (emphysema and/or chronic bronchitis), clinical pathologic correlations have indicated that these tests usually detect only relatively advanced disease. More recently, studies of the nitrogen concentration in exhaled gas after the patient breathes 100% oxygen (nitrogen washout studies) indicate that the closing volume is usually significantly increased before there is any appreciable change in FEV_1. A decrease in diffusing capacity for oxygen is found relatively early.

V. THERAPY

Treatment of the patient with chronic respiratory failure, particularly with superimposed acute pulmonary problems, should proceed in an orderly fashion, which will vary with the urgency of the situation (Table 12.3). Although an acute viral upper respiratory tract infection often is responsible for acute deterioration in COPD patients, a specific precipitating event is often not identified.

Most of these patients respond favorably to conservative treatment, including continuous supplemental oxygen administration, inhaled and intravenous bronchodilators, antibiotics, vigorous hydration, aggressive chest physical therapy and tracheal suctioning, avoidance of sedatives, physical stimulation as needed to keep them awake at appropriate times, and diuretics as needed to

Table 12.3

THERAPY FOR ACUTE RESPIRATORY FAILURE IN PATIENTS WITH CHRONIC OBSTRUCTIVE PULMONARY DISEASE	*Treat Any Precipitating Event*

Treat Any Precipitating Event
1. Respiratory infections
2. Congestive heart failure
3. Pulmonary emboli
4. Improper use of oxygen, sedatives, or tranquilizers
5. Pneumothorax

Conservative (Nonventilator) Measures
1. Oxygen
2. Bronchodilators
3. Corticosteroids
4. Removal of secretions
5. Chest physiotherapy
6. Aerosols
7. Intermittent positive-pressure breathing
8. Acid-base correction
9. Nutrition
10. Other therapy

Ventilatory Assistance

control pulmonary congestion. In one study of 91 consecutive hospitalized patients by Smith in 1968, 81 were managed successfully on this regimen with an acute mortality of only 13%.

A. CORRECTING PRECIPITATING PROBLEMS

The more common causes of acute respiratory failure in a patient with COPD include respiratory infections, acute heart failure, pulmonary thromboembolism, hypoxemia, and pneumothorax.

1. Respiratory Infection

AXIOM

Respiratory infection is the most common cause of an acute exacerbation of COPD.

Mycoplasma infection or viral infection (with respiratory syncytial virus, adenovirus, and/or influenza A_2 virus) is reported in more than half of these cases. Acute bacterial pneumonia caused by *Streptococcus pneumoniae* or *Hemophilus influenzae* is also a common cause of acute respiratory failure in this group.

Acute bacterial pneumonia should be suspected in patients who present with fever, a cough productive of purulent sputum, localized crackles or consolidation, leukocytosis, and radiographically demonstrated pulmonary infiltrate(s). Initial antibiotic therapy should be guided by the sputum Gram stain and modified according to sputum, pleural fluid, or blood culture results. Antibiotics are also indicated in those patients with a change in their sputum production, but without clear evidence of bacterial infection.

Initial parenteral therapy should include an IV broad spectrum antibiotic such as ampicillin, erythromycin, or cefazolin. In toxic patients, antibiotic coverage should be extended with an aminoglycoside to cover Gram-negative infections until the results of the sputum, pleural fluid, and blood cultures return. In less ill patients, antibiotic therapy can be initiated orally with either ampicillin, tetracycline, erythromycin, cephalexin, or trimethoprim/sulfamethoxazole.

2. Congestive Heart Failure

Acute congestive heart failure may be caused by ischemia, hypertension, pulmonary emboli, fluid overloading, arrhythmias, and various electrolyte disorders. In some instances, the changes of CHF may be difficult to differentiate from those of COPD. Congestive heart failure (CHF) can cause interstitial and alveolar edema, abnormal ventilation/perfusion (V/Q) ratios, and the subsequent development of hypoxemia, hypercapnia, and acidosis.

3. Pulmonary Thromboembolism

AXIOM

The most frequent cause of acute attacks of heart failure or hypoxemia of unknown origin is pulmonary emboli.

Acute pulmonary emboli are a frequent cause of acute respiratory failure, especially in patients with COPD. However, it may be difficult to rule out pulmonary emboli in such circumstances. Patients with acute exacerbations of obstructive airways disease have V/Q inequalities. Consequently, a routine ventilation/perfusion lung scan is not likely to be helpful in confirming or excluding a pulmonary embolus. Pulmonary angiography is necessary in most cases.

4. Improper Use of Oxygen, Sedatives, or Tranquilizers

Patients with rather severe COPD with hypercarbia may depend on hypoxic stimuli to maintain an adequate ventilation. If oxygen, hypnotics, or minor tranquilizers are given to such patients, an abrupt rise in the Pco_2 may occur due to hypoventilation.

5. Pneumothorax

AXIOM

All patients with acute respiratory symptoms should have a chest x-ray to look for new infiltrates or a hydropneumothorax.

Patients with COPD have a greatly increased chance of developing a pneumothorax by blowing out a bleb after a cough or Valsalva maneuver. In many instances, the pneumothorax in COPD patients is in an atypical location and can be quite small, but it can still cause severe symptoms. In many cases, a localized pneumothorax may be difficult to differentiate from a bleb. However, if the area in question is enlarging and the patient's symptoms are severe and/or getting worse, it may be less harmful to insert a small tube into the suspected pneumothorax under ultrasound or CT guidance. If the tube is small and the lesion is actually a bleb, a tube can still often relieve symptoms, even though a prolonged air leak may result.

6. Other Precipitating Factors

Beta-adrenergic receptor blockers, aspirin, nonsteroidal anti-inflammatory drugs, inhaled irritants, reflux esophagitis, sinusitis, cold, exercise, and emotional stress may all precipitate acute asthma or bronchospasm in selected COPD patients. These factors should be looked for and treated in any patient with increasing respiratory distress.

B. OXYGEN

Oxygen administration is important in COPD patients with respiratory distress, not only to improve oxygen delivery and cardiopulmonary function, but also to relieve hypoxic pulmonary vasoconstriction. However, the oxygen must be given very carefully, and the patient's ventilation monitored closely.

1. Methods of Administration

a. Devices

Several methods are available for administering oxygen, including nasal prongs, nasopharyngeal catheters, masks, nebulizers, and ventilators. Nasal prongs are usually well tolerated, but they are inefficient and seldom supply the patient with oxygen concentrations greater than 30% to 40%.

Nasopharyngeal catheters can provide inhaled oxygen concentrations up to 60% if large amounts of oxygen are given. However, if the nasal passage is narrowed or crooked, the catheter may cause discomfort. The tip of the catheter should be visible just above the soft palate; if it protrudes further into the pharynx, it may make the patient gag. When oxygen is given by nasal catheter, it may be wise to start with 1.0 liters/min, increasing it slowly by increments of 0.5 to 1.0 liters/min until reasonable oxygenation of the patient's blood is obtained.

Oxygen tents usually leak a great deal and seldom provide inhaled oxygen concentrations greater than 30%. Moreover, they tend to isolate the patient from the nurse and physicians. Some patients experience claustrophobia while others find the tents very comfortable, and the atmosphere inside can be well humidified if desired.

Masks can provide high oxygen concentrations (up to 80% to 100%) depending on the minute ventilation of the patient and the presence or absence of a rebreathing bag. However, anxious or restless patients may not tolerate the mask for more than a few minutes at a time.

Some physicians feel that the best method for supplying oxygen to a patient who has a reasonable minute ventilation is the Venturi mask, which can provide small, accurate increases in the F_{IO_2} to 0.24, 0.28, 0.35, or 0.40. Other physicians feel that since most patients frequently take off their masks, they are inferior to double nasal prongs with controlled low-flow oxygen. Both types of therapy, at least initially, should be guided by pulse oximetry or blood gas measurements.

In general, carbon dioxide retention is not a problem in these patients if the F_{IO_2} is kept at 0.40 or less. However, the least amount of oxygen needed should be used. Mental alertness is a good sign of adequate oxygenation, but arterial blood gas analysis showing an arterial oxygen saturation of at least 85% to 90% (which is equivalent to a P_{O_2} to 55 to 66 mm Hg) is often preferable.

b. Timing

In patients with hypoxemic chronic obstructive pulmonary disease, continuous proper use of oxygen therapy for 6 months may reduce pulmonary artery pressure and pulmonary vascular resistance (PVR) and improve stroke-volume index. Proper continuous use of oxygen for several years can lead to even greater improvement. Use of oxygen just at night also produces significant improvement but not to the degree achieved with continuous administration. Nevertheless, even with oxygen therapy, the 36-month survival rate in COPD patients with a PVR greater than 400 dyne·sec⁻¹·cm⁻¹ is only 15% (vs. 56% in those with a lower PVR).

pressure and pulmonary vascular resistance (PVR) and improve stroke-volume index. Proper continuous use of oxygen for several years can lead to even greater improvement. Use of oxygen just at night also produces significant improvement but not to the degree achieved with continuous administration. Nevertheless, even with oxygen therapy, the 36-month survival rate in COPD patients with a PVR greater than 400 dyne·sec^{-1}·cm^{-1} is only 15% (vs. 56% in those with a lower PVR).

pressure and pulmonary vascular resistance (PVR) and improve stroke-volume index. Proper continuous use of oxygen for several years can lead to even greater improvement. Use of oxygen just at night also produces significant improvement but not to the degree achieved with continuous administration. Nevertheless, even with oxygen therapy, the 36-month survival rate in COPD patients with a PVR greater than 400 dyne·sec^{-1}·cm^{-1} is only 15% (vs. 56% in those with a lower PVR).

2. Possible Harm From Oxygen Administration

AXIOM

Improperly monitored oxygen therapy in COPD can be fatal.

When oxygen is given to patients with COPD, the possible harm from oxygen administration must be kept in mind. These harmful effects may include depression of ventilation, pulmonary irritation, and atelectasis.

a. Depression of Ventilation

When oxygen is administered to patients with COPD and chronic elevation of their Paco$_2$, ventilation may become very slow and shallow, to the point of producing somnolence or coma. This phenomenon is relatively uncommon, and its exact cause, although unclear, may involve either carbon dioxide narcosis or oxygen coma.

Complete cessation of breathing following administration of oxygen is quite rare. It generally occurs only if relatively large amounts of oxygen are given to severely hypoxic patients whose respiratory centers are not responsive to changes in Paco$_2$. Such examples might include patients with severe CNS depression caused by morphine, cerebral trauma, or severe hypoxia. When the Po$_2$ of the arterial blood falls to less than 60 mm Hg, the chemoreceptors are maximally stimulated, but a sudden increase in the concentration of inhaled oxygen may occasionally stop ventilation for several minutes or longer.

Increased Pco$_2$ levels can alter the state of consciousness. Normal individuals breathing 10% carbon dioxide can become unresponsive, and 30% carbon dioxide may produce surgical anesthesia. Interestingly, giving oxygen to patients with a very high Paco$_2$ (75 to 100 mm Hg) may cause coma without any further rise of the Paco$_2$.

Oxygen coma does not usually occur unless the initial Paco$_2$ is greater than 50 mm Hg, the Pao$_2$ is less than 50 mm Hg, and the administration of oxygen raises the Paco$_2$ to rather high levels. Some of the theories on oxygen-induced coma include (1) spasm of cerebral vessels, (2) sudden withdrawal of anoxemic stimuli to the cerebral cortex, and (3) cerebral edema. Spasm of cerebral vessels due to inhalation of high concentrations of oxygen in most patients with acute respiratory failure is not important because the vessels are usually already maximally dilated due to the low Pao$_2$, which is usually present. Sudden withdrawal of the hypoxemic stimulus to the cerebral cortex may contribute to coma because the individual does not have to work as hard to maintain an adequate Pao$_2$ and now can rest. Some patients with chronic obstructive pulmonary disease have a cerebrospinal fluid (CSF) pressure that is high enough to produce papilledema; however, administering oxygen may cause the CSF pressure to temporarily increase further.

b. Pulmonary Irritation

It has been known for some time that chronic inhalation of oxygen concentrations of 80% to 100% for more than 24 hours may produce chest discomfort and a drop in vital capacity. If maintained for several days, the individual may show evidence of congestion, exudation, and edema in the lungs. On the other hand, inhalation of oxygen concentrations of less than 40%, even for prolonged periods, usually causes no apparent damage to the lungs.

c. Atelectasis

If a bronchus becomes temporarily blocked, the oxygen in the distal alveoli can be absorbed quite rapidly. If the patient is breathing 100% oxygen, the alveolus will collapse completely after the oxygen is absorbed, and it will be very difficult to expand the alveolus again. On the other hand, if the patient is breathing room air, the nitrogen will stay in the alveolus and help to maintain its diameter after the oxygen is absorbed, thereby reducing the tendency to atelectasis.

d. Hemodynamics

Degaute in 1981 found that administration of oxygen tends to increase arterial oxygen content but decreases arterial pH, oxygen delivery, cardiac output, and stroke volume. Interestingly, the most severely hypoxemic patients did not have a drop in cardiac output when oxygen was given.

C. MEASURES TO IMPROVE VENTILATION

Other measures to improve ventilation include removal of tracheobronchial secretions, use of bronchodilators, and increased alveolar ventilation with intermittent positive-pressure breathing (IPPB).

1. Bronchodilators

Bronchospasm is caused by increased tone in the circular muscles of the bronchi due either to abnormal neurogenic effects (excess stimulation of parasympathetic nerves and inhibition of sympathetic nerves) or to the adverse effects of various chemical mediators, such as histamine. For the past decade or so it has become increasingly clear that the intracellular (second) messenger (enzyme), 3′,5′- cyclic adenosine monophosphate(cAMP) is essential to produce dilatation of the airway. Most of the current drugs used as bronchodilators act to increase the level of cAMP either by increasing its production or by decreasing its breakdown. Anticholinergic agents may also be of value in selected patients.

a. Increased Production of cAMP

In bronchial smooth muscle, the beta$_2$ receptor sites for adrenergic agents are at a point where adenylate cyclase is bound to the cell membrane. Stimulation of this receptor site by catecholamines results in increased adenylate cyclase activity and increased conversion of ATP to cAMP. Corticosteroids may increase the production of cAMP by sensitizing or increasing the reactivity of the adenylate cyclase mechanism to catecholamines.

b. Catecholamines

(1) General Effects

Stimulation of beta$_1$-adrenergic receptors causes an increase in heart rate, myocardial contractility, myocardial oxygen consumption, and myocardial irritability. Stimulation of beta$_2$-adrenergic receptors causes bronchial and vascular smooth-muscle dilation, tremor, and decreased cellular release of inflammatory mediators.

The catecholamines that are frequently used as bronchodilators include epinephrine, racemic epinephrine, isoproterenol, isoetharine, metaproterenol, and ephedrine. Unfortunately, most of these agents have, in addition to their beta$_2$ (bronchodilating) effects, some beta$_1$ (cardiac) effects resulting in tachycardia and occasionally troublesome arrhythmias (Table 12.4).

Many catecholamines used as bronchodilators also have some alpha-adrenergic effects that cause vasoconstriction of the bronchial mucosal vessels. This helps to relieve inflammation and swelling of the bronchial mucosa, thereby further increasing the size of the lumen. However, increasing systemic vascular resistance may cause a drop in cardiac output.

Catecholamines may also reduce the release of histamine and other mediators at the bronchial level. There is a subset of COPD patients who are similar in some ways to asthmatics in that they have an exaggerated response to histamine or a challenge with inhaled mecholyl. This "bronchial hyperactivity" can often also be reversed, at least partially, by steroids.

These patients with bronchial hyperactivity do not demonstrate improvement in their FEV$_1$ after inhalation of beta-adrenergic agents, but maintenance bronchodilator therapy decreases the response to inhaled mecholyl. Mainte-

Table 12.4

ADRENERGIC EFFECTS OF CATECHOLAMINES

Tissue	Alpha	Beta₁	Beta₂
Myocardium	Reflex slowing	Increased rate; increased contractility	No effect
Arteries	Vasoconstriction	Slight vasodilation (especially in muscle)	Slight vasodilation (especially in muscle)
Bronchial muscle	Slight contraction	Unknown	Relaxation
Bronchial mucosa	Decreased swelling	Unknown	Possibly decreased swelling; possibly increased secretions

nance bronchodilator therapy is effective in this group of patients, not by producing immediate bronchodilation, but by decreasing the release of pre-formed histamine, and possibly other mediators, from mast cells.

(2) Specific Drugs

Epinephrine was the first beta-adrenergic agonist used to treat asthma and COPD. It remains useful, but it has undesired alpha-adrenergic and beta₁ cardiovascular side effects (Table 12.5).

Racemic epinephrine, an isomer of epinephrine, is believed to have more prolonged bronchodilator action and fewer beta₁ and other side effects than epinephrine. This agent can be given parenterally but not by aerosolization.

Ephedrine acts indirectly by causing release of norepinephrine from the ends of adrenergic nerves. It can be given orally, but it is not suitable for aerosol administration. It has significant beta₁ effects and, therefore, is best given in small doses in combination with small doses of theophylline. Since racemic epinephrine and ephedrine may cause excitement and restlessness, a tranquilizer, such as hydroxyzine or phenobarbital, is usually also given to reduce these side effects.

Isoproterenol was the first beta-adrenergic agonist developed for inhalation. It is also active sublingually and intravenously. Although it is an extremely powerful bronchodilator, it has strong beta₁ effects and has no alpha effect. Consequently, the bronchodilation it produces if given alone is short lived. In

Table 12.5

RELATIVE ADRENERGIC EFFECTS OF FREQUENTLY USED BRONCHODILATORS

	Alpha (Vasoconstriction)	Beta₁ (Cardiac Stimulation)	Beta₂ (Bronchodilatation)
Phenylephrine	++++		
Norepinephrine	++++	+	+
Epinephrine	+++	++++	++
Ethylnorepinephrine	++	++	++
Racemic epinephrine	++	++	+++
Ephedrine	+	+++	++++
Isoproterenol		++++	++++
Isoetharine		+	+++
Metaproterenol		+	+++
Salbutamol			++++
Terbutaline			++++

541

addition, it may cause some vasodilation of the vessels in the bronchial mucosa, thereby increasing the tendency to bronchial obstruction later. Some commercial preparations combine isoproterenol with a powerful vasoconstrictor, such as phenylephrine, to overcome this disadvantage. When given intravenously, isoproterenol may be very short acting (3 to 5 minutes), unless given by constant IV infusion at 1 to 2 μg/min. When given as an aerosol, the bronchodilator effect may last up to 30 to 45 minutes. For inhalation, 0.25 to 0.50 ml of a 1:200 solution can be given in 3 to 5 ml of saline through a nebulizer.

Isoetharine was developed as a β_2-selective agent; however it also has significant β_1 activity. It is usually combined with phenylephrine to increase its effectiveness.

The first true beta$_2$-selective drugs were metaproterenol, terbutaline, and albuterol. Metaproterenol is an aerosol bronchodilator that is not metabolized by catecholmethyl transferase. Consequently, it has a more prolonged effect than isoproterenol. However, a 3% incidence of tremor has been reported. Metaproterenol is administered by either a metered-dose inhaler or a gas-power nebulizer. The usual dose is 0.3 ml of a 5% solution diluted with 2.5 ml of normal saline.

Salbutamol and terbutaline are drugs with almost pure beta$_2$ properties. These drugs are very good bronchodilators and have the advantage that they can be given orally and by aerosols. Like metaproterenol, terbutaline can be administered by either a metered-dose inhaler or nebulizer. The dose for nebulization is 5 ml of a 0.1% solution administered every 4 hours.

c. Route of Administration

(1) Inhalation

Inhaled β_2-selective agonists are the cornerstone of treatment for severe bronchospasm in patients with asthma and COPD. Fears that frequent outpatient use of beta-agonist inhalation therapy prior to ER presentation might make subsequent use of these agents less effective are unfounded.

Metaproterenol, albuterol, and terbutaline are the ideal drugs to be delivered by inhalation. With acute severe asthma or COPD, one of these B$_2$-selective agonists is given every 15 minutes three or four times or until the patient shows significant improvement.

Inhaled albuterol is the most effective selective β_2 agonist. It has a slightly longer duration of action than metaproterenol and is administered by a metered-dose inhaler.

Salbutamol and terbutaline are also very good bronchodilators and can be given orally and by aerosols. However, when these agents are given parenterally or orally, they lose much of their β_2 selectivity.

With very severe bronchospasm, large doses of aerosolized bronchodilators must be administered because peripheral distribution is decreased by the high inspiratory frequencies and flow rates, low tidal volumes, and narrowed airways. Adequate delivery of beta agonists can be accomplished by a metered-dose inhaler during acute bronchospasm if proper technique is used and doses are increased. However, in the severe asthmatic, there is usually poor patient cooperation. It is advisable, therefore, to deliver the beta agonist by nebulization in the most acutely ill asthmatics because this requires minimal patient cooperation.

Two types of nebulizer systems are available for inhalation therapy, the face mask and the handheld nebulizer with a mouthpiece. The mouthpiece is preferred because it delivers more drug; however, more patient cooperation is required. In the severely ill asthmatic the face mask system may be necessary.

(2) Subcutaneous

Subcutaneous beta agonists (epinephrine, terbutaline) have a poor therapeutic/toxicity ratio when compared with inhaled β_2 agonists. However, subcutaneous epinephrine or terbutaline may be useful in children who have a reduced susceptibility to β_1 toxicity and do not take inhaled agents well. Moreover, the subcutaneous route induces greater bronchodilation than an equal amount of inhaled agent. The oral agents may be particularly helpful if the attack has lasted several days and mucus plugging is a possibility.

If subcutaneous adrenergic therapy is chosen, the epinephrine dose for adults is 0.3 to 0.5 ml of a 1:1000 dilution depending on age and weight. This may be repeated in the initial management every 15 minutes as many as three times. An alternative agent is subcutaneous terbutaline in 0.25-mg doses.

Agents with beta$_1$-adrenergic effects must be given subcutaneously with caution to the elderly and those with suspected coronary artery disease. Some clinicians feel that β_1 stimulation is less intense with terbutaline than with epinephrine. However, it is best to avoid parenteral adrenergic therapy in these patients if at all possible.

(3) Oral

Oral β_2-selective agents should not be used as primary treatment for patients with acute bronchospasm because the therapeutic/toxicity ratio is less than with inhaled agents.

d. Corticosteroids

Corticosteroids may increase the amount of cAMP by increasing the sensitivity of the adenylate cyclase receptors to beta$_2$ stimulators. These agents may also reduce inflammation and edema in the bronchial mucosa and decrease the release of various agents that can cause bronchospasm. In asthmatics, corticosteroids are an essential part of therapy, especially if mucosal edema and mucus plugging are prominent. Methylprednisolone given in doses of 60 to 125 mg every 4 to 6 hours enhances β_2-receptor responsiveness, interrupts arachidonic acid inflammatory pathways, decreases capillary basement membrane permeability, decreases leukocyte attachment, modulates calcium migration intracellularly, reduces airway mucus production, and suppresses IgE receptor binding.

Minimal or no side effects occur with a single large doses of intravenous corticosteroids. Some enhancement of beta-agonist effect may be seen in as little as 1 hour; however, 4 to 6 hours are required for anti-inflammatory activity. The argument for early use of steroids is therefore strong in asthmatics. In COPD without asthma, they may improve ventilatory dynamics, but more long-term clinical benefit is not clear.

e. Methylxanthines

Patients who present with very severe bronchospasm (PEFR <100 liter/min) and fail to respond to beta-agonist therapy should be given IV aminophylline. Theophylline, as a nonselective phosphodiesterase inhibitor, increases intracellular cyclic adenosine monophosphate (cAMP) levels, causing bronchial smooth muscle relaxation. Although this is an attractive mechanism to explain its beneficial effect in the asthmatic patient, it may not be totally correct because other phosphodiesterase inhibitors have not demonstrated significant bronchodilation.

The methylxanthines, including the drug theophylline, are found in beverages such as coffee, tea, and cola. Theophylline is only slightly soluble in water, whereas aminophylline, a close derivative, is readily soluble and can be given intravenously. Gastrointestinal absorption of most of these agents is erratic, but the alcoholic derivative (elixir) of theophylline is absorbed relatively well when given orally. Rectal suppositories of aminophylline are also well absorbed and can be extremely effective.

In addition to its pharmacologic relaxation of bronchial and vascular smooth muscle, theophylline augments cardiac rate and contractility, and acts as a respiratory stimulant. The decreased pulmonary and systemic vascular resistance and increased cardiac contractility can significantly enhance cardiac output.

The increased central respiratory drive produced by theophylline may be important in reducing the ventilatory depressant effects of oxygen therapy.

Theophylline also increases diaphragm strength and decreases fatigue in patients with stable COPD. An increase in FVC, FEV_1, and maximum transdiaphragmatic pressure can also be demonstrated. These effects are noted 7 days after therapy is initiated and persist for 30 days, suggesting that aminophylline has potent and long-lasting effects on diaphragmatic strength in patients with fixed airway obstruction.

AXIOM

Theophylline is to the diaphragm what digitalis is to the heart.

Theophylline can also act to improve mucociliary clearance and inhibit release of various mediators that can cause bronchospasm or mucosal edema. However, the clinical significance of many of these actions has not been established.

Although prolonged use of maintenance theophylline therapy in chronic obstructive lung disease remains controversial, evidence from well-designed studies indicates that it produces patient improvement as gauged by both objective and subjective measurements. Sustained-release theophylline may prevent episodes of bronchospasm by providing a smooth around-the-clock bronchodilator effect, thereby reducing the need for periodic aerosolized beta agonists.

If the patient has not been receiving a theophylline preparation, a loading dose of aminophylline, 6 mg/kg in the moderate attack and 7.5 mg/kg in the severe attack, should be given over 15 to 30 minutes. When patients have taken theophylline preparations chronically, but do not have evidence of toxicity, one half the loading dose should be administered. A half-loading dose (3 mg/kg) is also recommended in severely bronchospastic asthmatics who admit to poor or partial compliance in taking medications. Patients who routinely take theophylline preparations and have symptoms or signs of toxicity should not receive any methylxanthines until the serum theophylline level is known.

After the loading dose is given, aminophylline should be administered by continuous infusion at a rate of 0.5 to 0.7 $mg \cdot kg^{-1} \cdot h^{-1}$. The therapeutic range of serum theophylline is 10 to 20 $\mu g/ml$, and 12 to 15 $\mu g/ml$ is the ideal level. If blood levels are low, additional boluses of 1 mg/kg increase the serum level roughly 2 $\mu g/ml$. A 3 mg/kg bolus, therefore, is expected to raise serum levels about 6 $\mu g/ml$.

Theophylline is metabolized in the liver by the cytochrome P-450 system and the enzyme xanthine oxidase. The rate of metabolism is highly variable and may be affected by many factors. Regular cigarette smokers have a markedly increased theophylline clearance and often require a much higher dose of methylxanthines. Decreased clearance occurs in patients who are critically ill with COPD, pulmonary edema, CHF, cirrhosis, or pneumonia, and in patients receiving cimetidine or erythromycin. Because of the wide individual variation in theophylline metabolism, serum levels are extremely important for providing optimal patient management.

When the patient has improved and no longer requires IV aminophylline, the oral theophylline dose can be calculated from the required aminophylline infusion rate. The aminophylline infusion rate (mg/h) is multiplied by the desired dosage interval in hours. For example, if a patient requires 37.5 mg/h of aminophylline and a slow-release theophylline preparation is to be given twice daily, the 37.5 mg/h is multiplied by 12 hours to compute the dose. Theophylline should not be administered as a rectal suppository because of its unpredictable absorption.

Theophylline levels correlate rather poorly with toxicity, and symptoms are unreliable in predicting theophylline level. However, the longer acting the oral theophylline compound, the more likely it is to be associated with higher blood levels.

Because of theophylline's narrow therapeutic window, symptoms and signs of theophylline toxicity are common. Manifestations include nausea, vomiting, diarrhea, central nervous system stimulation, and cardiac stimulation (usually sinus tachycardia). Potentially serious manifestations include sinus tachycardia greater than 120 beats per minute with associated premature ventricular beats. Severe intoxication may be associated with frequent premature ventricular beats or tachycardia and grand mal seizures.

The current role of theophylline in reversible airway obstruction is becoming increasingly controversial. In a recent editorial, Newhouse pointed out that theophylline appears to be facing obsolescence because of major advances in the pharmacotherapy of obstructive airway diseases by means of improved aerosol therapy. The aerosol bronchodilators and prophylactic anti-inflammatory drugs are generally more effective than theophylline in the management of asthma and COPD, have a superior therapeutic ratio, and lower overall cost. Thus, they are likely, with rare exceptions, to replace theophylline in the treatment of reversible airflow obstruction.

In response, Jenne pointed out that (1) treatment with cromolyn or even high doses of inhaled corticosteroids usually produces improvement, but does not eliminate nonspecific airway hyperreactivity and the need for therapy with bronchodilators, particularly in the patient with more severe asthma; (2) 15 μg/ml theophylline is the equivalent of two puffs of albuterol at their peak effect (when the FEV_1 response to albuterol is averaged over 4 hours, theophylline is equivalent); (3) the supposed behavioral problems in children caused by theophylline are in the majority of cases due to the disease itself; (4) the asthma studies where theophylline was supposedly unnecessary were in patients already receiving some theophylline, and added theophylline with its possibility of overdosing was the issue.

f. Anticholinergics

(1) Atropine

Inhaled atropine is effective in treating bronchospasm in patients with asthma and COPD. Although anticholinergic agents may offer significant benefit to the asthmatic, they are probably even more useful in patients with COPD. The dose of atropine in patients with COPD or asthma is 0.025 mg/kg (1.75 mg in an average 70 kg man) in a total volume of 3 to 5 ml. It should be given by a hand-held nebulizer with a mouthpiece, not by face mask, to avoid atropine deposition in the eyes and the associated problems of glaucoma exacerbation or pupillary dilation. Few systemic side effects occur at the recommended dose. Drying or inspissation of airway secretions is usually not a problem. However, atropine is contraindicated in patients with glaucoma and bladder outlet obstruction.

(2) Ipratropium

A derivative of atropine, ipratropium is now available in the United States. It is as effective as atropine, but has fewer side effects. Ipratropium has a slow onset and prolonged duration of action. Fifty percent of its effect occurs at 3 minutes, 80% at 30 minutes, and 100% between 1.5 and 2 hours. Since its peak effect occurs 30 to 90 minutes after inhalation, it is often not very helpful for an acute attack. The ipratropium dose is 125 to 500 μg by nebulizer and 80 μg by metered-dose inhaler. It is primarily indicated for maintenance therapy of stable COPD.

Unless there is a contraindication to therapy (glaucoma or bladder outlet obstruction), inhaled anticholinergic therapy should be considered in most patients hospitalized with asthma and particularly in patients who still have significant bronchospasm after 3 to 4 hours of aggressive standard therapy, including inhaled beta agonists, IV aminophylline, and steroids.

545

2. Pulmonary Vasodilators

Although dilation of the bronchi in patients with severe asthma or COPD is vital, dilation of pulmonary arterioles, especially in patients with pulmonary hypertension and cor pulmonale, is also important.

a. Agents Available

Some of the more frequently used pulmonary vasodilators include oxygen, catecholamines, prostaglandins, ACE inhibitors, and calcium blockers. Oxygen and many of the bronchodilators reduce pulmonary hypertension by relief of the reversible pulmonary vasoconstriction caused by hypoxia.

Most catecholamines cause bronchoconstriction and an indirect vasodilation. However, isoproterenol can cause both systemic and pulmonary arterial vasodilation.

Some of the prostaglandins, such as PGE_1 and prostacyclin (PGI_2), can cause dilation of pulmonary arteries. However, the systemic side effects, such as hypotension, can be so marked that their use is still largely investigative.

Many agents used to treat systemic hypertension have an adverse effect on patients with chronic obstructive lung disease. However, recent studies on ACE inhibitors, such as captopril, have shown that they can reduce systemic vascular resistance while causing no pulmonary problems. In fact, it has been shown to decrease pulmonary artery pressure, pulmonary artery wedge pressure, and total pulmonary vascular resistance, and cause an increase in vital capacity. In particular, captopril appears to protect the pulmonary circulation from excess hypoxic pulmonary vasoconstriction.

Use of nifedipine, a calcium channel blocker, in patients with severe COPD and cor pulmonale, who are also receiving supplemental oxygen, appears to exert a strong vasodilating effect on the pulmonary circulation. This pulmonary vasodilation has been sustained over the course of 6 weeks of therapy.

b. Results with Pulmonary Vasodilators

Although it seems logical to focus on the pulmonary circulation in order to acquire a favorable outcome in pulmonary hypertension, it still remains unknown if reductions in the severity of the pulmonary hypertension by drugs correlates with improved and/or extended life.

AXIOM
Pulmonary vasodilators also dilate systemic arteries and can cause severe hypotension in hypovolemic patients.

Most of the agents that improve pulmonary hemodynamics by lowering pulmonary vascular resistance and increasing cardiac output have more significant effects on the systemic circulation. Major adverse effects, including systemic hypotension, arrhythmias, and heart failure, will occur in some patients.

AXIOM
Inhaled or systemic beta agonists may cause a paradoxical initial hypoxemia

Occasionally beta agonists will cause pulmonary vasodilation before bronchodilation. The resultant increased perfusion of lung segments that are still poorly ventilated results in a $\dot{V}/\dot{Q}$ imbalance and increased physiologic shunting in the lung. In patients who already have severe hypoxemia or marginal cardiac or cerebral blood flow, the further drop in Pao_2 can cause significant problems.

3. Anti-inflammatory Drugs

Since acute and chronic inflammation is important in the pathogenesis of asthma and COPD, efforts are made to suppress this process with agents such as corticosteroids and cromolyn.

a. Corticosteroids

Although corticosteroids are remarkably effective in suppressing inflammation associated with increased bronchial reactivity, they have many side effects, especially if used chronically. The development of steroid inhalants has been the greatest advance in those cases of asthma which are not due to bacterial infection.

(1) Mode of Action

Steroids probably act on components of the inflammatory response. Unlike beta-adrenergic agonists, steroids do not inhibit the release of mediators from mast cells, but they do inhibit the release of mediators from macrophages and eosinophils. This may explain why steroids in single doses do not block the early response to allergens, but do block the late response and the subsequent bronchial hyperresponsiveness. The reduction in bronchial hyperresponsiveness may take up to 3 months of steroid therapy. Steroids given by inhalation are more effective than those given orally, suggesting an action on cells close to the lumen of the airway. Long-term corticosteroids also reduce the immediate response to allergens and prevent exercise-induced asthma. These beneficial effects may be due to a reduction in the number of mast cells in the airway.

Steroids also inhibit the influx of inflammatory cells into the lung after exposure to allergens and reduce peripheral-blood eosinophilia. Steroids induce the synthesis of a 37-kd protein, lipocortin, which inhibits the production of phospholipase A_2, and thus leads to a decrease in the synthesis of prostaglandins, leukotrienes, and platelet-activating factor. Corticosteroids also prevent and reverse the down-regulation of pulmonary beta-adrenergic receptors, possibly by increasing the transcription of beta-adrenergic receptor protein.

(2) Clinical Use

Steroids such as beclomethasone diproprionate, budesonide, triamcinolone acetonide, and flunisolide are active when given by inhalation and can help control the disease without systemic effects or adrenal suppression. Steroids given by inhalation are as effective when given twice daily as when given four times daily. However, if the asthma becomes unstable, the four-dose regimen may be preferable.

The clinical response to steroids given by inhalation is dose related, and some patients respond only to higher doses ($> 500 \mu g$ daily). The introduction of "high-dose" inhalers, which deliver 200 to 250 μg of steroid per puff as compared with the conventional low-dose inhalers, which deliver 50 μg per puff, should ease the management of the more severe cases. Although steroids given by inhalation have been used traditionally as third-line therapy (after beta-adrenergic agonists and theophylline), increasing evidence suggests that they should be given at an earlier stage and should become first-line therapy for chronic asthma.

Orally administered steroids, such as prednisone, prednisolone, or methylprednisolone, are necessary to control asthma in only a minority of patients, but their use is associated with side effects when the daily dose exceeds 10 mg. A single dose in the morning to coincide with increased endogenous cortisol production, is associated with fewer side effects. Alternate-day dosing also produces fewer side effects, but it may not be as effective in controlling asthma. Short courses of orally administered steroids are indicated for exacerbations of asthma, particularly those following viral infections. Treatment with prednisone or prednisolone (30 mg daily) for 1 to 2 weeks is usually effective, and there is usually no need to taper the treatment when such short courses are used.

Some clinicians routinely use intravenous corticosteroids in advanced COPD patients, especially those who have severe bronchospasm for more than 3 days. After subjective and objective evidence of improvement in airflow has been demonstrated, one can switch to oral corticosteroids and taper off over several weeks.

(3) Side Effects

Side effects are uncommon when low doses of steroids ($< 400 \mu g$ daily) are given by inhalation. Inhaled doses of 1.5 to 2 mg a day may be given to adults, with no systemic effects or adrenal suppression. In children, low doses of steroids given by inhalation may be effective, but doses higher than 400 μg a day may cause some adrenal suppression.

Oral or IV steroids can produce well-known side effects, such as osteoporosis, weight gain, hypertension, diabetes, myopathy, psychiatric disturbances, skin fragility, and cataracts. Therefore, the minimal dose required should be used.

b. Cromolyn

Cromolyn given by inhalation is capable of preventing or controlling asthma in some patients, but it is less effective than steroids.

(1) Mode of Action

The mechanism of action of cromolyn is still unknown. At first, it was believed to inhibit the release of mediators from mast cells. It prevents the immediate and late response to allergens; however, other mast-cell–stabilizing drugs, such as oxatomide, do not, suggesting that cromolyn may also act on other inflammatory cells, such as macrophages or eosinophils. Cromolyn also prevents the bronchoconstriction induced by bradykinin, which may be neurally mediated, suggesting a possible effect on C-fiber sensory nerves in the airway. Such an effect may explain why cromolyn reduces the symptoms of asthma, particularly coughing, in some patients so effectively.

(2) Clinical Use

Cromolyn protects against various indirect bronchoconstrictor stimuli, such as exercise, but in only some patients. There seems to be no sure way of predicting which patients will respond. Although children with predominately allergic asthma have a better response to cromolyn therapy than adults, even adults with late-onset nonallergic asthma may benefit. Cromolyn is the anti-inflammatory drug of first choice in children (2 mg of aerosol or 20 mg of powder four times daily) because it has few side effects. Steroids given by inhalation are preferred in adults, because they are considerably more effective.

(3) Side Effects

Side effects with cromolyn are extremely rare, and the drug is very well tolerated, even by small children. The only side effect usually reported is throat irritation when the powder is inhaled. This is less common when the metered-dose aerosol is used.

4. Other Anti-inflammatory Drugs

a. Ketotifen

Ketotifen is an antihistamine that inhibits airway inflammation induced by platelet-activating factor in some primates. One double-blind study showed it to have marginal benefit in patients with asthma, but another showed no convincing effect. Long-term administration might be of benefit in mild childhood asthma.

b. Methotrexate

Methotrexate has long been used in the management of chronic rheumatoid arthritis. In low doses (15 mg weekly), it has a steroid-sparing effect in asthma, and may be indicated in patients who require high doses of orally administered steroids. Because the long-term side effects of methotrexate include pulmonary fibrosis and hepatic damage, such therapy is only indicated in patients with very severe asthma.

c. Gold

Gold salts have anti-inflammatory properties and have been used to treat rheumatoid arthritis for many years. In Japan, gold injections (chrysotherapy) have helped control asthma and have reduced the need for oral steroids.

d. Troleandomycin

The macrolide antibiotic troleandomycin has some steroid-sparing activity in asthma, but only in patients taking methylprednisolone. Its effect may be due to the prolongation of the half-life of methylprednisolone through its inhibition of cytochrome P-450 activity in the liver. It may also prolong the plasma half-life of theophylline through the same mechanism.

5. Removal of Tracheobronchial Secretions

Tracheobronchial secretions are removed most effectively by a good cough. Chest physiotherapy may be of great help in this regard. If the secretions are very thick, they may be liquified to some degree by various expectorants (such as potassium iodide), inhalation of steam from an ultrasonic nebulizer, mucolytic agents, and control of infection with antibiotics.

a. Nasotracheal Suction and Bronchoscopy

Excess secretions that the patient is unable to cough out adequately may be removed by nasotracheal suction or bronchoscopy. Nasotracheal suction, however, should be brief so as to prevent hypoxia and bronchospasm. Bronchoscopy is often best done in these patients through an endotracheal tube inserted under topical anesthesia. Ventilation and oxygenation can then be more reliably supported during the bronchoscopy. There should be minimal sedation so that the endotracheal tube can be removed as soon as possible after the procedure.

b. Chest Physiotherapy

Chest physiotherapy can be an important part of respiratory care, and it is being used increasingly throughout the country. When done properly with the patient in various positions, almost all portions of both lungs may be systematically inflated and cleared of secretions. The use of vibrators and gentle thumping or pounding on the patient's chest or back may help loosen and remove secretions that the patient might otherwise be unable to expectorate. Dependent drainage can also be extremely helpful in some patients, especially those with bronchiectasis.

c. Exercise Training

Coughing and deep breathing by normal subjects can be improved by exercise training of the inspiratory and expiratory muscles. The exercise capacity of many patients with COPD is ventilatory limited, but a number of studies have shown that their exercise performance can often be greatly improved by appropriate training.

d. Drugs

Some drugs may help improve the contractile strength and endurance of respiratory muscles, particularly the diaphragm. These agents may act by different mechanisms, either at the level of the excitation-contraction coupling process (digitalis and xanthines) or by improving respiratory muscle blood flow (dopamine, dobutamine, etc.).

e. Mucolytic Agents

Probably the best known mucolytic agent is acetylcysteine (Mucomyst), which apparently acts by "opening up" disulfide linkages in mucus, thereby liquefying it and lowering the viscosity of the tracheobronchial secretions. This agent may be administered by nebulization of 2 to 4 ml of the 10% or 20% solution every 4 to 6 hours. However, the physical trauma of the nebulization and/or excess heat can destroy part or all of its activity. Direct instillation into the trachea through an endotracheal tube may be performed, or a tracheotomy may also be done, starting with 1 ml of a 10% solution and increasing the dosage according to the patient's response.

PITFALL
Being unprepared to handle the increased pulmonary secretions that may develop after acetylcysteine.

Acetylcysteine, particularly after direct instillation into the tracheobronchial tree, may greatly increase the quantity of tracheobronchial secretions. If these secretions are not adequately removed by coughing or suction, they can seriously occlude the airway. Mucolytic agents can also cause severe bronchospasm and should generally be given with a bronchodilator. Some physicians feel that they should not be used during an acute asthmatic attack because of their tendency to cause bronchospasm. Rarely, mucolytic agents may cause sloughing or mucosa in the tracheobronchial tree.

AXIOM

As a general rule, a bronchodilator should be added whenever a mucolytic agent is used.

f. Aerosols

Aerosolization or nebulization refers to the introduction of droplets of fluid, mechanically mixed with air or oxygen, into the respiratory tract with or without other medications. The purposes of nebulization include humidification of the inhaled gases and transport of various medications into the lungs. Humidification may be of benefit by (1) reducing insensible water loss from the lungs; (2) decreasing (by dilution and absorption) the viscosity of mucoid material in the respiratory tract, thus permitting the cilia to function more efficiently; and (3) counteracting the drying effects of the gases introduced by a ventilator.

Although aerosolization and nebulization may be very beneficial, there are also some problems that may develop with their use. Ultrasonic nebulizers may provide large quantities of fluid particles of very small size (0.5 to 3.0 μm) that may be absorbed from the alveoli and cause fluid overload, especially in infants and older emphysematous patients.

Each nebulizer has its own advertised characteristic particle-size production. However, these instruments will vary in their output relative to the physical substance nebulized, gas flow through the instrument, fluid properties, temperature of gases, age of the instrument, and the mechanics used for nebulization or aerosolization. Widely differing estimates of the site of the ultimate deposition of particles of various sizes while breathing through the mouth have been reported. If the patient is breathing through an endotracheal or tracheostomy tube, larger particle sizes can penetrate into more peripheral areas of the lung.

The most important medications that may be introduced by aerosolization or nebulization include mucolytics (such as acetylcysteine, potassium iodide, and sodium ethasulfate), bronchodilators (such as isoproterenol or epinephrine), and surfactants (such as alcohol and propylene glycol).

6. Intermittent Positive-Pressure Breathing

IPPB may be very beneficial if used thoughtfully in selected patients to achieve specific results. Specific goals include stimulating the patient to breathe and cough more deeply and to bring moisture or medication down into the smaller bronchioles where it can be most effective. If these goals are not achieved, it is expensive and time consuming and may decrease other efforts to maintain a clear airway and optimal ventilation.

Some of the substances or medications that can be given with IPPB include water, saline, alcohol, mucolytic agents, and bronchodilators. Water and 3% saline are more irritating than normal saline and, therefore, tend to stimulate a better cough and more sputum production. Alcohol may reduce the stability of bubbles and help break them up; this may be particularly important in the treatment of pulmonary edema.

Mucolytic agents are indicated if the tracheobronchial secretions are too thick to be removed adequately by coughing or suction. A frequent drug combination used in IPPB treatments includes 2 to 4 ml saline, 0.5 to 1.0 ml acetylcysteine, and 0.25 to 0.5 ml of phenylephrine.

All drugs instilled directly into the tracheobronchial tree, except for sympathomimetic agents such as epinephrine and isoproterenol, have a bronchoconstrictive effect. It is, therefore, important to add bronchodilators when using such agents in inhalation therapy.

PITFALL

Failure to use a bronchodilator when administering an aerosol to patients with bronchospasm.

7. Acid-Base Corrections

If the pH is less than 7.10 and the patient is in shock or congestive heart failure, rapid correction of the acidosis to a pH of 7.20 to 7.25 should be considered. Prior to correction, however, an effort should be made to pinpoint the cause of the acidosis. Such acidosis may be due to an increased $Paco_2$ (i.e., a respiratory acidosis), decreased bicarbonate (i.e., a metabolic acidosis), or both. The increased $Paco_2$ might also be chronic and/or acute.

AXIOM
Chronic hypercarbia should not be reduced faster than 2 to 5 mm Hg per hour.

A sudden rise in the $Paco_2$ can usually be corrected rapidly by improving ventilation, but a chronically elevated $Paco_2$ should not be reduced faster than 2 to 5 mm Hg/h. If the patient has had a chronically elevated $Paco_2$, he will usually have a compensatory metabolic alkalosis. Thus, even if tissue perfusion is severely impaired and a lactic acidosis develops, the bicarbonate levels may still be greater than normal for some time. In some instances, the presence of a superimposed metabolic acidosis can also be inferred if there is an increased anion gap.

PITFALL
Administering bicarbonate to patients who cannot eliminate carbon dioxide properly.

If there is evidence of impaired tissue perfusion or cell metabolism causing a metabolic acidosis, and the $Paco_2$ is not elevated, bicarbonate may be given slowly (1 to 2 mEq/min) until the pH rises to at least 7.20. Unfortunately, if the patient's ventilation is poor and she or he cannot eliminate carbon dioxide properly, bicarbonate administration can raise the $Paco_2$ very rapidly to dangerous levels, and it will not be effective in raising the pH. In these rare circumstances, cautious administration of Tris-buffer may be indicated.

8. Nutrition

Malnutrition is a frequently encountered problem in patients with severe COPD. Although it is not an invariable accompaniment of chronic respiratory failure, it is a marker of severe disease and has an adverse effect on prognosis, independent of the usual measures of severity of disease. The reported prevalence of malnutrition varies according to the population surveyed and ranges from one third to one half of the patients.

PITFALL
Allowing muscle wasting in patients with COPD.

Maximum respiratory pressures have been reported to be lower in malnutrition, and diaphragmatic muscle mass at autopsy has been found to correlate with the muscularity of the subject, suggesting that inspiratory muscles may suffer the same degree of atrophy as skeletal nonrespiratory muscles. Inspiratory muscle failure is more likely to occur in COPD patients who are malnourished than in those who are not.

AXIOM
Proper nutrition and exercise must be maintained in COPD patients.

9. Other Measures

a. Treating Cor Pulmonale

Pulmonary hypertension and acute cor pulmonale are known complications of COPD. Cor pulmonale results in fluid retention and subsequent pulmonary congestion. A low-salt diet and diuretics should be used to reduce the fluid overload. The use of digitalis for cor pulmonale is controversial and probably should be reserved for patients with atrial fibrillation or cardiomegaly from CHF.

b. Prevention of Sleep Apnea

Many COPD patients become severely hypoxemic, hypercapnic, and acidotic when they fall asleep. Therefore, they should be watched carefully for sleep apnea and stimulated or awakened as needed. Hypnotics, minor tranquilizers, or other drugs with sedative properties should not be administered.

c. Preventing Deep Vein Thrombosis

The majority of patients with acute exacerbations or COPD are placed at bed rest initially. During this period, heparin should be administered subcutaneously in doses of 5000 units every 12 hours to try to prevent deep venous thrombosis and subsequent pulmonary thromboembolism. The effectiveness of this regimen is not proven; however, few side effects occur with low-dose heparin, and a number of studies have confirmed the effectiveness of low-dose heparin in other bedridden patients.

d. Respiratory Stimulants

Various respiratory stimulants have been tried in COPD without clear evidence of their efficacy. Doxapram acts through the peripheral carotid chemoreceptors, and at higher dosages it is a respiratory center stimulant. Medroxyprogesterone acetate has also been used in the treatment of certain types of respiratory failure.

Interestingly, Aubier found that COPD patients who had acute respiratory failure with hypoxemia, hypercapnia, an increased respiratory rate, and decreased tidal volume, actually had an inspiratory effort that averaged five times control levels, indicating a markedly increased respiratory drive. Even after treatment with oxygen, the inspiratory effort was still greater than normal. These data suggest that alveolar hypoventilation associated with acute exacerbations of COPD probably is not due to a decrease in respiratory drive and minute ventilation, but perhaps to an increase in either carbon dioxide production or dead space ventilation. Therefore, treatment with pharmacologically active respiratory stimulants has little physiologic basis in these patients.

e. Intensive Care Unit Admission

Patients with severe hypoxemia and acute respiratory acidemia should be admitted to an ICU for continuous cardioscopic monitoring of heart rate and rhythm. Frequent recording of vital signs, chest physical therapy, tracheal suctioning, and assessment of arterial blood gases and pH are more easily performed in this environment.

10. Mechanical Assistance with a Ventilator

a. Indications

Patients with chronic obstructive lung disease, even though they may have fairly severe hypoxemia, only occasionally require endotracheal intubation and mechanically assisted ventilation. However, if the patient with COPD is almost apneic, mechanical assistance with a ventilator should be started immediately. If minute ventilation is marginal and the patient has had severe trauma or has ongoing severe sepsis, early mechanical ventilatory support may be extremely important. Also, if the patient is severely hypoxemic ($Pao_2 < 40$ to 45 mm Hg) or acidotic (pH <7.20) and not easily corrected, endotracheal intubation and mechanically assisted ventilation are indicated.

b. Techniques of Applying Ventilatory Support

The best means of initial emergency resuscitation of any patient with severe hypoventilation is the self-inflating (Ambu) bag used with a mask to provide ventilatory support and oxygen. Later a definitive airway may be established with an endotracheal tube.

If mechanical ventilation is required, it should be done in an intensive care setting and should be supervised by physicians trained in respiratory care. This is best done in a special respiratory care unit, but it may also be done effectively in a general ICU in a community hospital.

Ventilation is generally begun with a tidal volume of only 6 to 8 ml/kg if the patient has CAO and 10 to 12 ml/kg if the patient does not. The optimal ventilatory rate is 10 to 14 per minute, but it is frequently difficult to get these patients to breathe that slowly unless excessive sedation is given. If the patient has chronic hypercarbia, the minute ventilation used may have to be relatively small, because the $Paco_2$ in such patients should probably not be reduced faster than 2 to 5 mm Hg/h.

AXIOM

If the $PaCO_2$ is reduced too rapidly, the resulting combined metabolic and respiratory alkalosis may cause severe arrhythmias or death.

When COPD is the dominant problem, positive end-expiratory pressure (PEEP) may be of little help and may cause the $Paco_2$ to rise significantly. In such patients, PEEP may overexpand relatively good alveoli rather than open up those that are atelectatic, thereby increasing the alveolar dead space.

AXIOM

PEEP should be avoided or used only with great caution in patients with advanced COPD.

Although the precise mechanisms remain unclear, there is a consensus that pulmonary rehabilitation with exercise training improves both the exercise performance and well-being of patients with severe CAO.

It has been proposed that resting the respiratory muscles, by using intermittent external negative pressure ventilation (ENPV) in patients with CAO thought to have a component of chronic inspiratory muscle fatigue, might improve their ventilatory muscle function. However, several uncontrolled and controlled studies have reached differing conclusions. Nevertheless, significant improvement may occur with ENPV in some patients with severe hypercarbia.

c. Monitoring

Intermittent negative pressure ventilation (NPV) for 8 hours per day for 2 consecutive days results in sustained improvement in gas exchange for 3 or more subsequent days in patients with COPD and carbon dioxide retention. Current data suggest that the sustained improvement in gas exchange after intermittent mechanical ventilation for 8 hours per day for 2 days is associated with improvement in respiratory center responsiveness to hypoxemia and hypercapnia.

Monitoring of patients with chronic respiratory failure, particularly while they are receiving mechanical ventilatory assistance, is extremely important and is the main reason to admit these patients to an intensive care unit.

(1) Clinical

Clinical monitoring of patients with severe CAO should include special attention to the lungs, vital signs, and CNS function. Breath sounds may be faint, but auscultation must be performed frequently and carefully to evaluate expansion of the lungs and to pick up any pneumothorax that may develop in its earliest phases. Patients with severe COPD often have some element of right heart failure and/or may be hypovolemic due to prior fluid and salt restriction or use of diuretics. Any drop in blood pressure or decreased tissue perfusion when the patient is initially put on a ventilator should suggest hypovolemia or a pneumothorax.

AXIOM

CNS function is a good guide to the adequacy of tissue perfusion and oxygenation.

A comfortable, awake, alert, and relaxed patient is one of the best indications that ventilation and cerebral perfusion are adequate. Restlessness and/or excessive lethargy should be considered as due to hypoxia or inadequate cerebral perfusion until proven otherwise.

AXIOM

The higher the hemoglobin level, the more valuable cyanosis can be as an index of tissue oxygenation.

Skin color can be a good guide to the adequacy of oxygenation and ventilation if the hemoglobin is 15.0 g/dl or higher. However, if the hemoglobin is less than 10.0 g/dl, cyanosis may not be noted even when cardiac output and/or the Pao_2 are severely reduced.

(2) Blood Gases

Arterial blood gases should be drawn before and within 30 minutes after the patient is placed on a ventilator. Once a Pao_2 of 50 to 60 mm Hg is achieved by adding oxygen in increments of only 2% to 5%, the minute ventilation can be gradually increased so that the $Paco_2$ will fall by only about 2 to 5 mm Hg per hour back to the $Paco_2$ that the patient maintains in his or her usual state of health. This is often the $Paco_2$ that provides an arterial pH of 7.35.

(3) Electrolytes

AXIOM

Patients with severe COPD often have hypokalemia and hypophosphatemia in spite of their acidosis.

Serum electrolyte levels should probably be drawn daily until the patient's condition is stable. Potassium levels are often low in these patients. Reduction of the $Paco_2$ and use of diuretics may further aggravate any tendency to hypokalemia.

Hypophosphatemia is frequent in patients with respiratory disorders and has been associated with ventilatory failure, possibly because of respiratory muscle weakness. In one study, patients with a mean serum phosphorus level of 0.55 mmol/liter had their diaphragmatic function studied before and after infusing 10 mmol of phosphorus as KH_2PO_4 over 4 hours. Raising the mean serum phosphorus levels to normal values increased diaphragmatic performance an average of 70%.

AXIOM

One should attempt to maintain normal phosphorus levels in patients with severe COPD.

(4) Chest X-Ray

The chest x-ray can help to confirm the adequacy of ventilation of both lungs and the position of the endotracheal tube. Atelectasis or hyperinflation of any area may also help determine the need for increased suction and/or changing the ventilator settings. It is also important to look for any infiltrate that might suggest pneumonitis or a pulmonary embolism.

(5) Electrocardiography

Continuous cardioscopic monitoring is important in patients with severe COPD on a ventilator because of the high incidence of arrhythmias, particularly if the patient has had severe hypercarbia. Over 50% of our patients with COPD put on a ventilator develop arrhythmias while their $Paco_2$ is being reduced.

d. Complications

Several major complications are frequently encountered in patients with chronic respiratory failure who require ventilatory assistance. These include pulmonary infections, pneumothorax, arrhythmias, pulmonary emboli, psychosis, ileus, and urinary tract infections.

(1) Pulmonary Infection

AXIOM

Most acute respiratory failure occurring in COPD patients is due to pulmonary infection.

Pulmonary infections are common even in the best functioning respiratory care units, and the longer a patient is on a ventilator, the more likely he or she is to develop pneumonitis. When it occurs, it should be recognized and treated promptly. Consequently, tracheal secretions should be smeared and cultured every 48 to 72 hours to determine which organisms may be present, even if there is no clinical evidence of infection. However, sputum samples should have less than 10 squamous epithelial cells and more than 25 polymorphonuclear leukocytes (PMNs) per high power field, as well as a predominance of one type of organism, to be reasonably reflective of an underlying pulmonary infection.

AXIOM

Of ICU patients with positive sputum cultures, about a third have only pneumonitis.

Positive tracheal cultures do not necessarily indicate the presence of clinically significant infection. Of the patients with positive sputum cultures, about a third have only bacterial colonization with no evidence of infection in the trachea or lung parenchyma. Only a small number of PMNs are present, and the bacterial count is only 10^1 to 10^2 per milliliter. Bacterial colonization of the tracheobronchial tree does not require antibiotic therapy unless the patient is severely immunosuppressed, as with granulocytopenia, and an organism such as pseudomonas is present.

In another third with positive sputum cultures, the tracheal secretions appear suppurative. Moderate numbers of PMNs and bacteria are present on smear and Gram stain. Quantitative culture produces approximately 10^3 to 10^4 organisms per milliliter, but there is no evidence of involvement of the pulmonary parenchyma. These patients are considered to have tracheobronchitis.

In the remaining third of ICU patients with positive sputum cultures, there is clinical and x-ray evidence of pneumonitis. Many PMNs and bacteria are present on Gram stain of the sputum. Quantitative cultures reveal 10^5 to 10^6 organisms per milliliter. Specific antibiotics, based on the culture and sensitivity reports, should generally be reserved for patients with severe tracheobronchitis or pneumonia.

(2) Pneumothorax

Development of a pneumothorax may be rapidly fatal in patients being mechanically ventilated for respiratory failure, particularly if they have COPD. The incidence of this complication is increased when ventilator pressures exceeding 50 cm H_2O are used, particularly if the patient has blebs or has had chest trauma. If the patient has a subclavian venous catheter inserted, the incidence of pneumothorax is increased even more. Consequently, the systems or peak inflation pressure on the ventilator should be noted frequently.

AXIOM

Any sudden rise in peak inspiratory pressure should be considered as due to an occluded endotracheal tube or a pneumothorax until proven otherwise.

Some of the problems with an endotracheal tube include kinking, displacement into the right mainstem bronchus, or occlusion by excessive secretions. If these problems have been ruled out and a hydrothorax or pneumothorax is definitely not present, it is likely that the lungs are becoming stiffer and less compliant.

Diagnosis of a pneumothorax can be extremely difficult at times. Auscultation of the chest may be deceptive. Some patients have rather large pneumothoraces with relatively good breath sounds on the affected side. An upright chest x-ray with the patient in expiration usually provides the most accurate diagnosis.

PITFALL
Relying on an AP chest x-ray on a supine patient to be used to rule out a pneumothorax.

In an emergency with a suspected tension pneumothorax, if a proper chest x-ray cannot be obtained almost immediately, a diagnostic and therapeutic pleural tap may be done using a large intracath or needle attached to a stopcock and a 50-ml syringe with a freely moving barrel. After the tip of the catheter or needle has entered the chest, a rapid outward movement of the barrel can be almost diagnostic of a tension pneumothorax. If a pneumothorax is found, a chest tube should be inserted and attached to a water seal and 20 to 30 cm H_2O suction.

(3) Pulmonary Emboli

Patients with chronic respiratory failure, especially if they also have congestive heart failure and/or are bedridden, have a greatly increased chance of developing pulmonary emboli.

AXIOM
Any sudden deterioration in pulmonary or cardiac function in a bedridden patient should be considered as due to pulmonary emboli until proven otherwise.

(4) Arrhythmias

Patients on ventilators, particularly if their blood gases or settings are changing rapidly, are prone to develop dangerous arrhythmias. Arrhythmias are particularly apt to occur if severe chronic hypercarbia is corrected rapidly, producing a severe combined alkalosis.

(5) Psychosis

"ICU psychosis" is a frequent and often extremely troublesome hazard, particularly in the aged, if the ICU patient is deprived of rest and is forced to remain relatively stationary because of multiple tubes and intravenous lines. A clock, radio, outside windows, and visits by family members are all helpful to the ICU patient. A confident, concerned physician and nursing staff who communicate well with the patient are probably most important.

(6) Ileus

Distention of the stomach and small bowel because of swallowed air occurs frequently in patients with respiratory problems, particularly in those with trauma or infection involving intra-abdominal organs. Nasogastric suction in such patients must be begun early and maintained until good gastrointestinal function is present.

AXIOM
Ileus is much easier to prevent with early placement of a well-functional nasogastric tube than it is to correct.

(7) Urinary Tract Infections

Many of the patients with COPD are elderly and have difficulty voiding, particularly if they are male and on ventilators. Indwelling urinary catheters are often inserted in such patients without first determining if they are really required. Even with the best closed techniques, urinary tract infections tend to occur if a urethral catheter is left in place for more than 5 to 10 days. Consequently, urine cultures should probably be taken at least once a week. Maintenance of an adequate urine output, frequent careful cleansing of the urethra and skin around the catheter, and removal of the catheter as soon as possible may help reduce the incidence of such problems.

(8) Weaning

Weaning patients with COPD from ventilatory assistance can be extremely difficult and complex, and there is no set prescription for success. In general, if the patient requires a fraction of inspired oxygen of less than 0.40, can maintain an adequate tidal volume off the ventilator, and can double it on command, she or he is probably ready to be weaned. Other indications that the patient may be weaned are the ability to generate negative inspiratory pressures of at least 20 and preferably 30 cm H_2O, to produce a vital capacity of at least 10 and preferably 15 ml/kg, and to maintain a normal $Paco_2$ with a minute ventilation of less than 10 to 12 liters/min and respiratory rate of less than 30 and preferably 20 per minute.

Elderly patients with COPD and severe trauma often can be weaned only over a period of several days or weeks. In contrast, younger patients in whom an underlying sepsis or cardiovascular problem has been controlled can often be weaned from a ventilator in 12 to 48 hours.

While the patient is off the ventilator, a T-piece supplying oxygen and moisture should be attached to the endotracheal or tracheostomy tube. In addition, it is important to "sigh" or hyperventilate the patient at least four to six times per hour.

In many patients, intermittent mandatory ventilation (IMV) with 5 to 10 cm H_2O pressure support can be very helpful and is being used successfully in many centers. Weaning in many of these patients may be accomplished more rapidly and effectively with IMV and pressure support than with standard assist-control ventilation.

VI. PREPARATION FOR AMBULATORY CARE

Most patients with COPD, except for periods of severe acute pulmonary decompensation, can be managed very well at home and in the office. Many of the features of ambulatory care, however, must be begun in the hospital.

A. PATIENT EDUCATION

Home maintenance management is essential so that the patient can intelligently manage the inhalation therapy devices, pharmacologic agents, and techniques of physical rehabilitation. Simple written directions and/or manuals reinforce instructions given in the hospital or office. The importance of avoiding smoking and air pollutants must be stressed.

PITFALL
Allowing a patient with COPD to come into contact with smokers.

Smokers with progressive chronic airflow obstruction show increased bronchial reactivity and atopic features similar to patients with asthma. Bronchial hyperactivity is not seen in all smokers, since only about 20% of smokers get COPD; however, smoking increases the incidence and severity of COPD.

There is a definite group of patients who have some biologic similarities to asthmatics and who will get bronchitis and COPD if they smoke. As a group they demonstrate an increased incidence of allergic rhinitis and history of allergy in the family. Further, cigarette-smoking COPD patients have increased concentrations of serum IgE compared to nonsmokers with COPD. Smokers also have increased levels of nonspecific serum IgE, white blood cell counts, and eosinophil counts than control groups of nonsmokers.

B. BRONCHIAL HYGIENE

It is important to combat impaired mucociliary clearance, mucus impaction, and increased airway resistance. Agents such as phenylephrine or racemic epinephrine can be started in doses of 1 drop per 10 kg body weight diluted 50/50 with water, to be given by hand bulb or pump-driven nebulizers. If the airway obstruction is severe, so that the FEV_1 is less than 1.0 liter, IPPB may be more effective for delivering the bronchodilators. Inhalation of moisture from a steam nebulizer should then be done for 10 minutes, followed by controlled expulsive coughing and/or use of postural drainage.

C. PROPER BREATHING

Patients should be taught to breathe with a relatively short relaxed inspiration, contraction of abdominal muscles during expiration, and slow prolonged exhalation against pursed lips.

D. PHYSICAL CONDITIONING

Patients should walk increasing distances two or three times a day. In this manner, improved exercise tolerance may be achieved even in patients who have irreversible airway disease.

E. PROPER NUTRITION

Many patients with COPD have moderate-to-severe anorexia and, consequently, develop increasing malnutrition and loss of muscle mass. This in turn results in progressive weakening of ventilatory and other muscles. Consequently, a proper diet, with special emphasis on adequate protein, at least 1.0 to 1.5 g/kg per day is important. However, carbohydrate loading (5 g/kg/d) can precipitate acute respiratory failure in chronically hypercapnic patients by causing an increased production of carbon dioxide. Oxygen therapy has limited value in this setting. In such individuals, a reduced carbohydrate intake can lower the Pco_2 and promote earlier weaning from a ventilator.

F. PHARMACOLOGIC THERAPY

Ephedrine, terbutaline, or methyl xanthines may be used to combat bronchospasm. Antibiotics should be given at the first clear indication of pneumonia, which is often due to *S. pneumoniae* or *H. influenzae*.

With chronic suppurative bronchitis, recommended antibiotics include tetracycline (2 g daily for 2 to 3 days and then 1 g daily for a total of 7 days) or ampicillin (2 to 4 g daily for 2 to 3 days and then 1 to 2 g daily for a total of 7 days). Erythromycin may be helpful if the patient is allergic to penicillin and the infection is not responding to tetracycline.

The use of corticosteroids in COPD is controversial, but in patients not responding to other therapy and where bronchospasm or bronchial edema play a significant role, prednisolone (30 mg daily for several weeks) may be helpful.

Digitalis and diuretics should be given if there is evidence of right heart failure. Small maintenance doses of digoxin, 0.125 to 0.250 mg daily, in the well-oxygenated heart are safe and effective. Thiazide diuretics are generally safer to use in these patients and cause less potassium loss than furosemide or ethacrinic acid.

Influenza virus vaccine given early in the autumn before the influenza season begins may significantly reduce the incidence of later pulmonary infections.

G. OXYGEN

Oxygen in the hypoxemic patient with right heart failure decreases reactive pulmonary arterial spasm and thereby reduces the resistance against which the right heart must pump. Care must be taken, however, to be sure that the patient continues to ventilate adequately while oxygen is being given. Patients with severe hypercarbia depend on hypoxia to drive the respiratory center, and administration of oxygen may remove this stimulus, greatly reducing the patient's efforts to breathe. The resultant hypoventilation may be rapidly fatal.

H. BRONCHODILATORS FOR PATIENTS WITH MYOCARDIAL ISCHEMIA

Myers and Bodgen recently reviewed the use of bronchodilators in patients with ischemic heart disease. These patients are at increased risk for complications, such as angina, arrhythmias, congestive heart failure, and myocardial infarction.

1. Beta$_2$ Agonists

To avoid arrhythmias and angina in patients with ischemic heart disease, an agent that minimizes beta$_1$-adrenergic receptor stimulation should be used. The most beta$_2$-selective bronchodilating agent is albuterol (Proventil, Ventolin), followed by terbutaline sulfate (Brethaire) and metaproterenol sulfate (Alupent, Metaprel). Isoproterenol (Isuprel) and epinephrine (Primatene) are relatively nonselective beta agonists and should be avoided.

2. Methylxanthines

Methylxanthine bronchodilating agents have inotropic and chronotropic effects on the heart, and these may lead to cardiac ischemia or arrhythmias, particularly if beta-agonist agents are used concurrently. Both classes of agents may also lower serum potassium levels. Theophylline has a narrow therapeutic window, and blood levels should be followed closely. This is especially important if the hepatic clearance is decreased because the patient is in CHF or is receiving erythromycin, propranolol, allopurinol, or histamine$_2$ (H$_2$) antagonists.

3. Ipratropium Bromide

Ipratropium bromide (Atrovent) metered-dose inhalant produces bronchodilation by anticholinergic action. When this agent is inhaled, systematic absorption is minimal and cardiac effects are negligible.

4. Cromolyn Sodium

Cromolyn sodium (Intal) in aerosol form is a mast cell stabilizer used to prevent bronchospasm induced by exercise or known extrinsic precipitating factors. Several weeks of treatment are usually needed before effects are evident. Therefore, this drug is not useful for acute exacerbations of asthma.

5. Corticosteroids

Corticosteroids do not produce cardiac irritability. However, hypokalemia and retention of sodium and water may result in arrhythmias or congestive heart failure.

I. RESULTS

Most deaths in asthma are probably related to an underlying COPD. Molfino, Nannini, and Martelli recently found that the majority of asthma-related deaths occur outside the hospital and are due to asphyxia with severe hypercarbia (Pco$_2$ 97 ± 31 mm Hg) and severe acidosis (pH 7.10 ± 0.11). Arrhythmias were not present, suggesting that undertreatment, rather than overtreatment, is the main cause of death.

SUMMARY POINTS

1. The most common cause of chronic respiratory failure is chronic airway obstruction (CAO), also called chronic obstructive pulmonary disease (COPD), which includes emphysema and chronic bronchitis.
2. Exposure to asbestos greatly increases the risk of pulmonary fibrosis, cancer of the lung, and mesothelioma.
3. The most characteristic lung volume change in COPD is an increased residual volume.
4. COPD patients with chronic hypercarbia depend on hypoxemia to maintain an adequate ventilation.
5. COPD patients receiving oxygen must be observed carefully for evidence of reduced ventilation or increasing respiratory acidosis.
6. Any tendency to hypoxemia or hypercarbia tends to become worse during sleep, especially in COPD patients.
7. Patients with COPD may develop a vicious cycle of increasing hypoxemia and pulmonary vasoconstriction.
8. A rise in pH of 0.10 tends to cause a 4% to 8% decrease in ionized calcium and magnesium levels, a 0.5 mEq/liter decrease in potassium, and a 10% drop in the PaO$_2$.
9. If the pH is less than 7.30 in a patient with COPD, the patient has developed either an additional acute respiratory problem or a superimposed metabolic acidosis due to sepsis or impaired tissue perfusion.
10. Closing volume and the tendency to develop atelectasis increases early in COPD.
11. The terminal phases of respiratory failure in patients with chronic pulmonary disease are most likely to be caused by superimposed acute pulmonary problems, such as pneumonia, pulmonary emboli, or cardiac failure.

12. The most frequent cause of acute attacks of heart failure or hypoxemia of unknown origin is pulmonary emboli.

13. All patients with acute respiratory symptoms should have a chest x-ray to look for new infiltrates or a hydropneumothorax.

14. Pulmonary vasodilators also dilate systemic arteries and increase vascular capacity.

15. The pulmonary vasoconstriction due to hypoxia in patients with COPD can often be reversed by careful, long-term administration of oxygen.

16. Inhaled or systemic beta agonists may cause a paradoxical initial hypoxemia.

17. When oxygen is given to patients with severe hypercarbia, care must be taken to give it slowly or in small amounts (only 1 to 2 liters of oxygen per minute or in concentrations of 24% to 28%), and the patient must be watched very carefully to be sure that he or she maintains adequate ventilation.

18. One must be prepared to handle the increased pulmonary secretions that may develop after acetylcysteine administration.

19. As a general rule, a bronchodilator should be added whenever a mucolytic agent is used.

20. One should use a bronchodilator whenever an aerosol is administered to a patient with bronchospasm.

21. Chronic hypercarbia should not be reduced faster than 2 to 5 mm Hg per hour.

22. One should not give bicarbonate to patients who cannot eliminate carbon dioxide properly.

23. One should not allow muscle wasting in patients with COPD.

24. Proper nutrition and exercise must be maintained in COPD patients.

25. Patients with COPD, even though they may have a moderately low $PaCO_2$ (50 to 55 mm Hg) and an elevated $PaCO_2$, only rarely require endotracheal intubation and mechanically assisted ventilation. However, if they have had severe trauma or sepsis or maintain a very low PaO_2 (less than 40 to 45 mm Hg) in spite of careful oxygen therapy, early mechanical ventilation support may be important.

26. A sudden rise in the $PaCO_2$ can usually be corrected rapidly by improving ventilation, but a chronically elevated $PaCO_2$ should generally not be reduced by more than 2 to 5 mm Hg per hour.

27. If chronic respiratory acidosis is corrected rapidly, the high bicarbonate levels will remain elevated for some time, and the resultant severe combined alkalosis may cause convulsions and/or dangerous arrhythmias.

28. In patients in whom COPD is the dominant problem, the FRC is often not reduced, and PEEP may impair pulmonary function.

29. CNS function is a good guide to the adequacy of tissue perfusion and oxygenation.

30. The higher the hemoglobin level, the more valuable cyanosis can be as an index of tissue oxygenation.

31. Patients with severe COPD often have hypokalemia and hypophosphatemia in spite of their acidosis.

32. One should attempt to maintain normal phosphorus levels in patients with severe COPD.

33. Most acute respiratory failure occurring in COPD patients is due to pulmonary infection.

34. Of ICU patients with positive sputum cultures, only about a third have pneumonitis.

35. The risk of pneumothorax is increased in patients with COPD who are given positive pressure ventilation. Any sudden rise in peak inspiratory pressure that cannot be readily explained and corrected should be considered as due to a pneumothorax until proven otherwise.

36. Any sudden rise in peak inspiratory pressure should be considered as due to an occluded endotracheal tube or a pneumothorax until proven otherwise.

37. One should not rely on an AP chest x-ray on a supine patient to rule out a pneumothorax.

38. Any sudden deterioration in pulmonary or cardiac function in a bedridden patient should be considered as due to pulmonary emboli until proven otherwise.

39. Ileus is much easier to prevent with early placement of a well-functional nasogastric tube than it is to correct.

40. One should try to prevent a patient with COPD from coming into contact with smokers.

BIBLIOGRAPHY

1. American Thoracic Society. Standards for the diagnosis and treatment of patients with chronic obstructive pulmonary disease (COPD) and asthma. Am Rev Respir Dis 136:225, 1987.
2. Aubier, M: Pharmacologic strategies for treating respiratory failure. Chest 97:98S, 1990.
3. Aubier, M, et al: Effect of hypophosphatemia on diaphragmatic contractility in patients with acute respiratory failure. N Engl J Med 313:420, 1985.
4. Barnes, PJ: A new approach to the treatment of asthma. N Engl J Med 321:1517, 1989.
5. Baum, GL: Differential diagnosis of chronic respiratory insufficiency. Med Clin North Am 57:623, 1973.
6. Belman, MT and Shadmehr, R: Targeted resistive ventilatory muscle training in chronic obstructive pulmonary disease. J Appl Physiol 65:2726, 1988.
7. Bertoli, L, et al: The influence of ACE inhibition on pulmonary haemodynamics and function in patients in whom beta-blockers are contraindicated. Postgrad Med J 62 (Suppl)1:47, 1986.
8. Block AJ and Circale, MJ: Acute respiratory failure in chronic pulmonary disease. Civetta, CJ, Taylor, RW, and Kirby, RR (eds). Critical Care. JB Lippincott, Philadelphia, 1988, p 1003.
9. Burke, CM, et al: Captopril and domiciliary oxygen in chronic airflow obstruction. Br Med J 290:1251, 1985.
10. Burrows, B, et al: The relationship of serum immunoglobulin E to cigarette smoking. Am Rev Respir Dis 124:523, 1981.
11. Celli, B: Controlled trial of external negative pressure ventilation in patients with severe chronic airflow obstruction. Am Rev Respir Dis 140:1251, 1989.
12. Celli, BR: Respiratory muscle function. Clin Chest Med 7:567, 1986.
13. Coleman, JJ, et al: Cardiac arrhythmias during the combined use of beta-adrenergic agonist drugs and theophylline. Chest 90:45, 1986.
14. Cropp, A and DiMarco, AF: Effects of intermittent negative positive pressure ventilation on respiratory muscle function in patients with severe chronic obstructive pulmonary disease. Am Rev Respir Dis 135:1056, 1987.
15. Dark, DS, Pingleton, SK, and Kerbu, GB: Hypercapnia during weaning: A complication of nutritional support. Chest 88:141, 1985.
15a. Degaute, JP, Domenighetti, G, Naeije, R, et al: Oxygen delivery in acute exacerbation of chronic obstruction pulmonary disease. Am Rev Respir Dis 124:26, 1981.
16. Efthimiou, J, et al: The effect of supplementary oral nutrition in poorly nourished patients with chronic obstructive pulmonary disease. Am Rev Respir Dis 137:1075, 1988.
17. Farber, MO, et al: Abnormalities of sodium and H_2O handling in chronic obstructive lung disease. Arch Intern Med 142:1326, 1982.
18. Ferris, B: Chronic bronchitis and emphysema: Classification and epidemiology. Med Clin North Am 57:637, 1973.
19. Fishman, DB and Petty, TL: Physical symptomatic and psychological improvement in patients receiving comprehensive care for chronic airway obstruction. J Chronic Dis 24:775, 1971.
20. Flenley, DC: Pathogenesis of pulmonary emphysema. Q J Med 234:901, 1986.
21. Foster, S, Lopez, D, and Thomas, HM: Pulmonary rehabilitation in COPD patients with elevated P_{CO_2}. Am Rev Respir Dis 138:1519, 1988.
22. Frank, MJ, et al: Left ventricular function, metabolism and blood flow in chronic cor pulmonale. Circulation 47:798, 1973.
23. Goodall, McC and Alton, H: Dopamine (3-hydroxytyramine) replacement and metabolism in sympathetic nerve and adrenal medullary depletions after prolonged thermal injury. J Clin Invest 48:1162, 1969.
24. Gutierrez, M, et al: Weekly cuirass ventilation improves blood gases and inspiratory muscle strength in patients with chronic airflow limitation and hypercarbia. Am Rev Respir Dis 138:617, 1988.
25. Herve, P, et al: Hypercapnic acidosis induced by nutrition in mechanically ventilated patients: Glucose versus fat. Crit Care Med 13:537, 1985.

26. Hill, NS: The use of theophylline in "irreversible" chronic obstructive pulmonary disease: An update. Arch Intern Med 148:2579, 1988.

27. Howell, S, Fitzgerald, RS, and Roussos, C: Effects of aminophylline, isoproterenol, and neostigmine on hypercapnic depression of diaphragmatic contractility. Am Rev Respir Dis 132:241, 1985.

28. Hudgel, DW and Weil, JV: Depression of hypoxic and hypercapnic ventilatory drives in severe asthma. Chest 68:498, 1975.

29. Hyman, AL and Kadowitz, RJ: Vasodilator therapy for pulmonary hypertensive disorders. Chest 85:145, 1984.

30. Jenne, JW: Theophylline is no more obsolete than "Two Puffs qid" of current beta$_2$ agonists. Chest 98:3, 1990.

31. Juan, G, et al: Effect of carbon dioxide on diaphragmatic function in human beings. N Engl J Med 310:874, 1984.

32. Kanner, RE: The relationship between airway responsiveness and chronic airflow limitation. Chest 86:54, 1984.

33. Kennedy, JI and Fulmer, JD: Pulmonary hypertension in interstitial lung disease. Chest 87:558, 1985.

34. Kundson, RJ and Rurrows, B: Early detection of obstructive lung diseases. Med Clin North Am 57:669, 1973.

35. Koretz, RL: Nutritional support: Whether or not some is good, more is not better. Chest 88:2, 1985.

36. Lam, A and Newhouse, MT: Management of asthma and chronic airflow limitation: Are methylxanthines obsolete? Chest 98:44, 1990.

37. Larson, JL, et al: Inspiratory muscle training with a pressure threshold breathing device in patients with chronic obstructive pulmonary disease. Am Rev Respir Dis 13:689, 1988.

38. Lesis, EM: Two simple tables for interpreting blood gas measurements. Postgrad Med J 53:195, 1973.

39. Lewis, MI, et al: Effect of nutritional deprivation on diaphragm contractility and muscle fiber size. J Appl Physiol 60:596, 1986.

40. Lisboa, C, et al: Inspiratory muscle function in patients with severe kyphoscoliosis. Am Rev Respir Dis 132:48, 1985.

41. Machlem, PT: The pathophysiology of chronic bronchitis and emphysema. Med Clin North Am 57:681, 1973.

42. Marks, A: Chronic bronchitis and emphysema: Clinical diagnosis and evaluation. Med Clin North Am 57:707, 1973.

43. Martin, JG: Clinical intervention in chronic respiratory failure. Chest 97:105S, 1990.

43a. Myers, KE, Bogden, PE: Bronchodilators for patients with ischemic heart disease. How to avoid complications. Postgrad Med 86:324, 1989.

44. Molfino, NA, Nannini, LJ, and Martelli, AN: Respiratory arrest in near-fatal asthma. N Engl J Med 324:285, 1991.

45. Murciano, D, et al: A randomized, controlled trial of theophylline in patients with severe chronic obstructive pulmonary disease. N Engl J Med 320:1521, 1989.

46. Newhouse, MT: Is theophylline obsolete? Chest 98:1, 1990.

47. Petty, TL and Nett, LM: After-crisis care in chronic airway obstruction. Chest 62:585, 1972.

48. Ramsdell, JW, Nachtwey, FJ, and Moser, KM: Bronchial hyperactivity in chronic obstructive bronchitis. Am Rev Respir Dis 126:829, 1982.

49. Ratto, D, et al: Are intravenous corticosteroids required in status asthmaticus? JAMA 260:527, 1988.

50. Remmers, JE: Sleeping and breathing. Chest 97:77S, 1990.

51. Rodenstein, DO, et al: Ventilatory and diaphragmatic EMG changes during negative-pressure ventilation in healthy subjects. J Appl Physiol 64:2272, 1988.

52. Rodenstein, DO, et al: Ventilatory and diaphragmatic EMG responses to negative-pressure ventilation in airflow obstruction. J Appl Physiol 65:1621, 1988.

53. Rounda, S and Hill, NS: Pulmonary hypertensive disease. Chest 85:397, 1984.

54. Salome, CM, et al: Effect of aerosolized fenoterol on the severity of bronchial hyperactivity in patients with asthma. Thorax 38:854, 1983.

55. Schnader, JY, et al: Arterial CO_2 partial pressure affects diaphragmatic function. J Appl Physiol 58:823, 1985.

56. Sharp, JT: Theophylline in chronic obstructive pulmonary disease. J Allergy Clin Immunol 78:800, 1986.

57. Schneider, SM: Chronic obstructive pulmonary disease. Emerg Med Clin North Am 7:237, 1989.

57a. Smith, JP, Stone, RW, and Muschenheim, C: Acute respiratory failure in chronic lung disease. Am Rev Respir Dis 97:791, 1968.

58. Stewart, BN, Hood, CL, and Block, AJ: Long-term results of continuous oxygen therapy at sea level. Chest 68:486, 1975.

59. Tashkin, DP, et al: Double-blind comparison of acute bronchial and cardiovascular effects of oral terbutaline and ephedrine. Chest 68:155, 1975.

562

CHRONIC RESPIRATORY FAILURE

60. Taylor, RG, et al: Bronchial reactivity to inhaled histamine and annual rate of decline in FEV_1 in male smokers and exsmokers. Thorax 40:9, 1985.
61. Thurlbeck, WM: Chronic bronchitis and emphysema. Med Clin North Am 57:651, 1973.
62. Tillman, CR: Hypokalemic hypoventilation complicating severe diabetic ketoacidosis. South Med J 73:231, 1980.
63. Timmis, RM, et al: Hemodynamic response to oxygen therapy in chronic obstructive pulmonary disease. Ann Intern Med 102:29, 1985.
64. Tirlapur, GV and Mir, MA: Effect of low calorie intake on abnormal pulmonary physiology in patients with chronic hypercapneic respiratory failure. Am J Med 77:987, 1984.
65. Unger, K, et al: Evaluation of left ventricular performance in acutely ill patients with chronic obstructive lung disease. Chest 68:135, 1975.
66. Varsano, S, et al: Hypophosphatemia as a reversible cause of refractory ventilatory failure. Crit Care Med 11:908, 1983.
67. Venables, KM, et al: Interaction of smoking and atopy in producing specific IgE antibody against a hapten protein conjugate. Br Med J 290:20, 1985.
68. Yan, K, Salome, CM, and Woolcock, AJ: Prevalence and nature of bronchial hyperresponsiveness in subjects with chronic obstructive pulmonary disease. Am Rev Respir Dis 132:25, 1985.
69. Zibrak, JD, et al: Evaluation of intermittent long-term negative pressure ventilation in patients with severe chronic obstructive pulmonary disease. Am Rev Respir Dis 138:1515, 1988.
70. Ziment, I: Pharmacology of airway dilators. Respir Ther 4:52, 1974.

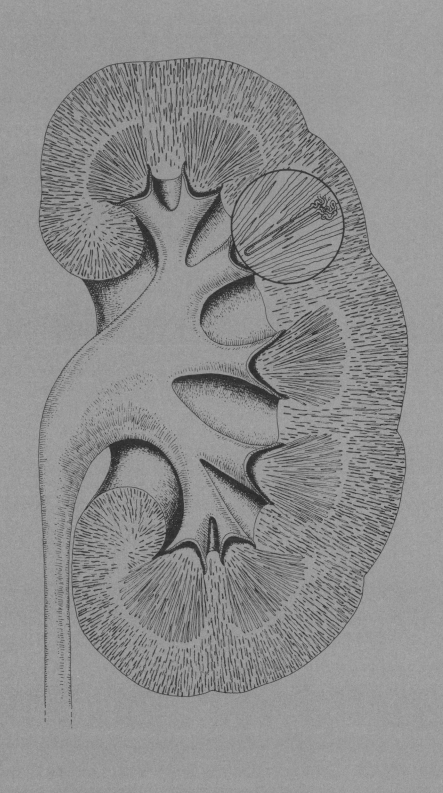

RENAL/FLUIDS

CHAPTER 13

Renal Anatomy and Physiology

I. FUNCTIONAL ANATOMY OF THE KIDNEY

A. LOCATION AND SIZE

The kidneys are paired retroperitoneal organs situated in the upper abdomen, on either side of the spinal column, and just above the level of the umbilicus (Fig. 13.1). They extend from the 11th or 12th thoracic vertebra down to about the second lumbar vertebra. The right kidney is usually lower because the right lobe of the liver lies above it. In the average 70-kg man, each kidney weighs 150 to 175 g. An average kidney is 10 to 12 cm long, 5 to 6 cm broad (from hilus to cortex), and 3 to 4 cm thick.

The kidney is surrounded by structures that protect it and tend to limit the amount of blood loss from trauma. The outermost layer is the tough renal fascia of Gerota. This extension of transversalis fascia surrounds a relatively thick layer of perirenal fat. The innermost layer, the fibrous renal capsule, is attached directly to the renal cortex, but at autopsy, it strips easily from the kidney unless inflammation or scarring is present.

B. CORTEX

A longitudinal section through the kidney shows that it is composed of an outer cortex and an inner medulla (Fig. 13.2). The renal medulla consists of 8 to 18 conical segments called pyramids. The apices of the pyramids are directed inward toward the renal pelvis in the hilus of the kidney. The renal cortex consists of two parts: (1) the cortex proper, which is about 10 to 12 mm thick and extends from the renal capsule to the bases of the pyramids; and (2) the renal columns, which run between the pyramids toward the renal pelvis.

C. MEDULLA

The renal medulla is composed of 4 to 14 pyramid-shaped structures called the renal pyramids, which can be divided into an outer zone (next to the cortex) and an inner zone (which forms the apices of the pyramids). The outer zone of the medulla, in turn, can be subdivided into an outer and an inner strip.

Each papilla projects into a cup-shaped minor calyx. Several minor calyces join to form a major calyx. The major calyces unite into the funnel-shaped renal pelvis.

Urine continuously exits the tip of the papilla and collects in the renal pelvis. From the renal pelvis, urine flows through the ureter to the urinary bladder for storage prior to intermittent voiding through the urethra. The structures from the minor calyces through the urethra are commonly termed the urinary tract.

D. THE NEPHRON

The primary functional unit of the kidney is the nephron. Each nephron is composed of a glomerulus, proximal tubule, loop of Henle, distal tubule, and collecting tubule (Fig. 13.3). Each kidney contains about 1.0 to 1.5 million nephrons, and up to 75% can be destroyed without serious ill effects to the patient.

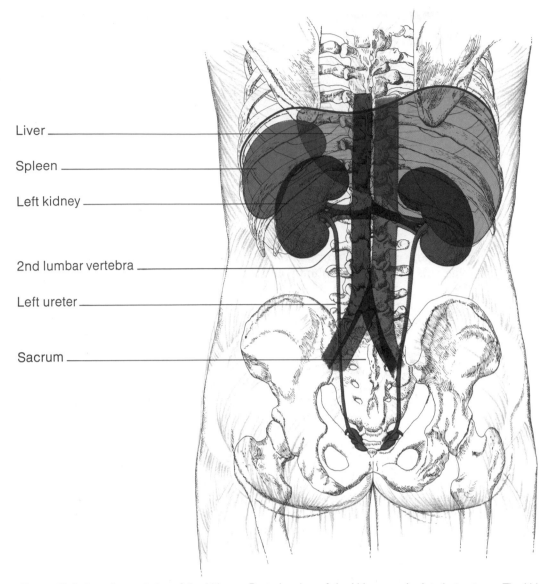

Liver

Spleen

Left kidney

2nd lumbar vertebra

Left ureter

Sacrum

Figure 13.1 Location and size of the kidneys. Posterior view of the kidneys and related structures. The kidney is well protected by the overlying bone (ribs and vertebral column) and heavy posterior musculature. The right kidney is slightly lower than the left, because of the liver. The kidneys normally extend from the eleventh or twelfth thoracic vertebra to the second lumbar vertebra. Normal kidneys in the 70-kg man average 160 to 175 g in weight, and are approximately 10 to 12 cm long and 5 to 6 cm wide.

1. Glomerulus

Each tubule begins as a small, spherical structure, referred to as a glomerulus, which is approximately 200 μm in diameter. The glomerulus consists of a spherical tuft of capillaries formed by the division of the afferent arteriole into two to eight branches that subdivide again into as many as 50 capillary loops. These loops have a supporting tissue called the mesangium. All of these structures are surrounded by an epithelial-lined membrane or capsule, often referred to as Bowman's capsule (Fig. 13.4). The multiple capillary loops provide a total glomerular filtration surface area of about 0.75 m² in each kidney. The capillary loops then join to form the efferent arteriole, which provides outflow for the blood from the glomerulus.

The glomerular capillaries are unique because they are interposed between two arterioles. The capillary loops are covered by the inner layer of the glomerular capsule. This single layer of endothelium is a continuation of the lining of the tubule to which it is attached. The glomerular filtrate leaving the capillaries is collected in the glomerular capsule before it passes into the proximal tubule.

Cortex

Renal pyramid

Minor calyx

Major calyx

Medulla

Renal pelvis

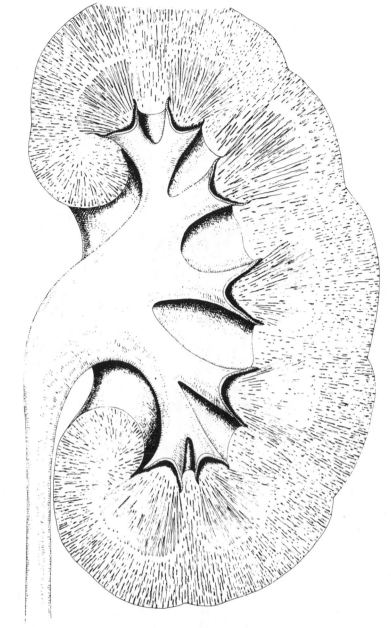

Ureter

Figure 13.2 Sagittal section of the kidney. The cortex is located peripherally with portions called the renal columns running centrally between the medullary pyramids. The cortex is composed mainly of glomeruli and the convoluted portions of the proximal and distal tubules. The medulla contains the loops of Henle and collecting system portions of the nephron. The core of the kidney is occupied by the renal pelvis into which the collecting system empties.

Two basic types of nephrons can be distinguished. Nephrons whose glomeruli lie in the outer two thirds of the cortex have short loops of Henle that remain completely in the cortex or only penetrate into the outer zone of the medulla. These nephrons are termed cortical nephrons. The other nephrons, which are called juxtamedullary nephrons, have their glomeruli in the inner cortex near the corticomedullary junction. These nephrons have long loops of Henle that descend deep into the inner zone of the medulla, before turning and ascending back up to the cortex. In man, approximately 85% of the nephrons are cortical, and the remaining 15% are juxtamedullary.

2. Proximal Convoluted Tubule

The proximal convoluted tubule, which receives the glomerular filtrate, is located in the renal cortex. It is a tortuous structure averaging 55 μm in diameter

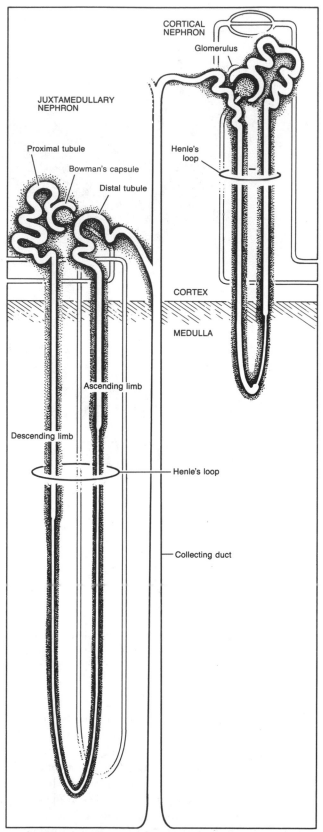

CORTICAL NEPHRON

Glomerulus

JUXTAMEDULLARY NEPHRON

Henle's loop

Proximal tubule

Bowman's capsule

Distal tubule

CORTEX

MEDULLA

Ascending limb

Descending limb

Henle's loop

Collecting duct

Figure 13.3 The nephron, the structural and functional unit of the kidney. Two types of nephrons, the cortical nephrons and juxtamedullary nephrons, are depicted. (From Dolan, JT: Critical Care Nursing. FA Davis, Philadelphia, 1991, p 401, with permission.)

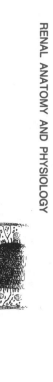

Proximal convoluted tubule

Capsule endothelium

Afferent arteriole

Capillary loop

Juxtaglomerular apparatus

Distal convoluted tubule

Macula densa

Bowman's capsule

Efferent arteriole

Mesangium cell

Bowman's space

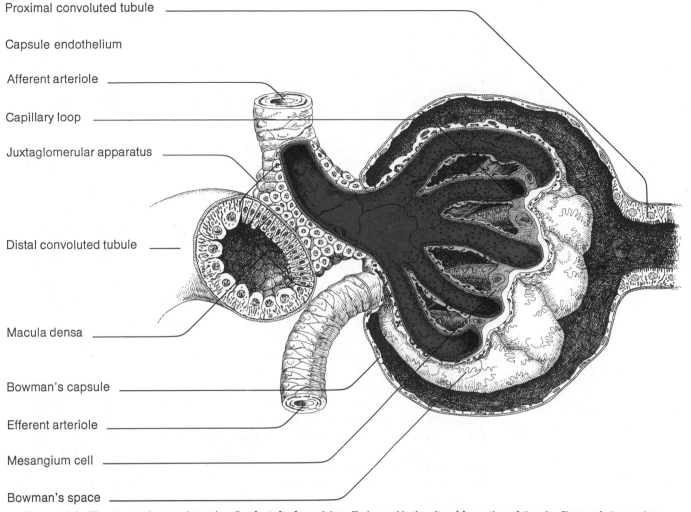

Figure 13.4 The glomerulus consists primarily of a tuft of special capillaries and is the site of formation of the ultrafiltrate of plasma that enters the proximal convoluted tubule. Blood enters at the afferent arteriole, passes through the multiple capillary loops, and back out the efferent arteriole. Filtration pressure is partially maintained within physiologic limits by the relative arteriolar muscular tone in both vessels. The blood is filtered as it passes through the capillary loops, which contain large specialized pores. The filtrate passes out into Bowman's space, whose integrity is maintained by a thin epithelium. The mesangium is the supporting tissue for the capillary loops. The filtrate collects in Bowman's space and enters the proximal convoluted tubule. The juxtaglomerular apparatus, formed by the macula densa of the distal tubule, specialized cells of the afferent arteriole, and a proliferation of mesangium called the polkissen, is believed responsible for the production and control of renin secretion by the kidney.

and 14 mm (14,000 μm) in length. The proximal tubule has traditionally been divided into the proximal convoluted tubule, which contorts itself in an apparently random fashion in the cortex, and the proximal straight tubule (pars recta), which dives toward the medulla as the descending limb of the loop of Henle. Recent studies suggest that the proximal convoluted tubule may be further subdivided on a functional basis into early and late convoluted segments, or part 1 and part 2, with the pars recta forming part 3 of the proximal tubule.

The cell border facing the tubular lumen has delicate filiform projections (microvilli) that constitute a brush border. They have large nuclei that are close to the basal surface. The cells have prominent basal and lateral processes and interdigitate extensively. Mitochondria are abundant, particularly in areas adjacent to the interdigitating processes.

The proximal tubule is responsible for the initial processing of the glomerular filtrate. Approximately two thirds of the filtered water and Na$^+$, and virtually all of the filtered glucose and amino acids, are reabsorbed in this region. Organic acids and bases, such as drugs and drug metabolites, are secreted into this area.

The epithelial cells of the proximal tubule are well adapted for the processes of reabsorption and secretion, with their large luminal surface area (created by the brush border), large basal surface area (created by the basal processes), and abundant mitochondria (which supply energy for the various transport processes). The numerous peritubular capillaries that surround the proximal tubule take up the reabsorbed water and solutes and deliver the substances to be secreted. The terminal portion of the proximal tubule descends into the renal medulla to become the descending limb of the loop of Henle.

3. Loop of Henle

The loop of Henle consists of a descending limb, a thin segment, and a thick ascending limb. As the descending limb enters the medulla, the limb's cuboidal cells are replaced by flattened cells in the thin segment. The length of a loop of Henle varies with the location of its glomerulus. About 80% to 85% of the glomeruli are located in the outer cortex and have short loops of Henle or no loop at all. Many of these do not reach the medulla or only reach its outer portion. The juxtamedullary glomeruli, in contrast, have long loops of Henle that penetrate deeply into the medulla, almost to the renal pelvis, before turning back.

There are also differences between the cortical and juxtamedullary nephrons in the ascending limb. In juxtamedullary nephrons, the ascending limb begins with a segment of flat, squamous epithelial cells, termed the thin ascending limb. Although these cells resemble the cells of the thin descending limb when viewed by light microscopy, structural differences are discernible with the electron microscope.

The thick ascending limb begins at the junction between the inner and outer zones of the medulla (Fig. 13.5). In this segment, the epithelial cells are cuboidal, extensively interdigitated, and contain numerous mitochondria. Although these cells lack a luminal brush border, a small number of short microvilli are present. The thick ascending limb traverses the outer zone of the medulla (the medullary portion of the thick ascending limb) and then ascends through the cortex to the level of its nephron's glomerulus. In cortical nephrons, the ascending limb consists entirely of cuboidal epithelial cells and does not have a thin ascending limb.

Like the proximal tubule, the loop of Henle both reabsorbs substances from the tubular fluid and secretes substances into it. In juxtamedullary nephrons, as much as 25% of the filtered water and Na^+ is reabsorbed in the loop of Henle, while urea is added to the tubular fluid. The loop of Henle also has an important role in urinary concentration.

4. Distal Convoluted Tubule

The distal convoluted tubule begins at the end of the ascending limb of the loop of Henle. The first part of the distal convoluted tubule contacts its originating glomerulus, where the afferent and efferent arterioles enter and leave. A specialized structure, the juxtaglomerular apparatus, is found at this point.

The distal tubule extends outward from its contact point with the glomerulus and continues toward the cortical surface. This part of the tubule is sometimes called the connecting tubule and has a somewhat convoluted shape.

The epithelial cells of the distal tubule, like those of the proximal tubule, are cuboidal, exhibit extensive basal and lateral interdigitations, and contain numerous mitochondria. Although these cells lack a luminal brush border, a small number of short microvilli are present (as in the thick ascending limb). The epithelial cells of the connecting tubule resemble those of the distal convoluted tubule, but are taller and have a more granular appearance.

5. Collecting Tubule

The connecting tubule (or most distal portion of the distal convoluted tubule) continues as the collecting tubule that descends into the medulla and joins with other tubules to form collecting ducts, which ultimately empty into the renal

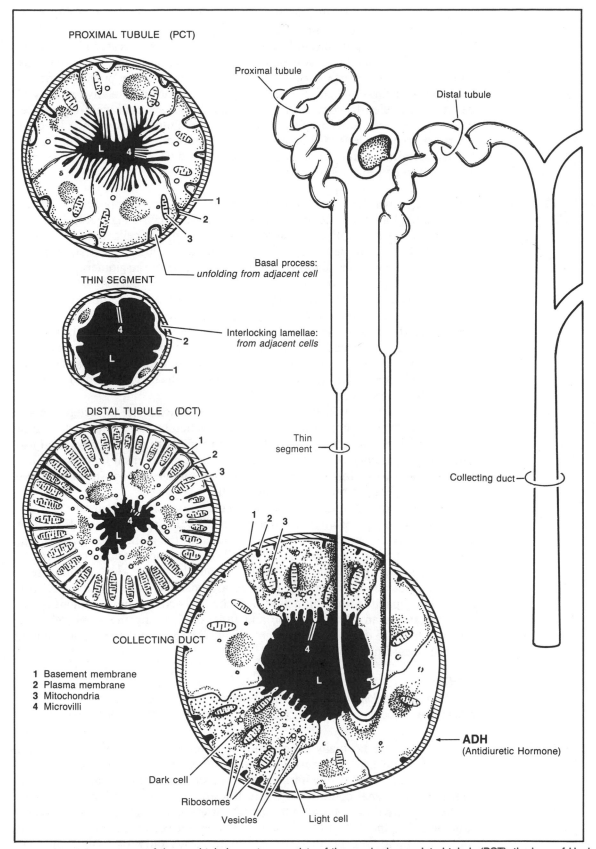

PROXIMAL TUBULE (PCT)

Proximal tubule

Distal tubule

1
2
3

Basal process:
unfolding from adjacent cell

THIN SEGMENT

4
2
L
1

Interlocking lamellae:
from adjacent cells

DISTAL TUBULE (DCT)

1
2
3
4
L

Thin
segment

Collecting duct

COLLECTING DUCT

1 Basement membrane
2 Plasma membrane
3 Mitochondria
4 Microvilli

1 2 3
4
L

← ADH
(Antidiuretic Hormone)

Dark cell
Ribosomes
Vesicles
Light cell

Figure 13.5 Microanatomy of the renal tubular system consists of the proximal convoluted tubule (PCT), the loop of Henle, the distal convoluted tubule (DCT), and the collecting duct. The structures of these various systems and their unique functions are depicted in cross section. (From Dolan, JT: Critical Care Nursing. FA Davis, Philadelphia, 1991, p 404, with permission.)

pelvis. In a longitudinal section of the kidney, the collecting tubules and ducts are evident as fanlike striations in the renal pyramids.

In the collecting tubule and duct, the epithelial cells increase in height until they are a columnar shape in the papillary collecting duct. Two basic cell types can be distinguished in the collecting tubules or ducts. The predominant cell type, the principal or light cell, stains lightly because of a relative paucity of cellular organelles. In contrast, the intercalated, or dark cells stain heavily because of abundant mitochondria. The distal convoluted tubules and collecting ducts are responsible for the final transformation of the tubule fluid into urine. Their functions include the reabsorption of Na^+ and Cl^-, the secretion of H^+ and K^+, and the concentration or dilution of urine.

E. JUXTAGLOMERULAR APPARATUS

The juxtaglomerular (JG) apparatus consists of three components: macula densa, extraglomerular mesangial cells, and granular cells (Fig. 13.4). The macula densa is a row of tightly packed, cuboidal epithelial cells, lining the distal convoluted tubule at the site of contact with its glomerulus. The extraglomerular mesangial cells are an extension of the mesangial cells of the glomerulus and are in the triangular region bounded by the afferent arteriole, efferent arteriole, and macula densa. This proliferation of mesangial cells is sometimes called the polkissen, or polar cushion. These mesangial cells are sometimes called agranular cells to distinguish them from the granular cells of the JG apparatus. The granular cells are located both in the region of the extraglomerular mesangial cells and in the walls of the adjacent afferent and efferent arterioles. They are believed to be specialized types of smooth-muscle cells that are derived from the walls of these arterioles.

The granular cells receive their name from the existence of secretory granules that contain renin, a proteolytic enzyme. When secreted into the lumen of the arterioles, renin acts on a specific protein in plasma, renin substrate (also called angiotensinogen), to produce a decapeptide, angiotensin I. Angiotensin I, in turn, has two amino acids removed by the angiotensin-converting enzyme (ACE) in the lung to produce angiotensin II.

Angiotensin II stimulates the adrenal cortex to secrete aldosterone and is a powerful constrictor of arteriolar smooth muscle. Thus, angiotensin II may be able to modulate the flow and pressure of blood in the glomerulus. In addition, the vasoconstrictor action of angiotensin II on systemic arterioles can increase systemic vascular resistance and thereby elevate the systemic blood pressure.

The association of vessels, glomerulus, and macula densa from one nephron in the JG apparatus, in conjunction with the vasoactive renin-angiotensin system, represents an ideal anatomic and functional arrangement, whereby the fluid reaching the distal nephron might "signal" the arterioles to alter glomerular blood flow and filtration.

AXIOM
The term *tubuloglomerular feedback* has been used to describe the regulation of glomerular blood flow and filtration by the fluid delivered to the distal nephron.

F. RENAL ARTERY AND BRANCHES

Each renal artery normally divides into an anterior and posterior branch and several segmental arteries, just before or soon after it enters the kidney (Fig. 13.6). These, in turn, divide into two or three smaller interlobar arteries, which run inside the renal columns of Bertin toward the junction of the cortex and medulla, where they give rise to the arcuate arteries. The arcuate arteries, which run parallel to the surface of the kidney between the cortex and medulla, divide into interlobular branches that pass up into the cortex and provide the numerous muscular afferent arterioles that supply the glomeruli. The efferent arterioles, which leave the glomeruli, are smaller in diameter, and are very responsive to changes in urine flow and sodium content in the distal tubule.

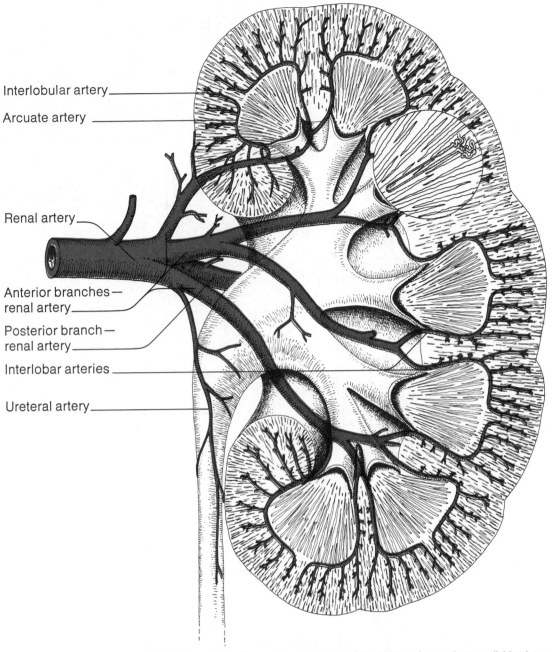

Interlobular artery

Arcuate artery

Renal artery

Anterior branches—
renal artery

Posterior branch—
renal artery

Interlobar arteries

Ureteral artery

Figure 13.6 Arterial supply to the kidney. Soon after entering the hilum of the kidney, the renal artery divides into several anterior and posterior branches. The branches then divide into interlobar arteries, which course between the medullary pyramids. The interlobar arteries then give off the arcuate arteries, which course between the cortex and medulla. From this arcuate complex arise the interlobular arteries, which give off the afferent arterioles to the glomeruli.

In the outer two thirds of the renal cortex, the efferent arterioles break up into a network of capillaries surrounding the renal tubules. However, the efferent arterioles from juxtamedullary glomeruli (those in the inner third of the renal cortex) do not feed into a peritubular capillary plexus. Instead, as straight vessels called the vasa recta, they continue into the medulla, following the long loops of Henle. They then form a capillary network around the ascending limb of the loop of Henle and return to the cortex, after which they enter the venous system (Fig. 13.7). Thus, the renal vessels for each nephron include two arterioles (afferent and efferent) and two capillary systems (the glomeruli and peritubular networks).

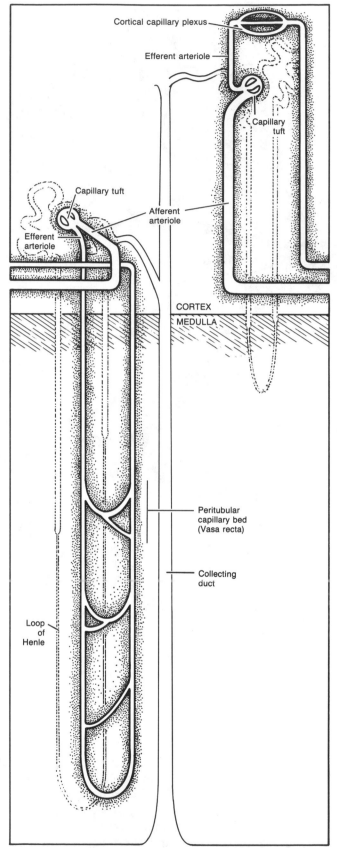

Figure 13.7 Vascular component of the nephrons. Blood supply to the cortical and juxtamedullary nephrons is differentiated. In each case, afferent arterioles carry blood to the glomeruli, where they give rise to the capillary tuft; these capillaries converge to form the efferent arterioles, which carry blood away from the glomeruli. Each efferent arteriole, in turn, gives rise to a second bed of capillaries: the cortical capillary plexus and the vasa recta, or pertibular capillaries. (From Dolan, JT: Critical Care Nursing. FA Davis, Philadelphia, 1991, p 405, with permission.)

G. RENAL BLOOD FLOW AND PRESSURES

1. Blood Flow through the Kidneys

Blood flow through both kidneys of a 70 kg man is approximately 1000 to 1200 ml/min. The portion of the cardiac output that passes through the kidneys is called the renal fraction. Since the normal cardiac output of a 70 kg adult man is 5 to 6 liters/min, the normal renal fraction can be calculated as about 20%.

In a healthy adult male weighing about 70 kg, the glomerular filtration rate (GFR) averages about 125 ml/min. The GFR is maintained at a relatively constant level by a system of "autoregulation" within the kidney that involves the afferent and efferent arterioles. When cardiac output, or blood pressure, falls, renal vascular resistance increases disproportionately, and causes an even greater decrease in renal blood flow (RBF). For example, normal cardiac output is 5 to 6 liters/min and normal renal blood flow is 1000 to 1250 ml/min. If the hematocrit is 45%, then the renal plasma flow (RPF) would be 550 to 688 ml/min or an average of 625 ml/min for a patient with a body surface area (BSA) of 1.73 m². If cardiac output falls by 10% to 4.5 to 5.4 liters/min, the decrease in RBF is often as much as 20% and the RPF may fall to 440 to 550 ml/min (Fig. 13.8).

If no other changes were to take place, the GFR would also fall by about 20%. However, renal autoregulation causes a rise in the efferent arteriolar resistance and a decrease in the afferent arteriolar resistance, which help to maintain a normal net glomerular filtration pressure. Since the GFR is maintained better than the RPF, the ratio of GFR to RPF, known as the filtration fraction, then rises above the normal value of 20% (125 ml GFR/625 ml RPF).

a. Special Aspects of Blood Flow through the Renal Vasculature

There are two capillary beds associated with each nephron: (1) the glomerulus, and (2) the peritubular capillaries. The glomerular capillary bed receives its blood from the afferent arteriole, and from this bed, the blood flows into the efferent arteriole and then into the peritubular capillary bed. The glomerular capillary bed is a high-pressure vascular bed, while the peritubular capillary bed is a low-pressure bed. Because of the high pressure in the glomerulus, fluid continually filters out of the glomerulus into a surrounding space called Bowman's capsule. The fluid is continually absorbed back into the capillaries because of the low pressure in the peritubular capillary system.

b. Blood Flow in the Vasa Recta

A special portion of the peritubular capillary system is the vasa recta, which are special vessels that descend around the loops of Henle. These vessels form capillary loops that surround the ascending limb of the loop of Henle, and then return to the cortex before emptying into the renal veins. The vasa recta play a special role in the formation of concentrated urine.

Only a small proportion of the total renal blood flow, normally about 1% to 2%, flows through the vasa recta. Thus, blood flow through the medulla of the kidney is much slower that the rapid blood flow in the cortex.

2. Pressures in the Renal Circulation

The intravascular pressure is approximately 80 to 100 mm Hg in the large arcuate arteries, and about 8 mm Hg in the veins into which the blood finally drains. The two major areas of resistance to blood flow through the nephron are (1) the small renal arteries and afferent arterioles, and (2) the efferent arterioles. In the small renal arteries and afferent arterioles the mean blood pressure falls from about 80 to 100 mm Hg at its arterial end to an estimated mean pressure of about 45 to 55 mm Hg in the glomerulus. As the blood flows through the efferent arterioles from the glomerulus to the peritubular capillary system, the pressure falls to a mean peritubular capillary pressure of 10 to 15 mm Hg.

3. Difference in Blood Flow between the Renal Cortex and Medulla

Blood flow to the renal cortex averages 2.0 ml/g of tissue per minute and accounts for approximately 90% of the total renal plasma flow. The outer medulla receives about 1.0 ml/g of tissue per minute and accounts for about 9% of the total renal plasma flow. Blood flow to the inner medulla accounts for only about 1.0% of total renal plasma flow. The relative distribution of blood flow

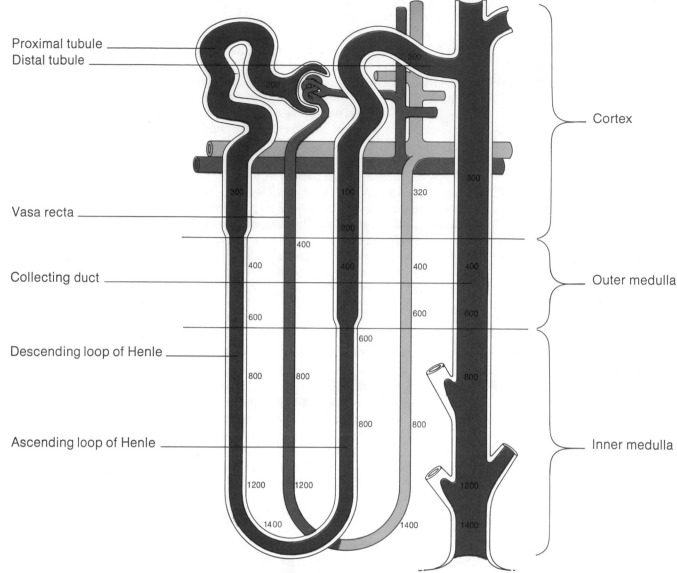

Proximal tubule
Distal tubule
Vasa recta
Collecting duct
Descending loop of Henle
Ascending loop of Henle

Cortex
Outer medulla
Inner medulla

Figure 13.8 Countercurrent multiplier. As the glomerular filtrate moves down the descending loop of Henle, it equilibrates osmotically with the ever-increasing osmotic pressure in the renal medulla created by the countercurrent mechanism. As the filtrate moves up the ascending loop of Henle, sodium is actively transported out of the nephron, and chloride follows passively, so the tubular fluid at the top of the loop of Henle is dilute. This fluid may be passed as urine without any osmotic change if the distal and collecting tubules are free of the influence of antidiuretic hormone (ADH). With increasing ADH effect, the distal tubule and collecting duct become increasingly permeable to water, and an increasingly concentrated urine is produced.

between the cortex and medulla is under metabolic control and may vary considerably under different conditions.

During water diuresis, renal blood flow increases, but a relatively greater increase occurs in flow to the outer medulla, as compared to the cortex. In contrast, increased sodium intake tends to elevate outer cortical blood flow. Decreased sodium intake or hypovolemia tends to divert blood flow to the juxtamedullary "sodium-retaining" nephrons.

The mechanisms controlling the intrarenal distribution of blood flow are not completely understood, but include the sympathetic nervous system, the renin-angiotensin system, the prostaglandins, and the antidiuretic hormone (ADH).

The reduced blood flow to the medulla is due to the relatively high vascular resistance in the vasa recta. The high resistance in these vessels may be partly due to the long length of these vessels and the increased viscosity of medullary blood. This low medullary blood flow is important for proper function of the urinary countercurrent concentrating mechanism (Fig. 13.8).

4. Function of the Peritubular Capillaries

Each day about 180 liters of fluid are filtered through the glomeruli and all but 1.0 to 1.5 liters of this is reabsorbed from the tubules into the renal interstitial spaces, and then into the peritubular capillaries. This is about four times as much fluid as is reabsorbed at the venous ends of all the other capillaries of the body.

II. RENAL OXYGEN CONSUMPTION

In most organs, blood flow is related to the oxygen requirements of the organ. Blood flow to the kidneys is very high relative to the oxygen needs of the kidneys. Indeed, the renal arteriovenous oxygen difference is only about 1.7 ml/dl, which is only 30% to 40% of what it is in other tissues.

In most organs, if the blood flow varies, the arteriovenous oxygen difference also changes, in order to meet the oxygen needs of the organ. However, the kidneys are unique in that changes in blood flow are generally accompanied by parallel changes in oxygen consumption, with the arteriovenous oxygen difference remaining relatively constant. The explanation for this is that a change in RBF is generally accompanied by a parallel change in GFR, and hence, in the quantity of ions and other solutes that must be reabsorbed. Solute reabsorption, in turn, requires oxygen for energy, with as much as 75% to 85% of the renal oxygen consumption being used to support the active reabsorption of ions and other solutes, particularly Na^+. In most instances, renal oxygen consumption is directly proportional to the amount of Na^+ reabsorbed.

AXIOM

Changes in GFR and solute reabsorption are responsible for much of the changes in oxygen consumption in the kidneys.

III. RENAL FUNCTION

The basic function of the nephron is to clean or "clear" the blood plasma of a variety of unwanted substances and regulate the concentration of various "wanted" substances. The substances that must be cleared include metabolic end products, such as urea, creatinine, and uric acid. In addition, there is daily intake of many other substances, such as sodium, potassium, chloride, and hydrogen ions, which will accumulate in excess quantities if they are not cleared appropriately from the plasma.

The principal mechanism by which the nephron clears the plasma of unwanted substances is filtration of a large proportion of the plasma through the glomerular membrane into the tubules of the nephron. Unwanted substances in the tubules are not reabsorbed, while desirable or needed substances, especially water and (certain) electrolytes, are reabsorbed back into the plasma of the peritubular capillaries. Thus, the needed portions of the tubular fluid are returned to the blood, and the unwanted portions pass out into the urine.

A second mechanism by which the nephron clears the plasma of unwanted or excess amounts of various substances is movement of these from the plasma into tubular epithelial cells that secrete them into the tubular fluid. Thus, the urine that is eventually formed is composed mainly of filtered substances, but also of small but important amounts of secreted substances.

A. GLOMERULAR FILTRATION

1. Forces Involved

The movement of fluid out of the glomerular capillaries into Bowman's space is determined by forces similar to those operating on any capillary. The factors involved in flow (F) or movement of water across any capillary membrane can be expressed by the following (Starling) equation:

$$F = K[(P_f - P_t) - (\sigma_p - \sigma_t)].$$

In the glomerulus, the filtration pressure (P_f) is quite high, often averaging 55 mm Hg. On the other hand, the tissue pressure (P_t), which in this case is the pressure of the fluid in Bowman's capsule, averages only about 10 mm Hg. However, if there is a urinary tract obstruction, pressure in Bowman's capsule may increase sufficiently to interfere with glomerular filtration.

The oncotic pressure of the plasma (σ_p) is normally about 22 to 25 mm Hg at the afferent end of the glomerulus and, because of loss of water from the glomerulus, about 30 to 35 mm Hg at the efferent end. The oncotic pressure in the tissue space of Bowman's capsule (P_t) is almost negligible. If the Staverman reflection coefficient for protein (σ) is less than 1.0, the oncotic pressure retarding filtration of fluid through the glomerulus will be correspondingly reduced.

In addition to a high net filtration pressure, glomerular filtration is also favored by the high permeability (K) of the glomerulus. Glomerular capillaries are about 100 times more permeable than capillaries in skeletal muscle.

2. Filtration Barriers

Blood enters the glomerular capillaries from the afferent arteriole. The glomerular capillary endothelial cell is the initial barrier. Fenestrae between the endothelial cells are approximately 61 angstroms (Å) in size, indicating that this potential route of diffusion or convection could hold back only cellular elements of blood, not dissolved proteins or electrolytes. However, the glomerular capillary basement membrane is produced by the mesangial cells of the glomerulus and is composed of glycoproteins with fixed negative charges. These negative charges serve to retard the passage of proteins. The estimated functional size of these pores is of such magnitude as to exclude large-size proteins, but not small solutes.

Thus, the basement membrane excludes macromolecules on the basis of both charge and size. The glomerular capillary basement membrane abuts the processes (podocytes) of the visceral epithelial cells. The physical space between the podocytes is large. The podocytes, however, are also lined by negatively charged proteins.

Because of the anatomic features just outlined, the glomerular capillary filtration apparatus acts as a very efficient, semipermeable membrane system that effectively excludes passage of molecules with a radius greater than 38 to 44 angstroms (Å) (3.8 to 4.4 nm) while allowing ready passage of molecules less than 20 Å (2 nm). It is important to note that these dimensions do not correspond to clearly identifiable structural pores, but rather reflect the functional characteristics of the filtration barrier.

3. Filtration Ratios

The filtrate/plasma ratio is 1.0 for substances with molecular weights less than 5000 and effective radii of less than 15 Å (1.5 nm), but falls sharply for larger molecules. For example, less than 1% of serum albumin (MW of 69,000 d and an effective radius of 3.6 nm) is filtered. The shape of the molecule is also important. The asymmetric shape and negative charge for albumin reduce its filtration through the glomerulus. In addition, substances such as bilirubin and calcium, which are bound to proteins, are also less apt to be filtered.

During the process of glomerular filtration, about a fifth of the plasma water, plus the filterable constituents of the blood (glucose, amino acids, sodium, potassium, chloride, bicarbonate, urea, creatinine, and other diffusible molecules), pass into Bowman's capsule. Nonfilterable molecules, such as protein, lipids, and formed elements of the blood, are retained by the capillary membrane and move with the remaining plasma into the efferent arteriole. The rate at which this ultrafiltrate of plasma is formed is called the glomerular filtration rate (GFR). This fluid is referred to as an ultrafiltrate because both cellular elements and proteins are retained by the filter (the glomerulus). A true filtrate would exclude only the cellular elements of the blood.

4. Regulation of Glomerular Filtration Rate

The two major factors governing GFR are the glomerular plasma flow and the hydraulic permeability of the filtration barrier. Each of these variables may be affected independently by diseases, hormones, and drugs. These, in turn, are affected by autoregulation and tubuloglomerular feedback. However, autoregulation of the GFR rate is similar to that observed for renal blood flow. Even when renal blood pressure varies over wide ranges, the GFR remains relatively constant.

The phenomenon of tubuloglomerular feedback regulation of GFR is manifested by decreases in the rate of glomerular filtration when there is an increased rate of flow of tubular fluid through Henle's loop. The reduction in GFR is largely due to decreased glomerular blood flow and decreased hydraulic conductivity. The tubuloglomerular feedback loop operates more efficiently to reduce glomerular filtration when tubular fluid flow is increased than to increase filtration in response to reductions in tubular flow.

B. FLUID AND SOLUTE CHANGES IN THE TUBULES

The renal tubules normally reabsorb over 99% of all the glomerular filtrate presented to them. At the normal GFR of 125 ml/min, about 180 liters of glomerular filtrate is produced each day. Because of tubular reabsorption, however, only about 1.0 to 1.5 liters of urine are actually excreted.

The constituents of the glomerular filtrate have traditionally been divided into three groups of substances according to their fate in the tubules: threshold substances; nonthreshold substances; and electrolytes, water, and other substances retained or excreted according to the needs of the individual.

1. Threshold Substances

Glucose, amino acids, phosphate, and sulfate are examples of threshold substances. They are entirely reabsorbed, unless present in greater than normal amounts. The maximum rate of reabsorption that can be achieved for each of these substances is termed its transport maximum (T_m). Therefore, these substances exhibit T_m-limited reabsorption. The affinity of the transport system of many substances with T_m-limited reabsorption is so high that the entire filtered load is reabsorbed from the tubular fluid as long as the transport system is unsaturated. For example, the reabsorption of glucose and amino acids is virtually complete if the filtered load does not saturate the transport system.

For glucose, the average normal value in men for T_m is approximately 2 mmol/min (375 mg/min). The average normal T_m in women is somewhat lower, about 1.7 mmol/min (303 mg/min). If the GFR is 125 ml/min, theoretically glucosuria should first occur at a plasma glucose of about 16 mmol/liter (300 mg/dl); that is, the renal threshold for glucose at a normal GFR is about 16 mmol/liter. However, the actual renal threshold for glucose for the entire kidney is approximately 11 mmol/liter (200 mg/dl) because the transport system of some tubules becomes saturated before others.

2. Nonthreshold Substances

Creatinine is not reabsorbed by the tubules. This holds true over wide ranges of plasma concentration. In fact, about 10% to 15% of the creatinine found in the urine is secreted into tubular fluid.

Urea is formed in the liver and is the major end product of protein metabolism and, like uric acid, is eliminated exclusively by the kidneys. The renal handling of urea represents an important example of passive reabsorption. No part of the tubule can actively reabsorb urea. However, urea will be passively reabsorbed whenever its concentration in the tubular fluid exceeds that in the surrounding peritubular fluid. As water is reabsorbed by the proximal tubule, the concentration of urea rises, thereby establishing a concentration gradient for the passive diffusion of urea from tubular lumen to peritubular space. By the end of the proximal tubule, about 40% of the filtered urea has been reabsorbed by this mechanism.

Because urea reabsorption occurs as a consequence of the reabsorption of water, urea reabsorption varies inversely with the rate of urine flow. In other words, the amount of urea excreted tends to increase proportionally to the rise in urine output.

3. Electrolytes and Water

The concentration of all the cations and most of the anions in the blood is largely determined by renal function. Except for some loss of electrolytes from the skin and in the feces, the kidneys regulate the concentration of all electrolytes brought into the body. All these substances are reabsorbed or excreted according to the needs of the individual (Table 13.1).

a. Sodium

Over 99% of the filtered sodium is removed by the tubules and returned to the blood. Normally, each liter of urine contains about 40 to 60 mEq of sodium. If renal perfusion or sodium intake is reduced, tubular reabsorption of sodium increases, and the concentration of sodium in the urine may fall to less than 10 to 20 mEq/liters. Renal salt excretion is also modified by changes in renin-angiotensin-aldosterone (RAA) activity and other renal mechanisms, referred to as *third factors*.

Approximately two thirds of the filtered Na^+ is reabsorbed by the proximal tubule. Na^+ must be accompanied by an anion to maintain electrical neutrality. Approximately 75% is accompanied by Cl^-, while the remaining 25% is accompanied by HCO_3^-. Three major mechanisms have been identified: unidirectional Na^+ transport (uniport), Na^+-H^+ exchange (antiport), and Cl^--driven Na^+ transport.

The renin-angiotensin-aldosterone(RAA) mechanism can be activated by a low pulse pressure in the afferent arterioles, increased catecholamine or sympathetic nervous activity, or hyperkalemia. Decreased quantities of sodium in the distal convoluted tubular fluid as it passes through the juxtaglomerular apparatus may also stimulate the renin production. Other factors that also stimulate aldosterone secretion, but to a lesser extent, are elevated plasma potassium concentrations and adrenocorticotropic hormone (ACTH).

As much as 8% to 10% of the glomerular filtrate is actively reabsorbed in the distal nephron. As in the proximal tubule, Na^+-K^+ ATPase provides the energy for the passive entry of Na^+, as well as for its active extrusion into interstitial fluid. Since the Cl^- permeability of the distal nephron is considerably lower than that of the proximal tubule, a substantial transepithelial potential difference can be generated.

An increased amount of Na^+ will be reabsorbed by the distal nephron if an increased load of Na^+ is delivered to this region. Thus, like the proximal tubule and thick ascending limb, the distal nephron exhibits load-dependent Na^+ reabsorption. It should be noted that, because of this load dependence of distal nephron Na^+ reabsorption, Na^+ resorption in the collecting tubules and ducts is also increased by aldosterone.

Table 13.1

FILTRATION, EXCRETION, AND "NET REABSORPTION" OF ELECTROLYTES IN THE KIDNEYS DURING A 24-HOUR PERIOD UNDER NORMAL CONDITIONS IN HEALTHY YOUNG ADULTS

Electrolytes	Filtered mEq	Excreted* mEq	Excreted* Percentage of Amount Filtered	Net Reabsorption mEq	Net Reabsorption Percentage of Amount Filtered
Sodium	25,200	90	0.36	25,110	99.64
Potassium	756	90	11.90	666	88.10
Chloride	18,000	120	0.67	17,880	99.33
Bicarbonate	4,320	0	0	4,320	100.00

Third factor is the term applied to mechanisms, other than changes in GFR and aldosterone concentration, that alter renal sodium excretion. For example, reabsorption of sodium in the proximal tubule is increased when extracellular fluid (ECF) volume is low, whereas expansion of the ECF tends to cause a natriuresis. Both events may occur even though GFR and aldosterone levels are kept constant. The mechanisms involved are not yet completely clear, but certainly involve atrial natriuretic factor (ANF).

Redistribution of intrarenal blood flow, from salt-conserving juxtamedullary nephrons to salt-losing superficial cortical nephrons, may play an important role in this response. Alteration of filtration fraction may also be important in controlling sodium and water absorption.

b. Potassium

The amount of potassium lost daily in the urine is determined to a large extent by the volume of urine, but may vary considerably, depending on potassium intake, acid-base changes, and sodium excretion. The excretion of potassium, in contrast to sodium, is almost obligatory. Even with acute hypokalemia, a large urine output will generally result in excretion of at least 30 to 40 mEq of potassium per liter, making the patient even more hypokalemic. If urine potassium levels are < 10 to 20 mEq/liter, there is usually a deficiency of aldosterone, or the patient has a severe chronic potassium deficit.

Normally, all of the filtered potassium is absorbed, but an amount equal to 10% to 15% of the quantity filtered is finally excreted in the urine. In renal disease with a low GFR, the excretion of potassium may even exceed the filtered load.

The renal handling of potassium is an important example of bidirectional transport. Potassium is almost completely reabsorbed in the proximal tubule, secreted in the thin descending limb of the loop of Henle, reabsorbed in the thin and thick ascending limbs of the loop of Henle, and both reabsorbed and secreted in the distal nephron. In the nephron as a whole, at least 93% of the potassium, which is filtered through the glomerulus, is usually reabsorbed; therefore, one can say that potassium undergoes net reabsorption. However, some net secretion also occurs under certain conditions because the calculated excretion of potassium is about 12% of the amount filtered by the glomerulus.

One of the major determinants for potassium secretion appears to be the concentration of potassium in the tubular fluid. When luminal flow is high, the secreted potassium is rapidly diluted, the gradient for potassium secretion is maintained, and increased amounts of potassium are secreted. In states of low flow, the cell-to-lumen potassium concentration gradient is rapidly decreased and the absolute rate of potassium secretion into the tubule lumen is diminished. Thus, flow rate in the distal tubule is a major factor influencing the urinary secretion and excretion of potassium.

AXIOM

Unless there is a moderate-severe potassium deficiency, increased urine output causes increased urinary potassium losses.

Another factor affecting potassium secretion into the distal tubule is the electric potential difference from the cell to the lumen of the distal tubule. The lumen's negative potential difference is generated by the tubule's reabsorption of sodium. The more sodium that is resorbed, the greater the potassium secretion into the tubule lumen.

Aldosterone increases the rate of potassium secretion by several mechanisms: (1) increased permeability of the luminal membrane to potassium; (2) enhanced rate of sodium reabsorption, rendering the tubule lumen more electronegative; and (3) increased activity of the Na^+-K^+ ATPase pump. The rate of aldosterone secretion is influenced by the renin-angiotensin system and by the plasma concentration of potassium.

c. Chloride

The amount of chloride that is absorbed passively depends primarily on the amount of sodium that has been actively absorbed. Chloride is the major anion accompanying sodium and its reabsorption is gradient and time limited. Vomiting (with significant loss of HCl) and decreased chloride in the glomerular filtrate causes urinary chloride excretion to fall rapidly. In fact, it may fall to almost zero, even when sodium excretion is still significant.

Chloride is extremely important in determining the kidney's ability to concentrate urine. In most of the tubule, chloride reabsorption occurs passively along with sodium transport. However, in the water-impermeable ascending thick limb of the loop of Henle, where up to 20% to 30% of sodium and chloride can be reabsorbed, chloride transport is active. This active transport of chloride apparently helps provide the crucial gradient needed to allow the "countercurrent" urine concentrating mechanism to function properly.

d. Bicarbonate

Sodium, bicarbonate, and chloride are absorbed in the proximal tubule, and hydrogen ions are secreted into the tubular lumen in exchange for sodium ions. However, if the extracellular fluid(ECF) is reduced, especially with chloride depletion, or if there is a potassium deficiency, increased amounts of sodium and bicarbonate are absorbed in the proximal tubule. This process produces what is sometimes referred to as contraction alkalosis. If saline is then given, thus re-expanding the ECF, proximal tubular absorption of sodium and bicarbonate is decreased to normal.

In the cells of the distal tubule, CO_2 (produced in the tubule cell or brought to the cell by the blood) is combined with H_2O (in the presence of the enzyme carbonic anhydrase) to form H_2CO_3. The H_2CO_3 is then dissociated into H^+ and HCO_3^-. The H^+ and K^+ inside the cell are then excreted into the tubular lumen in electroequivalent exchange for Na^+, which is absorbed into the tubule cells. The HCO_3^- then moves out through the other side of the cell into the bloodstream with the Na^+. This process of generating bicarbonate from H_2O and CO_2 occurs primarily in the distal tubule, but some secretion of hydrogen ions is also thought to occur in the proximal tubule by a similar mechanism.

Any situation that causes intracellular acidosis also increases the secretion of hydrogen ions into the tubular lumen, thereby increasing sodium and bicarbonate reabsorption. For example, in hypokalemia, potassium ions leave renal tubular cells in exchange for hydrogen ions, resulting in an intracellular acidosis and increased excretion of hydrogen ions. This causes increased bicarbonate generation and absorption, thereby tending to produce alkalosis in the blood.

AXIOM

Excretion of an acid urine, in spite of an alkalosis in the blood, is referred to as paradoxical aciduria and is usually due to hypokalemia.

Normally, bicarbonate is almost totally absorbed in the tubules and is absent from the urine. However, if the plasma bicarbonate levels rise above normal, if the ECF volume is expanded, or if hyperkalemia (which causes an intracellular alkalosis and decreased bicarbonate regeneration) is present, less bicarbonate is reabsorbed and bicarbonate may appear in the urine.

e. Reabsorption of Peptides and Proteins

Peptides and proteins that are smaller than serum albumin are filtered to a variable extent. Normally, these molecules are almost completely reabsorbed by the proximal tubule. The reabsorption of peptides and proteins from the proximal tubular fluid occurs predominantly by pinocytosis. Once inside the cells, they enter lysosomes, where they are degraded to their constituent amino acids, which then pass into the peritubular fluid. Insulin is also one of the peptides handled by the proximal tubule. When an insulin-requiring diabetic develops renal disease, the dose of insulin necessary to control the plasma glucose levels may decrease, since diseased kidneys degrade less insulin.

AXIOM

Decreased insulin requirements in a diabetic may be an indication of increasing renal dysfunction.

f. Organic Acids and Bases

The secretion of organic acids, such as para-amino hippurate (PAH), into urine occurs exclusively in the proximal tubule. The system that secretes PAH is nonselective. A large number of antibiotics and other drugs, such as the loop diuretics, are secreted into the proximal tubule lumen by the organic acid system.

A clinically useful competitive inhibitor of the organic acid secretory system, probenecid, can be administered in conjunction with rapidly secreted antibiotics, such as penicillin, to prolong their duration of action. A secretory system for organic bases is also present in proximal tubular cells.

The proximal tubule reabsorbs K^+, Ca^{++}, Mg^{++}, and phosphate. In addition, proximal tubular cells synthesize ammonia, a compound that is important in H^+ excretion.

C. CHANGES IN GLOMERULAR FILTRATE IN SPECIFIC PORTIONS OF THE TUBULES

1. Proximal Tubule

The proximal tubule reabsorbs about 80% to 85% of the glomerular filtrate. Glucose, sodium, potassium, and several other substances are actively absorbed, whereas chloride and water are passively reabsorbed. As water passively diffuses from the proximal tubular fluid, the concentration of other substances, such as urea, rises within the tubule. Urea, which becomes increasingly concentrated in the tubular fluid as water and electrolytes are absorbed, then passively diffuses from the proximal tubule to the peritubular blood. The 20 to 30 ml of fluid leaving the proximal tubule every minute to enter the more distal portions of the nephron is approximately isosmotic and has a pH similar to that of plasma.

As sodium chloride and bicarbonate leave the proximal tubule lumen and enter the lateral space on the nonluminal side of the tubule cells, the osmolality increase results in the movement of water from the tubular lumen into the lateral space. Some of the water goes from the lumen to the lateral space through the tubule cells, while the remainder moves from the lumen across the tight cell junctions into the lateral space. The increase in the volume of fluid in the lateral space produces an increase in the hydrostatic pressure. This, in turn, drives water and dissolved solutes from the lateral space to the peritubular space, from which they are returned to the body through the peritubular capillaries.

About 99% of the filtered glucose is normally reabsorbed by the proximal tubule. The carrier-mediated transport of glucose across the brush border is coupled to the passive entry of Na^+, and this helps to provide the energy for the transport of glucose across the brush border.

The proximal tubule also reabsorbs over 99% of the filtered amino acids. The normal plasma concentration of free amino acids is about 3 mmol/liter. Like glucose reabsorption, the reabsorption of amino acids by the proximal tubule is coupled to Na^+ reabsorption.

Following trauma, the GFR, and therefore the rate of flow in the proximal tubule, may decrease precipitously. Since reabsorption in the proximal tubule depends partly on the length of time the filtrate is exposed to its cells, the reabsorption of electrolytes and water is increased when the GFR is decreased. This reduces the volume of urine and its sodium content and helps to maintain the total body content of sodium and water at a normal level.

If the GFR rises as a result of fluid loading or an alteration of vascular dynamics, the rate of proximal tubular flow increases, and increased quantities of sodium and water are lost into the urine. The percentage of salt and water reabsorbed in the proximal tubule is relatively constant if other factors are held steady. This is known as glomerular-tubular balance.

Although the proximal tubule provides the bulk of salt and water regulation, fine adjustments in salt and water balance are made by aldosterone, antidiuretic hormones (ADH), atrial natriuretic factors (ANF), and several other factors acting on more distal portions of the tubule.

2. The Loop of Henle

In the loop of Henle, the Na^+Cl^--rich isotonic fluid that leaves the proximal tubule is reduced in volume and transformed into a hypotonic fluid in which urea is a major osmotically active solute. The loop of Henle accomplishes this by reabsorbing approximately 25% of the filtered Na^+ and 20% of the filtered water from the tubular fluid, while adding substantial amounts of urea.

a. The Medullary Gradient

The osmolality of the peritubular fluid in the renal cortex is essentially identical with that of plasma. However, the osmolality of the peritubular fluid in the medulla can increase to approximately 1200 to 1400 mOsm/kg H_2O at the tip of the papilla. In addition, although Na^+ and Cl^- are the predominant osmotically active solutes in the cortical peritubular fluid, a substantial fraction of the osmotically active solutes is urea. In fact, the concentration of urea in peritubular fluid increases from the corticomedullary junction, where its concentration is similar to that of plasma, to the tip of the papilla, where it accounts for about half of the osmotically active solutes. The term medullary gradient refers to the osmotic gradient that exists in the peritubular fluid between the corticomedullary junction and the tip of papilla. This may be as high as 900 to 1100 mOsm/liter.

The reabsorption of Na^+, Cl^-, and water in the loop of Henle is dependent upon the length of the loop. Thus, the juxtamedullary nephrons usually absorb more of these substances than the cortical nephrons.

b. Thin Descending Limb

The thin descending limb of the loop of Henle has a relatively low permeability to solutes, but is highly permeable to water. Thus, as the isotonic tubular fluid entering the thin descending limb flows downward through regions of increasingly hypertonic peritubular fluid, water is reabsorbed.

Because of the reabsorption of water, the tubular fluid osmolality may increase to 1200 to 1400 mOsm/kg H_2O at its termination at the hairpin turn. In cortical nephrons, whose loops only reach the junction between the outer and inner medulla, the tubular fluid osmolality increases to only about 600 mOsm/kg H_2O. In both juxtamedullary nephrons and cortical nephrons, the predominant solutes in the tubular fluid are Na^+ and Cl^-, but half or more of the solutes in the surrounding peritubular fluid is urea.

c. Ascending Limb

The ascending limb of the loop of Henle in juxtamedullary nephrons can be divided into two regions: the thin ascending limb, which begins at the hairpin turn; and the thick ascending limb, which begins at or near the junction between the inner and outer medulla. Cortical nephrons lack a thin ascending limb; their thick ascending limb, therefore, begins near the hairpin turn, at or above the junction between the inner and outer medulla.

(1) Thin Ascending Limb

The thin ascending limb is virtually impermeable to water, but is highly permeable to Na^+ and Cl^-, and moderately permeable to urea. Na^+ and Cl^- diffuse passively from the tubular lumen to the peritubular space, while urea can diffuse passively from peritubular space to the lumen, depending on its concentration gradient. In the juxtamedullary nephron the tubular fluid at the end of the thin ascending limb is estimated to contain about 400 mmol/liter of electrolytes and 100 mmol/liter of urea, for a total osmolality of approximately 500 mOsm/kg

H_2O. The thin ascending limb can secrete or absorb K^+ into the tubular fluid depending on peritubular blood concentrations.

(2) Thick Ascending Limb	The water permeability of the thick ascending limb is negligible and the urea permeability is quite low. The thick ascending limb actively transports Na^+ and Cl^- from lumen to peritubular space. The combination of low water permeability and active reabsorption of Na^+ and Cl^- means that the thick ascending limb lowers both the osmolality and the concentration of Na^+ and Cl^- in the tubular fluid to levels below those in the surrounding peritubular fluid. In the juxtamedullary nephrons, the tubular fluid at the end of the thick ascending limb is estimated to contain about 100 mmol/liter of electrolytes and 100 mmol/liter of urea, for a total of osmolality of approximately 200 mOsm/kg H_2O. In the cortical nephrons, the tubular fluid at the end of the thick ascending limb is estimated to contain approximately 100 mmol/liter of electrolytes and 40 mmol/liter of urea, for a total osmolality of 140 mOsm/kg H_2O.

3. Distal Nephron

a. Solute Concentrations

The average tubular fluid entering the distal nephron contains approximately 100 mmol/liter of electrolytes and other nonurea solutes and 50 mmol/liter of urea, for a total osmolality of approximately 150 mOsm/kg H_2O. Whereas Na^+ and Cl^- are the primary nonurea solutes entering the distal nephron, other nonurea solutes become increasingly important as the fluid moves more distally in the nephron. Tubular reabsorption in the distal nephron reduces Na^+ and Cl^- concentrations to such low levels that the concentration of solutes, such as creatinine, uric acid, K^+, NH_4^+, Ca^{++}, Mg^{++}, and phosphate, becomes increasingly important.

4. Water Reabsorption

a. ADH Effect

In the presence of maximal ADH secretion, the high water permeability of the collecting tubule and duct prevents the establishment of an osmotic gradient across the tubular epithelium. Since the osmolality of the tubular fluid entering the collecting tubule and duct is only about 150 mOsm/kg H_2O and the osmolality of the surrounding peritubular fluid ranges from approximately 300 mOsm/kg H_2O in the cortex to 1200 to 1400 mOsm/kg H_2O at the tip of the papilla, over 70% of the water entering the collecting tubule and duct can be absorbed. Because of the high water permeability, the urea concentration can increase from about 50 mmol/liter to about 175 mmol/liter.

(1) Cortical-Medullary Gradients

In the medullary collecting ducts, water continues to be reabsorbed as the tubular fluid flows downward through regions of increasingly hypertonic peritubular fluid, and additional Na^+ and Cl^- can also be reabsorbed. Over 50% of the water entering the medullary collecting duct is reabsorbed in this region, and the urea concentration can increase from about 175 to 400 mmol/liter. The concentration of nonurea solutes also increases (from about 125 mmol/liter to about 200 mmol/liter) as Na^+ and Cl^- are absorbed. Consequently, under normal circumstances, the osmolality of the tubular fluid at the end of the medullary collecting duct will be approximately 600 mOsm/kg H_2O.

Additional water is absorbed in the papillary collecting duct as the tubular fluid continues flowing downward through the medullary gradient. However, ADH causes the papillary collecting tubule and the medullary collecting duct to increase their permeability to both urea and water. It is estimated that approximately two thirds of the water entering the papillary collecting duct can be absorbed there, and the concentration of nonurea solutes increases approximately three-fold, from about 200 to 500 mmol/liter. Since urea is reabsorbed, its concentration increases less markedly, from approximately 400 to 600 mmol/liter.

(2) Glomerular-Tubular Balance

At least some of these changes in each distal tubule are regulated by that tubule's juxtaglomerular apparatus's production of renin, which may influence the GFR in that nephron. The control mechanisms for this are not yet completely clear, but may include the volume of fluid in the distal tubule, the rate of sodium transport in the distal tubule, and the pressure and flow relationships in the afferent arteriole. It has been suggested that the juxtaglomerular apparatus may allow each nephron to control its own filtration rate by a local feedback loop, thereby preventing too wide a variation in the delivery of salt to the distal nephron. This local control mechanism has been referred to as glomerular-tubular balance.

(3) Other Factors

In the normal kidney, the tubular fluid delivered to the collecting tubule and duct is always hypotonic, and the final urine osmolality is determined by the effect of ADH on water permeability. However, the osmolality of urine is not solely dependent upon the ADH level. Most important, the concentrating and diluting mechanisms in the collecting tubules and ducts are markedly dependent on the proper function of the thick ascending limb to produce the corticomedullary osmotic gradient. Even if plasma ADH is high, a concentrated (hypertonic) urine can be excreted only in the presence of a proper osmotic medullary gradient.

Some other factors that affect the concentrating and diluting mechanisms of the kidney include the following:

1. *Availability of urea.* A protein-deficient diet or severe liver disease will provide less urea for maintaining maximum peritubular fluid osmolality.

2. *Rate of flow through the collecting duct.* A rapid flow, such as with a diuretic or water diuresis, will tend to wash out the medullary gradient.

3. *Presence of prostaglandins.* Some prostaglandins increase blood flow through the vasa recta, thereby reducing the maximum osmolality gradient. Prostaglandins also impair the formation of concentrated urine by inhibiting adenylate cyclase, thereby inhibiting the effect of ADH on the water permeability of the collecting tubule and ducts. Since ADH stimulates prostaglandin synthesis by the kidneys, this inhibition is a form of negative feedback.

IV. CONTROL OF RENAL ACTIVITY

Renal activity is controlled by the volume and pressure in the vascular system, the autonomic nervous system, various hormones, and the levels of various electrolytes.

A. BLOOD VOLUME AND PRESSURE

Decreases in intravascular volume or pressure cause renal vascular constriction, which, in turn, reduces RPF. As a consequence, the GFR falls, and increased amounts of water and sodium are absorbed in the proximal tubule. In addition, decreased urine flow and sodium in the distal tubule stimulate the juxtaglomerular apparatus to secrete renin. This, in turn, results in increased levels of angiotensin, which causes more vasoconstriction and less renal artery flow and stimulates secretion of aldosterone by the adrenal cortex. Aldosterone increases the absorption of sodium, bicarbonate, and water, and decreases absorption of potassium and chloride.

B. AUTONOMIC NERVOUS SYSTEM

Stimulation of the sympathetic nervous system results in renal arterial and arteriolar constriction, thereby decreasing RPF. Efferent arteriolar vasoconstriction, however, generally prevents as much of a decrease in GFR.

The nerves to the kidney seemingly also play some role in regulating the amount of vasoconstriction in the afferent and efferent arterioles. This helps to keep the GFR relatively constant under wide ranges of pressure and flow. However, even a denervated kidney will respond to changes in flow and pressure by autoregulation, suggesting the presence of an intrinsic control mechanism that may be related to stretch receptors in the renal vasculature.

C. HORMONES

The primary hormones affecting the function of the kidneys are antidiuretic hormones, adrenocortical hormones, parathyroid hormones, and atrial natriuretic peptides.

1. Antidiuretic Hormone

Verney first demonstrated that certain receptors in the brain (referred to as osmoreceptors) were extremely sensitive to changes in the osmolarity of the blood. Injection of hypotonic solutions into a carotid artery stimulates a water diuresis, whereas injection of hypertonic saline or glucose prevents the water diuresis. Hypophysectomy also stimulates a water diuresis and blocks the antidiuretic effects of hypertonic solutions. Later studies show that hypovolemia could also abolish the water diuresis caused by injection of hypotonic solutions into the carotid artery. This demonstrates that decreases in the effective intravascular volume have a more powerful effect on ADH secretion than does decreased plasma osmolarity.

The concentration of the urine depends critically on the presence of antidiuretic hormones. Arginine vasopressin (the other name for ADH) is produced in the supraoptic nucleus of the hypothalamus and is translocated to the posterior pituitary gland for storage and release. The regulation of ADH release is normally under the control of the osmolality of the immediate extracellular fluid environment near the osmole receptors in the supraoptic and paraventricular nuclei of the hypothalamus. ADH secretion is almost completely suppressed when plasma osmolality is less than 270 to 280 mOsm/kg of water, and is progressively increased as plasma osmolality exceeds 290 mOsm/kg of water.

Although the osmolality of the plasma is the usual determinant of ADH release, there are several stronger stimuli including nausea and vomiting, pain (particularly abdominal), and hypovolemia.

AXIOM
In patients with hyponatremia and hypovolemia, ADH secretion will be increased and water retention will occur, tending to cause more hyponatremia.

The ability of ADH to increase water permeability in the collecting tubule and duct involves the binding of ADH to receptors on the surfaces of the epithelial cells, the activation of adenylate cyclase, and the generation of cyclic AMP, which in turn leads to the insertion of protein-containing aggregates into the luminal membrane. These aggregates apparently function as channels for water movement.

ADH is essential for the reabsorption of water from the distal tubule and collecting ducts. If there is an absence of ADH, as may occur with hypothalamic or posterior pituitary disease or with intracranial trauma, the cells of the distal tubule and the collecting tubules are rendered impermeable to water. These portions of the tubules are then unable to reabsorb water, and large volumes of dilute urine are excreted, even if the patient needs to conserve water. This process is called diabetes insipidus.

If adequate ADH is produced, but the kidney becomes unresponsive to the ADH, the patient is said to have nephrogenic diabetes insipidus. Some causes of nephrogenic diabetes insipidus include severe hypercalcemia or hypokalemia and various drugs, including aminoglycosides, amphotericin, and lithium.

AXIOM
Aminoglycosides can cause direct tubular damage and reduced response to ADH.

589

Since the final urine is identical with the tubular fluid leaving the papillary collecting duct, the final urine in diabetes insipidus has an osmolality of approximately 70 mOsm/kg H_2O, of which about 50 mmol/liter is urea and about 20 mmol/liter represents nonurea solutes. With a GFR of 125 ml/min (180 liters/d), the rate of urine flow theoretically would be greater than 15 ml/min (26 liters/d). However, even in the absence of ADH, the water impermeability of the collecting tubule and duct is relative, not absolute, so that some of the water flowing through that area will be reabsorbed. Therefore, the actual urine flow is slightly less than the flow rate of tubular fluid at the tip of the loop of Henle.

2. Adrenocortical Hormones

The adrenocortical hormones with mineralocorticoid activity, of which aldosterone is the most important and most powerful, tend to increase the reabsorption of sodium and bicarbonate in the distal tubule. At the same time, these hormones promote the excretion of potassium and hydrogen ions. In hyperaldosteronism, the increased total body sodium is seldom reflected by a rise in the serum sodium concentration because of the concomitant retention of water. Patients with hyperaldosteronism tend to develop hypokalemic, hypochloremic metabolic alkalosis. Adrenal insufficiency, in contrast, results in a decrease in extracellular fluid, hyponatremia, hypochloremia, and hyperkalemia.

3. Parathyroid Hormone

Parathyroid hormone mobilizes calcium from bones, increases the absorption of calcium from the intestinal tract and renal tubular fluid, and increases urinary phosphate excretion. In patients with chronic renal insufficiency, abnormalities in calcium and phosphorus metabolism result in hyperphosphatasemia and hypocalcemia, which may then produce a secondary hyperparathyroidism with bone demineralization. If the hyperparathyroidism persists after a successful renal transplant, the patient is said to have tertiary hyperparathyroidism.

4. Atrial Natriuretic Factor

Atrial natriuretic factor(ANF) or peptide is a substance liberated by the atria of the heart when they are distended. Apparently this is interpreted as hypervolemia, and ANF acts on the kidneys to promote a salt and water diuresis. Normal plasma values for ANF vary between laboratories, but probably range between 2 and 30 pmol/liter. Although plasma ANF levels may approach 300 to 500 pmol/liter in severe congestive heart failure or renal failure, many experimental studies have employed much higher plasma or tissue bath concentrations. ANF effects in such studies must be regarded as pharmacologic, rather than physiologic or pathophysiologic, until confirmed at appropriately low ANF concentrations.

Studies with atrial extracts and synthetic peptides have shown that ANF promotes a diuresis and natriuresis by several methods. It directly increases glomerular filtration rate and has several important actions on the collecting tubules, including inhibition of ADH.

In addition to its direct and indirect effects on tubular sodium transport processes, ANF may also alter intrarenal hydrostatic forces. Several studies have also confirmed the ability of infused ANF to suppress juxtaglomerular cells and reduce aldosterone secretion in anesthetized animals and in humans. The inhibition of the renin-aldosterone axis by ANF is greater when the body has an excess of sodium.

Cogan, in a recent review of ANF, notes that its potency as a pharmacologic agent in altering cardiovascular and renal function makes it an attractive candidate for treating patients with hypertension, congestive heart failure, or glomerular hypofiltration and antinatriuresis. So far, however, the overall benefit from short-term, parenteral administration of ANF in diseases associated with edema has been relatively unimpressive and often limited by hypotension.

In patients with congestive heart failure, infusion of large amounts of ANF temporarily augments cardiac output but results in little natriuresis. Even in pharmacologic concentrations, ANF lacks the potency to overcome the more potent renal salt-retaining effects of the renin-angiotensin-aldosterone and sympathetic nervous systems, which are activated in congestive heart failure. In patients with the nephrotic syndrome, ANF infusion augments both sodium and protein excretion in parallel with a reduction in blood pressure. Variable short-term benefits also have been reported in patients with systemic hypertension, pulmonary hypertension, and cirrhosis.

An exciting therapeutic prospect for ANF is possible reversal of acute renal failure by increasing GFR. In various models of acute renal failure in rats, ANF administered after hemodynamic insults partially restored GFR. Assessment of the efficacy of ANF in humans is obviously needed.

5. Prostaglandins

In patients with impaired renal blood flow, local vasodilating prostaglandins, such as prostacyclin (PGI_2) and PGE_2 may help to maintain perfusion of the tubules. One significant source of renal problems in the elderly is the use of nonsteroidal anti-inflammatory drugs (NSAIDs). These powerful prostaglandin inhibitors have been associated with acute renal failure, particularly in patients with congestive heart failure or cirrhosis, which tend to impair renal perfusion.

AXIOM

NSAIDs should be avoided in patients with cardiac, liver, or renal disease.

NSAIDs are believed to prevent renal synthesis of the prostaglandins needed to maintain adequate renal perfusion. Thus, an older patient's renal function may become seriously impaired when on NSAIDs. By inhibiting prostaglandins, NSAIDs can cause hyperkalemia because of reduced renin and aldosterone secretion, or they may potentiate the effect of ADH and lead to hyponatremia.

D. EPIDERMAL GROWTH FACTOR

Epidermal growth factor (EGF) belongs to an extensive class of molecules, referred to as growth factors, that mediate cell growth and differentiation. These factors also may stimulate acute cell responses. Their effects may be mediated through autocrine, paracrine, and/or endocrine mechanisms.

Current information indicates that the mammalian kidney is a significant site of EGF synthesis, second only to the salivary gland in the rodent, and probably exceeding most other tissues in humans. Limited evidence suggests a role of EGF on tubular function. EGF peptides processed intracellularly or by membrane-localized peptidases appear to be continuously excreted and secreted into urine from the apical membrane surface of the cells of the thick ascending loop of Henle and distal convoluted tubule cells. This urinary EGF is constantly bathing urinary tract epithelial surfaces and could play a role in maintaining surface integrity. It is also possible that a precursor or some other form of EGF is anchored in the apical membrane, where it can function as a receptor to help regulate membrane transport events.

V. ACID-BASE CONTROL BY THE KIDNEYS

A normal diet generally contains some nonvolatile acids, such as phosphate and sulfate, which must be excreted by the kidneys. The breakdown of protein in critically ill or injured patients further adds to the acid load presented to the kidneys.

Ordinarily, the kidneys excrete only about 70 mEq of acid per day, but in acidosis this may be increased more than fourfold. The excretion of acid and regulation of acid-base balance are accomplished by three mechanisms: (1) direct excretion of hydrogen ion; (2) excretion of hydrogen ion with urine buffers, such as Na_2HPO_4; and (3) excretion of hydrogen ion with ammonia.

A. DIRECT EXCRETION OF HYDROGEN ION

Only a very small amount of hydrogen ion, as titratable free acid, is present in the urine. Even at a pH of 4.5 to 5.0, which is usually the most acidic that urine can become, the kidneys directly excrete less than 1 mEq of hydrogen ion per day.

B. EXCRETION WITH URINE BUFFERS

Within the tubule, carbonic acid (H_2CO_3) normally combines with dibasic sodium phosphate (Na_2HPO_4) to form sodium bicarbonate ($NaHCO_3$) and monobasic sodium phosphate (NaH_2PO_4):

$$H_2CO_3 + Na_2HPO_4 \rightarrow NaHCO_3 + NaH_2PO_4.$$

The $NaHCO_3$ is then absorbed and the NaH_2PO_4 is excreted in the urine.

C. EXCRETION WITH AMMONIA

Another mechanism of nonvolatile acid excretion occurs through the renal production of ammonia (NH_3) from the metabolism of glutamine and other amino acid precursors. Ammonia is a gas that diffuses into both the tubule lumen and the peritubular capillary blood. In the lumen, NH_3 is protonated to NH_4, and in this state it is trapped in the lumen because of the lower permeability of ionized substances in the lipids of tubule cell walls. This process is known as ionic diffusion trapping.

Increased renal ammonia production is the major mechanism for eliminating fixed acid from the body, and may, in severe metabolic acidosis, account for excretion of up to 400 to 500 mEq of fixed acid per day. Ammonium is formed by

$$NH_3 + H_2CO_3 \rightarrow NH_4^+ + HCO_3^-.$$

The ammonium ions may be excreted with anions, such as sulfate:

$$2NH_4HCO_3 + Na_2SO_4 \rightarrow 2NaHCO_3 + (NH_4)_2SO_4.$$

The $NaHCO_3$ is then absorbed, and the ammonium sulfate is excreted in the urine. This mechanism normally accounts for excretion of 40 to 50 mEq of acid per day.

VI. TESTS OF RENAL FUNCTION

The most frequently used tests of renal function include urinalysis, BUN, and serum creatinine. Various clearances, filtration fractions, and tubular maximums are less frequently measured, but are more accurate and informative.

A. URINE OUTPUT

The measurement of urine output is probably the most frequently performed renal function test. As a single measure of renal function, however, the urine flow rate is not a very specific test. Patients with severe renal failure may have normal urine flow rates. Urine flow depends on the intake of water, the glomerular filtration rate, the tonicity of the medullary interstitium, the concentration of ADH, the response of the kidney to ADH, and the tubular absorption of sodium.

Although a low urine output, in spite of fluid loading and inotropic support in critically ill or injured patients, is a bad sign and indicates renal impairment, a high urine output may be present, in spite of severe renal dysfunction.

B. URINALYSIS

Examination of a urine specimen includes evaluation of its specific gravity, osmolarity, chemical constituents, and formed elements.

1. Specific Gravity

The specific gravity of normal urine varies from 1.010 to 1.035, but may be less than 1.005 with diabetes insipidus or a large water load. A low specific gravity, identical to or lower than glomerular filtrate, may also be seen with renal failure with few functioning nephrons.

This is a relatively simple test to perform and can provide important information on the renal concentrating ability. However, the specific gravity can be a difficult or inaccurate method of measuring tubular function, especially if only small amounts of urine are available. In addition, many substances in the urine affect specific gravity, yet have nothing to do with renal function.

AXIOM
Protein, mannitol, and other high molecular weight substances, such as dextran or soluble contrast agents, may give the urine a high specific gravity, even if the kidneys have a poor concentrating ability.

2. Osmolality

Urine osmolality, as determined by its freezing point, is an excellent measure of renal tubular function, especially if the patient can be dehydrated safely. Urine osmolality may be lower than serum osmolality or it may be as high as 1400 mOsm/liter in young, healthy dehydrated individuals. In older patients, or in those who have recently undergone trauma or surgery, the kidney may be unable to concentrate urine to more than 600 mOsm/liter.

Whenever possible, the urine osmolality should be compared with the plasma osmolality. If plasma osmolality is low, urine osmolality should be very low (<50 to 100 mOsm/kg). In contrast, if the tubules are working well and there is reduced renal perfusion due to dehydration, urine osmolality may be very high. In the oliguric patient, a urine/plasma osmolality ratio of less than 1.1:1 generally indicates the presence of vasomotor nephropathy, whereas a ratio exceeding 1.5:1 suggests that the oliguria is due to hypovolemia.

To use the urine osmolality most effectively as a guide to tubular function, one must place the patients in a situation in which they will be maximally concentrating their urine. This was formerly done by water deprivation but is now commonly done by injecting exogenous ADH followed by hourly urine collections. If the tubules are normal, a young adult eating a normal diet should reach urine osmolarity of at least 1000 mOsm/liter.

AXIOM
A high urine osmolality suggests that nephron function is relatively intact.

When the urine output is low and urine osmolality should be elevated, such as in dehydration or hypovolemia, the finding of an iso-osmolar urine suggests that the kidney is incapable of producing a concentrated urine. Other factors that may alter the ability of the kidneys to concentrate urine include congestive heart failure, hypothyroidism, chronic diuretic use, chronic renal failure, glucosuria, and fasting (especially protein deprivation). Severe hypokalemia or hypercalcemia also reduces the ability of the kidney to concentrate urine.

3. Chemical Constituents

The main chemical constituents of urine that are tested routinely in the laboratory include pH, glucose, ketones, bilirubin, and occult blood.

a. pH

Urine is usually acid, with a pH of 4 to 6 in a patient on a normal diet. An alkaline urine suggests that the patient has an alkalemia or a urinary tract infection with urea-splitting organisms. If the urine is acid in the presence of alkalemia, a paradoxical aciduria is said to be present. This is usually associated with hypokalemia or severe chloride depletion. A relatively alkaline urine is found in patients with renal tubular acidosis, a condition caused by incomplete reabsorption of bicarbonate or insufficient secretion of hydrogen ions.

b. Glucose

Under most circumstances, urine contains less than 0.25% glucose. If the level is higher, the tubular maximum for glucose (about 180 to 250 mg/200 ml) reabsorption has been exceeded because of an excessive intake of glucose, the presence of diabetes mellitus, an increase in GFR, or a reduction in tubular transport function because of drugs or disease. Glycosuria, in the absence of high exogenous carbohydrate loads and stress, usually means that a patient has diabetes mellitus.

Urine glucose levels are generally reported as 1+, 2+, 3+, or 4+, which indicate urine glucose concentrations exceeding 0.25%, 0.5%, 1.0%, and 2.0%, respectively. The two common tests for urine glucose are copper reduction, which detects many substances other than glucose, and glucose oxidase, which is much more specific. False-positive glucose oxidase results may be seen if the specimen is contaminated with hydrogen peroxide or hypochlorites, and false-negative results may occur in the presence of L-dopa or aspirin.

c. Ketones

The presence of ketone bodies in the urine suggests excessive metabolism of fat with increased quantities of acetone, acetoacetic acid, and/or beta-hydroxybutyric acid in the blood. Ketone bodies in the urine without glycosuria suggest an inadequate carbohydrate intake (starvation ketosis), whereas ketonuria with glycosuria suggests the presence of diabetes mellitus with acidosis.

d. Protein

A small amount of protein, less than 100 mg/liter, is filtered by the normal glomerulus. However, if most of this protein were not reabsorbed in the tubule, the protein loss would be about 18 g/d. The assessment of the significance of protein in the urine depends on the measurement of its 24-hour excretion.

By definition, proteinuria refers to excretion of more than 100 mg of protein in 24 hours. A small amount of protein, especially of low molecular weight, is filtered by the glomerulus, but the bulk of it is reabsorbed in the proximal tubule. When found in the urine, protein usually reflects glomerular disease, but may also indicate renal tubular defects, polycystic kidneys, infection, hypertension, or renal vein thrombosis. The molecular weight of the protein may also be helpful in determining its etiology. Urinary protein of large molecular weight (>55,000 d) generally indicates glomerular basement membrane injury (glomerulonephritis), whereas low molecular weight urinary protein tends to indicate renal tubular injury (acute tubular necrosis or infection). When protein excretion exceeds 3.5 g/d, the diagnosis of nephrotic syndrome is often made.

e. Bilirubin

Bile is not usually detectable in urine. If bilirubin is found in the urine, there is generally some abnormality of the biliary or hepatic excretory system, resulting in an excessive amount of conjugated bilirubin in the plasma.

f. Occult Blood

If there has been any bleeding in the urinary tract, the urine will usually be positive for occult blood. It is more reliable to examine the urine microscopically for red cells. Red blood cell casts are not seen in the sediment of patients with otherwise normal kidneys. A markedly positive test for occult blood, especially if associated with a deep brown urine and no red cells on the microscopic exam, is suggestive of myoglobinuria.

AXIOM

If the urine is positive for occult blood but there are no red blood cells in the urine, one should suspect myoglobinuria.

g. Urinary Sodium

In an oliguric patient, a spot urine sodium can be helpful in determining its etiology. If the urine sodium, is <10 mEq/liter under such circumstances, there is usually impaired renal perfusion. However, urine sodium >40 mEq/liter in the presence of oliguria suggests renal failure.

h. Urinary Potassium

Measurement of either a spot or 24-hour urinary K$^+$ concentration has limited use in the clinical situation. Increased urinary K$^+$ excretion confirms the kidneys as the source of loss of this important electrolyte. The two most common causes for high urinary K^+ are hyperaldosteronism and acidosis with increased excretion of ketone bodies. Since the body can lose K^+ by means other than the kidney, as well as shift K^+ in and out of cells, the absolute measurement of renal loss provides only a crude estimate of potassium balance.

4. Formed Elements

Urine should be examined under the microscope for red blood cells (RBC), white blood cells (WBCs), bacteria, casts, and crystals (Fig. 13.9). There are ordinarily about 2 to 3 WBCs, 0 to 2 RBCs, and no bacteria per high-power field when unspun, undiluted urine is examined under the microscope. Normally, occasional hyaline casts can be seen. If the initial microscopic examination is negative, the urine is centrifuged at 1500 to 2500 rpm for 5 minutes, the supernatant is removed, and the sediment is resuspended and examined.

The presence of casts containing cellular elements implies parenchymal renal disease, whereas red blood cells can come from any part of the urinary

Formed elements in urine

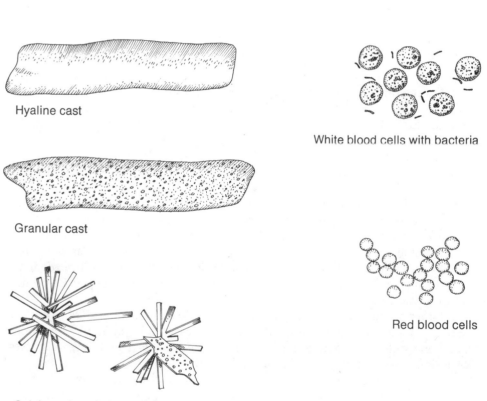

Hyaline cast

White blood cells with bacteria

Granular cast

Red blood cells

Calcium phosphate crystals

Calcium oxalate crystals

Epithelial cells

Figure 13.9 Formed elements in urine.

tract. White blood cell casts indicate inflammatory renal disease, and casts composed of epithelial cells are associated with tubular damage. Oval fat bodies are suggestive of the nephrotic syndrome.

Crystals of calcium oxalate or calcium phosphate may indicate hypercalcemia or calcium-containing renal calculi. Uric acid crystals reflect hyperuricosuria, and uric acid stone formation may indicate that the patient has gout or another disease associated with hyperuricemia. Cystine crystals indicate that the patient probably has cystinuria, since such crystals are almost never found in the urine under normal conditions. Triple-phosphate crystals often indicate the presence of urinary tract infection caused by urea-splitting organisms.

Multiple polymorphonuclear leukocytes, with or without bacteriuria, indicate a urinary tract infection or nearby irritative focus. The presence of eosinophils, when the urinary sediment is appropriately stained, may indicate the presence of interstitial nephritis.

C. BLOOD UREA NITROGEN

Although an elevated BUN is usually considered to be characteristic of renal dysfunction, many nonrenal factors can alter the BUN level. If the patient has severe liver disease, the BUN tends to be lower than normal because the liver is unable to synthesize urea at a normal rate from the amino acid remnants brought to it.

AXIOM

A BUN <5 mg/dl should make one suspicious of hepatic dysfunction.

On the other hand, dehydration, bleeding into the intestinal tract, or tissue necrosis can raise the BUN to 50 mg/100 ml, even when renal function is normal. Since food in the intestinal tract may also elevate the BUN, blood for this test should be drawn while the patient is in a fasting state.

As a general rule, a 10:1 ratio exists between the blood levels of urea nitrogen and creatinine. Mild-moderate plasma volume water deficits will produce low rates of urine flow, increasing blood urea levels with little or no elevation of the serum creatinine. Consequently, the BUN/creatinine ratio in such patients will tend to be greater than 10:1 because of diffusion of urea from the tubules into the blood. A ratio of BUN to creatinine greater than 20:1 strongly suggests that the elevated BUN has a prerenal cause, such as water and salt depletion, or a high rate of protein catabolism. Severe ECF volume deficits, causing a significant reduction in GFR, will tend to raise both the BUN and serum creatinine.

Other circumstances that can lead to a BUN/serum creatinine ratio greater than 20:1 include hypoalbuminemia and decreased left ventricular function. Catabolic states, gastrointestinal bleeding, steroid therapy, and large abscesses with tissue destruction are additional causes of a high ratio.

Situations that are associated with low BUN/creatinine ratios include inanition, liver disease, vigorous dialysis, severe diarrhea, and enzyme abnormalities, such as ornithine transcarbamoylase deficiency.

D. SERUM CREATININE

The serum creatinine level is generally a much better indicator of renal function than the BUN. However, mild elevations of the serum creatinine may be caused by ingestion of large quantities of meat, vigorous exercise, tissue destruction, or moderate-severe ECF volume deficits.

AXIOM

A high-normal serum creatinine in thin, inactive, elderly individuals is often associated with modern-severe reductions in creatinine clearance.

Serum creatinine levels may remain deceptively normal in older, thinner individuals in spite of a significant reduction in creatinine clearance, because of the decrease in muscle mass, meat intake, and exercise. Although a serum creatinine concentration of 1.2 or 1.4 mg/100 ml may be consistent with a normal GFR in a muscular young male, a similar plasma value in an elderly, thin, inactive female may indicate a 50% to 75% reduction in GFR.

The relationship between serum creatinine levels and creatinine clearance is especially poor in septic patients. In severe sepsis, the renal excretion of creatinine may fall from a normal of 1000 to 1500 mg/day to less than 300 to 600 mg/day.

In one of our intensive care unit (ICU) studies, evidence of renal failure by clinical examination and the usual laboratory tests correlated very poorly with creatinine clearance. Of the ICU patients with a good urine output (>1.0 $ml \cdot kg^{-1} \cdot h^{-1}$), normal BUN, and normal serum creatinine, 40% had a creatinine clearance of <40 ml/min, which is evidence of moderate-severe renal dysfunction.

AXIOM

Creatinine clearance may be very low in septic patients with normal serum creatinine levels.

E. RENAL CLEARANCE

The term *clearance* was first used by Van Slyke to denote the volume of plasma that was "cleared" or emptied of urea per minute. Since then, the concept of renal clearance has come into wide use as a quantitative description of the rate at which the kidneys excrete various substances in relation to their concentration in the plasma.

Plasma clearance of a substance may be calculated as UV/P, where U is the concentration of the substance in the urine (usually in mg/dl), V is the volume (ml) of urine excreted per minute, and P is the concentration of the substance in the plasma (usually in mg/dl).

It is important to emphasize that the clearance formula simply produces a number that describes the rate at which the kidney removes a substance from the plasma. Clearance refers to the volume of plasma that will provide the quantity of the substance excreted in the urine in 1 minute. The clearances that are most frequently measured include creatinine, inulin, osmol, and para-amino hippurate (PAH).

1. Creatinine Clearance (Cl_{cr})

The basic requirements for a substance that can be used to measure GFR are (1) that it is present in the blood at a constant level, (2) that it is freely filterable at the glomerulus, and (3) that it is neither secreted nor absorbed by the tubules. Creatinine is the endogenous substance that most closely approximates these requirements; however, some creatinine is also secreted in the urine by the tubules, so that the creatinine in the urine is about 10% to 15% more than that which is filtered. This would make Cl_{cr} 10% to 15% more than the GFR. However, other substances in the blood are also measured as creatinine, which tends to lower the calculated Cl_{cr}. Thus, the two errors tend to partially balance each other.

AXIOM

The creatinine clearance is probably the best single test for following renal function serially.

To evaluate renal function, creatinine clearances, rather than urea clearances, are used, because some of the filtered urea diffuses back through the tubule into the blood stream. At urine flow rates of over 1.0 ml/min, urea clearance will normally be about 75 ml/min, while normal creatinine clearance in young adults is about 125 ml/min.

The usual creatinine clearance test involves collecting the patient's urine for a period of 12 to 24 hours and drawing a sample of the patient's blood midway through the collection period to measure the plasma creatinine levels. If the urine concentration of creatinine (U) is 150 mg/dl, the urine volume (V) is 0.8 ml/min (48 ml/h), and the serum creatinine is 1.0 mg/dl, then the creatinine clearance (Cl_{cr}) can be calculated as

$$Cl_{cr} = \frac{UV}{P}$$

$$= \frac{(150 \text{ mg/dl}) (0.8)}{1.0 \text{ mg/dl}}$$

$$= \frac{120}{1} = 120 \text{ ml/min.}$$

Although creatinine clearance in young healthy adults is about 125 ml/min, values above 80 ml/min are generally considered satisfactory. To compare individuals of various sizes, clearance values are often contrasted with a normal value for an individual with a body surface of 1.73 m². Nomograms are available for determining surface area from height and weight. Women tend to have a GFR about 10% to 15% lower than men, even after a correction is made for any difference in surface area.

The following formula was developed by Cockcroft and Gault to estimate creatinine clearance in normal men receiving renal toxic drugs:

$$Cl_{cr} = \frac{(140 - \text{age}) \times \text{lean body weight in kg}}{72 \times \text{serum creatinine}}.$$

If the patient is female, the result is multiplied by 0.85.

We have found that this technique for estimating Cl_{cr} from serum creatinine levels can be extremely inaccurate, especially in septic patients who may have a severely reduced creatinine excretion. Similar findings were recently reported by Martin and colleagues.

AXIOM

In renal disease, the creatinine clearance calculated from urine and plasma creatinine levels and urine flow tends to be higher than results from other more accurate tests of glomerular filtration rate.

In humans, creatinine levels in the urine are increased by tubular secretion, particularly if GFR is low. In addition, measurement of serum creatinine can be falsely elevated by various endogenous chromogens. These problems can contribute to significant errors in the estimation of GFR. As serum creatinine rises above 3.0 mg/dl, the Cl_{cr} may overestimate GFR by 30% or more.

2. Inulin Clearance

Since inulin is excreted solely by filtration through the glomeruli and is neither absorbed nor secreted, its clearance is a more accurate indicator of glomerular filtration rate than Cl_{cr}. During the test, inulin must be infused intravenously at a rate that will keep plasma levels constant. Even though it is the test against which all other methods are compared, it is not usually practical for clinical purposes.

The normal value for GFR, assessed by inulin clearance, is influenced by sex, age, and body size. For men up to 30 years of age, the normal value is 130 ± 18 ml·min^{-1}·1.73 m^{-2} (mean $\pm$ SD). Thereafter, inulin clearance declines with advancing age by approximately 10 ml/m per decade. Consequently, the normal inulin clearance for an 80-year-old man is approximately 80 ml·min^{-1}·1.73 m^{-2}. The precise reason for the decline in GFR is unknown; however, aging is also accompanied by a decline in renal plasma flow and development of glomerular sclerosis and arteriolar medial sclerosis.

3. Osmolar and Free-Water Clearance

Free-water clearance (Cl_{H_2O}) is defined as the difference between the rate of urine flow (V) (in ml/min) and the osmolar clearance (Cl_{osm}):

$$Cl_{H_2O} = V - Cl_{osm}.$$

The osmolar clearance is a standard clearance, except that it refers to the total number of osmotically active solute particles instead of a single substance; thus Cl_{osm} represents the volume of plasma completely cleared of all osmotically active solute particles per unit time and is calculated as $U_{osm}·V/P_{osm}$. It is important to note that Cl_{osm} also represents the hypothetical rate of urine flow that would be measured if urine were isotonic to plasma.

Cl_{osm} is relatively independent of the urine tonicity. This is because an average of 650 mOsm of electrolytes and other solutes must be excreted per day by a normal man to eliminate waste products, such as creatinine and urea, and to maintain a normal electrolyte balance; thus the average $U_{osm}·V$ equals 650 mOsm/day or 0.45 mOsm/min. If serum osmolality is 300 mOsm/liter, C_{osm} will average about 1.5 ml/min.

Free-water clearance (Cl_{H_2O}) is calculated by the following formula:

$$Cl_{H_2O} = V - Cl_{osm}.$$

If the urine output is 1.0 ml/min, the equation above reads as follows:

$$Cl_{H_2O} = 1.0 - 1.5 = -0.5 \text{ ml/min}.$$

Since urine usually has a higher osmolality than plasma, the free-water clearance will be negative. A positive free-water clearance is abnormal under most circumstances and especially if the patient is dehydrated.

4. Para-amino Hippurate Clearance

PAH, if infused at a rate that will produce plasma levels of about 2 mg/100 ml, will be almost completely removed in a single passage through the kidney. It is filtered and secreted by the tubules so completely during one passage that calculation of its clearance generally reflects the RPF quite well. However, a steady state is necessary, and its determination is useful only in clinical units specially set up to handle the technical problems of performing such measurements. Reductions in PAH clearance may be caused by decreases in renal plasma flow as well as tubular secretory function.

RPF studies with hippuran can be particularly deceptive in patients with severe trauma or sepsis. It is usually assumed that at least 85% to 90% of the renal plasma flow will go to glomeruli and tubules. However, Lucas and colleagues, using renal vein catheterization studies in some septic and trauma patients, showed that more than 50% of the RPF may bypass the glomeruli and tubules. Thus hippuran studies may provide data on "effective" RPF rather than total RPF.

Renal blood flow can also be estimated by various radiologic methods, including angiography and scans of the kidney using radioisotopes. However, these are seldom used on ICU patients without trauma or suspected renal artery stenosis.

F. FILTRATION FRACTION (GFR/RPF)

In the normal kidney, the relationship between the glomerular filtration rate (GFR) and renal plasma flow (RPF) is relatively constant; the ratio of the two (the filtration fraction) is maintained at about 0.2. However, if the RPF decreases by more than 30%, the GFR does not fall as much, because of compensatory dilatation of the afferent arterioles and constriction of the efferent arterioles.

AXIOM
Major decreases in RPF tend to increase the filtration fraction.

If the glomerular membrane becomes sclerotic or damaged, the filtration fraction may fall to 0.10 to 0.15, or less. In contrast, in hypertensive individuals with a reduced RPF, the filtration fraction may rise to 0.3 or higher, because of the increased hydrostatic pressure in the glomeruli.

The level of filtration fraction affects the oncotic pressure of the peritubular blood to some extent. If the filtration fraction is high, thereby removing a higher percentage of plasma water than normal, the oncotic pressure of peritubular blood will be high. This will produce a more favorable gradient for reabsorption of salt and water from the proximal tubule. The converse is also true.

AXIOM
An increased filtration fraction tends to increase salt and water resorption by the kidneys.

G. TUBULAR MAXIMUMS (T_m)

The secretory capacity of the tubules, as reflected by the T_m, indicates their integrity and functional capacity. For example, the T_m for PAH (T_mPAH) is normally about 85 mg/min. In malignant hypertension, it may be reduced by half; in severe nephritis, it may be reduced to 10 mg/min or less.

PAH is excreted partly by glomerular filtration and partly by tubular secretion. If a large quantity of PAH is infused, the amount delivered to the kidneys will exceed the ability of the tubules to secrete it (i.e., it will exceed the T_m). If inulin is given at the same time as the PAH, the maximum rate of tubular excretion can be calculated by subtracting the inulin GFR from the PAH clearance. The difference represents the amount of PAH that the tubules can secrete. When this value is constant, the T_m has been determined.

1. Calculation of Fractional Excretion

Tests of tubular function include determinations of the fractional rates of excretion of a solute, the concentration of the solute in the urine, and the urinary osmolality. The term fractional excretion is defined as the ratio of the amount of a substance filtered at the glomerulus that is excreted in the urine. The fractional excretion rate can be calculated as the clearance of a substance divided by the clearance of a glomerular filtration marker, such as creatinine. Thus the fractional excretion (FE) of a solute(s) can be determined from the following equation:

$$FE_s(\%) = \frac{Cl_s}{Cl_{cr}} \times 100\%$$

$$= \frac{(U_s \times V) - P_s}{(U_{cr} \times V) - P_{cr}} \times 100\%$$

$$= \frac{U_2/P_s}{U_{cr}/P_{cr}} \times 100\%.$$

U_s and P_s are the urine and ultrafiltrable plasma concentrations of the solute; U_{cr} and P_{cr} are the urine and plasma concentrations of the glomerular filtration marker, creatinine (cr); and V is the urine flow rate.

2. Urate

In normal human beings, the FE or urate is approximately 7% to 10% of the filtered load. In patients with tubular defects in the absorption of urate or in individuals receiving a drug that inhibits the absorption of urate, the FE of urate rises. Since urate and phosphate are handled predominantly in the proximal convoluted tubule, calculation of the FE of these two substances can be used to reflect transport activity in that segment of the nephron.

3. Sodium

AXIOM

FE_{Na} is often considered the best test to differentiate between prerenal oliguria and acute tubule necrosis.

In normal individuals, the FE of sodium is less than 1%. The FE of sodium increases when sodium is ingested, diuretics are administered, or renal tubular disease is present. In a patient with signs of fluid overload, a low FE rate of sodium is inappropriate. In a patient with normal hydration or in a patient who is volume depleted, a FE of sodium greater than 3% is inappropriate and may indicate renal tubular disease or the administration of diuretics.

With prerenal oliguria, the urine sodium tends to be low (<10 to 20 mEq/liter), the serum sodium is relatively normal (140 mEq/liter), the urine creatinine tends to be high (80 to 120 mg/dl), and plasma creatinine tends to be normal (1.0 to 1.3 mg/dl). Therefore,

$$FE_{Na} = \frac{U_{Na}/P_{Na}}{U_{cr}/P_{cr}} \times 100\%$$

$$= \frac{15/140}{100/1.2} \times 100\%$$

$$= \frac{0.107}{83.3} \times 100\%$$

$$= 0.00128 \times 100\% = 0.128\%.$$

With renal failure, the urine sodium is about 40 to 80 mEq/liter, the serum sodium tends to be low (?130 mEq/liter), the serum creatinine tends to be low (?40 to 60 mg/dl), and the plasma creatinine tends to be slightly elevated (?2.0 mg/dl). Therefore,

$$FE_{Na} = \frac{60/130}{50/2.0} \times 100\%$$

$$= \frac{0.462}{25} \times 100\%$$

$$= 1.85\%.$$

4. Renal Failure Index

The renal failure index (RFI) is similar to the FE_{Na}, but does not use urine creatinine in the equation. Thus,

$$RFI = \frac{U_{Na}}{U_{cr}/P_{cr}}.$$

For prerenal oliguria:

$$RFI = \frac{15}{100/1.2} = \frac{15}{83.3}$$

$$= 0.18.$$

For renal failure:

$$RFI = \frac{60}{50/2.0} = \frac{60}{25}$$

$$= 2.4.$$

As with FE_{Na}, a RFI <1 implies prerenal oliguria, and a RFI >2 or 3 implies renal failure.

5. Synthesis of Erythropoietin

In response to renal hypoxia, the kidneys synthesize erythropoietin, a glycoprotein hormone that regulates the production of red blood cells in the bone marrow. It is thought that the elevated hematocrit, often seen in patients who live at high altitudes or have chronic lung disease, can be attributed, at least in part, to increased production of erythropoietin. Furthermore, many diseases of the kidneys are associated with an erythropoietin deficiency and anemia.

The exact site of erythropoietin synthesis in the kidney is not yet established. In fact, some investigators believe that the kidneys do not synthesize erythropoietin, but produce an enzyme that acts on a plasma globulin to form erythropoietin.

AXIOM

With normochromic anemia of unknown etiology, one should rule out renal failure.

VII. CHANGES IN THE ELDERLY

A. GLOMERULAR CHANGES

Renal mass declines progressively with age. Studies have shown that the normal kidney loses about 20% of its mass between the ages of 40 and 80 years. This loss is much greater in the cortex than in the medulla, with vascular changes accompanying the loss of tissue.

With the progressive loss of renal tissue, renal plasma flow decreases from 600 ml/min at age 40 to 300 ml/min at age 85. There is a corresponding decrease in the glomerular filtration rate, which falls from 120 ml/min at age 40 to about 50 to 70 ml/min at age 85.

Creatinine clearance, which closely parallels glomerular filtration rate, also decreases with age. This decrease begins in the fourth decade and continues in a more or less linear fashion at the rate of 8 ml·min^{-1}·1.73 m^{-2} of body surface area per decade.

B. TUBULAR CHANGES

Anatomic and physiologic changes in the renal tubular system also occur with age. First, the renal tubular mass is reduced. Studies on the renal secretion of iodopyracet (Diodrast), an indicator of total tubular mass, show that the decrease in tubular mass is comparable in magnitude to the changes that occur in renal blood flow and glomerular filtration rate.

TABLE OF NORMAL VALUES

Urine volume: 0.6 to 1.5 liters/d
BUN: 10 to 20 mg/100 ml
Serum creatinine: 0.4 to 1.2 mg/100 ml
Creatinine clearance: 80 to 125 ml/min
Osmolarity:
  serum: 275 to 295 mOsm/liter
  urine (with fluid restriction): 600 to 1400 mOsm/liter
Urinalysis:
  pH: 4 to 7
  albumin: <100 to 150 mg/d
  glucose: $<0.25\%$
  formed elements:
    RBC: 0 to 2/HPF
    WBC: 2 to 3/HPF
    no bacteria
    occasional hyaline casts/HPF
Electrolytes
  sodium: 40 to 80 mEq/liter

potassium: 40 to 80 mEq/liter
chloride: 80 to 120 mEq/liter
RPF (PAH clearance): 625 ml/min
GFR: 125 ml/min
Filtration fraction: (GFR/RPF) 0.2

SUMMARY POINTS

1. Each kidney contains about 1.0 to 1.5 million nephrons, and up to 75% can be destroyed without serious ill effects to the patient.
2. The kidneys consist of an outer cortex (containing the glomeruli and proximal and distal convoluted tubules) and an inner medulla (containing the loops of Henle and the collecting ducts and tubules).
3. There are two types of nephrons. Outer cortical nephrons make up 85% of the total and lie almost completely within the cortex. The remaining 15% are juxtamedullary (salt-saving nephrons), with long loops of Henle extending into the medulla.
4. The nephron consists of a glomerulus, proximal convoluted tubule, loop of Henle, distal convoluted tubule, and collecting tubule and ducts.
5. The juxtaglomerular apparatus is located at the junction of the distal convoluted tubule and the afferent and efferent arterioles. It consists of a macula densa (special cells of the distal tubule), extraglomerular mesangial cells, and granular cells containing renin.
6. The juxtaglomerular apparatus can be stimulated by the sympathetic nervous system, decreased renal perfusion, hyperkalemia, or decreased sodium in the distal tubule to release renin. Renin converts angiotensin into angiotensin I, which is then converted to angiotensin II by ACE. Angiotensin II is a powerful vasoconstrictor that increases the release of aldosterone from the adrenal cortex.
7. Renal *blood* flow averages 1000 to 1200 ml/min. This results in an average renal *plasma* flow (RPF) of 625 ml/min and an average glomerular filtration rate (GFR) of 125 ml/min. The ratio of GFR/RPF is called the filtration fraction, and it averages 0.2.
8. When cardiac output or blood pressure falls, renal vascular resistance increases disproportionately, causing an even greater decrease in renal blood flow.
9. Stimulation of the sympathetic nervous system results in renal arterial and arteriolar constriction, thereby decreasing RPF. Efferent arteriolar vasoconstriction, however, generally prevents a corresponding decrease in GFR.
10. Renal oxygen consumption is proportional to renal blood flow and the amount of sodium absorbed in the tubule.
11. Decreased effective intravascular volume can override the effect of increased osmolarity on ADH secretion.
12. Glucose, amino acids, phosphate, and sulfate are examples of threshold substances. They are entirely reabsorbed by the tubules, unless they are present in greater than normal amounts in the plasma.
13. If urinary tract obstruction occurs, pressure in Bowman's capsule may increase enough to interfere with glomerular filtration.
14. If renal perfusion is reduced, tubular absorption of sodium increases, and the concentration of sodium in the urine may fall to less than 10 to 20 mEq/liter.
15. Over 99% of the filtered sodium is removed by the tubules and returned to the blood.
16. *Third factor* is the term applied to mechanisms, other than changes in GFR and aldosterone concentration, that alter renal sodium excretion.
17. Any situation, such as hypokalemia or impaired perfusion, that results in intracellular acidosis causes an increase in the secretion of hydrogen ions

into the tubular lumen, thereby increasing sodium and bicarbonate re-absorption.

18. The excretion of potassium, unlike sodium, is obligatory and will increase with the amount of urine, until or unless the patient has been hypokalemic for several days.

19. The excretion of an acid urine in spite of an alkalosis in the blood is referred to as paradoxical aciduria, and is usually caused by hypokalemia.

20. Decreased insulin requirements in a diabetic may be an indication of increasing renal dysfunction.

21. The osmolality in the glomerular filtrate at the end of the proximal tubule is about 280 to 300 mOsm/kg. At the end of the loop of Henle, because of active excretion of sodium, osmolality is reduced to about 140 to 200 mOsm/kg.

22. Urine is concentrated in the distal nephron and collecting tubules and ducts by the medullary osmotic gradient and ADH.

23. Increased ADH activity decreases urine volume and increases urine solute concentration.

24. Atrial natriuretic factor(ANF) is released by the atria when they are distended, as in heart failure, and causes a salt and water diuresis.

25. NSAIDs should be avoided in patients with cardiac, liver, or renal disease.

26. The specific gravity is generally a relatively inaccurate method of measuring urinary renal concentrating and tubular function.

27. About 70 mEq of nonvolatile acid is excreted by the kidneys daily. This includes 1 mEq of free acid, 20 to 30 mEq with buffers such as NaH_2PO_4, and 40 to 50 mEq with ammonium ion.

28. Urine osmolarity is an excellent method for measuring concentrating and tubular function, especially in dehydrated individuals.

29. In the oliguric patient, a urine plasma osmolarity ratio of less than 1.1 generally indicates the presence of vasomotor nephropathy, whereas a ratio exceeding 1.2 suggests that the oliguria is due to prerenal causes.

30. The finding of a high urine osmolality suggests that nephron function is relatively intact.

31. If the urine is positive for occult blood, but there are no red blood cells in the urine, one should suspect myoglobinuria.

32. Excretion of more than 150 mg of protein per day usually implies either a significant abnormality in the glomeruli or a urinary tract infection.

33. BUN often reflects renal function rather poorly. Many nonrenal factors, such as gastrointestinal bleeding or dehydration, can raise the BUN, whereas cirrhosis and other liver diseases may cause the BUN to fall.

34. A BUN <5 mg/dl should make one suspicious of hepatic dysfunction.

35. Creatinine clearance may be very low in patients with normal serum creatinine levels if they have decreased creatinine excretion because of sepsis.

36. A ratio of BUN to creatinine greater than 20:1 suggests that the cause of the elevated BUN may be prerenal, such as water and salt depletion, or a high rate of protein catabolism.

37. The creatinine clearance is probably the best single test for following renal function serially.

38. The fractional excretion of sodium is often considered the best test to differentiate between prerenal oliguria and acute tubular necrosis.

39. With normochromic anemia of unknown etiology, one should rule out renal failure.

BIBLIOGRAPHY

1. Arendshorst, WJ and Gottschalk, CW: Glomerular ultrafiltration dynamics: Historical perspective. Am J Physiol 248:F163, 1985.
2. Barger, AC and Hear, JA: The renal circulation. N Engl J Med 284:482, 1971.

3. Berliner, RW and Bennett, CM: Concentration of urine in the mammalian kidney. Am J Med 42:777, 1967.

4. Berry, CA: Heterogeneity of tubular transport process in the nephron. Annu Rev Physiol 44:181, 1982.

5. Brech, WJ, et al: The influence of renin on the intrarenal distribution of blood flow and autoregulation. Nephron 12:44, 1973.

6. Brenner, BM, et al: Quantitative importance of changes in postglomerular colloid osmotic pressure in mediating glomerular tubular balance in the rat. J Clin Invest 52:190, 1973.

7. Burg, M and Good, D: Sodium chloride coupled transport in mammalian nephrons. Annu Rev Physiol 465:533, 1983.

8. Clive, DM and Stoff, JS: Renal syndromes associated with nonsteroidal anti-inflammatory drugs. N Engl J Med 310:563, 1984.

9. Cockcroft, DW and Gault, PH: Prediction of creatinine clearance from serum creatinine. Nephron 16:31, 1976.

10. Cogan, MG: Atrial natriuretic peptide. Kidney Int 37:1148, 1990.

11. Fretler, SP, et al: The physiologic approach to renal tubular acidosis. J Urol 102:665, 1969.

12. Evans, DW: Renal function in the elderly. Am Fam Pract 38:147, 1988.

13. Fisher, DA, Salido, EC, and Barajas, L: Epidermal growth factor and the kidney. Annu Rev Physiol 51:67, 1989.

14. Goldstein, MH, Lenz, PR, and Levitt, MF: Effect of urine flow rate on urea reabsorption in man: Urea as a "tubular marker." J Appl Physiol 26:594, 1969.

15. Ives, HE and Rector, FC, Jr: Proton transport and cell function. J Clin Invest 73:285, 1984.

16. Jamison, RL: Intrarenal heterogeneity: The case for two functionally dissimilar populations of nephrons in the mammalian kidney. Am J Med 54:281, 1973.

17. Jamison, RL and Hall, DA: Collecting duct function and sodium balance. Annu Rev Physiol 33:241, 1982.

18. Kanwar, YS: Biophysiology of glomerular filtration and proteinuria. Lab Invest 51:7, 1984.

19. Kassirer, JP: Clinical evaluation of kidney function—glomerular function. Current concepts. N Engl J Med 285:385, 1971.

20. Kassirer, JP: Clinical evaluation of kidney function—tubular function. Current concepts. N Engl J Med 285:499, 1971.

21. Kriz, W and Lever, AF: Renal countercurrent mechanisms: Structure and function. Am Heart J 78:101, 1969.

22. Levey, AS, Perrone, RD, and Madias, NE: Serum creatinine and renal function. Annu Rev Med 39:465, 1988.

22a. Lucas, CE, et al: Altered renal hemostasis with acute sepsis: Clinical significance. Arch Surg 106:444, 1973.

22b. Lucas, CE: The renal response to acute injury and sepsis. Surg Clin N Am 56:621, 1976.

23. Manitius, A, et al: On the mechanism of impairment of renal concentrating ability in potassium deficiency. J Clin Invest 39:684, 1960.

24. Martin, C, et al: Assessment of creatinine clearance in intensive care patients. Crit Care Med 18:1224, 1990.

25. Pelkington, LA, et al: Intrarenal distribution of blood flow. Am J Physiol 208:1107, 1965.

26. Raine, AEG, Firth, JG, and Ledingham, JGG: Renal actions of atrial natriuretic factor. Clin Sci 76:1, 1989.

27. Relman, AS and Schwartz, WB: The nephropathy of potassium depletion: A clinical and pathological entity. N Engl J Med 225:195, 1956.

28. Smith, HW: Principles of Renal Physiology. Oxford University Press, New York, 1956.

28a. Van Slyky, DD, et al: The clearance extraction percentage and estimated filtration of sodium ferrocyanide in the mammalian kidney: Comparison with insulin, creatinine and urea. Am J Physiol. 113:611, 1935.

29. Verney, EB: Absorption and excretion of water. The antidiuretic hormone. Lancet 2:739, 1946.

30. Wolf, AV and Pillay, VKG: Renal concentration tests: Osmotic pressure, specific gravity, refraction and electrical conductivity compared. Am J Med 46:837, 1969.

CHAPTER 14

Oliguria and Acute Renal Failure

I. CONCERNS

AXIOM

An ounce of renal failure prevention is worth several pounds of cure.

Preservation of renal function is extremely important. The usual renal function tests may not be significantly abnormal until 75% of the functioning nephrons are lost. If more than 50% of renal function is lost, fluid balance is less well maintained, white blood cell (WBC) and platelet function become impaired, and red blood cell (RBC) production decreases. The incidence of pneumonia and gastrointestinal bleeding increase. The overall mortality rate of acute oliguric renal failure is at least 50%, but in patients with severe trauma or sepsis, it may be 90% or greater, especially if any other organ failure is present.

The simplest overall screening tests for acute renal failure in intensive care unit (ICU) patients include (1) hourly urine output (should be at least 0.5 $ml \cdot kg^{-1} \cdot h^{-1}$), (2) careful measurement of all fluid intake and output, and (3) serum creatinine levels at least every other day.

One should watch renal function especially closely if the patient (1) has had trauma with extensive muscle damage or multiple transfusions, (2) is to undergo a procedure that could cause hypotension, or (3) is to receive any potentially nephrotoxic drug. Myoglobinuria or hemoglobinuria in oliguric patients is a particularly severe threat to renal function. Hypotension lasting only 10 minutes can have a severe impact on splanchnic blood flow. Medications, such as aminoglycosides, are frequently used for many days; during that time, the loss of kidney function may be subtle, but progressive and profound.

Renal function loss may occur without oliguria and may present as a polyuric state in its early stages, especially after aminoglycoside therapy. Other clues to loss of renal function include development of refractoriness to previously effective doses of diuretics, or urinary sodium (Na^+) concentrations between 40 and 80 mEq/liter in a patient with renal hypoperfusion or oliguria. Grossly abnormal-appearing urine from pigments, such as bile, myoglobin, and hemoglobin, can warn of a state predisposing to the loss of renal function. Urine that is particularly frothy is often indicative of heavy proteinuria.

AXIOM

At least half of all in-hospital cases of acute renal failure can be prevented or decreased in severity by careful attention to renal perfusion and potentially nephrotoxic agents.

II. DEFINITIONS

Renal failure may be defined as the inability of the kidneys to excrete the by-products of cell metabolism in adequate quantities. Consequently, urea and other nitrogenous substances accumulate in the blood; oliguria may or may not be present. Other manifestations of renal failure include disturbances of acid-base and electrolyte and water balance.

A. ABNORMALITIES IN URINE VOLUME

1. Oliguria

Oliguria, which is often the first clinical sign of acute impairment of renal function, may be loosely defined as a urine output less than that required to excrete the products of metabolism. A urine volume of less than 400 ml/day in an average-size adult male is usually considered to be oliguria. Oliguria might also be more precisely defined as a urine output of less than $0.25 \text{ ml} \cdot \text{kg}^{-1} \cdot \text{h}^{-1}$ or $240 \text{ ml} \cdot \text{m}^{-2} \cdot \text{d}^{-1}$. The advantage of defining oliguria in terms of the hourly urine volume is the relatively quick diagnosis of oliguria. A urine output less than 25 to 30 ml/h in an adult should be investigated and corrected promptly.

AXIOM

Oliguria lasting more than 2 to 3 hours in a critically ill patient may be irreversible.

In critically ill or injured ICU patients, the definition of oliguria may have to be changed, because the minimal urine output required to excrete the by-products of metabolism and catabolism in such patients may be more than 1.5 to 2.0 times greater than normal. The total osmolal load for an adult 70-kg man averages about 600 to 800 mOsm per day or about $10 \text{ mOsm} \cdot \text{kg}^{-1} \cdot \text{d}^{-1}$. This is equivalent to an osmolar excretion rate of about $0.4 \text{ mOsm} \cdot \text{kg}^{-1} \cdot \text{h}^{-1}$. If the patient can concentrate the urine to $1200 \text{ mOsm/kg } H_2O$, it would take a urine rate of $0.33 \text{ ml} \cdot \text{kg}^{-1} \cdot \text{h}^{-1}$ to excrete the osmolal load.

In critically ill or injured patients, the osmolal load on the kidney may be increased to 1000 to 1400 mOsm or about 40 to 60 mOsm/h. Since maximal urinary concentration in critically ill patients is only about 600 mOsm, each milliliter of urine is capable of excreting about 0.6 mOsm. Consequently, in the critically ill, a urine output of at least $1.0 \text{ ml} \cdot \text{kg}^{-1} \cdot \text{h}^{-1}$ is probably needed, and if the patient is hypercatabolic, the minimal urine output may be $1.5 \text{ ml} \cdot \text{kg}^{-1} \cdot \text{h}^{-1}$.

AXIOM

Although a low urine output in a critically ill patient is often a harbinger of impending renal failure, the presence of a "normal" urine output is no guarantee that renal function is normal.

In healthy individuals, the kidney normally reabsorbs 98% to 99% of the glomerular filtrate. Thus there is a fractional excretion of only 1% to 2% of the glomerular filtrate. If the fractional excretion rises to 10%, a glomerular filtration rate (GFR) of only 10 ml/min results in an apparently "normal" urine output of 1.0 ml/min or 60 ml/h. Since the excretion of catabolic products depends primarily on GFR, most of the chemical and clinical abnormalities of oliguric renal failure will occur in patients with a greatly reduced GFR, no matter how high the urine output is.

Initially, especially in shock or trauma, oliguria may represent an appropriate defense mechanism to conserve water and salt. However, if the oliguria is marked or persistent, it greatly increases the risk of developing acute renal failure. A kidney producing a concentrated urine at low flow rates is much more vulnerable to damage by nephrotoxins or pigments than a kidney with a high urine flow.

Oliguria should be differentiated from anuria, which is generally defined as urinary output of less than 2 ml/h or 50 ml/day. Complete anuria is unusual except in patients with obstruction of the lower urinary tract. Even with very severe acute renal failure, there is usually at least 2 to 3 ml of urine per hour.

B. ACUTE VASOMOTOR NEPHROPATHY

1. Terminology

Acute renal failure developing in critically ill or injured patients was often called *acute tubular necrosis* in the past. Physicians at that time felt that tubular damage, with consequent tubular obstruction and backdiffusion of tubular fluid, was the primary cause of the acute renal failure and oliguria. This concept was based on observation of tubular casts and degenerative changes at autopsy. However, it is now clear that tubular necrosis does not necessarily occur in acute renal failure. Micropuncture studies have shown that neither tubular obstruction nor passive backdiffusion of glomerular filtrate accounts for the oliguria. It has been suggested that a more appropriate term is *acute vasomotor nephropathy*, because the common underlying abnormality in both ischemic and toxic renal damage appears to be related to a marked decrease in GFR and maldistribution of blood flow within the kidney.

This severe afferent arteriolar constriction can occur as a result of tubular damage initiated by ischemia or tubular toxins through a tubuloglomerular feedback mechanism. Since the pathophysiology of acute renal failure is still unresolved, the term *acute intrinsic renal failure* is also appropriate.

2. Pathophysiology

a. Reduced Glomerular Filtration Rate

Measurements of GFR in oliguric patients by classic clearance techniques are unreliable. However, GFR and renal blood flow (RBF) in nonoliguric patients with acute vasomotor nephropathy are consistently depressed to extremely low levels, even if urine output is normal or increased. However, the histologic changes seen in biopsy material or at autopsy do not appear sufficiently severe to explain the reductions in GFR or RBF. Most observers now feel that internal alterations in the RBF are due to functional, rather than anatomic, pathological changes.

A marked increase in tone of some of the afferent arterioles, for example, may cause such a severe reduction in glomerular capillary pressure that filtration will cease in the involved nephrons. If many or most of the nephrons are affected, the total GFR can be reduced and renal vascular resistance will be increased. As a result, RBF will decline. Persistence of these abnormalities beyond a few hours is not easily explained because vasospasm in most vascular systems does not usually persist for such prolonged periods. Experiments now suggest that vascular endothelial swelling may contribute to these prolonged changes.

b. Altered Blood-Flow Distribution

In chronic renal disease, renal blood flow may be reduced to less than 10% of normal, yet renal function remains adequate to sustain life. In a patient with acute vasomotor nephropathy, a similar reduction in RBF may be lethal. The main difference between these two conditions appears to be the distribution of blood flow. In chronic renal failure the blood flow perfuses a portion of the outer cortex at a rate that provides enough glomerular filtration to maintain a stable state. In acute renal failure, most of the blood flow goes to the inner cortical and medullary areas, so that relatively few glomeruli are perfused. Thus, the total renal blood flow may be the same, but the GFR and functional effects are quite different.

The mechanisms by which the changes in blood flow distribution in acute vasomotor nephropathy are produced are still conjectural. Some of the factors that may play a role include local feedback loops, renin-angiotensin-aldosterone (RAA), prostaglandins, vasodilating substances, oliguria, increased pigments in the blood, and various drugs.

(1) Local Feedback Loops

Changes in blood flow distribution may be mediated by local feedback loops involving tubular flow rates, the juxtaglomerular apparatus, and local renin release. This concept implies individual nephron control of SNGFR as determined by tubular fluid transport rates.

Under normal circumstances, according to this theory, high rates of flow in the distal tubule, with increased salt flux across the macula densa, cause the local release of renin and the generation of angiotensin. This constricts the afferent arteriole and reduces the SNGFR and the tubular fluid flow. The reverse is true under conditions of low rates of sodium delivery to the distal tubule. It is possible that impaired tubular-glomerular feedback may occur in vasomotor nephropathy, causing even further reductions in GFR.

(2) Renin

Renin is produced at the juxtaglomerular apparatus, a convenient location for causing afferent vasoconstriction. This, in turn, could lead to virtual cessation of filtration in the cortical nephrons. Such an interpretation is supported by the facts that peripheral plasma renin levels are usually increased during the early stages of acute renal failure and that patients with pre-existing high plasma renin levels are more susceptible to vasomotor nephropathy.

Infusion of angiotensin II into rabbits can produce vasomotor nephropathy; however, attempts to prevent the vasomotor nephropathy by immunization against renin or angiotension II have produced conflicting results. These immunization studies do not, however, invalidate the possibility that local release of renin at the juxtaglomerular apparatus acts directly on its own glomerulus. This possibility is supported by the observation that long-term salt loading, which depletes intrarenal renin, protects animals against vasomotor nephropathy. Comparable protection is not afforded by acute volume expansion, which depresses peripheral but not renal parenchymal renin levels.

(3) Prostaglandin

The severe vasoconstriction seen in acute renal failure may be offset by local release of prostaglandin E, which acts as a vasodilator. Prostaglandin release may explain some of the variable effects of angiotensin in the production of acute vasomotor nephropathy (AVN) in intact experimental animals. A balance between renin and vasodilating prostaglandins in the renal parenchyma may control the distribution of RBF. The intrarenal roles of renin and prostaglandin are still being studied.

c. Tubular Changes

In most cases of acute renal failure, the urine will be low in sodium and moderately concentrated. If RBF and/or redistribution of blood progresses to a point where the GFR becomes very low, the filtered load of solute per nephron becomes so great that the tubules can no longer reabsorb much of the salt and water. The tubular fluid is then relatively high in sodium, and physiologic changes characteristic of nonoliguric renal failure can develop. Although histologic evidence of tubular damage is seen, the severity of the azotemia often does not correlate with the degree of histologic change.

3. Platelet-Activating Factor

The role of platelet-activating factor (PAF) in the etiology of renal failure and the possible role of PAF antagonists was recently reviewed by Pirotzky and colleagues. PAF is a phospholipid mediator produced by a variety of inflammatory cells, including neutrophils, monocytes, eosinophils, macrophages, and platelets, as well as endothelial cells. PAF infusions can cause severe cardiovascular collapse associated with marked extraction of fluid from capillaries into the interstitial fluid space. PAF may also cause a drop in cardiac output by constricting coronary arteries. These infusions can reduce GFR, RBF, urine output, and sodium extraction. Even with very low dose infusions, which do not lower GFR, there was increased Na^+, Ca^{++}, and Mg^{++} reabsorption by the tubules.

Additional evidence of the role of PAF in the genesis of renal failure has come from several experiments in which PAF antagonists prevented or reduced the severity of several types of experimental acute renal failure.

III. ETIOLOGY OF OLIGURIA AND ACUTE RENAL FAILURE

A number of factors that were thought to be important in the pathogenesis of acute vasomotor nephropathy include reduced RBF, a marked decline in GFR, altered blood flow distribution in the kidneys, oliguria, pigments in the blood, and various drugs. In at least 50% of cases, ischemic damage to renal parenchyma is apparent. In another 45%, sepsis or various drugs appear to be important factors. In the remaining 5%, other causes, such as urinary tract obstruction, vasculitis, or nontoxic interstitial nephritis, are present.

The various causes of acute renal failure or oliguria are often classified as prerenal, renal, and postrenal.

A. PRERENAL OLIGURIA

Oliguria due to prerenal conditions is, in most instances, caused by inadequate renal perfusion secondary to a reduction in plasma volume, cardiac output, or blood pressure. Occasionally, however, prerenal failure or oliguria may be caused by excessive vasoconstriction, increased intra-abdominal pressure, or plasma electrolyte or protein abnormalities.

The clinical presentation of prerenal failure is usually oliguria. This is an extremely important sign that must not be overlooked in critically ill or injured patients. The urine output in such individuals should be closely monitored, and whenever oliguria or a rising BUN develops, an immediate search for the cause should be undertaken.

1. Hypovolemia

Hypovolemia, even when mild, can greatly reduce both renal perfusion and urine output. However, fluid deficits in critically ill or injured patients are often greatly underestimated, particularly if sepsis is present. The capillary leak and third-space fluid losses associated with sepsis may greatly increase fluid needs, but peripheral edema, weight gain, and increased central venous pressure (CVP) are also often present, making it appear as if the patient were overloaded with fluid.

A slight fall in arterial blood pressure has numerous cardiovascular and hormonal effects. It stimulates aortic arch and carotid-sinus baroreceptors to increase sympathetic nervous system activity and antidiuretic hormone (ADH) release through vagal and sympathetic nerve pathways. It also increases plasma renin and aldosterone concentrations through intrarenal changes.

A loss of 10% to 15% of the blood volume will generally not affect the systolic arterial pressure, but it may lower atrial pressures by 3 to 6 cm H_2O. This decreases vagal afferent impulses detected by subendocardial stretch receptors present in both atria. The reduction in vagal impulses allows the hypothalamic centers to release ADH from the posterior pituitary, which, in turn, influences the kidney to retain water. This very sensitive regulatory mechanism rapidly alters renal function to maintain maximal urinary concentration and conserve plasma volume.

2. Cardiac Failure

During cardiac failure, the cardiac output is often less than that necessary to support the metabolic requirements of the patient. Vasoconstriction proportional to the severity of the heart failure tends to occur in the splanchnic and renal vascular beds. Initially, intrarenal (autoregulatory) adjustments of afferent and efferent arteriolar tone will sustain the glomerular filtration rate (GFR). However, with severe reductions in renal blood flow (RBF), the intrarenal adjustments are no longer adequate, and the GFR declines, urine flow rates are reduced, and urinary sodium concentrations fall below 10 to 20 mEq/liter.

A relatively normal GFR in the face of a reduced RBF (i.e., a higher filtration fraction) can be an important cause of the salt and water retention seen in cardiac failure. Researchers have proposed that the higher filtration fraction increases peritubular oncotic pressure, which in turn increases proximal tubular reabsorption of sodium.

3. Hypotension

Although GFR is usually not severely reduced unless the mean arterial pressure falls below 40 mm Hg, patients with as little as 10 minutes of decreased blood pressure at a level two thirds of their normal value have been known to progress to severe oliguric acute renal failure lasting 7 to 10 days. Furthermore, in some patients with chronic severe hypertension, reduction of the blood pressure to less than 150/90 may result in a significant reduction in GFR. It appears that the thick ascending limb of the loop of Henle may be particularly vulnerable to ischemic injury.

Following a hypotensive episode, a normal urine output can be present for 12 to 18 hours before oliguria supervenes. Patients suffering from ischemic renal damage are rarely anuric. Those with no urine output should be evaluated for possible obstructive lesions in the renal vasculature and collecting system and for intrarenal clotting.

AXIOM
Oliguria may be delayed for 12 to 18 hours after an episode of hypotension.

4. Excessive Vasoconstriction

Excessive vasoconstriction of the renal arterial system is usually associated with hypovolemia or cardiac failure. Such vasoconstriction may persist for several hours or days after the blood volume and cardiac output have been returned to normal. Vasodilators may dramatically improve urine output in such patients, even without producing major changes in blood volume or cardiac output.

AXIOM
Renal vasoconstriction may persist for up to 24 to 48 hours after severe trauma or hypotension.

5. Increased Intra-abdominal Pressure

Patients with severe abdominal distention due to postoperative hemorrhage may develop severe progressive oliguria. This "abdominal compartment syndrome" appears to be caused by compression of the renal veins and inferior vena cava. Interestingly, after operative decompression of the abdomen, many of these patients develop polyuria and rapid complete resolution of their renal failure.

In experimental studies of the vascular dynamics, renal failure is consistently caused by increased intra-abdominal pressure produced by intraperitoneal instillation of graded amounts of saline. Oliguria occurred at intra-abdominal pressures of 15 to 20 mm Hg, and anuria occurred at pressures greater than 20 mm Hg. However, as soon as the intra-abdominal pressure was reduced, inferior caval pressure fell and urine output increased.

AXIOM
Increased intra-abdominal pressure can cause oliguria and renal failure.

6. Vascular Occlusion

a. Arterial

Occlusion of major portions of the renal arterial tree can cause oliguria, flank pain, hematuria, and proteinuria. Similar vascular occlusion may occur because of cholesterol, blood clot, fat, and marrow emboli. Large or small vessel occlusion may occur. A patient with known atrial fibrillation or a ventricular aneurysm is much more likely to have large emboli. Patients with recent abdominal vascular trauma or surgery are more likely to develop cholesterol emboli, sometimes heralded by cutaneous necrotic lesions below the level of the umbilicus and by blue toes. Initially, the fractional excretion of sodium (FE_{Na}) will be low, but within 6 to 12 hours, it may begin to rise as increasing areas of the kidney become dysfunctional.

b. Venous

Venous occlusive disease as a cause of acute renal failure is relatively uncommon. One should suspect this problem if there is impaired renal function plus proteinuria and lower extremity swelling. It is also seen with pressure on the vena cava from a malignancy. Hypercoagulable patients have an increased incidence of renal vein thrombosis. A pulmonary embolus associated with these symptoms and signs indicates the need for venography to exclude clots in the renal veins and inferior vena cava.

7. Altered Blood Chemistry

Severe hyponatremia or hypoproteinemia may occassionally be associated with severe oliguria that will not improve until relatively large quantities of sodium or albumin are administered. The mechanisms by which these abnormalities cause severe oliguria are unknown, but may be mediated by osmoreceptors or the juxtaglomerular apparatus.

8. Hypercalcemia

Severe hypercalcemia can cause acute renal failure. Initially, the urine output will be normal or high. However, because hypercalcemia blocks the antidiuretic hormone (ADH) effect on the renal tubules, producing a nephrogenic diabetes insipidus, patients with hypercalcemia can quickly become dehydrated and oliguric. This problem may also be associated with some hypertension due to the effects of hypercalcemia on vascular smooth muscle.

9. Hypokalemia

Hypokalemia to levels less than 2.0 mEq/liter can cause nephrogenic diabetes insipidus and vacuolization of tubule cells with a modest azotemia. Serum creatinine is rarely higher than 3.0 mg/dl and the BUN seldom exceeds 60 mg/dl. Such individuals are not oliguric initially, but may later become dehydrated because of the reduced ability to concentrate urine. This entity can be an important factor in accelerating the development of renal failure.

AXIOM
Severe hypercalcemia and hypokalemia can cause nephrogenic diabetes insipidus and severe dehydration.

B. RENAL (PARENCHYMAL) FAILURE

There are many conditions that can cause acute renal failure. The most important of these include sepsis, trauma, and various drugs.

1. Sepsis

a. Causes of Renal Failure in Sepsis

Sepsis can cause renal failure in a wide variety of ways. Certainly, hypotension and the associated reduced tissue perfusion may be an important precipitating factor. However, renal failure can occur in sepsis without hypotension or any apparent hypoperfusion.

Both clinically and experimentally, acute vasomotor nephropathy with ischemia alone can be very difficult to produce. For example, patients with bleeding duodenal ulcers may have prolonged periods of renal ischemia, but they rarely develop acute renal failure. In contrast, patients who suffer massive trauma or sepsis are much more likely to develop acute renal failure with relatively modest renal ischemia.

(1) Reduced Renal Blood Flow

For many years it was assumed that sepsis was associated with increased renal vascular resistance and decreased renal blood flow, even if the cardiac output was normal or high. Indeed, because of the fluid sequestration (third spacing of fluid) in sepsis, very large quantities of fluid are often needed to maintain an adequate urine output. This apparent reduction in RBF was a convenient explanation for the high incidence of renal failure in patients with severe sepsis. Studies of RBF in such patients were few, but those that were performed generally showed a reduced clearance of para-amino hippurate (PAH). This seemed to confirm the hypothesis that RBF was reduced in sepsis, even in the hyperdynamic state.

In newer studies, however, measurements of PAH extraction ratios (which are used to measure renal plasma flow) by Lucas and others, using a catheter in the right renal vein of patients with hyperdynamic sepsis, provided some very interesting data. Normally 85% to 91% of the PAH reaching the kidney will be excreted in the urine and only 9% to 15% will reach the renal veins. However, in some of the septic patients, up to 70% of the PAH reaches the renal veins. This means that the usual PAH clearance, which assumes almost 100% extraction of PAH by the kidney, underestimates the actual RBF by as much as 300%. When the calculations of RBF are corrected for the greatly reduced extraction ratios, the total RBF in sepsis is generally well maintained at about 20% of the cardiac output.

(2) Damage Caused by the Infection Itself

Recent studies show that total renal blood flow during severe sepsis may, in fact, be normal in individuals who subsequently develop severe renal failure. This suggests the presence of circulating toxins that affect kidney function. Much of the renal damage in sepsis is probably related to excessive activation of the complement, coagulation, and kinin systems, plus release of a wide variety of cytokines from activated macrophages. The most important of these cytokines are the tumor necrosis factor (TNF) and interleukin 1 (IL-1). Complement can cause leukostasis in a variety of organs, especially the lungs, where the polymorphonuclear leukocytes (PMNs) can release toxic radicals and lysosomal enzymes. Excess activation of clotting, especially in the face of low antithrombin levels, may cause fibrin to occlude capillaries in vital organs.

Horl and colleagues recently demonstrated that neutrophil activation is increased in patients with acute renal failure, and it is increased further by superimposed sepsis. They also found that cellulose-containing dialysis membranes cause a further activation of neutrophils.

(3) Intrarenal Blood Flow

It is now clear that the kidneys participate in the hyperdynamic circulatory changes of sepsis. Whether the reduced PAH extraction ratios are due to anatomic shunting, redistribution of blood flow, or failure of cellular transport mechanisms is still not clear. Many observers have suggested that a reduced PAH extraction ratio is an index of the diversion of blood flow away from the cortex to the medulla; however, evidence is conflicting on this point. Nevertheless, at least two experimental methods have demonstrated that, in sepsis, flow is diverted from the cortex toward the medulla. In experimental animals, radioactive microspheres large enough to be trapped in capillary vessels have demonstrated that administration of pyrogens or vasodilators alter blood flow in the direction of the medulla. The use of xenon-133 and krypton-85 washout studies in both animals and humans have confirmed these observations.

Thus, although the GFR may be maintained at relatively normal levels, there appears to be hyperperfusion of the juxtamedullary nephrons, a high rate of blood flow in the medulla, and a reduced filtration fraction.

(4) Urine Concentration

The ability of the kidney to concentrate urine is usually greatly reduced during severe sepsis. This may be related to the redistribution of blood flow within the kidney and the decrease in filtration fraction. If less of the filterable crystalloids and water are removed from the glomerulus, the postglomerular blood surrounding the tubules will have a lower protein content and osmolarity than normal. If blood flow in the postglomerular vessels is greater than normal, the hydrostatic pressure in the peritubular blood rises. Both of these alterations will discourage transport of salt and water out of the proximal tubule. High flow rates in the vasa recta also tend to wash out the osmolar gradient in the medullary interstitium, thereby reducing the concentrating ability of the kidney. In the septic patient, sodium absorption also tends to be less efficient, and tubular fluid tends to contain increased sodium and water.

(5) Urine Volume
(a) Oliguria

Most patients with sepsis will have a reduced urine output as increased amounts of fluid are sequestered in an expanding third space. Indeed, if more than 200 ml of IV fluid is needed each hour to maintain an adequate urine flow, one should assume that sepsis is present until proven otherwise.

Surprisingly, large fluid losses can sometimes occur after the ingestion of diuretics and before the extent of the volume depletion is recognized. The severe hypovolemia that may rapidly follow the diuretic, especially if it is in a patient who is already hypovolemic, can rapidly result in acute vasomotor nephropathy.

(b) Polyuria

Although true polyuria is usually defined as a urine output greater than 300 ml/h, the excretion of high urine volumes in spite of a relative or absolute hypovolemia in an occasional patient with severe sepsis has been referred to as the *inappropriate polyuria of sepsis*. In these patients, the volume of urine and sodium excreted is excessive relative to the circulating blood volume.

The polyuria in some of these patients appears to be associated with an expanded extracellular fluid (ECF) volume. However, the increased ECF found in such patients is largely due to an obligatory third-space loss. The phenomenon of inappropriate polyuria may also be related to the generalized vasodilation and increased blood flow often seen in sepsis. The reduced filtration fraction and resulting reduction in peritubular oncotic pressure may also contribute to this polyuria.

In some cases of sepsis, the clinician fails to adequately replace the large urine loss because of a fear that the patient is already overloaded with fluid. The feeling that the patient is overloaded with fluid is often reinforced by the presence of lung congestion and an elevated CVP. However, both of these changes may be due to alterations within the lungs and may occur in spite of a marked hypovolemia.

The first indication that a polyuric patient is becoming hypovolemic is often a fall in the sodium concentration of urine to less than 10 to 20 mEq/liter. In most patients with polyuria due to fluid overload, the urine sodium will be greater than 40 mEq/liter (unless the fluid overload is due to pure water). Unless aggressive fluid replacement is begun rapidly at that point, the diminished circulating volume can rapidly result in acute oliguric vasomotor nephropathy, a condition that few severely injured or septic patients survive.

2. Trauma

Trauma can cause renal failure, not only because of hypovolemia and hypoperfusion of the kidneys, but also by release of hemoglobin, myoglobin, and other substances that can severely damage the nephrons. Indeed, the worst renal damage occurs when all of these factors (hypovolemia, pigments, and trauma) are present.

a. Physiologic Changes

(1) Renal Blood Flow

In studies of severely injured patients, RBF is found rather consistently reduced —on occasion to less than 30% of normal—in spite of adequate fluid loading and a normal cardiac output. The increased catecholamine release associated with trauma may cause renal arteriolar vasoconstriction, elevated renal vascular resistance, and reduced RBF.

In general, the RBF varies inversely with the extent of the injury and the number of blood transfusions. This reduction in RBF often persists for several days after injury. If recovery is uneventful, RBF usually returns to normal by the sixth day after injury.

(2) Blood Pressure

Any reduction in BP can cause a severe reduction in RBF after trauma. However, reduced renal perfusion can occur without hypotension following trauma, and is part of the physiologic response to injury.

(3) Increased Cortical Vascular Resistance

Radioactive xenon-133 washout studies in patients with acute injury (as well as in micropuncture studies in rats) have indicated that the oliguric phase of trauma is associated with a reduction in total RBF by at least 30% and an increased vascular resistance in the outer renal cortex. This redistributes renal blood flow to the juxtamedullary cortex and medulla. Increased blood flow to the medulla and juxtamedullary nephrons, which have long loops of Henle, will generally result in a lower volume of more concentrated urine with lower sodium concentrations.

(4) Glomerular Filtration

Although the RBF in trauma may be rather low, the GFR in injured nonhypotensive patients is usually maintained above 40 ml/min, because of autoregulation and changes in resistance in the afferent and efferent arterioles. With hypovolemia, the reduction in RBF is proportionally much greater than that of the GFR. Consequently, filtration fraction is increased and oncotic pressure in the postglomerular capillary rises. In turn, the osmotic gradient between the tubules and the surrounding plasma increases, and salt and water are more easily transported out the tubule, adding to salt and water retention in the body.

As might be expected, with a decline in the GFR and increased endogenous protein breakdown, many patients with severe trauma and sepsis have elevated BUN and serum creatinine levels in spite of a normal or increased urine output. As the GFR returns to normal, the BUN and serum creatinine tend to gradually fall back to normal.

AXIOM

Little or no correlation exists between urine volume and the GFR and RBF in critically ill or injured patients after fluid resuscitation.

In some trauma patients with severe reductions in GFR, the urine output may be normal or high. If the GFR is significantly reduced, but blood flow is poorly distributed so that most of it goes to the renal medulla and juxtamedullary nephrons, the increased flow rates in the vasa recta can cause a washout of the medullary concentrating gradient. This process interferes with the renal concentrating mechanisms so that an inappropriately high volume of relatively dilute urine may result. Even when the low GFR is recognized and an adequate fluid resuscitation is provided, it may take several days for the GFR to recover to normal.

(5) Urine Concentration

With severe dehydration, young adult kidneys can usually concentrate urine to about 1200 to 1400 mOsm/liter. This ability diminishes to about 600 mOsm/liter at 50 years of age. This degree of concentrating ability is maintained until relatively late in life.

During major surgery, and for a variable period of time after all types of trauma, many patients are unable to concentrate their urine to levels previously possible, even if pharmacologic doses of vasopressin (antidiuretic hormone) are given. Consequently, a larger volume of urine is required to excrete the same solute load, and the solute load may be greatly increased after trauma or sepsis. If an increased urine volume cannot be achieved, azotemia may develop. Such a combination of events occurs frequently.

AXIOM

The definition of oliguria, arbitrarily set at a volume of less than 400 ml/d, should probably be revised upward to 800 to 1000 ml/d in patients with severe trauma or sepsis. Any lesser volume requires early investigation and treatment.

This inability of the kidneys to respond to vasopressin after trauma or surgery may be related to toxic agents (such as anesthetics), aberrations in blood flow distribution, or unknown factors. If no medullary osmotic gradient is produced, ADH is ineffective. If tubular cells are unable to pump sodium ion, no gradient can be produced, and urinary concentrating ability will be disturbed. Whatever the reason, urine usually cannot be concentrated above 600 mOsm/liter during the intraoperative or postoperative period.

AXIOM

Although a decreased urine output can be an important indication of a fluid deficit or renal failure in injured patients, a normal urine output does not rule out a significant reduction in renal function.

In one study, many resuscitated patients with a normal or increased urine output had a GFR that was 25% less than normal and an RBF that was 50% less than normal.

(6) Pigments

Myoglobin or hemoglobin casts in urine and on histologic sections of renal tubules suggest that tubular plugging with such pigment may be an important cause of acute renal failure. However, such findings are inconsistent and generally rather limited. Although the casts may be the end result of low rates of urine flow associated with high pigment loads from transfusion reactions or muscle damage, they are probably not the sole cause of acute renal insufficiency.

In a recent review of traumatic rhabdomyolysis, Better and Stein noted that the damaged muscle cells liberate a wide variety of potentially nephrotoxic substances into the blood stream. These include potassium, purines, phosphate, lactic and other organic acids, myoglobin, thromboplastin, creatine kinase, and creatinine. Movement of water, sodium, chloride, and calcium into the damaged muscle cells may contribute to a simultaneous reduction in RBF and GFR. Within hours, while the plasma urea and creatinine levels are still normal, dangerous degrees of hyperkalemia, hyperphosphatemia, hyperuricemia, hypocalcemia, and metabolic acidosis may develop.

3. Antibiotics

Antibiotics are the principal exogenous toxins or drugs that can cause loss of renal function in critically ill patients. Patients with decreased renal function, advanced age, unstable blood pressure, diabetes mellitus, and hepatic insufficiency are particularly prone to loss of renal function with antibiotic therapy.

a. Aminoglycosides

Aminoglycosides have been shown to be nephrotoxic, particularly in postoperative patients and when given in association with diuretics such as furosemide. Eisenberg and associates found a 7.3% incidence of nephrotoxicity due to aminoglycosides in 1756 patients treated at six Philadelphia area hospitals. The average cost of treating each nephrotoxic patient was $2,501 or $183 for each of the 1756 patients receiving aminoglycosides. Certainly this cost, plus the cost of pharmacokinetic studies, must be considered when ordering gentamicin or tobramycin.

Experimental studies in rats indicate that gentamicin can concentrate in the renal cortex to levels 10 to 50 times greater than plasma, and this increases the susceptibility of the kidneys to acute ischemic injury, even before any overt nephrotoxicity is apparent. The nephrotoxic effect is directly related to the duration of gentamicin administration. Gentamicin induces similar lesions in other animals and in man. Tobramycin is probably less nephrotoxic than many of the other aminoglycosides. Certainly, kanamycin and streptomycin should be avoided, if possible, in individuals with oliguria or early AVN.

Aminoglycosides can be nephrotoxic even if given in the proper dosage, based on the patient's lean body weight, creatinine clearance, and measured peak and trough levels. On occasion a clue to early aminoglycoside toxicity is the development of polyuria and K^+ wasting. Many patients have moderate-to-severe aminoglycoside nephrotoxicity without a significant decrease in urine output. Although the prognosis is better for this group than for those who have loss of renal function with no urine output, the problems presented during the episode of acute renal failure are almost identical.

b. Amphotericin

When given in large doses for a protracted period, amphotericin has caused nephrogenic diabetes insipidus and impaired renal function in many individuals. However, the newer, purer forms of amphotericin are less nephrotoxic.

c. Penicillin

Penicillin may lead to loss of renal function in several ways. Some patients develop acute glomerulonephritis with microscopic hematuria, RBC casts, 3+ to 4+ proteinuria, modest hypertension, and azotemia. An interstitial nephritis with a low fractional Na^+ excretion can also occur. Patients with interstitial nephritis may develop flank discomfort from kidney swelling. Fever, eosinophilia, and increased eosinophils in the urinary sediment are typically present, and an allergic reaction is common. The diagnosis of interstitial nephritis is important, since withdrawal of the offending drug and administration of steroids lead to return of renal function.

d. Other Antibiotics

Some of the first generation cephalosporins, especially cephalothin and cephaloridine, plus the tetracyclines (with the exception of doxycycline), may also induce or exacerbate acute renal failure in patients with pre-existing renal disease, especially if loop diuretics are also being given.

4. Angiotensin-Converting Enzyme Inhibitors

Captopril and Enalapril are associated with acute loss of renal function, especially in patients with severe congestive heart failure (CHF) or renal artery stenosis. This entity is reversible after withdrawal of the drugs.

5. Nonsteroidal Anti-inflammatory Medications

Nonsteroidal anti-inflammatory medications are a significant cause of acute renal function loss, especially in elderly patients with decreased renal perfusion (volume depletion from any cause, congestive heart failure, nephrotic syndrome, or bilateral renal artery stenosis). Many of the features of penicillin-induced interstitial nephritis are present. Less commonly, they cause acute glomerulonephritis. Fortunately, the loss of renal function is reversible with the withdrawal of medication.

6. Hyperuricemia

Although renal failure from hyperuricemia is not common in traumatized patients, it is extremely important in those with a hypermetabolic or tissue-destructive state resulting from problems such as cancer chemotherapy. Serum uric acid levels usually exceed 15 mg/dl, and urate crystals are usually found in the urine. An intense delayed nephrogram may be seen on an IV pyelogram (IVP). This problem can be aborted with an alkaline diuresis, and it responds well to hemodialysis.

2. Radiocontrast Agents

Typically, radiocontrast agents have osmolalities higher than 1000 mOsm/kg of water and routinely produce an osmotic diuresis. Damage to the proximal tubule with decreased sodium reabsorption can also cause an osmotic diuresis. The iodine in radiocontrast agents may also cause reactions that can damage the kidneys. Dye toxicity is particularly likely in patients with decreased left ventricular function who receive greater than 150 ml of contrast material for a single study.

With osmotic diuresis, the proximal tubule fails to reabsorb the bulk of the filtered solute, and polyuria may result. Osmotic diuretics increase medullary blood flow, which reduces the solute concentration in the medullary interstitium. Whereas approximately 50% of the volume entering the descending limb is normally reabsorbed, less than 10% may be reabsorbed during an osmotic diuresis. In the collecting duct, water reabsorption is limited by the lack of a hypertonic medullary interstitium. The presence or absence of ADH becomes less important in these circumstances and the urine will approach isosmolality.

8. Diabetes Insipidus

Central diabetes insipidus (due to head trauma or neurosurgical procedures) and nephrogenic diabetes insipidus (due to various drugs or electrolyte abnormalities) can cause severe polyuria. In contrast to an osmotic diuresis, in which the urinary osmolality is relatively isotonic, water diuresis and diabetes insipidus produce a very dilute urine (urine osmolality of 50 to 100 mOsm/kg water). A water diuresis may result either from a lack of ADH or from an inability of the collecting duct to respond to ADH. In the normal kidney with a GFR of 100–125 ml/min, 60 to 70 ml of the filtrate will be reabsorbed by the proximal tubule. Half of the remaining fluid, or 15 to 25 ml/min, will be reabsorbed in Henle's loop. If no further reabsorption occurs, as with diabetes insipidus, as much as 15 ml/min (or 900 ml/h) could be excreted as urine. Urine flow rates of this magnitude are not usually observed, however, since diabetes insipidus can rapidly cause hypovolemia, a reduction in GFR, and an increase in the percentage of electrolytes and fluid reabsorbed in the proximal tubule.

AXIOM

A continued urine output in excess of 900 ml/h suggests that mechanisms other than diabetes insipidus are present.

If the large quantities of urine excreted with diabetes insipidus are not replaced, the patient may become hypovolemic, and oliguric renal failure may supervene. To avoid this, fluid intake and output, blood pressure, and pulse must be carefully monitored.

9. Anesthesia

Total renal blood flow, as measured by PAH clearance, falls by 20% to 40% during general anesthesia with potent inhalation anesthetics, or with balanced techniques using nitrous oxide, narcotics, and muscle relaxants. The same anesthetics generally cause a somewhat lower reduction (15% to 30%) in GFR. With deeper levels of anesthesia, hydration has no effect on the decrease in blood flow and filtration rate. The urine flow rate decreases even more than the GFR. The decrease in urine flow rate is usually accompanied by a modest increase in urine osmolality to less than 700 to 800 mOsm/kg of water.

The mechanisms responsible for the decrease in RPF, GFR, and urine output following induction of anesthesia are unclear. Well-conducted general anesthesia is not associated with significant elevations in plasma-renin activity or in vasopressin. Furthermore, almost all modern general anesthetics cause a reduction in sympathetic activity and in catecholamine concentrations in plasma.

Methoxyflurane, which generates inorganic fluoride, has been reported to be an indirect renal toxin that causes renal injury. The typical patient has a polyuria that is resistant to therapy with vasopressin. The only other anesthetic that releases significant amounts of fluoride is enflurane. Very prolonged and deep anesthesia with this agent can also produce fluoride levels that impair renal function. Except for these two agents, no other general anesthetics cause direct renal toxicity.

10. Liver Disease and the Kidney

Patients with advanced liver failure (especially with encephalopathy, jaundice, and ascites) may develop a characteristic type of renal dysfunction, termed hepatorenal syndrome (HRS). This renal dysfunction is characterized by oliguria, a reduction in GFR, and severe sodium retention (urine sodium, usually <10 mEq/liter). Interestingly, the severity of the renal failure may not correlate well with the degree of renal dysfunction. Small amounts of protein are found in the urine, and hyaline and granular casts are typical of HRS. Renal concentrating ability is usually impaired, but the urine osmolality can often be modestly elevated.

The most characteristic abnormality in the HRS is the extremely low concentration of sodium found in the urine. This has been attributed primarily to a reduction in distal delivery of sodium to the tubules because of reduced filtration and enhanced proximal reabsorption.

In patients with cirrhosis and HRS, renal angiography reveals severe attenuation of interlobar arteries, with loss of visualization of arcuate and interlobular arteries. Xenon scans reflect diminution in flow, particularly to the superficial cortex. This renal vasoconstriction is not reversed by alpha-adrenergic blockade.

The GFR is severely reduced in HRS, and serum creatinine levels are usually in the range of 4 to 6 mg/dl. Cirrhotic patients, with or without HRS, tend to have elevated plasma-renin activity and aldosterone concentrations. The concept of a reduced "effective circulating blood volume" has been used to explain the apparent paradox of an increased extracellular fluid volume with renal responses characteristic of volume depletion.

Bilirubin per se does not cause the renal functional abnormalities seen in HRS, but bile salts do induce vasodilation, hypotension, and sodium retention when administered chronically. The treatment of HRS is unsuccessful unless hepatic function improves.

11. Acute Pyelonephritis

Significant loss of renal function in acute pyelonephritis is unusual. However, severe bilateral infection with organisms, such as *Staphylococcus aureus*, can lead to azotemia, especially if papillary necrosis with subsequent ureteral plugging results.

12. Renal Cortical Necrosis

Most episodes of acute renal failure, caused by ischemia or nephrotoxins, are not associated with acute tissue necrosis. However, renal cortical necrosis may occur in sepsis, late pregnancy with abruptio placentae or septic abortion, uncontrolled hypertension, and disease entities that lead to a microangiopathic hemolytic anemia. Microangiopathic hemolytic anemia with damage to red cells by strands of fibrin in small vessels can be seen in disseminated intravascular coagulation (DIC), thrombotic thrombocytopenic purpura, and hemolytic uremic syndrome. Concurrent abnormalities in liver and brain function are frequently seen, along with fever and consumptive coagulopathy in some cases.

13. Malignant Hypertension

A diastolic pressure greater than 110 mm Hg may be a cause of acute renal function loss in a patient critically ill from some other disease entity. Evidence of organ failure that may be caused by hypertension requires emergency therapy, often with alpha- and beta-adrenergic blocking agents.

14. Thrombotic Thrombocytopenic Purpura (Hemolytic Uremic Syndrome)

In a recent review, Murphy has pointed out that thrombotic thrombocytopenic purpura (TTP) and hemolytic uremic syndrome (HUS) are now known to be the same disease process and are characterized by thrombocytopenia, microangiopathic hemolytic anemia, neurologic abnormalities, fever, and renal dysfunction. The renal failure is due to obliteration of glomerular capillaries. Most of these patients are jaundiced. Therapy is nonspecific and involves corticosteroids, plasmapheresis, and exchange-plasma infusions.

15. Vasculitis

It is unusual to develop vasculitis in the critical care setting. However, patients with microscopic hematuria, RBC casts, and 3+ to 4+ proteinuria should be evaluated for an underlying vasculitis. Other features suggesting an underlying vasculitis include hypertension, hemorrhages and exudates in the optic fundi, skin rashes, splinter hemorrhages in the nail beds, arthritis, and a sedimentation rate over 80 mm/h.

16. Multiple Myeloma

Multiple myeloma occurs with increasing frequency in the elderly population and is associated with acute renal failure from several causes. These patients are particularly prone to develop acute renal failure from radiocontrast dyes, especially if they have a high concentration of light-chain proteins in their urine. In addition, multiple myeloma is associated with hypercalcemia, which by itself can cause renal problems. Clues to the diagnosis of multiple myeloma include anemia of inappropriate severity, increased globulins, and a sedimentation rate over 75 mm/h.

17. Postrenal Failure

Possible obstruction to urine flow must be considered in the initial evaluation of any patient with acute renal function loss. A rectal and pelvic examination and placement of a Foley catheter in the urinary bladder can usually exclude obstruction of the lower urinary tract rather quickly.

There are many intrinsic and extrinsic causes of obstructive renal failure. Many patients with obstructive uropathy initially have a totally normal urine output with unremarkable urinary sediment. In the first 24 hours of obstructive uropathy leading to azotemia, the laboratory picture may suggest a prerenal oliguria. The urinary Na^+ concentration may be low, with a fractional Na^+ excretion less than 1%. However, after this initial phase, the fractional excretion of Na^+ gradually increases to levels greater than 3%. On occasion, with a subtotal obstruction, the urine output increases as the kidneys develop a form of nephrogenic diabetes insipidus. Patients with obstructive uropathy are rarely hypertensive from this problem.

Intraluminal obstruction to urine flow from a new or pre-existing problem must be considered in all patients with acute renal failure. Since 5% of the population has only one functioning kidney, the possibility of movement of a pre-existing kidney stone, sloughed papilla, or collecting system clot must be considered. Collecting duct abnormalities, due to tumor infiltration or stricture, should also be considered. The potential problem with a hypertrophied prostate may be avoided by placing a Foley catheter in patients who have frequent, small voidings, modest azotemia, and/or a palpable bladder.

Relief of obstruction may bring about a major diuresis, which may be due to an osmotic diuresis (from excretion of excess urea, salt, and water), a refractoriness to ADH, and/or an intrinsic insult to the renal tubules allowing an uncontrolled diuresis. Careful monitoring of intravascular volume at the time of relief of obstructive uropathy is important. If the obstruction is present for less than 2 weeks, a prompt return to normal renal function may be expected. With obstruction of several months' duration, maximum improvement in renal function may take weeks. The creatinine clearance may never return to a normal value.

18. Chronic Renal Failure

A pre-existing chronic renal failure, especially if mild, can be unsuspected, but potentially very dangerous in critically ill patients. Serum creatinine levels may be deceptively normal despite impaired renal function in elderly, sedentary, and poorly muscled individuals. The urinalysis may be normal or may have minimal changes, such as a trace of protein on the urinary dipstick and/or a few hyaline and granular casts.

Diabetes mellitus, hypertension, hypercholesterolemia, peripheral vascular disease, and a heavy smoking history are commonly associated with chronically abnormal kidney function. Subtle, chronic lower urinary tract obstruction in older men also can lead to a decreased GFR.

Patients with chronic renal function impairment tend to have a decreased GFR, which poses a number of potential problems when they become critically ill. Renal drug toxicity is much more common because of an unanticipated decreased excretion of antibiotics and other potentially nephrotoxic agents.

A patient with decreased kidney function is more likely to retain fluid, not only because of changes in renal function, but also because of increased ADH and aldosterone release. Compounding this problem is a refractoriness to diuretics because of the decreased GFR. Diminished kidney function also carries with it a greater risk of hyperkalemia, both from intrinsic release of intracellular K^+ and inappropriate handling of administered K^+. An increased sensitivity to radiocontrast dye is also present, with a greater likelihood of temporarily decreased function after angiography. Previously impaired kidneys improve much more slowly after acute renal failure than previously normal kidneys, partly because of their decreased ability to clear the toxins that accumulated during the acute episode.

If a critically ill patient is found to have a chronic impairment of renal function, creatinine clearance should be determined with proper factoring for body surface area. In addition, a renal ultrasound study to exclude an obstructive uropathy and determine the amount of renal parenchyma present is indicated. Vascular lesions are a less common cause of subclinical chronic renal failure; consequently, nuclear medicine studies are usually not necessary.

IV. DIAGNOSIS

A. DIFFERENTIATING PRERENAL AND POSTRENAL OLIGURIA FROM AVN

Probably the most important entity to be distinguished from acute vasomotor nephropathy is prerenal oliguria due to hypovolemia (Table 14.1). Some of the other more important problems that should be ruled out include cardiac failure, renal vascular occlusion, and urinary tract obstruction.

1. Prerenal Oliguria

a. Clinical Criteria

The most frequent cause of oliguria is inadequate renal perfusion due to hypovolemia. However, the clinical picture can sometimes be very deceptive. If the patient appears to have an increased *total* extracellular fluid volume, but has a greatly reduced urinary excretion of sodium and high urinary osmolality, the kidney may be sensing a reduced *effective* circulating volume. In such a patient, hemodynamic monitoring often indicates that the blood volume or cardiac output is lower than suspected clinically.

In critically ill or injured patients, low blood pressure, low central venous pressure (CVP), and/or low pulmonary artery wedge pressure (PAWP) suggest that hypovolemia may be present, but the converse is not necessarily true. In spite of a normal or high blood pressure and CVP, such patients may be hypovolemic. However, if the PAWP is more than 18 to 20 mm Hg, heart failure may be developing, and it is unlikely that additional fluids will be very helpful. In some patients, the central volume is appropriate or overexpanded and the renal response reflects hormonal or nervous system override of normal volume regulatory mechanisms.

Severe hypoalbuminemia may also be a contributing factor. Other problems may include severe acidosis, which can cause profound venodilatation, decreased cardiac output, and hypotension refractory to catecholamines. In the

Table 14.1

TESTS TO DIFFERENTIATE OLIGURIA DUE TO HYPOVOLEMIA FROM THAT DUE TO ACUTE VASOMOTOR NEPHROPATHY (AVN)	*Hypovolemia*	*AVN*
Urine specific gravity	>1.016	<1.010
Urine/plasma osmolarity	>1.2	<1.1
Urine sodium	10–20 mEq/L	>40 mEq/L
BUN/serum creatinine ratio	>20	<10
Urine/plasma creatinine	>20	<10
Fractional excretion of sodium	<1%	>3%
Renal failure index	<1	>2

traumatized patient, cardiac tamponade and myocardial contusion should also be considered when cardiovascular failure is present.

Emboli can cause decreased tubular perfusion. Parenchymal swelling associated with interstitial nephritis can also decrease glomerular blood flow. Patients with hepatorenal syndrome typically have low urine sodium levels that are usually strongly suggestive of prerenal azotemia. However, in these patients, the low urine sodium may be due to a circulating toxin that decreases intrarenal blood flow.

2. Laboratory Tests

a. Specific Gravity

The urine specific gravity is a relatively inaccurate measure of urine concentration, and it is difficult to use the hygrometer if there are only small amounts of urine. Furthermore, high molecular weight substances, such as protein and dextran, may raise the urine specific gravity to high levels without much change in osmolarity. Nevertheless, a urine specific gravity greater than 1.020 plus a low urine output suggest that the patient is hypovolemic, especially if the urine is protein-free. A specific gravity less than 1.010 under the same circumstances suggests renal insufficiency.

b. Urine Osmolarity

A high urine osmolarity in the presence of oliguria suggests that the patient is dehydrated, and a low urine osmolarity with oliguria suggests that renal failure is present. The urine/plasma osmolarity ratio can also be helpful. If the urine/plasma (U/P) osmolarity ratio is 1.2:1 or higher, hypovolemia is a probable cause. However, if the ratio is 1.1:1 or less in an oliguric patient, it is probably due to vasomotor nephropathy.

c. Urine Sodium

A urine sodium concentration that is falling or is less than 10 to 20 mEq/liter suggests that renal tubular function is intact, but that there is impaired renal perfusion, usually due to hypovolemia. A urine sodium of 40 mEq/liter or higher in a patient who is oliguric suggests one of several possibilities: acute renal failure, an inappropriate ADH effect, action of a potent diuretic (such as furosemide), or adrenocortical insufficiency.

d. Blood Urea Nitrogen

The BUN tends to rise rapidly in patients with severe prerenal azotemia, since there is usually greatly increased reabsorption of filtered urea by the renal tubules. Any situation that increases tissue breakdown, such as gastrointestinal bleeding, can also result in a high BUN. High-protein feedings, either intravenously or by mouth, can overwhelm the kidney's ability to excrete urea.

A rapidly rising BUN with little or no change in the serum creatinine suggests upper gastrointestinal hemorrhage, accelerated tissue breakdown, or blood volume deficit. All these situations can result in a BUN/serum creatinine ratio greater than 20:1.

e. Serum Creatinine

In the early stages of acute renal failure, serum creatinine levels will often be normal in spite of a progressive decrease in creatinine clearance. This occurs, at least partly, because of the relatively wide normal range for serum creatinine levels. For example, if a thin, inactive elderly patient has a normal serum creatinine of 0.6 mg/dl, a 50% reduction in renal function will result in an increase to about 1.2 mg/100 ml, which is still within normal limits for most laboratories. In the patient who has suffered severe trauma or is septic, accelerated tissue destruction often leads to a much more rapid rise in BUN than in creatinine.

f. Urine Creatinine

During hypovolemia, the urine concentration of creatinine tends to rise above 100 mg/dl, whereas during acute renal failure it usually falls rapidly to levels below 40 mg/dl. Thus if the urine/plasma creatinine ratio exceeds 20, the patient is probably hypovolemic. A ratio of less than 10 is more characteristic of acute renal failure.

g. Creatinine Clearance

A normal young adult excretes approximately 1500 mg of creatinine a day in 1000 to 1500 ml of urine. Consequently, U_{cr} levels normally average 100 to 150 mg/dl. If the urine output is 1000 ml/day (0.7 ml/min) and the serum creatinine (S_{cr}) is 0.8 mg/dl, the

$$Cl_{cr} = \frac{UV}{P} = \frac{(150)(0.7)}{(0.8)} = 131 \text{ ml/min.}$$

With AVN, the U_{cr} tends to fall rapidly and cause an abrupt fall in Cl_{cr}.

AXIOM

Cl_{cr} is usually the most accurate, readily available test to follow renal function.

h. Free-Water Clearance

Free-water clearance (Cl_{H_2O}) is defined as urine flow per minute minus osmolar clearance and is normally negative. Isosthenuria (urine osmolarity the same as plasma) is one of the earliest and most consistent functional characteristics of renal ischemia. As urine osmolality falls, osmolar clearance also falls and free-water clearance becomes less negative. If urine osmolality falls below that of serum, free-water clearance becomes positive, a fall in osmolar clearance may occur, even before a fall in Cl_{cr}, in some patients as AVN is developing.

In a patient with prerenal oliguria, the urine flow may be 0.5 ml/min, serum osmolarity 300 mOsm/liter, and urine osmolarity 600 mOsm/liter:

$$Cl_{osm} = \frac{(600)(0.5)}{(300)} = 1.0 \text{ ml/min}$$

$$Cl_{H_2O} = \text{urine flow (ml/min)} - Cl_{osm}$$
$$= 0.5 - 1.0 = -0.5 \text{ ml/min.}$$

In AVN, the urine flow may also be 0.5 ml/min, but serum osmolarity is apt to be normal or low (e.g., 280 mOsm/liter) and urine osmolarity close to that of serum, or even lower. If urine osmolarity is 200 mOsm/liter,

$$Cl_{osm} = \frac{(0.5)(200)}{(280)} = 0.36 \text{ ml/min}$$

$$Cl_{H_2O} = 0.5 - 0.36 = 0.14 \text{ ml/min.}$$

AXIOM

The Cl_{H_2O} is less negative or may even become positive with AVN.

i. Fractional Excretion of Sodium (FE_{Na})

AXIOM

The FE_{Na} is the most accurate method for differentiating between prerenal and renal oliguria.

The fractional excretion of sodium compares the renal clearance of sodium to the renal clearance of creatinine by the following formula:

$$FE_{Na} = \frac{U_{Na}/P_{Na}}{U_{cr}/P_{cr}} \times 100\%.$$

In general a FE_{Na} less than 1.0 implies prerenal oliguria, and a FE_{Na} greater than 3 implies acute renal failure.

With prerenal oliguria, we can expect the urinary sodium (U_{Na}) to be less than 10 to 20 mEq/liter and the P_{Na} plasma sodium to be relatively normal. The urine creatinine (U_{cr}) should be about 100 mg/dl and the plasma creatinine (P_{cr}) about 1.0 mg/dl. Thus, using these numbers, the FE_{Na} with prerenal oliguria will be

$$FE_{Na} = \frac{10/140}{100/1} \times 100\% = \frac{7.14}{100} = 0.07\%.$$

In contrast, with acute renal failure, the likely numbers will be

$$FE_{Na} = \frac{80/130}{40/2} \times 100\% = \frac{61.5}{20} = 3.1\%.$$

Interestingly, in hemoglobinuric and myoglobinuria-induced renal failure, the FE_{Na} is frequently less than 1%. This may be due to the effect of production of a pronounced tubuloglomerulary feedback reaction by ferrihemate, which would result in diffuse constriction of afferent arterioles.

j. Renal Failure Index

The renal failure index is calculated by

$$RFI = \frac{U_{Na}}{U_{Cr}/P_{cr}}.$$

An RFI of less than 1.0 implies prerenal oliguria, and an RFI greater than 2.0 implies renal failure. Using the same numbers as in the prerenal example for FE_{Na}, one would expect

$$RFI = \frac{10}{100/1.0} = 0.1.$$

In acute renal failure, one might expect

$$RFI = \frac{80}{40/2} = 40.$$

3. Problems with Laboratory Indices

The characteristic laboratory changes seen with prerenal oliguria include a decreased Cl_{cr}, $U_{Na} < 20$ mEq/liter, and FE_{Na} ($<1\%$) with an increased BUN, S_{cr}, BUN/Cr ratio, and urine osmolality >600 to 800 mOsm/kg water. However, these urine indices of volume depletion may be nondiagnostic with (1) the administration of diuretics; (2) the presence of high rates of excretion of non-electrolyte osmoles, such as glucose, mannitol, or urea; or (3) renal disease.

4. Recent Studies

AXIOM

Readily reversible oliguria in ICU patients may be due to hypovolemia (treated with fluid) or ADH excess (treated with diuretics).

In a recent prospective study of ICU patients, Zaloga and Hughes found an 18% incidence of oliguria (<0.33 ml·kg^{-1}·h^{-1}). On clinical assessment, 7 (39%) were thought to be hypovolemic and 11 (61%) were considered normovolemic. Compared with the hypovolemic patients, the normovolemic oliguric patients had significantly lower serum osmolalities (278 ± 3 vs. 290 ± 5 mOsm/kg H$_2$O) and serum sodium concentrations (138 ± 3 vs. 132 ± 1 mEq/liter). In addition, normovolemic patients had significantly higher urine sodium concentrations (83 ± 12 vs. 13 ± 2 mEq/liter), fractional excretions of sodium (1.14 ± 0.2 vs. 0.15 ± 0.03), and renal failure indices (1.5 ± 0.3 vs. 0.21 ± ± 0.04). ADH concentrations were increased in six hypovolemic and six normovolemic patients. The hypovolemic patients increased their urine output from 17 ± 2 ml/h to greater than 0.5 ml·kg^{-1}·h^{-1} following a 500-ml bolus of normal saline. The normovolemic oliguric patients remained oliguric following the saline bolus (13 ± 2 to 19 ± 3 ml/h), but responded well to diuretics. The authors concluded that oliguria is common in critically ill patients and can result from renal hypoperfusion or ADH excess. Urine sodium, fractional excretion of sodium, and renal failure index were not useful for predicting renal failure in these patients, but were useful for separating the two prerenal etiologies for oliguria.

The patients with normovolemic oliguria responded to furosemide therapy, and the hypovolemic patients responded to fluid therapy. None of these patients developed renal failure, and all were discharged alive from the ICU.

5. Fluid Challenge

Even if all these renal function tests indicate probable renal failure, hypovolemia may still be a possible cause of continued oliguria. A fluid challenge of a crystalloid solution may be given at 10 to 20 ml/min for 20 to 30 minutes while noting the renal response and watching for signs of fluid overload. A balanced electrolyte solution containing no potassium should generally be used, but should be modified for any abnormalities in the electrolyte composition of the patient. The blood pressure, pulse, and CVP must be watched closely. If the CVP or PAWP rises abruptly, or if rales appear, the fluid challenge should be discontinued. Otherwise, about 500 ml of fluid should be given in 20 to 30 minutes. If the oliguria is due to hypovolemia, an increase in urinary flow rate should be noted within 10 to 20 minutes of beginning the infusion, with a maximum response within 30 to 45 minutes of completing the infusion.

The fluid balance in oliguric patients must be checked very carefully to be sure that no hypovolemia is present. Serial CVP or PAWP determinations may be very helpful in this regard. If the CVP and PAWP are low, there is a good chance that the patient is hypovolemic. In critically ill or injured patients, however, respiratory failure may cause a deceptive elevation in the CVP, despite persistent hypovolemia.

a. Dopamine

If hypotension or a reduced cardiac output persist in spite of adequate fluid loading (as gauged by an abrupt increase in the CVP or PAWP to a fluid challenge or a PAWP exceeding 18 mm Hg), some element of cardiac failure is probably present. In such circumstances, an agent such as dopamine may be of help. At dosages of 1 to 3 $\mu g \cdot kg^{-1} \cdot min^{-1}$, it is a renal vasodilator and may improve renal blood flow and urine output. At dosages of 5 to 15 $\mu g \cdot kg^{-1} \cdot min^{-1}$, it can increase cardiac output and blood pressure and further improve renal blood flow.

b. Diuretics

(a) Furosemide

When there is convincing evidence of fluid overload or cardiac failure without vasomotor nephropathy, a trial of diuretics may be in order. However, the use of diuretics to stimulate an increased urine output in patients who are oliguric secondary to hypovolemia is to be condemned. Furosemide in doses of 20 to 40 mg, depending on the severity of the fluid overload, may stimulate a greatly increased urine flow rate. If the GFR is reduced, as it often is in these patients, much larger doses may be required. However, there is no convincing evidence that the use of furosemide in high doses has any therapeutic benefit once vasomotor nephropathy is established. Furthermore, it may actually do harm by direct nephrotoxic effects, by potentiating the nephrotoxic actions of other drugs, or by exacerbating ECF volume deficits.

(2) Mannitol

Mannitol, in dosages of 6.25 to 12.5 g/h after a loading dose of 50 g, may also be used to help stimulate a diuresis. However, since mannitol is hypertonic, it may temporarily increase blood volume. Consequently, it should be administered cautiously in the elderly or in those with suspected cardiac failure.

Mannitol, if not excreted promptly, may cause a nephrosis that is transient and characterized by tubular cell vacuolation. These changes have been ascribed to intense stimulation of the tubuloglomerular feedback mechanism that modulates the single-nephron glomerular filtration rate.

c. Nuclear Medicine Studies

If there is serious consideration of major loss of perfusion, nuclear medicine blood flow studies may be useful. Such studies may also help one to look sequentially at renal blood flow after renal artery repair, or during suspected renal transplant rejection.

B. POSTRENAL FAILURE

1. Clinical

Postrenal failure should be suspected if the patient is completely anuric or has had trauma or surgery near or involving the ureters, bladder, or urethra. Most postrenal causes of oliguria can be evaluated with a Foley catheter and/or pyelography.

2. Foley Catheter

If a Foley catheter is not already present in a patient who is anuric, it should be inserted. Obstruction of the bladder outlet may then be eliminated as a cause of anuria, and urinary flow rates should be measured. Once it is clear that bladder or urethral obstruction is not present and that the patient will be able to void spontaneously, the catheter should be removed.

3. Renal Ultrasound

Renal ultrasound studies can be very helpful in excluding urinary tract obstruction, even in patients with major renal insufficiency. It allows the determination of residual renal mass and excludes unexpected problems, such as renal tumors or perinephric collections of blood or pus in critically ill patients. It is the most valuable anatomic study from the standpoint of information obtained, ease of performance, and expense.

4. Computed Tomography

Computed tomography (CT) allows an even more precise look at the kidneys than does ultrasound. The renal parenchyma, collecting system, and vasculature can often be seen without the use of contrast material. Giving IV contrast to a patient with already diminished renal function can be a problem because it can cause complete oliguric renal failure.

5. Pyelography

If anuria is confirmed with a properly placed and patent Foley catheter and if the patient had an operative procedure or trauma in which the ureter(s) might have been injured or occluded by ligatures, pyelography is indicated. High-dose (drip-infusion) pyelography (IVP) with delayed films often reveals a reasonable nephrogram that shows whether or not the calyces are distended. It is also frequently possible to see the bladder. If this procedure is done in a reasonably short period of time after a possible ureteral obstruction, retrograde pyelography can sometimes be avoided. However, if the possibility of an obstructive lesion of the ureter still exists after the IVP, retrograde pyelography is indicated.

C. DIAGNOSIS OF ACUTE VASOMOTOR NEPHROPATHY

1. Clinical

If all volume deficits are more than adequately corrected, cardiac output is restored, hypotension is corrected, serum sodium, protein, and acid-base composition are reasonably normal, and yet the urine flow does not respond to osmotic or loop diuretics, acute vasomotor nephropathy is a likely diagnosis, provided that the urinary composition is compatible with that diagnosis.

AXIOM

If one assumes that renal function is good because the urinary output is normal or high in a critically ill or injured patient, the diagnosis of acute vasomotor nephropathy may be greatly delayed.

Although the rate of urine flow is usually monitored closely in critically ill or injured patients, it has serious limitations as an index of the functional status of the kidney. It is becoming increasingly apparent that complex changes occur in the kidney following trauma or sepsis, and sophisticated studies are usually required to demonstrate the functional abnormalities early when treatment or preventative measures are more apt to be successful.

Patients with acute renal failure often have an altered level of consciousness and are more sensitive to the soporific effects of drugs. However, these patients are unlikely to manifest localizing neurologic signs.

Renal failure patients often hypoventilate. Consequently, atelectasis and pulmonary infection are common. Patients with acute respiratory failure tend not to tolerate excess fluid, and with advancing uremia have even more of a tendency to exude fluid across their leaky pulmonary capillaries.

The qualitative platelet defect that occurs when the BUN level is more than 100 mg/dl may lead to occult bleeding, particularly in the gastrointestinal tract. This in turn may cause a disproportionately high BUN level.

Healing is slowed in patients with acute renal failure. Appropriate enteral nutrition may be helpful in this regard.

2. Laboratory Tests

a. Oliguric Renal Failure

The urine from patients with acute vasomotor nephropathy (AVN) may contain tubular epithelial cells, pigmented casts, 1^+ to 2^+ proteinuria, and red cells. However, none of these findings are constant, and patients with severe trauma or sepsis and normal renal function may have similar findings. The specific gravity in AVN is usually low, but it may be deceptively high because of increased quantities of protein or sugar in the urine.

The BUN is greatly influenced by protein metabolism and intake, and the rate of urea synthesis. However, BUNs over 100 mg/dl tend to correlate with obtundation in many patients with acute renal failure. Similar levels are also associated with decreased platelet adhesiveness due to the accumulation of guanidinosuccinic acid. In uncomplicated cases, the BUN can increase at a rate of 10 to 20 $mg \cdot dl^{-1} \cdot d^{-1}$, but in hypercatabolic states, the rise in BUN often exceeds 25 $mg \cdot dl^{-1} \cdot d^{-1}$.

Plasma creatinine concentrations in severe acute vasomotor nephropathy may increase at the rate of 2 to 3 $mg \cdot dl^{-1} \cdot d^{-1}$. A rise in serum creatinine of greater than 1 to 2 $mg \cdot dl^{-1} \cdot d^{-1}$ usually indicates a creatinine clearance of less than 10 ml/min. For reasons that are unclear from a biochemical standpoint, critically ill patients frequently decrease their production and excretion of creatinine after a certain degree of renal failure has developed. As a consequence, in acute renal failure, the serum creatinine may rise to only 5 to 6 mg/dl, even if almost no urine output is present. However, measurement of creatinine clearance will more accurately indicate the severity of the patient's renal failure.

The urine sodium concentration in the oliguric phase of acute renal failure is usually greater than 40 mEq/liter; the ratio of urine to plasma creatinine concentration is usually less than 20; and the ratio of BUN-to-plasma urea creatinine concentration is usually less than 10. Urine osmolarity is approximately the same as that of plasma in both oliguric and nonoliguric renal failure. Unfortunately, exceptions to these findings are frequent.

Since potassium excretion is usually closely related to urine volume, serum potassium levels may rise rapidly in oliguric patients, particularly in those with sepsis or extensive trauma.

AXIOM

An $FE_{Na} > 3\%$ in a patient with a rising BUN and creatinine is highly suggestive of AVN.

The best test for differentiating prerenal oliguria from AVN is the fractional excretion of sodium (FE_{Na}), which requires measuring serum and urine sodium and creatinine.

$$FE_{Na} = \frac{U_{Na}/P_{Na}}{U_{Cr}/P_{Cr}} \times 100\%.$$

Values less than 1% suggest the presence of intact tubular function with inadequate renal perfusion. Values of 1% to 3% are indeterminate and values $> 3\%$ usually indicate significant renal tubular dysfunction.

There is considerable evidence for varying degrees of persisting tubular function, even in patients with severe acute vasomotor nephropathy. Urinary acidification, for example, is a function of the distal tubule. The fact that many patients with acute renal failure have an acid urine, even with severe oliguria, supports the concept that tubular function may be intact and that the most important abnormality is a reduction in the GFR. This is also supported by the fact that potassium secretion, which is also a distal tubular function, is maintained, and the concentration of potassium in the urine in oliguric patients is usually relatively normal.

b. Nonoliguric Renal Failure

Nonoliguric vasomotor nephropathy is seldom recognized until there is a rise in the BUN, serum creatinine, or serum potassium levels. It is important, therefore, to measure the BUN, serum creatinine, and electrolytes daily during the first few days after any major trauma and during sepsis. Because elderly, debilitated, or septic patients may have serum creatinine levels that are normal and rise very slowly in spite of rather severe renal impairment, creatinine clearance studies may be very helpful in selected cases. Approximately 40% of our surgical ICU patients, who have had a normal urine output, BUN, and serum creatinine, have a creatinine clearance of less than 40 ml/min, indicating at least a moderate degree of AVN.

Although a 12- to 24-hour creatinine clearance study is more accurate, a 2-hour study, particularly if fluid intake through IVs and output through a Foley catheter are constant and the study is repeated daily, may provide important trending data.

The urinary constituents in nonoliguric renal failure may be quite variable. Urinary sodium is usually high in AVN, but it may be low if there is a salt deficiency, particularly in patients with massive burns. Formed elements are less prominent in the urine of the nonoliguric patients, perhaps because of the dilutional effect of the high urinary flow rates. Urine-to-plasma ratios of osmolarity, urea, and creatinine, however, are usually quite similar to those found in patients with oliguric renal failure.

V. TREATMENT OF RENAL FAILURE

A. TREATMENT OF OLIGURIA

The diagnosis and treatment of oliguria are closely related. In some instances, re-establishing an increased renal blood flow can help reduce the severity of the renal dysfunction. An organized plan should include correction of renal perfusion and chemical abnormalities and use of various diuretics as appropriate (Table 14.2).

1. Correction of Hypovolemia

Hypovolemic patients often respond favorably to a fluid challenge with increases in blood pressure, cardiac output, and urine output, but show little or no increases in the CVP or PAWP, initially. If this occurs, additional fluids should be given until the vital signs stabilize and the hourly urine flow rates exceed $0.5 \text{ ml} \cdot \text{kg}^{-1} \cdot \text{h}^{-1}$, or there is evidence of fluid overload.

Although cardiac output, systemic (peripheral) vascular resistance, and systemic (BP) are all important, renal blood flow seems to correlate best with left atrial pressure measurements, as reflected by the pulmonary artery wedge pres-

---

Table 14.2

TREATMENT OF OLIGURIA	1. Correct hypovolemia
	2. Improve cardiac output
	3. Correct hypotension
	4. Use of vasodilators
	5. Correct acidosis
	6. Correct hyponatremia
	7. Correct hypoproteinemia
	8. Use of diuretics

sures (PAWP). This relationship is thought to be due to a vasoconstrictive neural reflex that occurs in the kidneys when left ventricular preload is inadequate. Thus, "normalization" or a mild-moderate increase in the PAWP may help optimize blood flow to the kidneys.

Whenever possible, the patient's blood pressure should be maintained at or slightly above the patient's usual levels. Elderly people frequently have inadequate renal perfusion with a systolic pressure of less than 140 mm Hg.

a. Inotropoic Agents

(1) Dopamine

If systemic BP or cardiac output are not normal or are slightly greater than normal in spite of optimal fluid loading, inotropic support should be attempted. Dopamine, in dosages of 1 to 3 $\mu g \cdot kg^{-1} \cdot min^{-1}$, may significantly improve splanchnic and renal blood flow and increase urine output without increasing BP or cardiac output. At dosages of 5 to 10 $\mu g \cdot kg^{-1} \cdot min^{-1}$, BP and cardiac output usually rise and urine output may increase further. At dosages exceeding 20 to 50 $\mu g \cdot kg^{-1} \cdot min^{-1}$, there is an increasing vasoconstrictor response, which may also further increase urine flow.

In a study of adult cardiac surgical patients with postoperative oliguria and left ventricular dysfunction, dopamine infusions at 100 $\mu g/min$ improved creatinine clearance from 70 to 115 ml/min, osmolar clearance from 3.7 to 9.3 ml/min, and free-water clearance from -1.5 to -3.7 ml/min. Urinary sodium concentration increased from 15 to 20 mEq/liter. Overall, urine flow increased from 22 ml/h to 54 ml/h; however, 9 of 15 patients continued to have a urine output of less than 0.5 $ml \cdot kg^{-1} \cdot h^{-1}$. Increasing the dopamine infusions further to 200 $\mu g/min$ in these nine patients improved urine output to more than 0.5 $ml \cdot kg^{-1} \cdot h^{-1}$, and also improved all other renal function variables.

In one study of eight patients who were unresponsive to extracellular volume expansion and furosemide, the combination of dopamine, 1 to 3 $\mu g \cdot kg^{-1} \cdot min^{-1}$, and furosemide, 100 to 200 mg, as an IV bolus every 6 to 8 hours induced a brisk, lasting diuresis in all eight patients. Urine output rose from a mean of 0 to 10 ml/h before treatment to more than 100 ml/h immediately after the start of therapy. Substantial diuresis occurred for at least 48 to 72 hours and persisted when treatment was finally discontinued.

AXIOM

The renal vasodilatory action of dopamine may enhance delivery of furosemide to certain critical intrarenal areas.

(2) Use of Vasopressors

Production of an adequate volume of glomerular filtrate usually requires a mean arterial blood pressure of at least 40 to 50 mm Hg. In older patients with arteriosclerosis and extensive narrowing of renal arteries, a much higher perfusion pressure may be required. If oliguria and hypotension persist in spite of an adequate extracellular fluid (ECF) volume and the administration of inotropic agents, vasoconstrictor agents, such as dopamine in high doses or norepinephrine, may be tried. The use of such agents to raise the mean arterial pressure to 90 to 110 mm Hg may occasionally improve the urine flow rate. However, vasopressors are potentially hazardous, because they may reduce renal perfusion rather than improve it.

AXIOM

As a general rule, vasopressors should be used only as a last resort. However, they may be needed in individuals who have not responded to other therapy and require a high central aortic pressure to maintain vital organ perfusion.

b. Vasodilators

Not infrequently, especially after trauma, the RBF may be very low, in spite of adequate fluid volume and the use of inotropic agents. When persistent severe vasoconstriction is present, careful administration of a vasodilator may be indicated. An intra-arterial line to accurately monitor the blood pressure and a CVP or PAWP line to monitor filling pressures in the heart should be in place before a potent vasodilator is given to critically ill patients.

The systemic vasodilators used most frequently in critically ill patients are nitroprusside and nitroglycerin. The initial dose is usually $0.3 \, \mu g \cdot kg^{-1} \cdot min^{-1}$, or less. This may be cautiously increased, but the dose should probably not exceed $3.0 \, \mu g \cdot kg^{-1} \cdot min^{-1}$. Response to vasodilators may be judged by the warmth and color of the skin, blood pressure, and arteriovenous oxygen differences. If the skin becomes warmer and drier, diastolic pressure falls, pulse pressure increases, and the arteriovenous oxygen difference narrows, significant vasodilation has occurred. Since all vasodilators increase vascular capacity, they should be given only if the patient has an adequate ECF and plasma volumes, and if large intravenous lines are available to give fluid rapidly should the blood pressure fall.

2. Correction of Chemical Abnormalities

Although water restriction is generally the preferred method for treating dilutional hyponatremia, this method is often ineffective in the acutely injured patient because of a reduced functional ECF volume. Under such circumstances, careful administration of hypertonic (3%) saline may produce dramatic benefit and diuresis. It should be emphasized that the administration of hypertonic saline to a patient with vasomotor nephropathy can be somewhat hazardous, and most nephrologists prefer to correct the severe electrolyte abnormalities of AVN with peritoneal dialysis or hemodialysis.

3. Severe Acidosis

If a severe metabolic acidosis (pH < 7.10 to 7.15) persists in spite of adequate tissue perfusion, and if the patient is not overloaded with water and sodium, sodium bicarbonate in doses of 0.3 mEq per milliequivalent base deficit per kilogram may be given. For example, a 70-kg man with a base deficit of 9 mEq/liter can be given $0.3 \times 9 \times 70$ (i.e., 189) mEq of bicarbonate. Usually, sodium bicarbonate should not be administered faster than 3 to 5 mEq/min.

An acute respiratory acidosis should be corrected by improving ventilation, using ventilatory assistance if necessary. If the patient has a chronic respiratory acidosis, the Pco_2 should not be lowered faster than 5 mm Hg/h.

4. Hypoproteinemia

Plasma proteins of less than 2.0 to 2.5 g/dl may occasionally be associated with severe oliguria, which will persist until the protein levels are improved. In oliguric patients, it may be helpful to raise serum albumin levels above 2.5 g/dl. This may be done with intravenous albumin or plasma; however, more than 100 to 200 g of albumin may be required daily to maintain adequate plasma albumin concentrations. The use of albumin, especially in large quantities, is extremely controversial in these situations.

5. Use of Diuretics

There is much controversy concerning the value of diuretics in critically ill patients who are oliguric in spite of adequate fluid loading and vital signs. There is experimental evidence that high urine flow rates protect against many types of acute lung injury. Furthermore, patients with nonoliguric renal failure generally do much better than patients with oliguric renal failure requiring dialysis. Consequently, many clinicians believe that it is extremely important to maintain an adequate urine flow, even if large doses of diuretics are required. Others think that diuretics have a very limited role in preventing renal failure, and do not reduce the incidence, duration, or severity of acute renal failure. However, there is general agreement in the fact that nonoliguric patients are much easier to care for than oliguric patients. There is also agreement that diuretics should not be given unless oliguria persists despite adequate administration of fluid and good tissue perfusion. The diuresis that may result from these agents should not be allowed to cause hypovolemia. An adequate or increased blood volume and

Table 14.3

ACTION OF THE DIURETICS ON THE KIDNEY

	Mannitol, IV	Furosemide and Ethacrynic Acid, Oral or IV	Thiazides, Oral	Acetazolamide, Oral
Major action site	Proximal tubule ascending limb of loop of Henle	Ascending limb of loop of Henle	Loop of Henle distal tubule	Proximal tubule
Sodium reabsorption	I	IIII	III	I
Relative potency	Dose related	++++	+++	+
Clinical indications	Prerenal azotemia; cerebral edema	Pulmonary edema; edema with	BUN	Edema	Metabolic cor pulmonale

cardiac output must be maintained at all times. This may require the replacement of urine output volume for volume.

a. Agents Available

The diuretics used most frequently in intensive care units are furosemide and mannitol. Occasionally, ethacrynic acid, thiazides, or acetazolamide may be used (Table 14.3).

(1) Furosemide

Furosemide is an extremely potent loop diuretic, and it can increase urinary output in many patients about to develop acute vasomotor nephropathy. *Loop-acting diuretics* gain access to tubular fluid by the organic anion secretory system and, depending on the degree of binding to plasma proteins, by filtration. These agents act on the luminal side of the tubule to inhibit sodium chloride cotransport systems in the luminal membrane of the thick ascending limb of Henle's loop. Failure to observe a response to loop diuretics may be due to (1) failure of the drug to be secreted in patients with renal failure, or (2) a greatly increased rate of sodium reabsorption in the proximal convoluted tubule with reduced delivery of filtrate to the thick ascending limb. Relative degrees of impaired diuretic response may be overcome by administration of higher doses of the drug. However, some nephrologists believe that furosemide will not increase urinary output in established vasomotor nephropathy and may directly damage tubule cells and divert blood flow away from the renal cortex.

The recommended initial dose of furosemide is 20 to 40 mg intravenously. If an adequate response is not obtained, an 80-mg dose may be given. We often then double the dose until a bolus of at least 300 to 400 mg of furosemide has been given. If there is still severe oliguria, one can generally assume that acute renal failure is established.

(2) Mannitol

Mannitol is an osmotic diuretic that occasionally may be very helpful in establishing and maintaining an adequate rate of urine flow. It can be given in a variety of ways. Our current technique consists of a loading dose of 25 to 50 g given over a 15- to 30-minute period, followed by a constant infusion of 6.25 to 12.5 g/h for 6 to 8 hours or longer, depending on the patient's response.

The mechanisms by which this osmotic diuretic may reverse impending renal insufficiency are not known; however, it is thought that high rates of urine flow in the distal tubule may favorably influence the juxtaglomerular apparatus and the feedback loop controlling glomerular blood flow. Mannitol may also improve renal cortical blood flow and help to prevent the cortical ischemia that develops in severely injured or septic patients during hyponatremia. More important, mannitol may function as a free-radical scavenger.

Since mannitol may rapidly expand the blood volume prior to its diuretic effect, it should be used cautiously in the presence of heart disease or evidence of possible fluid overload. It is important to remember that the kidney is the sole route of excretion of mannitol. Administration of mannitol to a patient whose GFR is severely reduced may result in retention of a large amount of unwanted osmoles in the plasma.

(3) Ethacrynic Acid

In an occasional patient who is unresponsive to furosemide, 100 to 200 mg of ethacrynic acid intravenously may produce significant diuresis. Although it acts in a fashion similar to furosemide, ethacrynic acid is used infrequently because its side effects have included deafness and abnormal liver function tests. However, these reactions are usually seen only in patients with renal or hepatic failure, who were given large doses of this agent. Because of its toxicity and because it is so unlikely to be effective if furosemide has failed, some nephrologists do not use ethacrynic acid at all.

(4) Thiazides

The various thiazide diuretics act by interfering with renal tubular reabsorption of sodium and chloride. These agents are less potent than furosemide or ethacrynic acid and are generally given for long-term outpatient oral therapy of hypertension and congestive heart failure.

(5) Acetazolamide

Acetazolamide (Diamox) is an enzyme inhibitor. It acts specifically on carbonic anhydrase, which catalyzes the reversible reaction as follows:

$$H_2O + CO_2 \rightleftharpoons H_2CO_3.$$

Interference with this reaction decreases the kidney's ability to acidify urine and results in a diuresis of bicarbonate, sodium, and potassium. This is manifested in the blood as a hyperchloremic acidosis. Consequently, acetazolamide may be particularly useful in the presence of metabolic alkalosis, especially if the kidney can excrete bicarbonate. Acetazolamide is nontoxic and must be given by mouth. It is not very potent and loses its effectiveness in a few days.

6. Reduce Metabolite and Pigment Load

A thorough and immediate debridement of nonviable tissue and drainage of any suppurative collections are essential to reduce the quantity of vasoactive materials, nitrogenous substances, and pigments presented to the kidney. It may even be wise to remove any injured tissue whose viability is in doubt. Overly prolonged efforts to save an extremity in patients with severely impaired renal function may result in loss of life.

AXIOM

If the BUN rises faster than 25 mg·dl⁻¹·d (hypercatabolic renal failure), special efforts must be made to find and eradicate necrotic tissue or infected foci.

Myoglobin or hemoglobin can make urine appear dark red and the sediment may contain highly pigmented casts. These pigments are easily detected on the occult blood portion of the urinalysis dipstick and can be confirmed by lack of red blood cells on microscopic examination of the urine. If this test is not positive, neither substance is probably present in significant amounts.

Early alkaline diuresis may be effective in preventing acute renal failure from hemoglobinuria. Alkalinization is not effective for myoglobinuria, but high-volume diuresis (intravenous fluids and diuretics) is in order. Myoglobinuria most often follows traumatic muscle damage, but rhabdomyolysis may occur with various drugs (especially alcohol), heat stress, muscle disease, and various toxins.

Better and Stein point out that prevention of the systemic and renal complications of the crush syndrome requires early, vigorous treatment to sustain the circulation, with infusion of up to 1.5 liters of fluid per hour after the limbs have been freed. The urine pH should be kept above 6.5, using bicarbonate as needed for up to 36 hours. The urge to explore limbs and perform fasciotomy is discouraged except for compartment syndrome with high compartment pressures due to ischemia.

In a recent study, a special effort was made to maintain a urinary pH above 6.5 and diuresis of at least 300 ml/h in seven patients with severe crush injuries of the extremities. A solution containing sodium chloride, 75 mEq/liter, in 5% dextrose was rapidly infused through a central venous line. Sodium bicarbonate, 44 mEq/liter, was added to alternating 500-ml bottles. If an adequate urine output was not obtained, but the CVP rose by more than 5 cm H_2O, a 20% mannitol solution was given in a dose of 1 g/kg. An average of 568 ml of fluid was needed each hour to maintain an adequate diuresis. However, renal failure did not occur in any of these patients.

7. Anemia and Transfusions

Anemia frequently accompanies renal failure, and a hematocrit of 25% is not unusual. If complications require blood transfusions, the blood should be cross-matched carefully to prevent even minor incompatibilities, particularly if the patient has previously been given O-negative or type-specific blood. The transfused blood should also be as fresh as possible.

If a patient receiving a blood transfusion develops oliguria, the possibility of a mismatched transfusion must be considered and appropriate steps taken immediately. These usually include stopping the transfusion, increasing urine volume with fluid and/or diuretics, and rendering the urine alkaline with sodium bicarbonate.

8. Fluid Intake

a. Oliguric Renal Failure

The most frequent error in the management of patients with established oliguric renal failure is failure to adequately restrict fluid intake. In a patient with extensive tissue destruction, fluid shifts, and blood losses, the proper volume of fluid to administer can be very difficult to accurately determine. Therefore, it is imperative that the patient's fluid balance and vital signs be closely monitored. In some instances, continuous monitoring of the CVP of PAWP may be required for several days.

The patient's weight should also be monitored daily. Any increase in body weight must be considered due to fluid accumulations, whereas a weight loss greater than 0.3 to 0.5 kg/d implies inadequate fluid replacement. Some patients with excessive catabolism due to severe trauma, burns, or sepsis, however, may lose more than 1.5 kg/d of body weight unless adequate nutrition is given. These weight changes must be considered when evaluating the fluid needs of the patient. Attempts to prevent weight losses greater than 0.5 kg/d in patients with severe catabolism by giving fluid can easily cause fluid overload.

Most patients with oliguric renal failure require only 400 to 500 ml of fluid (about 250 ml/m² of body surface area), in addition to replacement of all measured external losses to sustain a proper fluid balance. However, much larger quantities of fluid may be required to maintain normal vital signs in patients with trauma or sepsis who have large ongoing external or third-space fluid losses. When third-space fluid is mobilized during recovery, the danger of an expanded plasma volume is great. In such instances, continuous arteriovenous hemofiltration (CAVH) or dialysis may be required to remove the excess fluid.

b. Nonoliguric Renal Failure

Patients with acute vasomotor nephropathy have a better chance for survival if a normal or increased rate of urine flow can be maintained. The same general fluid formula applies to patients with either oliguric or nonoliguric renal failure, that is, $250 \text{ ml} \cdot \text{m}^{-2} \cdot \text{d}^{-1}$, plus measured fluid losses. However, if the urine flow rate declines, it is important to be certain that it has not fallen because of hypovolemia.

9. Nutritional Support

There is increasing evidence of improved survival in patients given early adequate caloric intake plus essential amino acids during the treatment of renal failure. The caloric requirements of some critically ill and injured patients may exceed 30 to 35 nonprotein $cal \cdot kg^{-1} \cdot day^{-1}$. If these calories are not supplied by exogenous sources, the patient's own fat and muscle will be used to supply them, and weight loss, muscle wasting, and increasing azotemia will result. If the patient's gastrointestinal tract is functioning, high-calorie, low-water-content foods can be given by mouth to supply at least 25 to 30 g nonprotein $cal \cdot kg^{-1} \cdot d^{-1}$ and 0.5 to 1.0 g $protein \cdot kg^{-1} \cdot d^{-1}$.

Intravenous hyperalimentation of fluids containing 10% to 40% glucose and 4.2% to 8.4% amino acids may be administered by injection into large central veins. Intravenous hyperalimentation is probably the most important single advance in the treatment of these patients. In patients with oliguric renal failure, who are sustaining minimal external losses, it is difficult to provide adequate caloric intake unless intravenous fat emulsions are used. In nonoliguric renal failure, fluid intake restrictions are less confining, and it is easier to provide the needed calories.

With parenteral nutrition, equal amounts of essential and nonessential amino acids can be used. Over a period of several days, the concentration of dextrose is increased from 10% to as high as 40%, and the amino acids may be given in concentrations of 4.2% to 8.4%.

The electrolyte composition of the total parenteral nutrition (TPN) is important, and a typical solution has an Na^+ concentration of approximately 75 mEq/liter with 50 mEq/liter Cl^- and 25 mEq/liter acetate. Calcium (8.1 mEq/liter) is almost always given. Magnesium replacement depends on serum magnesium levels. Potassium chloride, acetate, or phosphate may or may not be necessary depending on blood levels. Phosphorus is usually not administered in large amounts in acute renal failure. However, when anabolic, such patients may use a great deal of phosphorus in protein synthesis and become hypophosphatemic, even when they are anuric.

Amino acid administration may quickly cause a metabolic acidosis, while excessive acetate can cause metabolic alkalosis.

10. Prevention of Gastric Erosions

Since there is an increased frequency of gastric erosions and peptic ulceration in patients with renal failure, particularly if sepsis or acute respiratory failure has developed, antacids and/or H_2 antagonists are indicated to maintain the gastric pH above 4.5. One or two ounces of antacid or food may also be given every hour through a nasogastric tube, aspirating the stomach for 5 to 10 minutes, and checking the gastric pH before the next dose. Antacids containing magnesium should be avoided in renal failure, because serum magnesium levels may rise rapidly to dangerous levels in such patients. Aluminum hydroxide may be particularly useful because it can also help to control the hyperphosphatemia often seen with acute renal failure.

11. Hyperkalemia

If acute oliguric vasomotor nephropathy (Table 14.4) develops, hyperkalemia and fluid retention are the biggest threats to the patient's life. With severe

Table 14.4

TREATMENT OF OLIGURIC ACUTE VASOMOTOR NEPHROPATHY

1. Reduce renal load (of pigments and metabolites)
2. Reduce fluid intake to 400 to 500 ml/d plus measured losses
3. Supply adequate calories and protein
4. Provide antacids and manage electrolytes (especially potassium)
5. Administer cation exchange resins p.r.n.
6. Provide peritoneal dialysis or hemodialysis p.r.n.

a. Etiology

trauma or sepsis, the blood potassium level may rise rapidly to levels exceeding 6.0 mEq/liter, in spite of hemodilution. This is predominantly the result of movement of intracellular potassium into the ECF. It is even more severe if the patient is also acidotic.

Since large quantities of potassium are released from tissue cells in patients with severe trauma or sepsis, and since the main route of excretion of potassium is through the kidneys, serum potassium levels may rise very rapidly in these patients if they become oliguric. If the patient is receiving multiple transfusions of old blood (which may contain up to 35 mEq potassium per liter) or large amounts of aqueous (potassium) penicillin, which contains 1.67 mEq of potassium per million units, the serum potassium will rise even faster.

The serum levels of potassium must be followed closely, and blood samples for these determinations may have to be drawn every 4 to 6 hours. Trauma to blood, while it is being drawn, can cause hemolysis of red blood cells, resulting in a false elevation of potassium levels in the sample.

b. Effects of Hyperkalemia

High concentrations of potassium can cause conduction blocks initially in the atria, then in the AV node, and finally in the ventricles, with the heart eventually stopping in diastole. Continuous cardioscopic monitoring is very important in patients with acute renal failure, because ECG changes are often manifested prior to the onset of serious arrhythmias. Initially, elevated levels of intracellular potassium are often shown on the ECG by high, peaked T waves. Increasingly, severe hyperkalemia can cause widening of the QRS complex, and sine waves usually herald a cardiac arrest.

c. Emergency Treatment of Hyperkalemia

The emergency management of hyperkalemia with arrhythmias should proceed rapidly (Table 14.5). If cardiac toxicity is severe, calcium infusion is the most effective measure for correction. Intravenous infusions of 10 to 20 ml of 10% calcium gluconate or calcium chloride may be administered in 15 to 20 minutes and repeated every 4 to 6 hours, or more often as needed. Extreme caution is necessary in the digitalized patient, because calcium increases the incidence and risk of digitalis toxicity.

It is generally felt that alkalinization of the plasma by intravenous infusion of sodium bicarbonate may rapidly lower plasma potassium levels by causing potassium to shift into the cells. However, a recent letter to the editor by Battle, Salem, and Levin, and an article by Blumberg and colleagues, noted that sodium bicarbonate may not work at all or may take several hours to have an effect. Nevertheless, one can try one to two ampules of sodium bicarbonate (each ampule containing 44.6 mEq), administered slowly intravenously at about 2 to 5 mEq/min. The sodium infused may also counteract hyperkalemic toxicity, especially in hyponatremia or volume-depleted patients, because of the opposing effects of sodium and potassium on cardiac function.

Infusions of glucose with insulin can also be helpful. A number of nephrologists believe that rapid correction of life-threatening hyperkalemia is best accomplished by infusion of insulin, which rapidly translocates potassium into

---

Table 14.5

EMERGENCY TREATMENT OF HYPERKALEMIA

1. Calcium gluconate or chloride (10%): 5 to 20 ml in 10 to 20 min
2. Sodium bicarbonate: 1 to 2 ampules intravenously in 10 to 20 min
3. Glucose and insulin (50 ml 50% G/W or with 5 to 10 units of insulin followed by 20% G/W with 40 to 80 units of insulin per liter
4. Cation exchange resins (sodium polystyrene sulfonate) 40 to 80 g/d in divided doses
5. Peritoneal dialysis or hemodialysis

cells. Fifty milliliters of 50% glucose with 5 to 10 units of insulin is given rapidly followed by 100 to 200 ml of 20% glucose with 40 to 80 units of insulin. The transport of glucose into the cell and its transformation to glycogen causes binding of potassium. This effectively removes some of the serum potassium from the blood.

Inhalation of beta$_2$-adrenergic agonists, such as albuterol, that are usually used to treat asthma, can also lower serum potassium levels. Infusions of epinephrine may also lower serum potassium levels in about half the patients. Alpha-adrenergic agonists tend to raise serum potassium levels.

Potassium can be removed from the body by the use of cation exchange resins such as sodium polystyrene sulfonate (K-exalate). This technique, however, is much slower than the emergency methods described above and may require 4 to 12 hours to lower serum potassium levels significantly. If the gastrointestinal tract is functioning, up to 20 g can be given by mouth three or four times a day. To potentiate the effect of the resin and to prevent fecal impaction, 20 ml of a 70% sorbitol solution is usually administered with each dose of resin. In patients who cannot take medications by mouth, or when a more rapid effect is desired, the resin can be administered as a retention enema. The enema consists of 50 g of resin suspended in a mixture of 50 ml of 70% sorbitol and 100 to 150 ml of tap water. The enema should be retained for at least half an hour and may be repeated three or four times a day.

If extensive tissue necrosis or hemolysis is present, acute dialysis should be provided in addition to hourly sorbitol enemas. Such a patient may require hemodialysis two or three times a day for 3 to 4 hours at a time.

12. Hypokalemia

Hypokalemia is most apt to occur during the polyuric (recovery) phase of acute renal failure. Patients who develop acute renal failure may already be K$^+$ depleted because of long-term diuretic therapy. If potassium levels fall below 3.0 mEq/liter, they should be increased to greater than 4 mEq/liter, or a level at which no dysrhythmias related to hypokalemia are likely. However, such replacement must be given very cautiously, using increments at one half the usual rate of replacement. No specific formula for K$^+$ replacement in this situation is available, but if the patient has a normal serum pH and a serum K$^+$ less than 3 mEq/liter, the total body K$^+$ deficit is usually greater than 200 mEq.

13. Metabolic Acidosis

The kidneys normally excrete about 70 mEq of nonvolatile acid per day. This acid load is derived from food metabolism and bicarbonate losses from the gastrointestinal tract. The acidosis of acute renal failure is rarely life threatening, and serum HCO$_3^-$ is usually not less than 15 mEq/liter. However, lower values suggest an additional cause of the acidosis and may require hemodialysis.

If the serum HCO$_3^-$ is 15 mEq/liter, or greater, in patients who have acute renal failure and an increased anion gap acidosis, specific treatment without the administration of large amounts of NaHCO$_3^-$ is preferred; however, if the HCO$_3^-$ is less than 15 mEq/liter, some bicarbonate may be needed to correct the HCO$_3^-$ to at least 20 mEq/liter. In instances of severe, combined metabolic acidosis, hemodialysis may be necessary to maintain a serum pH above 7.25 to 7.30.

14. Hyponatremia

Hyponatremia is common in acute oliguric renal failure, but is not usually a serious problem. The most common cause is the administration of fluids, such as 5% dextrose in water, that are too dilute, especially if the patient cannot excrete the water excess. Unless the patient is perspiring excessively, only gastrointestinal losses require replacement with sodium-containing fluids. The administration of maintenance fluids to a patient with oliguric renal failure is best achieved by 5% dextrose in one half normal saline. This fluid can be adjusted to nearly normal saline by the addition of one ampule of NaHCO$_3^-$ per liter, when indicated.

Serum sodium concentrations in oliguric renal failure usually rise or fall because of changes in total water content, not because of changes in the total body content of sodium. However, in nonoliguric renal failure, the sodium losses in the urine must be carefully monitored and replaced. In some individuals, urine sodium losses may exceed 150 to 200 mEq/d.

15. Hypocalcemia

Patients with acute renal failure to tend to develop low total and ionized calcium levels. The formation of 1,25-dihydrocholecalciferol, which is the active metabolite of vitamin D, is reduced, and serum calcium levels are further depressed as the serum phosphorus rises. However, tetany is unusual.

An unusual source of hypocalcemia may occur in patients with rhabdomyolytic renal failure as calcium is deposited within the damaged muscle.

16. Hypermagnesemia

In acute renal failure, magnesium levels may rise along with potassium, and extremely high levels could be lethal. However, values greater than 4 mEq/liter are usually avoidable, if the patient is not given any magnesium in the form of cathartics or antacids.

17. Hyperphosphatemia

Phosphate retention and hyperphosphatemia, by lowering serum calcium levels, can aggravate the secondary hyperparathyroidism that often develops rather early in most patients with chronic renal failure. Hyperphosphatemia rarely develops before renal function has declined to about 25% of normal, and consequently, the absence of hyperphosphatemia in early renal failure does not mean that phosphate metabolism is unaltered. Normal or low serum phosphorus levels are often found in mild renal insufficiency because the secretion of parathyroid hormone has already increased and has led to decreased reabsorption of phosphate in the renal tubules.

Because of the adverse effects of phosphate retention, major therapeutic efforts should be directed toward the control of serum phosphorus levels in patients with severe renal failure. Such patients are commonly given aluminum or calcium salts to bind phosphorus in the intestine, and thereby reduce serum concentrations of phosphorus. Potentially, such salts may bind either dietary or endogenous phosphorus.

In a recent study, Shiller and associates found that calcium acetate increased fecal excretion of phosphorus by binding both dietary and endogenous phosphorus, but the binding of dietary phosphorus was quantitatively more important. For the most efficient phosphorus binding, calcium should be given with enteral feedings.

18. Decreased Thyroxine

Thyroid function in patients with acute renal failure is often decreased, resulting in low levels of T_3 and T_4. However, reversed T_3 levels (rT_3) may be elevated. This combination of findings has been referred to as the sick euthyroid syndrome. If a patient with acute renal failure has decreased thyroxine (T_4) levels, thyroid function may still be adequate as long as the level of thyroid-stimulating hormone (TSH) is normal.

19. Hyperglycemia

Critically ill patients with renal failure tend to have insulin resistance and hyperglycemia. In addition, increased hepatic glucose production and growth hormone are present. If blood glucose levels are greater than 250 mg/dl, a continuous IV drip of low-dose insulin may be helpful. However, in diabetics, as renal function deteriorates, there is less loss of insulin in the kidney, and it may deceptively appear as if the diabetes is improving.

20. Antibiotics

In the absence of any identifiable infection, prophylactic antibiotics are probably contraindicated. If antibiotics are required, the dosages must be carefully monitored with peak and trough levels, particularly if they are excreted by the kidneys.

Table 14.6

INDICATIONS FOR DIALYSIS IN RENAL FAILURE	1. Uremia 2. Fluid overload 3. Hypertension 4. Electrolyte disturbances, especially hyperkalemia 5. Acid-base disturbances, especially metabolic acidosis 6. Pericardial effusions 7. Hemostasis abnormalities

21. Dialysis

Despite major improvements in dialysis techniques and in the management of critically ill or injured patients, the mortality rate in patients developing acute vasomotor nephropathy often exceeds 70%. Although it is generally believed that vigorous, early dialysis improves the survival of patients with acute renal failure, the mortality figures with acute renal failure are not markedly different from those of 20 years ago. The mortality rates in patients referred for dialysis for renal failure associated with severe sepsis still often exceed 90%.

Hemodialysis (HD) and peritoneal dialysis (PD) came into wide use for the treatment of renal failure in the 1960s. Although the basic principles of dialysis have remained the same, many refinements have improved dialysis therapy during the past decade. These include the use of new "high-efficiency" dialyzers and continuous long-term ultrafiltration.

a. Indications for Dialysis

There are specific indications for dialysis (Table 14.6), but the physicians must also make a clinical judgment in each case regarding its potential benefits and risks. In an ICU setting, fluid overload is the most frequent reason to institute dialysis. However, this problem is increasingly being treated with ultrafiltration, whereby extracellular fluid is removed without exposure to dialysate.

In patients with normal renal function, hyponatremia is usually treated with fluid restriction or diuretics, but these steps may not be adequate in patients with oliguric renal failure. Altered sensorium or seizures in patients with acute renal failure and hyponatremia may be a manifestation of hypo-osmolality and increased brain water, rather than uremia. This may also be treated by dialysis or ultrafiltration.

Hyperkalemia sufficient to produce cardiac conduction or rhythm disturbances is a frequent complication of acute renal failure. In instances where other measures are ineffective or not feasible, hemodialysis provides a rapid means of removing potassium. However, other methods of correcting the hyperkalemia should not be withheld while waiting for dialysis to become effective.

Metabolic acidosis with an enlarged anion gap may be seen in association with lactic acidosis, ketoacidosis, and renal failure. Dialysis in those circumstances can provide a buffer, in the form of acetate or lactate, both of which can be metabolized into bicarbonate.

Occasionally, uremic patients develop a coagulopathy caused by impaired platelet aggregation, especially when the BUN exceeds 75 to 100 mg/dl. Dialysis may be very helpful in reversing this problem; however, the heparin for hemodialysis may temporarily make the platelet problem worse. DDAVP, a synthetic analogue of arginine vasopressin (ADH), may control such bleeding quite effectively.

Very large pericardial effusions may be seen with chronic renal failure. Occasionally, pericardiocentesis, or a pericardial window, is required, but dialysis will usually help relieve this problem. However, 6% to 18% of patients undergoing dialysis develop pericarditis.

Table 14.7

COMPARISON OF TYPICAL
VALUES FOR HEMODIALYSIS
AND PERITONEAL DIALYSIS

Type of Dialysis	Clearance		Inulin/ Urea Ratio	Blood Flow (ml/min)	Dialysate Flow (ml/min)	Total Surface Area (m²)
	Urea (ml/min)	Inulin (ml/min)				
Hemodialysis	150	5	0.03	200–300	350–500	0.7–2
Peritoneal dialysis	20–25	5	0.25	?60–80	30–40	1–2

Adapted from Nolph, KD, et al: Determinants of low clearance of small solutes during peritoneal dialysis. Kidney Int 13:117, 1978.

b. Peritoneal Dialysis

There are many similarities between hemodialysis (HD) and peritoneal dialysis (PD) (Table 14.7). Both rely on diffusion of a solute down a concentration gradient. The ability of a solute to diffuse through a peritoneal membrane depends on its molecular weight and ability to bind to protein. Convective transfer also plays a role in PD. HD has a higher clearance rate for low molecular weight substances such as urea, but PD is equally effective for the clearance of middle molecules in the weight range of inulin. Furthermore, if continuous PD is used, the cumulative clearance of larger molecular weight substances exceeds that of HD. Since the middle molecules may include uremic toxins, PD may be in some instances a more effective therapy. As with HD, peritoneal solute clearance is limited by its permeability to various solutes, peritoneal blood flow rate, and dialysate flow rate.

The ultrafiltration rate is highest at the initiation of the PD. This accounts for the fact that dwell time can be greatly reduced if rapid fluid removal is needed. However, if the dwell time is increased from 1 hour to 4 to 8 hours and 4.25% dextrose solution is used, one can achieve very effective ultrafiltration. With the longer dwell times, ultrafiltration slows, and after osmotic equilibration is reached, absorption of the dialysate fluid into the body may occur.

Peritoneal dialysis is much simpler to perform than hemodialysis. Since there is no extracorporeal blood circulation and the dialysate is readily available in bags or bottles, attention need only be given to peritoneal access and sterility. The dialysate infuses into the peritoneum by gravity, is allowed to dwell within the abdomen, and is then gravity drained into another bag and discarded. With shorter dwell times and more frequent dialysis cycles, extensive nursing attention is required.

There are a number of advantages to peritoneal dialysis. A dialysis machine and technically trained personnel are not required. The likelihood of disequilibrium symptoms and hypotension is decreased. Patients with borderline low blood pressure or severely compromised left ventricular function tend to tolerate fluid removal with peritoneal dialysis better than with hemodialysis. The technique does not require systemic heparinization, and there is less risk of bleeding.

However, there are some disadvantages. The presence of the peritoneal catheter may be associated with bowel perforation, intra-abdominal bleeding, or major infections. "Third spacing" of fluid into the peritoneal cavity can lead to intravascular depletion. A large volume of intra-abdominal fluid can cause pleural effusions and elevated diaphragms, with an increased likelihood of atelectasis and pneumonia.

Peritoneal dialysis is protein depleting, and with recent abdominal surgery, dialysis may be ineffective. The reduced splanchnic blood flow in hypotensive patients, makes this form of dialysis inefficient. Because of its low efficiency, patients with increased metabolism or marked catabolism may not be adequately dialyzed.

Manji and colleagues recently pointed out another problem with peritoneal dialysis that occurs if the dialysate has high glucose levels. Using indirect calorimetry and analysis of the dialysis effluent for its dextrose concentrations, it was found that four of five patients absorbed more than 500 g of dextrose from the dialysate in 24 hours. This could cause hyperglycemia, worse respiratory failure, and hepatic steatosis. Consequently, the dextrose from dialysis fluid must be taken into account when determining the nutritional needs and status of patients on peritoneal dialysis.

c. Hemodialysis

Hemodialysis is the preferred treatment of most patients with acute severe oliguric renal failure. Laboratory abnormalities and volume excess can be corrected rapidly in the early part of a 3- or 4-hour treatment. Because they are treated for only a portion of the day, the patients are readily available for other therapy.

(1) Physiologic Principles

Solute removal during hemodialysis depends primarily on passive diffusion across a semipermeable membrane. The solute concentration gradient across the membrane is the major driving force for transfer of the solutes. As equilibrium between the concentrations of solute in the blood and dialysate is approached, there is decreased net movement of solute.

Blood and dialysate flow rates are adjusted to replenish the supply of incoming solute available for diffusion. Higher flow rates also increase the turbulence of flow through the artificial kidney and break up areas of decreased flow, which tend to occur near the membrane. The relatively high viscosity of blood (3.5 to 4.0 times that of water) predisposes to the creation of a "boundary layer" at the blood-membrane interface. As these layers are broken up, fresh blood with higher solute levels can be carried to the membrane surface for exchange. High hematocrit and plasma protein levels increase blood viscosity and may adversely affect mass transfer.

The relation between blood flow rate and solute removal, expressed as clearance, is not a straight line. The curve plateaus at a point at which membrane area and solute permeability limit diffusion. For urea (molecular weight 60), the maximum flow-dependent dialysance for most artificial kidneys is reached at a blood flow rate of 300 ml per minute. Beyond that, there is little additional increase in transfer of urea. Most systems try to use a dialysate flow of 450 to 500 ml/min to maintain efficiency of mass transfer and economy of dialysate.

The dialytic removal of protein-free water, ultrafiltration, is the result of the hydrostatic pressure gradient applied across membrane. The ease with which a device ultrafilters depends on its water permeability and surface area.

If the ultrafiltration rate is sufficiently high (>30 ml/min), poorly diffusible solutes with molecular weights in the range of 300 to 5000 (middle molecules) are removed by convective mass transfer. Solvent drag, the friction between water and solute, permits these larger substances to cross the membrane. The large volumes of water ultrafiltered across the membrane help increase the net mass transfer of these poorly diffusible solutes.

The type of membrane used can be important. Most commercially available artificial kidneys are made of cuprophane, a specially treated cellulose material. Early and striking formation of C3a, C5a, and terminal complement complexes occur in chronic uremia patients who are undergoing regular hemodialysis treatment with dialyzers made of cuprophane. In contrast, noncellulosic membranes (e.g., polysulfane, polyacrylonitrile, or polymethylmethacrylate) do not cause significant complement activation. Neutrophil activation is increased more in patients with acute (vs. chronic) renal failure undergoing dialysis, and it is increased even further by superimposed sepsis. Cellulose-containing dialysis membranes cause even further activation of neutrophils.

(2) Access

HD requires access to the patient's vascular space. The vessels used should be large enough to permit blood flow rates of at least 300 ml per minute. Direct cannulation of an artery and a nearby vein can be achieved by surgical cutdown. This approach, however, sacrifices the vessels used and is limited by local thrombosis or infection. The availability of polytetrafluoroethylene or polytef (Teflon), a relatively bioinert material, led to the development of a variety of indwelling arteriovenous shunts.

Femoral vein catheterization can provide quick and simple access for dialysis. Initially, both the femoral vein and artery were catheterized using the Seldinger technique. With mechanical devices available to allow the use of a single cannula with separate internal openings to two fused catheters, catheterization of only the vein is possible.

More recently, flexible, radiopaque double-lumen catheters have been inserted into the subclavian vein, and these can be used to provide immediate dialysis. Catheter patency is maintained by heparin-saline infusion or by flushing the catheter twice daily (every 12 hours) with 2 to 3 ml (2000 to 3000 units) of heparin. The latter technique allows the patient to be free of an IV connection. The catheter can be easily changed weekly.

Patients with chronic renal failure will probably have some form of permanent vascular access. This is generally an arteriovenous fistula, which is a surgically created direct anastomosis between an artery (usually the radial) and a nearby vein (usually the cephalic). Occasionally, because of either poor vessels or repeated loss of fistulas due to thrombosis, prosthetic materials, such as polytetrafluoroethylene (Gore Tex), are used to connect an artery and vein in the arm or forearm.

(3) Hemodialysis Machines

The dialysis machine delivers blood and dialysate to the artificial kidney. The machine consists of a blood pump, a dialysate delivery system, and a number of safety devices. The speed of the blood pump can be used to adjust blood flow rate. Concentrated dialysate is diluted with water to a ratio of 34:1. It can be mixed either in a large (100 to 200 liters) tank (batch method) or by an on-line proportioning system. The batch system, often used for coil dialyzers, requires that the solution be discarded and remixed during the treatment, as the dialysate solute concentration is raised and the concentration gradient diminishes. The on-line proportioning system provides a continuous supply of fresh dialysate to the artificial kidney. Because mixed dialysate is not stored, the machine is small and readily portable, allowing easy mobility from the dialysis unit to the intensive care unit.

d. Dialysate Composition

Dialysate is an electrolyte solution with solute concentrations designed to correct the patient's abnormal physiologic state (Table 14.8). Because one of the major

Table 14.8

COMPOSITION OF FREQUENTLY USED DIALYSATES

Component	Hemodialysis	Peritoneal Dialysis
Na^+	130–146 mEq/L	132 mEq/L
K^+	0–3 mEq/L	0
Cl^-	96–115 mEq/L	96 mEq/L
Acetate	36 mEq/L	—
Lactate	—	40 mEq/L
Ca^{++}	3.25 mEq/L	3.5 mEq/L
Mg^{++}	1.5 mEq/L	0.5, 1.5 mEq/L
Glucose	0–250 mg/dL	1.5%, 347 mOsm/L
		2.5%, 398 mOsm/L
		4.3%, 486 mOsm/L

functions of dialysis is to correct metabolic acidosis, the dialysate must contain a source of alkali. Lactate is the alkali source for most PD solutions, although acetate has also been used. There is no significant difference in peritoneal clearance of either base. The sodium (Na^+) and potassium (K^+) concentrations in the dialysate are chosen to cause a net removal of these cations.

Due to a low concentration gradient from dialysate to blood, there is minimal magnesium (Mg^{++}) transfer during dialysis, and a safe physiologic blood level is maintained. However, exogenous Mg^{++} intake may occasionally necessitate the use of low Mg^{++} peritoneal dialysates.

The dialysate concentration of ionized calcium of 3.5 mEq/liter causes a positive calcium balance during dialysis. Glucose may be added to hemodialysis dialysate to protect diabetics from hypoglycemia and reduce the loss of amino acids. In peritoneal dialysis, glucose provides the osmotic driving force for ultrafiltration and is a significant source of calories.

In certain instances, drugs may be added to the peritoneal dialysate. When an HD catheter is first used, heparin is often added to the dialysate for the first three to five exchanges to help prevent clotting of the catheter.

e. General Care

Patients should be weighed carefully before and after dialysis, because actual measurement of fluid loss on HD is not easily performed. Electrocardiographic monitoring and supplemental oxygen should be used, because of the known changes in cardiac output, oxygen transport, and complement activation that occur with hemodialysis.

No medications should be given during dialysis unless everyone is aware of their potential impact. Procedures, such as endoscopy or bronchoscopy, may cause dysrhythmias or hypotension and should not be performed during dialysis. Although there is a tendency for patients to become hypotensive during hemodialysis, this should be prevented and/or corrected rapidly with fluid and/or infusions of albumin or another colloid. Patients with nonoliguric renal failure may develop oliguria because of hemodialysis-associated hypotension.

f. Hemodialysis Hypotension

Hypotension during hemodialysis may be due to hypovolemia, decreased cardiac reserve, autonomic insufficiency (especially in elderly diabetics), rapid decrease in plasma osmolality, and acetate-induced decreases in systemic vascular resistance. The hypotension can be prevented or treated by making sure the patient is not hypovolemic prior to or during the hemodialysis. This may be helped by using isovolemic dialysis (i.e., not removing fluid), initially. Increasing dialysate sodium concentrations from 140 to 150 mEq/liter may help. One should also withhold antihypertensive or negative inotropic drugs before dialysis. The dialysate temperature can also be set 1° to 2°C below the patient's core temperature to help prevent vasodilation. In women and patients with decreased muscle mass, bicarbonate rather than acetate should be used in the dialysate.

g. Hemodialysis Modifications

Patients undergoing conventional HD are usually dialyzed for 4 to 6 hours, three times per week, using a dialysis membrane with a surface area of 1 to 2 m². Blood flow rates are 200 to 300 ml/min, and dialysate flow rates are 350 to 500 ml/min. Although many patients do reasonably well on this regimen, unexplained clinical deterioration, or suboptimal relief of symptoms, is generally treated with an empiric trial of increased solute removal. This can be achieved by increasing blood flow rate, membrane size or permeability, or time on dialysis.

(1) Sequential Ultrafiltration and Dialysis

The removal by ultrafiltration of more than 2.0 liters of fluid per treatment, using conventional HD techniques, is frequently accompanied by hypotension, nausea or vomiting, or muscle cramps. Researchers have presumed that these effects are the result of depletion of intravascular volume that is more rapid than its replenishment by mobilization of extravascular fluid.

Because of its efficacy, the technique of isolated ultrafiltration is commonly used in fluid-overloaded patients who tolerate other types of fluid removal poorly. However, ultrafiltration must be followed by an appropriate period of standard HD (to restore dialysate flow and lower the hydrostatic pressure gradient) to achieve adequate solute removal. Even at an ultrafiltration rate as high as 35 ml/min, the clearance of urea is only 35 ml/min. This is much less than the 150 ml/min usually attained with routine HD.

(2) Hemofiltration

This procedure involves the use of a high hydrostatic pressure gradient and a membrane with increased water and solute permeability. The net effect is a high ultrafiltration rate. Essentially all of the ultrafiltrate is replaced with a physiologic electrolyte solution to prevent volume depletion. Dialysate is not necessary with hemofiltration because no diffusion takes place and solute removal occurs entirely by ultrafiltration. The major potential advantages of hemofiltration are better control of fluid balance and hypertension.

(3) Continuous Arteriovenous Hemofiltration (CAVH)

CAVH has now been successfully applied to the treatment of a rather large number of critically ill patients. A small, hollow fiber filter made of a polysulfone membrane (Amicon Diafilter) permits continuous ultrafiltration at an average rate of 10 liters per day. Sufficient hydrostatic pressure for ultrafiltration can be generated in most patients by connecting the device to an artery and a vein through an AV shunt or fistula. Continuous heparin infusion to prevent clotting of the filter and fluid replacement is required.

This technique can be substituted for HD or PD, and is particularly desirable when hemoaccess and hemodialysis equipment is not readily available. It is also useful in patients with fluid overload or large fluid requirements, as in IV hyperalimentation, in which fluid removal is a major objective. Furthermore, there is often sufficient urea removal to prevent severe azotemia, except in hypercatabolic patients. Continuous arteriovenous hemofiltration is also valuable for patients with hemodynamic instability or decreased serum proteins.

Patients with high hematocrit, atherosclerotic peripheral arteries, or hypercoagulability may not do well with hemofiltration. The technique also requires a reasonably sophisticated knowledge of heparin use, blood flow calculation, and fluid volume management.

With the increasing emphasis on nutritional support, many renal units now use continuous AV hemofiltration to prevent fluid overload, while administering calories and essential amino acids by the intravenous route. Bartlett and colleagues found that using continuous arteriovenous hemofiltration to achieve a positive energy balance resulted in a significant increase in survival rate (38% versus 9%) compared to patients with persisting energy deficits.

Voerman and associates recently emphasized the safety and efficacy of slow, continuous arteriovenous hemodiafiltration (CAVHD). In 13 patients who had acute renal failure but were apparently too unstable to be treated with standard hemodialysis, CAVHD was used with five survivors. With a dialysis rate of 1600 ml/h, urea clearance was adequate. The only problems found with CAVHD were thrombocytopenia and a tendency to hyponatremia.

(4) Hemoperfusion

Another means of removing solutes is to perfuse the blood through a column of activated charcoal or resin adsorbents rather than a standard dialyzer. In this procedure solutes are removed by adherence to the column. Although hemoperfusion has been tried in patients with end-stage renal failure, its role appears to be limited by its variable removal of urea and failure to remove water.

h. Prolonged Hemodialysis

Spurney and colleagues recently pointed out that prolonged need for hemodialysis for acute renal failure does not necessarily imply a poor prognosis. Dialysis support for acute renal failure is required for >4 weeks in only about 8% of

Table 14.9

COMPLICATIONS OF HEMODIALYSIS	
	1. Problems with vascular access
	2. Cardiovascular, especially hypotension
	3. Neurologic
	a. Disequilibrium syndrome
	b. Subdural hematoma
	c. Dialysis dementia
	4. Infections
	a. Vascular access
	b. Hepatitis
	c. Contamination of dialysis equipment
	5. Nutritional: loss of vitamins, amino acids, and trace elements
	6. Hematologic
	a. Anemia
	b. Leukopenia
	c. Antinuclear antibodies
	7. Hypoxemia
	8. Metabolic
	a. Metabolic acidosis or alkalosis
	b. Respiratory alkalosis
	c. Hypokalemia
	9. Other
	a. Muscle cramps
	b. Nausea and vomiting

patients. However, the prognosis in these patients can be fairly good. Spurney and colleagues found that 88% of 26 patients requiring prolonged dialysis support (>4 weeks) for acute renal failure recovered enough renal function to come off dialysis after an average of 8.4 ± 0.7 weeks.

i. Complications of Hemodialysis

A variety of complications may occur with HD (Table 14.9). Almost invariably, the mean arterial pressure falls somewhat during hemodialysis, and in 25%, actual hypotension occurs. This appears to be the result of several factors, including the volume of plasma removed during the procedure, osmotically related shifts of fluid, and depression of myocardial contractility, possibly caused by components of the dialysate.

Hemodialyzed patients are subject to increased CNS abnormalities, sometimes referred to as disequilibrium syndrome. A patient with disequilibrium syndrome may become confused or somnolent, or have seizures. This phenomenon is most likely related to osmotic shifts of fluid and abrupt changes in K^+, magnesium, calcium, and acid-base status.

Vascular access sites may bleed or become infected. Errors in technique may lead to hemolysis, hypothermia or hyperthermia, and embolization of clot or air. Hemodialysis acutely lowers the blood levels of many major antibiotics and makes proper dosage more difficult.

j. Results of Hemodialysis

It has been reported that aggressive early hemodialysis may significantly reduce the mortality rate from acute renal failure in surgical patients. In one series, where patients were dialyzed to keep the BUN below 70 mg/100 ml and the serum creatinine below 5.0 mg/100 ml, the incidence of major sepsis was reduced from 83% to 63%, bleeding episodes were reduced from 60% to 36%, and the mortality rate was reduced from 80% to 36%. Although most nephrologists believe in prophylactic dialysis, these figures have not been confirmed in most other large series.

22. Management of the Diuretic Phase

The oliguric phase of renal failure is followed by a diuretic phase during recovery. The period of oliguria may last for a few days or many weeks, with a median duration of 10 to 20 days. If renal function does not return within 28 days, renal cortical necrosis may have developed. This should be confirmed or ruled out by a renal biopsy.

During the phase of increasing urine volumes, the urine-to-plasma ratios of creatinine and urea differ little from those found during the oliguric phase. The urinary electrolyte content is quite variable and must be monitored closely. The losses of water, sodium, potassium, and bicarbonate during the diuretic phase may be excessive and may quickly lead to ECF volume deficits if replacement is inadequate.

Measurements of urinary volume and electrolyte concentrations, under these circumstances, allow more precise replacement. Replacement of slightly less than the losses may be helpful, because quite a bit of extra water may accumulate during the oliguric phase. However, failure to replace the massive fluid and electrolyte losses that may occur during the diuretic phase may also result in death.

During the diuretic phase, azotemia may continue to increase in spite of the high urine volumes. Impaired concentrating ability, tubular transport maximum for PAH, and inulin clearance may persist for many weeks. Dialysis for azotemia at this time may be just as important as in the nonoliguric phase. Renal function usually recovers after 1 year, but sophisticated testing of renal function has seldom been performed on those patients in the late recovery phases.

23. Renal Transplantation

Persons with end-stage renal disease have a number of options, which can include in-center or home hemodialysis, intermittent peritoneal dialysis at home, continuous ambulatory peritoneal dialysis, or transplantation of a cadaver kidney or a kidney from a living related donor.

The chances of successful renal transplantation from a cadaver donor have risen because of (1) improvements in tissue typing and organ preservation, (2) the discovery that blood transfusions prior to transplantation enhanced the likelihood of successful kidney grafting, and (3) the discovery of cyclosporine. The nature of the nephrotoxic action of cyclosporine is still not known. It is hoped that a derivative may be found that retains the immunosuppressive properties of cyclosporine, but minimizes its nephrotoxic side effects.

The decision as to whether a dialysis patient should receive a cadaver kidney should be based on evaluation of the complications associated with the two procedures and their potential effects on the patient's general life-style, opportunity for rehabilitation, and family and social responsibilities. Transplantation repeatedly and reliably gives better long-term results. Also, informed consent concerning the long-term risks of hemodialysis is as important as informed consent concerning the early risks of renal transplantation.

The constant death rate with the use of hemodialysis far exceeds the death rate from transplantation. Even the 1-year survival with transplantation is better than that with dialysis, although most patients who reach transplantation have already survived a period of dialysis. Cadaver transplantation is not likely to reach the success rates of living related donor transplantation. The long-term studies of unilaterally nephrectomized patients in Sweden still give the best evidence that donation of a kidney from a normal person is not deleterious to the donor's long-term health.

Renal transplant recipients are not placed at an increased risk of death when returned to hemodialysis after transplant failure. Most transplant surgeons prefer to make no undue attempts to prolong allograft survival by administering massive doses of immunosuppressive agents. Patients can return to maintenance dialysis with no increase in the risk of death, and an independent decision can then be made regarding subsequent transplantation.

SUMMARY POINTS

1. The definition of oliguria, arbitrarily set at 400 ml/d, should probably be revised to 800 ml/d in patients with severe trauma or sepsis. Lower urine volumes require early investigation.

2. Although a decreased urine output may be an important indication of hypovolemia in an injured individual, a normal urine output does not rule out a significant reduction in renal blood flow or renal function.

3. The most frequent cause of oliguria is impaired renal perfusion due to hypovolemia.

4. Acute renal failure seldom causes complete anuria. Complete anuria generally implies mechanical occlusion of both renal arteries, or complete obstruction of the lower urinary tract.

5. Fluid deficits in critically ill or injured patients are often greatly underestimated, particularly if sepsis is present.

6. Diuretics should be used very cautiously in patients with severe trauma or sepsis, because oliguria in these patients is often due to inadequate fluid replacement. Furthermore, surprisingly large fluid losses can occur after diuresis and before the extent of volume depletion is recognized.

7. The primary treatment of renal failure is prevention. Once oliguric renal failure becomes established in critically ill or injured patients, the mortality rate approaches 80% to 90%, in spite of vigorous therapy.

8. The diagnosis and treatment of acute vasomotor nephropathy may be greatly delayed in a critically ill or injured patient, if one assumes that renal function is good because the urinary output is normal or high.

9. Although urine-specific gravity is not a very accurate measure of urine concentration, a specific gravity greater than 1.020 and a low urine output suggest that the patient is hypovolemic, especially if the urine is free of protein or other unexpected solute.

10. A rapidly rising BUN, with little or no change in the serum creatinine, suggests upper gastrointestinal hemorrhage, accelerated tissue breakdown, or a blood volume deficit.

11. In the early stage of acute renal failure, the urine output, BUN, and serum creatinine may be normal, in spite of a progressive decrease in creatinine clearance.

12. If the urine/plasma creatinine ratio exceeds 20, the patient is probably hypovolemic.

13. In the presence of oliguria, a urine/plasma osmolar ratio greater than 1.2 suggests that the patient is hypovolemic, whereas a ratio less than 1.1 suggests renal failure.

14. A urine sodium concentration that is decreasing or is less than 10 to 20 mEq/liter suggests intact renal tubular function, but impaired renal perfusion, usually due to hypovolemia.

15. Measurement of creatinine clearance in the postoperative or post-traumatic period is probably the best single, readily available method for following early vasomotor nephropathy.

16. A kidney producing concentrated urine at low flow rates is more vulnerable to nephrotoxins (such as aminoglycosides, hemoglobin, and myoglobin) and is more likely to develop acute renal failure than a kidney with high urine flow.

17. A thorough and early debridement of nonviable tissue and drainage of suppurative collections is essential in oliguric patients to reduce the entry into the blood of vasoactive materials, nitrogenous substances, and pigments.

18. One should avoid the use of diuretics to stimulate an increased urine output in patients who may be oliguric secondary to hypovolemia. A diuresis under such circumstances can aggravate hypovolemia and renal damage by further depleting an inadequate ECF volume.

19. Mannitol should be used cautiously in the presence of severe heart disease or fluid overload.
20. Patients in nonoliguric renal failure seldom develop hyperkalemia, unless excessive potassium is administered or there is extensive tissue breakdown.
21. If oliguric vasomotor nephropathy develops, hyperkalemia and fluid retention are generally the greatest threats to the patient's life.
22. Hyponatremia in patients with acute renal failure is usually due to water retention. Administration of sodium to such patients may be extremely dangerous.
23. Failure to replace the massive fluid and electrolyte losses that may occur during the diuretic phase of renal failure may be rapidly fatal.

BIBLIOGRAPHY

1. Abel, RM, et al: Improved survival from acute renal failure after treatment with intravenous essential L-amino acids and glucose: Results of a prospective double-blind study. N Engl J Med 288:695, 1973.
2. Alfred, HJ and Cohen, AJ: Use of dialytic procedures in the intensive care unit. In Rippe, JM, et al (eds): Intensive Care Medicine. Little, Brown & Co, Boston, 1985, p 562.
3. Arieff, AI and Guisado, R: Effects on the central nervous system of hypernatremic and hyponatremic states. Kidney Int 10:104, 1976.
4. Baer, PG and Navar, LG: Renal vasodilatation and uncoupling of blood flow and filtration rate autoregulation. Kidney Int 4:12, 1973.
5. Bailey, RR, et al: Protective effect of furosemide in acute tubular necrosis and acute renal failure. Clin Sci 45:1, 1973.
6. Barsotti, G, et al: Reversal of hyperparathyroidism in severe uremics following very low-protein and low-phosphate diet. Nephron 30:310, 1982.
7. Bartlett, RH, et al: Continuous arteriovenous hemofiltration: Improved survival in surgical acute renal failure? Surgery 100:400, 1986.
8. Battle, DC, Salem, M, and Levin, ML: More on therapy for hyperkalemia in renal insufficiency (letter to the editor). N Engl J Med 320:1496, 1989.
9. Better, OS and Stein, JH: Early management of shock and prophylaxis of acute renal failure in traumatic rhabdomyolysis. N Engl J Med 12:825, 1990.
10. Bingham, CT: Thrombotic thrombocytopenic purpura. JAMA 265:91, 1991.
11. Blumberg, A, et al: Effect of various therapeutic approaches on plasma potassium and major regulating factors in terminal renal failure. Am J Med 85:507, 1988.
12. Brech, WJ, et al: The influence of renin on the intrarenal distribution of blood flow and autoregulation. Nephron 12:44, 1973.
13. Cantarovich, F, et al: High-dose furosemide in established acute renal failure. Br Med J 4:449, 1973.
14. Chenoweth, DE, Cheung, AK, and Henderson, IW: Anaphylatoxin formation during hemodialysis: Effects of different dialyzer membranes. Kidney Int 24:764, 1983.
15. Coburn, JW and Salusky, IB: Control of serum phosphorus in uremia (editorial). N Engl J Med 320:1140, 1989.
16. Corwin, HL, Schreiber, MJ, and Fang, LST: Low fractional excretion of sodium: Occurrence with hemoglobinuric and myoglobinuric-induced acute renal failure. Arch Intern Med 144:981, 1984.
17. Cumming, AD, Kline, R, and Linton, AL: Association between renal and sympathetic responses to nonhypotensive systemic sepsis. Crit Care Med 16:1132, 1988.
18. Danielson, RA: Differential diagnosis and treatment of oliguria in post-traumatic and postoperative patients. Surg Clin North Am 55:697, 1975.
19. Davenport, A and Roberts, NBC: Serum aluminum levels in acute renal failure. Lancet ii, December 13, 1986, p 1397.
20. Davis, RD et al: Acute oliguria after cardiopulmonary bypass: Renal functional improvement with low-dose dopamine infusion. Crit Care Med 10:852, 1982.
21. Deppish, R, et al: Dialysis membranes generate terminal complement complexes (abstr). Blood Purif 6:351, 1988.
23. Diamond, JR and Yoburn, DC: Nonoliguria acute renal failure with low fractional excretion of sodium. Ann Intern Med 96:597, 1982.
24. Druml, W, et al: Elimination of amino acids in acute renal failure. Nephron 42:62, 1986.
25. Eisenberg, E and Gotch, FA: Normocalcemic hyperparathyroidism culminating in hypercalcemic crisis: Treatment with hemodialysis. Arch Intern Med 122:258, 1968.
26. Eisenberg, JM, et al: What is the cost of nephrotoxicity associated with aminoglycosides? Ann Intern Med 107:900, 1987.

27. Ganeval, D, Kleinknecht, D, and Gonzales-Duque, LA: High-dose furosemide in renal failure. Br Med J 1:244, 1973.

28. Gauer, OH: Osmocontrol versus volume control. Fed Proc 27:1132, 1968.

29. Gelfand, MC and Winchester, JR: Hemoperfusion: Results in uremia. Clin Nephrol 11:107, 1979.

30. Hercz, G and Coburn, JW: Prevention of phosphate retention and hyperphosphatemia in uremia. Kidney Int (Suppl) 22:S215, 1987.

31. Hermreck, AS and Thal, AP: Mechanisms for the high circulatory requirements in sepsis and shock. Ann Surg 170:677, 1969.

32. Hermreck, AS, et al: Renal response in sepsis. Arch Surg 107:169, 1973.

33. Holick, MF: Vitamin D and the kidney. Kidney Int 32:912, 1987.

34. Hollenberg, NK, et al: Acute renal failure due to nephrotoxins: Renal hemodynamic and angiographic studies in man. N Engl J Med 282:1329, 1970.

35. Horl, WH, et al: Neutrophil activation in acute renal failure and sepsis. Arch Surg 125:651, 1990.

36. Horl, WH, et al: Different complement and granulocyte activation in patients dialyzed with PMMA dialyzers. Clin Nephrol 25:304, 1986.

37. Iqbal, Z and Friedman, EA: Preferred therapy of hyperkalemia in renal insufficiency: Survey of nephrology training-program directors. N Engl J Med 320:60, 1989.

38. Jochimsen, F, et al: Impairment of renal function in medical intensive care: Predictability of acute renal failure. Crit Care Med 18:480, 1990.

39. Kennedy, AC, et al: Factors affecting the prognosis in acute renal failure. Q J Med 42:73, 1973.

40. Kleinknecht, D, et al: Uremic and nonuremic complications in acute renal failure: Evaluation of early and frequent dialysis on prognosis. Kidney Int 1:190, 1972.

41. Krakauer, H, et al: Recent U.S. experience in treatment of end-stage renal disease by dialysis and transplantation. N Engl J Med 308:1558, 1983.

42. Kumar, SM and Lesh, M: Pericarditis in renal disease. Prog Cardiovasc Dis 22:357, 1980.

43. Lauer, A, et al: Continuous arteriovenous hemofiltration in the critically ill patient. Clinical use and operational characteristics. Ann Intern Med 99:455, 1953.

44. Leone, MR, et al: Early experience with continuous arteriovenous hemofiltration in critically ill pediatric patients. Crit Care Med 14:1058, 1986.

45. Lindner, A: Synergism of dopamine and furosemide in diuretic resistant, oliguric acute renal failure. Nephron 33:121, 1983.

46. Linton, AL, Bailey, RR, and Turnbull, DI: Relative nephrotoxicity of cephalosporin antibiotics in an animal model. Can Med Assoc J 107:414, 1972.

47. Lopez-Hilker, S, et al: Hypocalcemia may not be essential for the development of secondary hyperparathyroidism in chronic renal failure. J Clin Invest 78:1097, 1986.

48. Lordon, RE and Borton, JR: Post-traumatic renal failure in military personnel in Southeast Asia. Am J Med 53:137, 1972.

49. Lucas, CE, et al: Altered renal homeostasis with acute sepsis. Arch Surg 106:444, 1973.

50. Luke, RG: Renal replacement therapy. N Engl J Med 380:1593, 1983.

51. Luke, RG, et al: Factors determining response to mannitol in acute renal failure. Am J Med Sci 259:168, 1970.

52. Luke, RG, et al: Mannitol therapy in acute renal failure. Lancet 1:980, 1965.

53. Manji, N, et al: Peritoneal dialysis for acute renal failure: Overfeeding resulting from dextrose absorbed during dialysis. Crit Care Med 18:29, 1990.

54. Matas, AJ, et al: Fate of the patient returned to hemodialysis after losing a renal transplant. JAMA 250:1053, 1983.

55. McDonald, FD: The prevention of acute renal failure in the rat by long-term saline loading: A possible role of the renin-angiotension axis. Proc Soc Exp Biol Med 131:610, 1969.

56. Menashe, P, Ross, SA, and Gottlieb, JE: Acquired renal insufficiency in critically ill patients. Crit Care Med 16:1106, 1988.

57. Mukau, L and Latimer, RG: Acute hemodialysis in the surgical intensive care unit. Am Surg 54:548, 1988.

57a. Murphy, WG, Moore, JC, Barr, RD, et al: Relationship between platelet aggregating factor and von Willebrand factor in thrombotic thrombocytopenic purpura. Brit J Hematol 66:509, 1987.

58. Narins, RG and Chusid, P: Diuretic use in critical care. Am J Cardiol 57:26A, 1986.

59. Nolph, KD, et al: New directions in peritoneal dialysis concepts and applications. Kidney Int (Suppl 10)18:S111, 1980.

60. Ogden, DA: Consequences of renal donation in man. Am J Kidney Dis 2:501, 1983.

61. Oken, DE: Hemodynamic basis for human acute renal failure (vasomotor nephropathy). Am J Med 76:702, 1984.

62. Oken, DE: Nosologic considerations in the nomenclature of acute renal failure. Nephron 8:505, 1971.

63. Parker, A and Nolph, KD: Magnesium and calcium mass transfer during continuous ambulatory peritoneal dialysis. Trans Am Soc Artif Intern Organs 26:194, 1980.

64. Pirotzky, E, et al: Involvement of platelet-activating factor in renal processes. Adv Lipid Res 23:277, 1989.

65. Popovach, RP and Moncreif, JW: Kinetic modeling of peritoneal transport. Contrib Nephrol 17:59, 1979.
66. Prough, DS and Zaloga, GP: Monitoring of renal function. Crit Care Med 4:573, 1988.
67. Rasmussen, HH and Ibels, LS: Acute renal failure: Multivariate analysis of causes and risk factors. Am J Med 73:211, 1982.
68. Rector, FE, et al: Sepsis: A mechanism for vasodilation in the kidney. Ann Surg 178:222, 1973.
69. Richards, WO, et al: Acute renal failure associated with increased intra-abdominal pressure. Ann Surg 197:183, 1983.
70. Ron, D, et al: Prevention of acute renal failure in traumatic rhabdomyolysis. Arch Intern Med 144:277, 1984.
71. Rosenberg, JC: Dialysis as a substitute for renal function in surgical patients. Curr Probl Surg 13:1, 1972.
72. Rubin, J, et al: Comparison of the effects of lactate and acetate on clinical peritoneal clearance. Clin Nephrol 12:145, 1979.
73. Schiller, LR, et al: Effect of the time of administration of calcium acetate on phosphorus binding. N Engl J Med 320:1110, 1989.
74. Shusterman, N, Strom, BL, and Murray, TG: Risk factors and outcome of hospital-acquired acute renal failure. Am J Med 83:65, 1987.
74a. Spurney, RF, Fulkerson, WJ, and Schwab, SJ: Acute renal failure in critically ill patients: Prognosis for recovery of kidney function after prolonged dialysis support. Crit Care Med 19:8, 1991.
75. Stannat, S, et al: Complement activation during hemodialysis. Contrib Nephrol 46:102, 1985.
76. Stein, JH, et al: Effect of renal vasodilatation on the distribution of cortical blood flow in the kidney of the dog. J Clin Invest 50:1429, 1971.
77. Steiner, RW: Interpreting the fractional excretion of sodium. Am J Med 77:699, 1984.
78. Stone, JK: Renal failure in the trauma patient. Crit Care Clin 6:111, 1990.
79. Stott, RB, et al: Why the persistently high mortality in acute renal failure? Lancet 2:75, 1972.
80. Thorburn, GD, et al: Intrarenal distribution of nutrient blood flow determined with krypton[85] in the unanesthetized dog. Circ Res 13:290, 1963.
81. Voerman, HJ, et al: Continuous arterial-venous hemodiafiltration in critically ill patients. Crit Care Med 18:911, 1990.
82. Wilmore, DW, and Dudrick, SJ: Treatment of acute renal failure with intravenous essential L-amino acids. Arch Surg 99:669, 1969.
83. Zager, RA and Sharma, HM: Gentamicin increases renal susceptibility to an acute ischemic insult. J Lab Clin Med 101:670, 1983.
84. Zaloga, GP and Hughes, SS: Oliguria in patients with normal renal function. Anesthesiology 72:598, 1990.
85. Zarich, S, Fang, LST, and Diamond, JR: Fractional excretion of sodium. Arch Intern Med 145:108, 1985.
86. Zimmerman, JE: Respiratory failure complicating post-traumatic acute renal failure: Etiology, clinical features, and management. Ann Surg 174:12, 1971.

CHAPTER 15

Fluid and Electrolyte Problems

| I. GENERAL APPROACH | Fluid, electrolyte, and acid-base problems frequently occur in critically ill patients. To provide a general approach to these problems a series of axioms have been developed. |

AXIOM
Never completely trust the laboratory.

Some of the worst complications of fluid and electrolyte or acid-base management have occurred when aggressive therapy was based on an erroneous laboratory result. Laboratory errors do occur, especially at night and on weekends. Not only are there errors in obtaining the sample and labeling it, but also in performing the test and reporting the result. Instead of blindly accepting an erroneous result, the physician should, whenever possible, try to decide what each test will probably show before the result comes back. If the laboratory result does not seem to correlate properly with the patient's condition or other data, three things should be done:

1. The patient and the record should be carefully re-examined.

2. If the laboratory result still does not seem to fit, the test should be repeated.

3. If there is still a question about the laboratory result, a sample from a normal individual should be analyzed. In some instances, an abnormal result on an apparently normal individual provides the first evidence that a laboratory error exists. Occasionally, laboratory errors are suspect because all the results of a particular test at a certain time are higher or lower than expected.

AXIOM
Biologic systems react primarily to rate of change and not to absolute concentrations.

Whenever patients develop abnormalities, they tend to adapt to the abnormalities gradually, so that they become increasingly "normal" for them. Attempts to correct long-standing or slowly developing electrolyte abnormalities rapidly may cause more harm than good.

AXIOM
Abnormalities should be treated at approximately the rate at which they developed.

A not infrequent example is the patient who has been on a low-salt diet and diuretics for years and requires urgent surgery. A serum sodium concentration of less than 110 mEq/liter may now be well tolerated and relatively "normal" for this patient. Administration of normal or hypertonic saline solutions in an effort to rapidly return the patient's serum sodium levels to at least 130 mEq/liter prior to emergency surgery is likely to cause severe congestive heart failure. On the other hand, if a patient has cardiac arrest, the severe metabolic acidosis that can develop within a few minutes can be at least partially corrected rather rapidly with sodium bicarbonate.

PITFALL
Rapid correction of a chronic asymptomatic abnormality.

Even when an abnormality has developed rather rapidly, we tend to correct only half the calculated deficit at a time. We then re-evaluate the patient and repeat the laboratory tests to determine the rate and amount of correction still required.

AXIOM
The highest priority in treatment is maintenance of intravascular volume and tissue perfusion.

In correcting multiple fluid, electrolyte, and acid-base abnormalities, the highest priority, generally, should be given to correction of fluid volume and perfusion deficits; the second priority is correction of pH; the third priority is potassium, calcium, and magnesium abnormalities; and the fourth priority is correction of sodium and chloride abnormalities. If blood volume and tissue perfusion are restored to normal, many electrolyte and acid-base abnormalities will correct themselves spontaneously.

PITFALL
Correcting pH levels without also considering the effect on potassium, calcium, and magnesium.

Changes in pH affect potassium, calcium, and magnesium levels. In no instance should one be corrected without considering the effect that it may have on the others. For example, acidosis is often associated with hyperkalemia and increased plasma levels of ionized calcium and magnesium. In contrast, alkalosis tends to lower plasma levels of potassium and ionized calcium and magnesium. If a severely acidotic patient has a low serum potassium level, one should suspect that a laboratory error has occurred or that the patient has a severe potassium deficiency.

AXIOM
If all the measured electrolyte levels are low, symptoms are apt to be less severe than if only one electrolyte were decreased.

A. ORDERING ELECTROLYTES

As a general rule, electrolytes are ordered rather indiscriminately. Civetta and others have shown that unnecessary electrolyte tests are often ordered in an ICU. Lowe, Arst, and Ellis have recently shown that rational ordering of electrolytes in an emergency department will pick up 94% of significant electrolyte abnormalities and reduce the ordering of electrolyte studies by 76%. Their suggested criteria include poor oral intake, vomiting, chronic hypertension, diuretic use, recent seizure, muscle weakness, age 65 years or more, alcoholism, abnormal mental status, and recent history of an electrolyte abnormality. Other guidelines for ordering laboratory tests have also been suggested (Table 15.1).

II. ATOMIC WEIGHTS

Proper correction of electrolyte abnormalities may be facilitated by some knowledge of the atomic weights of the elements most likely to be involved in fluid and electrolyte problems (Table 15.2). The equivalent weight is the atomic weight divided by its usual electric charge or valence. For example, if the plasma level of ionized calcium, which has an atomic weight of 40 and an equivalent weight of

Table 15.1

SUGGESTED GUIDELINES FOR ORDERING LABORATORY TESTS

To confirm a clinical diagnosis or impression with additional information

To stage a disease for therapeutic or prognostic purposes

To use as a screening test, if evidence suggests that finding the condition in an asymptomatic state can alter the long-term outcome of the patient

To provide data that may indicate whether or not a disease might develop at some future time

To effectively monitor drug therapy

To rule out treatable or life-threatening disease that, although somewhat unlikely, is of such potential danger that one cannot afford to miss it

To use as part of a protocol for a research project

Source: Adapted from Corman, IC: The interpretation of laboratory tests. Prim Care 7:691, 1980.

20, is 4.0 mg, the concentration of ionized calcium can also be expressed as 2.0 mEq/liter or 1.0 mmol/liter. Magnesium sulfate is usually stocked and given in terms of grams, without indicating how many milliequivalents of magnesium are present. If one knows the atomic weights, one can readily calculate the molecular weight of $MgSO_4 \cdot 7\,H_2O$ as $24 + 32 + (4)(16) + 7(18) = 246$. Thus, a gram of $MgSO_4$ contains 4.06 mmol or 8.1 mEq of magnesium.

III. WATER

Normally, about 55% to 60% of the body weight of an adult is water. In the newborn, there is relatively more water, usually equivalent to 70% to 80% of the body weight. Fat is relatively anhydrous, and muscle is about 77% water. Consequently, obese adult women may have less than 50% of their weight as water, while muscular men may have more than 60% to 65% of their weight as water.

A. OSMOLARITY AND OSMOLALITY

Alterations in the amount of water present in the various fluid spaces are primarily related to the number of particles present. Colligative properties refer to physiologic effects entirely due to the number of particles present in a given volume of solvent. Osmotic pressure is one of the colligative properties with which we are most concerned. The osmotic pressure of serum is largely regulated by antidiuretic hormone (ADH), which increases water reabsorption in the collecting ducts of the kidney. The most important stimuli to ADH secretion, in descending order of potency, are nausea, pain, hypovolemia, and hyperosmolarity.

AXIOM

Hypovolemia is a much stronger stimulus to ADH secretion than hyposmolarity is an inhibitor to ADH. Consequently, increased ADH secretion tends to perpetuate hyponatremia in hypovolemic patients.

Table 15.2

ATOMIC AND EQUIVALENT WEIGHTS

Element	Symbol	Atomic Weight	Equivalent Weight
Calcium	Ca	40	20
Carbon	C	12	3
Chlorine	Cl	35.5	35.5
Hydrogen	H	1	1
Magnesium	Mg	24	12
Oxygen	O	16	8
Phosphorus	P	31	6.2
Potassium	K	39	39
Sodium	Na	23	23
Sulfur	S	32	5.3

Serum osmolarity can be measured directly by determining the freezing point of the serum. Serum osmolarity can also be calculated from the sodium, glucose, and blood urea nitrogen (BUN) levels, using the following formula:

$$\text{Osmolarity} = 2(\text{Na}) + \frac{\text{glucose}}{18} + \frac{\text{BUN}}{2.8}.$$

Note that the glucose (mg/dl) and BUN (mg/dl) are divided by their respective molecular weights divided by 10 (because we are working with deciliters and not liters).

Thus, normal serum osmolarity, which is about 275 to 295 mOsm/liter can usually be calculated as

$$S_{Osm} = 2(140) + \frac{90}{18} + \frac{14}{2.8}$$

$$= 280 + 5 + 5 = 290.$$

The contributions from mannitol (18 mg/dl), glycerol (9 mg/dl), and ethanol (4.6 mg/dl) can also be included. This equation will not provide an accurate estimate of ECF osmolality if other (unexpected or unknown) solutes are present in significant quantity. Thus, a difference or "gap" between measured and calculated osmolality of more than 10 mOsm/kg should suggest the presence of another solute, such as lactate, ethanol, methanol, and so forth. An osmolar gap of more than 50 mOsm/liter is often fatal.

The terms osmolarity, osmolality, oncotic pressure, and tonicity are often confused. Osmolarity refers to the number of particles per liter of solution (e.g., plasma), whereas osmolality refers to the number of particles per liter of solvent (e.g., plasma water). Since plasma is about 91% to 93% water, osmolality reflects osmotic pressure better and is usually 7% to 9% higher than the osmolarity.

The plasma oncotic pressure is the difference in osmotic pressure created by the presence of protein or other relatively nonpermeable substances, assuming that the plasma is equilibrated against a solution having the same ionic composition as plasma, but lacking protein. Because of the Donnan equilibrium and various ions kept in the vascular system by plasma proteins, the concentration of diffusible ions in the plasma is 0.43 mmol/liter higher than in the interstitial fluid. The sum of 0.43 mmol/liter and the protein concentration, which is 0.8 mmol/liter, determines the plasma oncotic pressure. Since each millimole per liter generates 19.3 mm Hg of oncotic pressure, the average total oncotic pressure of plasma is 1.23 × 19.3 mm Hg, or 23.7 mm Hg.

When the extracellular osmolality is increased by solutes restricted to the extracellular fluid, the intracellular osmolality is increased by a shift of water from the cell to the extracellular fluid. The osmols, that can cause a shift of water out of the cells are called *effective* or *impermeant* osmols, and those that distribute across the cell membrane equally, and therefore do not cause a shift of water out of the cell, may be termed *ineffective* or *permeant* osmols.

The osmolality produced by effective osmols is referred to as tonicity, or the effective osmolality. The principal extracellular electrolytes, sodium, chloride, and bicarbonate, are all effective osmols. Glucose is an effective osmol for most, but not all, cells. For example, it can easily enter red blood cells, hepatocytes, and osmoreceptor cells in the brain; hence, it does not draw water from them. Thus, when we consider a substance as an effective osmol, it is usually in reference to muscle, the organ that represents the greatest bulk of the body's tissues.

Some solutes (e.g., urea, ethanol, methanol, ethylene glycol, etc.) pass freely across cell membranes and do not exert a force for water movement between the two major body fluid compartments. Such noneffective solutes contribute to body fluid osmolality, but not to tonicity. Tonicity cannot be measured, but it can be estimated, under normal circumstances, as follows:

$$2 \times [Na^+] + \frac{[glucose]}{18} = [2 \times 140] + \frac{90}{18} = 285 \text{ mOsm/kg } H_2O.$$

Mannitol, glycerol, and sorbitol would have to be included in this calculation if they are present in the ECF. Urea, ethanol, methanol, and ethylene glycol, no matter how severe the azotemia or the intoxication, would not.

B. FLUID SPACES

The total body water is normally divided into the intracellular fluid (ICF) and extracellular fluid (ECF). Classically, it has been taught that the ICF is 40% of the body weight and the ECF (which includes water in interstitial fluid, plasma, bone, connective tissue, and transcellular fluid) is equal to about 20% of the body weight. It is now clear, however, that the ECF is actually about 25% to 30% of the body weight and the ICF is equal to about 30% to 35% of the body weight (Table 15.3).

1. Extracellular Fluid

Some of the fluid markers (such as sodium, chloride, and bromide) used to estimate the size of the extracellular fluid (ECF) space also penetrate cells to varying degrees. Thus, they overestimate the ECF. Conversely, other ECF markers (such as inulin, mannitol, and sucrose) do not penetrate certain parts of the extracellular fluid space and, therefore, underestimate the ECF. As a result, depending on the type of marker used, the extracellular fluid volume could be calculated to vary from 27% to 45% of the total body water.

AXIOM
Malnutrition and sepsis tend to increase the extracellular fluid space and decrease the intracellular fluid space.

Normally, the intracellular water (ICW) is about 55% of the total body water (TBW), and the exchangeable potassium (K_e), which is primarily in ICW, is about 80 mEq/liter in the TBW. In malnutrition, the ICW falls, the ECF increases, and the exchangeable potassium (K_e) can fall to about 50 mEq/liter in the TBW. In contrast, the total exchangeable sodium (Na_e), which is normally about 75 mEq/liter of TBW, can rise with malnutrition, trauma, or sepsis to about 95 mEq/liter of TBW. Thus, the ratio of K_e/Na_e which is normally about 1.05 to 1.10 (80/75) can fall to about 0.55 (50/95) in severe malnutrition. In sepsis, the K_e/Na_e can fall even lower.

The electrolyte concentrations of extracellular fluid (ECF) are thought, by some scientists, to resemble that of the earth's seas millions of years ago; how-

Table 15.3

SIZE AND SODIUM AND POTASSIUM CONTENT OF VARIOUS FLUID SPACES	Percentage of Body Weight as Water	Percentage of Total Body Sodium	Percentage of Total Body Potassium
Plasma	4.5	1.2	0.4
Interstitial fluid (lymph)	12.0	20.0	1.0
Dense connective tissue and cartilage	4.5	11.7	0.4
Bone	4.5	43.1	7.6
Transcellular	1.5	2.6	1.0
Total extracellular	27.0	97.6	10.4
Total intracellular	33.0	2.4	89.6
Total body	60.0	100.0	100.0

Table 15.4

Solution	Sea Water	Extracellular Fluid	Interstitial Fluid	Intracellular Fluid
THE ELECTROLYTE CONCENTRATION OF BODY FLUIDS (mEq/L)				
Cations				
Sodium	425	142	144	10
Potassium	15	4.5	4.5	150
Magnesium	105	2	1.0	40
Calcium	35	4.5	2.5	
Total	580	153	152	200
Anions				
Chloride	500	102	113	
Phosphates	10	2	2	120
Sulfates	45	1	1	30
Bicarbonate	25	27	30	10
Protein		16	1	40
Organic acids		5	5	
Total	580	153	152	200

ever, the concentrations of magnesium and sulfate in sea water are now so high (105 and 45 mEq/liter, respectively), that this seems unlikely.

The electrolyte concentrations in the plasma and interstitial fluid (ISF) are approximately the same except for protein-bound electrolytes, such as calcium and magnesium. Cellular fluid has much more potassium, magnesium, phosphate, and protein than the ECF, but has relatively little sodium and very little calcium or chloride (Table 15.4).

2. Interstitial Fluid

a. Characteristics of Interstitial Fluid

The interstitial fluid space is not physiologically uniform. It consists of a small liquid and large gel phase invested by a fibrous meshwork, the latter largely made up of collagen fibers that hold the cells together. The ground substance between the collagen fibers consists largely of anionic polymers, referred to as glycosaminoglycans, which bind cations selectively and limit their mobility to varying degrees. Glycosaminoglycans also limit the mobility of water, holding some of the bound water in an icelike lattice.

Only a small part of the interstitial fluid is freely movable, and this portion is felt to have the following characteristics:

1. The ion concentrations are predictable by the Donnan equilibrium.
2. Interstitial protein is dissolved in this portion.
3. This portion exchanges water with the capillary fluid.
4. This is the route for water to move from capillaries to lymphatics.

The electrolyte concentrations of interstitial fluid, obtained primarily by the analysis of lymph fluid, probably reflect the average composition of the freely movable interstitial fluid fairly accurately.

b. Donnan Equilibrium

The concentrations of electrolytes in the interstitial fluid are different from those in the plasma, because the concentration of proteins is much lower in interstitial fluid (Table 15.5). When two solutions are separated by a membrane permeable to water and small ions, and when one of the solutions contains more nonpermeable ions than the other, the distribution of permeable or diffusible ions occurs in a predictable manner that can be calculated from the products of the diffusible cations and anions in each solution according to the requirements of the Donnan equilibrium, that is,

$$(C^+ \text{ plasma}) (A^- \text{ plasma}) = (C^+ \text{ ISF}) (A^- \text{ ISF}).$$

Table 15.5

DISTRIBUTION OF ELECTROLYTES ACROSS THE CAPILLARY ACCORDING TO THE DONNAN EQUILIBRIUM	Plasma mEq/L	Interstitial Fluid mEq/L
Diffusible cations	156	152
Diffusible anions	140	144
Protein Anions	16	8
Total	312	304

On the average, the proteinate anion concentration in plasma is 16 mEq/liter, and in interstitial fluids the proteinate anion is 8 mEq/liter. If the concentrations of diffusible cations and anions in the plasma are 156 and 150 mEq/liter, respectively, the concentrations of diffusible cations and anions in the interstitial fluid can be calculated from the equation

$$156 \times 140 = c \times (c - 8),$$

where c is the diffusible cation concentration in the interstitial fluid and $c - 8$ the concentration of diffusible anions. Thus, $c^2 - 8c - 21,840 = 0$, and $c = 152$ mEq/liter. Thus, the concentration of diffusible anions is 144 mEq/liter.

3. Intracellular Fluid

Intracellular fluid has much more potassium, magnesium, phosphate, and protein than ECF, but has relatively little sodium and almost no calcium or chloride. However, the electrolyte concentration of intracellular fluid varies greatly from tissue to tissue. For example, in muscle, the concentration of chloride is 2 to 3 mEq/liter, and the resting membrane potential of the cell membrane is about −90 mV. In contrast, in erythrocytes, the concentration of chloride is about 70 mEq/liter and the cell membrane potential is only about −7 mV.

The potassium concentration in muscle cells is about 160 mEq/liter, whereas in platelets it is only 118 mEq/liter. The concentration of sodium in muscle cells and in red blood cells is 12 to 17 mEq/liter, but the sodium concentration in leukocytes is about 34 mEq/liter. Because muscle represents the bulk of the body cell mass, it is customary to use the electrolyte concentration of muscle cells as representative of the total body's intracellular electrolyte concentration.

C. DAILY FLUID REQUIREMENTS

Daily fluid requirements include (1) *basic needs* for urine and insensible water loss; (2) *current losses* for gastrointestinal loss, sweat, or increased loss of insensible water; and (3) *correction* for any defects or excesses.

1. Basic Needs

Basic needs include urine loss of about 600 to 1000 $ml \cdot m^{-2} \cdot d^{-1}$ and an insensible water loss of about 350 to 700 $ml \cdot m^{-2} \cdot d^{-1}$. In an average-size 70-kg adult man, this amounts to about 1000 to 1500 ml of urine and 600 to 1200 ml of insensible water loss per day. It includes about 300 ml from the skin and 700 ml from the lungs per day. Insensible water loss is pure water of evaporation and contains essentially no electrolytes. In contrast, sweat has an electrolyte content equivalent to about 0.2 to 0.3 normal saline.

2. Current Losses

Current losses can include (1) about 500 ml of increased sensible water loss per 1°C fever; (2) 500 to 1500 ml extra for mild, moderate, or severe sweating; and (3) gastrointestinal fluid. The electrolyte contents of the various fluids that may be lost from the body can vary greatly, but certain average values can be used (Table 15.6).

Table 15.6

AVERAGE ELECTROLYTE CONTENTS OF VARIOUS BODY FLUIDS (mEq/L)	Sodium	Potassium	Chloride	Bicarbonate	Volume/d
Saliva	10–60	10–20	15–40	30–15	1000–2000
Stomach	40–100	5–15	15–20	—	1500–2500
Bile	130–140	4–6	95–105	30–40	50–1000
Pancreas	130–140	4–6	40–60	80–100	1000–2000
Small intestine	130–140	4–6	40–60	80–100	1000–2000
Colon	80–140	25–45	80–100	30–50	100–600
Sweat	40–50	5–10	45–60	—	200–1500

3. Deficits

Water deficits can be estimated from weight loss, thirst, and physical signs. Severe thirst usually indicates a fluid deficit of at least 2% of the body weight. Soft eyes, tachycardia, severe oliguria, or organ dysfunction usually indicate severe dehydration. If an adult patient appears slightly, moderately, or severely dehydrated, she or he has lost fluid equal to 6%, 8%, or 10% of the body weight, respectively. Thus, a severely dehydrated 70-kg man has lost at least 7.0 liters of fluid. If an infant has mild, moderate, or severe dehydration, the amount of water lost is equivalent to 5%, 10%, and 15% of the body weight, respectively.

Oliguria is generally due to hypovolemia and impaired renal perfusion causing a "prerenal azotemia." Occasionally, however, oliguria may be caused by "renal" disease or injury. Some of the tests used to differentiate these two entities are listed below:

Test	Prerenal Azotemia	Renal Failure
$FE_{Na} = \dfrac{U_{Na}/P_{Na}}{U_{Cr}/P_{Cr}} \times 100\%$	<1%	>3%
BUN/Cr ratio (S_{Cr} <4.0 mg/dl)	>20:1	<10:1
Urine osmolarity	>450	<300
Urine specific gravity	>1.015	<1.010

In general, a urine output of $0.5\ \text{ml}\cdot\text{kg}^{-1}\cdot\text{h}^{-1}$ or more indicates adequate fluid repletion, except in the presence of high output renal failure, glycosuria, or diuretics.

IV. SODIUM

The total body sodium content is normally about 40 mEq/kg of body weight or about 2800 mEq in the average normal 70-kg man. Almost 98% is present in extracellular fluid, where the concentration is about 140 mEq/liter. About one third is fixed in bone and the other two thirds is readily exchangeable in isotopic studies. However, intracellular sodium levels are usually less than 10 to 12 mEq/liter.

A. HYPONATREMIA

1. Etiology

a. General Causes

(1) Dilution

AXIOM

Hyponatremia is usually due to hemodilution by too much total body water.

Hyponatremia is usually due to hemodilution by too much total body water. The total body sodium content tends to be kept rather constant by the kidneys, and consequently, the most frequent cause of hyponatremia is too much total body water, producing a dilutional hyponatremia. The tendency to retain water can be greatly increased in patients with severe trauma, sepsis, cardiac failure, cirrhosis, renal failure, or chronic malnutrition.

(2) Sodium Loss

Occasionally, hyponatremia is due to sodium loss. Some of the more frequent causes of sodium loss include excessive vomiting, diarrhea, and sweating. If these losses are not corrected, the ECF and urine sodium concentration will fall. However, if these losses are treated with fluids that do not contain adequate sodium, a severe hyponatremia may develop. Increased urine sodium losses occur with diuretics, adrenal insufficiency, salt-losing nephritis, cystic disease of the renal medulla, the postoliguric phase of acute vasomotor nephropathy, and after renal transplantation or relief of urinary obstruction. Other less obvious causes of increased urine sodium loss include ketoacidosis and metabolic alkalosis with hypokalemia.

(3) Factitious Hyponatremia

Factitious hyponatremia may occur because of severe hyperglycemia, hyperlipidemia, or hyperproteinemia. Because glucose tends to stay in extracellular fluid, hyperglycemia tends to draw water out of cells into the ECF. Each 100 mg/dl increase in plasma glucose levels decreases the serum sodium concentration by about 1.6 mEq/liter. Thus, in a previously normal patient, the serum sodium concentration would fall to about 124 mEq/liter, if the blood glucose levels rise rapidly to 1100 mg/dl.

AXIOM

In "true" hyponatremia, plasma osmolarity is reduced; in "factitious" hyponatremia, plasma osmolality is usually normal or increased.

Mannitol, if present in excessive quantities, can produce factitious hyponatremia in a manner and quantity almost identical to that of glucose. If 100 g of mannitol is given rapidly and almost none is excreted, theoretically, its concentration in the ECF of a 70-kg man may be as high as 7.0 g or 7000 mg/liter (700 mg/dl). This could lower serum sodium levels by about 11.2 to 12.6 mEq/liter, but would leave a normal plasma osmolarity.

Normally, plasma water occupies approximately 910 to 930 ml of each liter of plasma. High levels of plasma lipids or proteins increase plasma volume, decreasing the percentage that is water. This can be important if sodium determinations are performed with flame emission spectrophotometry (FES), which measures the mass of sodium in a given volume of serum. If the serum sodium concentration measured by FES is 140 mmol/liter and if serum water occupies 93% of the serum volume, the concentration of sodium in serum water will be 140 mmol/liter divided by 0.93 to equal 150 mmol/liter, which is normal. If the plasma contained only 86% water, the serum sodium reported by FES would be only 129 mEq/liter, even though the concentration of sodium in the serum water is still 150 mEq/liter.

In states of hyperproteinemia (e.g., multiple myeloma) or hyperlipidemia (familial, idiopathic, or secondary), there is an increased mass of the nonaqueous components of serum and a concomitant decrease in the proportion of serum composed of water. The serum water fraction can be estimated from the following equation adapted from Waugh:

$$S_W = 99.1 - 0.1(S_L) - 0.07(S_P),$$

where S_W is the percentage of serum volume occupied by water, S_L is the serum lipid concentration (grams per liter), and S_P is the serum protein concentration (grams per liter). Normally, the total serum lipids (triglycerides of 40 to 150 mg/dl and cholesterol of 140 to 220 mg/dl) are about 2 to 4 g/liter and serum proteins are about 60 to 75 g/liter. If a patient has an abnormally high serum lipid concentration of 50 g/liter and a normal protein concentration of 74 g/liter, only 88% of the serum volume will be occupied by water. If the concentration of sodium in serum water is normal (150 mmol/liter), the serum sodium concentration will be 150 mmol/liter $\times$ 0.88 = 132 mmol/liter, which is clearly below the normal range.

Ion-selective electrodes measure only sodium activity in serum water. That activity is unaffected by the proportion of serum occupied by water. Thus, in the aforementioned case, the sodium activity in the undiluted specimen would be about 150 mmol/liter, a normal value for the sodium concentration in serum water.

Hyperlipidemia is seen in 20% to 70% of persons with diabetes mellitus, and in up to 50% of patients admitted to the hospital with diabetic ketoacidosis. Hyperlipidemia is more common and severe in patients with poor glucose control, and such patients are prone to ketoacidosis or hyperosmolar hyperglycemic nonketotic states. In one series, 38% of patients with severe diabetic ketoacidosis had factitious hyponatremia.

b. Classification of Hyponatremia by the Size of the Functional Extracellular Fluid

The major causes of hyponatremia can be classified according to functional ECF volume and urine sodium concentrations (Table 15.7). Once it is clear that the hyponatremia is "real," because plasma osmolality is less than 280 mOsm/kg, one should make a clinical estimate of the ECF volume of the patient. This estimation can be assisted by looking for predisposing factors, such as vomiting or diarrhea, diuretic use, and pre-existing disease, such as primary nephropathy, liver or heart disease, and central nervous system disorders. A careful review of the fluid intake and output, as well as their composition over the past few days, is important. The physical examination should emphasize findings that define the patient's state of hydration. Certain laboratory tests that may be useful include serum electrolytes, urea nitrogen, creatinine, glucose, urine electrolytes, and osmolality. With these data, one can usually classify the patient's hyponatremia into one of three categories: (1) hypotonic hyponatremia associated with hypovolemia, (2) hypotonic hyponatremia associated with normal or only slightly increased ECF volume, and (3) hypotonic hyponatremia associated with hypervolemia or edema.

Table 15.7

CAUSES OF HYPONATREMIA	1. Hyponatremia with decreased ECF
	a. Extrarenal losses; urinary sodium <20 mEq/L
	(1) Sweating, vomiting, diarrhea
	(2) Third space sequestration (burns, peritonitis, pancreatitis)
	b. Renal losses; urinary sodium >20 mEq/L
	(1) Loop or osmotic diuretics
	(2) Aldosterone deficiency (Addison's disease)
	(3) Ketonuria
	(4) Salt-losing nephropathies; renal tubular acidosis
	2. Hyponatremia with normal ECF; urinary sodium >20 mEq/L
	a. Inappropriate antidiuretic hormone secretion
	b. Sick cell or "reset osmostat" syndromes
	c. Physical and emotional stress or pain
	d. Myxedema, Addison's, or Sheehan's syndromes
	3. Hyponatremia with increased ECF
	a. Urinary sodium >20 mEq/L
	(1) Renal failure
	b. Urinary sodium <20 mEq/L
	(1) Cirrhosis
	(2) Cardiac failure
	(3) Renal failure
	4. Pseudohyponatremia = hypoproteinemia, hyperlipidemia, hyperglycemia

ECF = extracellular fluid.

(1) Hypovolemic Hyponatremia

These conditions are associated with loss of both water and sodium, but involve replacement with relatively more water than sodium. In hypovolemic patients with healthy kidneys not receiving diuretics, the urine sodium concentration is usually less than 20 mEq/liter; however, in severe metabolic alkalosis secondary to vomiting, increased amounts of sodium are lost in the urine along with increased urine bicarbonate.

By far, the most common cause of hypovolemic hyponatremia in children is a viral gastroenteritis that causes vomiting and/or diarrhea. Fistulas and various types of gastrointestinal tubes occasionally cause this condition. Among other causes is excessive sweating, especially in patients with cystic fibrosis and adrenal insufficiency. A similar disturbance occurs when isotonic body fluid is translocated within the body to a "third space." The unequal balance of electrolyte and water loss produces a contracted ECF and hyponatremia that is maintained by the inability of the kidneys to excrete free water. The impairment of water excretion to defend ECF volume at the expense of tonicity is accomplished by (1) decreased glomerular filtration, (2) increased proximal tubular reabsorption of solute and water, (3) decreased delivery of fluid to the diluting segment of the nephron, and (4) the presence of ADH released by nonosmotic stimuli.

AXIOM

Hyponatremia, with hypovolemia and increased urine sodium losses in adults, is usually due to diuretics, Addison's disease, or renal disorders.

Excessive renal loss of sodium can be caused by a number of drugs, and by endogenous (osmotic) diuretics, mineralocorticoid deficiency, and certain primary kidney disorders. In these conditions the urine sodium concentration is greater than 20 mEq/liter. Under the influence of loop diuretics, the kidneys cannot appropriately dilute or concentrate the urine. Loop diuretics can also cause volume depletion and hypokalemia. The hypokalemia, in turn, tends to cause an intracellular movement of sodium, further contributing to the hyponatremia.

Osmotic diuretics cause increased urinary losses of sodium and water, resulting in ECF volume depletion and hyponatremia. Other causes of increased urinary sodium losses in concentrations that are at least half isotonic are glucosuria associated with uncontrolled diabetes mellitus, urea diuresis after relief of urinary tract obstruction, and mannitol administration for the treatment of cerebral edema. Hyperglycemia and mannitol also make hyponatremia worse by causing the movement of water from the intracellular space to the ECF compartment.

The combination of hyponatremia, ECF volume contraction, hyperkalemia, and renal sodium wasting without renal failure suggests the possibility of adrenal insufficiency. Decreased mineralocorticoid secretion impairs the reabsorption of sodium in exchange for potassium and hydrogen ions in the distal tubule.

Salt wasting, sufficient to cause hyponatremia, occurs in certain renal disorders, such as medullary cystic disease, polycystic kidney disease, and obstructive uropathy, even in the absence of any renal excretory impairment. Patients with advanced renal failure have an impaired ability to conserve sodium, but the defect is usually mild and does not cause hyponatremia unless the patient is severely sodium restricted. Proximal renal tubular acidosis (type 2 RTA) may also cause sodium wasting, because the bicarbonate ion, which is lost in greatly increased quantities, obligates the excretion of sodium. Hyperkalemic renal tubular acidosis (type 4 RTA) is characterized by aldosterone insensitivity of the renal tubules, high aldosterone levels, hyperkalemia, metabolic acidosis, and hyponatremia. In all of these disorders the urinary sodium concentration is relatively high despite the presence of hypovolemia.

For the most part, extrarenal sodium losses are associated with a low urinary sodium concentration. Conversely, primary renal disorders and drug- and hormone-induced renal dysfunction are associated with renal salt wasting and a high urinary sodium concentration.

Patients described as having a combination of euvolemia and hyponatremia actually usually have a slightly increased ECF volume; however, these patients do not have ascites, are not edematous, and have a near normal total body sodium content despite the presence of hyponatremia. If symptoms are present, they are usually central nervous system manifestations of hypotonicity. Urinary sodium concentration is usually greater than 20 mEq/liter and may be much higher in states of ADH excess, which is the most important factor in the initiation and perpetuation of most cases of euvolemic hyponatremia.

The syndrome of inappropriate (excess) secretion of ADH (SIADH) is the most common cause of euvolemic hyponatremia in children. The chronic hyponatremia of this syndrome is sustained by a constant or intermittent secretion of ADH, which is inappropriate in relation to both osmotic and volume stimuli. The diagnostic criteria are

1. Hypotonicity and hyponatremia (plasma osmolality <280 mOsm/kg H_2O)
2. Inappropriately concentrated urine (i.e., urine osmolality >100 mOsm/kg H_2O)
3. High urine sodium concentration (except during sodium restriction)
4. No clinical evidence of hypervolemia or hypovolemia
5. Normal renal, cardiac, hepatic, adrenal, and thyroid function
6. Correction by (severe) water restriction

AXIOM

If the serum osmolality is less than 270 to 280 mOsm/kg, the urine osmolality should be less than 50 to 100 mOsm/kg.

It should be noted that, as serum osmolality progressively rises above 300 mOsm/liter, urine osmolality will progressively rise from 600 to 1200 mOsm/liter. However, if serum osmolality is less than 270 to 280 mOsm/liter, there should be almost no ADH secretion, and urine osmolality will be 50 mOsm/liter or less.

AXIOM

Whenever serum osmolality is low and urine osmolality is high, one should look for SIADH; however, the diagnosis of SIADH is primarily one of exclusion.

The diagnosis of SIADH is primarily one of exclusion. The diagnosis should be considered only in the absence of hypovolemia, hypervolemia (edema), endocrine dysfunction, renal failure, and drugs that may impair water excretion. Drugs that tend to cause hypotonic hyponatremia either stimulate the release of ADH centrally or potentiate its effect on the kidney, or both. The most frequent other causes of SIADH are malignancies, pulmonary diseases, and infections or other disorders of the central nervous system (Table 15.8).

SIADH in children is very common with central nervous system infections, and the situation is made worse by the administration of excess volumes of parenteral fluids. Because the CNS symptoms and signs caused by hyponatremia may be obscured by the primary central nervous system disease, hyponatremia itself may be the first clue to the diagnosis. Since SIADH is a problem of water retention, not sodium depletion, aggressive sodium administration is appropriate only to relieve neurologic symptoms. Attempts to correct the hyponatremia of SIADH with sodium-rich solutions will cause an increase in urinary sodium excretion, but little change in the serum sodium.

Table 15.8

CAUSES OF THE SYNDROME OF INAPPROPRIATE SECRETION OF ANTIDIURETIC HORMONE		
Central Nervous System Disorders	*Drugs*	
Head trauma	Narcotics	
Brain tumors/abscesses	Chlorpropamide	
Meningitis/encephalitis	Nonsteroidal antiinflammatory agents	
Subarachnoid hemorrhage	Vincristine, vinblastine	
Delirium tremens	Cyclophosphamide, phenothiazines	
	Monoamine oxidase inhibitors	
Tumors	Tricyclic antidepressants	
Cancer, lung (especially small cell)	Thiazide diuretics	
Cancer, pancreas, ovary		
Lymphoma	*Endocrine Disorders*	
Thymoma	Hypothyroidism	
	Glucocorticoid insufficiency	
Pulmonary Disorders		
Tuberculosis	*Miscellaneous*	
Pneumona/empyema	Porphyris	
Lung abscess	Pain, nausea	
Cystic fibrosis/COPD	Idiopathic	

COPD = chronic obstructive pulmonary disease.

AXIOM

Attempts to correct the hyponatremia or SIADH with sodium-rich solutions will usually cause an increase in urinary sodium excretion, but little change in the serum sodium.

A variant of SIADH is not infrequently seen in chronically ill or malnourished individuals. This condition is referred to as a *reset osmostat* and identifies a clinical state of hyponatremia that is characterized by a resetting downward of the plasma osmolality at which ADH is released. These patients have a chronic hyponatremia that is usually asymptomatic. They respond to water loading by decreasing ADH secretion and by diluting the urine. Likewise, sodium loading results in an increase in ADH secretion and hypertonic urine. Other than treatment of the underlying disease, no therapy is specifically indicated to correct the hyponatremia.

AXIOM

Chronic asymptomatic mild-moderate hyponatremia may require no therapy except to look for its etiology.

Endocrinologic disturbances that can cause hypotonic hyponatremia include glucocorticoid deficiency and hypothyroidism. Adrenal insufficiency allows increased ADH secretion and increased water reabsorption in the renal collecting ducts. The condition resembles SIADH, except that these patients respond to exogenous glucocorticoid by abruptly increasing urine volume and decreasing urine osmolality. Severe hypothyroidism causes hyponatremia by promoting increased ADH secretion.

Recently Oelkers presented data on five women with hypopituitarism (previously undiagnosed in four) who presented to the hospital with severe symptomatic hyponatremia (111 to 118 mEq/liter), pale skin, and complete, or almost complete, absence of axillary and pubic hair. Hypopituitarism was later proven in all five. Plasma vasopressin levels were inappropriately high (1.3 to 25.8 pmol/liter or 1.4 to 28 ng/liter) in relation to plasma osmolality (236 to 260 mOsm/kg water). All five patients had normal renal function and had no signs of volume depletion. Infusions of isotonic or hypertonic saline were relatively ineffective, but the hyponatremia was resolved within a few days of starting hydrocortisone. Thus, ACTH deficiency can cause SIADH. It was also clear that, when one is considering hypopituitarism as a cause of hyponatremia, one should not rely on plasma cortisol levels alone, but should also evaluate the response of plasma sodium levels to hydrocortisone therapy.

Acute water intoxication accounts for the diagnosis of hyponatremia in a few patients with impaired free water excretion. Since infants are unable to excrete a water load with the same efficiency as older children, they are at somewhat greater risk of developing hyponatremia from water loading. Postoperative patients are also at increased risk, owing to their high ADH secretion secondary to pain and stress.

Other cases of acute water intoxication have been reported secondary to ingestion of low solute formula in infants, use of tap water enemas, and intake of swimming pool water. Chronic water intoxication or *psychogenic polydipsia* is rare, except in mentally disturbed patients. The renal mechanisms that result in hyponatremia in these patients include the "washing out" of the normal renal medullary concentrating gradient.

(3) Hypervolemic Hyponatremia

AXIOM

The most frequent cause of hyponatremia is administration of too much water to patients with cardiac, liver, or renal disease.

Patients with hypervolemic hyponatremia usually have total body water in great excess and often present with pulmonary or peripheral edema. They generally have an impaired ability to excrete a water load. This allows retention of more water than sodium. These patients may be subcategorized into two groups: (1) the generalized edematous states of congestive heart failure, cirrhosis of the liver, and the nephrotic syndrome; and (2) advanced acute or chronic renal insufficiency.

In the generalized edematous patients, hyponatremia is often the result of a decreased effective arterial blood volume. In heart failure, the decreased effective blood volume is caused by a low cardiac output, whereas in cirrhosis of the liver, the decreased effective arterial blood volume is related to decreased peripheral resistance with arteriovenous shunting and splanchnic venous pooling. The low blood volume found in the nephrotic syndrome is a result of low capillary oncotic pressure, with resultant loss of fluid from the intravascular to the interstitial space. In each of these disorders, a decline in the effective arterial blood volume activates baroreceptors, leading to increased ADH release, renal water retention, dilution of ECF solutes, and hyponatremia. Furthermore, the edematous disorders are characterized by a decreased glomerular filtration rate and an enhanced proximal tubular reabsorption of fluid. The avid retention of sodium causes the urinary sodium concentration to be less than 20 mEq/liter, unless diuretics are being used.

Patients with oliguric acute or chronic renal failure may develop extreme salt and water overload through intravenous fluid administration. The decrease in glomerular filtration largely determines the extent of the impairment of water excretion. Urinary sodium concentration is variable but usually exceeds 40 mEq/liter.

2. Pathophysiology

The pathophysiologic changes of hyponatremia are most apparent when serum sodium levels fall below 120 mEq/liter in less than 12 to 24 hours. The effects on the central nervous system are usually the most obvious, but dysfunction in the cardiovascular and musculoskeletal systems may also occur.

a. Central Nervous System

AXIOM

Whenever a patient develops CNS changes, one should immediately look for hypoxemia, hypoglycemia, hyponatremia, and sepsis.

As serum sodium concentrations fall, the osmotic gradient that develops across the blood-brain barrier causes water to move into the brain, causing apathy, agitation, headache, altered consciousness, seizures, and even coma. The severity of symptoms is dependent not only on the rapidity, but also on the magnitude of the fall in the serum sodium concentration. Acute hyponatremia, occurring in 24 hours or less and resulting in a serum sodium concentration of less than 120 mEq/liter or a rate of fall of 0.5 mEq/liter or more per hour, can cause muscular twitching, seizures, and coma. The mortality rate with acute severe hyponatremia with CNS changes has been reported to be as high as 50% in adults. In animals in whom serum sodium is reduced to 110 mmol/liter in 2 hours, there is gross evidence of brain edema and the mortality rate is 88%.

When plasma sodium is lowered slowly over several days or weeks by a combination of sodium depletion and water ingestion, patients are usually less symptomatic, but even patients with chronic hyponatremia may experience focal weakness, hemiparesis, ataxia, and a positive Babinski sign.

AXIOM

Sudden, severe hyponatremia can cause severe brain swelling and neurologic symptoms.

As hyponatremia develops, the osmotic equilibrium between brain and plasma allows movement of increased amounts of water into the brain. However, brain swelling is less than would be predicted on the basis of the osmotic shifts alone. The brain's adaptation to hyponatremia is accomplished by two mechanisms: (1) movement of interstitial fluid into the cerebrospinal fluid, and (2) loss of cellular potassium and organic osmolytes. With acute hyponatremia, water moves into the brain from the plasma, causing an increase in the hydrostatic pressure of the cerebral interstitial fluid. The increased interstitial pressure accelerates the clearance of interstitial fluid into the cerebrospinal fluid, which is returned to the systemic circulation through the arachnoid villi. The movement of sodium-rich interstitial fluid out of the brain reduces brain sodium, which, in turn, reduces the osmotic gradient for the movement of water into the brain.

The loss of sodium, potassium, and chloride from the brain provides most of the protection against cerebral edema in the first hours of hyponatremia; however, when hyponatremia is sustained, the brain slowly loses other intracellular osmolytes, mainly amino acids. Loss of organic osmolytes during prolonged or severe hyponatremia is especially important in defending the brain against swelling.

The adaptive changes that protect the brain from excessive swelling also render it susceptible to dehydration during correction of the fluid and electrolyte problem. Indeed, there is often more risk of brain damage during treatment than before treatment. The rate of recovery of brain intracellular potassium and organic osmolytes during correction of the hyponatremia is much slower than the rate of loss of these substances during the development of the problem.

PITFALL

If correction of hyponatremia occurs more rapidly than the brain can recover solute, the higher plasma osmolality may dehydrate and injure the brain, producing what is now called the osmotic demyelination syndrome, or central pontine myelinolysis.

b. Cardiovascular

The cardiovascular response to hyponatremia depends primarily on the effective arterial blood volume, which may increase, decrease, or remain normal, depending on the underlying disorder. Intravascular volume is determined in part by the distribution of water between the intracellular and extracellular fluid (ECF) compartments. Thus, in the volume-depleted patient, hyponatremia can cause a further decrease in the intravascular volume by allowing movement of water out of the ECF compartment into the intracellular fluid space.

AXIOM

Shock occurs at lesser degrees of total body water depletion in hyponatremic patients.

AXIOM

If a patient is hypovolemic, increased ADH secretion will tend to enhance water reabsorption by the kidneys, even if the patient is quite hyponatremic.

Antidiuretic hormone (ADH) is one of the main factors opposing the hypovolemic effect of fluid shifts induced by hyponatremia. The ADH is released primarily as a response to the decreased effective arterial blood volume, which often accompanies hyponatremic edematous disorders. Nonosmotic stimulation of ADH release overrides the hyposmotic suppressive effect of hyponatremia, and increased ADH is present in almost all hyponatremic conditions. Initially, the function of ADH in this setting may seem paradoxic, because it potentiates the hyponatremic state by increasing water reabsorption by the renal tubules. ADH can also be a potent vasoconstrictor, however, and even at the low ADH concentrations, which are characteristic of clinical hyponatremia, it increases peripheral vascular resistance, thereby increasing blood flow to the liver and kidneys at the expense of the skin and muscle.

c. Musculoskeletal

Most patients with hyponatremia have normal muscle tone and function. However, muscle cramps and weakness can occur during strenuous exercise, especially if excess sweating is replaced with water. These symptoms are usually resolved rapidly when the serum sodium concentration is corrected back to normal.

d. Renal

The usual renal response to hyponatremia is production of dilute urine; however, this process is abrogated to some extent by the presence of increased concentrations of ADH. The amount of ADH present depends on the primary disease process and the effective arterial blood volume.

A urine sodium concentration of less than 10 mEq/liter usually indicates that the renal handling of sodium is intact and that the effective arterial blood volume is contracted. In contrast, a urine sodium concentration greater than 20 mEq/liter often indicates intrinsic renal tubular damage or a natriuretic response to hypervolemia. The urine sodium concentration will also vary somewhat, according to the ongoing gains and losses of salt and water. Urine sodium will tend to increase if the underlying disease significantly impairs renal function.

3. Diagnosis

AXIOM

Most hyponatremia is due to dilution.

The excess total body water may be iatrogenic or due to disease such as congestive heart failure, hepatic failure, or nephrotic syndrome. A decrease in the total body sodium due to excess diuresis, vomiting, diarrhea, or sweating is less common. The importance of each factor can usually be determined by careful review of the patient's history and his or her intake and output. Additional information can be obtained by comparing the sodium concentration and osmolarity of the serum and urine. A urine sodium of less than 10 to 20 mEq/liter suggests that either the ECF or the body content of sodium is low (if renal perfusion is adequate). If the urine sodium concentration is high, the patient usually has a water overload, is on diuretics, or has renal disease. If the serum sodium is less than 120 to 125 mEq/liter, there is often a decreased total body

666

content of sodium, as well as hemodilution. The patient may also have the syndrome of inappropriate antidiuretic hormone secretion (SIADH), but this is less common.

4. Treatment

a. Water Restriction

AXIOM

Fluid restriction is usually the best treatment for hyponatremia in stable asymptomatic patients.

While the water intake is being restricted, however, one must attempt to correct the underlying process and maintain an adequate tissue perfusion. If the effective ECF volume is depleted, strict water restriction can cause severe complications.

b. Hypertonic Saline

AXIOM

Hypertonic (3%) saline is generally used to treat hyponatremia that is severe, acute, and symptomatic.

If the hyponatremia is severe (less than 120 mEq/liter) and develops rapidly ($0.5 \text{ mEq} \cdot \text{liter}^{-1} \cdot \text{h}^{-1}$ decrease in serum sodium levels), and the patient is restless, administration of 3% saline solution is usually indicated. The 3% saline solution (which contains 513 mEq of sodium per liter) can be given at 25 to 100 ml/h, with careful observation for fluid overload and too rapid a rise in serum sodium levels. Attention should also be given to changes in urine sodium levels.

PITFALL

Failure to follow serum (and urine) sodium levels closely when giving hypertonic saline.

Unfortunately, hypertonic saline often increases either serum levels too rapidly or the serum sodium concentration only transiently, because much of the administered sodium is rapidly excreted in the urine. Consequently, in many patients, it may be helpful to give furosemide as well to reduce the amount of water present in the body.

c. Calculating Sodium Deficits

AXIOM

One should not use the total body water to calculate and treat sodium deficits in patients who have an expanded ECF.

Methods of calculating sodium deficits are somewhat controversial. Most authors calculate sodium deficits using total body water (60% of the body weight) as the sodium space, because sodium tends to equilibrate with the total body water even though most of the sodium is in the ECF. Thus, a euvolemic 80-kg man with a serum sodium of 120 mEq/liter would have a total sodium deficit of $(80 \text{ kg} \times 60\%) (140 - 120) = (48)(20) = 960$ mEq. However, most patients with hyponatremia are hypervolemic, and replacement based on such calculations could result in administration of too much sodium. Accordingly in hypervolemic hyponatremic patients, we usually calculate sodium deficits using a sodium space equivalent to 20% of the body weight. Thus, a hypervolemic 80-kg man with a serum sodium of 120 mEq/liter would be assumed to have a sodium deficit equal to $(20\% \times 80 \text{ kg}) \times (140 - 120)$ or $(16)(20) = 320$ mEq. However, if the patient's response indicates that the amount of sodium is inadequate, more can be given as needed. It must be stressed that, unless there is a history or other evidence of sodium loss from the body, most patients with hyponatremia have a normal or even increased total body content of sodium, and fluid restriction is usually the only treatment required.

d. Treatment of Pseudohyponatremia

Treatment of pseudohyponatremia, when due to hyperglycemia, is directed at its cause. Once an adequate urine output is obtained and insulin becomes effective, glucose levels fall and serum sodium levels will usually correct spontaneously. Regardless of the type of hyponatremia present, no treatment is usually necessary if serum osmolality is normal and the patient is asymptomatic.

e. Complications of Therapy

AXIOM

Slowly developing chronic severe hyponatremia is often safer than its treatment.

Complications with the treatment of acute hyponatremia, especially if there is no underlying CNS, hepatic, or renal disorder, are uncommon and occur in less than 2% of such patients. In chronic hyponatremia, brain edema is usually not severe and little evidence exists that chronic hyponatremia itself causes brain damage. Nevertheless, these patients appear to be at greatest risk for brain injury during the correction process.

The injury that occurs during or after correction of the hyponatremia progresses in a predictable manner and has been called the osmotic demyelination syndrome or central pontine myelinolysis (CPM). These neurologic changes are believed to be due to correction of the serum sodium at a rate faster than the brain can adapt to the higher osmolality. Other factors contributing to CPM in patients with chronic hyponatremia may include alcoholism, malnutrition, toxins, and metabolic imbalance.

Brain histology in fatal cases of central pontine myelinolysis shows myelinolysis and demyelination of central pontine and extrapontine myelin-bearing neurons. In typical cases, the clinical findings include fluctuating levels of consciousness, behavioral disturbances, dysarthria, dysphagia, or convulsions, progressing to pseudobulbar palsy and quadriparesis. Improvement may occur after several weeks of severe debilitation, but some patients are permanently impaired.

AXIOM

Treatment of severe, chronic hyponatremia is safest when done slowly and with diuretics.

The threshold for the production of CPM in patients with severe, chronic hyponatremia is a rate of correction of serum sodium levels faster than $0.5 \text{ mEq} \cdot \text{liter}^{-1} \cdot \text{h}^{-1}$ ($12 \text{ mEq} \cdot \text{liter}^{-1} \cdot \text{d}^{-1}$). In patients with severe, acute hyponatremia, correction at rates exceeding 0.5 to $1.0 \text{ mEq} \cdot \text{liter}^{-1} \cdot \text{h}^{-1}$, with or without diuretics, does not usually cause any problems. Severe neurologic complications have occurred almost exclusively in clinically hypernatremic patients treated with hypertonic or isotonic saline without the addition of furosemide or an osmotic diuretic. Similar patients treated with the same fluids, but with furosemide almost uniformly, have done well. Patients with chronic hyponatremia corrected at a rate less than $0.5 \text{ mEq} \cdot \text{liter}^{-1} \cdot \text{h}^{-1}$ have also done well.

B. HYPERNATREMIA

1. Etiology

AXIOM

Hypernatremia is usually due to inadequate water intake.

The most frequent cause of hypernatremia is a decrease in total body water because of reduced intake or excessive loss. The more common causes of hypotonic fluid losses are diarrhea, vomiting, hyperpyrexia, and excessive sweating. Less frequently, hypernatremia is caused by use of oral lactulose, osmotic diuresis with mannitol or glycerol, or increased intake of salt (Table 15.9). One can also classify the causes of hypernatremia according to the status of the blood volume (Table 15.10).

Table 15.9

CAUSES OF HYPERNATREMIA	1. Loss of water
	a. Reduced water intake
	(1) Defective thirst
	(2) Unconsciousness
	(3) Inability to drink water
	(4) Lack of acess to water
	b. Increased water loss
	(1) Vomiting, diarrhea
	(2) Sweating, fever
	(3) Hyperventilation
	(4) Diabetes insipidus, osmotic diuresis
	(5) Thyrotoxicosis
	(6) Severe burns
	2. Gain of sodium
	a. Increased intake
	(1) Hypertonic saline ingestion or infusion
	(2) Sodium bicarbonate administration
	b. Renal salt retention (usually because of poor perfusion)

a. Decreased Water Intake

Probably the main defense against hypernatremia is thirst. Although increased ADH secretion occurs before thirst, thirst is generally a far more important defense. However, patients who are in coma or are paralyzed will be unable to obtain adequate fluids.

b. Excess Water Excretion

Failure of ADH mechanisms is an important cause of hypernatremia, and it may be central or renal in origin. Neonates with immature kidneys, and adults with certain types of renal disease, such as obstructive uropathy or renal dysplasia, may be unable to excrete sodium properly. Consequently, their urine osmolality may be fixed between 200 to 300 mOsm/kg with a urine sodium of 60 to 100 mOsm/kg.

c. Increased Sodium Intake

The body tends to keep its total content of sodium remarkably constant, and if excessive sodium is given, the kidney will usually excrete it quite rapidly. However, if renal function is impaired, a dangerous expansion of the ECF may occur. One source of excessive sodium administration is the use of sodium-containing antibiotics, such as ticarcillin, which has an average of 5.2 mEq of sodium per gram.

Table 15.10

CAUSES OF HYPERNATREMIA RELATED TO BLOOD VOLUME	1. Hypovolemia
	a. Nonrenal H_2O losses (U_{Na} <10 mEq/L, U_{osm} >400 mOsm/L) from skin, GI, or respiratory tracts
	b. Renal H_2O losses (U_{Na} >20 mEq/L, U_{osm} <300 mOsm/L) from diuretics, renal disease, relief of urinary obstruction, adrenal failure, osmoreceptor failure
	2. Euvolemia
	a. Impaired thirst (coma)
	b. Nonrenal H_2O losses (GI, skin, respiratory)
	c. Renal H_2O losses from diabetes insipidus, reset osmostat, relief of urinary obstruction, renal disease, osmotic diuretics
	3. Hypervolemia
	a. Iatrogenic (hypertonic saline therapy)
	b. Mineralocorticoid excess (U_{Na} >20 mEq/L, U_{osm} >300 mOsm/L) from hyperaldosteronism, Cushing's disease, congenital adrenal hyperplasia, exogenous corticosteroids

GI = gastrointestinal.

d. Diabetes Insipidus

A particularly interesting cause of hypernatremia is diabetes insipidus (DI), which results in excessive loss of hypotonic urine. DI may be central in origin (due to a failure of secretion of ADH) or nephrogenic (due to renal unresponsiveness to ADH). About 30% of central DI is idiopathic and about 60% is secondary to neoplasms (25%), pituitary surgery (20%), or trauma (15%). Most of the remaining 10% is due to various granulomas (tuberculosis, sarcoidosis, eosinophilic granuloma) or local vascular problems (aneurysms, thrombosis, Sheehan's syndrome). Nephrogenic DI may be primary (familial) or secondary to a wide variety of causes, including hypercalcemia, hypokalemia, renal disorders, various drugs (including lithium, demeclocycline, amphotericin B, aminoglycosides, cisplatin), hematologic disorders (sickle cell disease, myeloma), malnutrition, or amyloidosis.

PITFALL
Failure to anticipate the triphasic swings in ADH levels in traumatic diabetes insipidus.

Traumatic DI is typically triphasic. After an initial polyuria from insufficient ADH secretion by hypothalamic cells, there is a transient second phase with a relatively normal urine flow lasting 1 to 7 days, due to release of previously formed hormone from the posterior pituitary. In the third phase, central DI returns after the released hormone has been utilized. The DI then gradually improves over a period of weeks or months as ADH-secreting cells gradually regenerate. The ADH-secreting cells have their cell bodies in the hypothalamus, and these are not usually completely destroyed by trauma.

Differentiation between central and nephrogenic DI is best achieved by noting (1) the response of serum and urine osmolarity to water deprivation (trying to reach a serum osmolarity greater than 295 mOsm/liter) and (2) the response to 5 units of subcutaneous aqueous vasopressin. Patients with central DI show little or no response to dehydration, but respond well to vasopressin ($U_{osm} \geq 800$ mOsm/liter). Nephrogenic DI shows little or no response to dehydration or vasopressin.

2. Pathophysiology

AXIOM
Shock is unusual in hypernatremic dehydration.

Because sodium does not freely penetrate tissue cell membranes, ECF and plasma volume tend to be relatively well maintained in hypernatremic dehydration until the water loss is greater than 10% of the body weight. Although there may be rather profound dehydration in some patients with severe hypernatremia, shock is an infrequent occurrence. When the severity of dehydration results in a loss of 10% of body weight, skin turgor becomes reduced, and a characteristic "doughy" feel can be appreciated when the skin of the abdomen is pinched between the fingers.

Acute symptomatology is seen in many patients once serum sodium concentrations exceed 158 mEq/liter. Patients tend to become irritable, and infants may have a high-pitched cry or wail, alternating with periods of severe lethargy. As dehydration and hypernatremia become more severe, one may see increased muscle tone or even coma with eventual seizures. Fever can be a contributing cause and a result of hypernatremic dehydration.

Permanent sequelae are not uncommon in children when serum sodium concentrations exceed 160 to 165 mEq/liter. Up to 16% of children with hypernatremia develop chronic neurologic deficits as a consequence. The overall mortality of hypernatremia is above 10%. If the plasma osmolality exceeds 350 mOsm/kg, the incidence of severe morbidity or mortality may exceed 25% to 50%.

Hypocalcemia, which is frequently seen in patients with hypernatremia, may contribute to the CNS symptomatology. However, the mechanism of the hypocalcemia is unclear.

Massive brain hemorrhage, or multiple small hemorrhages and thromboses, may occur when hypernatremia causes enough cellular dehydration and resultant brain shrinkage to cause tearing of cerebral blood vessels. This has been observed most frequently in neonates following acute administration of a large sodium load. As a consequence, the amount of sodium bicarbonate administered to acidotic infants must be limited.

If the hypernatremia persists for more than a few days, the brain dehydration may resolve, and brain water content may return to normal or near normal levels due to accumulation in the brain cells of "idiogenic osmoles," which are amino acids, particularly taurine. The formation of these idogenic osmoles increases intracellular osmolality, attracts water back into the brain cells, and restores their cellular volume. If the hypertonicity develops gradually, this protective mechanism tends to prevent severe brain cell shrinkage.

3. Treatment

PITFALL

Using glucose in water to aggressively treat hypernatremia, especially if it has been present for a few days.

Initially, when dehydration is severe, plasma volume should be restored with plasma-expanding fluids, such as normal saline or Ringer's lactate, which is administered until blood pressure and tissue perfusion are adequate. Once adequate perfusion is re-established, fluid containing 75 to 80 mEq/liter of sodium (i.e., 0.45% saline) should be given until the urine output is at least 0.5 $ml \cdot kg^{-1} \cdot h^{-1}$. Moderately hypotonic fluids (0.2% to 0.3% saline) can then be given with the aim of restoring normal hydration and bringing serum sodium concentrations down to normal in 48 to 72 hours. The reduction of serum sodium concentration should not exceed 10 to 15 $mEq \cdot liter^{-1} \cdot d^{-1}$.

The amount of water needed to correct hypernatremia can be estimated by the following equation:

$$\text{Water deficit (liters)} = TBW \left(1 - \frac{Na_2}{Na_1}\right).$$

TBW is normally expected to be about 60% of the body weight. Thus, if Na_1 is 160 mEq/liter and the Na_2 (desired serum sodium) is 145 mEq/liter, the water deficit in a 70-kg man is as follows:

$$\text{water deficit} = (60\% \times 70 \text{ kg}) \left(1 - \frac{145}{160}\right)$$

$$= \frac{(42)(15)}{160} = \frac{630}{160} = 3.9 \text{ L.}$$

As a general rule, each liter of water deficit results in a rise of serum sodium of 3 to 5 mEq/liter or 8 to 15 mOsm/liter. If there is any evidence of cardiac failure, rehydration must be done more slowly and with careful attention to changes in the CVP and/or PAWP. If the patient has significant ongoing fluid losses, these must be included in replacement therapy.

The sodium to be given can be calculated as 80 to 100 mEq/liter of estimated fluid deficit. Maintenance sodium needs can usually be disregarded. The sodium is given primarily as chloride, but sodium lactate or acetate can be given if the patient is acidotic.

In hypernatremia, with an excess of total body sodium, the restoration of a normal ECF volume often initiates a substantial natriuresis. However, if this does not occur promptly, sodium should be removed with diuretics, such as furosemide, while 0.45% saline is administered.

Because of the predilection of children with hypernatremia to also develop hyperglycemia, glucose should probably be given only as a 2.5% solution until glucose levels fall to relatively normal levels. Calcium gluconate may also be added, depending on plasma-ionized calcium levels. Once an adequate urine output is established, 20 to 40 mEq of potassium chloride should be added to each liter of fluid. Potassium aids water entry into cells.

AXIOM

Rapid correction of hypernatremia, especially if it is chronic, can cause seizures and severe neurologic sequelae.

Unless the hypernatremia is of short duration, idiogenic osmoles are presumed to be present in brain cells. Consequently, rehydration and lowering of serum sodium concentration too rapidly can cause brain cells to swell, resulting in cerebral edema and an increased likelihood of seizures, permanent neurologic sequelae, or even death. Serum electrolyte levels should be monitored frequently to ensure that the appropriate rate of decline of serum sodium concentration occurs.

In the case of acute hypernatremia, correction of serum sodium levels can be achieved rather rapidly with little fear of cerebral edema because idiogenic osmoles will not yet be present in the brain cells. However, rapid fluid administration in patients with hypernatremia due to excessive sodium administration may result in hypervolemia and pulmonary edema.

In children with acute severe sodium excess and a serum sodium concentration of more than 180 to 200 mEq/liter, peritoneal dialysis using a high-glucose (7.5%) low-sodium dialysate may be life saving. However, this must be done with frequent monitoring of serum electrolyte levels. Whenever the duration of the hypernatremia is unclear, rapid correction of serum sodium levels down to about 155 mEq/liter is recommended. This can be followed by slower correction of the serum sodium levels until they approach 145 mEq/liter.

Hypercalcemia is a common, unexplained finding in hypernatremia, and the addition of calcium gluconate to rehydration fluids is often indicated. Hyperglycemia also tends to accompany the hypernatremia. However, insulin treatment is not recommended because it may increase brain "idiogenic osmole" content.

In the case of central diabetes insipidus, administration of vasopressin or 1-desamino-(8-D-arginine)-vasopressin (DDAVP) must be undertaken carefully and fluid intake should be regulated so that the serum sodium concentrations do not drop too rapidly.

V. POTASSIUM

Elemental potassium was discovered in 1807 by Sir Humphrey Davy, who obtained it from caustic potash (KOH). It is now recognized as the major intracellular cation in the body. Chemical analysis of cadavers with radioactive $K40$ reveals a total body potassium content of about 50 to 55 mEq/kg or a total of about 3500 mEq in a young, healthy 70-kg man. However, "exchangeable potassium" measured with $K42$ provides somewhat lower values averaging about 45 mEq/kg.

Over 70% to 75% of the total body potassium is in muscle. Thus, protein malnutrition with muscle wasting may be associated with severe total body deficiencies in potassium. In women with severe muscle wasting, the total exchangeable body potassium content may be as low as 20 to 25 mEq/kg of body weight.

AXIOM

Severe hemolysis or muscle damage can cause serum potassium to rise rapidly to lethal levels.

Almost 98% of the total body potassium is within cells where the concentration is 110 to 150 mEq/liter. In contrast, the concentration of potassium in the ECF is normally only 3.5 to 5.0 mEq/liter. This large K^+ gradient across cell membranes is critical for normal neuromuscular function.

The normal total daily potassium intake is about 50 to 150 mEq. Meat contains about 1 mEq of potassium for each gram of protein. Some of the fruits and vegetables with a high potassium content include oranges, grapefruit, tomatoes, bananas, avocados, and raisins. Of the average 100 mEq of potassium ingested daily, 5 to 10 mEq is lost in the feces and a similar amount in sweat, leaving 80% to 90% to be excreted by the kidneys.

A. HYPOKALEMIA

The most frequent causes of hypokalemia are intracellular shifts and increased losses of potassium, especially in urine (Table 15.11).

1. Etiology
a. Intracellular Shifts

AXIOM

Metabolic alkalosis tends to cause hypokalemia; metabolic acidosis tends to cause hyperkalemia.

(1) Increased Bicarbonate

Potassium tends to move inside cells and hydrogen ions tend to move out of cells whenever the pH of the ECF rises, especially if the rise in pH is due to increased bicarbonate levels. A rise in the pH of 0.10 due to increased plasma bicarbonate levels generally causes a 0.5 (0.3 to 0.8) mEq/liter fall in serum potassium levels. Thus, if a patient with a serum potassium level of 4.2 mEq/liter and a pH of 7.40 is given bicarbonate and the pH is raised to 7.60, the serum potassium level will tend to fall to about 3.2 mEq/liter. Interestingly, immediately after an elevation in the P_{CO_2}, plasma potassium levels rise transiently, but then return to baseline values fairly rapidly.

(2) Loss of Gastric Acid

Hypokalemia seen with excessive vomiting is primarily due to the metabolic alkalosis that develops, not the loss of potassium present in the vomitus, even though the potassium content of highly acid gastric juice may exceed 10 mEq/liter. The alkalosis, in turn, causes a shift of potassium ions into cells in exchange for hydrogen ions. The mild hypovolemia that also frequently develops when there is excess loss of gastric juice stimulates an increased secretion of aldosterone, which further contributes to the potassium loss and increases absorption of sodium and bicarbonate. Hypercalcemia can also cause increased potassium loss in the urine.

During the treatment of severe diabetic ketoacidosis, potassium follows glucose into the cells and a very dangerous hypokalemia may develop rapidly as

---

Table 15.11

CAUSES OF HYPOKALEMIA
1. Shift into the cell
   a. Raising the pH of blood
   b. Administration of insulin and glucose
2. Reduced intake
3. Increased loss
   a. Renal loss
      (1) Primary hyperaldosteronism
      (2) Secondary hyperaldosteronism associated with diuretics, malignant hypertension, Bartter's syndrome, renal artery stenosis
      (3) Miscellaneous
         (a) Hypercalcemia
         (b) Liddle's and Bartter's syndromes
         (c) Magnesium deficiency
         (d) Renal tubular acidosis
         (e) Acute myelocytic and monocytic leukemia
   b. Gastrointestinal loss (vomiting, diarrhea, fistulas)

insulin begins to become effective, unless potassium is given as soon as glucose levels begin to fall. Although the glucose movement into cells brings potassium in with it, insulin by itself also directly increases the cellular uptake of potassium. Furthermore, as the pH rises toward normal and urine volumes increase, serum potassium levels can fall even further, because of increasing shift into the cells and loss in the urine.

PITFALL

As diabetic ketoacidosis is treated, if potassium is not given as soon as plasma glucose levels begin to fall, severe hypokalemia may develop rapidly, causing dangerous arrhythmias.

b. Diuresis

AXIOM

Hypokalemia plus hypochloremia, hyponatremia, and hypovolemia are due to excess diuresis until proven otherwise.

Although normal kidneys can retain needed sodium very well, it is much more difficult to conserve potassium. Indeed, potassium losses in urine are almost "obligatory" and are usually directly proportional to the volume of urine. Urine potassium normally averages about 40 to 80 mEq/liter. Even with severe, acute potassium deficits, urine potassium losses will often exceed 30 mEq/liter for at least several days.

AXIOM

A urine potassium of less than 10 mEq/liter usually indicates a severe chronic potassium deficit.

Use of loop diuretics, such as furosemide (Lasix), may cause urine potassium losses to exceed 100 mEq/liter. Indeed, loop diuretics are the most common cause of severe hypokalemia. Renal losses of potassium are also increased by alkalosis, hypochloremia, and hypomagnesemia. Renal tubular acidosis (type I) causes hypokalemia because there is impaired hydrogen ion excretion in the distal tubule.

c. Hyperaldosteronism

AXIOM

Hypertension plus hypokalemic, hypochloremic metabolic alkalosis is due to excess corticosteroids until proven otherwise.

Adrenal corticosteroids, especially aldosterone, cause the kidneys to excrete potassium and chloride and retain sodium and bicarbonate. This can cause a significant hypokalemic metabolic alkalosis. The combination of hypertension and hypokalemic metabolic alkalosis can be an important clue to hyperaldosteronism. Chronic or excessive ingestion of licorice can cause hypokalemia by a similar effect. Bartter's syndrome, occurring mostly in children, is characterized by hypokalemic metabolic alkalosis, juxtaglomerular hyperplasia, hyperreninemia and hyperaldosteronism, kaliuresis, and sodium and bicarbonate retention, without hypertension or edema. Liddle's syndrome is a familial type of pseudohyperaldosteronism. The electrolyte changes are characteristic of hyperaldosteronism, but aldosterone levels are normal.

The normal colon conserves about 500 to 1000 ml of water a day along with significant quantities of sodium, chloride, and bicarbonate (Table 15.12). Because of the high concentrations of potassium (up to 90 mEq/liter) and bicarbonate (30 to 74 mEq/liter) in stool, severe diarrhea can result in the loss of large quantities of these substances, producing a hypokalemic metabolic acidosis. Correction of only the metabolic acidosis will tend to cause an even worse hypokalemia.

Table 15.12

DAILY WATER AND ELECTROLYTES DELIVERED TO AND FROM THE NORMAL COLON

Fluid and Electrolyte	Delivered to Colon		Delivered to Stool	
	Amount	Concentration (mEq/L)	Amount	Concentration (mEq/L)
Water	600 ml		100 ml	
Sodium	76 mEq	125	4 mEq	40
Potassium	5 mEq	9	9 mEq	90
Chloride	36 mEq	60	2 mEq	15
Bicarbonate	44 mEq	74	3 mEq	30

PITFALL

Failure to anticipate potassium deficits in patients with severe diarrhea.

d. Epinephrine Infusions

An interesting cause of hypokalemia is the infusion of epinephrine, which can cause serum potassium levels to fall by more than 0.5 mEq/liter. This may be an important cause of arrhythmias in some patients with acute myocardial infarction. It is now known that beta$_2$-adrenergic receptors are involved in the regulation of extrarenal potassium disposal. The generation of cyclic AMP activates $Na^+K^+ATPase$, which augments intracellular/extracellular exchange of K^+ for Na^+. This increases intracellular potassium levels and hyperpolarizes the cell membrane. Theophylline potentiates this tendency of epinephrine to increase potassium influx into cells.

2. Physiologic Effects

AXIOM

Hypokalemia can cause severe muscle weakness.

Severe hypokalemia with levels below 2.0 to 2.5 mEq/liter may cause muscle weakness and increase the tendency to intestinal ileus. Indeed, respiratory paralysis has been seen with levels below 1.5 to 2.0 mEq/liter.

AXIOM

Severe hypokalemia can cause nephrogenic diabetes insipidus and severe dehydration, which must be considered when correcting the electrolyte abnormalities.

Most patients with hypokalemia are dehydrated because of its effect on renal tubules causing a nephrogenic diabetes insipidus. Hypokalemia tends to cause a metabolic alkalemia, not only through contraction alkalosis, but also through increased acid excretion in the urine (paradoxical aciduria). It also increases the tendency to glycosuria.

AXIOM

The most frequent cause of paradoxical aciduria is hypokalemia.

The sensitivity of the heart to digitalis and the likelihood of digitalis toxicity with arrhythmias or an AV block are increased in the presence of hypokalemia. In patients treated with hydrochlorothiazide, there is a direct relationship between the severity of the hypokalemia, concomitant hypomagnesemia, and the incidence of ventricular ectopy. Administration of both potassium and magnesium are important parts of the treatment of arrhythmias due to digitalis toxicity.

Hypokalemia increases renal tubular production of ammonia, and this may aggravate hepatic encephalopathy in patients with advanced cirrhosis.

3. Diagnosis

The diagnosis of hypokalemia is made primarily on serum electrolyte studies. However, serum potassium levels should be interpreted relative to the arterial pH. A low serum potassium level may be expected in an alkalotic patient, but hypokalemia in an acidotic patient is either a laboratory error or evidence of a severe potassium deficit. In some instances, the patients can act as if they are hypokalemic even with normal blood levels, particularly after cardiopulmonary bypass and with metabolic alkalosis. In patients with metabolic alkalosis, paradoxic aciduria strongly suggests a functional hypokalemia.

On ECG, hypokalemia less than 3.0 mEq/liter may cause low voltage QRS complexes, flattened T waves, depressed ST segments, prominent P and U waves, and prolonged QT and PR intervals (Fig. 15.1). A small U wave (between the T and P waves) can be seen in some normal individuals in the early precordial leads (V_1 to V_3), but it is more prominent and frequent with diastolic hypertension and coronary artery disease. The U wave may become especially prominent as potassium levels fall below 2.5 mEq/liter. Potassium levels below 2.0 mEq/liter also tend to widen the QRS complex.

Urine potassium levels can give some indication of the duration of hypokalemia and the severity of the total body deficit. Urine potassium levels that are normal (40 to 80 mEq/liter) in the presence of hypokalemia usually suggests that the potassium deficit is new and relatively mild. Hypokalemia with urine potassium levels less than 10 mEq/liter suggests a severe, chronic potassium deficiency. However, if the hypokalemia is due to primary aldosteronism, urine potassium levels may be elevated despite severe, chronic hypokalemia.

Urine potassium levels less than 10 mEq/liter suggest a chronic and severe potassium deficit that is not apt to respond well to attempts at rapid correction.

HYPOKALEMIA

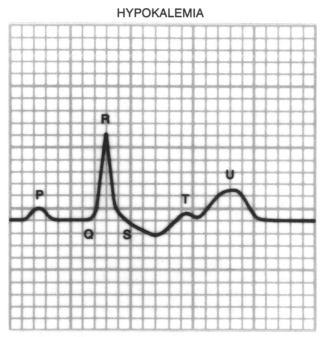

Figure 15.1   Hypokalemia. (From Dolan, JT: Critical Care Nursing. FA Davis, Philadelphia, 1991, p 826, with permission.)

4. Treatment

Acute severe hypokalemia is treated by infusing 10 to 15 mEq of KCl/h in 50 to 100 ml of 5% dextrose in water (D_5W) or 0.9% normal saline by IV piggyback for 3 to 4 hours. The ECG should be continuously monitored during potassium infusions. As a general rule, no more than 40 mEq of potassium should ever be put in a liter of IV fluids (except by careful IV piggyback) and no more than 40 mEq should ever be given in an hour.

Potassium equilibrates in the total body water, and it generally takes at least 40 to 50 mEq to raise the serum potassium level by 1.0 mEq/liter. Chronic deficits usually require much larger amounts of potassium in order to maintain an increase in serum levels, and not infrequently, much of the infused potassium is promptly excreted in the urine.

AXIOM
Relatively mild-moderate hypokalemia may be associated with large total body deficits.

Chronic hypokalemia may be associated with very severe potassium deficits, which often exceed 300 to 500 mEq. One way to estimate total body potassium deficits is from pH-corrected plasma potassium levels. The percentage by which serum levels (corrected for pH) are below 4.2 mEq/liter is twice as large as the percentage of total body potassium deficit. Thus, a patient with a serum potassium of 1.6 mEg/liter at a pH of 7.5 should have a serum potassium level of about 2.1 mEq/liter at a pH of 7.4. This indicates a 50% reduction in serum potassium. The percent deficit in total body potassium is half of the percent deficit in the plasma. Total body potassium ranges between 20 mEq/kg in a markedly muscle-wasted woman to 45 mEq/kg in a normal muscular man. Thus, if the patient is a 50-kg muscle-wasted woman, her total potassium content should be (20 mEq/kg)(50kg) = 1000 mEq.

B. HYPERKALEMIA

1. Etiology

There are many causes of hyperkalemia and it is easy to hemolyze blood as it is being drawn to produce a pseudohyperkalemia. Other causes of pseudohyperkalemia include leukocytosis, especially greater than 600,000/mm³, or thrombocytosis, especially greater than 1,000,000/mm³. These are particularly apt to cause hyperkalemia if the blood is not analyzed within 30 minutes of being drawn.

PITFALL
Excessive opening and closing of a fist below a tourniquet prior to drawing electrolyte levels.

Don and colleagues recently showed that excessive opening and clenching of the fist for several minutes while a tourniquet is applied raises potassium levels in the veins below the tourniquet 0.4 to 1.6 mEq/liter (average of 1.0 mEq/liter). The presence of the tourniquet by itself did not raise serum potassium levels. The more common causes of hyperkalemia are listed in Table 15.13.

AXIOM
Renal failure with oliguria is the most common cause of dangerous hyperkalemia.

Normally, 90% to 95% of the potassium taken in is excreted in the urine. Thus, anuria or severe diguria can cause a severe progressive rise in serum potassium levels.

Since each kilogram of lean muscle tissue may contain over 100 mEq of potassium, breakdown of muscle from trauma or sepsis may release large quan-

Table 15.13

ETIOLOGY OF HYPERKALEMIA	1. Factitious
	a. Laboratory error
	b. Pseudohyperkalemia: hemolysis, thrombocytosis, leukocytosis
	2. Metabolic acidemia (acute)
	3. Increased intake into the plasma
	a. Exogenous: diet, salt substitutes, low-sodium diet, medications
	b. Endogenous: hemolysis, GI bleeding, catabolic states, crush injury
	4. Inadequate distal delivery of sodium and decreased distal tubular flow
	5. Oliguric renal failure
	6. Impaired renin-aldosterone axis
	a. Addison's disease
	b. Primary hypoaldosteronism
	c. Other (heparin, beta blockers, prostaglandin inhibitors, captopril)
	7. Primary renal tubular potassium secretory defect
	a. Sickle cell disease
	b. Systemic lupus erythematosus
	c. Postrenal transplantation
	d. Obstructive uropathy
	8 Inhibition of renal tubular secretion of potassium
	a. Spironolactone
	b. Digitalis
	9. Abnormal potassium distribution
	a. Insulin deficiency
	b. Hypertonicity (hyperglycemia)
	c. Beta-adrenergic blockers
	d. Exercise
	e. Succinylcholine
	f. Digitalis

tities of potassium into the bloodstream. Patients with myoglobinemia are apt to develop renal failure, and, if that occurs, fatal hyperkalemia can develop very rapidly. Occasionally, succinylcholine can raise serum potassium levels abruptly in patients with severe crush injuries or burns. A similar problem may develop with hemolysis due to transfusion reactions.

Excessive intake of potassium is an infrequent cause of hyperkalemia, but can occur with IV administration of potassium-containing drugs. Aqueous (potassium) penicillin, for example, contains about 1.7 mEq of potassium per million units. Rapid injection of large dose of IV penicillin can cause cardiac arrest, especially in children.

2. Physiologic Effects

As potassium levels rise above 6.0 to 6.5 mEq/liter, cardiac conductivity and contractility may be impaired. With severe hyperkalemia, above 6.5 to 7.0 mEq/liter, an intracardiac block can be produced, first in the atria, then in the AV node, and finally in the ventricles, with the heart eventually stopping in diastole. Occasionally, hyperkalemia may cause such weakness that ventilatory failure may develop. The effects of hyperkalemia are increased if the patient has hyponatremia and hypocalcemia.

3. Diagnosis

AXIOM

Lethal hyperkalemia is most apt to develop in patients with severe tissue damage and oliguric renal failure.

One should suspect hyperkalemia in patients with oliguric renal failure, severe hemolysis, or excessive tissue breakdown. Since acidosis by itself can cause serum potassium levels to rise, potassium levels should be correlated with the arterial pH. It is unusual for a moderate-severe hyperkalemia to exist without acidosis.

HYPERKALEMIA

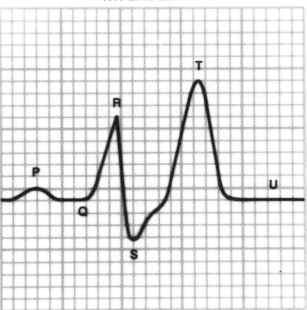

Figure 15.2 Hyperkalemia. (From Dolan, JT: Critical Care Nursing. FA Davis, Philadelphia, 1991, p 825, with permission.)

Mild hyperkalemia brings the membrane potential closer to threshold, and conduction in the heart is initially improved. As the serum K^+ level rises above 5.6 to 6.0 mEq/liter, the first ECG sign of hyperkalemia, as a result of speeded repolarization, is usually tall, peaked T waves, best seen in the precordial leads (Fig. 15.2). With further increases in serum potassium levels to 6.0 to 6.5 mEq/liter, impulse conduction decreases, often resulting in prolonged PR and QT intervals. At levels above 6.5 to 7.0 mEq/liter, diminished P waves and depressed ST segments can occur. This finding is not specific for hyperkalemia, however, and may be seen with massive cerebrovascular accidents and myocardial ischemia. Although ST segments are usually depressed with moderately severe hyperkalemia, elevation resembling acute myocardial ischemia may be seen occasionally.

At serum potassium levels of 7.0 mEq/liter or greater, impulses may still be conducted from the SA node to the ventricle because the intra-atrial conduction fibers are less sensitive to hyperkalemia than are atrial muscle fibers. Delayed conduction in the interventricular conducting system can produce patterns resembling bundle branch block.

As the levels exceed 7.5 to 8.0 mEq/liter, P waves disappear, the QRS complex widens, the S and T waves tend to merge, and the ventricular rhythm becomes irregular. At levels exceeding 10 to 12 mEq/liter, a classic sine wave is usually seen.

Death from hyperkalemia is usually the result of a diastolic arrest caused by block of the distal Purkinje fibers, or of ventricular fibrillation caused by re-entrant circuits that develop because of prolonged ventricular conduction.

4. Treatment

AXIOM

Mild-moderate hyperkalemia can usually be managed by stopping all potassium intake and increasing urine output.

If serum potassium levels rise above 5.0 to 5.5 mEq/liter, one must begin to look for factors predisposing to oliguric renal failure or increased red cell or other tissue breakdown. Whenever possible, all potassium-containing solutions and drugs should be discontinued. Diuresis is extremely helpful. Even when renal function is severely impaired, each liter of urine usually contains at least 30 to 40 mEq of potassium per liter.

If serum potassium levels rise above 5.5 to 6.0 mEq/liter, or there is extensive tissue damage and diuresis is not possible, one should consider using an ion exchange resin. Kayexalate (sodium polystyrene sulfonate) is an ion exchange resin that may be administered by mouth or by retention enemas. Each gram of sodium resin exchanges with and removes about 1.0 mEq of potassium from the plasma. When given orally, 15 to 25 g of Kayexalate is given with 50 ml of a 20% sorbitol solution every 4 to 6 hours. Kayexalate tends to be constipating, and the sorbitol increases the speed of evacuation of bowel contents. Rectal administration is 20 g of Kayexalate in 200 ml of a 20% sorbitol solution every 4 hours. The enema should be retained at least 30 minutes, if at all possible.

PITFALL

In patients with fluid overload or impaired cardiac function, the absorption of sodium from Kayexalate may precipitate acute heart failure.

If serum potassium levels are less than 6.5 mEq/liter and there are no ECG changes due to the hyperkalemia, treatment efforts may be directed primarily at reducing potassium intake and increasing potassium loss in the urine.

If serum potassium levels rise above 6.5 mEq/liter, one should consider giving glucose and insulin, and possibly also sodium bicarbonate. As glucose enters cells, it "pulls" potassium, magnesium, and phosphorus in with it. After an initial 50 ml of 50% IV glucose with 5 to 10 units of regular insulin, a liter of 20% glucose with 40 to 80 units of insulin may be given over the next 2 to 6 hours.

Sodium bicarbonate causes an alkalosis that tends to reduce serum potassium levels. It also increases the serum concentration of sodium, which also helps oppose the potassium effects. Each ampule (50 ml of a 7.5% solution) should be given relatively slowly by continuous IV infusion over at least 15 to 30 minutes, depending on the urgency of the situation. Hypertonic (3%) sodium chloride in doses of 50 to 100 mEq IV over 30 to 60 minutes may be helpful in hyponatremic patients; the sodium may also antagonize the effects of high potassium levels.

Calcium gluconate, or calcium chloride, is usually given only for severe hyperkalemia with levels >7.0 to 7.5 mEq/liter. The calcium opposes the cell membrane effects of the hypervolemia and does not alter the blood levels of potassium. Ten milliliters of 10% calcium gluconate contains 4.6 mEq of calcium, while a similar ampule of calcium chloride contains 13.4 mEq of calcium. The calcium is also more rapidly available from the chloride than from the gluconate. One ampule is given by slow IV infusion over at least 10 to 20 minutes. Additional calcium is given much more slowly, as needed.

AXIOM

Calcium must be given very cautiously to patients on digitalis.

If calcium has to be given to patients on digitalis, it must be done with great caution, since hypercalcemia potentiates the toxic effects of digitalis on the heart. Therefore, if calcium must be given on an emergency basis to patients taking digitalis, an ampule should be added to 100 ml of 5% dextrose in water and infused slowly over at least 20 to 30 minutes to permit a more even distribution throughout the extracellular space.

Table 15.14

EMERGENCY THERAPY OF HYPERKALEMIA

	Mechanism	Dose	Onset of Action	Duration of Hypokalemic Effect
Calcium gluconate (10%)	Antagonism	10–20 ml IV	1–3 min	30–60 min
Sodium bicarbonate	Antagonism and redistribution	50–100 mEq IV	5–10 min	1–2 h
Insulin plus glucose	Redistribution	20 U reg insulin with 50 g glucose IV over 1 h	30 min	4–6 h
Diuretics, furosemide	Excretion	40–80 mg IV	With diuresis	With diuresis
Cation exchange resin (Kayexalate)	Excretion	15–50 g p.o. or per rectum with sorbitol	1–2 h	While in intestine
Peritoneal dialysis or hemodialysis	Excretion	—	Within minutes	During dialysis

AXIOM

Calcium is the initial drug of choice if a patient develops dangerous arrhythmias due to hyperkalemia.

If a dangerous tachyrhythmia develops in a hyperkalemic patient, all of the above steps may have to be done together and rapidly. Such emergency treatment must proceed rapidly according to a predetermined program (Table 15.14). If the patient is in acute oliguric renal failure, hemodialysis and/or peritoneal dialysis should be set up while the above measures are being used.

VI. CALCIUM

A. CONTENT, INTAKE, AND OUTPUT

Calcium is the most abundant mineral in the human body. The total body calcium content is 15 to 20 g/kg of body weight or about 1.0 to 1.5 kg in a normal-size adult. About 99% is in bone as the mineral apatite, which has the general formula $Ca_5(F,Cl, OH, H_2CO_3)(PO_4)_3$. The average daily calcium intake is about 800 to 1000 mg primarily from milk and milk products. About one third of this calcium (300 to 350 mg) is absorbed, primarily in the small bowel, by both active (vitamin D dependent) and passive (concentration dependent) absorption. Loss of calcium into the GI tract (150 to 200 mg/d) and urine (150 mg/day) usually balances the GI absorption quite closely.

B. CONTROL OF CALCIUM LEVELS

Calcium homeostasis is under the control of parathyroid hormone (PTH), calcitonin, and vitamin D metabolites, especially calcitrol (1,25-dihydroxy-vitamin D).

1. Parathyroid Hormone

PTH is secreted by the parathyroid gland, primarily in response to low ionized calcium or magnesium levels. Parathormone raises serum calcium levels by several mechanisms, but especially by stimulating osteoclasts to increase bone resorption. It has less activity in the intestine, where it works in combination with calcitrol to indirectly stimulate calcium absorption. It also has an indirect action in the kidney, through adenylate cyclase stimulation, whereby it increases calcium resorption and increases phosphorous excretion. PTH also stimulates conversion of 25(OH) D to the much more metabolically active 1,25 $(OH)_2$ D.

2. Calcitonin

Calcitonin is secreted in response to influence by elevations in serum calcium and epinephrine, glucagon, and gastrin. It decreases the release of calcium from bone by inhibiting the activity of the osteoclasts. It also has a limited role in increasing calcium loss through the kidney.

3. Vitamin D

Vitamin D can be produced nonenzymatically by ultraviolet irradiation of skin, or it can be absorbed directly from the GI tract, particularly from fortified milk products. Since it is a fat-soluble vitamin, its absorption requires bile salts and micelle formation. Vitamin D is hydroxylated in the liver to 25-hydroxycholecalciferol [25(OH)D], and in the kidney it is further hydroxylated to either $1,25(OH)_2 D$ or $24,25(OH)_2 D$. The synthesis of $1,25(OH)_2 D$, which is much more potent metabolically, increases with hypocalcemia or hypophosphatemia. During hypercalcemia there is a reversal of the above sequence, so that more $24,25(OH)_2 D$, which is much less active, is formed.

C. FUNCTIONS OF CALCIUM

Calcium is vital to a wide variety of bodily functions, including neutrophil chemotaxis, lymphocyte activation, and membrane stability of a wide variety of cells. It is a required factor in the clotting cascade for activation or conversion of factors IX, VII, VIII, prothrombin, and fibrinogen. It is also necessary for platelet aggregation and granule release. However, very small amounts of calcium, probably less than 0.3 to 0.4 mEq/liter, are needed for clotting.

AXIOM

Hypocalcemia probably does not cause coagulation defects because cardiovascular function would be so severely impaired by the hypocalcemia before calcium levels got low enough to affect clotting.

Calcium is also essential for the release of neurotransmitters in the central and peripheral nervous systems, and it plays a critical role in muscle depolarization. Calcium ion influx into the depolarized myocardial cell prolongs depolarization. This is represented by the plateau or phase 2 portion of the cardiac action potential.

Stimulation of skeletal muscle causes calcium ions to be released from the sarcoplasmic reticulum into the cytoplasm, where it binds to, and alters, troponin. This alteration of troponin allows actin and myosin to interact, which causes the muscle to contract.

D. IONIZED AND PROTEIN-BOUND CALCIUM

Total plasma calcium levels average 8.5 to 10.5 mg/dl. The calcium present in the plasma is in three forms: (1) protein-bound calcium (normally 4.0 to 4.5 mg/dl), (2) complexed (nonprotein-bound, nonionized) calcium (normally 0.5 to 1.0 mg/dl), and (3) ionized calcium (normally 4.2 to 4.8 mg/dl). Increasingly, calcium levels are being reported as milliequivalents per liter, which is one half the number expressed as milligrams per deciliter. Thus, 4.4 mg/dl of ionized calcium is the same as 2.2 mEq/liter or 1.1 mmol/liter. The ionized calcium fraction, which is normally 2.1 to 2.4 mEq/liter or 1.05 to 1.2 mmol/liter, is responsible for virtually all the physiologic effects of calcium, of which the neuromuscular changes are most obvious.

AXIOM

If plasma protein levels are low, total calcium levels will also be low, even if ionized calcium levels are normal.

On average, each gram of protein binds 0.8 mg of calcium. Thus, if the non-protein–bound calcium is 4.9 mg/dl, and the total protein is 7.0 mg/dl, the total calcium is

$$Ca^{tot} = 4.9 + (0.8)TP = 4.9 + (0.8)(7.0) = 4.9 + 5.6 = 10.5 \text{ mg/dl}.$$

If the albumin (alb) and globulin (glob) concentrations are unusual, one can estimate the normal total calcium (mg/dl) by the following formula:

$$Ca^{tot} = 4.9 + (1.1)(alb) + (0.2)(glob).$$

Thus, if the albumin is 3.0 mg/dl and globulin is 4.0 mg/dl,

$$Ca^{tot} = 4.9 + (1.1)(3.0) + (0.2)(4.0) = 4.9 + 3.3 + 0.8 = 9.0 \text{ mg/dl.}$$

Because the relationship between total calcium, ionized calcium, and the plasma proteins varies so much, these formulas provide only a gross estimation of the relationship between ionized calcium and total calcium.

E. HYPOCALCEMIA

1. Definition

Hypocalcemia is often defined as an ionized calcium below 2.0 mEq/liter or 1.0 mmol/liter. Total calcium levels, especially in the presence of hypoalbuminemia, may be very low and yet be associated with normal ionized calcium levels. Some of the more common causes of ionic hypocalcemia are shock, sepsis, renal failure, and pancreatitis (Table 15.15). Hypocalcemia is unusual in ambulatory patients, except those with chronic renal disease or chronic hypoparathyroidism following thyroid or parathyroid surgery.

2. Etiology

a. Movement into "Sick" Cells

AXIOM

A rapid drop in ionized calcium levels in the blood usually indicates that cell membrane function is impaired.

The concentration of ionized calcium in the ECF is about 1.0 mmol/liter or 10^{-3} mol/liter. The concentration of ionized calcium in the cytoplasm of most cells is about 10^{-7} mol/liter. This gradient of 10^4 or 10,000:1 is maintained by active metabolic processes. Any problem that interferes with cell metabolism, such as shock or sepsis, will tend to reduce ionized calcium levels by allowing increased net movement of calcium across the cell membrane into the cytoplasm of the poorly functioning cells.

By the time ionized calcium levels in plasma have fallen to less than two thirds of normal, ionized calcium levels in the cytoplasm of many cells may have risen 200-fold. Following trauma, serum calcium levels may be low, especially with the fat embolism syndrome. This occurs not only because of cell dysfunction and calcium binding to free fatty acids, but also because of fatty acid inhibition of cell membrane calcium pumps.

b. Pancreatitis

AXIOM

Low calcium levels in pancreatitis may be the first indication that complications are developing.

Table 15.15

CAUSES OF HYPOCALCEMIA	Shock or sepsis
	Impaired production of 1,25-dihydroxyvitamin D
	Malabsorption
	Severe hepatic failure
	Renal failure
	Anticonvulsant therapy
	Pancreatitis
	Hypomagnesemia
	Alkalosis
	Decreased serum albumin levels
	Hypoparathyroidism
	Idiopathic
	Postsurgical
	Pseudohypoparathyroidism
	Osteoblastic metastases
	Fat embolism syndrome

Acute pancreatitis is an important cause of hypocalcemia. Pancreatic lipase breaks down fat into fatty acids and glycerol. The fatty acids combine with calcium to form insoluble calcium soaps and reduce serum calcium levels. The combination of necrotic fat plus calcium soaps makes up much of what is recognized as the fat necrosis of pancreatitis. In addition, as protein moves into the inflammatory exudate, the resultant hypoproteinemia may cause total calcium levels to fall. Pancreatitis not only reduces parathormone secretion, but also the response of tissues to it. If total calcium levels fall below 8.0 mg/dl, the chance of severe complications from pancreatitis is increased.

c. Drugs

AXIOM
One of the causes of hypocalcemia in ICU patients may be the use of cimetidine to prevent stress gastric bleeding.

A large number of drugs can cause hypocalcemia (Table 15.16). One of the most frequently used is cimetidine. This histamine (H_2) receptor-blocking agent apparently lowers serum calcium levels by decreasing the synthesis or secretion of parathyroid hormone.

d. Postoperative Hypocalcemia

(1) Hypoparathyroidism

Currently, the incidence of postoperative hypocalcemia after surgery for hyperparathyroidism ranges from 13% to 30%. Up to 10% of postparathyroidectomy patients may have hypoparathyroidism, as defined by a fasting calcium of less than 8.5 mg/dl and a simultaneous inorganic phosphorus of greater than 4.5 mg/dl. Postoperative hypocalcemia can be due to hypoparathyroidism from the permanent surgical removal of parathyroid tissue, transient ischemia of the parathyroid glands in patients who have extensive bilateral neck surgery, or long-term hypercalcemic suppression of nonadenomatous parathyroid glands.

(2) Hungry Bone Syndrome

The term *hungry bone syndrome* was coined by Albright and now indicates postparathyroidectomy hypocalcemia due to rapid remineralization of the skeleton. During this accelerated remineralization, a persistent hypocalcemia and hypophosphatemia may be severe enough to cause tetany. These patients may require vigorous calcium and vitamin D supplementation for prolonged periods of time.

AXIOM
A patient with hyperparathyroidism and an elevated alkaline phosphatase is particularly apt to develop hypocalcemia following parathyroid surgery.

Table 15.16

DRUGS THAT CAN CAUSE HYPOCALCEMIA	Cimetidine
	Phosphates (e.g., enemas, laxatives)
	Dilantin, phenobarbital
	Gentamicin, tobramyin
	Cisplatin
	Heparin
	Theophylline
	Protamine
	Glucagon
	Norepinephrine
	Citrate (blood)
	Loop diuretics
	Glucocorticoids
	Magnesium sulfate
	Sodium nitroprusside

In a recent study, Brasier and Nussbaum found the hungry bone syndrome in 13% of their patients after parathyroid surgery. Patients were thought to have this problem if they had a fasting calcium level less than 8.5 mg/dl and a simultaneous inorganic serum phosphorus of less than 3.0 mg/dl on postoperative day 3 or later.

e. Renal Failure

Hypocalcemia is a frequent finding in renal failure. This may be partially due to the resulting hyperphosphatemia, but there is also decreased production of $1,25(OH)_2$ D in the kidney, which, in turn, causes decreased intestinal absorption of calcium.

Secondary hyperparathyroidism with increased PTH levels often results from the hypocalcemia of chronic renal failure. If PTH levels remain elevated and hypercalcemia develops in spite of cure of the renal failure by renal transplantation, the patient is said to have tertiary hyperparathyroidism.

f. Phosphate Overload

Phosphate overload from nonrenal causes may also lead to hypocalcemia. This is the presumed mechanism in acute rhabdomyolysis of hyperpyrexia and major trauma. Excessive use of phosphate cathartics and sodium phosphate (Fleets) enemas can cause significant hyperphosphatemia in patients with renal disease, in children with Hirschsprung's disease, or in small infants.

g. Hypomagnesemia

AXIOM

Whenever one sees hypocalcemia, one should also look for hypomagnesemia.

Hypomagnesemia as a cause of, or in association with, hypocalcemia may be seen in alcoholism, excess diuretic use, epilepsy, and renal failure. Neonatal hypomagnesemia leads to low parathyroid hormone secretion, decreased responsiveness of bone cells to parathyroid hormone, and decreased calcium mobilization from bone.

h. Idiopathic Hypoparathyroidism

Idiopathic hypoparathyroidism is probably an autoimmune disorder in which pernicious anemia, exostoses, moniliasis, Hashimoto's disease, sterility, and Addison's disease may be seen. This syndrome may also be associated with cataracts, mental retardation, intracranial calcification, and papilledema due to increased intracranial pressure.

i. Nonsurgical Primary Hypoparathyroidism

Hypocalcemia with primary hypoparathyroidism has been reported from parathyroid infarction, metastases to the parathyroids, and hemochromatosis of the parathyroids.

j. Pseudohypo-parathyroidism

Pseudohypoparathyroidism is a familial disorder characterized by decreased end-organ responsiveness to parathormone resulting in hypocalcemia, hyperphosphatemia, parathyroid hyperplasia, and excessive serum parathormone concentrations. These patients usually have a very low urinary cyclic AMP excretion that only slightly increases with infusion of parathormone. This condition may be inherited as an X-linked dominant trait with variable penetrance. Patients are short in stature, have round facies, brachycephaly, a short thick neck, short pudgy fingers and toes, and growth failure of the fourth and fifth metacarpals. Mental retardation, seizures, subcutaneous soft-tissue calcification, and a male-to-female ratio of 2:1 can be seen. The skin can be dry and coarse, and the hair is often brittle.

k. Vitamin D Deficiency

Hypocalcemia due to vitamin D deficiency is rare in the United States. Infants born to vitamin D deficient mothers who lack sunlight exposure and receive no vitamin D supplementation may have rickets. Breast milk has low vitamin D content, and breast milk feeding without sunshine exposure in unsupplemented infants may result in infantile rickets.

3. Physiologic Effects

AXIOM

The physiologic effects of hypocalcemia are usually due to acute reductions in ionized calcium levels.

Although normal ionized calcium levels are 2.1 to 2.4 mEq/liter, (1.05 to 1.2 mmol/liter), serious physiologic changes do not usually occur until ionized levels in serum are less than 1.4 mEq/liter (0.7 mmol/liter). Below those levels, hypocalcemia can cause a wide variety of signs and symptoms (Table 15.17).

The severity of the signs and symptoms of hypocalcemia depend greatly on the rapidity of the fall in calcium. The more acute the drop in the serum calcium, the more likely the significant pathophysiologic changes. As serum calcium levels fall, neuronal membranes become increasingly more permeable to sodium, enhancing excitation. Potassium and magnesium have an antagonizing effect on this excitation.

Decreased ionized calcium levels reduce the strength of myocardial contraction, primarily by inhibiting relaxation and decreasing the sensitivity of the heart to digitalis. Hypocalcemia should be considered as a possible etiologic factor in patients with refractory heart failure.

Low ionized calcium levels increase parathormone (PTH) secretion, which mobilizes calcium from bone and decreases renal tubular absorption of phosphate and bicarbonate. This, in turn, may cause an increased absorption of chloride, producing a tendency to hyperchloremic hypophosphatemic renal tubular acidosis. A ratio of chloride to phosphate greater than 35 to 1 mEq/mg in the plasma is sometimes considered to be highly suggestive of hyperparathyroidism.

Table 15.17

SYMPTOMS AND SIGNS OF HYPOCALCEMIA	
	General
	Weakness, fatigue
	Neurologic
	Tetany
	Chvostek's and Trousseau's signs
	Paresthesias circumorally and in digits
	Impaired memory, confusion
	Hallucinations, dementia, seizures
	Extrapyramidal disorders
	Dermatologic
	Hyperpigmentation
	Course brittle hair
	Dry scaly skin
	Cardiovascular
	Heart failure; hypotension
	Vasoconstriction
	Muscular
	Spasms/cramps
	Weakness
	Skeletal
	Osteodystrophy
	Rickets
	Osteomalacia
	Miscellaneous
	Dental hypoplasia
	Cataracts
	Decreased insulin secretion

Increased cytoplasmic calcium activates phospholipase, which increases prostaglandin production and alters cell lipids. Increased cytoplasmic calcium also interferes with cell metabolism. Efforts by mitochondria to pump the excess calcium from the cytoplasm into the mitochondrial matrix greatly reduce adenosine triphosphate(ATP) formation. Consequently, giving calcium during shock or sepsis may transiently improve hemodynamics. However, if cell metabolism does not also improve, some of the additional calcium moves into the cytoplasm within 30 to 40 minutes. This further increases cytoplasmic calcium levels and causes additional improvement of cell metabolism and cardiovascular function.

Movement of calcium into ischemic cerebrovascular smooth-muscle cells may cause persistent cerebral vasoconstriction, with resultant failure of cerebral reperfusion after strokes or cardiac arrest. This may be a major cause of the poor results in management of these problems. Consequently, there has been some interest in the use of calcium blockers for cerebral resuscitation. In a recent study of cardiac arrest victims, nimodipine, one of the new calcium-channel blockers, improved the early CNS response.

4. Diagnosis

Hypocalcemia causes a wide array of signs and symptoms (Table 15.17).

a. Symptoms

PITFALL

Failure to ask about perioral or digital paresthesias in patients who have just had thyroid or parathyroid surgery.

The most characteristic initial symptom of hypocalcemia following thyroid or parathyroid surgery is parasthesias around the mouth or in the fingertips. Hypocalcemia should be suspected in any patient who is irritable and has hyperactive deep tendon reflexes following thyroid or parathyroid surgery. It should also be suspected in patients who have seizures, particularly if they ever had thyroid surgery, even if it was many years previously.

b. Signs

A positive Chvostek's or Trousseau's sign is usually considered to be fairly good clinical evidence of hypocalcemia. A positive Chvostek's sign is a twitch at the corner of the mouth when the examiner taps over the facial nerve just in front of the ear. However, it is present in about 10% to 30% of normal individuals. Nevertheless, eyelid muscle contraction with the Chvostek maneuver is said to be almost diagnostic of hypocalcemia.

Trousseau's sign, which is generally a more reliable indicator of hypocalcemia, is positive if carpopedal spasm is produced when the examiner applies a blood pressure cuff to the upper arm and maintains a pressure above systolic for 3 minutes. The fingers are spastically extended at the interphalangeal joints and flexed at the metacarpophalangeal joints. The wrist is flexed and the forearm is pronated.

c. Laboratory Findings

AXIOM

Severe alkalosis can cause clinical signs of hypocalcemia even when total calcium levels in blood are normal.

Signs of hypocalcemia may be found with normal total serum calcium levels if the patient is very alkalotic. Each 0.1 rise in pH lowers ionized calcium levels by about 3% to 8%. Consequently, a very alkalotic patient may have normal total serum calcium levels with ionic hypocalcemia. Similar signs and symptoms may be caused by hypomagnesemia, strychnine, or tetanus toxin.

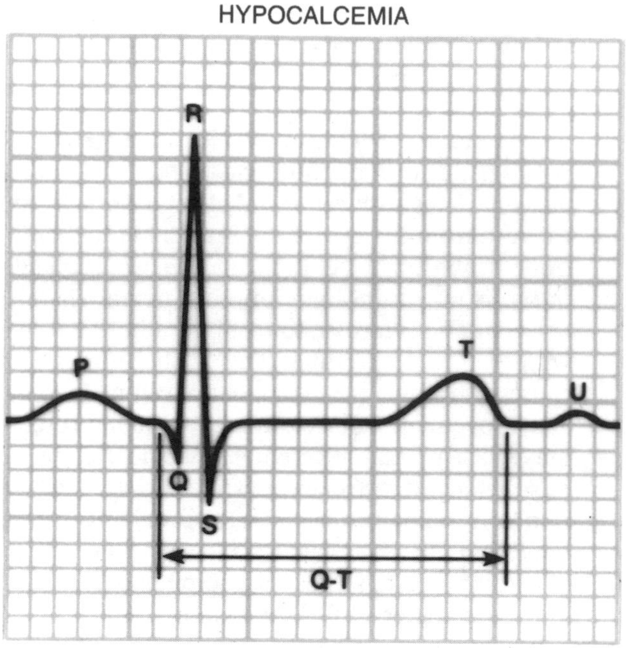

HYPOCALCEMIA

Figure 15.3 Hypocalcemia. (From Dolan, JT: Critical Care Nursing. FA Davis, Philadelphia, 1991, p 827, with permission.)

Decreased plasma levels of ionized calcium are diagnostic, but ionic hypocalcemia should be suspected if the patient has decreased levels of total calcium in the presence of normal plasma proteins. Primary hypoparathyroidism is characterized by a low serum parathyroid hormone concentration, hyperphosphatemia, and hypocalcemia.

d. Electrocardiography

The most characteristic ECG findings in hypocalcemia are prolonged QT intervals (Fig. 15.3); however, the QRS and T waves are of normal width, and it is the ST segment that is really prolonged. These findings are usually seen with serum calcium levels less than 6.0 mg/dl.

e. X-Rays

Radiologically, rickets is characterized by craniotabes, frontal skull bossing, rachitic rosary ribs, widened rib cage (Harrison's groove), and bowed legs. Healed fractures are also often present. Other radiographic changes include cupping and splaying of the metaphyseal ends of long bones, widening between the metaphyses and epiphysis, bone demineralization, and thinning of cortical bone.

5. Treatment

Treatment of hypocalcemia is tailored to the individual and directed toward the underlying cause. If the patient is asymptomatic, oral calcium therapy with or without vitamin D may be all that is required. Calcium lactate, calcium glubionate, calcium ascorbate, calcium carbonate, and calcium gluconate are available in oral preparations. Milk, because of the large amount of phosphate present, is not really a good source of calcium, except in growing children, who also need the phosphate.

PITFALL

Administering calcium rapidly IV for mild-moderate hypocalcemia without symptoms can cause unnecessary cardiovascular, neuromuscular, and renal complications.

Symptomatic patients following thyroid or parathyroid surgery are often treated with parenteral calcium (Table 15.18). With severe acute hypocalcemia,

Table 15.18

TREATMENT OF HYPOCALCEMIA

	Preparations	Amount of Calcium	Usual Doses
Parenteral			
Ca²⁺ gluconate (10%)	10-ml ampules	93 mg Ca²⁺ (4.6 mEq)	10–20 ml in 100 ml D₅W over 10–15 min
Ca²⁺ chloride (10%)	10-ml ampules	272 mg Ca²⁺ (13.6 mEq)	2.5–10 ml in 100 ml D₅W over 10–20 min
Oral			
Ca²⁺ gluconate tablets	1000 mg	92 mg Ca²⁺ (4.5 mEq)	1–4 g/d in divided doses q. 6 h
Ca²⁺ gluconate (neocalglucon)	5-ml syrup	23 mg Ca²⁺/ml	1–4 tsp/d in divided doses q. 6 h
Ca²⁺ lactate tablets	650 mg	79 mg Ca²⁺	1–4 g/d in divided doses q. 6 h

10 ml of 10% calcium chloride or calcium gluconate may be given IV over 10 to 20 minutes, followed by a continuous IV drip that provides a gram of calcium chloride over a period of 6 to 12 hours. If the patient is not symptomatic, or if the hypocalcemia is not severe and prolonged for more than 10 to 14 days, treatment with calcium may not be indicated. One should not administer calcium rapidly IV to asymptomatic patients with mild-moderate hypocalcemia because it can cause severe unnecessary cardiovascular, neuromuscular, and renal complications. For chronic hypoparathyroidism, use of oral calcium salts and rather high doses of vitamin D may be required.

During massive transfusions, if the patient is in shock or heart failure, in spite of adequate volume replacement therapy, and blood is being given faster than 1 unit every 5 minutes, 10 ml of 10% calcium chloride can be given after every 4 to 6 units of blood. Calcium is seldom required at a slower rate during transfusions or for elective surgery.

AXIOM

Calcium is seldom required during resuscitation unless large amounts of blood are being given very rapidly and the patient is in shock or heart failure.

Although it has been recognized for some time by us and others that clinical sepsis is often associated with hypocalcemia, it is not clear whether giving calcium is of any benefit. Although administration of calcium to hypocalcemic patients with septic shock may temporarily improve blood pressure and cardiac output, the effect is usually short lived.

Recently, Steinhorn, Sweeney, and Layman have shown that calcium supplementation fails to improve the outcome of experimental sepsis. This underscored the previous findings of Malcolm, Zaloga, and Holaday, and Zaloga, Chernow, and Lake that calcium administration increases mortality rate in endotoxin-treated rats and animals with endogenous sepsis due to cecal ligation. Chernow, in an accompanying editorial, reviewed this data, and to the question of whether calcium has a therapeutic role in sepsis, he answered, "probably—sometimes."

Although, in the past, the use of calcium had been advocated for the treatment of asystole or electromechanical dissociation, it has now been shown that the chances of successful resuscitation are reduced by giving calcium. On the other hand, patients with bradyasystolic arrest and chronic renal failure are apt to have hyperkalemia and hypocalcemia and may benefit from calcium administration.

For the prevention of rickets, 400 IU of vitamin D is the recommended daily intake. Treatment of established rickets may involve a daily dose of vitamin D as high as 5000 to 10,000 IU until the electrolyte and bone changes are corrected.

F. HYPERCALCEMIA

1. Etiology

Hypercalcemia may be defined as a total calcium level exceeding 10.5 mg/dl or an ionized calcium level exceeding 2.7 mEq/liter. This abnormality has been found in 0.3% to 5.0% of patients studied in various biomedical profiles. There are many causes of hypercalcemia (Table 15.19). A mnemonic sometimes used to remember some of the more common causes of hypercalcemia is "Pam P. Schmidt" for parathormone, Addison's disease, multiple myeloma, Paget's disease, sarcoidosis, cancer, hyperthyroidism, milk-alkali syndrome, immobilization, excess vitamin D, and thiazides.

a. Malignancies

AXIOM

The most frequent cause of severe hypercalcemia (>14 mg/dl) is malignant neoplasms with either extensive metastases or parathormonelike activity.

Hypercalcemia is quite common in women with carcinoma of the breast who are being treated with estrogens. Hypercalcemia is also seen with increased frequency in lung cancer (especially of the squamous cell type) and renal carcinomas. Other malignancies associated with hypercalcemia, but which are less frequent, include multiple myeloma, pheochromocytoma, and some acute

---

Table 15.19

CAUSES OF HYPERCALCEMIA	*Malignancy*
	Lung (squamous cell carcinoma)
	Breast
	Kidney
	Myeloma
	Leukemia
	Endocrinopathies
	Primary hyperparathyroidism
	Hyperthyroidism
	Pheochromocytoma
	Adrenal Insufficiency
	Acromegaly
	Drugs
	Hypervitaminosis D and A
	Thiazides
	Lithium
	Hormonal therapy for breast cancer
	Granulomatous Disease
	Sarcoidosis
	Tuberculosis
	Histoplasmosis
	Coccidiomycosis
	Immobilization
	Miscellaneous
	Paget's disease of bone
	Postrenal transplantation
	Recovery from acute renal failure
	Phosphate depletion syndrome

leukemia. In general, the higher the serum calcium level, especially above 14.0 mg/dl, the more likely the hypercalcemia will be due to malignancy.

b. Primary Hyperparathyroidism

The most common overall cause of hypercalcemia, particularly in ambulatory care settings, is primary hyperparathyroidism, which accounts for 25% to 50% of all hypercalcemia. Primary hyperparathyroidism is caused by a parathyroid adenoma in about 80% of cases and parathyroid hyperplasia in the remaining 20%. With very high calcium levels and no evidence of a malignancy, an enlarged parathyroid gland can sometimes be palpated in the neck. Parathyroid carcinoma is a rare cause of hyperparathyroidism.

c. Multiple Endocrine Adenomas

PITFALL
Failure to look for pancreatic, pituitary, adrenal, and thyroid neoplasms in patients with primary hyperparathyroidism.

Parathyroid adenomas may be sporadic or familial. The familial type may be part of a multiglandular endocrinopathy, and one should look for associated pancreatic, pituitary, adrenal, and thyroid neoplasms in any patient with primary hyperparathyroidism. The combination of parathyroid, pituitary, and pancreatic islet adenomas is known as multiple endocrine adenomatosis type I (MEA-I) or Wermer's syndrome. MEA-IIA (Sipple's) syndrome consists of hyperparathyroidism combined with pheochromocytoma and medullary cell carcinoma of the thyroid. In infants, parathyroid hyperplasia may be inherited as a familial autosomal dominant or recessive trait. It is sometimes seen in infants of hypoparathyroid mothers in response to chronic intrauterine hypocalcemia.

d. Immobilization

AXIOM
Critically ill patients, especially those with sepsis, tend to develop ionic hypocalcemia, but this may be masked or occasionally overbalanced by the tendency to hypercalcemia with immobilization.

In patients who are immobilized, the parathyroid-vitamin D axis is suppressed and calcium may leave bone rapidly, producing hypercalcemia, at least temporarily. Urinary excretion of calcium in such patients may exceed 200 to 300 mg/d, and there is an increased tendency to nephrolithiasis. Patients with Paget's disease, especially if they are at bed rest because of their pain, may have severe hypercalcemia, because of rapid bone turnover. Astronauts, due to their weightlessness, may rapidly lose large amounts of calcium from their bones and may develop a severe, prolonged negative calcium balance.

e. Hyperthyroidism

Although intestinal absorption of calcium is reduced in hyperthyroidism, up to one third of patients with thyrotoxicosis will concurrently have hypercalcemia, which resolves with treatment of the thyroid disorder. The source of excess calcium is presumed to be bone, but the exact mechanism is not known.

f. Addison's Disease

Hypercalcemia has been seen in patients with Addison's disease and adrenal crisis, perhaps because of a lack of the hypocalcemic effect of corticosteroids.

g. Hypervitaminosis

Hypervitaminosis A and D can cause hypercalcemia. In vitamin A toxicity, the patient will present with arthralgias, alopecia, a desquamating pruritus, and signs and symptoms of hypercalcemia. Both vitamins A and D cause increased osteoclastic resorption of bone, but vitamin D toxicity also causes increased intestinal absorption of calcium. Vitamin A toxicity usually subsides after discontinuation of vitamin A intake, but vitamin D toxicity may require treatment with corticosteroids.

h. Milk-Alkali Syndrome

Milk-alkali syndrome is now an extremely uncommon cause of hypercalcemia, but it was reported in the past in patients with peptic ulcer disease who drank excessive quantities of milk and took large amounts of antacids.

i. Granulomas

Many granulomatous diseases may be associated with hypercalcemia. Hypercalcemia occurs in up to 17% of patients with sarcoidosis because of increased sensitivity to vitamin D in the intestine, which results in increased absorption of calcium. This hypercalcemia responds to corticosteroids or vitamin D restriction. Hypersensitivity to vitamin D can also be seen in tuberculosis. There also are a number of reports of hypercalcemia in patients with disseminated coccidioidomycosis, silicon granulomas, berylliosis, and histoplasmosis.

AXIOM
Hypercalcemia with lung lesions may be due to malignancy or granulomas.

j. Thiazide Diuretics

Hypercalcemia can be seen with the use of thiazide diuretics, which increase the renal tubular reabsorption of calcium and decrease plasma volume. It is one of the more common causes of hypercalcemia in ambulatory patients. Virtually all other diuretics, especially the loop diuretics, increase urinary calcium excretion and tend to cause hypocalcemia.

k. Syndromes in Infancy

Hypercalcemia may be seen in Williams syndrome, which is characterized by supravalvular aortic stenosis and elfin facies. Blue diaper syndrome, in which excessive amounts of indole derivatives cause blue urine because of an error in tryptophan metabolism, may also be associated with hypercalcemia.

2. Pathophysiologic Effects

The effects of hypercalcemia can be neuromuscular, cardiovascular, gastrointestinal, renal, and skeletal. Neuromuscular changes include decreased sensitivity, responsiveness, strength of muscular contraction, and nerve conduction. This causes increasing weakness and fatigue, which may progress to ataxia and altered mental status.

In mild hypercalcemic states, cardiac conduction is slowed, automaticity is decreased, and the refractory period is shortened. There is also increased sensitivity to digitalis preparations. Gastrointestinal mortality is impaired, but there is increased acid secretion with gastrin.

AXIOM
Patients with severe hypercalcemia are usually severely dehydrated.

Loss of renal concentrating ability, as might be expected with nephrogenic diabetes insipidus, is the most frequent renal effect of hypercalcemia. This is a reversible tubular defect, which results in polyuria and dehydration in spite of polydipsia. Sodium, potassium, and magnesium reabsorption are reduced in the proximal tubule. Potassium wasting results in hypokalemia in up to one third of patients. Nephrocalcinosis and nephrolithiasis are caused by the hypercalcemia and are aggravated by dehydration. As the hypercalcemia persists, increasing microscopic calcium deposits in the kidney may result in progressive renal insufficiency.

With serum concentrations greater than 16 mg/dl, calcium salts may be deposited in the myocardium, kidneys, lungs, subcutaneous tissue, blood vessel walls, conjunctiva, and cornea. If phosphate is given, calcium phosphate can rapidly precipitate in tissues. Hypertension is seen with increased frequency in hypercalcemic patients, probably as a result of increased arteriolar vasoconstriction.

Table 15.20

SYMPTOMS AND SIGNS OF HYPERCALCEMIA	*General*
	Malaise/weakness
	Polydipsia, dehydration
	Neurologic
	Confusion
	Apathy, depression, stupor
	Decreased memory
	Irritability
	Ataxia
	Hyporeflexia, hypotonia
	Metastatic Calcification
	Band keratopathy
	Conjunctivitis
	Pruritus
	Cardiovascular
	Hypertension
	Arrhythmias
	Vascular calcification
	ECG abnormalities:
	QT shortening
	Widening of T wave
	Digitalis sensitivity
	Gastrointestinal
	Anorexia, weight loss
	Nausea, vomiting
	Constipation
	Peptic ulcer disease
	Pancreatitis
	Urologic
	Polyuria, nocturia
	Renal insufficiency
	Nephrolithiasis
	Skeletal
	Fractures
	Bone pain

3. Diagnosis

Hypercalcemic patients with plasma total calcium levels below 12.0 mg/dl are usually asymptomatic, but higher levels can cause a wide variety of symptoms and signs (Table 15.20).

Patients with total calcium levels above 14 to 16 mg/dl are usually very weak, lethargic, and confused. Frank coma is uncommon, but calcium levels should probably be drawn in any patient with a coma of unknown etiology. Polyuria, in spite of polydipsia, tends to cause increasing dehydration.

A mnemonic sometimes used for the signs and symptoms of hypercalcemia is stones (renal calculi), bones (osteolysis), psychic moans (psychiatric disorders), and abdominal groans (peptic ulcer disease and/or pancreatitis). The most common gastrointestinal symptoms are anorexia and constipation, but these are very nonspecific.

AXIOM

Failure to closely monitor calcium levels in patients with extensive bone metastases.

Hypercalcemia should be suspected in patients with extensive metastatic bone disease, particularly if the primary tumor involves the breast, lungs, or kidneys. It should also be suspected in individuals with combinations of clinical problems, such as renal calculi, pancreatitis, or ulcer disease. As with hypocalcemia, ionized calcium levels should be measured and/or total calcium levels should be correlated with serum proteins. If the patient is hypoproteinemic, total calcium levels may be normal or low in spite of increased ionized calcium levels.

AXIOM

The most frequent ECG finding with hypercalcemia is a shortened QT interval.

On ECG, hypercalcemia may be associated with depressed ST segments, widened T waves, and shortened ST segments and QT intervals (Fig. 15.4). Bradyarrhythmias may occur, and bundle-branch patterns may progress to second-degree block, and then complete heart block. Levels above 20 mg/dl may cause cardiac arrest.

The diagnosis of primary hyperparathyroidism is classically based on two laboratory findings: (1) elevated serum calcium levels on at least three different occasions, and (2) a serum PTH level that is disproportionately high for a simultaneously measured serum calcium level. A serum chloride/phosphorus ratio exceeding 35:1 can help confirm the diagnosis.

4. Treatment

Treatment of hypercalcemia is particularly important for patients with (1) calcium levels greater than 12 mg/dl, (2) symptoms, (3) inability to maintain a good fluid intake, or (4) abnormal renal function. Treatment is aimed at correcting the dehydration, promoting urinary calcium excretion, and decreasing calcium influx into the extracellular fluid from the skeletal system and gastrointestinal tract.

PITFALL

Failure to adequately correct the dehydration associated with hypercalcemia, especially before giving diuretics.

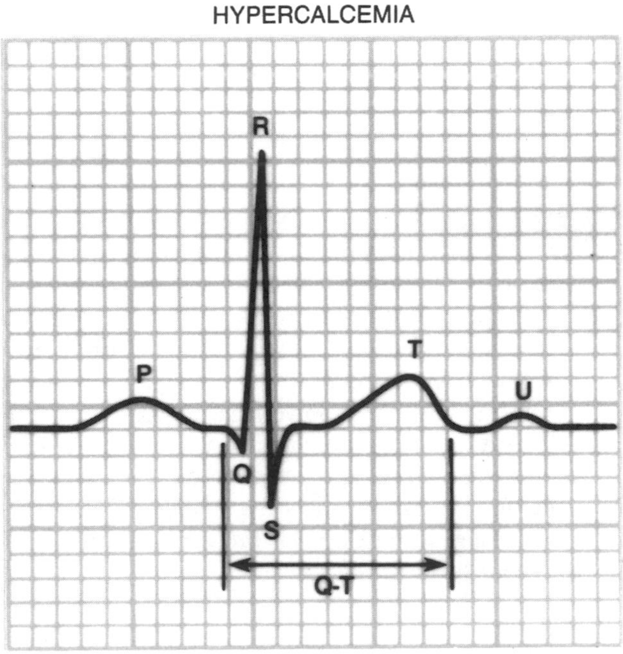

HYPERCALCEMIA

Figure 15.4 Hypercalcemia. (From Dolan, JT: Critical Care Nursing. FA Davis, Philadelphia, 1991, p 826, with permission.)

Patients with hypercalcemia tend to be dehydrated because high calcium levels interfere with ADH and the ability of the kidney to concentrate urine. Consequently, the initial and safest treatment is restoration of the ECF with relatively large amounts of saline. More than 5 to 10 liters of normal saline may be required in the first 24 hours to correct the dehydration. Some authors attempt to achieve a urine output as high as 250 $ml \cdot m^{-2} \cdot h^{-1}$ to facilitate calcium excretion and ensure continued adequate hydration. In patients with cardiac or renal disease, such fluid therapy may be dangerous, and peritoneal dialysis or hemodialysis may be required.

Once the ECF has been restored, a wide variety of diuretics (but not thiazides) may further increase renal excretion of calcium. Furosemide in doses of 1 to 3 mg/kg has been advocated. Up to a third of patients with hypercalcemia have hypokalemia, and in those with malignant disease, more than half the patients may have hypokalemia. Some patients will also have hypomagnesemia. The tendency to develop hypokalemia and hypomagnesemia will be aggravated by the diuresis and should be watched carefully and promptly corrected or prevented with appropriate electrolyte therapy.

PITFALL

Failure to adequately watch for potassium and magnesium deficiencies while treating hypercalcemia.

A wide variety of other modalities are also available to treat hypercalcemia. Mithramycin is a cytotoxic drug that suppresses bone resorption and calcium release from bone. It may be particularly helpful in patients with metastatic bone disease. Small daily doses of 15 to 25 μg/kg in 5% dextrose IV over a period of 3 hours for 3 days can lower serum calcium levels within 24 to 48 hours; however, the mithramycin often suppresses bone resorption for only 5 to 7 days. It must be used with caution in patients with bone marrow problems, thrombocytopenia, or renal or hepatic insufficiency.

Calcitonin (Calcimar) is also an osteoclast inhibitor and is less toxic than mithramycin. The dosage is usually 0.5 to 4 MRC units per kilogram given intramuscularly every 12 hours. The dose may be increased to a maximum of 8 MRC units per kilogram every 6 hours. Effects are usually seen within the first 12 hours, but patients often become refractory to it within 2 days. When calcitonin is used in conjunction with corticosteroids, the action of calcitonin is more prolonged.

Glucocorticoids may reduce serum calcium levels in patients with sarcoidosis, vitamin A or D intoxication, multiple myeloma, leukemia, or breast cancer. Glucocorticoids work by inhibiting bone resorption and gastrointestinal absorption of calcium. Steroids may also cause a shift of calcium inside cells, where it may be bound to mitochondria. The dosage of hydrocortisone in adults is 25 to 100 mg every 6 to 8 hours IV. The effect of this treatment may not be apparent until after the first 12 hours. If no effect is seen after 7 to 10 days, the therapy may be discontinued.

Intravenous phosphates and EDTA are rarely used now because they can cause a very rapid fall in plasma calcium levels. This can cause tissue deposition of calcium phosphate, renal cortical necrosis, and even shock.

When possible, irradiation or resection of neoplasms producing PTH-like activity should be considered. If parathyroid hyperplasia or adenoma is suspected, it should be treated surgically as soon as possible.

VII. MAGNESIUM

Magnesium is a vital element in all biologic systems and is the key element in chlorophyll, the basic producer of the world's food chain. The total body content of magnesium averages about 2000 mEq (24 g), with about 50% to 70% present in bone. The majority of the remaining magnesium is intracellular, with only 1% present in the ECF. The serum concentration of magnesium is about 1.8 to 2.4 mg/dl or 1.5 to 2.0 mEq/liter. About 25% to 35% of the magnesium present in the blood is protein bound, 10% to 15% is complexed, and 50% to 60% is ionized. The concentration of magnesium intracellularly is thought to be about 40 mEq/liter, making it the second most abundant intracellular cation.

The usual daily requirement is about 24 to 28 mEq (288 to 336 mg), usually from vegetables and cereals. About 40% is excreted in the urine and 60% in feces. Renal excretion protects against hypermagnesemia, but not hypomagnesemia, which will develop if intake is consistently less than 3.0 mg·kg^{-1}·d^{-1}.

A. HYPOMAGNESEMIA

1. Etiology

AXIOM

Hypomagnesemia is usually seen with poor oral intake or excessive loss of body fluids.

A wide variety of problems can cause hypomagnesemia (Table 15.21). In adults, magnesium deficiencies are most frequently seen in patients with alcoholism, cirrhosis, malnutrition, pancreatitis, or excessive gastrointestinal fluid losses. Diarrhea is usually more of a problem (Mg^{++} content of 10 to 14 mEq/liter) than upper gastrointestinal loss (1 to 2 mEq/liter). Chronic hyperparathyroidism increases urinary losses of magnesium and will eventually cause hypomagnesemia.

Intravenous hyperalimentation or treatment of diabetic ketoacidosis without providing adequate magnesium, especially in a previously malnourished patient, can cause an abrupt fall in plasma magnesium levels. This is largely due to magnesium that is "pulled" into cells with glucose or new lean body mass that is synthesized. Hypophosphatemia, which can also develop with IV hyperalimentation, can contribute to the hypomagnesemia.

Table 15.21

CAUSES OF HYPOMAGNESEMIA	*Gastrointestinal*
	Protein-calorie malnutrition
	Hyperalimentation after malnutrition
	Malabsorption
	Alcoholic cirrhosis
	Pancreatitis
	Renal
	Glomerulonephritis/pyelonephritis
	Diuretic phase of acute tubular necrosis
	Hypercalcemia
	Endocrine
	Hyperaldosteronism
	Hyperparathyroidism/hyperthyroidism
	Drug-induced
	Diuretics
	Aminoglycosides
	Cisplatin
	Vitamin D intoxication
	Alcohol
	Citrate (blood)
	Miscellaneous
	Lactation
	Hungry bone syndrome
	Burns
	Sepsis

Renal wasting of magnesium can be seen with loop diuretics, hypophosphatemia, ketoacidosis, aminoglycosides, and nephrotoxic chemotherapeutic agents.

The normal renal threshold for magnesium (1.5 to 2.0 mEq/liter) is significantly decreased by cisplatin, diuretics, hypercalcemia, growth hormone, thyroid hormone, and calcitonin. Cisplatin causes dose-dependent, cumulative, reversible renal tubular injury. Even when GFR is not diminished by cisplatin, renal magnesium wasting, along with a secondary hypocalcemia and hypokalemia, may develop.

AXIOM
Potassium and magnesium deficiencies frequently coexist.

Potassium wasting with hypomagnesemia is thought to occur as a result of impaired ATP production. This, in turn, impairs the function of the membrane Na^+/K^+ transport system and causes loss of the normal Na^+/K^+ gradient. The accompanying hypocalcemia may be due to (1) impaired PTH release by the parathyroid gland, (2) decreased peripheral sensitivity to PTH, or (3) abnormal blood-bone calcium balance independent of PTH.

2. Physiologic Effects

Magnesium is essential to a large number of vital enzymes, including membrane-bound adenosine triphosphatase(ATPase). Consequently, hypomagnesemia may result in a wide variety of neuromuscular, gastrointestinal, and cardiovascular changes (Table 15.22).

Hypomagnesemia may cause increased muscular irritability similar to that seen with hypocalcemia. It can also cause many central nervous system signs and symptoms, including depression, vertigo, ataxia, and seizures. In severe chronic alcoholics, delirium tremens is associated with moderate-severe total body magnesium deficiencies, but often with relatively normal plasma magnesium levels.

Cardiac arrhythmias, particularly in patients on digitalis, are often due to combined potassium and magnesium deficiencies. In the setting of an acute myocardial infarction, the administration of magnesium has been shown to reduce the incidence of malignant dysrhythmias and mortality.

Magnesium is a potent smooth-muscle relaxant, which has also been used

Table 15.22

SYMPTOMS AND SIGNS OF HYPOMAGNESEMIA	*Neuromuscular*
	Tetany, seizures, irritability
	Muscle weakness
	Ataxia, nystagmus, vertigo
	Confusion, obtundation, coma
	Apathy, depression
	Paresthesias
	Gastrointestinal
	Dysphagia
	Anorexia, nausea
	Cardiovascular
	Heart failure, hypotension
	Arrhythmias
	Miscellaneous
	Hypokalemia
	Hypocalcemia

successfully to treat asthmatic bronchospasm and stop uterine contractions during labor (tocolysis).

AXIOM

If a digitalis-toxicity arrhythmia is not corrected by giving IV potassium, one should also give magnesium.

Some metabolic manifestations of magnesium deficiency include difficulties in treating hypokalemia, impaired PTH secretion, decreased response to thiamine, and vitamin D resistant hypocalcemia. Other manifestations include hypothermia, hypotension, nephropathy, incomplete distal (type I) renal tubular acidosis, dysphagia, and anemia due to shortened red blood cell survival.

It has been noted that patients with severe, acute pancreatitis and hypocalcemia usually have normal serum magnesium levels; however, their mononuclear cell magnesium content may be significantly low and their retention of magnesium with a loading test may be significantly increased. This implies that, in spite of the normal serum magnesium levels, there is an intracellular and total body magnesium deficiency. This may contribute to the severity of the pancreatitis and the pathogenesis of the hypocalcemia.

3. Diagnosis

PITFALL

Relying on serum magnesium levels to diagnose magnesium deficiency.

One cannot rely on plasma levels to diagnose magnesium deficiencies because it is not unusual to have total body magnesium content fall rather severely before plasma levels decrease. The diagnosis of magnesium deficiency is suggested by increased neuromuscular irritability (hyperreflexia, positive Chvostek's or Trousseau's signs, tremor, tetany, or even convulsions) in the presence of normal serum calcium levels. Hypomagnesemia, or total body magnesium deficits, should be suspected in alcoholics, cirrhotics, and patients on IV fluids for prolonged periods. Hypomagnesemia may develop rapidly during IV hyperalimentation, especially when anabolism begins.

The ECG changes seen with magnesium deficiencies include prolonged PR and QT intervals, widened QRS complexes, depression of ST segments, and inversion of T waves, especially in the precordial leads. The changes may be somewhat similar to those caused by hypokalemia and/or hypocalcemia, and many of these changes may be related to Mg^{++} deficiency altering cardiac intracellular potassium content.

4. Treatment

PITFALL

Failure to consider and simultaneously correct potassium, calcium, and phosphate deficiencies when treating magnesium deficiency.

Hypokalemia, hypocalcemia, and hypophosphatemia are often present with hypomagnesemia and must be monitored carefully, especially if magnesium is being given rapidly by IV. It must be emphasized that, whenever one is treating a magnesium deficiency, one should look for and correct any associated potassium, calcium, or phosphate deficiencies.

Patients with a magnesium deficiency may require more than 50 mEq of oral magnesium (6 g $MgSO_4$) per day. In chronic alcoholics with delirium tremens and in patients with severe, proven hypomagnesemia, up to 8 to 12 g of IV or IM $MgSO_4$ may be required the first day. The first 10 to 15 mEq (1.5 to 2.0 g) of IV $MgSO_4$ can be given over 1 to 2 hours, and the rest should be given somewhat more slowly. This may be followed by up to 4 to 6 g/d thereafter. If IV alimentation is being given to a hypomagnesemic patient, 12 to 16 mEq (1.5 to 2.0 g) should be added to each liter of TPN.

If magnesium is being given rapidly, as in the treatment of eclampsia, the deep tendon reflexes (which disappear at about 3 to 4 mEq/liter) should be checked frequently, and blood levels should be measured once or twice daily. If deep tenden reflexes decrease or disappear, magnesium administration should stop, at least temporarily.

B. HYPERMAGNESEMIA

AXIOM

Hypermagnesemia is usually associated with some degree of renal dysfunction.

1. Etiology

Hypermagnesemia occurs rather infrequently, except in patients with renal failure who are given magnesium-containing drugs, particularly antacids such as Maalox. Other less frequent causes include untreated diabetic acidosis and adrenal insufficiency. Hypermagnesemia may also be seen with tumor lysis, rhabdomyolysis, burns, hyperparathyroidism, hypothyroidism, and ECF volume contraction, all of which lead to decreased magnesium clearance.

2. Physiologic Effects

Progressively increasing magnesium levels above 3.0 to 4.0 mEq/liter can reduce neuromuscular irritability and cause the disappearance of deep tendon reflexes. Increasing muscular weakness is noted with levels above 4.0 mEq/liter, and levels above 5.0 to 6.0 mEq/liter may cause increasing vasodilation and hypotension. Levels above 8.0 to 10.0 mEq/liter can cause cardiac conduction abnormalities and neuromuscular paralysis with hypotension and/or ventilatory failure and death.

3. Diagnosis

Elevated serum magnesium levels are usually diagnostic; however, the possibility of hypermagnesemia should also be considered in patients with hyperkalemia or hypercalcemia. Hypermagnesemia should also be suspected in patients with renal failure, particularly in those who are on magnesium-containing antacids, such as Maalox.

4. Treatment

PITFALL

Failure to frequently monitor deep tendon reflexes in individuals receiving magnesium, especially if it is given faster than 1 gram every 2 to 4 hours.

The initial treatment of hypermagnesemia is similar to that used for hypercalcemia and includes dilution by administering IV fluids, and then using diuretics, especially furosemide, as needed. Any acidosis should be corrected, and a slow infusion of calcium gluconate can also help to control symptoms. Peritoneal dialysis and hemodialysis are thought by some to be relatively ineffective with divalent cations, but removal of up to 700 mg of magnesium with one hemodialysis treatment has been reported.

VIII. PHOSPHORUS (PHOSPHATE)

The normal adult man contains about 700 g of phosphorus, of which about 80% is present in bones. Phosphorus is essential to a wide variety of reactions, especially energy metabolism in the form of high-energy phosphates and phosphocreatine. Serum phosphorus levels drop with age, from a high of 4.0 to 7.0 mg/dl in the newborn to 3.0 to 5.0 mg/dl in adults. Serum calcium and phosphorus levels generally change inversely to each other, and the product of their two concentrations in milligrams per deciliter usually averages about 30 to 40. The normal oral intake is about 10 to 12 mmol, with urinary excretion largely regulated by PTH.

A. HYPOPHOSPHATEMIA

1. Etiology

Because phosphorus is available in so many foods and is so easily absorbed, hypophosphatemia is unusual unless there is (1) reduction in oral intake, (2) excess loss of phosphorus, or (3) excessive movement of PO_4 from the ECF into cells (Table 15.23).

Table 15.23

CONDITIONS ASSOCIATED WITH HYPOPHOSPHATEMIA	
	Intake
	Deficiency of dietary phosphate
	Dialysis alcohol
	Total parenteral alimentation (TPN)
	Redistribution
	Glucose infusion
	Respiratory alkalosis
	Beta-adrenergic agents
	Osteoblastic metastases
	Nutritional recovery syndrome
	Androgens, estrogens
	Diuretic phase of severe burns
	Renal Causes
	Multiple renal tubular transport defect
	Idiopathic Fanconi syndrome
	Cystinosis
	Hereditary fructose intolerance
	Galactosemia
	Wilson's disease
	Oculocerebrorenal (Lowe's) syndrome
	Primary or secondary hyperparathyroidism
	Miscellaneous Causes
	Tumor-induced hypophosphatemia
	Post-transplantation hypophosphatemia
	Hypercalciuric nephrolithiasis

PITFALL
Failure to look carefully for hypophosphatemia in patients on TPN or with low potassium or magnesium levels or hypercalcemia.

Hypophosphatemia is being increasingly recognized, especially in patients on IV hyperalimentation, which increases phosphate movement into cells as anabolism occurs. Phosphorus is also consumed during phosphorylation of glucose as it moves into cells. Intracellular shifts occur as well in the presence of respiratory alkalosis and with the administration of anabolic steroids, sodium bicarbonate, epinephrine, or glucagon.

AXIOM
Metabolic alkalosis tends to lower plasma levels of phosphate, potassium, and magnesium.

Hypophosphatemia may be seen with metabolic alkalosis, especially after prolonged antacid therapy. Antacids with calcium and magnesium bind to phosphate and impair its intestinal absorption. Metabolic or respiratory alkalosis also increases phosphate loss in the urine. Respiratory alkalosis may increase phosphate movement into cells. Hyperparathyroidism and alcoholism are additional causes of hypophosphatemia.

Other causes of hypophosphatemia include malignancies with hypercalcemia (due to phosphaturia), renal tubular defects, hypokalemia, hypomagnesemia, and use of phosphate-binding antacids.

PITFALL
Failure to look for hypophosphatemia during rapid healing or anabolism.

During recovery from starvation or after severe burns, the body requirement for phosphate can greatly increase. The phosphate and potassium requirement of patients who undergo a partial hepatectomy may be particularly large, especially if more than 60% of the liver has been resected. In general, 5.0 mmol of phosphate is used to generate 1.0 g of protein; therefore, phosphate requirements may be as high as 30 to 60 mmol/d. Thus, extensive tissue repair or healing can quickly lead to severe phosphorus deficiency if there is inadequate intake.

2. Physiologic Effects

AXIOM

The neuromuscular changes of hypophosphatemia are usually noted clinically, but hematogenic changes in hypophosphatemia may be much more important.

Hypophosphatemia may be associated with depletion of ATP in platelets, red blood cells, and white blood cells, reducing their survival time and function. Platelet membrane changes may result in a bleeding tendency because of impaired aggregation. Severe phosphate deficiency can decrease the red cell content of 2,3-DPG and cause red blood cells to become rigid spherocytes, thereby impairing capillary perfusion.

Decreased, 2,3-diphosphoglycerate (2,3-DPG) increases the affinity of hemoglobin for oxygen, thereby reducing the arterial Po_2 and oxygen availability to tissues. Phosphate depletion in macrophages may impair chemotaxis, phagocytosis, and intracellular killing, resulting in decreased resistance to infection.

Progressive weakness and tremors may be noted as blood phosphate levels fall below 0.5 to 1.0 mg/dl. Circumoral and fingertip paresthesias may be present along with absent deep-tendon reflexes. Mental obtundation, anorexia, and hyperventilation may also occur. Patients may become so weak that they cannot be weaned from a ventilator or ambulated. Myocardial function, as measured by left ventricular stroke work, may also be impaired.

3. Diagnosis

Patients with diabetic or alcoholic ketoacidosis, or severe malnutrition, are particularly prone to develop hypophosphatemia. This problem should be anticipated within 12 to 48 hours of early treatment of diabetic ketoacidosis, within 24 to 96 hours of treatment for alcoholic ketoacidosis, and within 5 to 10 days of beginning IV hyperalimentation.

PITFALL

Relying completely on blood phosphorus levels to rule out phosphorus deficiency.

The ratio of intracellular to extracellular phosphorus concentration is approximately 100:1. Since 80% of the total body phosphorus is in bone, serum phosphorus levels may not reflect total body stores, and the magnitude of the total body deficit cannot be estimated adequately from blood levels, particularly if there are acute changes.

4. Treatment

Treatment of hypophosphatemia should be primarily preventive and must be an integral part of any nutrition program. At least 7 to 9 mmol of phosphate, usually as a combination of KH_2PO_4 and K_2HPO_4 (dibasic and monobasic phosphates), should be given with each 1000 calories. In some instances, more than double that amount of phosphate may be required to bring phosphate levels up to normal.

Because phosphate administration may cause a precipitous fall in serum calcium levels, calcium should also be given, usually as calcium gluconate, in doses of 0.2 to 0.3 $mEq \cdot kg^{-1} \cdot d^{-1}$. Other hazards of phosphate therapy include soft tissue calcification, hypotension, and hyperosmolality. If potassium phosphate is used, the therapy may also cause hyperkalemia.

For severe hypophosphatemia with blood levels of less than 1.0 mg/dl (0.32 mmol/liter) or symptoms, immediate intravenous replacement is required. Otherwise oral preparations can be used often.

AXIOM
Administration of phosphate IV must be done very cautiously and with close attention to associated electrolytes.

If the hypophosphatemia is recent and uncomplicated, the initial recommended daily dose is 2.5 mg/kg. Prolonged or multifactorial hypophosphatemia may require 5 mg/kg. Up to 25% to 50% more phosphorus is needed if the patient is symptomatic; however, less is required in the presence of hypercalcemia. Each dose is administered IV over 6 hours, and serum phosphorus is checked after each dose. To minimize the risks of hyperphosphatemia, a total dose of no more than 7.5 mg/kg should be administered. Risks of phosphate therapy include hypocalcemia, metastatic calcification, hypotension, and hyperkalemia from the potassium salts.

B. HYPER-PHOSPHATEMIA

Hyperphosphatemia is most apt to be seen with renal dysfunction. However, it may also be caused by increased phosphate movement out of cells into the ECF, increased phosphorus or vitamin D intake, hypoparathyroidism, or any problem associated with hypocalcemia or hypomagnesemia (Table 15.24).

1. Etiology

2. Physiologic Effects

Problems due to hyperphosphatemia are usually those associated with renal failure, hypocalcemia, or hypomagnesemia, which is usually present.

3. Therapy

PITFALL
Attempting to lower high phosphate levels without adequately considering its primary cause or associated electrolyte abnormalities.

Therapy is aimed at treating the underlying cause and restricting PO_4 intake to less than 200 mg/d. With normal renal function, PO_4 excretion can be increased with saline (1 to 2 liters every 4 to 6 hours) and acetazolamide (500 mg every 6 hours). PO_4 absorption from the GI tract is decreased with oral PO_4 binders (i.e., aluminum carbonate or hydroxide 30 to 45 ml q.i.d.). These binders also absorb PO_4 secreted into the gut lumen and are of benefit even if no oral PO_4 is given. If clinically significant hypocalcemia exists, calcium should be

---

Table 15.24

CONDITIONS ASSOCIATED WITH HYPERPHOSPHATEMIA	*Intake*
	Phosphate-containing enema or laxative
	Redistribution
	Respiratory acidosis
	Lactic acidosis
	Chemotherapy for neoplasms
	Rhabdomyolysis
	Septic shock
	Renal Causes
	Decreased glomerular filtration rate
	Hypoparathyroidism
	Miscellaneous Causes
	Hyperthyroidism
	Vitamin D intoxication
	Acromegaly

cautiously administered. If renal failure is present, hemodialysis may be required.

IX. CHLORIDE

A. GENERAL CHARACTERISTICS

Chloride is the major anion in the extracellular fluid. It fulfills several important physiologic functions. It is an important factor in maintaining (1) urine concentration in the renal countercurrent mechanisms, (2) ECF volume, (3) acid-base and potassium balance, and (4) a normal anion gap.

1. Intake and Excretion

Chloride is readily absorbed in the large and small bowel by active and passive transport mechanisms, which are either sodium or bicarbonate dependent. Stomach parietal cells possess the unique capacity to secrete chloride plus hydrogen ions (H^+). However, in the small bowel, much of the chloride is exchanged for bicarbonate. About 90% of the chloride ingested is excreted in the urine, with the remainder lost in the stool and in sweat.

2. Distribution in the Body

Chloride is almost entirely extracellular, where its concentration is usually about 70% to 75% that of sodium. There is little chloride in bone, and virtually all the chloride in the body is diffusible and metabolically active.

3. Chloride Role in the Kidney

PITFALL

Failure to consider the possible role of hypochloremia in patients with renal dysfunction.

Chloride is extremely important in determining the kidney's ability to concentrate urine. In most of the tubule, chloride reabsorption occurs passively along with sodium transport. However, in the water-impermeable ascending thick limb of the loop of Henle, where up to 20% to 30% of sodium and chloride can be reabsorbed, chloride transport is active. This active transport of chloride apparently provides the crucial gradient needed so that the "countercurrent" urine-concentrating mechanism functions properly. In the absence of ADH, this mechanism can also allow absorption of solute without water in the collecting ducts, allowing urine to be more dilute if needed.

Chloride is significantly involved in plasma acid-base regulation. Although not directly responsible for regulation of H^+ ion concentration, reciprocal changes in plasma bicarbonate and chloride concentrations occur during renal adjustments of ECF pH, when hydrogen and chloride are secreted, and when bicarbonate is reabsorbed. Renal acid excretion and bicarbonate reabsorption can be greatly modified by an insufficient quantity of readily reabsorbable anion, particularly chloride, in the glomerular filtrate.

4. Normal Levels and Factors Affecting Its Measurement

The range for normal serum chloride is 96 to 108 mEq/l. It can be measured in serum, plasma, urine, sweat, cerebrospinal fluid (CSF), and occasionally stool and other body fluids. Serum determinations are most commonly done, but heparinized (or EDTA) plasma may also be analyzed.

AXIOM

If the clinical picture does not support a laboratory finding of hyperchloremia, it may be factitious or caused by other halides.

Hemolysis can produce pseudohypochloremia secondary to a dilutional effect by red blood cell (RBC) water; therefore, serum should be promptly separated from red cells. As with sodium, an increase in total serum protein may produce pseudohyperchloremia as a result of water displacement. Because all of the chemical methods for analyzing chloride also pick up the other halides, the presence of bromide and iodide can falsely elevate serum chloride levels.

Table 15.25

HYPOCHLOREMIA	*Metabolic Alkalosis*
NaCl responsive (U_{Cl} <10 mEq/L)	
GI losses	
Vomiting/gastric drainage	
Villous adenoma	
Diuretics	
Cystic fibrosis	
Rapid correction of chronic hypercapnia	
NaCl resistant (U_{Cl} >20 mEq/L)	
Excess mineralocorticoid activity	
Primary hyperaldosteronism	
Cushing's syndrome	
Bartter's syndrome	
Severe potassium depletion	
Miscellaneous (variable urine chloride)	
Massive blood transfusions	
Alkali administration	
Large doses of synthetic penicillins	

B. HYPOCHLOREMIA

1. Etiology

AXIOM

Hypochloremia is usually due to diuretics, loss of gastric acid, or hemodilution.

The most frequent causes of hypochloremia (<95 mEq/liter) are excessive diuresis, especially after administration of loop diuretics, and loss of highly acid gastric secretions through vomiting or nasogastric suction (Table 15.25).

Diuretic use promotes natriuresis, kaliuresis, and chloruresis. Vomiting and external gastric drainage lead to a complex series of events. Gastric parietal cells secrete hydrogen and chloride into gastric fluid while bicarbonate is generated into the circulation. Acid-base balance is maintained by secretion of an equivalent amount of bicarbonate and hydrogen absorption in the more distal GI tract. Metabolic alkalosis results when this balance is upset by vomiting or any other external loss of hydrochloric acid. This alkalosis is maintained by increased renal absorption of sodium and bicarbonate due to ECF volume depletion.

If metabolic alkalosis is present, sodium conservation and volume maintenance take precedence over acid-base and potassium balance, and the kidney is influenced by aldosterone to accelerate the exchange of sodium for potassium and hydrogen ions. However, if abundant chloride is provided, the pattern is reversed, leading to bicarbonate diureses and correction of the alkalosis.

AXIOM

Diarrhea may have very high levels of potassium and bicarbonate.

In contrast to gastric contents, stool is usually low in chloride and rich in bicarbonate and potassium. Consequently, diarrheal diseases, unless vomiting is a prominent feature, are usually associated with metabolic acidosis rather than alkalosis. An exception is found with villous adenoma of the colon and in a rare congenital disorder known as chloride diarrhea, which arises from a defect in the ileal and colonic $Cl-HCO_3$ exchange mechanism. In both these situations, metabolic alkalosis is caused primarily by a loss of chloride without bicarbonate, and is augmented by ECF volume contraction.

Serious chloride depletion can occur from the skin, secondary to severe sweating that is replaced with just water. Sweat usually has less than 30 mEq of sodium chloride per liter; however, patients with cystic fibrosis may have much higher salt levels in their sweat. Patients with cystic fibrosis can easily develop metabolic alkalosis in hot weather because of a marked loss of chloride with their excess perspiration.

AXIOM
If a child's sweat tastes salty, the diagnosis of cystic fibrosis should be considered.

2. Physiologic Effects

The most frequent physiologic effects of hypochloremia are those due to the metabolic alkalosis and hypokalemia with which it is usually associated. Numerous studies have implicated chloride depletion in both the generation and maintenance of metabolic alkalosis. Because chloride is the only anion other than bicarbonate that is readily reabsorbed with sodium, chloride depletion accelerates Na-H exchange all along the tubule. Loss of H$^+$ generates new bicarbonate and results in alkalosis. In addition, because low blood chloride levels impair active chloride transport and the associated sodium reabsorption in the ascending limb, more sodium is delivered to the distal nephron for H$^+$ and potassium exchange. This exchange removes increased amounts of H$^+$ and potassium, making the alkalosis more severe.

PITFALL
Failure to evaluate urine chloride levels in patients with hypochloremia.

Chloride-responsive alkalosis (with a urine chloride less than 10 mEq/liter) is established and maintained by ECF volume depletion and chloride deficits. Volume depletion supplies the stimulus for sodium retention, but chloride is not available in sufficient quantity to maintain electrical neutrality. Therefore, the exchange of sodium for hydrogen and potassium ions is accelerated and bicarbonate is generated. There is minimal urinary chloride excretion (less than 1 mmol/liter), because there is nearly complete reabsorption of filtered chloride in the sodium-avid tubule.

3. Diagnosis

No signs or symptoms are specifically characteristic of hypochloremia. A history of vomiting, excessive nasogastric suction, or diuretic therapy, together with evidence of volume depletion, should signal the possible presence of hypochloremia and an associated metabolic alkalosis. Metabolic alkalosis may cause muscle weakness, neuromuscular irritability, and hypoventilation. This hypoventilation may be especially dangerous in patients already hypoxic secondary to chronic obstructive pulmonary disease.

If a patient has a metabolic alkalosis and the urinary chloride levels are low (less than 10 mEq/liter), the patient is said to have a chloride-responsive alkalosis. Such patients usually have a relatively simple chloride deficit and will often respond to chloride administration alone. If urine chloride levels are 40 mEq/liter or higher, the hypochloremia is frequently due to hemodilution. However, if the patient is not overloaded with fluids, the hypochloremia is apt to be due to, or associated with, excessive corticosteroids and/or hypokalemia.

Hypochloremia with increased urine chloride can be due to excess mineralocorticoid activity, which causes Na$^+$ and HCO$_3^-$ retention and increased excretion of H$^+$, K$^+$, and Cl$^-$ (Table 15.25). The associated ECF volume expansion results in diminished proximal tubule sodium chloride reabsorption and, therefore, an increased delivery of sodium to the distal tubule. The exchange of sodium for potassium and hydrogen ions is also enhanced, resulting in an even greater loss of H$^+$ and K$^+$ in the urine.

It has been noted that metabolic alkalosis with severe potassium depletion may be resistant to correction with sodium chloride alone. Severe potassium depletion may directly alter the renal tubular handling of chloride, resulting in chloride wasting. To reverse this chloride-wasting nephropathy, correction of at least part of the potassium deficit is required.

4. Treatment

Chloride-responsive metabolic alkalosis will usually respond to IV administration of 0.9% sodium chloride alone. Chloride-resistant metabolic alkalosis usually also requires potassium and, in severe cases, may require hydrogen ions. Hypochloremia, due to dilution from excess total body water, is usually best treated by cautious dehydration.

As a general rule, deficits in total body chloride are best treated by giving one fourth of the calculated chloride deficit as potassium chloride and three fourths as sodium chloride. The total body chloride deficit can be estimated rapidly by multiplying 20% of the body weight by the serum chloride deficit. Thus, an 80-kg patient with a serum chloride of 60 mEq/liter has a total deficit of $(80 \text{ kg} \times 20\%)(100 - 60) = 16 \times 40$ or 640 mEq/liter.

If the patient is severely dehydrated, the total additional chloride deficit may be estimated by assuming that the mild, moderate, or severe dehydration involves a 6%, 8%, or 10% loss, respectively, of body weight as ECF containing 100 mEq of chloride per liter. Thus, if an 80-kg man is severely dehydrated, one can assume that he has lost at least 8 liters of ECF containing 100 mEq of chloride per liter or a total of 800 mEq of chloride. Since he can be assumed to have only 8 liters of ECF left, the deficit in the remaining ECF is 8×40, or 320 mEq. Thus, the total chloride deficit in a severely dehydrated 80-kg man with a serum chloride of 60 mEq/liter would be $800 + 320$, or 1120 mEq.

If the patient has renal dysfunction, so that potassium cannot be given, if the metabolic alkalosis is very severe, or if the metabolic alkalosis does not respond to sodium chloride plus potassium chloride, 0.1 N hydrogen chloride or amino acid hydrochlorides may be useful. If 0.1 N hydrogen chloride is used, it should be given slowly through a central IV line, watching carefully for any leakage into tissues.

C. HYPERCHLOREMIA

1. Etiology

Hyperchloremia is usually due to dehydration, administration of excessive amounts of sodium chloride, or various problems that can cause a normal anion gap metabolic acidosis (Table 15.26). The most frequent causes of normal anion gap acidosis are gastrointestinal losses of bicarbonate (small bowel or pancreatic fistulas or diarrhea) or renal bicarbonate losses (Table 15.26). Excess administration of chloride as saline, potassium chloride, and amino acid hydrochlorides can also cause hyperchloremia. All of these substances readily dissociate and consume bicarbonate, resulting in hyperchloremic metabolic acidosis.

2. Pathophysiology

The physiologic effects of hyperchloremia are primarily due to the underlying dehydration or metabolic acidosis. Clinically, most changes in plasma chloride concentration parallel those of sodium. Primary hypernatremic states are, for the most part, predictably accompanied by hyperchloremia. In addition, changes in serum chloride accompany reciprocal changes in serum bicarbonate. As a result, hypochloremia usually accompanies metabolic alkalosis, and hyperchloremia accompanies normal anion gap metabolic acidosis.

The systemic effects of acute and severe metabolic acidosis are well known and include Kussmaul (slow, very deep) respirations, decreased myocardial contractility, and a drop in peripheral resistance. In children, bone disease associated with chronic acidosis, such as that seen in RTA, may manifest itself as stunted growth (secondary to acidosis-induced bone mineral loss), rickets, and osteomalacia.

Table 15.26

ETIOLOGY OF HYPERCHLOREMIA ASSOCIATED WITH PRIMARY HYPERNATREMIC STATES	*Administration of Hypertonic or Excess NaCl*
	Normal Anion-Gap Metabolic Acidosis
	GI losses of bicarbonate
	Diarrhea
	Small bowel fistulas
	Biliary or pancreatic fistulas
	Ureterosigmoidostomy/obstructed ileal loop conduit
	Cholestyramine ingestion
	Renal losses of bicarbonate
	Renal tubular acidosis
	Hypoaldosteronism
	Hyperparathyroidism
	Carbonic anhydrase inhibitors
	Miscellaneous
	Dilutional acidosis
	Hyperalimentation acidosis
	Compounds with chloride anion
	Compensation of chronic respiratory alkalosis
	Low Anion-Gap States
	Hypoalbuminemia
	Halide toxicity (bromide or iodide)

3. Diagnosis

Clinical features of hyperchloremia are difficult to list independently, because the presentation is usually a manifestation of the primary underlying disorder and associated metabolic abnormalities. Elevated serum chloride and sodium levels usually indicate dehydration. Elevated chloride levels with normal or low serum sodium levels usually indicate either excess chloride administration as potassium chloride or amino acid hydrochlorides, or excess loss of bicarbonate from the body.

PITFALL
Failure to determine anion gap and arterial pH in patients with hyperchloremia.

Anion gap and arterial pH can be extremely helpful in determining the cause and treatment of hyperchloremia. A low anion gap (less than 10 mEq/ liter) can be associated with hyperchloremia in several pathologic states. When reduced concentration of unmeasured anions exists, as in cirrhosis or nephrosis with hypoalbuminemia, the normally unmeasured anion albumin is partially replaced with the measured anions chloride and bicarbonate, so that the anion gap will tend to fall. Unmeasured nonsodium cations, such as cationic proteins in multiple myeloma or severe hypercalcemia, hypermagnesemia, and acute lithium overdose, obligate an increased chloride or bicarbonate to counterbalance the positive charge.

AXIOM
Very high serum chloride levels, especially in outpatients, should make one suspect iodide or bromide toxicity.

An overestimation of serum chloride occurs when bromide (or other halide) is present because it interferes with all laboratory determinations of chloride. Bromism should be suspected when the anion gap is very small or negative.

4. Treatment

If there is excess administration of chloride or excessive losses of bicarbonate, this should be corrected. Hyperchloremia due to dehydration is best treated by slowly administering increased amounts of isotonic fluids with little or no chloride. However, if too much hypotonic fluid is given too rapidly, seizures due to cerebral edema may develop.

SUMMARY POINTS

1. Never completely trust the laboratory.
2. Biologic systems react primarily to rate of change and not to absolute concentrations.
3. Abnormalities should be treated at approximately the rate at which they develop.
4. One should not correct a chronic asymptomatic abnormality rapidly.
5. Highest priority in treatment is maintenance of a normal or increased blood volume and adequate tissue perfusion.
6. One should not correct pH levels without also considering the effects on potassium, calcium, and magnesium.
7. If all the measured electrolyte levels are low, symptoms are apt to be less severe than if only one electrolyte were decreased.
8. Hypovolemia is much stronger as a stimulus to ADH secretion than hyposmolarity is as an inhibitor. Consequently, increased ADH secretion tends to perpetuate hyponatremia in hypovolemic patients.
9. Malnutrition and sepsis tend to increase the extracellular fluid space and decrease the intracellular fluid space.
10. Hyponatremia is usually due to hemodilution by too much total body water.
11. In "true" hyponatremia, plasma osmolarity is reduced; in "factitious" hyponatremia, plasma osmolality is usually normal or increased.
12. Hyponatremia with hypovolemia and increased urine sodium losses in adults is usually due to diuretics, Addison's disease, or renal disease.
13. If the serum osmolality is less than 270 to 280 mOsm/kg, the urine osmolality should be less than 50 to 100 mOsm/kg.
14. Whenever serum osmolality is low and urine osmolality is high, one should look for SIADH; however, the diagnosis of SIADH is primarily one of exclusion.
15. Attempts to correct the hyponatremia of SIADH with sodium-rich solutions will usually cause an increase in urinary sodium excretion, but little change in serum sodium levels.
16. Chronic asymptomatic mild-moderate hyponatremia may require no therapy, except to look for its etiology.
17. The most frequent cause of hyponatremia is administration of too much water to patients with cardiac, liver, or renal disease.
18. Whenever a patient develops CNS changes, one should immediately look for hypoxemia, hypoglycemia, hyponatremia, and sepsis.
19. Sudden, severe hyponatremia can cause severe brain swelling and neurologic symptoms.
20. If correction of hyponatremia occurs more rapidly than the brain can recover solute, the higher plasma osmolality may dehydrate and injure the brain, producing what is now called the "osmotic demyelination syndrome" or "central pontine myelinolysis."
21. Shock occurs at lesser degrees of total body water depletion in patients who are hyponatremic.
22. If a patient is hypovolemic, increased ADH secretion will tend to increase water reabsorption by the kidney, even if the patient is already hyponatremic.
23. Each 100 mg/dl that blood glucose levels are above 100 mg/dl reduces serum sodium levels by about 1.6 mEq/liter.
24. Fluid restriction is usually the best treatment for hyponatremia in stable asymptomatic patients.

25. Hypertonic (3%) saline is generally used to treat hyponatremia only if it is severe, acute, and symptomatic.
26. One should follow serum (and urine) sodium levels closely when giving hypertonic saline.
27. One should not use the total body water to calculate and treat sodium deficits in patients who have an expanded ECF.
28. Developing chronic severe hyponatremia slowly is often safer than its treatment.
29. Treatment of severe chronic hyponatremia is safest when done slowly and with diuretics.
30. Hypernatremia is usually due to inadequate water intake.
31. One should anticipate a triphasic swing in ADH levels in traumatic diabetes insipidus.
32. Shock is unusual in hypernatremic dehydration.
33. One should not use glucose-in-water to aggressively treat hypernatremia, especially if it has been present for a few days.
34. Rapid correction of hypernatremia, especially if it is chronic, can cause seizures and severe neurologic sequelae.
35. Severe hemolysis or muscle damage can rapidly raise the serum potassium to lethal levels.
36. Metabolic alkalosis tends to cause hypokalemia, and metabolic acidosis tends to cause hyperkalemia.
37. If potassium is not given as soon as plasma glucose levels begin to fall as diabetic ketoacidosis is treated, severe hypokalemia may develop rapidly, causing dangerous arrhythmias.
38. Hypokalemia plus hypochloremia, hyponatremia, and hypovolemia are caused by excess diuresis until proven otherwise.
39. A urine potassium of less than 10 mEq/liter usually indicates a severe chronic potassium deficit.
40. Hypertension plus hypokalemic hypochloremic metabolic alkalosis is due to excess corticosteroids until proven otherwise.
41. One should anticipate potassium deficits in patients with severe diarrhea.
42. Hypokalemia can cause severe muscle weakness.
43. Severe hypokalemia can cause nephrogenic diabetes insipidus and severe dehydration, which must be considered when correcting electrolyte abnormalities.
44. The most frequent cause of paradoxical aciduria is hypokalemia.
45. Serum potassium levels are extremely responsive to changes in pH.
46. One should not attempt to correct hypovolemia rapidly if the urinary potassium is very low.
47. Whenever potassium is given, it should be looked upon as a potentially lethal drug.
48. Relatively mild-moderate hypokalemia may be associated with large total body deficits of potassium.
49. Renal failure with oliguria is the most common cause of dangerous hyperkalemia.
50. Lethal hyperkalemia is most apt to develop in patients with severe tissue damage and oliguric renal failure.
51. Mild-moderate hyperkalemia can usually be managed by stopping all potassium intake and increasing urine output.
52. In patients with fluid overload or impaired cardiac function, the absorption of sodium from Kayexalate may precipitate acute heart failure.
53. Calcium must be given very cautiously to patients on digitalis.
54. Calcium is the initial drug of choice if a patient develops dangerous arrhythmias due to hyperkalemia.
55. Hypocalcemia probably does not cause coagulation defects because car-

diovascular function would be impaired before calcium reached such levels.

56. If plasma protein levels are low, total calcium levels will also be low, even if ionized calcium levels are normal.

57. A rapid drop in ionized calcium levels in blood usually indicates that cell membrane function is impaired.

58. Low calcium levels in pancreatitis may be the first indication that complications are developing.

59. One of the causes of hypocalemia in ICU patients may be the use of cimetidine to prevent gastric bleeding from stress.

60. A patient with hyperparathyroidism and an elevated alkaline phosphatase is particularly apt to develop hypocalcemia following parathyroidectomy.

61. Whenever one sees hypocalcemia, one should also look for hypomagnesemia.

62. The physiologic effects of hypocalcemia are usually due to acute reductions in ionized calcium levels.

63. A rapid fall in ionized calcium levels in blood may be associated with severe, complex cellular changes.

64. One should ask about perioral and digital paresthesias in patients who have just had thyroid or parathyroid surgery.

65. Severe alkalosis can cause clinical signs of hypocalcemia, even when total calcium levels in blood are normal.

66. Administering calcium rapidly IV for mild-moderate hypocalcemia without symptoms can cause unnecessary cardiovascular, neuromuscular, and renal complications.

67. Calcium is seldom required during resuscitation, unless large amounts of blood are being given very rapidly and the patient is in shock or heart failure.

68. The most frequent cause of severe hypercalcemia (≥ 14 mg/dl) is malignant neoplasms with either extensive metastases or parathormonelike activity.

69. One should look for pancreatic, pituitary, adrenal, and thyroid neoplasms in patients with primary hyperparathyroidism.

70. Critically ill patients, especially those with sepsis, tend to develop ionic hypocalcemia, but this may be masked or occasionally overbalanced by the tendency to hypercalcemia with immobilization.

71. Hypercalcemia with lung lesions may be due to malignancy or granulomas.

72. Patients with severe hypercalcemia are usually severely dehydrated.

73. One should closely monitor calcium levels in patients with extensive bone metastases.

74. The most frequent ECG finding with hypercalcemia is a shortened QT interval.

75. The initial treatment of hypercalcemia is correction of the dehydration, particularly before giving any diuretics.

76. While treating hypercalcemia, one can easily cause or aggravate hypokalemia and hypomagnesemia.

77. Hypomagnesemia is usually seen with poor oral intake or excessive loss of body fluids.

78. Potassium and magnesium deficiencies frequently coexist.

79. If a digitalis-toxicity arrhythmia is not corrected by giving IV potassium, one should also give magnesium.

80. One should not rely on serum magnesium levels to diagnose magnesium deficiency.

81. One should consider, and simultaneously correct, potassium, calcium, and phosphate deficiencies when treating a magnesium deficiency.

82. Hypermagnesemia is usually associated with some degree of renal dysfunction.
83. One should frequently monitor deep tendon reflexes in individuals who are receiving magnesium, especially if it is given faster than 1 g every 2 to 4 hours.
84. One should look carefully for hypophosphatemia in patients who are on TPN, have low potassium or magnesium levels, or are hypercalcemic.
85. Metabolic alkalosis tends to lower plasma levels of phosphate, potassium, and magnesium.
86. One should anticipate hypophosphatemia during rapid healing or anabolism.
87. The neuromuscular changes of hypophosphatemia are what is usually noted clinically, but the hematogenic changes may be much more important.
88. One should not rely completely on blood phosphorus levels to rule out phosphorus deficiency.
89. Administration of phosphate IV must be done very cautiously and with close attention to associated electrolytes.
90. One should not attempt to lower high phosphate levels without adequately considering the primary cause or associated electrolyte abnormalities.
91. One should consider the possible role of hypochloremia in patients with renal dysfunction.
92. If the clinical picture does not support a laboratory finding of hyperchloremia, it may be factitious or caused by other halides.
93. Hypochloremia is usually due to diuretics, loss of gastric acid, or hemodilution.
94. Diarrhea may have very high levels of potassium and bicarbonate.
95. If a child's sweat tastes salty, the diagnosis of cystic fibrosis should be considered.
96. One should evaluate urine chloride levels in patients with hypochloremia.
97. Failure of metabolic alkalosis to improve rapidly with saline infusions should make one look for severe hypokalemia or excess corticosteroids.
98. One should consider dehydration in determining the total chloride deficits.
99. One should determine anion gap and arterial pH in patients with hyperchloremia.
100. Very high serum chloride levels, especially in outpatients, should make one suspect iodide or bromide toxicity.

BIBLIOGRAPHY

1. Abraham, AS: Magnesium therapy for acute myocardial infarction. Compr Ther 14:64, 1988.
2. Aldinger, KA and Samaan, NA: Hypokalemia with hypercalcemia: Prevalence and significance of treatment. Ann Intern Med 87:571, 1977.
3. Arieff, A, Llach, F, and Massry, SG: Neurological manifestations and morbidity of hyponatremia correlation with brain water and electrolytes. Medicine (Baltimore) 55:121, 1976.
4. Auffant, RA, Dunns, JG, and Amicite, R: Ionized calcium concentration and cardiovascular function after cardiopulmonary bypass. Arch Surg 116:1072, 1981.
5. Baltarowich, LL: Chloride. Emerg Med Clin North Am 4:175, 1986.
6. Barker, GL: Hyperkalemia presenting as ventilatory failure. Anesthesia 35:885, 1980.
7. Bartter, FC and Schwartz, WB: The syndrome of inappropriate secretion of antidiuretic hormone. Am J Med 42:790, 1967.
8. Berry, PL: Hyponatremia. Pediatr Clin North Am 37:351, 1990.
9. Bohrer, H, Fleischer, F, and Krier, C: Hyperkalemic cardiac arrest after cardiac surgery following high-dose glucose-insulin-potassium infusion for inotropic support. Anesthesiology 69:949, 1988.
10. Brasier, AR and Nussbaum, SR: Hungry bone syndrome: Clinical and biochemical predictors of its occurrence after parathyroid surgery. Am J Med 84:654, 1988.
11. Braunwald, E: The mechanism of action of calcium-channel blocking agents. N Engl J Med 307:1611, 1982.

12. Brem, AS: Disorders of potassium homeostasis. Pediatr Clin North Am 37:419, 1990.
13. Burtis, WJ, et al: Humoral hypercalcemia of malignancy. Ann Intern Med 108:454, 1988.
14. Chawla, RK, et al: Electrocardiographic changes stimulating acute myocardial infarction caused by hyperkalemia: Report of a patient with a normal coronary arteriogram. Am Heart J 95:637, 1978.
15. Chernow, B: Calcium: Does it have a therapeutic role in sepsis? Crit Care Med 18:895, 1990.
16. Chernow, B, et al: Hypomagnesemia with implications for the critical care specialist. Crit Care Med 10:193, 1982.
17. Chernow, B, et al: Hypocalcemia in critically ill patients. Crit Care Med 10:848, 1982.
17a. Civetta, JM, Hudson-Civetta, JA, and Nelson, LD: Evaluation of Apache II for cost containment and quality assurance. Annals of Surg 212:266–274, 1990.
18. Cluitmans, FHM and Meinders, AE: Management of severe hyponatremia: Rapid or slow correction? Am J Med 88:161, 1990.
19. Cohen, HC, Rosen, KM, and Pick, A: Disorders of impulse conduction and impulse formation caused by hyperkalemia in man. Am Heart J 89:501, 1975.
20. Conley, SB: Hypernatremia. Pediatr Clin North Am 37:365, 1990.
21. Connor, TB, et al: Hypocalcemia precipitating congestive heart failure. N Engl J Med 307:869, 1982.
22. Cox, RE: Hypoparathyroidism: An unusual case of seizures. Ann Emerg Med 12:314, 1983.
23. Craddock, PR, et al: Acquired phagocytic dysfunction: A complication of the hypophosphatemia of parenteral hyperalimentation. N Engl J Med 290:1403, 1974.
24. Daugirdas, JT, Kronfol, NO, and Tzamaloukas, AH: Hyperosmolar coma: Cellular dehydration and serum sodium concentration. Ann Intern Med 110:855, 1989.
25. DeCristofaro, JD and Tsang, RC: Calcium. Emerg Med Clin North Am 4:207, 1986.
26. Desai, TK, Carlson, RW, and Geheb, MA: Hypocalcemia and hypophosphatemia in acutely ill patients. Crit Care Clin 5:927, 1978.
27. Don, BR, et al: Pseudohyperkalemia caused by fist clenching during phlebotomy. N Engl J Med 322:1290, 1990.
28. Edwards, H, Zinberg, J, and King, TC: Effect of cimetidine on serum calcium levels in an elderly patient. Arch Surg 116:1088, 1981.
29. Ellman, H, Dembin, H, and Seriff, N: The rarity of shortening of the Q-T interval in patients with hypercalcemia. Crit Care Med 10:320, 1982.
30. Ettinger, PO, Reyan, TJ, and Oldewurtel, HA: Hyperkalemia, cardiac conduction, and the electrocardiogram: A review. Am Heart J 88:360, 1974.
31. Ferris, TF, et al: Renal potassium induced by vitamin D. J Clin Invest 41:1222, 1962.
32. Fiaccadori, E, et al: Muscle and serum magnesium in pulmonary intensive care unit patients. Crit Care Med 16:751, 1988.
33. Fiskin, RA, Heath, DA, and Bold, AM: Hypercalcemia: A hospital survey. Q J Med 49:405, 1980.
34. Fitzgerald, F: Clinical hypophosphatemia. Am Rev Med 29:1779, 1979.
35. Garella, S, Chazan, JA, and Cohen, JJ: Saline-resistant metabolic alkalosis or "chloride wasting nephropathy." Ann Intern Med 73:31, 1970.
36. Goldman, RS and Finkbeiner, SM: Therapeutic use of magnesium sulfate in selected cases of cerebral ischemia and seizure. N Engl J Med 319:1224, 1988.
37. Harrington, JT and Cohen, JJ: Measurements of urinary electrolytes: Indications of limitations. N Engl J Med 293:1241, 1975.
38. Hartman, F, et al: Rapid correction of hyponatremia in the syndrome of inappropriate secretion of antidiuretic hormone. Ann Intern Med 78:870, 1973.
39. Heining, MPD and Jordan, WS: Heparinization of samples for plasma ionized calcium measurement. Crit Care Med 16:67, 1988.
40. Hensen, J, et al: Effects of incremental infusions of arginine vasopressin on adrenocorticotropin and cortisol secretion in man. J Clin Endocrinol Metab 66:668, 1988.
41. Hollifield, JW: Electrolyte disarray and cardiovascular disease. Am J Cardiol 63:21B, 1989.
42. Horvath, B, Pecci, J, and Gay, W: Fewer tests may cost more. N Engl J Med 312:1645, 1985.
43. Inaba, H, Hirasawa, H, and Mizuguchi, T: Serum osmolality gap in postoperative patients in intensive care. Lancet ii: 1331, 13 June, 1987.
44. Iseri, LT, Freed, J, and Bures, AR: Magnesium deficiency and cardiac disorders. Am J Med 58:837, 1975.
45. Kaplan, EB, et al: The usefulness of preoperative laboratory screening. JAMA 253:3576, 1985.
46. Kassirer, JP and Schwartz, WB: The response of normal man to selective depletion of hypochloric acid. Am J Med 40:10, 1966.
47. Katz, AM: Is calcium beneficial or deleterious in patients with cardiac arrest? Ann Intern Med 109:91, 1988.
48. Katz, MD: Hyperglycemia-induced hyponatremia: Calculation of the expected serum sodium depression. N Engl J Med 289:843, 1973.
49. Kreusser, W, et al: Effects of phosphate depletion on magnesium metabolism in rats. J Clin Invest 61:573, 1978.

50. Kurtzman, NA, et al: Renal grand rounds: A patient with hyperkalemia and metabolic acidosis. Am J Kidney Dis 15:333, 1990.
51. Lafferty, FW and Hubay, CA: Primary hyperparathyroidism: A review of the long-term surgical and nonsurgical morbidities as a basis for a rational approach to treatment. Arch Intern Med 149:989, 1989.
52. Lang, RM, et al: Left ventricular contractility varies directly with blood-ionized calcium. Ann Intern Med 108:524, 1988.
53. Leibman, J and Edelman, IS: Inter-relations of plasma potassium concentration, plasma sodium concentration, arterial pH and total exchangeable potassium. J Clin Invest 38:2176, 1959.
54. Lim, M, Linton, RAF, and Ban, DM: Early changes in plasma potassium after acute alterations in Paco$_2$ in anesthetized dogs, monitored continuously with intravascular potassium selective electrodes. Crit Care Med 10:747, 1982.
55. Lowe, RA, Arst, HF, and Ellis, BK: Rational ordering of electrolytes in emergency department. Ann Emerg Med 20:16, 1991.
56. Lowe, RA, et al: Rational ordering of serum electrolytes: Development of clinical criteria. Ann Emerg Med 16:260, 1987 [Errata. Ann Emerg Med 16:816, 1987].
57. Malcolm, DA, Zaloga, GP, and Holaday, JW: Calcium administration increases the mortality of endotoxic shock in rats. Crit Care Med 17:900, 1989.
58. Martin, ML, Hamilton, R, and West, MF: Potassium. Emerg Med Clin North Am 4:131, 1986.
59. McMahon, MJ, Woodhead, JS, and Hayward, RD: The nature of hypocalcemia in acute pancreatitis. Br J Surg 65:216, 1978.
60. McNamara, RM, et al: Intravenous magnesium sulfate in the management of acute respiratory failure complicating asthma. Ann Emerg Med 18:197, 1989.
61. Miller, CE and Remenchik, AP: Problems involved in accurately measuring the K content of the human body. Ann NY Acad Sci 110:175, 1965.
62. Oelkers, W: Hyponatremia and inappropriate secretion of vasopressin (antidiuretic hormone) in patients with hypopituitarism. N Engl J Med 321:492, 1989.
63. Okayama, H, et al: Bronchodilating effect of intravenous magnesium sulfate in bronchial asthma. JAMA 257:1076, 1987.
64. Olinger, ML: Disorders of calcium and magnesium metabolism. Emerg Med Clin North Am 7:795, 1989.
65. Peak, W, Carpenter, MA, and Trunkey, D: Ionized calcium: The effect of septic shock in the human. J Surg Res 26:605, 1979.
66. Pine, RW, Vincenzi, FF, and Larrico, CJ: Apparent inhibition of the plasma membrane Ca^{2+} pump by oleic acid. J Trauma 23:366, 1983.
67. Pinto, IJ, et al: Tall upright T waves in the precordial leads. Circulation 36:708, 1968.
68. Podrid, PJ: Potassium and ventricular arrhythimias. Am J Cardiol 65:33E, 1990.
69. Raff, H: Glucocorticoid inhibition of neurohypophysial vasopressin secretion. Am J Physiol 252:R635, 1987.
70. Rasmussen, H: The calcium messenger system: I. N Engl J Med 314:1094, 1986.
71. Rasmussen, H: The calcium messenger system: II. N Engl J Med 314:1164, 1986.
72. Robertson, GJ Jr, et al: Inadequate parathyroid response in acute pancreatitis. N Engl J Med 294:512, 1976.
73. Rogers, EM, Cheng, LC, and Zierler, K: Beta-adrenergic effect on Na$^+$-K$^+$ transport in rat skeletal muscle. Biochem Biophys Acta 464:347, 1977.
74. Ryzen, E and Rude, RK: Low intracellular magnesium in patients with acute pancreatitis and hypocalcemia. West J Med 152:145, 1990.
75. Schulman, M and Narins, RG: Hypokalemia and cardiovascular disease. Am J Cardiol 65:4E, 1990.
76. Scribner, BH and Burnell, JH: Interpretation of the serum potassium concentration. Metabolism 5:468, 1956.
77. Seller, RH, et al: Digitalis toxicity and hypomagnesemia. Am Heart J 79:57, 1970.
78. Siesjo, BK: Calcium, ischemia, and death of brain cells. Ann NY Acad Sci 522:638, 1988.
79. Snyder, NA, Feigal, DW, and Arieff, AI: Hypernatremia in elderly patients: A heterogeneous, morbid, and iatrogenic entity. Ann Intern Med 107:309, 1987.
80. Steinhorn, DM, Sweeney, MF, and Layman, LK: Pharmacodynamic response to ionized calcium during acute sepsis. Crit Care Med 18:851, 1990.
81. Stenven, H, et al: Use of calcium in prehospital cardiac arrest. Ann Emerg Med 12:136, 1983.
82. Sterns, RH: The treatment of hyponatremia: Unsafe at any speed? AKF Nephrol Letter 6:1, 1989.
83. Stewart, AF, et al: Calcium homeostasis in immobilization: An example of reportive hypercalciuria. N Engl J Med 306:1136, 1982.
84. Surawicz, B: Relationship between electrocardiogram and electrolytes. Am Heart J 73:814, 1967.
85. Surawicz, B and Gettes, LS: Two mechanisms of cardiac arrest produced by potassium. Circ Res 12:415, 1963.

86. Swaminathan, R, et al: Hypophosphatemia in surgical patients. Surg Gynecol Obstet 148:448, 1979.
87. Vann, PW, Coulter, M, and Wasserberger, JS: Use of calcium in brady-asystolic arrest. Ann Emerg Med 11:590, 1982.
88. Vincent, JL: Should we still administer calcium during cardiopulmonary resuscitation? Intensive Care Med 13:369, 1987.
89. Waugh, WH: Utility of expressing serum sodium per unit of water in assessing hyponatremia. Metabolism 18:706, 1969.
90. Weisberg, LS: Pseudohyponatremia: A reappraisal. Am J Med 86:315, 1989.
91. White, BC, et al: The possible role of calcium blockers in cerebral resuscitation: A review of the literature and synthesis for future studies. Crit Care Med 11:202, 1983.
92. Wilson, RF, Soullier, G, and Antonenko, D: Ionized calcium levels in critically ill surgical patients. Am Surg 45:485, 1979.
93. Zaloga, GP, and Chernow, B: The multifactorial basis for hypocalcemia during sepsis: Studies of the parathyroid hormone-vitamin D axis. Ann Intern Med 107:36, 1987.
94. Zaloga, GP, Chernow, B, and Lake, CR: The Pharmacologic Approach to the Critically Ill Patient. Williams & Wilkins, Baltimore, 1983, p 530.
95. Zaloga, GP, et al: Low dose calcium administration increases mortality during septic peritonitis. Crit Care Med 18:S209, 1990.

CHAPTER 16

Acid-Base Problems

I. INTRODUCTION

A. THE TERMS ACID AND BASE

The Latin *acidus*, meaning sour tasting, refers to the sour taste of acid substances, such as vinegar. The term *base* was introduced in 1774 by Rouelle, who defined it as a substance that reacts with an acid to form a salt. Bronsted defined an acid as any substance that could supply a hydrogen ion; a base was any substance that could accept a hydrogen ion. The acidity of any solution, whether blood, interstitial fluid, or cell water, is a measure of the hydrogen ion activity of that solution.

B. pH

The concentration of hydrogen ions, even in a very acid solution, is extremely low. In a so-called neutral solution, the number of hydrogen ions (H^+) equals the number of hydroxyl ions (OH^-); in water, at 25°C the number of hydrogen ions is 1/10,000,000 or 10^{-7} mol/liter. The term pH refers to the negative logarithm of the hydrogen ion concentration. Hasselbalch coined the term after Sorensen referred to a hydrogen ion concentration of 10^{-7} as "7 puissance hydrogen." Thus, a solution with a pH of 1 has a hydrogen ion concentration of 1×10^{-1} and is extremely acidic, whereas a solution with a pH of 13 has a hydrogen ion concentration of 1×10^{-13} and is extremely alkaline.

C. HENDERSON-HASSELBALCH EQUATION

The Henderson-Hasselbalch equation states that the pH is equal to the pK (the negative log of the dissociation constant, or the pH at which half of the compound is ionized) plus the log of the ratio of the concentration of a base to its related acid:

$$pH = pK + \log \frac{\text{proton acceptor (base)}}{\text{proton donor (acid)}}.$$

About 80% of the buffering for the extracellular fluid is in the bicarbonate-carbonic acid system. The average normal concentration of bicarbonate is 24 mEq/liter, and the average normal concentration of carbonic acid is 1.2 mEq/liter. Thus, the ratio of bicarbonate to carbonic acid is normally 20:1. The log of 20 is 1.3, and the addition of 1.3 to 6.1 (the pK of the bicarbonate-carbonic acid system) results in a pH of 7.4, or the normal arterial pH:

$$pH = 6.1 + \log \frac{HCO_3^-}{H_2CO_2}$$

$$= 6.1 + \log \frac{24}{1.2}$$
$$= 6.1 + \log 20$$
$$= 6.1 + 1.3 = 7.4.$$

AXIOM

If the ratio of bicarbonate to carbonic acid is doubled or reduced by half, the pH changes by 0.3.

The normal ratio of HCO_3^- to H_2CO_3 is 20:1, and the log of 20 is 1.3. Since the log of 2 is 0.301, whenever the ratio of HCO_3^- to H_2CO_3 is reduced by one half, the pH falls by 0.3. On the other hand, if the $HCO_3^-:H_2CO_3$ ratio increases from 20:1 to 40:1, the pH rises from 7.40 to 7.70.

The H_2CO_3 can be calculated by multiplying the Pco_2 by 0.03. Thus, with a HCO_3^- of 12 and Pco_2 of 40 mm Hg, the H_2CO_3 is 1.2, the ratio of HCO_3^- to H_2CO_3 is 10 (log of 1.0), and the pH is 7.1. If the HCO_3^- falls to 6 and the Pco_2 is still 40 mm Hg, the ratio of HCO_3^- to H_2CO_3 is 5 (log of 0.7) and the pH is 6.8.

D. HYDROGEN ION CONCENTRATIONS

Some investigators prefer to use hydrogen ion concentration, rather than pH, when discussing or calculating acidity (Table 16.1). At a pH of 7.40, the hydrogen ion activity is equivalent to 40 mmol/liter. The relationship between $[H^+]$ (expressed as mmol/liter) and Pco_2 and HCO_3^- can be expressed clinically by the following formula:

$$[H^+](mmol/L) = \frac{(24)(Pco_2)}{(HCO_3^-)}.$$

If a table relating H^+ to pH is available, it is easy to calculate the pH, Pco_2, or HCO_3^-, if the other two are known.

Thus, if the Pco_2 is 25 and the HCO_3^- is 12,

$$H^+ = \frac{(24)(25)}{(12)}$$

$$H^+ = \frac{600}{12} = 50 \text{ mmol/L}.$$

An H^+ activity of 50 mmol/liter is equivalent to a pH of 7.30 (Table 16.1).

E. INTRACELLULAR pH

Many difficulties are encountered in measuring intracellular pH (pH_i) especially in humans. Measurements from the human quadriceps muscle by Sahlin in 1978 revealed a pH_i of 7.00 ± 0.06 in 13 studies. In 20 studies of human red blood cells by Warth and Desforges in 1978 the pH_i was found to be 7.06 to 7.10. Thus, the pH_i is 0.30 to 0.40 units less than the arterial pH.

To maintain a chronic stable pH_i, acid must be extruded from the cell relatively soon after it is formed. However, the initial handling of acid in the cell is much more complex. When responding to an acute internal acid load, the cell first recruits several relatively rapid mechanisms that consume or bind H^+, thereby minimizing the magnitude of the pH_i decrease. Later, the pH_i slowly returns to normal as acid is extruded from the cell.

Table 16.1

ESTIMATING BASE DEFICIT FROM THE pH AND BICARBONATE	pH	Sum of Base Deficit and Bicarbonate	Base Deficit if Bicarbonate Is 24 mEq/L
	7.00–7.09	32	8
	7.10–7.19	30	6
	7.20–7.29	28	4
	7.30–7.34	26	2
	7.35–7.45	24	0
	7.45–7.49	23	−1
	7.50–7.59	22	−2

The initial mechanisms for handling an acid load intracellularly include (1) physicochemical buffering, (2) cellular consumption of nonvolatile acids, and (3) the transfer of acid or alkali between the cytosol and organelles. In the broadest sense, all three are buffering mechanisms, since they reversibly consume H^+. In combination, they neutralize more than 99.99% of the acid or alkali introduced into a cell. For example, the addition of 10^{-3} mol of H^+ to 1 liter of cell content might lower pH_i from 7.1 to 7.0, representing an increase of only about 2×10^{-8} mol in free $[H^+]$. All the rest of the H^+ is "consumed" or "buffered" by the three mechanisms described above.

The conversion of a weak acid (e.g., lactic acid) to a neutral product (e.g., glucose) or to one that can readily leave the cell (e.g., carbon dioxide) results in the loss of intracellular H^+. Internal pH can also be influenced by other reactions, such as the hydrolysis of ATP (which releases H^+) or phosphocreatinine (which consumes H^+). Folbergrova and colleagues show that intracellular acid loading (accomplished by increasing P_{CO_2}) leads to a reduction in the levels of several acidic metabolic intermediates (pyruvate, lactate, citrate, alpha-ketoglutarate, maleate, glutamate, and aspartate). Intracellular acid loading also causes an elevation of glucose and glucose 6-phosphate levels. This pattern suggests that reducing pH_i inhibits a step (possibly the phosphofructokinase reaction) in the glycolytic pathway. The maximum amount of H^+ that can be neutralized through these acidic intermediates is about 50% of that taken up by physicochemical buffers. Other evidence of metabolic consumption of acid comes from Cohen and associates, who show that increased lactate uptake by the isolated, perfused rat liver is associated with a rise in pH_i, as would be expected if lactate ions enter the cell and are converted to neutral products.

Intracellular alkalosis (produced by decreasing P_{CO_2}) leads to increased levels of pyruvate, lactate, and other acidic metabolic intermediates in rat brain, and these metabolic changes thereby partially neutralize an alkaline load.

It must be recognized that physicochemical, biochemical, and organelle buffering mechanisms offer only partial and short-term solutions to acid loading. They can only minimize the decrease in pH_i and are of limited capacity. The restoration of a normal pH_i after an acute acid load requires the eventual extrusion of all added acid. As this extrusion proceeds, buffers release the H^+, which they previously consumed, and are thereby restored to their initial state.

F. ACID PRODUCTION, TRANSPORT, AND EXCRETION

1. Carbon Dioxide (Volatile Acid)

With an average carbon dioxide production of 200 to 300 ml/min, the body's total carbon dioxide production is 288,000 to 432,000 ml/d. Since 22.4 ml carbon dioxide is equivalent to 1.0 mEq of acid, about 12,000 to 20,000 mEq of volatile acid is produced each day by the body's metabolism of carbohydrate, protein, and fat, and is excreted by the lungs. Most carbon dioxide transport to the lungs from peripheral tissues is provided by plasma bicarbonate and red cell hemoglobin. Carbon dioxide present as carbonic acid in arterial blood averages about 1.2 (1.05 to 1.35) mEq/liter, equivalent to a P_{CO_2} of 40 mm Hg.

2. Nonvolatile Acid Excretion

Ordinarily the kidney excretes about 70 mEq of acid each day, but in acidotic patients, acid excretion may be increased fourfold to sixfold. Renal tubular excretion of acid is normally accomplished by three mechanisms: (1) direct excretion of hydrogen, which accounts for only about 0.1 mEq of acid per day; (2) excretion with urine buffers, including the NaH_2PO_4 system, which accounts for about 20 mEq of acid per day; and (3) excretion with ammonia (produced in the distal tubal cells from glutamine and other precursors), which accounts for about 50 mEq of acid per day.

AXIOM

Dehydration (without shock) increases sodium and bicarbonate absorption in the kidney and tends to cause a metabolic alkalosis.

In the proximal tubule, sodium and bicarbonate are absorbed independent of the effects of aldosterone, and hydrogen is secreted into the tubular lumen in exchange for sodium ions. If the extracellular fluid volume is reduced or "contracted," increased amounts of sodium and bicarbonate are absorbed in the proximal tubule, which may cause a "contraction metabolic alkalosis." If saline solution is given to expand the extracellular fluid, proximal tubular absorption of sodium and bicarbonate is decreased. Sodium deficiency, increased aldosterone production, or decreased aldosterone metabolism by the liver also increase the absorption of sodium and bicarbonate in the proximal tubule.

In the distal tubule cells, H_2CO_3 is dissociated into H^+ and HCO_3^-. Here H^+ and K^+ are excreted into the urine in exchange for Na^+. The HCO_3^-, which was formed in the cell, and the Na^+, which is absorbed out of the tubule lumen, move out the other side of the tubule cell into the bloodstream as $NaHCO_3$.

Anything that increases the intracellular concentration of hydrogen or potassium ions also increases the secretion of hydrogen and/or potassium ions into the distal tubular lumen and the reabsorption of sodium. When a potassium deficiency develops in the extracellular fluid, potassium ions leave tissue cells in exchange for hydrogen, resulting in an intracellular acidosis and an extracellular alkalosis. Increased potassium is also absorbed in the distal tubule in exchange for hydrogen ions, and increased hydrogen ions are then excreted in the urine. Thus, a hypokalemic alkalemic patient may put out a paradoxically acid urine.

AXIOM

Hypokalemia is the most frequent cause of alkaline urine excretion by the acidotic patient.

Renal tubular acidosis may be classified as proximal or distal depending on the nephron segment primarily involved in the generation of this defect. In proximal tubular acidosis, urinary pH is increased at normal rates of bicarbonate filtration, denoting a failure of the proximal nephron to reabsorb the normal load of bicarbonate. However, when the filtered load of bicarbonate is decreased, urinary pH decreases to normal levels, indicating that the distal nephron is able to take care of the distal bicarbonate loads that remain within the normal range.

When the distal nephron is predominately involved (distal tubular acidosis), the ability to create transepithelial pH gradients, and thus to produce an acid urine, is impaired at any filtered load of bicarbonate because of an intrinsic defect of the acidification capacity of the last tubule segments.

A widely used model for distal acidosis is based on treatment with amphotericin B, a polyene antifungal antibiotic, which is incorporated into cell membranes and is responsible for the formation of cation-selective "pores," that is, channels that markedly increase the permeability for Na^+ and K^+.

Acidification of urine by the distal nephron can be evaluated clinically by measuring urine and arterial PCO_2, after making the urine alkaline by bicarbonate loading. The urine-blood (U-B) PCO_2 difference indicates the amount of urine carbon dioxide generation that is due to distal hydrogen ion secretion. When distal hydrogen ion secretion is impaired, as in distal tubular acidosis, urine PCO_2 falls, and U-B PCO_2 differences are reduced.

G. BUFFERS

A wide variety of metabolic and respiratory factors produce or take up hydrogen ions. These changes in hydrogen ion concentration could cause wide swings in the pH, if it were not for a group of substances referred to as buffers, which are capable of partially neutralizing acids and bases. The acid-buffering capacity of any agent or solution is determined by the number of hydrogen ions that the agent can take up for each unit change in pH. In general, for each 1000 to 10,000 mEq of acid added to the body, only about 1 mEq remains unbuffered or free to produce a change in pH.

AXIOM

About 99.99% of an acid load is buffered or combined with other compounds to prevent sudden pH changes.

The average adult man has a total buffer base, or buffering capacity, of about 1000 mEq. The chief buffers in blood are the hemoglobin in red blood cells and the bicarbonate and protein in plasma. Most of the total buffering against carbon dioxide is provided by hemoglobin, but moment-to-moment buffering of the blood and interstitial fluid is provided primarily by the bicarbonate-carbonic acid system. The most important intracellular buffers are phosphate and protein. Patients with anemia, low plasma protein levels, or decreased muscle mass have a reduced buffering capacity and are apt to have wide swings in pH when they become ill or injured. In such individuals, impaired tissue perfusion of relatively short duration may cause severe acidosis.

AXIOM

The body generally tolerates an acid load much better than a base excess.

Most of the body's buffer systems are designed to neutralize acid. Mortality and morbidity tend to be much worse in patients with alkalosis than in those with a corresponding amount of acidosis.

1. Buffer Base

To recognize and quantify nonrespiratory (metabolic) acidosis or alkalosis, changes in plasma bicarbonate concentrations are traditionally evaluated. However, since bicarbonate concentration in plasma is also affected by changes in Pco_2 (the respiratory disturbances), several Pco_2-independent indexes of the nonrespiratory acid-base disturbance have been proposed, such as standard bicarbonate concentration or eucapnic pH (both standardized for a Pco_2 of 40 mm Hg) and buffer base (BB), either in whole blood or in plasma; base excess or deficit is a measure of the deviation of BB from its normal value.

Conceptually, all the Pco_2-independent indicators of the metabolic acid-base disturbances are meant to parallel the differences among the sums of all strong (i.e., completely dissociated) cations and anions in plasma. This was recognized in 1948 by Singer and Hastings, who coined the term *plasma buffer base*, meaning the difference between what they called fixed acids and bases in plasma, a quantity corresponding to the strong ion difference (SID) later described by Stewart. Singer and Hastings also identified that Pco_2 and BB operate as two independent variables that can change independently of each other.

2. Base Excess

An increase in the amount of buffer base present is referred to as a base excess, and a decrease may be referred to as a base deficit or a negative base excess.

The appropriate respiratory (ventilatory) component of the acid-base status of a patient is fairly predictable. A sudden increase of 10 mm Hg in Pco_2 (with bicarbonate staying constant) causes the pH to decrease by about 0.10 unit, whereas a sudden decrease of 10 mm Hg in Pco_2 (with bicarbonate staying constant) causes the pH to increase by about 0.13. Thus, the difference between the actual pH and the pH predicted from the Pco_2 represents a deviation from the normal buffer base status.

The metabolic component may also be estimated, because a rise in bicarbonate of 5.0 mEq/liter (with Pco_2 staying constant) raises the pH about 0.08, and a fall in bicarbonate of 5.0 mEq/liter (again with Pco_2 staying constant) lowers the pH about 0.10.

As a general rule, the base deficit (negative base excess) represents the mEq/liter of bicarbonate required to restore the total buffer base of the extracellular fluid (ECF) to normal. There are a number of ways to determine the base deficit. One can estimate it by (1) subtracting the actual bicarbonate from 26 mEq/liter at a pH of 7.30 to 7.34 or from 28 mEq/liter at a pH of 7.20 to 7.29, (2) using a nomogram, (3) using a table (Table 16.1), or (4) using a technique described by Shapiro.

AXIOM

As a general rule, the lower the pH, the greater the base deficit, even if bicarbonate levels are held constant.

Thus, if the pH is 7.04, P_{CO_2} is 76, and HCO_3^- is 19.9 mEq/liter, the base deficit should be about $32 - 19.9 = 12.1$ mEq/liter.

If the pH is 7.47, P_{CO_2} is 18, and HCO_3^- is 12.7 mEq/liter, the base deficit should be $23 - 12.7 = 10.3$ mEq/liter.

Shapiro has described three steps for estimating the metabolic component (i.e., base deficit) of an acid-base abnormality:

1. Determine the P_{CO_2} variance difference between measured P_{CO_2} and 40; move decimal point two places to the left.

2. Determine the predicted pH from the P_{CO_2} variance. If the P_{CO_2} is over 40, subtract half of the P_{CO_2} variance from 7.40. If P_{CO_2} is under 40, add the P_{CO_2} variance to 7.40.

3. Estimate the base excess/deficit from the pH variance. Determine the difference between the measured and predicted pHs. Move the decimal point two places to the right and multiply by two thirds.

> *Example A:* pH 7.04, P_{CO_2} — 76 mm Hg, HCO_3^- 19.9 mEq/L
> $76 - 40 = 36 \times \frac{1}{2} = 0.18$
> $7.40 - 0.18 = 7.22$
> $7.22 - 7.04 = 18.0 \times \frac{2}{3} = 12$ mEq/L base deficit

> *Example B:* pH 7.47, P_{CO_2} — 18 mm Hg, HCO_3^- 12.7 mEq/L
> $40 - 18 = 0.22$
> $7.40 + 0.22 = 7.62$
> $7.62 - 7.47 = 15.0 \times \frac{2}{3} = 10$ mEq/L base deficit.

3. Nonvolatile Weak Acids

Stewart ascertained that, in addition to P_{CO_2} and plasma buffer base (SID), a third independent variable exists in body fluids, which is the total concentration of nonvolatile weak acids, designated as $[A_T]$. In plasma, the main constituent of $[A_T]$ is the protein (predominately albumin). The contribution of phosphate is less than one tenth of the total $[A_T]$.

P_{CO_2} and buffer base are the controlled quantities in the biological regulation of acid-base balance. However, any abnormality in the amount of nonvolative weak acids $[A_T]$, especially plasma proteins, will produce an acid-base disturbance. Thus, hypoproteinemia tends to cause a nonrespiratory alkalosis, and abnormally high concentrations of plasma albumin can give rise to a nonrespiratory acidosis.

If the anion gap is normal in a hypoproteinemic patient, unidentified anions must be present. This increase in unidentified anions would be missed if the plasma protein level was not known.

AXIOM

Plasma proteins are nonvolatile weak acids and should be measured as part of the evaluation of acid-base status.

Base excess or deficit does not distinguish strong acids (e.g., lactic, keto) from weak nonvolatile acids (plasma proteins, phosphate). The existing nomograms for the estimation of BB are based on data obtained in blood with normal concentrations of plasma proteins. Therefore, a deficit of nonvolatile weak acids appears as an apparent increase in plasma buffer base.

H. CARBON DIOXIDE CONTENT

Carbon dioxide content refers to the total of all carbon dioxide present in the blood (normally 24 to 31 mEq/liter). In the plasma, carbon dioxide content includes carbonic acid, bicarbonate, and carbamino compounds. The amount of carbonic acid present (averaging about 1.05 to 1.35 mEq/liter) can be estimated by multiplying the P_{CO_2} by 0.03. The arterial bicarbonate concentration normally is 24 mEq/liter. The concentration of the carbamino compounds, which consist of various forms of carbon dioxide combined with amino groups on proteins, averages about 0.5 to 1.0 mEq/liter, depending on total carbon dioxide and protein concentrations.

II. EVALUATING ACID-BASE ABNORMALITIES

A. CHECKING THE CONSISTENCY AND ACCURACY OF LABORATORY REPORTS

PITFALL

Failure to correlate arterial bicarbonate levels with the carbon dioxide level obtained from electrolyte studies.

When obtaining blood for blood gas studies in patients with complicated acute problems, additional blood for electrolyte determinations should be drawn. The bicarbonate present can then be estimated from the carbon dioxide content, as well as from the pH and P_{CO_2}.

1. Correlating Carbon Dioxide Content and Bicarbonate

Under ordinary circumstances, the arterial bicarbonate concentration is approximately 1.5 to 2.0 mEq/liter less than the arterial carbon dioxide content reported as part of an electrolyte analysis. Since the venous P_{CO_2} is normally about 6 mm Hg higher than the arterial P_{CO_2} and venous bicarbonate is 1.1 mEq/liter higher than arterial bicarbonate, the venous carbon dioxide content is usually about 1.0 to 1.5 mEq/liter higher than the arterial carbon dioxide content. Thus, if arterial blood is drawn for blood gas determinations and venous blood is drawn for electrolytes, the carbon dioxide content in venous blood should be about 2.5 to 3.0 mEq/liter more than the arterial bicarbonate.

AXIOM

One should not accept an arterial bicarbonate that is higher than the venous carbon dioxide found on an electrolyte study.

2. Correlating pH and Electrolytes

Correlating pH with potassium and other electrolyte values can help estimate acid-base status. Patients with severe acidosis tend to have high serum potassium levels, and patients with a severe alkalosis tend to have low serum potassium levels. In general, a rise or fall of 0.10 in the pH is associated with a corresponding fall or rise of about 0.5 (0.3 to 0.8) mEq/liter in serum potassium. Thus, a patient with a pH of 7.30 and a plasma potassium of 4.8 mEq/liter tends to have a plasma potassium level of 3.8 if the pH is raised to 7.50. The potassium level in serum is slightly higher than that in plasma because the clotting process releases some potassium.

3. Correlating Chloride and Bicarbonate Levels

Plasma chloride and bicarbonate concentrations tend to move in opposite directions. Thus, patients who have a metabolic alkalosis (and high plasma bicarbonate levels) tend to have low plasma chloride levels, whereas those with metabolic acidosis (and low plasma bicarbonate levels) tend to have normal or elevated chloride levels. However, if there are increased amounts of unmeasured anions, such as lactate, present (causing an increased anion gap), bicarbonate may be very low and chloride may be normal or even low.

4. Effect of P_{CO_2} and HCO_3^- on pH

With mild-moderate acidosis (pH 7.25 to 7.35), a 10.0 mm Hg rise in the P_{CO_2} produces a decrease of about 0.10 in pH while a 5.0 mEq/liter decrease in bicarbonate produces a pH decrease of about 0.10 (Table 16.2). Note that a 10

Table 16.2

pH CORRELATED WITH PCO₂ AND BICARBONATE	HCO_3^- (mEq/L)					
	5	9	14	19	24	29
P_{CO_2} (mm Hg)	pH					
60	6.54	6.80	6.99	7.12	7.22	7.31
50	6.62	6.88	7.07	7.20	7.30	7.39
40	6.72	6.98	7.17	7.30	7.40	7.48
30	6.84	7.10	7.29	7.42	7.53	7.61
20	7.02	7.28	7.47	7.60	7.70	7.78
10	7.32	7.58	7.77	7.90	8.00	8.09

mm Hg increase in P_{CO_2} (with bicarbonate staying normal) or a 5 mEq/liter decrease in bicarbonate (with P_{CO_2} staying normal) will drop the pH from 7.40 to 7.30. In other words, a 1.0 mEq/liter change in bicarbonate causes about twice as much change in pH as does a 1.0 mm Hg change in the P_{CO_2}. Thus, a patient whose bicarbonate falls from 24.0 to 19.0 mEq/liter and whose P_{CO_2} falls from 40 to 30 mm Hg will still have a pH of approximately 7.40. This "quick and dirty" way to estimate bicarbonate from the pH and P_{CO_2} can also be used as a check on the consistency and accuracy of the laboratory results.

B. CATEGORIZING THE ABNORMALITY

1. Simple Disorders

Acid-base abnormalities can often be defined in terms of the pH and the relative amounts of arterial bicarbonate and carbonic acid. The normal average concentration of bicarbonate in arterial blood is 24 mEq/liter with a normal range of about 21 to 26 mEq/liter. If the arterial bicarbonate is greater than 26 mEq/liter and the pH is greater than 7.40, the patient is said to have a metabolic alkalosis. If the arterial bicarbonate is less than 21 mEq/liter and the pH is less than 7.40, the patient is said to have metabolic acidosis.

The P_{CO_2} is normally 35 to 45 mm Hg. If the arterial P_{CO_2} is lower than 35 mm Hg and the pH is greater than 7.40, the patient is said to have respiratory alkalosis. In contrast, if the arterial P_{CO_2} is greater than 45 mm Hg and the pH is less than 7.40, the patient is said to have respiratory acidosis. In some centers, especially in Europe, the P_{CO_2} is reported in kPa (kilopascals). One can convert P_{CO_2} to kPa by multiplying it by 0.1333. Thus, the normal P_{CO_2} in kPa is 4.7 to 6.0.

2. Mixed Disorders

AXIOM

If the pH is relatively normal, but the P_{CO_2} and bicarbonate are abnormal, one can assume that a mixed acid-base disorder is present.

In many instances, more than one acid-base problem is present at a time. For example, if a patient with chronic respiratory acidosis (pH = 7.35; P_{CO_2} = 50 mm Hg; HCO_3^- = 26.7 mEq/liter) develops pyloric stenosis and is vomiting large amounts of highly acidic fluid (which would ordinarily cause a metabolic alkalosis), the patient could develop a pH of 7.40 with a P_{CO_2} of 55 mm Hg and an HCO_3^- of 32 mEq/liter. This might be confusing under many clinical circumstances. However, in general, if the arterial pH is relatively normal (7.36 to 7.44) and the P_{CO_2} and/or HCO_3^- are abnormal, one can assume that a mixed abnormality is present. The mixed abnormality should also be detectable from the history and physical examination, or other laboratory data. In this regard, the anion gap and BB may be helpful.

3. Different Disorders in Arterial and Venous Blood

Weil and colleagues and Adrogue and associates have emphasized the big differences that can occur between arterial and central or mixed venous blood in patients with severe circulatory failure or cardiac arrest, especially if the patient is on a ventilator. In such patients, the arterial blood often reveals a mild-to-moderate metabolic acidosis with partial respiratory compensation (pH = 7.25 to 7.35; P_{CO_2} = 25 to 35 mm Hg; HCO_3^- = 15 to 20 mEq/liter). The venous blood may show essentially the same or a slightly higher bicarbonate, but a much lower pH and much higher P_{CO_2} (pH = 7.20 to 7.10; P_{CO_2} = 50 to 70 mm Hg; HCO_3^- = 17 to 23 mEq/liter). Under such circumstances, it is thought that the arterial blood reflects the adequacy of pulmonary function, but the venous P_{CO_2} reflects the adequacy of tissue perfusion.

AXIOM

In patients with a very low cardiac output or severe hypermetabolism, the arterial PCO_2 reflects pulmonary function and the venous PCO_2 reflects tissue metabolism and blood flow.

C. COMPENSATORY CHANGES

Any abnormality that disturbs the normal ratio between arterial bicarbonate and carbonic acid tends to immediately stimulate a compensating metabolic or respiratory response to try to bring the ratio back to 7.35, if the primary problem is an acidosis, or 7.45, if the problem is an alkalosis.

1. Respiratory Compensation

a. Metabolic Acidosis

Respiratory compensation for a primary metabolic acidosis can occur very rapidly. For example, if patients develop a metabolic acidosis with a bicarbonate of 14 mEq/liter, they will tend to hyperventilate rather rapidly, producing a compensatory respiratory alkalosis. The P_{CO_2} would have to fall to 20 mm Hg to produce complete compensation to a pH of 7.40; however, the acute compensation (within 1 to 2 hours) may be only about 50% of that, and the compensation over 24 hours may be only 75% complete.

b. Metabolic Alkalosis

Compensation for alkalosis is seldom as good as for acidosis. Furthermore, the compensatory hypoventilation for a metabolic alkalosis is restricted by the hypoxemia that develops along with the hypoventilation.

AXIOM

The PCO_2 seldom rises above 50 to 55 mm Hg to compensate for a metabolic alkalosis unless oxygen is given.

If a patient develops a metabolic alkalosis with an HCO_3^- of 36 mEq/liter, the P_{CO_2} would have to rise to 60 mm Hg for a complete compensation to a pH of 7.40. The acute compensation would be only about 25% to 40%, raising the P_{CO_2} to about 45 to 48 mm Hg. Even after 48 hours, the respiratory compensation is often only about 60% complete.

c. Metabolic Compensations

During acute and chronic hypocapnia and hypercapnia, the changes in HCO_3^- are almost linear over the range of Pa_{CO_2} (20 to 100 mm Hg) encountered in altered pathologic states (Table 16.3). Thus, one can predict to some degree what the HCO_3^- "should be" for any Pa_{CO_2}. This observation leads to certain rules of thumb to characterize various acid-base abnormalities:

1. During each hypercapnia, HCO_3^- increases 1 mmol/liter for each 10-mm Hg increase in Pa_{CO_2} above 40 mm Hg.

2. During chronic hypercapnia, HCO_3^- increases 4 mmol/liter for each 10-mm Hg increase in Pa_{CO_2} above 40 mm Hg.

3. During acute hypocapnia, HCO_3^- decreases 2 mmol/liter for every 10-mm Hg decrease in Pa_{CO_2} below 40 mm Hg.

4. During chronic hypocapnia, HCO_3^- decreases at least 5 mmol/liter for every 10-mm Hg decrease in Pa_{CO_2} below 40 mm Hg.

Table 16.3

ACUTE pH AND BICARBONATE RESPONSE TO CHANGES IN P_{CO_2}	P_{CO_2}	pH	HCO_3^-
	15	7.73	19
	20	7.62	20
	25	7.54	21
	30	7.49	22
	35	7.44	23
	40	7.40	24
	50	7.32	25
	60	7.26	26
	70	7.21	27
	80	7.16	28

Example 1: Shortly after respiratory arrest and endotracheal intubation of an otherwise healthy adult male, an arterial blood gas reveals a pH of 7.21, P_{CO_2} of 70 mm Hg, and HCO_3^- of 27 mEq/liter. Obviously, the primary problem is respiratory acidosis, but is there any associated metabolic problem? Application of the rule of thumb indicates that the HCO_3^- should have risen by $30 \div 10 = 3$ mEq/liter, which it did. Therefore, this is a pure respiratory acidosis.

Example 2: An otherwise healthy man sustains an acute airway obstruction. An endotracheal tube is inserted and an arterial blood sample is drawn simultaneously. The laboratory reports as follows:

$$pH = 7.20; \ Pa_{CO_2} = 60 \text{ mm Hg}; \ HCO_3^- = 21 \text{ mEq/L}.$$

The patient is acidemic, and because the Pa_{CO_2} is 60 mm Hg, at least a portion of the acidemia is respiratory. Application of the rule of thumb for acute hypercapnia suggests that the HCO_3^- should be 26 mmol/liter (at least 2 mmol above normal) (Table 16.3). Since the actual HCO_3^- in this patient is 21 mmol/liter, a deficit of 5 mmol/liter exists. Thus, a combined respiratory and metabolic acidosis is present.

Example 3: A 60-kg woman with COPD has an acute myocardial infarction. Arterial blood gas analysis shows the following:

$$pH = 7.35; \ P_{CO_2} = 60 \text{ mm Hg}; \ HCO_3^- = 32 \text{ mm Hg}.$$

The patient apparently has a chronic respiratory acidosis due to the elevation of both the P_{CO_2} and bicarbonate. Since the HCO_3^- rose 4 mEq/liter for each 10 mm rise in the P_{CO_2}, this is a pure respiratory acidosis.

Example 4: A patient with chronic COPD has an acute myocardial infarction. Arterial blood gas analysis:

$$pH = 7.20; \ Pa_{CO_2} = 60 \text{ mm Hg}; \ HCO_3^- = 21 \text{ mEq/L}.$$

The arterial pH of 7.20 confirms acidemia, and the Pa_{CO_2} of 60 mm Hg reveals that respiratory factors are present. However, when one is dealing with chronic hypercapnia, a P_{CO_2} of 60 mm Hg should have an HCO_3^- of 32 mmol/liter (Table 16.4). The actual HCO_3^- is only 21 mmol/liter, a deficit of 11 mmol/liter, indicating that there is also a metabolic component to the acidosis.

Example 5: An extremely anxious patient with some vague abdominal pain has an arterial blood gas drawn revealing

$$pH = 7.35; \ P_{CO_2} = 25 \text{ mm Hg}; \ HCO_3^- = 21 \text{ mEq/L}.$$

Table 16.4

CHRONIC pH AND BICARBONATE RESPONSE TO CHANGES IN P_{CO_2}	P_{CO_2}, mm Hg	pH	HCO_3^-, mmol/L
	20	7.47	14
	30	7.45	20
	40	7.40	24
	50	7.37	28
	60	7.35	32
	70	7.33	36
	80	7.32	40

Since the HCO_3^- fell approximately 2.0 mEq/liter for each 10-mm Hg fall in the P_{CO_2}, this is a pure respiratory alkalosis.

AXIOM

As a compensatory response to respiratory alkalosis the bicarbonate seldom falls below 18.0 mEq/liter, acutely, or 15.0 mEq/liter, chronically.

d. Failure of Compensatory Mechanisms

Failure of compensatory mechanisms, or a combination of primary processes driving the pH in the same direction so that it rapidly falls and stays below 7.10 or rises above 7.60, is frequently lethal.

AXIOM

Inability to at least partially compensate for an acid-base abnormality usually means a severe disturbance of ventilatory, renal, or general cellular function.

D. ANION GAP IN BLOOD

1. Definition

The concept of the anion gap was described in 1939 by Gamble. It was believed that the law of electroneutrality required that the number of positive charges contributed by serum cations should equal the number of negative charges contributed by serum anions.

Sodium (Na^+), chloride (Cl^+), and bicarbonate (HCO_3^-) are considered the measured ions. Potassium is ignored because its value changes so little. Thus, the concept of electroneutrality can be expressed by the simple equation:

$$Na^+ + UC = Cl^+ + HCO_3^- + UA,$$

where UC (unmeasured cations) indicates the sum of the charges of the cations other than sodium and UA (unmeasured anions) equals the sum of the charges of all of the anions other than chloride and bicarbonate. As can be seen from Table 16.5, the sum of the unmeasured cations (Ca^+, K^+, and Mg^{++}) is usually about 12.0 mEq/liter and the sum of the unmeasured anions is about 23 mEq/liter.

Table 16.5

ANION AND CATIONS IN PLASMA	Cations		Anions	
	Na^+	142	Cl^-	103
	Ca^{++}	5	CO_2	27
	K^+	4	Protein	16
	Mg^{++}	3	HPO_4^-	2
		153	SO_4^-	1
			Lactic acid	1
			Organic acids	3
				153

The term anion gap (AG) was coined to indicate the difference between the measured sodium level and the measured chloride and bicarbonate (really carbon dioxide content) levels.

$$AG = Na^+ - (Cl^- + HCO_3^-).$$

The equation can also be written as

$$UA - UC = Na^+ - (Cl^- + HCO_3^-) = AG,$$

indicating that a rise in UA and/or a decrease in UC will cause an increase in the AG, independent of the presence or absence of an acid-base disorder. The reverse is also true. In other words, a decrease in UA and/or rise in UC will cause a decrease in the AG.

Ordinarily, the sodium concentration is about 142 mEq/liter and the sum of the carbon dioxide content and chloride anions is about 130 mEq/liter. Thus the difference (or anion gap) between the sodium concentration and the sum of these two anions averages about 12 mEq/liter. In patients with excessive acid production, the anion gap tends to be increased. On the other hand, in patients with metabolic acidosis due to loss of bicarbonate, the anion gap usually stays relatively normal (12 ± mEq/liter).

2. Unmeasured Cations and Anions

Assigning numerical values for the charges of the serum constituents is accomplished easily for sodium, potassium, bicarbonate, and chloride. It is more difficult to assign values for phosphate and protein, which can have multiple charges. The total concentration of serum calcium and magnesium, rather than just the ionized fraction, is used in the calculation of unmeasured cations because the nonionized portions of those cations are bound to protein (especially albumin, which is a polyanion) or are complexed with bicarbonate, phosphate, sulfate, lactate, or citrate. Thus, they "cover" or balance an equivalent number of negative charges on these anions. In other words, protein-bound and complexed calcium and magnesium contribute to the charge balance in the serum.

The difficulty in establishing the precise charge contributions of sulfate and organic acid anions arises because clinical laboratories do not measure these serum constituents routinely. At least 29 acid anions are detectable in plasma; however, in normal individuals the combined contribution to the serum anions by lactate, pyruvate, acetoacetate, 3-hydroxybutyrate, and citrate is only 1.8 to 2.6 mEq/liter.

Although the concentration of serum phosphate is readily measured in the clinical laboratory, it is not a simple matter to derive its charge, which is a function not only of phosphate concentration but also of serum pH. Serum phosphorus concentration in mg/dl is converted to mmol/liter by multiplying by 10 and dividing by 31, the atomic weight of phosphorus. At a pH of 7.4, the ratio of HPO_4^- to $H_2PO_4^-$ is about 4 to 1. Thus, 80% of the phosphate contributes two negative charges as HPO_4^-, and 20% contributes one charge as $H_2PO_4^-$; thus, the charge contribution of phosphate in milliequivalents per liter at a pH of 7.4 is equal to the mmol/liter of phosphate multiplied by 1.8.

Normal serum proteins are polyanions. Although their net contribution to overall charge balance is difficult to assess exactly, a normal mixture of serum proteins is about 2.3 mEq/liter per gram of protein at pH 7.40. This charge reflects a number of variables: the type of protein, the concentration of protein, and serum pH.

Albumin contributes about 2.6 mEq/liter for each gram per deciliter, and globulin provides approximately 1.7 mEq/liter for each gram per deciliter. However, in metabolic alkalosis, the proteinate charge increases. Both Van Slyke and Van Leeuwen report a 4% to 5% increase in the negative charge of protein for each 0.10 unit rise in pH. Thus, if the proteinate charge is 16.1 mEq/liter at a pH of 7.40, the proteinate charge would be 17.4 to 17.7 at a pH of 7.60. In other words, the anion gap should increase about 1.5 mEq/liter.

3. Types of Abnormalities

Lolekha and Lolekha evaluated 7466 sets of electrolyte studies. They found a normal AG in 50.4% and an increased AG in 46.7%. Among the latter, 90% ranged from 19 to 28 mEq/liter, with a mean of 25 mEq/liter; most frequently, the level was from 19 to 21 mEq/liter. Only 2.8% of elevated values exceeded 30 mEq/liter. A decrease in AG (3 to 8 mEq/liter, mean 6 mEq/liter) was observed in only 2.9% of the cases.

AXIOM

It should be remembered that, although the anion gap can help diagnose an acid-base abnormality, changes in the anion gap are usually more informative than anion gap levels themselves.

4. Etiology of Increased Anion Gap

An increased anion gap may be caused by (1) artifacts; (2) an accumulation of organic acids, such as that seen in lactic acidosis, ketoacidosis, acute renal failure, and toxic ingestions; (3) exogenous anions; (4) reduced inorganic acid excretion, such as in chronic renal failure; (5) an increase in the anionic contribution of unmeasured weak acids; (6) a decrease in unmeasured cations; or (7) a combination of these factors.

a. Changes Due to Artifacts

A spurious increase in the AG (even in the presence of normal concentrations of the individual electrolytes) may result from excessive exposure of the serum to air. When serum, placed in small measuring vessels for microautomated chemical analysis, is not analyzed promptly, the percentage of increase in sodium, potassium, and chloride are similar, but HCO_3^- decreases due to escape of carbon dioxide. After 2 hours, the absolute increases in the concentrations of sodium and chloride are 6.9 ± 1.9 and 4.2 ± 1.8 mEq/liter, respectively, while the decrease in HCO_3^- is 3.5 ± 1.2 mEq/liter. As a result, AG increases an average of 6.2 ± 2.3 mEq/liter.

False elevations of serum chloride may result from the presence of other halide ions, as in patients who have taken in excessive quantities of bromide or iodide. These elevations occur because bromide and iodide interfere with both colorimetric and "ion-selective" techniques, resulting in reported values for chloride that exceed the sum of the true chloride concentration plus that of the other halides. Minimal interference with chloride measurement occurs with the use of chloridimetry, which should be used if halide poisoning with bromide or iodide is suspected.

Spurious hyperchloremia (with an equivalent apparent decrease in the AG) may also occur from the technical artifact caused by hypertriglyceridemia using colorimetric (but not titrimetric or potentiometric) techniques. In a prospective study by Graber and colleagues, every patient with a triglyceride level exceeding 1000 mg/dl had a spurious elevation of chloride ranging from 9 to 93 mEq/liter. This artifact would be independent of any change induced by displacement of the water phase of the plasma (i.e., pseudohyponatremia).

PITFALL

Drawing blood for arterial gas analysis into syringes with too much heparin.

If there is excess heparin in the syringe in which arterial blood is drawn, the heparin will tend to cause an acidosis and lower the pH, Pco_2, and bicarbonate, producing a picture of metabolic acidosis with partial respiratory compensation.

b. Increased Organic Acids

The organic acids most likely to increase the anion gap are lactic acid, keto acids, and a variety of other organic acids apt to increase in renal failure. Although an increase in unmeasured anions theoretically could result from increased phosphate, protein, sulfate, or organic anions, for practical purposes, only increases in organic anions or major toxic ingestions account for large increases in the anion gap.

Patients with anion gaps greater than 35 mEq/liter usually have ethylene glycol or methanol intoxication, hyperglycemic hyperosmolar coma, or lactic acidosis. In fact, such patients can have anion gaps greater than 50 mEq/liter. Severe ischemia (pH <7.00) occurs most commonly in such patients.

AXIOM
The most severe high anion gap metabolic acidosis is seen with ingestions (methanol or ethylene glycol), lactic acidosis (severe shock or cardiac arrest), or hyperglycemic coma.

(1) Lactic Acidosis

PITFALL
Assuming that all lactic acidosis is due to inadequate tissue oxygenation.

The causes of lactic acidosis have been divided into those due to inadequate tissue oxygenation (type A) and those due to other factors, such as diabetes mellitus, hypercarbia, tumors, and so forth (type B) (see Table 16.6).

The presence of acidosis with an increased anion gap in a patient in severe shock is most often due to lactic acidosis. In less dramatic clinical settings, however, the diagnosis of lactic acidosis is more difficult to document. In Gabow's studies, lactic acidosis was confirmed biochemically in only 43% of the patients in whom it was suspected on clinical grounds.

AXIOM
With any tendency to lactic acidosis, other, often unidentifiable, organic acids will also increase and usually to a much greater extent.

Unfortunately many patients with lactic acidosis will not show an elevated anion gap. Indeed, recently, Iberti and associates found that 57% of the patients with elevated lactate levels did not have an increased anion gap.

(2) Ketoacidosis and Hyperglycemic Coma

AXIOM
A tendency to ketoacidosis is less apparent in patients with a good urine output.

In the presence of adequate hydration and a normal or increased urine output, ketoacidosis tends to be minimal because the increased ketones are rapidly excreted. However, if the extracellular fluid volume is reduced, as is usually the case in ketoacidosis, the excretion of keto anions is retarded, producing a ketoacidosis with an increased anion gap. However, if the patient maintains an adequate salt intake and preserves normal or nearly normal extracellu-

---

Table 16.6

COHEN AND WOOD'S CLASSIFICATION OF LACTIC ACIDOSIS	*Type A (Tissue Hypoxia)* Shock states Profound anemia Massive catecholamine excess
	Type B (Tissue Oxygenation Appears Normal) Diabetes mellitus Liver failure Renal failure Carcinoma Seizures Alkaloses Drugs/toxins Inborn errors of metabolism Hypoglycemia

lar fluid volume, renal perfusion, and glomerular filtration rate, keto anions are excreted almost as fast as they are produced. Under these circumstances, chloride is retained by the kidney in place of ketones, a rise in the serum chloride balances the fall in the serum bicarbonate concentration, and the serum anion gap remains or becomes normal. The increase in serum chlorides will be even greater if the patient is resuscitated with 0.9% saline solution, rather than with Ringer's lactate.

Although some ketonemia probably occurs in all spontaneously occurring instances of hyperglycemic coma, even those described as being nonketotic, increases in neither plasma beta-hydroxybutyrate nor lactate are sufficient to explain the elevated AG levels, which some investigators have reported to average as high as 34 mEq/liter. Thus, the cause of the greatly increased anion gap in hyperosmolar comas is not clear.

(3) Other Organic Acids

A wide variety of organic acids may be released into the blood in increased amounts in critically ill or injured patients. These may include fatty acids, amino acids, pyruvic acids, and a number of other acid metabolites of incomplete cell metabolism.

c. Toxic Ingestions

Intoxications with salicylate, methanol, ethylene glycol, paraldehyde, toluene, sulfur, and formaldehyde lead to the formation of acid metabolites and/or organic acids that result in an increase in the AG. Some of these poisonings can be suspected clinically because of the presence of an increased osmolal gap (measured serum osmolality minus calculated serum osmolality).

If the patient has a high AG-metabolic acidosis without chronic renal failure, shock, or diabetic ketoacidosis, intoxication with methanol or ethylene glycol should be the first consideration. If the osmolal gap is increased, intoxication with methanol or ethylene glycol poisoning is even more likely.

d. Exogenous Anions

The influence of the poorly reabsorbable anion carbenicillin on the AG is a good example of the effect of the addition of unmeasured anion to the extracellular fluid. Lipner and colleagues observed these renal tubular effects (a decrease in pH value and enhanced excretion of ammonium) and detected an increase in the AG from the control value of 11.2 to 18.3 mEq/liter as well. In contrast, the administration of polymyxin B, a cationic antibiotic, has been reported as a cause of hyperchloremia and a fall in anion gap, sometimes to negative levels.

e. Reduced Inorganic Acid Excretion

In renal failure, increased quantities of sulfuric and phosphoric acid may accumulate in the bloodstream. With muscle damage, a number of sulfur-containing compounds may greatly increase the anion gap. Thus, crush injury to muscle with renal failure can cause a rapid severe rise in anion gap.

f. Increased Unmeasured Weak Acids

In septic shock increased quantities of pyruvic acid, beta-hydroxybutyric acid, fatty acids, and citric acid accumulate, but they add only slightly to the anion gap. However, in sepsis, the known compounds, including lactic acid, only account for 25% to 50% of the anion gap that develops. Thus, the etiology of a large part of the anion gap of shock, especially septic shock, is unknown.

g. Decreased Unmeasured Cations

The unmeasured cations are relatively constant in value. However, calcium could conceivably fall from 10 to 7 mg/dl (5 to 3.5 mEq/liter). Potassium could fall from 5.0 to 3 mEq/liter, and magnesium could fall from 2.0 to 1.5 mEq/liter without the patient's becoming extremely ill. Thus, these changes combined would only result in a decrease of about 4.0 mEq/liter in the unmeasured cations without obvious severe changes in the patient's condition.

h. Alkalemia

AXIOM

Although there may be great variations in unmeasured anions, the levels of unmeasured cations is quite constant.

Alkalemia itself can induce an increase in organic acid production. However, an increased anion gap and alkalemia can coexist in the absence of a demonstrated increase in organic acids. First, alkalemia tends to increase the net negative charge of serum proteins and, second, certain exogenously administered anions (citrate, lactate, and acetate) can, through their metabolism, generate metabolic alkalosis and, by partial persistence in the circulation, elevate the anion gap. In Gabow's study of patients with an increased anion gap, 10 of the 42 subjects were alkalemic, and nine had a normal serum pH.

AXIOM

Since alkalosis itself can cause an increased anion gap, the value of the anion gap in diagnosis of mixed acid-base disorders decreases as the pH rises above normal.

Alkalemia occurs in up to 50% of patients with alcoholic ketoacidosis or salicylate intoxication. Similarly, in one study, 42% of patients with rhabdomyolysis and an increased anion gap were alkalemic. Four of seven normotensive patients with classic heat stroke had an increased anion gap. Alkalemia in alcoholic ketoacidosis, salicylate intoxication, rhabdomyolysis, and classic heat stroke is usually accounted for by enough respiratory and/or metabolic alkalosis to counteract the acidifying effect of organic acid overproduction.

AXIOM

In combined metabolic and respiratory alkalosis, one can estimate the metabolic component by adding the increase in anion gap to the bicarbonate levels.

Respiratory alkalosis frequently occurs in patients undergoing alcohol withdrawal. If one adds the increase in the anion gap to the actual serum bicarbonate concentration, a measure of the true extent of the metabolic alkalosis can be obtained. One can think of this value as the level of serum bicarbonate concentration that would have been present had the newly formed organic acids not titrated away a portion of the bicarbonate.

The interpretation of an increased anion gap in patients with alkalemia is complicated because alkalemia itself can increase the anion gap. Alkalemia can increase both organic acid generation and the negative charge on protein. In acute respiratory alkalosis, lactic acid production can increase modestly and thereby raise plasma lactate levels by 2 to 3 mEq/liter. This increase in lactic acid production appears to result from an increased activity of phosphofructokinase, which enhances glycolysis through the Embden-Meyerhof pathway and thereby increases the conversion of glucose to lactate.

Two interrelated factors are responsible for the increase in the net negative charge on serum proteins by alkalemia. First, alkalemic states are often associated with a reduced blood volume and hemoconcentration. Second, proteins surrender protons when titrated in an alkaline direction, thereby uncovering additional negative charges.

Utilizing Van Leeuwen's formula, one can anticipate that alkaline titration alone can increase anion gap by about 0.6 mEq/liter per 0.10 pH rise. Some investigators have reported that, by combining all of these factors, severe metabolic alkalosis due to loss of gastric acid may increase AG by 8 to 12 mEq/liter. About 25% of the total increase results from the above-mentioned effect of pH, and about 75% results from hemoconcentration. Before this phenomenon was recognized more generally in 1979, increases in AG in hypotensive patients with severe gastric alkalosis were usually attributed (without confirmation) to lactic acidosis.

In summary, an anion gap greater than 30 mEq/liter usually indicates the presence of an organic acidosis. Values between 23 and 30 mEq/liter are also suggestive of an organic acidosis, but, frequently, the nature of the retained anion cannot be established. In acidotic patients with values between 16 and 22 mEq/liter, uremia or mild organic acidosis may be present. If the patient is alkalemic, hemoconcentration or administration of an exogenous anion may be the cause of an increased anion gap.

5. Decreased Anion Gap

An anion gap of seven or less is unusual. The main causes of a decreased anion gap are decreased unmeasured anions, increased unmeasured cations, and various analytical errors causing falsely low sodium levels or falsely high chloride levels (Table 16.7).

a. Decreased Unmeasured Anions

AXIOM

Hypoalbuminemia is probably the most common cause of a decreased anion gap in hospitalized patients.

For each 1.0 g/dl reduction in serum albumin the anion gap will fall approximately 2.5 to 3.0 mEq/liter and the standard bicarbonate (the bicarbonate that would be present if the Pa_{CO_2} were 40 mm Hg) will increase by an average of 3.4 mmol/liter.

Rossing, Maffeo, and Fend, based on their study, presented somewhat larger corrections in anion gap (AG) and smaller corrections in bicarbonate due to decreases in albumin levels:

$$HCO_3^- = (\text{albumin in g/dl}) \ (-2.63)$$
$$AG = (\text{albumin in g/dl}) \ (+4.20).$$

In other words, if the albumin falls from 4.5 to 2.5 g/dl, bicarbonate should rise by 5.3 mEq/liter and AG should fall by 8.4 mEq/liter. Due to hypoalbuminemia, these changes are the most likely explanation for the decreased anion gap frequently observed in patients with nephrotic syndrome or advanced liver disease.

Some reduction in the anion gap occurs in hypoosmolar states, presumably as a result of dilution. This change is most apparent in the syndrome of inappropriate secretion of antidiuretic hormone (SIADH). Almost 25% of patients with SIADH have an anion gap of less than 6 mEq/liter.

Table 16.7

CAUSES OF A DECREASED ANION GAP	*Decreased Unmeasured Anions* Hypoalbuminemia Hemodilution *Increased Unmeasured Cations* IgG multiple myeloma Increased calcium, magnesium, or potassium levels Acute lithium intoxication Polymyxin B administration *Nonrandom Analytic Error* Hypernatremia (severe) Hyperviscosity Bromide intoxication Iodide ingestion Hyperlipidemia

b. Increased Unmeasured Cations

The decreased anion gap in multiple myeloma is due to an increased serum concentration of cationic IgG paraproteins. Hypercalcemia and hypoalbuminemia also can contribute to a low plasma anion gap in patients with multiple myeloma.

c. Analytic Errors

AXIOM
Severe dehydration associated with hypernatremia can cause falsely low serum sodium levels and decreased anion gap.

Among the causes of nonrandom laboratory errors leading to artifactual reduction in the anion gap, hypernatremia and hyperviscosity are the most important. When the actual serum sodium concentration exceeds 170 mEq/liter, certain flame photometers yield artifactually low values. Hyperviscosity also can lead to falsely low values for serum sodium and, hence, anion gap, because the flame photometer apparatus may fail to aspirate a proper aliquot of hyperviscous serum.

AXIOM
Bromide and iodide ingestions lower anion gap.

Because bromide reacts very strongly with the reagents utilized to measure chloride by the Autoanalyzer method, artifactually high values for serum chloride concentration are frequently seen in bromide-intoxicated patients. Indeed, this laboratory error may be sufficient to actually produce a negative anion gap.

Iodine, another halogen capable of accumulating in the serum, can also cause an artificial increase in serum chloride concentration and, hence, a decrease in the anion gap. Overestimation of serum chloride concentration can also occur in the presence of hyperlipidemia, because lipids scatter light in such a way as to falsely elevate the concentration of chloride when determined by the calorimetric method.

6. Ratio of Change of Anion Gap (Delta AG) to Change in Plasma Bicarbonate (Delta HCO$_3^-$)

In uncomplicated, increased anion gap metabolic acidosis, the decrease in plasma bicarbonate should be roughly equal to the increase in the anion gap (i.e., delta AG/delta HCO$_3^-$ = 1.0). This ratio is also called the *delta gap*.

AXIOM
Whenever the AG changes much more or less than the bicarbonate, one should be suspicious of a coexisting or mixed acid-base disorder.

In classical diabetic ketoacidosis (DKA) and lactic acidosis, the rise in AG is similar, quantitatively, to the decrease in bicarbonate. The ratio of the change in anion gap and bicarbonate, therefore, is close to 1.0. However, since excretion of the ketoanions tends to reduce the AG, while not directly affecting the bicarbonate, some patients with DKA, whose ketoanion excretion is greater than usual, may have metabolic acidosis that is primarily of the hyperchloremic variety. The hyperchloremic acidosis so frequently observed during the treatment of DKA is also believed to be largely explainable on the same basis. In a pure hyperchloremic metabolic acidosis, delta gap is close to zero. Ratios between 0.3 and 0.7 or greater than 1.2, usually, but not always, indicate a mixed acid-base disorder or a pre-existing low AG.

In renal failure, there is no cause-and-effect relationship between the AG and the bicarbonate. The fall in bicarbonate is related largely to a failure of ammoniagenesis and seldom exceeds 8 to 12 mEq/liter, whereas the rise in the AG is related to the reduction in the glomerular filtration rate (GFR) and rarely leads to an anion retention of more than 4.0 mEq/liter. Thus, reciprocal stoichiometry between AG and bicarbonate should not be expected. However, even in end-stage chronic renal failure, the AG rarely exceeds 23 mEq/liter. Indeed, in patients with mild-to-moderate chronic renal failure (serum creatinine concentration between 2 and 4 mg/dl), the AG is usually normal. In patients with more severe chronic renal failure, the AG averages about 16 mEq/liter with an average delta AG/delta HCO_3 of only 0.4.

Thus, the delta gap is helpful in the diagnosis of mixed acid-base disorders because this ratio is usually close to 1.0 in typical organic acidoses.

AXIOM

A delta gap greater than 1.2 or less than 0.8 suggests the presence of a mixed acid-base disorder.

7. Urinary Anion Gap

AXIOM

Calculation of the urine anion gap helps one to determine if ammonium production is adequate in patients with an acidemia.

According to Hilton and colleagues, the urinary AG (in milliequivalents per liter), is determined by $Na^+ + K^+ - Cl^-$. Potassium is included in the formula because its concentration in urine is large and highly variable. The value for bicarbonate is not included because it is not easily measured in the urine in most clinical laboratories, and if the pH of the urine is <6.4 the bicarbonate concentration will be trivial.

The major ionic species in bicarbonate-free urine are $Na^+ + K^+ + Ca^{++} + Mg^{++} + NH_4^+ = H_2PO_4 + SO_4 + OA$ (organic anion). Excretion of phosphate, sulfate, and organic anions, does not generally change importantly when acid-base status is modified. The normal mean AG in a 24-hour collection of urine from a patient ingesting a normal diet is approximately 40 mEq (Table 16.8).

In an acidemic patient with an acidic urine, a markedly negative AG (i.e., chloride much greater than the sum of sodium and potassium) indicates a high (appropriate) level of ammonium ion (NH_4^+). On the other hand, finding a positive urine AG (chloride less than the sum of sodium and potassium) in an acidemic patient suggests that ammonium production by the kidneys is inappropriately low.

Currently, it appears that the clinical use of urinary AG involves (1) the differential diagnosis (renal versus extrarenal origin) of hyperchloremic metabolic acidosis by providing an estimate of urinary ammonium levels, and (2) assessment of the cause of renal potassium wasting by providing a clue to the excretion of large amounts of nonreabsorbable anion resulting in a kaliuresis. Examples of nonreabsorbable anions in an acid urine include carbenicillin, salicylate, and ketoanions. Since most clinical laboratories cannot provide a

Table 16.8

AVERAGE DAILY URINARY EXCRETION OF CATIONS AND ANIONS IN FOUR NORMAL SUBJECTS EATING A NORMAL DIET*

Cations	mEq/d	Anions	mEq/d
Na^+	127 ± 6	Cl^-	135 ± 5
K^+	49 ± 2	SO_4^-	34 ± 1
Ca^{++}	4 ± 1	H_2PO_4	20 ± 1
Mg^{++}	11 ± 1	Organic anions	29 ± 1
NH_4^+	28 ± 2		
Total	219 ± 3		218 ± 6

*Values are shown as mean ± SE. Modified by Goldstein and coworkers:
Urine AG = $(Na^+ + K^+) - Cl^-$ = (127 + 49) − 135 = 41
or
$NH_4^+ = (Na^+ + K^+) - Cl^- + 13)$ = (127 + 49) − (135 + 13)
= 176 − 148 = 28 mEq.

733

measurement of urinary ammonium, the urinary AG can, in a sense, provide the clinician with a "poor man's" ammonium measurement.

In general, when the cause of hyperchloremic metabolic acidosis is extrarenal, the normal kidney responds by markedly increasing the excretion of ammonium. In contrast, ammonium excretion will be low (less than 40 to 80 mmol/d) in distal renal tubular acidosis (RTA) or with decreased ammonia availability to the collecting tubule.

If the urinary AG is markedly negative (i.e., high ammonium content), the differential diagnosis of a hyperchloremic metabolic acidosis includes (1) gastrointestinal alkali loss (e.g., secretory diarrhea), (2) proximal RTA with an acidic urine, (3) administration of extra chloride, and (4) high AG-type metabolic acidosis masquerading as hyperchloremic metabolic acidosis of renal origin (e.g., patients with hypoalbuminemia, halide poisoning, etc.).

If the urinary AG is positive, or has a small negative value (e.g., representing a low rate of ammonium excretion) in a patient with hyperchloremic metabolic acidosis, the different diagnoses include (1) distal RTA, (2) reduced ammonium production, and (3) acid gain plus urinary excretion of the conjugate base (e.g., ketoanionuria). If ammonium excretion is very low, urinary pH may be low (i.e., high in free H^+) even if the rate of distal tubular H^+ secretion is subnormal.

If ammonium is expressed in terms of milligrams per milligrams of creatinine in the urine (and the urine creatinine excretion is assumed to be $20 \text{ mg} \cdot \text{kg}^{-1} \cdot \text{d}^{-1}$), one can estimate the 24-hour ammonium excretion from data obtained from a random urine specimen.

a. Summary

The urinary AG appears to be helpful in the differential diagnosis of hyperchloremic metabolic acidosis by providing an estimation of urinary ammonium levels. Highly negative values for the urinary AG suggest an extrarenal loss of alkali. Positive values are seen in patients with impaired renal ammonium excretion and organic aciduria.

8. Venous Studies

PITFALL
In critically ill patients with a puzzling acid-base picture or poor response to therapy, one should analyze venous pH, PCO_2, and bicarbonate.

If, for some reason, it is difficult to obtain arterial blood or, if a percutaneous sample is obtained and it is not clear whether the sample is arterial or venous, central venous blood from a subclavian or pulmonary artery catheter can be used to advantage. In patients with a normal cardiac output, arterial values can usually be obtained by adding 0.05 to the central venous pH, by subtracting 6 or 7 mm Hg from the venous PCO_2, and subtracting 1.1 mEq/liter from the venous bicarbonate. However, during shock or severe heart failure, the differences between the arterial and mixed venous values may be more than three to four times normal. Under such circumstances, the arterial PCO_2 provides information on how well the lungs are working. However, the central venous, or mixed venous PCO_2, is a much better reflector of overall tissue metabolism. This impression is supported by the studies of Falk, Rackow, and Weil in cardiac arrest patients and Adrogue and associates in patients with circulatory failure.

III. METABOLIC ACIDOSIS

AXIOM
Metabolic acidosis is usually due to increased acid production or loss of bicarbonate.

A. ETIOLOGY

The causes of metabolic acidosis can be divided into two main groups: those associated with increased production of organic acids (increased anion gap metabolic acidosis) and those associated with a loss of bicarbonate or addition of chloride (normal anion gap metabolic acidosis).

Table 16.9

CAUSES OF HIGH ANION GAP METABOLIC ACIDOSIS	*Lactic Acidosis*
	Type A—decrease in tissue oxygenation
	Type B—no decrease in tissue oxygenation
	Renal Failure
	Acute
	Chronic
	Ketoacidosis
	Diabetes
	Alcoholism
	Prolonged starvation (mild acidosis)
	High-fat diet (mild acidosis)
	Ingestion of Toxic Substances
	Elevated osmolar gap
	Methanol
	Ethylene glycol
	Normal osmolar gap
	Salicylate
	Paraldehyde

1. Increased Anion Gap Metabolic Acidosis

The most frequent causes of increased production of organic acids and an increased anion gap metabolic acidosis are lactic acidosis, ketoacidosis, uremia, and drug intoxication (especially methanol, ethanol, ethylene glycol, and salicylates). Ketoacidosis may be caused by diabetes, starvation, or alcoholism (nondiabetic) (Table 16.9).

The most frequent cause of an organic acidosis in critically ill or injured patients, especially those with impaired blood flow or sepsis, is lactic acidosis. The causes of lactic acidosis, in turn, can be divided into those associated with poor tissue oxygenation (type A) and those with normal oxygenation (type B) (Table 16.6).

The immediate precursor of lactic acid is pyruvic acid. This three-carbon acid may be transformed into fat or amino acids, or it may be transported into mitochondria, where it is incorporated into the Krebs cycle after being oxidized to acetyl-CoA. Liver and kidney cortex contain enzymes that catalyze the conversion of pyruvate back to glucose (i.e., cause gluconeogenesis).

Lactic acid, in sharp contrast to its immediate precursor, pyruvic acid, represents a metabolic dead end. Its only means of metabolic transformation is through the lactic dehydrogenase (LDH) reaction, which regenerates pyruvate and at the same time converts nicotinamide-adenine dinucleotide (NAD) to its reduced form (NADH).

An important cause of lactic acidosis in patients with a heavy alcoholic intake is thiamine deficiency. The severity of the lactic acidosis in some of these individuals, who have usually stopped drinking 1 to 5 days earlier, is the reason this problem is called acute pernicious or fulminating beriberi. A similar problem can occur with TPN, if adequate thiamine is given with large amounts of glucose.

2. Normal Anion Gap (Hyperchloremic) Metabolic Acidosis

The most frequent causes of bicarbonate loss, resulting in normal anion gap (hyperchloremic) metabolic acidosis, include severe diarrhea, pancreatic fistulas, renal tubular acidosis, adrenal insufficiency, and therapy with carbonic anhydrase inhibitors, ammonium chloride, arginine hydrochloride, or amino acid hydrochlorides (as in TPN). The causes of normal anion gap metabolic acidosis can be further divided into those with normal or high serum potassium levels and those with hypokalemia (Table 16.10).

735

Table 16.10

CAUSES OF NORMAL ANION GAP METABOLIC ACIDOSIS	*With a Tendency to Normal or Elevated Potassium Levels*
	Subsiding diabetic ketoacidosis
	Early uremic acidosis
	Early obstructive uropathy
	Renal tubular acidosis—type 4
	Hypoaldosteronism (Addison's disease)
	Infusion or ingestion of HCl, NH_4Cl, lysine-HCl, and arginine-HCl
	Potassium-sparing diuretics
	With a Tendency to Hypokalemia
	Renal tubular type 1 (classical distal) acidosis and type 2 (proximal) acidosis
	Acetazolamide
	Acute diarrhea with losses of HCO_3^- and K^+
	Ureterosigmoidostomy with increased resorption of H^+ and Cl^-, and losses of HCO_3^- and K^+
	Obstruction of artificial ileal bladder
	Dilution acidosis

AXIOM

Normal anion gap metabolic acidosis due to loss of gastrointestinal fluid tends to be associated with hypokalemia.

There are three main types of RTA designated as RTA I, RTA II, and RTA IV. RTA I involves failure of the distal renal tubules to excrete acid properly, and RTA II involves wasting of bicarbonate in the proximal renal tubules. Both RTA I and RTA II tend to cause a normal anion gap metabolic acidosis with hypokalemia. RTA IV usually causes hyperkalemia. Most of the acute gastrointestinal losses of bicarbonate (diarrhea and pancreatic or small bowel fistulas) are associated with significant losses of potassium.

B. PATHOPHYSIOLOGY

1. Compensatory Changes

Any increase in the quantity of hydrogen ions in the bloodstream almost immediately results in an increase in alveolar ventilation. As a general rule, each 1.0 mEq/liter fall in bicarbonate tends to cause a relatively rapid 0.5 to 1.0 mm Hg fall in the Pco_2. Thus, if the bicarbonate falls to 14 mEq/liter, the Pco_2 would be expected to fall rapidly to about 30 to 35 mm Hg. Within 6 to 24 hours, the Pco_2 would be expected to fall about 1.0 to 1.5 mm Hg for each 1.0 mEq/liter decrease in bicarbonate. If the fall in Pco_2 after 6 to 24 hours is less than 1.0 mm Hg per 1 mEq fall in bicarbonate, respiratory compensation is inadequate. Further compensation is provided during the next several days by increased renal excretion of acid.

AXIOM

After 6 to 24 hours, the PCO_2 should fall about 1.0 to 1.5 mm Hg for each 1.0 mEq/liter decrease in bicarbonate.

2. Muscle Function

In general, mild acidosis is often associated with an increase in the strength of muscular contraction. This is known as the staircase phenomenon or treppe, in which an isolated muscle, which is rapidly and repetitively stimulated, progressively increases its strength of contraction. However, a pH of less than 7.20 to 7.25 tends to impair muscular and cardiovascular function unless there is a corresponding increase in (stimulatory) catecholamines.

3. Catecholamines and Vascular Reactivity

Acidosis increases the secretion of catecholamines, which, at mild degrees of acidosis, can offset the depressant effect of the acidosis. However, if the acidosis is very severe (pH <7.00 to 7.10), response to the catecholamines is markedly impaired.

Severe acidosis also tends to cause systemic arterial vasodilation and venous constriction, increasing the tendency to capillary stasis. Acidosis tends to cause pulmonary vasoconstriction with increased strain on the right heart as well. Beta-adrenergic receptors are particularly prone to develop rapid desensitization and uncoupling in the presence of severe lactic acidosis.

4. Oxygen Delivery and Availability

Oxygen availability to tissues is affected differently by acute and chronic metabolic acidosis. Acute acidosis shifts the oxyhemoglobin dissociation curve to the right, thereby reducing the affinity of hemoglobin for oxygen and increasing oxygen availability to tissues. However, acidosis for more than 12 to 36 hours results in impaired erythrocyte glycolysis, reducing the intraerythrocytic concentration of 2,3-diphosphoglyceric acid (2,3-DPG). This shifts the oxyhemoglobin dissociation curve to the left, reducing the release of oxygen from hemoglobin into plasma, thereby decreasing oxygen availability to tissues. Chronic acidosis may also make red blood cells more rigid, thereby reducing their flow through nutrient capillaries.

C. DIAGNOSIS

The diagnosis of metabolic acidosis is usually based on a low pH with low bicarbonate levels. Calculation of the anion gap can help determine the cause of the metabolic acidosis. Severe metabolic acidosis, regardless of its origin, tends to cause nausea, vomiting, abdominal distress, and varying degrees of CNS dysfunction.

1. Increased Anion Gap Metabolic Acidosis

The mnemonic "muksleep" is used by some students to remember the first letters of some of the more common causes of increased anion gap metabolic acidosis: methanol, uremia, ketoacidosis, salicylates, lactate, ethanol, ethylene glycol, and paraldehyde (Table 16.9). Patients examined in the emergency department can have any one of these problems. However, if the problem develops in the hospital, toxic drug ingestions are much less likely. Another mnemonic that is used is "mudpiles" in which the "i" represents iron or isoniazid. Other causes of increased anion gap include toluene, carbon monoxide, and cyanide.

a. Lactic Acidosis

In type A lactic acidosis, there is poor tissue oxygenation and perfusion. In type B, however, there is no evidence of decreased tissue perfusion, and the mechanism of the acidosis is unknown.

Patients with lactic acidosis may have nonspecific findings of nausea, vomiting, restlessness, Kussmaul respirations, and stupor or coma. The serum lactic acid level (as lactate) is elevated but usually does not account for more than a small fraction of the increased anion gap acidosis. Other laboratory abnormalities include hyperuricemia, hyperphosphatemia, and leukocytosis.

It is generally assumed that the development of metabolic acidosis during sepsis is secondary to lactic acidosis. However, Rackow and associates assessed the composition of the anion gap during severe sepsis induced by cecal perforation in rats. They found that the lactate concentration in the septic animals rose to only 2.2 ± 0.3 mEq/liter as compared to 0.9 ± 0.2 mEq/liter in the sham animals ($P<0.001$). This 1.3 mEq/liter increase in lactate accounted for only 15% of the increase in the anion gap in the septic animals. The other measured metabolic intermediates (such as pyruvate, citrate, betahydroxybutyrate, acetoacetate, anionic amino acids, and albumin) could not account for the entire anion gap as well.

An increase in unmeasured strong acids in sepsis could arise from several etiologies, including renal failure and ketoacidosis. Various organic and inorganic anions from skeletal muscle can occur as a result of septic proteolysis. Elevated purine nucleotide degradation products include uric acid and free fatty acids.

It has been obvious since Peretz and colleagues noted a direct relationship between mortality rate and increased levels of lactate in critically ill patients, that lactate is an important prognostic factor. An elevated lactate level should also make one suspect inadequate tissue perfusion in at least part of the body. Iberti and associates recently noted that hyperlactemia was associated with an increased mortality rate at all levels above normal: 100% with lactate levels ≥ 10 mmol/liter, 75% between 5.0 and 9.9 mmol/liter, and 36% between 2.5 and 4.9 mmol/liter.

Unfortunately, in the study by Iberti and associates the anion gap was an insensitive screen for picking up hyperlactemia. Although all of Iberti's patients with a lactate ≥ 10 mmol/liter had an AG ≥ 16 mmol/liter, 50% of those with lactates of 5.0 to 9.9 mmol/liter and 79% of those with lactates of 2.5 to 4.9 mmol/liter did not.

b. Ketoacidosis

Ketoacidosis can be caused by either an increase in the free fatty acid load to the liver or an increased conversion of free fatty acids to keto acids. The increased free fatty acid load may result either from stress (causing increased catecholamine-induced lipolysis) or, occasionally, from a high-fat diet. Increased conversion of fatty acids to keto acids may occur in diabetic ketoacidosis, alcoholism, or, to a lesser degree, prolonged starvation or a high-fat diet.

The most common keto acid formed is betahydroxybutyrate, followed by acetoacetate and hydroxybutyric acid. The nitroprusside test is commonly used to document the presence of ketones in serum and urine. This test is positive with increased levels of acetoacetate or acetone, but not with betahydroxybutyric acid. The more acidotic the patient, the more betahydroxybutyric acid formed from acetoacetate. Therefore, the test may reveal relatively little of the ketoacidosis present in an severely acidotic patient.

AXIOM

A negative ketone test does not rule out ketosis in a severely acidotic patient.

(1) Diabetic Ketoacidosis

The patient with diabetic ketoacidosis is usually an insulin-dependent diabetic who is out of control and has developed polydipsia, polyuria, and polyphagia. On physical examination, the patient tends to be hyperventilating, with acetone breath and an altered mental status. The laboratory definition of diabetic ketoacidosis is a serum glucose level greater than 300 mg/dl (16.7 mmol/liter), increased serum ketones, and a pH of less than 7.30.

In ketoacidosis, the retained ketoanions are betahydroxybutyrate and acetoacetate and the usual ratio of betahydroxybutyrate to acetoacetate is $3:1$ to $4:1$. Ketonuria occurs in almost all cases of diabetic ketoacidosis, but it is also common in alcoholic ketoacidosis, and it occurs in approximately 25% of patients with salicylate intoxication. With increasing acidosis, the amount of betahydroxybutyrate increases and the amount of acetoacetate decreases. Since only acetoacetate reacts with nitroprusside (the key reagent in Acetest tablets and Ketostix), the severity of the ketosis may be underestimated. This occurs typically in patients with severe acidosis from tissue hypoxia and/or lactic acidosis.

Other laboratory findings in diabetic ketoacidosis may include leukocytosis and an increased serum osmolality and osmolal gap. Serum sodium is often low, secondary to hyperglycemia. Serum potassium is often elevated because of the acidosis, in spite of total body potassium deficits of up to 10 mEq/kg body weight.

Although elevated glucose levels are considered characteristic of diabetic ketoacidosis, they can be deceptive. Modestly elevated serum glucose levels, 150 to 250 mg/dl, can occur in alcoholic ketoacidosis and salicylate intoxication. Conversely, hypoglycemia usually suggests starvation ketosis, but may also be seen in alcoholic ketoacidosis, where serum glucose levels are lower than 50 mg/dl in about 13% of patients.

AXIOM

Alcoholic ketoacidosis can be associated with high, normal, or low glucose levels, but seldom above 250 to 300 mg/dl.

Depending upon the amount of hydration and ability of the kidneys to excrete the increased keto acids in the blood, there may be a wide spectrum of acid-base patterns in diabetic ketoacidosis ranging from pure high anion gap (HAG) metabolic acidosis to pure hyperchloremic normal anion gap (NAG) metabolic acidosis. Severe dehydration tends to result in increased retention of ketones and an increased anion gap. After 4 to 8 hours of therapy with saline solution, many patients will develop a hyperchloremic (normal anion gap) acidosis because of retention of chloride in excess of sodium and excretion of ketones by the kidneys.

(2) Alcoholic Ketoacidosis

Except for alcohol, the patient with alcoholic ketoacidosis has generally not eaten for at least 24 to 36 hours. The patients tend to be dehydrated and malnourished with epigastric pain, ethanol odor, and altered mental status. The increased anion gap is usually due to betahydroxybutyrate. Laboratory studies usually reveal ketones; high, normal, or low glucose levels; elevated amylase levels; and hyperuricemia. A variable ethanol level may be present.

(3) Starvation Ketosis

The patient has a history of starvation and is usually cachectic, hypoglycemic, and ketotic. There is accelerated gluconeogenesis with depletion of liver glycogen stores, hypoinsulinemia, and lipolysis. In prolonged starvation (4 to 6 weeks), ketogenesis serves to supply ketones for the brain.

(4) High Fat Diets

A diet with a high fat content may cause a mildly elevated anion gap due to ketosis from increased betaoxidation of free fatty acids in the liver.

c. Renal Failure

In acute renal failure, the glomerular filtration rate is decreased. As a consequence, organic acids, phosphates, and sulfates (from endogenous metabolism) are retained, producing a metabolic acidosis with a high anion gap. In chronic renal failure, ammonia excretion is diminished, causing a further increase in anion gap. However, the AG in uremic acidosis is usually less than 24 mEq/liter, and there is a poor correlation between the change in AG and the change in bicarbonate.

If there is severe muscle damage, it may greatly increase the tendency to renal failure. The resulting myoglobinuric renal failure can produce a severe metabolic acidosis with a strikingly increased AG level. At least part of this acidosis is caused by the metabolism of large amounts of the sulfur-containing amino acids released from myoglobin.

d. Toxic Ingestions

Whenever one sees a patient with a severe metabolic acidosis of unknown etiology, the anion and osmolar gaps should be evaluated.

Methanol, ethylene glycol, salicylate, and paraldehyde poisoning can cause metabolic acidosis with a high anion gap. Ethylene glycol and methanol can also cause an increased osmolar gap.

(1) Methanol

Methanol is known as wood alcohol and is a clear liquid found in solvents, shellacs, and varnishes. It is sometimes ingested by alcoholics as a substitute for ethanol. The usual lethal dose is 30 ml of absolute methanol, but deaths have been reported after ingestion of as little as 6 ml. Peak methanol levels develop 30 to 60 minutes after ingestion, but there is usually a 12- to 24-hour latent period before symptoms start.

Classically, the patient with methanol poisoning describes cloudy, blurred, or misty vision. The person may see yellow spots or may develop a central scotoma or blindness, which may or may not be reversible. These symptoms are caused by formaldehyde, a metabolite, or methanol. Other symptoms include nausea, vomiting, weakness, epigastric pain, headache, dizziness, and central nervous system depression. Examination of the eyes may disclose optic disc hyperemia, edema, and decreased pupillary reaction to light.

AXIOM
A severe high anion gap metabolic acidosis with visual problems suggests a diagnosis of methanol intoxication.

Laboratory studies reveal metabolic acidosis with a high anion gap and an elevated osmolar gap. The high anion gap is mainly caused by formic acid, a metabolite of methanol.

(2) Ethylene Glycol

This odorless substance is present in antifreeze, hydraulic brake fluid, cellophane softeners, and solvents for paints and plastics. The minimal lethal dose is 1.0 to 1.5 ml/kg. Peak ethylene glycol levels are reached after 1 to 4 hours, but toxic manifestations are delayed from 4 to 12 hours.

The three stages of ethylene glycol toxicity are central nervous system injury (during the first 12 hours), respiratory depression and cardiopulmonary failure (at 12 to 24 hours), and renal failure (at 24 to 72 hours). The toxic effects of ethylene glycol poisoning are produced by metabolites of ethylene glycol, including glycoaldehydes, glycolic acid, glyoxylic acid, and oxalate. Glycolic acid and lactic acid are responsible for the high anion gap. Oxalate is the primary factor in renal toxicity.

The diagnosis of ethylene glycol poisoning is supported by a urine sediment with calcium oxalate crystals. The maximum production of oxalate occurs 8 hours after ingestion, so there may be no crystalluria if the patient presents soon after ingestion.

AXIOM
A severe high anion gap metabolic acidosis with oxalate crystals in the urine suggests ethylene glycol ingestion.

Other laboratory findings include hypocalcemia, leukocytosis, and an elevated osmolal gap. The osmolal gap may be normal if it is measured many hours after ingestion, when ethylene glycol is no longer present in the serum.

(3) Salicylates

The usual toxic dose of salicylates is 200 to 300 μg/kg, with blood levels of 500 mg/dl reported as potentially lethal. Peak levels occur 2 to 4 hours after ingestion of most preparations.

The first manifestation of salicylate poisoning includes tinnitus and hearing impairment. These symptoms occur at an average adult dose of 4.5 g/d. In mild toxicity, there might also be vomiting 3 to 8 hours after ingestion. In moderate toxicity, symptoms include severe hyperpnea and marked lethargy or excitability. Severe toxicity is frequently manifested by coma and seizures.

AXIOM
Respiratory alkalosis going on to or combining with a high anion gap metabolic acidosis suggests salicylate toxicity.

Salicylates directly stimulate the respiratory center, causing respiratory alkalosis. Later, an increased metabolic rate with the production of more carbon dioxide may result in respiratory acidosis. Eventually, the direct toxic effect on carbohydrate metabolism produces the classic high anion gap metabolic acidosis.

(4) Paraldehyde

This sedative and antiseizure medication is rarely used now. The average minimal lethal blood level is approximately 500 $\mu g/ml$. Manifestations of toxicity include gastritis, renal failure, fatty changes in the liver, pulmonary hemorrhages, edema, and congestive heart failure. These patients tend to have a mild-to-moderate dehydration, hypotension, and Kussmaul respirations. The characteristic offensive odor is usually the obvious clue to diagnosis.

The elevated anion gap with paraldehyde ingestion is caused by acetic acid and chloracetic acid. Diagnosis is made by detection of paraldehyde in the serum and acetaldehyde in the urine and blood. When a nitroprusside reaction test is used, paraldehyde may cause a false-positive reaction for ketones called *pseudoketosis*.

(5) Other Substances

Severe intoxication with lithium or magnesium reduces the anion gap by increasing the level of unmeasured cation.

2. Rapid Laboratory Evaluation of Patients with High Anion Gap Metabolic Acidosis

A urine dipstick test that is positive for both ketones and glucose rapidly confirms diabetic ketoacidosis. If the test is negative for glucose, alcoholic or starvation ketoacidosis should be considered. If there is a history of paraldehyde ingestion, and/or the urine contains acetaldehyde, paraldehyde poisoning is possible, and the finding of ketonuria may represent a false-positive reaction.

If the urine dipstick test is negative for ketones, the serum osmolality should be tested to determine whether there is an elevated osmolar gap. Causes of a high osmolar gap include ethylene glycol and methanol poisoning and diabetic ketoacidosis. If calcium oxalate crystals are found in the urine, ethylene glycol poisoning should be suspected. If there is a history of visual impairment, or an abnormal funduscopic examination, methanol poisoning is the most likely cause.

When the osmolar gap is normal, the urine should be tested with ferric chloride. If a purple color develops, salicylate poisoning should be considered, although it is important to remember that the test is very sensitive and may be positive with only modest amounts of salicylates.

Renal failure is diagnosed when blood urea nitrogen and creatinine levels are elevated. Lactic acidosis is confirmed by elevated lactic acid levels. If there is no renal failure or drug intoxication, an increased anion gap is usually due to ketoacidosis or lactate accumulation. In patients without uremia, drug intoxication, or diabetic ketoacidosis, an increased anion gap is usually due to lactate accumulation.

An anion gap of 30 mEq/liter or more usually indicates an organic (lactic or keto) acidosis, even in the presence of uremia. With anion gaps of 20 to 29 mEq/liter, 60% to 75% of patients will have an organic acidosis. Of those with no identified organic acidosis, changes in total proteins, phosphate, potassium, or calcium will account for about 50% of the increased anion gap.

According to Gabow and colleagues, if the anion gap exceeds 0.5 times the serum bicarbonate concentration plus 16.0, the diagnosis of an organic acidosis is justified. Thus, a patient with a bicarbonate of 6 mEq/liter and an anion gap of 22 mEq/liter probably has an organic acidosis, because the Gabow factor $(HCO_3^- \times 0.5) + 16 = (0.5)(6) + 16 = 3 + 16 = 19$, which is less than the anion gap of 22. On the other hand, if the bicarbonate is 18 mEq/liter and the AG is still 22 mEq/liter, the Gabow factor will be $(18)(0.5) + 16 = 9 + 16 = 25$. Since this is more than the anion gap of 22, the cause of the anion gap is probably not an organic acidosis.

3. Normal Anion Gap Metabolic Acidosis

Normal anion gap metabolic acidosis is caused primarily by a loss of bicarbonate, with little or no increase in organic acids. A mnemonic for the causes of NAG-MAc is USED CARP. These include ureteroenterostomy, small bowel fistulas, extra chloride (such as in NH_4Cl or amino acid hydrochlorides), diarrhea, carbonic anhydrase inhibitors (Diamox and Sulfamylon), adrenal insufficiency, renal tubular acidosis, and pancreatic fistula. These and other causes of NAG-MAc can be subdivided into those that tend to cause hyperkalemia and those that cause hypokalemia (Table 16.10).

In most of these problems, a careful history and routine laboratory studies should clarify the cause.

D. Treatment

The treatment of metabolic acidosis, should be directed at (1) improvement of tissue perfusion and ventilation, (2) correction of the underlying problem, and (3) administration of sodium bicarbonate, if needed.

1. Improved Tissue Perfusion and Ventilation

Almost every type of metabolic acidosis will be improved by restoration of an adequate or increased blood volume, cardiac output, and tissue oxygenation. If there is any problem with ventilation, so that the respiratory compensation is inadequate, early ventilatory assistance should be strongly considered.

2. Correction of the Primary Process

As the patient is being resuscitated, a strong effort should be made to determine the primary process causing the metabolic acidosis and to correct it. An adequate fluid resuscitation should correct most shock, but inotropes may occasionally be required. Sepsis may require eradication of the focus of infection plus antibiotics. For diabetic ketoacidosis, insulin and, later, glucose and potassium will be needed.

Treatment of toxic ingestions may require specific therapy. The treatment of severe methanol poisoning is administration of enteral or parenteral ethanol, because alcohol dehydrogenase (the enzyme that metabolizes ethanol, ethylene glycol, and methanol) has a significantly greater affinity for ethanol than for the other alcohols. Ethanol levels should be maintained at approximately 100 mg/dl. Hemodialysis is often required if the methanol blood concentration is greater than 50 mg/dl.

Ethylene glycol poisoning is treated with supportive measures (e.g., respiratory support) and administration of ethanol. If ethylene glycol levels exceed 50 mg/dl, or if renal failure is present, hemodialysis is indicated. Some authors also recommend thiamine, 100 mg IM, and pyridoxine, 100 mg IV or IM.

Therapy for salicylate poisoning consists initially of emesis with syrup of ipecac or, in a comatose patient, gastric lavage coupled with activated charcoal. Increasingly, it appears that activated charcoal may be most effective. Salicylate excretion may be enhanced through alkalinization of the urine with or without concomitant diuresis. For severe poisoning (salicylate levels greater than 100 mg/dl), hemodialysis is indicated.

Treatment of paraldehyde poisoning includes lavage, activated charcoal, and supportive measures. Emesis should not be promoted, since paraldehyde is locally corrosive to the gastrointestinal tract and is rapidly absorbed.

3. Bicarbonate Therapy

If a severe metabolic acidosis persists after maximal efforts to improve tissue perfusion with fluid, inotropics, and vasodilators, as needed, sodium bicarbonate therapy to raise the pH from less than 7.10 to at least 7.20 to 7.25 should be considered. Sodium bicarbonate should probably also be given if the arterial bicarbonate falls below 5.0 mEq/liter, because any additional decrease in bicarbonate could cause a precipitous fall in pH.

If the patient is not in severe shock, bicarbonate can be given at about 2.5 mEq/min. The amount of bicarbonate given should not exceed 1.0 mEq/kg at a time or raise the pH to more than 7.25 to 7.30 to prevent alkaline overshoot. For each 0.1 pH rise, oxygen availability to tissue drops by about 10% because of the shift of the oxyhemoglobin dissociation curve to the left. Giving bicarbonate to patients with hypoxemia due to pulmonary dysfunction or a right-to-left cardiopulmonary shunt may rapidly lower the arterial Pco_2 to dangerous levels. In patients with severe diabetic ketoacidosis, rapid bicarbonate administration can cause severe CNS changes.

Bicarbonate deficits are usually calculated using 30% to 50% of the body weight as the bicarbonate space. In patients with bicarbonate deficits of less than 10 mEq/liter, calculations using 30% of the body weight as the bicarbonate space seem to provide adequate correction. For moderate bicarbonate deficits of 10 to 15 mEq/liter, 40% of the body weight can be used as the bicarbonate space. However, in patients with severe acidosis with base deficits exceeding 15 mEq/liter, the bicarbonate space involves almost the entire total body water and should be considered to be equal to 50% of the body weight.

Thus, in an acutely ill 80-kg man with a bicarbonate concentration of 10 mEq/liter (i.e., a deficit of 14 mEq/liter), one can assume a bicarbonate space of 40%, or 32 liters. As a consequence, he would have a total bicarbonate deficit of (80 kg $\times$ 40%) $\times$ 14 mEq/liter = 448 mEq. However, we correct only half the deficit initially and administer only about 1.0 mEq/kg over a 30-minute period. The rest of the bicarbonate is given much more slowly and is guided by frequent ABG analyses. If the patient is hemodynamically unstable, more rapid infusion of bicarbonate might be desirable.

PITFALL
Routine use of bicarbonate during CPR without following arterial (and mixed venous) blood gases.

The American Heart Association now urges restraint in the use of sodium bicarbonate during cardiopulmonary resuscitation. Experimentally, HCO_3^- administered to correct severe hypoxic lactic acidosis actually increases lactate production. Part of the difficulty may be related to the fact that carbon dioxide (elaborated by the reaction of H^+ and bicarbonate) diffuses rapidly across cell membranes, creating intracellular acidosis while the extracellular acidosis is decreasing. If the patient cannot excrete the carbon dioxide produced by the bicarbonate, an increasing respiratory acidosis may occur.

If the arterial Pco_2 is normal or low but the venous Pco_2 is very high, as it can be in patients with cardiac arrest or a very low cardiac output, the administration of bicarbonate for low levels of bicarbonate is controversial. If the venous Pco_2 is high, bicarbonate may cause a paradoxic acidosis in brain and other tissues. The increased carbon dioxide generated by the bicarbonate rapidly crosses the blood-brain barrier, while the bicarbonate crosses the blood-brain barrier very slowly. The increased cerebrospinal fluid carbon dioxide generates carbonic acid, which causes a cerebrospinal fluid acidosis in spite of an increasing alkalemia.

Nevertheless, Bleich, in an editorial, and Narius and Cohen, in an important paper, feel that if the arterial bicarbonate is less than 10.0 mEq/liter, it is reasonable to give 100 to 150 mEq of bicarbonate to "stop the next flood of lactic acid from bankrupting the body's bicarbonate stores."

4. New Directions

Kearns and Wolfson have called attention to dichloroacetate and carbicarb as two new approaches to the treatment of metabolic acidosis. The proposed mechanism of action of dichloroacetate (DCA) is stimulation of pyruvate dehydrogenase, the rate-limiting enzyme in the oxidation of pyruvate and lactate. DCA has been used by Stacpoole in human trials, with significant improvement in serum lactate, pH, and bicarbonate levels. However, outcome was not significantly improved.

Carbicarb is a mixture of sodium carbonate and sodium bicarbonate (Na_2CO_3/$NaHCO_3$), which buffers hydrogen ion without the net generation of carbon dioxide. Hydrogen ion is buffered preferentially by Na_2CO_3, producing additional bicarbonate ion. When excess carbon dioxide accumulates, or is generated, carbonic acid is formed. This dissociates into H^+ and HCO_3^-, and the hydrogen ion combines with sodium carbonate to form additional bicarbonate. Thus, carbicarb not only buffers excess hydrogen ion but consumes carbon dioxide to yield more bicarbonate buffer, and it offers a means of avoiding the increase in tissue Pco_2 that is thought to be a deleterious effect of the use of bicarbonate. It would be a particular advantage in patients with inadequate ventilation or very poor tissue perfusion.

IV. METABOLIC ALKALOSIS

A. ETIOLOGY

AXIOM

The two most frequent causes of metabolic alkalosis are excessive diuresis (with loss of potassium, hydrogen, and chloride) and excessive loss of gastric secretions (with loss of hydrogen and chloride).

1. Loss of Gastric Acid

Normally the stomach makes 2 to 5 mEq of free acid per hour. This may be increased twofold to fourfold in patients with an active duodenal ulcer. Thus, a patient who is vomiting large amounts of acid, because of pyloric stenosis from duodenal ulcer disease, is particularly apt to develop a severe metabolic alkalosis. Removal of large amounts of gastric acid with a nasogastric tube may also produce the same effect.

2. Excessive Diuresis

Hypokalemia due to diuresis with excessive loss of potassium in the urine is probably the most common cause of metabolic alkalosis. Since potassium loss in urine averages 30 to 60 mEq/liter, use of diuretics can easily produce a severe hypokalemia, along with an excessive loss of chloride. Potassium will tend to come out of tissue cells to correct the hypokalemia, and hydrogen ions will tend to go back into the cells, causing an alkalemia. In addition, the kidney will tend to excrete hydrogen ions to conserve potassium. Diarrhea or excessive colostomy or ileostomy drainage may contain more than 25 to 50 mEq of potassium per liter and may also cause severe hypokalemia.

PITFALL

Failure to appreciate the amount of potassium and bicarbonate that can be lost with diarrhea.

3. Mineralocorticoids

Mineralocorticoids tend to cause metabolic alkalosis by promoting the renal absorption of bicarbonate and sodium and by increasing the excretion of potassium, hydrogen, and chloride ions. Hypokalemia can produce a vicious cycle, because the depletion of potassium causes even more excretion of hydrogen ions, which aggravates the metabolic alkalosis. Reabsorption of potassium appears to be independent of aldosterone, but an aldosterone deficiency markedly reduces the ability of the distal tubule to secrete hydrogen ions and reabsorb bicarbonate.

AXIOM
Hypokalemia increases the tendency to metabolic alkalosis; the reverse is also true.

4. Increased Intake of Citrate or Lactate

AXIOM
Patients receiving massive blood transfusions and large amounts of Ringer's lactate will tend to become alkalotic over the next 12 to 48 hours.

Massive transfusions of bank blood can greatly increase the quantity of citrate in the body (17 mEq from each unit of whole blood and 5 mEq from each unit of packed red blood cells). As this citrate is metabolized over the next 24 to 48 hours, plasma bicarbonate levels rise proportionally, producing an increasing alkalosis. Ringer's lactate has a pH of about 5.5. However, after it is given, about half of it (L-lactate) is metabolized in the liver into bicarbonate, which tends to cause a metabolic alkalosis. The D-lactate is excreted unchanged in the urine.

5. Antacids

Clinicians often attempt to prevent stress gastric ulceration and bleeding in critically ill patients by maintaining a pH inside the stomach of 5.0 or higher with antacids and/or hydrogen-receptor antagonists, such as cimetidine. In some instances, large quantities of antacid are required. Absorption of these antacids and/or removal of the excess acid that they neutralize may significantly contribute to a metabolic alkalosis.

6. Dehydration

PITFALL
One should not attempt to correct a severe metabolic alkalosis without first correcting any coexistent dehydration.

Dehydration that is not severe enough to interfere with tissue perfusion may cause a "contraction alkalosis," because sodium and bicarbonate absorption in the kidney is increased. However, if the extracellular fluid is expanded, sodium and bicarbonate reabsorption in the kidney is reduced, and this may cause a "dilution acidosis."

Since the kidney is the organ responsible for excreting excess bicarbonate when the plasma concentration is high, renal failure may make it very difficult to eliminate bicarbonate. However, if the renal failure is only mild to moderate, the ability to excrete bicarbonate is still relatively well preserved.

7. Excretion of Nonresorbable Anions

The newer synthetic penicillins, such as ticarcillin, when excreted into the tubular lumen, have a negative charge and are not resorbed. This causes an increased loss of hydrogen ions in the urine. Increased excretion of phosphates may cause a similar problem.

8. Posthypercapnia

After a period of respiratory acidosis, a compensatory rise in bicarbonate will tend to occur until the arterial pH is about 7.35. For example, with a chronic Pco_2 of 60 to 70 mm Hg, the arterial bicarbonate will tend to rise to levels of 32 to 37 mEq/liter, respectively. Even after the hypercapnia has been corrected, the bicarbonate levels will remain elevated for some time.

9. Severe Hypoproteinemia

To maintain electrical neutrality, a fall in serum proteins, especially albumin, tends to cause a rise in bicarbonate. A fall in albumin levels from 4.5 g/dl to 1.5 g/dl can cause serum bicarbonate levels to rise by up to 9.6 mEq/liter.

AXIOM

Hypoalbuminemia tends to increase plasma bicarbonate levels.

10. Other Problems

Other situations that tend to maintain high serum bicarbonate concentrations include hypokalemia, hypercarbia, and secondary hypoparathyroidism. Chloride deficiency is often listed as a cause of persistently high plasma bicarbonate levels, but chloride deficiency will only raise the renal bicarbonate threshold if it is accompanied by a reduced effective arterial volume. Resistant metabolic alkalosis may also be seen with secondary hypoparathyroidism, milk-alkali syndrome, or malignancy-induced hypercalcemia.

B. PHYSIOLOGIC EFFECTS

Although alkalosis tends to inhibit sympathetic nervous system activity and decrease adrenergic effects, it also tends to increase endogenous catecholamine release and accentuate adrenergic vasodilator effects.

Metabolic alkalosis reduces the amount of potassium in the blood by about 0.5 mEq/liter for each 0.10 rise in pH. Ionized calcium and magnesium levels in the plasma also fall, about 4% to 8% for each 0.1-pH rise. This tends to increase neuromuscular irritability and may impair cardiovascular function, particularly if plasma ionized calcium levels fall below 1.6 to 1.7 mEq/liter. The alkalosis also reduces oxygen availability by about 10% for each 0.1-pH rise. Alkalosis may also cause tachyarrhythmias, probably due to potassium and/or calcium changes. The hypokalemia that develops secondary to an alkalosis may also interfere with muscle function, causing weakness and/or ileus.

AXIOM

Failure to compensate adequately for a metabolic alkalosis may be the first indication of an occult hypoxemia.

The usual pulmonary compensation for a metabolic alkalosis is hypoventilation with slow, shallow breathing. As the Pco_2 rises because of hypoventilation, the Po_2 falls, but the chemoreceptors will usually not allow the arterial Po_2 to fall much below 60 mm Hg. Thus, the $Paco_2$ will not usually rise above 50 to 55 mm Hg unless the associated hypoxemia is corrected by giving oxygen.

With alkalosis, there is usually some degree of cerebral dysfunction. Blood ammonia levels tend to rise in metabolic alkalosis, and this may be part of the cause of the CNS changes.

PITFALL

One should probably not allow patients to remain severely alkalotic, even if they appear to be doing well otherwise.

If there is a combined metabolic and respiratory alkalosis, the arterial pH can rise rapidly to above 7.55. In a study at Detroit General Hospital, we found that the mortality rate of critically ill or injured patients was increased significantly if their arterial pH rose above 7.55. Almost all patients maintaining an arterial pH above 7.70 died.

C. DIAGNOSIS

The diagnosis of a metabolic alkalosis is made from laboratory studies revealing a bicarbonate level exceeding 26 mEq/liter and a pH above 7.45. In most instances, there is also an associated hypokalemia and hypochloremia. Clinically, metabolic alkalosis is characterized by slow, shallow respiration (in contrast to the hyperventilation generally seen with metabolic acidosis). Determining the cause of the alkalosis can be facilitated by determining if urine chloride levels are above 20 mEq/liter or below 10 mEq/liter.

The causes of metabolic alkalosis are often divided into those causing "saline-responsive alkalosis" and those causing "saline-resistant alkalosis." Saline-responsive alkalosis is characterized by low urine chloride levels

Table 16.11

CHLORIDE-RESPONSIVE AND CHLORIDE-RESISTANT METABOLIC ALKALOSIS	Chloride Responsive*	Chloride Resistant
	Loop diuretics	Exogenous corticosteroids, including licorice
	Pyloric stenosis†	Increased endogenous corticosteroids
	Excess nasogastric suction†	Cushing's syndrome
	Excess antacids	Hyperaldosteronism
	Posthypercapnia	Adrenal cortical lesions
		Cirrhosis
		Bartter's syndrome
		Liddle's syndrome

*Urine chloride <10 mEq/L.
†Assuming normal gastric acidity.

($<$10 mEq/liter) and will usually respond well to saline. In saline-resistant alkalosis, urine chloride levels exceed 20 mEq/liter and there is a poor response to saline alone.

Saline-resistant alkalosis is most frequently caused by increased endogenous or exogenous adrenal corticosteroids, or severe hypokalemia. Bartter's syndrome (hypertrophy and hyperplasia of the cells of the juxtaglomerular apparatus) and Liddle's syndrome (pseudohyperaldosteronism with a clinical picture of hyperaldosteronism, but normal aldosterone secretion) are interesting examples of saline unresponsive alkaloses (Table 16.11).

D. TREATMENT

Chloride-responsive alkalosis, such as that caused by vomiting or excessive nasogastric suction, usually responds adequately to administration of fluid and chloride. If the patient is adequately hydrated, the chloride deficit can be calculated on the basis of 20% of the body weight. Thus, if the patient weighs 80 kg and has a serum chloride of 60 mEq/liter, the chloride deficit can be calculated as $(20\%)(80kg)(100 - 60$ mEq/liter$) = 640$ mEq/liter. If the patient is severely dehydrated, one can use 60% of the body weight to calculate the chloride deficit.

Half the chloride deficit is corrected over a period of 4 to 12 hours. Approximately one fourth of the chloride is given as potassium chloride and three fourths as sodium chloride. Normally, the potassium is not given faster than 15 mEq/h and is not given if serum potassium levels exceed 5.0 mEq/liter.

If the patient is hypokalemic, the kidneys tend to excrete H^+ and retain HCO_3^-, and this may result in a paradoxical aciduria (excretion of acid urine in the presence of an alkalemia). If adequate chloride is administered to patients with a chloride-responsive alkalosis, the increased chloride in the glomerular filtrate allows increased sodium absorption in the proximal tubule. As less sodium is presented to the distal tubule, less H^+ is excreted, less HCO_3^- is absorbed, and the metabolic alkalosis begins to resolve.

Chloride-resistant alkalosis is usually not associated with hypovolemia. Consequently, relatively large quantities of Na^+ and Cl^- are filtered, and increased H^+ and K^+ are excreted as the Na^+ is reabsorbed in the distal tubule. These patients may require very large quantities of potassium to correct the alkalosis.

If the alkalosis is severe (the carbon dioxide content exceeds 40 mEq/liter, the pH exceeds 7.55, or the patient has tetany), one half of the chloride deficit is given as sodium chloride, one fourth as potassium chloride, and one fourth as some type of hydrochloride (NH_4Cl, arginine hydrochloride, or 0.1 N hydrochloric acid). Theoretically, ammonium chloride should be helpful, but many of these patients have renal or hepatic problems that increase the risk of giving ammonium compounds. Arginine hydrochloride may be helpful with hepatic insufficiency but is contraindicated in severe renal dysfunction. Interestingly, some investigators feel that these chlorides may acidify the ECF but not the cells, and are therefore not really very helpful.

If hydrochloric acid (0.10 N) is used, it must be given cautiously by slow infusion into a large vein at approximately 25 to 50 ml/h. The hydrochloric acid can be administered with amino acids to provide a higher pH and "gentler" solution than hydrochloride alone.

In some instances, Diamox (acetazolamide), which inhibits carbonic anhydrase and thereby increases renal bicarbonate excretion, may be given by mouth, or through a nasogastric tube, to correct a mild-to-moderate metabolic alkalosis.

V. RESPIRATORY ALKALOSIS

A. ETIOLOGY

In stressful situations, such as shock, sepsis, or trauma, there is a tendency to hyperventilate and develop respiratory alkalosis with a Pco_2 of 25 to 35 mm Hg, or less. If hypoxia or metabolic acidosis develops, the tendency to hyperventilation is increased even further.

B. PHYSIOLOGIC EFFECTS

AXIOM
Severe respiratory alkalosis tends to perpetuate itself because it causes cerebral vasoconstriction and CSF acidosis.

Severe respiratory alkalosis tends to perpetuate itself. If the $Paco_2$ falls, cerebral vasoconstriction occurs. In fact, each 1.0 mm Hg drop in the arterial Pco_2 reduces cerebral blood flow by about 2% to 4%. Thus, a severe respiratory alkalosis, especially if the Pco_2 is less than 20 mm Hg, can reduce cerebral blood flow enough to cause cerebral metabolic acidosis. This cerebral metabolic acidosis will then cause the respiratory center to increase ventilation even more, producing a progressively more severe respiratory alkalosis.

The initial response to hypocapnia is a shift of hydrogen chloride and lactate ions out of the cell. In severe respiratory alkalosis, lactic acid levels may increase by 2.0 to 3.0 mmol/liter. This buffering is rapid and may be complete within 15 minutes of the initiation of the hypocapnia. The renal compensation will also begin to take effect within 2 to 4 hours after the onset of hypocapnia.

AXIOM
In spite of an increased Po_2, respiratory alkalosis may actually reduce oxygen availability to tissues.

Alkalosis shifts the oxyhemoglobin dissociation curve to the left, causing hemoglobin to hold oxygen more tightly. Each 0.10-pH rise lowers the Po_2 about 10% and reduces oxygen availability to tissues by about 10% for each pH increase of 0.10.

C. DIAGNOSIS

Respiratory alkalosis is diagnosed by a rise in pH above 7.40 and a decrease in $Paco_2$ below 35 mm Hg. Occasionally, it may be difficult to differentiate hyperventilation of psychogenic origin from compensatory hyperventilation or hyperventilation due to sepsis or pulmonary emboli. In such patients, careful continued observation of the patient and the blood gases is essential. It should be remembered that the Pao_2 may be 80 mm Hg or higher in 12% of the patients with proven pulmonary emboli. Although the Po_2 may be relatively normal initially, with continued sepsis, the Po_2 will eventually fall.

D. TREATMENT

PITFALL
Attempting to correct respiratory alkalosis without first ruling out hypoxia, pulmonary embolism, and sepsis.

The treatment of respiratory alkalosis is correction of the primary problem, and, in particular, one must look for underlying hypoxia, pulmonary embolism, and sepsis. If the problem is hysterical hyperventilation, treatment is best accomplished by having the patient rebreathe his or her expired air, which has a P_{CO_2} about two thirds that in arterial blood. Not infrequently, the most convenient rebreathing device is a paper bag. Once the P_{CO_2} begins to rise toward normal, the cerebral blood flow usually improves enough to correct the intracerebral acidosis and return the pattern of ventilation toward normal.

In critically ill patients who have severe respiratory alkalosis (P_{CO_2} less than 20 to 25 mm Hg and pH more than 7.55 to 7.60) and are not on a ventilator, sedation may be given, but very cautiously. One must be sure that patients do not reduce their ventilation to the point of developing hypoxia.

If patients are on ventilators, they may be placed on intermittent mandatory ventilation (IMV). While on IMV, the respirator rate may be progressively reduced as long as (1) the P_{CO_2} does not exceed 45 mm Hg, (2) the pH is not below 7.35, and (3) the patient's respiratory rate is less than 30 per minute.

VI. RESPIRATORY ACIDOSIS

A. ETIOLOGY

A P_{CO_2} elevated above 45 mm Hg is usually caused by inadequate minute ventilation and/or increased dead space. However, increased carbohydrate metabolism may contribute to hypercarbia if pulmonary function is marginal. This is most apt to occur in patients who are on a ventilator and are receiving three or more liters of 20% to 25% IV glucose per day. Fever can also increase carbon dioxide production about 13% for each 1°C rise in temperature.

Inadequate minute ventilation is most frequently due to head trauma, pulmonary disease, or excess sedation. The chronic hypoventilation seen in extremely obese patients is often referred to as the Pickwickian syndrome, because of reference to such an individual (fat boy Joe) in Charles Dicken's *Pickwick Papers*. Patients with severe chronic obstructive pulmonary disease (COPD) have increased dead space and frequently have a decreased minute ventilation.

In general, a rise in the P_{CO_2} stimulates the respiratory center to increase respiratory rate and minute ventilation. Rebuck and Slutsky have found that ventilation normally increases about 1.0 to 4.0 liters/min for each 1.0-mm Hg increase in the P_{CO_2}. The average response to hypoxemia is a 0.6 to 2.8 liters/min increase in ventilation for each 1% decrease in arterial oxygen saturation. However, if the arterial P_{CO_2} chronically exceeds 60 to 70 mm Hg, as may occur in up to 5% to 10% of patients with severe emphysema, the respiratory acidosis may depress the respiratory center. Under such circumstances, the stimulus for ventilation is provided primarily by hypoxemia acting on chemoreceptors in the carotid and aortic bodies. Giving the patient oxygen could take away the main stimulus the patient has to breathe, causing the P_{CO_2} to rise abruptly to extremely dangerous levels.

PITFALL

One should not administer oxygen to patients with COPD without carefully watching for the development of apnea or hypoventilation.

B. PATHOPHYSIOLOGY

Multiple consequences of hypercapnia involving the ventilatory system, kidneys, CNS, and cardiovascular system have been described. With a sudden severe decrease in minute ventilation, the P_{CO_2} rises rapidly and the pH may fall abruptly because bicarbonate compensation by the kidney is very slow. In completely apneic patients, the Pa_{CO_2} rises by about 2.0 to 3.0 mm Hg/min. A rapid increase of the Pa_{CO_2} to 60 mm Hg can cause the pH to fall to about 7.22. However, over the next few hours or days, a rise in bicarbonate will gradually restore the pH to about 7.30 to 7.32. After several days, the bicarbonate usually rises enough to raise the pH to 7.33 to 7.35. A high bicarbonate level in an ambulatory patient should make one suspicious of chronic respiratory acidosis.

Neurologic signs or symptoms usually accompany acute, severe respiratory acidosis. The risk of brain acidemia is higher in respiratory acidosis than in metabolic acidosis. Carbon dioxide penetrates lipid structures, such as the blood-brain barrier, very readily, and can markedly decrease the pH of the brain. Bicarbonate, which is water soluble, penetrates much more slowly. Coma can occur at a P_{CO_2} exceeding 65 to 70 mm Hg; however, if the respiratory acidosis develops very slowly, it may not develop until the P_{CO_2} exceeds 100 to 110 mm Hg.

C. DIAGNOSIS

Respiratory acidosis, by definition, is present when the Pa_{CO_2} exceeds 45 mm Hg and the pH is 7.39 or less. If the pH is less than 7.30, the respiratory acidosis is usually acute or there is a superimposed metabolic acidosis. If the carbon dioxide content of an electrolyte study is high, one should suspect chronic respiratory acidosis or metabolic alkalosis. If the chloride and potassium levels are normal or high, the patient is likely to have respiratory acidosis. In contrast, metabolic alkalosis is usually associated with hypokalemia and hypochloremia.

AXIOM

In a mixed acid-base picture, hypocalcemia tends to indicate that the primary process is a metabolic alkalosis and not a respiratory acidosis.

D. TREATMENT

Treatment of respiratory acidosis is primarily designed to improve alveolar ventilation. In general, if the minute ventilation is doubled, the P_{CO_2} will be reduced by 50%. In patients with COPD, various bronchodilators (such as aminophylline, metaproterenol [Alupent], and albuterol [Ventolin]), together with careful administration of small amounts of oxygen, may substantially improve ventilation. However, ventilatory assistance may be required in some patients who do not respond adequately to lesser measures, particularly if the pH falls below 7.20 to 7.25. Unfortunately, it may be extremely difficult to extubate such patients later.

In patients with a chronic respiratory acidosis, reduction of the P_{CO_2} should generally proceed slowly. The minute ventilation for a 70-kg man is normally about 6 liters/min, and in COPD patients it may be less than 4 liters/min. In a patient with COPD and severe hypercarbia, it may be wise to start treatment with a minute ventilation of about 5 liters/min and then gradually increase it according to the clinical response and changes in P_{CO_2}.

PITFALL

Reducing the P_{CO_2} of a chronic respiratory acidosis faster than 5 mm Hg/h can cause sudden development of a severe combined metabolic and respiratory alkalosis with resulting arrhythmias.

A rapid rise in pH can cause an abrupt fall in ionized calcium. The resulting ionic hypocalcemia can then cause dangerous arrhythmias or seizures.

More recently, the problems with ventilation in malnourished individuals has been explored in depth. Increased carbohydrate metabolism increases carbon dioxide production and can cause a respiratory acidosis. On the other hand, administration of adequate amounts of glucose may enable previously exhausted subjects to continue work. In malnourished individuals, increased protein intake can also gradually increase muscle mass and improve the maximal ventilatory response.

SUMMARY POINTS

1. The acidity of a solution is equal to the ratio of the activities of the acid to its corresponding base multiplied by its dissociation constant.
2. If the ratio of bicarbonate to carbonic acid is doubled or reduced by half, the pH changes by 0.3.
3. Normal intracellular pH (pH_i) is about 7.00 to 7.10.
4. The initial mechanisms for handling an acid load intracellularly include (a) physicochemical buffering, (b) cellular consumption of nonvolatile acids, and (c) the transfer of acid or alkali between the cytosol and organelles.
5. Normally the body excretes 12,000 to 20,000 mEq of acid as carbon dioxide from the lungs and 70 mEq of nonvolatile acid from the kidneys each day.
6. The normal daily renal excretion of acid includes 0.1 mEq of free acid, 20 to 30 mEq of NaH_2PO_4, and 40 to 50 mEq of NH_4^+.
7. In severe metabolic acidosis, renal excretion of acid may rise to about 300 to 400 mEq/d.
8. Dehydration (without shock) increases sodium and bicarbonate absorption in the kidney and tends to cause a metabolic alkalosis.
9. Hypokalemia is the most frequent cause of excretion of an alkaline urine in an acidotic patient.
10. About 99.99% of an acid load in the ECF is buffered or combined with other compounds to prevent sudden pH changes.
11. Most of the body's buffer systems are designed to neutralize acid, not alkali.
12. As a general rule, the lower the pH, the greater the base deficit, even if bicarbonate levels are held constant.
13. Plasma proteins should be measured as part of the evaluation of acid-base status.
14. One should not accept laboratory reports of a venous carbon dioxide content lower than the arterial bicarbonate.
15. In mild-to-moderate acidosis, an acute 1.0-mm Hg rise in PCO_2 without a change in HCO_3^- reduces pH by 0.01. An acute fall in HCO_3^- of 1.0 mEq/liter without a change in PCO_2 reduces pH by 0.02.
16. If the pH is relatively normal but the PCO_2 and bicarbonate are abnormal, one can assume that a mixed acid-base disorder is present.
17. The PCO_2 seldom rises above 50 to 55 mm Hg to compensate for a metabolic alkalosis unless oxygen is given.
18. Inability to compensate for an acid-base abnormality usually means a severe disturbance of ventilatory, renal, or other cellular functions.
19. As a compensatory response to respiratory alkalosis, bicarbonate seldom falls below 18.0 mEq/liter, acutely, or 15.0 mEq/liter, chronically.
20. Inability to at least partially compensate for an acid-base abnormality usually means a severe disturbance of ventilatory, renal, or general cellular function.
21. Anion gap (AG) in blood = $Na^+ - (Cl^- + CO_2)$ and is normally 12 mEq/liter.
22. Although the anion gap can help diagnose an acid-base abnormality, changes in the anion gap are usually more informative than isolated anion gap levels.
23. Drawing arterial blood gases into syringes with too much heparin will tend to cause an erroneous acidosis.
24. The most severe high anion gap metabolic acidoses are seen with ingestions (methanol or ethylene glycol), lactic acidosis (severe shock or cardiac arrest), or hyperglycemia coma.
25. One should not assume that all lactic acidosis is due to inadequate tissue oxygenation.
26. With any tendency to lactic acidosis, other, often unidentifiable, organic acids will also increase and usually to a much greater extent.

27. A tendency to ketoacidosis will be less apparent in patients with a good urine output.
28. Although there may be great variations in unmeasured anions, the levels of unmeasured cations are quite constant.
29. Since alkalosis itself can cause an increased anion gap, the value of this parameter in diagnosing mixed acid-base disorders decreases as the pH rises above normal.
30. In combined metabolic and respiratory alkalosis, one can estimate the metabolic component by adding the increase in anion gap to the bicarbonate levels.
31. Hypoalbuminemia is probably the most common cause of a decreased anion gap in hospitalized patients.
32. One should not assume that reported laboratory values are always accurate.
33. Severe dehydration associated with hypernatremia can cause falsely low serum sodium levels and can decrease anion gap.
34. Bromide and iodide ingestions lower anion gap.
35. Calculation of the urine anion gap helps one to determine if ammonium production is adequate in patients with an acidemia.
36. Simultaneous analysis of arterial and venous pH, PCO_2, and bicarbonate in critically ill patients allows one to evaluate pulmonary function and cardiac output to some extent.
37. Metabolic acidosis is usually due to increased acid production or loss of bicarbonate.
38. Normal anion gap metabolic acidosis is usually due to loss of gastrointestinal fluid and tends to be associated with hypokalemia.
39. One should raise the pH to 7.20, or higher, if a shock patient has a poor response to catecholamines.
40. One should not assume that a 90% to 95% arterial oxyhemoglobin saturation indicates that adequate oxygen is available to the tissues.
41. The more common causes of high anion gap metabolic acidosis (HAG-MAc) include lactic acidosis, ketoacidosis, renal failure, and toxic ingestions (especially ethanol, methanol, salicylates, and paraldehyde).
42. The more common causes of a normal anion gap metabolic acidosis include ureteroenterostomy, small bowel or pancreatic fistula, diarrhea, administration of extra chlorides, carbonic anhydrase inhibition, Addison's disease, and renal tubular acidosis.
43. One should not assume that oxygen availability and consumption are satisfactory just because arterial oxyhemoglobin saturation is 90% to 95%.
44. One cannot assume that ketones are absent, or only minimally present, if the nitroprusside test is negative in patients with severe acidosis.
45. Alcoholic ketoacidosis can be associated with high, normal, or low glucose levels, but seldom above 250 to 300 mg/dl.
46. One should evaluate anion and osmolar gaps in patients admitted with a metabolic acidosis of unknown etiology.
47. A respiratory alkalosis combined with a high anion gap metabolic acidosis suggests salicylate toxicity.
48. One should not use bicarbonate during CPR without following arterial (and mixed venous) blood gases.
49. The two most frequent causes of metabolic alkalosis are excessive diuresis (with loss of potassium, hydrogen, and chloride) and excessive loss of gastric secretions (with loss of hydrogen and chloride).
50. In evaluating metabolic alkalosis, one must be aware of the large amount of bicarbonate and potassium that can be lost with diarrhea.
51. Hypovolemia increases the tendency to metabolic alkalosis.
52. Patients receiving massive blood transfusions and large amounts of Ringer's lactate will tend to become alkalotic over the next 12 to 48 hours.

53. One should not attempt to correct a metabolic alkalosis without first correcting any coexistent dehydration.
54. Hypoalbuminemia tends to increase plasma bicarbonate levels.
55. Failure to compensate adequately for a metabolic alkalosis may be the first indication of an otherwise inapparent hypoxemia.
56. One should not allow patients to remain severely alkalotic, even if they appear to be doing well otherwise.
57. Chloride-resistant alkalosis is usually due to excess corticosteroids or severe hypokalemia.
58. One should not correct hypocarbia without first ruling out hypoxia, pulmonary embolus, sepsis, or metabolic acidosis.
59. One should not administer oxygen to patients with COPD without carefully watching for the development of apnea or hypoventilation.
60. Rapid correction of a chronic respiratory acidosis can cause sudden development of a severe combined metabolic and respiratory alkalosis.
61. In treating patients with a chronic respiratory acidosis, one should generally not allow the reduction of $PaCO_2$ by more than 5.0 mm Hg/h.

BIBLIOGRAPHY

1. Adrogue, HJ, Wilson, H, and Boyd, AE, III: Plasma acid-base patterns in diabetic ketoacidosis. N Engl J Med 307:1603, 1982.
2. Adrogue, HJ, et al: Assessing acid-base status in circulatory failure: Differences between arterial and central venous blood. N Engl J Med 320:1312, 1989.
3. Adrogue, HJ, et al: Influence of Steady-State Alterations in Acid-Base Equilibrium on Fate of Administered Bicarbonate in the Dog. (Tufts Univ.)
4. American Heart Association: Standards and guidelines for cardiopulmonary resuscitation and emergency cardiac care: Part III. Adult advanced cardiac life support. JAMA 255:2933, 1986.
5. Askanazi, J, et al: Nutrition and the respiratory system. Crit Care Med 10:163, 1982.
6. Askanazi, J, et al: Nutrition for the patient with respiratory failure: Glucose vs fat. Anesthesiology 54:373, 1981.
7. Askanazi, J, et al: Effects of parenteral nutrition on ventilatory drive. Anesthesiology 53:5185, 1980.
8. Aubier, M, et al: Respiratory Muscle Contribution to Lactic Acidosis in Low Cardiac Output. McGill University Press, Montreal.
9. Barton, M, et al: Is catecholamine release pH mediated? Crit Care Med 10:751, 1982.
10. Bleich, HL: The clinical implications of venous carbon dioxide tension. N Engl J Med 320:1345, 1989.
11. Boron, WF: Intracellular pH regulation in epithelial cells. Ann Rev Physiol 48:377, 1986.
12. Brackett, NC, Jr, Cohen, JJ, and Schwartz, WB: Carbon dioxide titration curve of normal man. N Engl J Med 272:6, 1965.
13. Brackett, NC, Jr, et al: Acid-base response to chronic hypercapnia in man. N Engl J Med 280:124, 1969.
14. Brenner, RJ, et al: Incidence of radiologically evident bone disease, nephrocalcinosis and nephrolithiasis in various types of renal tubular acidosis. N Engl J Med 307:217, 1982.
15. Campbell, CH: The severe lactic acidosis of thiamine deficiency: Acute pernicious or fulminating beriberi. Lancet 2:446, 1984.
15a. Cohen, RD, et al: The techniques and uses of intracellular pH measurements. Ciba Found Symp 87:20, 1982.
16. Davies, AO: Rapid desensitization and uncoupling of human β-adrenergic receptors on an in vitro model of lactic acidosis. Metabolism 59:398, 1984.
17. Emmett, ME and Narins, RG: Clinical use of the anion gap. Medicine 56:38, 1977.
18. Falk, JL, Rackow, EC, and Weil, MH: End-tidal carbon dioxide concentration during cardiopulmonary resuscitation. N Engl J Med 318:607, 1988.
19. Felig, PU and McCurdy, DK: The hypertonic state. N Engl J Med 297:1444, 1977.
20. Felig, P, Havel, RJ, and Smith, LH: Metabolism. In Smith, LH, Jr and Thier, SO (eds): Pathophysiology: The Biological Principles of Disease, ed 2. WB Saunders, Philadelphia, 1985, p 364.
21. Figueras, J, et al: Relationship between pulmonary hemodynamics and arterial pH and carbon dioxide tension in critically ill patients. Chest 70:466, 1976.
21a. Folbergrov, AJ, et al: Phosphorylase alpha and labile metabolites duirng anoxia: correlation to membrane fluxes of K+ and Ca2+. J Neurochem 55:1690, 1990.

22. Foster, DW and McGarry, JD: The metabolic derangements and treatment of diabetic keto-acidosis. N Engl J Med 309:159, 1983.

23. Fulop, M: Ventilatory response in patients with acute lactic acidosis. Crit Care Med 10:173, 1982.

24. Gabow, PA: Disorders associated with altered anion gap (discussion). Kidney Int 27:472, 1985.

25. Gabow, PA, et al: Diagnostic importance of an increased serum anion gap. N Engl J Med 303:854, 1980.

25a. Gamble, JL: Chemical anatomy, physiology, and pathology of extracellular fluids: A lecture syllabus. ed 6, Harvard University Press, 1960, p 131.

26. Garella, S, Dana, CL, and Chazan, JA: Severity of metabolic acidosis as a determinant of bicarbonate requirements. N Engl J Med 289:121, 1973.

27. Goldenheim, PD and Kazemi, H: Cardiopulmonary monitoring of critically ill patients. N Engl J Med 311:776, 1984.

27a. Goldstein, MB, et al: The urine anion gap: A clinically useful index of ammonium excretion. Am J Med Sci 292:198, 1986.

28. Graf, H, Leach, W, and Arieff, AI: Evidence for a detrimental effect of bicarbonate therapy in hypoxic lactic acidosis. Science 227:754, 1985.

28a. Graber, ML, et al: Spurious hyperchloremia and decreased anion gap in hyperlipidemia. Ann Intern Med 98:607, 1983.

29. Grundler, W, Weil, MH, and Rackow, EC: Arteriovenous carbon dioxide and pH gradients during cardiac arrest. Circulation 74:1071, 1986.

30. Hale, RJ, Crase, J, and Nattrass, M: Metabolic effects of bicarbonate in the treatment of diabetic ketoacidosis. Br Med J 289:1035, 1984.

31. Heistad, DD and Kontos, HA: Cerebral circulation. In Berne, RM (ed): The Cardiovascular System, Vol III, Shephert, JT and Abboud, FM (eds): Peripheral Circulation and Organ Blood Flow, part I. Williams & Wilkins, Baltimore, 137:82, 1983.

32. Hertford, JF, McKenna, JP, and Chamovitz, BN: Metabolic acidosis with an elevated anion gap. Am Fam Physician 39:159, 1989.

32a. Hilton, JG, et al: The urine anion gap: The critical clue to resolve a diagnostic dilemma in a patient with ketoacidosis. Diabetes Care 7:486, 1984.

33. Hoffman, RS and Goldfrank, LR: Ethanol-associated metabolic disorders. Emerg Med Clin North Am 7:943, 1989.

34. Hood, I and Campbell, ENM: Is pK ok? N Engl J Med 306:864, 1982.

35. Iberti, TJ, et al: Low sensitivity of the anion gap as a screen to detect hyperlactatemia in critically ill patients. Crit Care Med 18:275, 1990.

36. Isreal, RS: Diabetic ketoacidosis. Emerg Med Clin North Am 7:859, 1989.

37. Kazemi, H and Johnson, DC: Regulation of cerebrospinal fluid acid-base balance. Physiol Rev 66:953, 1986.

38. Kearns, T and Wolfson, AB: Metabolic acidosis. Emerg Med Clin North Am 7:823, 1989.

39. Korner, PI: Central nervous control of autonomic cardiovascular function. In Berne, RM (ed): The Cardiovascular System, Vol I, The Heart. Williams & Wilkins, Baltimore, 1979, p 691.

40. Krupp, MA: Fluids and electrolyte disorders. In Schroeder, SA (ed): Current Medical Diagnosis and Treatment 1988. Appleton & Lange, Norwalk, CT, 1988, p 34.

41. Kwun, KB, et al: Treatment of metabolic alkalosis with intravenous infusion of concentrated hydrochloric acid. Am J Surg 146:328, 1983.

42. Lever, E and Jaspan, JB: Sodium bicarbonate therapy in severe diabetic ketoacidosis. Am J Med 75:263, 1983.

43. Lieber, CS: Biochemical and molecular basis of alcohol-induced injury to liver and other tissues. N Engl J Med 319:1639, 1988.

43a. Lipner, HI, et al: The behavior of carbenicillin as a nonreabsorbable anion. J Lab Clin Med 86:183, 1975.

43b. Lolekha, PH and Lolekha, S: Value of the anion gap in clinical diagnosis and laboratory evaluation. Clin Chem 29:279, 1983.

44. Luft, D, et al: Definition of clinically relevant lactic acidosis in patients with internal diseases. Am J Clin Pathol 80:484, 1983.

45. Malchoft, CD, et al: Determinants of glucose and ketoacid concentrations in acutely hyperglycemic diabetic patients. Am J Med 77:275, 1984.

46. Malnic, G: Role of the kidney in controlling acid-base balance. Clin Nephrol Urol 9:241, 1988–1989.

47. Man, S, Oh, MS, and Carroll, HJ: The anion gap. N Engl J Med 297:814, 1977.

48. Mathias, DW, Clifford, PS, and Klopfenstein, HS: Mixed venous blood gases are superior to arterial blood gases in assessing acid-base status and oxygenation during acute cardiac tamponade in dogs. J Clin Invest 82:833, 1988.

49. McCurdy, DK and Feig, PU: Hyperosmolar coma. N Engl J Med 15:855, 1977.

50. Mehta, K, Krause, JA, and Carlson, RW: The relationship between anion gap and elevated lactate (abstr). Crit Care Med 14:405, 1986.

51. Molloy, DW, et al: Use of sodium bicarbonate to treat tricyclic antidepressant-induced arrhythmias in a patient with alkalosis. Can Med Assoc J 130:1457, 1984.

52. Moore, SE and Good, JT: Mixed venous and arterial pH: A comparison during hemorrhagic shock and hypothermia. Ann Emerg Med 11:300, 1982.

53. Moxham, J: Aminophylline and the respiratory muscles: An alternative view. Clin Chest Med 9:325, 1988.

54. Murray, JF: The Normal Lung. WB Saunders, Philadelphia, 1986, p 176.

55. Narins, RG and Cohen, JJ: Bicarbonate therapy for organic acidosis: The case for its continued use. Ann Intern Med 106:615, 1987.

56. Narins, RG and Emmet, M: Simple and mixed acid-base disorders: A practical approach. Medicine, 59:161, 1980.

57. Narins, RG and Goldberg, M: Renal tubular acidosis: Pathophysiology, diagnosis and therapy. Disease-a-Month 13:6, 1977.

58. Natelson, S and Nobel, D: Effect of the variation of pK of the Henderson-Hasselbalch equation on values obtained for total CO_2 calculated from P_{CO_2} and pH values. Clin Chem 23:767, 1977.

59. Ordog, GJ, Easserberger, J, and Balasubramaniun, S: Effect of heparin on arterial blood gases. Ann Emerg Med 14:233, 1985.

60. Parot, S, et al: Hypoxemia, hypercapnia, and breathing pattern in patients with chronic obstructive pulmonary disease. Am Rev Respir Dis 126:882, 1982.

61. Peretz, DI, et al: The significance of lacticacidemia in the shock syndrome. Ann NY Acad Sci 119:1133, 1965.

62. Pichette, C, et al: Elevation of the blood lactate concentration by alkali therapy without requiring additional lactic acid accumulation: Theoretical considerations. Crit Care Med 10:323, 1982.

63. Pope, DW and Dansky, D: Hyperosmolar hyperglycemic nonketotic coma. Emerg Med Clin North Am 7:849, 1989.

64. Price, HL: Effects of carbon dioxide on the cardiovascular system. Anesthesiology 21:652, 1960.

65. Prys-Roberts, CH: Hypercapnia. In Gray, TC and Nunn, JF (eds): General Anesthesia, ed 3, Vol I, Basic Sciences. Appleton-Century-Crofts, New York, 1971, p 164.

66. Rackow, EC, et al: Unmeasured anion during severe sepsis with metabolic acidosis. Circ Shock 30:107, 1990.

66a. Rebuck, AS, et al: A mathematical expression to describe the ventilatory response to hypoxia and hypercapnia. Respir Physiol 31:107, 1977.

67. Relman, AS: "Blood gases": arterial or venous? N Engl J Med 315:183, 1986.

68. Ross, A and Boron, WF: Intracellular pH. Physiol Rev 61:296, 1981.

69. Rossing, TH, Maffeo, N, and Fencl, V: Acid-base effects on altering plasma protein concentration in human blood in vitro. J Appl Physiol 61:2260, 1986.

70. Schwartz, WB, Brackett, NC, Jr, and Cohen, JJ: The response of extracellular hydrogen ion concentration to graded degrees of chronic hypercapnia: The physiologic limits the defenses of pH. J Clin Invest 44:291, 1965.

71. Schwartz, WB and Relman, AS: A critique of the parameters used in the evaluation of acid-base disorders. N Engl J Med 268:1382, 1963.

71a. Shapiro, BA: Arterial blood gas monitoring. Crit Care Clin 4:479, 1988.

72. Seki, S: Clinical features of hyperosmolar hyperglycemia nonketotic diabetic coma associated with cardiac operations. J Thorac Cardiovasc Surg 91:867, 1986.

73. Settergren, G, Soderland, S, and Eklof, A: Blood oxygen tension and oxyhemoglobin saturation in hypoxemia due to right-to-left shunt or low inspired oxygen concentration. Crit Care Med 10:163, 1983.

74. Shaffer, MA: Acid-base homeostasis. In Rosen, P (ed): Emergency Medicine: Concepts and Clinical Practice, ed 2. CV Mosby, St. Louis, 1988, p 1956.

75. Sutton, RN, Wilson, RF, and Walt, AJ: Differences in acid-base levels and oxygen-saturation between central venous and arterial blood. Lancet 2:748, 1967.

76. Tenney, SM and Reese, RE: The ability to sustain great breathing efforts. Respir Physiol 5:187, 1968.

76a. Van Leeuwen, AM: Net cation equivalency of the plasma proteins: A study of ion-protein interaction in human plasma by means of in vivo ultrafiltration and equilibrium dialysis. Acta Med Scand (Suppl) 422:1, 1964.

76b. Van Slyke, DD, et al: Studies of gas and electrolyte equilibria in blood. The amounts of alkali bound by serum albumin and globulin. J Biol Chem 79:769, 1928.

77. Velez, RJ, Myers, B, and Guber, MS: Severe acute metabolic acidosis (acute beriberi): An avoidable complication of total parenteral nutrition. JPEN 9:216, 1985.

78. Wahren, J, et al: Glucose metabolism during leg exercise in man. J Clin Invest 50:2715, 1971.

79. Walmsley, RN and White, GH: Normal "anion gap" (hyperchloremic) acidosis. Clin Chem 31:309, 1985.

80. Weil, MH, et al: Difference in acid-base state between venous and arterial blood during cardiopulmonary resuscitation. N Engl J Med 315:153, 1986.
81. Weinberger, SE, Schwartzstein, RM, and Weiss, JW: Hypercapnia. N Engl J Med 321:1223, 1989.
82. Wilson, A and Vulcano, B: A double-blind, placebo-controlled trial of magnesium sulfate in ethanol withdrawal syndrome. Alcoholism 8:542, 1984.
83. Wilson, RF, et al: Severe alkalosis in critically ill patients. Arch Surg 104:551, 1972.

Index

Numbers followed by an "f" indicates figures; numbers followed by a "t" indicate tabular material.

hypernatremia in, 668
hypokalemia in, 674–675, 675t
hyponatremia in, 661
metabolic acidosis in, 735–736
metabolic alkalosis in, 744
secretory, 734
Diastasis, 31, 31t
Diastole, 30–31, 30f, 31t
coronary blood flow during, 9–10, 10f
time in, 68
Diastolic dysfunction, 189
Diastolic filling, interference with, 190
Diastolic pressure, 40
Diastolic pressure time index (DPTI), 107
Diazepam (Valium)
in cerebral resuscitation, 343
in subarachnoid hemorrhage, 331
Dibenzyline, 54
DIC. See Disseminated intravascular
coagulation
Dichloroacetate, in metabolic acidosis, 744
Diet
in acute myocardial infarction, 99–100
high fat, 739
Diffusion of gas
through fluids, 391–392
impaired, 423, 426
through respiratory membrane, 381,
392–394
through tissue, 392
Digital paresthesia, in hypocalcemia, 687
Digitalis. See also Digoxin
in acute myocardial infarction, 110
in advanced cardiac life support, 307
in ARDS, 457
in arrhythmias, 102, 153
calcium administration with, 680–681
cardioversion in patient taking, 134
in COPD, 558
in cor pulmonale, 551
effect on electrocardiogram, 120
in heart failure, 212–213, 212t
Digitalis intoxication, 636, 675, 698
arrhythmias in, 131–132, 135–137,
140–141, 148, 155, 179, 212–213
cardioversion in, 137, 162
vagal maneuvers in, 134
Digoxin. See also Digitalis
in acute myocardial infarction shock,
105
adverse effects of, 179, 213
in ARDS, 457
in arrhythmias, 135, 137–138, 179–180
in COPD, 558
dosage of, 179, 212
in heart failure, 212–213, 216
indications for, 178
mode of action of, 178
in pulmonary edema, 217
in pulmonary embolism, 517
in shock, 262–263
Dihydroergotamine, in prevention of deep
vein thrombosis, 499
Dilantin. See Diphenylhydantoin
Diltiazem, in acute myocardial infarction,
98–99
Dilution acidosis, 745
Dilutional hyponatremia, 631, 658–659
Diphenylhydantoin (Dilantin, phenytoin)
adverse effects of, 171, 684t
in arrhythmias, 137, 149, 170–171
in cerebral resuscitation, 343
dosage of, 165t, 170
indications for, 170
IV administration of, 171

mode of action of, 170
in subarachnoid hemorrhage, 331
2,3-Diphosphoglycerate (2,3-DPG)
in banked blood, 256, 408
in hypophosphatemia, 701
in metabolic acidosis, 736
oxyhemoglobin dissociation and, 406,
408
Diplopia, 321t
Dipyridamole. See Persantine
Direct mechanical ventricular assistance,
305
Direct-current countershock, 162
Disequilibrium syndrome, 645
Disopyramide
adverse effects of, 168
in arrhythmias, 150, 167–168
dosage of, 168
mode of action of, 167–168
Dissecting aortic aneurysm, 81
Disseminated intravascular coagulation
(DIC)
ARDS and, 439, 444
correction of, 274–275
development of, 238
in shock, 244–245, 273–275
Distal convoluted tubule, 567, 570–571f,
572, 573f, 587
Distribution of gas, impaired, 426
Diuresis
excessive, metabolic alkalosis in, 744
hypokalemia in, 674
osmotic, 618–619, 621
water, 589, 619
Diuretic(s)
in acute myocardial infarction shock,
106
in acute renal failure, 631–633
in advanced cardiac life support, 309–
310
adverse effects of, 661, 684t, 692
in ARDS, 456–457
in cerebral resuscitation, 340
in coma, 326
in COPD, 558
in heart failure, 204–205, 216
in hypercalcemia, 695
in hyperkalemia, 681t
hypochloremia caused by, 704
intracranial pressure reduction, 326
in oliguria, 626
in pulmonary embolism, 517
in sepsis, 615
in shock, 271
in trauma, 615
Diving reflex, 134
Dobutamine
in acute myocardial infarction shock,
105
in advanced cardiac life support, 307
dosage of, 213, 263
in heart failure, 212t, 213
in pulmonary embolism, 517
in shock, 263
stimulation of adrenergic receptors by,
45t
Donnan equilibrium, 656–657, 657t
Dopamine
in acute myocardial infarction shock,
105
in acute renal failure, 630
in advanced cardiac life support, 307
adverse effects of, 263
dosage of, 213, 263, 630
in heart failure, 212t, 213

in oliguria, 626
in pulmonary embolism, 517
in shock, 263, 268–269, 271
Dopamine receptor(s), 43t, 45, 45t
Dopexamine, 45t
Doppler ultrasonography, in deep vein
thrombosis, 495–496
Doxapram, in COPD, 552
2,3-DPG. See 2,3-Diphosphoglycerate
DPTI. See Diastolic pressure time index
Dual oximetry, 415
Duodenal ulcer, 744
Dust cell. See Alveolar macrophage
DVT. See Deep vein thrombosis
Dynamic hyperinflation. See Auto-PEEP
Dysarthria, 321t
Dysconjugate ocular mobility disorder,
331
Dysphagia, 321t
Dyspnea
in ARDS, 448
in COPD, 533–534
in fat embolism syndrome, 433
in heart failure, 197–198
in pulmonary embolism, 510, 510t

ECG. See Electrocardiogram
Echocardiogram
in heart failure, 200–201
measurement of cardiac contractility,
27
in pulmonary embolism, 516
transmitral pulsed-Doppler, 22
Eclampsia, 699
ECMO. See Extracorporeal membrane
oxygenation
Ectopic beat(s)
atrial, 129, 131f, 160t
ventricular, 130, 142, 142f
Ectopic focus, 126
theory of atrial fibrillation, 138
Ectopic supraventricular tachycardia,
135–137
Edecrin. See Ethacrynic acid
Edema. See also Pedal edema; Peripheral
edema; Pulmonary edema
of heart failure, 192f
hyponatremia and, 664
EDRF. See Endothelium-derived relaxing
factor
Edrophonium, in arrhythmias, 135
Effective compliance, 376
Effective osmol, 654
Effective resistance, 376
Efferent arteriole, 571f, 574–575, 576f,
577
Efficiency of cardiac contraction, 29
EGF. See Epidermal growth factor
Ejection click, 32
Ejection fraction, 26–27, 202
Elastase, 240, 444
Elastic stockings, 497–498
Elderly, weaning parameters in, 477
Electrocardiogram (ECG). See also specific
disorders
correlation with venous pressure waves,
20f
His bundle, 121, 121f
in mechanically-ventilated patient, 554
normal, 119–124, 120–123f
relationship to action potential, 13,
13f
"sawtooth" pattern, 138, 138f
vectorial analysis of, 121–123, 123f

765

Narcotic(s)
in hypotensive patient, 84–85
in hypovolemic patient, 84–85, 235–236
Nasal prongs, 538
Nasogastric suction, 704
Nasogastric tube, 427, 439, 455, 556, 744
Nasopharyngeal catheter, 538
Nasopharynx, 355
Nasotracheal suctioning, 425, 427, 549
Nausea and vomiting. See Vomiting
Near drowning, 332, 334, 342
Nebulization, 542
in ARDS, 459
in COPD, 550
Neck pain, in acute myocardial infarction, 72
Neck vein(s), distended, 18, 20, 198, 200, 511, 534
Necrotic tissue, eradication of, 633
Necrotizing pancreatitis, 82
Negative inspiratory pressure, in ventilatory weaning, 477
Neonate. See Infant
Nephritis, interstitial, 618, 623
Nephrogenic diabetes insipidus, 589, 613, 618–619, 670, 675
Nephron, 567–574, 570f
cortical, 569, 570f, 572
juxtamedullary, 569, 570f, 572
Nephrotic syndrome, 591, 596, 664, 731
Neurogenic control
of blood flow, 39–40
of coronary blood flow, 10–11
of pulmonary vascular resistance, 35
of renal activity, 588–589
Neurogenic pulmonary edema, 439–440
Neurogenic shock, 224, 225t, 226
Neutrophil(s), in ARDS, 442–444
Nicotine, 126
Nifedipine
in acute myocardial infarction, 99
in COPD, 546
in heart failure, 206t, 209, 209t
Nimodipine
in cerebral resuscitation, 344
in subarachnoid hemorrhage, 329–330
Nitrate
in acute myocardial infarction, 98
in advanced cardiac life support, 309
effect on coronary blood flow, 11
in heart failure, 205–208, 206t
oral, 206–208
Nitric oxide, 56
Nitrite
in advanced cardiac life support, 309
in heart failure, 205–206, 206t
Nitroglycerin
in acute myocardial infarction, 98
in acute myocardial infarction shock, 106
in acute renal failure, 631
in advanced cardiac life support, 307, 309
dosage of, 207, 631
in heart failure, 206t, 207
mode of action of, 207
in shock, 271
sublingual, 207
tolerance to, 207
transdermal, 208
Nitroprusside
in acute myocardial infarction shock, 106
in acute renal failure, 631
in advanced cardiac life support, 307
adverse effects of, 206–207, 684t

dosage of, 206, 631
in heart failure, 206–207, 206t
mode of action of, 206
in shock, 271
Nitroprusside test, 738
Nodal rhythm, 132
Nonsteroidal anti-inflammatory agent(s)
in acute renal failure, 618
adverse effects of, 591
in shock, 271
No-reflow phenomenon, 335–336
Norepinephrine (Levophed)
in acute myocardial infarction shock, 106
in acute renal failure, 630
in advanced cardiac life support, 307
adverse effects of, 684t
in arrhythmias, 135
blood pressure and, 41–42
in COPD, 541t
effect on coronary blood flow, 11
in heart failure, 192–193
in pulmonary embolism, 517
in shock, 268–269
stimulation of adrenergic receptors by, 43, 45, 45t
Normal saline, in resuscitation, 250
Nose
anatomy of, 355, 356f
occlusion of, 425
Nuclear medicine study, in acute renal failure, 626
Nursing care, in ARDS, 453–454
Nutrition
in acute renal failure, 635
in COPD, 551, 558

O antigen, 272
Obesity, 454, 494
Obstructive pulmonary defect, definition of, 370–371
Obstructive renal failure, 621, 627
Ohmeda CPU 1 ventilator, 471
Oliguria
definition of, 608
diagnosis of, 622–629
due to antidiuretic hormone excess, 625
due to hypovolemia, 625–626
etiology of, 610–622
prerenal, 601, 611–613, 622–626
renal, 613
in sepsis, 614–615
treatment of, 629t
Oncotic pressure
interstitial, 58
plasma, 654
Open-chest cardiac massage, 304
Opioid(s), endogenous, 236
Opsonin, 247
Optimal PEEP, 466
Oral contraceptive(s), 492
Organic acid(s)
increased production of, 734
plasma, 725t, 726
increased, 727–729, 742
renal handling of, 585
Organic base(s), renal handling of, 585
Oropharyngeal airway, 301
Oropharynx, 355
aspiration of contents of, 427–428
Orthopnea, in heart failure, 198
Osmol(s)
effective, 654
ineffective, 654

Osmolality
definition of, 653–655
of plasma, 593
of serum, 662
of urine, 588, 593, 662
Osmolar clearance, 599
Osmolar gap, 654
Osmolarity
definition of, 653–655
of serum, 456, 654
of urine, 623, 628
Osmoreceptor(s), 589
Osmotic demyelination syndrome, 665, 668
Osmotic diuresis, 618–619, 621
Osmotic pressure, 654
Otic ganglion, 42f
Overdose, 225t, 226–227, 320, 424
Overdrive pacing, 161
Oximetry
dual, 415
pulmonary, 261
pulse, 415–416, 461
Oxygen
availability in metabolic acidosis, 736
concentration and partial pressure in alveoli, 395
content of arterial blood, 412
control of ventilation, 367–368
diffusion coefficient of, 392
diffusion in lungs, 381
diffusion into tissues from capillary, 403
renal consumption of, 578
solubility coefficient of, 391
toxic products of, 233–234, 240, 337–338, 440, 443–444
Oxygen coma, 539
Oxygen consumption index, in shock, 262
Oxygen debt, in shock, 262
Oxygen delivery, 412
in metabolic acidosis, 736
in shock, 266
Oxygen extraction
increase in heart failure, 193
index, 415
Oxygen mask, 538
Oxygen reserve, 10, 413
Oxygen saturation in mixed venous blood, 261
Oxygen tent, 538
Oxygen therapy
in acute myocardial infarction, 85
in acute myocardial infarction shock, 103–104
adverse effects of, 539–540
in chronic hypercarbia, 368
in COPD, 531–532, 537–540, 546, 558, 749
in CPR, 301
in heart failure, 210–211
methods of administration of, 538–539
in pulmonary edema, 216
in pulmonary embolism, 516
in shock, 249
Oxygenation
monitoring of, 402
ventilatory parameters, 476–477
Oxyhemoglobin dissociation, 400–401
factors affecting, 405–408, 405–408t, 406–407f
in metabolic acidosis, 736
normal, 405
in respiratory alkalosis, 748
shift to left, 405–406, 406f, 408
shift to right, 405–406, 406f, 408